Operative Pediatric Surgery

Operative Pediatric Surgery

SEVENTH EDITION

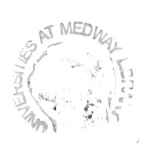

Edited by

Lewis Spitz MBChB PhD MD(Hon) FRCS (Edin, Eng) FRCSI(Hon) FAAP(Hon) FCS(SA)(Hon) FACS(Hon)
Emeritus Nuffield Professor of Paediatric Surgery, Institute of Child Health, University College London and Consultant Paediatric Surgeon, Great Ormond Street Hospital for Children NHS Trust, London, UK

Arnold G Coran MD
Emeritus Professor of Pediatric Surgery, The University of Michigan Medical School and the C.S. Mott Children's Hospital, Ann Arbor, Michigan; Professor of Pediatric Surgery, New York University School of Medicine, New York, New York, USA

Associate editors

Daniel H Teitelbaum MD
Professor of Surgery, Section of Pediatric Surgery, University of Michigan, Ann Arbor, Michigan, USA

Hock Lim Tan MBBS MD FRACS FRCS(Eng)
Visiting Paediatric Surgeon, Prince Court Medical Centre, Kuala Lumpur, Malaysia, and Adjunct Professor of Surgery, Faculty of Medicine, University of Indonesia, Jakarta

Agostino Pierro MD FRCS(Eng) FRCS(Ed) FAAP
Nuffield Professor of Paediatric Surgery, Institute of Child Health, University College, London and Great Ormond Street Hospital for Children NHS Trust, London, UK

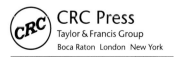

CRC Press
Taylor & Francis Group
Boca Raton London New York

CRC Press is an imprint of the
Taylor & Francis Group, an **informa** business

Typesetting by Phoenix Photosetting, UK

CRC Press
Taylor & Francis Group
6000 Broken Sound Parkway NW, Suite 300
Boca Raton, FL 33487-2742

Visit the Taylor & Francis Web site at
http://www.taylorandfrancis.com

and the CRC Press Web site at
http://www.crcpress.com

Contents

SECTION IV: THORACIC

SECTION V: ABDOMINAL

SECTION VI: TUMORS

SECTION VII: ENDOCRINE

SECTION VIII: UROLOGY

SECTION IX: NEURAL TUBE DEFECTS

SECTION X: TRAUMA

SECTION XI: SPECIAL SECTION

Contributors

Ian A Aaronson MA FRCS
Professor of Urology and Pediatrics and Director of Pediatric Urology, Medical University of South Carolina, Charleston, SC, USA

Niyi Ade-Ajayi MPhil FRCS(paed)
Department of Paediatric Surgery, King's Hospital, London, UK

Craig T Albanese MD
Stanford University-Lucile Packard Children's Hospital, Stanford, CA, USA

Richard J Andrassy MD FACS
Denton A Cooley MD Chair in Surgery; Jack H Mayfield MD Distinguished University Chair in Surgery; Professor and Chairman, Department of Surgery, The University of Texas Medical School at Houston, Houston, TX, USA

C Martin Bailey BSc FRCS FRCSEd
Honorary Consultant Paediatric Otolaryngologist, Great Ormond Street Hospital for Children, London, UK

Sean J Barnett MD MS
Assistant Professor of Surgery and Pediatrics, Division of Pediatric General and Thoracic Surgery, Cincinnati Children's Hospital Medical Center, Cincinnati, OH, USA

Spencer W Beasley MS FRACS
Clinical Professor of Paediatrics and Surgery, Christchurch School of Medicine and Health Sciences, University of Otago, and Clinical Director, Department of Paediatric Surgery, Christchurch Hospital, Canterbury District Health Board, Christchurch, New Zealand

Adrian Bianchi MD FRCS(Eng) FRCS(Ed)
Specialist Paediatric Reconstructive Surgeon, Royal Manchester Children's Hospital, Manchester, UK

Deborah F Billmire MD
Riley Hospital for Children, Indiana University School of Medicine, Indianapolis, IN, USA

Robert Bingham MB BS FRCA
Consultant Paediatric Anaesthetist, Anaesthetic Department, Great Ormond Street Hospital, London, UK

Andrea Bischoff MD
Colorectal Center for Children, Cincinnati Children's Hospital Medical Center, Cincinnati, OH, USA

David A Bloom MD
Jack Lapides Professor of Urology and Chair, Department of Urology, University of Michigan Health System and Medical School, Ann Arbor, MI, USA

Su-Anna M Boddy MS FRCS
Consultant Paediatric Urologist, St George's Hospital, London, UK

John Boutros MD
Hospital for Sick Children, Department of Pediatric Surgery, Toronto, Canada

Steven W Bruch MD MSc FACS FAAP
Associate Clinical Professor of Surgery, University of Michigan, Mott Children's Hospital, Ann Arbor, MI, USA

Matias Bruzoni MD
Stanford University-Lucile Packard Children's Hospital, Stanford, CA, USA

Casey M Calkins MD
Associate Professor of Pediatric Surgery, Division of Pediatric Surgery, Medical College of Wisconsin, Milwaukee, WI, USA

Nicholas Sy Chao
Associate Consultant, Queen Elizabeth Hospital, Hong Kong

Robert E Cilley MD
Professor of Surgery and Pediatrics, Division of Pediatric Surgery, Department of Surgery, Pennsylvania State University College of Medicine, Penn State Hershey Children's Hospital, Hershey, PA, USA

Emily Christison-Lagay MD FACS
Fellow, Division of Pediatric General and Thoracic Surgery, Hospital for Sick Children, Toronto, Ontario, Canada

Paolo De Coppi MD MR PhD
Senior Lecturer Consultant, UCL Institute of Child Health and Great Ormond Street Hospital, London, UK

Arnold G Coran MD
CS Mott Children's Hospital, University of Michigan, Ann Arbor, MI, USA

Peter Cuckow MB BS FRCS(Paed)
Consultant Paediatric Urologist, Department of Paediatric Surgery, Institute of Child Health, London, UK

Joe Curry MBBS FRCS(Eng) FRCS (Paed Surg)

Specialty Lead for Neonatal and Paediatric Surgery, Department of Paediatric Surgery, Great Ormond Street Hospital for Children Institute of Child Health, London, UK

Mark Davenport ChM FRCS(Paeds) FRCS(Glas) FRCS(Eng)

Consultant Paediatric Hepatobiliary Surgeon, Department of Paediatric Surgery, King's College Hospital, London, UK

Delphine Demède MD

Department of Pediatric Urology, Hôpital Mère-Enfants – GHE, Lyon, France

Bryan J Dicken MD

Assistant Professor of Surgery, Stollery Children's Hospital, Edmonton, Alberta, Canada

Peter W Dillon MD MS

Professor of Surgery and Pediatrics, Division of Pediatric Surgery, Department of Surgery, Pennsylvania State University College of Medicine, Penn State Hershey Children's Hospital, Hershey, PA, USA

Patricia K Donahoe MD

Marshall K Bartlett Professor of Surgery, Chief of Pediatric Surgical Services, Emeritus, Director of Pediatric Surgical Research Laboratories, Massachusetts General Hospital, Boston MA, USA

Alexander Dzakovic MD

Children's Memorial Hospital, Chicago, IL, USA

Scott A Engum MD

Professor of Surgery, Department of Surgery, Indiana University School of Medicine, Division of Pediatric Surgery, James Whitcomb Riley Hospital for Children, Indianapolis, IN, USA

Steven J Fishman MD

Senior Associate in Surgery and Co-Director, Vascular Anomalies Center, Children's Hospital Boston, Associate Professor of Surgery, Harvard Medical School, Boston, MA, USA

Alan Flake MD

Professor of Surgery and Obstetrics, University of Pennsylvania, School of Medicine, Ruth and Tristram C Colleet, Jr. Chair in Pediatric Surgery, Director, Department of Surgery, Children's Hospital of Philadelphia, Abramson Research Center, Philadelphia, PA, USA

John Foker MD PhD

Department of Surgery, University of Minnesota, Minneapolis, MN, USA

Michel François MD

Department of Pediatric Urology, Hôpital Mère-Enfants – GHE, Lyon, France

Michael WL Gauderer MD

Professor of Pediatric Surgery and Pediatrics, University of South Carolina School of Medicine (Greenville); Children's Hospital, Greenville Hospital System University Medical Center, Greenville, SC, USA

James D Geiger MD

Professor of Surgery, Section of Pediatric Surgery, School of Medicine, University of Michigan Medical School, Ann Arbor, MI, USA

Marina George BSc MBBS FRCA

Consultant Paediatric Anaesthetist, Anaesthetic Department, Great Ormond Street Hospital for Children, London, UK

Prasad Godbole MS FRCS(Paeds) FEAPU

Consultant Paediatric Urologist and Honorary Senior Lecturer, Sheffield Children's NHS Trust, Sheffield, UK

Michael J Goretsky MD

Associate Professor of Clinical Surgery and Pediatrics at Eastern Virginia Medical School and Surgeon at Children's Hospital of the King's Daughters, Norfolk, VA, USA

Joe Grainger MMedSci FRCS

Consultant Paediatric ENT Surgeon, Birmingham Children's Hospital NHS Foundation Trust, Birmingham, UK

Jay L Grosfeld MD

Professor of Pediatric Surgery, Emeritus, Indiana University School of Medicine, Indianapolis, IN, USA

Erica R Gross MD

Research Fellow, Columbia University, College of Physicians and Surgeons, and Pediatric ECMO Fellow, Morgan Stanley Children's Hospital, New York-Presbyterian, New York City, New York, USA

Miguel Guelfand MD

Associated Professor and Consultant in Paediatric and Neonatal Surgery, Hospital Exequiel Gonzalez Cortez y Clinica Las Condes, Santiago, Chile

Munther Haddad MD

Chelsea and Westminster Hospital, London, UK

Nigel J Hall MRCPCH FRCS(Paed Surg) PhD

Clinical Lecturer Department of Paediatric Surgery, Institute of Child Health, London, UK

Ben Hartley BSc FRCS

Consultant Pediatric Otolaryngologist, Great Ormond Street Hospital for Children, London, UK

David M Heimbach MD

Emeritus Professor of Surgery, University of Washington Burn Center, Harborview Medical Center, Seattle, WA, USA

Shawn L Hervey-Jumper MD

Resident Surgeon, Department of Neurosurgery, University of Michigan Health System, Ann Arbor, MI, USA

Melanie Hiorns MD

Consultant Paediatric Radiologist, Great Ormond Street Hospital for Children, London, USA

Ronald B Hirschl MD

Arnold G Coran Collegiate Professor of Surgery, CS Mott Children's Hospital, University of Michigan, Section of Pediatric Surgery, Ann Arbor, MI, USA

George W Holcomb III MD MBA

Surgeon-in-Chief, Children's Mercy Hospital, Katharine Berry Richardson Professor of Surgery, Kansas City, MO, USA

Michael E Höllwarth
Department of Paediatric and Adolescent Surgery, Medical University of Graz, Graz, Austria

John M Hutson AO BS MD DSc(Melb) MD(Monash) FRACS FAAP(Hon)
Professor of Paediatric Surgery, University of Melbourne, Royal Children's Hospital, Melbourne, Victoria, Australia

Thomas H Inge MD PhD
Associate Professor of Surgery and Pediatrics and Surgical Director, Surgical Weight Loss Program for Teens, Division of Pediatric General and Thoracic Surgery, Cincinnati Children's Hospital Medical Center, Cincinnati, OH, USA

Saleem Islam MD
Associate Professor of Surgery, Division of Pediatric Surgery, University of Florida College of Medicine, Gainesville, FL, USA

Kishore Iyer FRCS(Eng)
Director, Intestinal Transplantation and Rehabilitation Program, Mount Sinai Medical Center, New York, New York, USA

Tom Jaksic MD Phd
W Hardy Hendren Professor of Surgery, Department of Surgery, Children's Hospital Harvard Medical School, Boston, MA, USA

Marcus Jarboe MD
Assistant Professor of Surgery, Section of Pediatric Surgery, Mott Children's Hospital, University of Michigan, Ann Arbor, MI, USA

Paul RV Johnson MBChB MA MD FRCS(Eng) FRCS(Edin) FRCS(Paed Surg)
Professor of Paediatric Surgery, University of Oxford; Consultant Paediatric Surgeon, John Radcliffe Hospital, Oxford, UK

Frederick M Karrer MD
Professor of Surgery and Pediatrics, The David R and Kiku Akers Chair in Pediatric Surgery, The Children's Hospital, The University of Colorado School of Medicine, Aurora, CO, USA

Naziha Khen-Dunlop MD
Necker-Enfants Malades Hopsital, Paris Descartes University, Paris, France

Edward Kiely FRCS(I) FRCS FRCPCH
Consultant Paediatric Surgeon, Department of Paediatric Surgery, Great Ormond Street Hospital for Children, London, UK

Peter Kim MD PhD FRCSC
Professor, Department of Surgery, University of Toronto, Hospital for Sick Children, Toronto, Ontario, Canada

Shaun M Kunisaki MD
Pediatric Surgery Section, Department of Surgery, CS Mott Children's Hospital, University of Michigan, Ann Arbor, MI, USA

Tom R Kurzawinski MD
Consultant Pancreatic and Endocrine Surgeon, University College London Hospitals, Royal Free Hospital and Great Ormond Street Hospital, London, UK

Bhanumathi Lakshminarayanan
Specialist Registrar, Department of Paediatric Surgery, Great Ormond Street Hospital for Children Institute of Child Health, London, UK

Jacob C Langer MD
Hospital for Sick Children, Division of Pediatric Surgery, Toronto, Canada

Joseph L Lelli Jr MD
Assistant Professor of Surgery, Wayne State University Medical School, The Children's Hospital of Michigan, Detroit, MI, USA

Marci M Lesperance MD FACS FAAP
Professor and Division Chief, Pediatric Otolaryngology; Department of Otolaryngology-Head and Neck Surgery, CS Mott Children's Hospital, University of Michigan Health System, Ann Arbor, MI, USA

Phillip A Letourneau MD
General Surgery Resident, Department of Surgery, University of Texas Medical School, Houston, TX, USA

Marc A Levitt MD
Director, Colorectal Center for Children, Professor of Surgery, Colorectal Center for Children, Cincinnati Children's Hospital Medical Center, University of Cincinnati, Cincinnati, OH, USA

Nguyen Liem MD
Professor, National Hospital of Pediatrics, Dong da Hanoi, Vietnam

David A Lloyd MChir FRCS FCS(SA)
FAC Emeritus Professor, University of Liverpool; Emeritus Consultant Paediatric Surgeon, Alder Hey Children's Hospital, Liverpool, UK

Pedro-José Lopez MD
Associated Professor and Consultant Paediatric Surgery and Urology, Hospital Exequiel Gonzalez Cortes y Clinica Alemana, Santiago, Chile

John Magee MD
Professor of Surgery, Section of Transplantation, Department of Surgery; Director, Pediatric Abdominal Transplantation, University of Michigan Medical School, Ann Arbor, MI, USA

Padraig SJ Malone MB MCh FRCSI FRCS FEAPU
Consultant Paediatric Urologist, Department of Paediatric Urology, Southampton University Hospitals NHS Trust, Southampton General Hospital, Southampton, UK

Mark V Mazziotti
Assistant Professor of Surgery in the Pediatric Surgery Division of the Michael E DeBakey Department of Surgery and Assistant Professor of Pediatrics at Baylor College of Medicine, Houston, TX, USA

Alastair JW Millar MBChB FRCS (Eng) FRACS (Paed Surg) FCS (SA) DCH (Roy Coll Phys & Surg Eng)
Charles FM Saint Professor of Surgery, Department of Paediatric Surgery, Red Cross War Memorial Children's Hospital, Cape Town, South Africa

Pierre Mouriquand MD FRCS(Eng) FEAPU
Department of Pediatric Urology, Hôpital Mère-Enfants – GHE, Lyon, France

Karin M Muraszko MD
Professor and Chair, Department of Neurosurgery, University of
Michigan Health System, Ann Arbor, MI, USA

Feilim L Murphy FRCSI
Consultant Paediatric Urologist, St George's Hospital, London, UK

Imran Mushtaq MB ChB MD FRCS(Glas) FRCS(Paed)
Consultant Paediatric Urologist, Great Ormond Street Hospital for
Children, London, UK

Alp Numanoglu MBChB FCS(SA)
Principal Specialist and Associate Professor, Department of
Paediatric Surgery, Red Cross War Memorial Children's Hospital,
University of Cape Town, Cape Town, South Africa

Donald Nuss MB ChB
Professor of Clinical Surgery and Pediatrics at Eastern Virginia
Medical School, Children's Hospital of the King's Daughters,
Norfolk, VA, USA

Mikko P Pakarinen MD PhD
Associate Professor and Consultant in Pediatric Surgery,
Children's Hospital, University of Hesinki, Helsinki, Finland

John M Park MD
Cheng-Yang Chang Professor of Pediatric Urology, Director of
Pediatric Urology, Department of Urology, University of Michigan
Health System and Medical School, Ann Arbor, MI, USA

Emma Parkinson
Specialist Registrar, Department of Paediatric Surgery, Great
Ormond Street Hospital for Children Institute of Child Health,
London, UK

Alberto Peña MD
Founding Director, Colorectal Center for Children, Professor of
Surgery, Cincinnati Children's Hospital Medical Center, University
of Cincinnati, Cincinnati, OH, USA

Rafael V Pieretti MD
Lecturer in Pediatric Surgery, Chief of Pediatric Urology,
Massachusetts General Hospital, Boston, MA, USA

Agostino Pierro MD FRCS(Eng) FRCS(Ed) FAAP
Professor of Paediatric Surgery, Paediatric Surgery Unit, Institute
of Child Health, University College London, London, UK

Garrett D Pohlman MD
Resident, University of Colorado, Denver, Anschutz Medical
Campus, Division of Urology, Aurora, CO, USA

Kristina M Potanos MD
Department of Surgery, Children's Hospital Boston and Harvard
Medical School, Boston, Massachusetts

Thomas Pranikoff MD
Professor of Surgery and Pediatrics, Section of Pediatric Surgery,
Wake Forest School of Medicine, and Pediatric Surgeon, Brenner
Children's Hospital, Winston-Salem, NC, USA

Prem Puri MS FRCS FRCS(ED) FACS FAAP (HON)
Newman Clinical Research Professor, University College Dublin,
President, National Children's Research Centre, Our Lady's
Children's Hospital, Consultant Paediatric Surgeon, Beacon
Hospital, Dublin, Ireland

Frederick J Rescorla MD
Professor, Section of Pediatric Surgery, Attending Surgeon,
Indiana University School of Medicine, James Whitcomb Riley
Hospital for Children, Indianapolis, IN, USA

Yann Révillon MD
Professor, Necker-Enfants Malades Hopsital, Paris Descartes
University, Paris, France

Risto J Rintala MD PhD
Professor of Pediatric Surgery, Children's Hospital, University of
Helsinki, Helsinki, Finland

Jonathan P Roach MD
Resident in Pediatric Surgery, The Children's Hospital, The
University of Colorado School of Medicine, Aurora, CO,
USA

Heinz Rode MMed(Surg) FCS(SA) FRCS(Ed)
Emeritus Professor of Paediatric Surgery, Red Cross War
Memorial Children's Hospital, University of Cape Town, South
Africa

Derek Roebuck FRCR FRANZCR
Consultant Interventional Radiologist, Department of Radiology,
Great Ormond Street Hospital, London, UK

Steven S Rothenberg MD FACS
Clinical Professor of Surgery, Columbia University College of
Physicians and Surgeons, New York, NY and Chief of Pediatric
Surgery, The Rocky Mountain Hospital for Children, Denver, CO,
USA

Shawn D St Peter MD
Director, Center for Prospective Clinical Trials, Children's Mercy
Hospital, Kansas City, MO, USA

John A Sandoval MD
Assistant Member of Surgery, Department of Surgery, St. Jude
Children's Research Hospital, Memphis, TN, USA

Marshall Z Schwartz MD
Professor of Surgery and Pediatrics, Department of Surgery, St
Christopher's Hospital for Children, Philadelphia, PA, USA

Robert C Shamberger MD
Robert E Gross Professor of Surgery, Harvard Medical School,
Chief of Surgery, Children's Hospital, Boston, MA, USA

Neil J Sherman MD FACS FAAP
Associate Clinical Professor of Surgery, Keck University of
Southern California School of Medicine, West Covina, CA, USA

Naima Smeulders MA MD FRCS(Paeds)
Consultant Paediatric Urologist, Great Ormond Street Hospital
and UCLH Hospitals NHS Trusts, London, UK

Stig Sømme MD
Children's Hospital, Department of Pediatric Surgery, University of
Colorado, Aurora, CO, USA

Lewis Spitz MBChB PhD MD(Hon) FRCS (Edin, Eng) FRCSI(Hon) FAAP(Hon)
FCS(SA)(Hon) FACS(Hon)
Emeritus Nuffield Professor of Paediatric Surgery, Institute of
Child Health, University College London; Consultant Paediatric
Surgeon, Great Ormond Street Hospital for Children, London, UK

James E Stein MD FACS FAAP
University of Southern California-Keck School of Medicine, Attending Pediatric Surgeon, Children's Hospital of Los Angeles, Los Angeles, CA, USA

Charles JH Stolar MD
Professor of Surgery, Columbia University, College of Physicians and Surgeons, and Attending Surgeon, Morgan Stanley Children's Hospital, New York-Presbyterian, New York City, New York, USA

Steven Stylianos
Chief, Division of Pediatric Surgery, Associate Surgeon-in-Chief, Cohen Children's Medical Center of NY, North Shore – LIJ Health System, New York, NY, USA

Ian Sugarman MB ChB FRCS(Paed Surg)
Consultant Paediatric Surgeon, Leeds General Infirmary, Leeds, UK

Riccardo A Superina MD CM FRCS(C) FACS
Professor of Surgery, Feinberg School of Medicine, Northwestern University, Director, Transplant Surgery and Co-Director Siragusa Transplant Center, Children's Memorial Hosital, Chicago, IL, USA

Jonathan Sutcliffe MB ChB FRCS(Paed Surg)
Consultant Paediatric Surgeon, Leeds General Infirmary, Leeds, UK

Paul KH Tam MD
Chair, Professor of Pediatric Surgery, The University of Hong Kong, Queen Mary Hospital, Hong Kong

Hock Lim Tan MBBS MD FRACS FRCS(Eng)
Visiting Paediatric Surgeon, Prince Court Medical Centre, Kuala Lumpur, Malaysia, and Adjunct Professor of Surgery, Faculty of Medicine, University of Indonesia, Jakarta

Bayani B Tecson MD FPCS FPSPS FPALES
Associate Professor of Surgery, School of Medicine, Saint Louis University, Baguio City. Chairman, Department of Surgery, Notre Dame De Chartres Hospital, Baguio City, Philippines

Daniel H Teitelbaum MD
CS Mott Children's Hospital, University of Michigan, Ann Arbor, MI, USA

Jessica Ternier MD
Consultant Neurosurgeon, Great Ormond Street Hospital for Children, London, UK

Dominic NP Thompson MBBS BSc FRCS(SN)
Consultant Neurosurgeon, Great Ormond Street Hospital for Children NHS Trust, London, UK

Shaheen J Timmapuri MD
Assistant Professor of Surgery and Pediatrics, Department of Surgery, St Christopher's Hospital for Children, Philadelphia, PA, USA

Benno Ure MD PhD
Professor of Paediatric Surgery and Chairman, Hannover Medical School, Hannover, Germany

Julian Wan
Clinical Associate Professor, Pediatric Urology, Department of Urology, University of Michigan Medical Center, Ann Arbor, MI, USA

Thomas R Weber MD
Rush University School of Medicine, Chicago, IL, USA

John R Wesley MD
Adjunct Professor of Surgery, Northwestern University Feinberg School of Medicine, Ann & Robert H. Lurie Children's Hospital of Chicago, Chicago, IL, USA

Duncan T Wilcox MD FRCS FEAPU
Chair of Pediatric Urology, Professor of Pediatric Urology – University of Colorado, The Ponzio Family Chair in Pediatric Urology, Children's Hospital Colorado, Aurora, CO, USA

Atsuyuki Yamataka MD Phd FAAP(Hon)
Department of Pediatric General and Urogenital Surgery, Juntendo University School of Medicine, Tokyo, Japan

Augusto Zani MD
Department of Paediatric Surgery, King's College Hospital, London, UK

David C van der Zee MD PhD
Professor of Pediatric Surgery, Department of Pediatric Surgery, University Medical Centre Utrecht, The Netherlands

Contributing medical artists

Graeme Chambers
50 Ballymartin Road, Killinchy, Co. Down

Peter Cox
Crown Hill, High Street, Newent, Gloucestershire

Emily Evans
Unit 1, 10–28 Millers Avenue, London

Oxford Designers and Illustrators
Aristotle House, Aristotle Lane, Oxford

Phoenix Photosetting
Chatham, Kent

Preface

The seventh edition of *Operative Pediatric Surgery* has been extensively updated and revised. It follows the well-established format of previous editions with the focus being on limited and concise text accompanying simple clear black and white line drawings. We have attempted to maintain the consistency of style and a high standard of artwork which has characterised previous editions. All the artwork has been done by a single group of medical artists thereby maintaining a unified conformity for all the operative drawing.

Each chapter commences with a short historical review, followed by the principles and justification for the procedure, preoperative investigations and preparation and the operative procedure in well-defined stages from incision, through the surgical details to wound closure. This is followed by notes on postoperative care, complications and outcome. Finally, there is a short list of recommended further reading related to the actual operation.

A new departure, reflecting the advances in minimal invasive surgery, is that, where relevant, each chapter comprises the open alongside the laparoscopic/thoracoscopic technique. Minimal invasive surgery offers significant advantages in cosmesis, reduced postoperative pain and shorter hospital stay which has obvious economic implications. There are new sections on operating room requirements for minimal invasive surgery and the ergonomics of laparoscopic surgery.

Other new chapters include thyroidectomy, management of varicocele, soft tissue and thoracic trauma, surgical procedures for dialysis and exposure for spinal surgery.

We wish to thank all authors for their efforts at achieving the highest standards with their contributions. They were all selected for their established expertise and international reputation in their particular field. We are confident that they will be proud of being involved in this publication.

The textbook is aimed primarily at trainees in pediatric surgery but provides a useful resource for established surgeons when performing wide-ranging and uncommon procedures. It is generally recognised as the operative surgery manual of choice for pediatric surgeons around the world and incorporates the varying practice of surgeons in different countries by including urology, myelomeningocele repair and transplantation.

We welcome the three new co-editors, Daniel Teitelbaum, Agostino Pierro and Hock Tan.

Operative Pediatric Surgery uniquely compliments the two volume textbook, *Pediatric Surgery*, also now in its seventh edition, in covering the full range of neonatal and general pediatric surgery.

Lewis Spitz and Arnold G Coran
January 2013

Preface from the sixth edition

This is the sixth edition of *Operative Pediatric Surgery* and the second in which the two editors have collaborated. The new edition encompasses all the major advances in the specialty that have occurred in the past decade since the previous edition was published in 1995.

The most noteworthy advance in pediatric surgery has been the development of minimal invasive surgery, which has the advantages, in addition to obvious cosmetic superiority, of reduced postoperative pain, reduced metabolic response to operative trauma, and significant reduction of postoperative hospitalization. Numerous new authors have been recruited to contribute to this developing field of minimal invasive surgery.

Other new sections include congenital vascular malformations, the Nuss procedure for pectus excavatum, the Bianchi bowel-lengthening procedure, interventional radiology, and bariatric surgery. We have omitted sections that do not fall within the purview of the pediatric surgeon, such as cleft lip and palate, protruding ears, and congenital hand deformities.

We have retained the format of previous editions of initial principles and justification for the procedure, followed by preoperative investigations and preparation, the operative procedure, and postoperative management. All illustrations are simple black and white line drawings, which have maintained the consistently high standard demanded by Gillian Lee and her associates. A limited number of recommendations for further reading are included at the end of each chapter. These may not always appear to be up to date, but have been included as the operative technique may have remained unaltered over the years.

We wish to thank all authors for their efforts at achieving the highest standard of contribution. They were selected because of their established expertise in their fields and their international reputations, and we are grateful for their time and patience. We are confident that they will be pleased with and proud of the ultimate publication.

This textbook has succeeded in being generally accepted as the operative manual of choice for pediatric surgeons around the world and takes into account the varying practices of pediatric surgery in different countries. The previous edition completely sold out within a few years of publication, and we are confident that this expanded, up-to-date new volume will be as successful.

We trust that trainees as well as established pediatric surgeons will find this textbook useful as a guide when performing a wide range of procedures.

Lewis Spitz
Arnold G. Coran

List of abbreviations used

ACC	adrenocortical carcinoma		ECLS	extracorporeal life support
ACE	antegrade continence enema		ECMO	extracorporeal membrane oxygenation
ADH	anti-diuretic hormone		ECW	extracellular water
AFP	alfa fetoprotein		EES	Ethicon endosurgery
AFP	alfa-fetoprotein		EGD	esophagogastroduodenoscopy
AGB	adjustable gastric band		EHL	electrohydraulic lithotripsy
AGC	advanced gastric cancer		EKG	electrocardiogram
AGIR	autologous gastrointestinal reconstruction		EMR	endomucosal resection
APSA	American Pediatric Surgical Association		ERCP	endoscopic retrograde
ASIS	anterior superior iliac spine			cholangiopancreatography
AVF	arteriovenous fistulas		ESWL	extracorporeal shock-wave lithotripsy
AVM	arteriovenous malformation		ETV	endoscopic third ventriculostomy
b-hCG	beta-human chorionic gonadotropin		EXIT	*ex utero* intrapartum treatment
b-HCG	beta-human chorionic gonadotropin		FAST	focused abdominal sonography for trauma
BA	biliary atresia		FDA	Food and Drug Administration
BMI	body mass index		FEV1	forced expiratory volume in the first second
BVT	basilic vein transposition		FISH	fluorescent hybridization
BXO	balanitis xerotica obliterans		FISH	fluorescent *in situ* hybridization
CAM	cystic adenomatoid malformations		FNH	focal nodular hyperplasia
CCAM	congenital cystic adenomatoid malformation		FRC	functional residual capacity
CDH	congenital diaphragmatic hernia		FVC	forced vital capacity
CF	cystic fibrosis		GA	general anesthesia
CGRP	calcitonin gene-related peptide		GE	gastroesophageal
CHI	congenital hyperinsulinism		GFR	glomerular filtration rate
CI	calcineurin inhibitors		GI	gastrointestinal
CI	confidence interval		GTN	glyceryl trinitrate
CMV	cytomegalovirus		GU	genitourinary
CNS	central nervous system		HB	hepatoblastoma
COG	Children's Oncology Group		HCC	hepatocellular carcinoma
CPAP	continuous positive airway pressure		hCG	human chorionic gonadotrophin
CRP	C-reactive protein		HCG	human chorionic gonadotropin
CSF	cerebrospinal fluid		HD	high definition
CT	computed tomography		HDMI	high-definition multimedia interface
CTA	computed tomography angiography		HEHE	hepatic epithelioid hemangioendothelioma
CVC	central venous catheters		HIV	human immunodeficiency virus
CVP	central venous pressure		HMD	hyaline membrane disease
DEXA	dual energy x-ray absorptiometry analysis		IBD	inflammatory bowel disease
DMSA	dimercaptosuccinate		ICP	intracranial pressure
DPL	diagnostic peritoneal lavage		ICU	intensive care unit
DSD	disorders of sexual development		ICW	fetal intracellular water
EA	esophageal atresia		IFALD	intestinal failure-associated liver disease
EBV	Epstein–Barr virus		IIR	internal inguinal ring
ECG	electrocardiogram		INR	international normalization ratio
ECG	electrocardiography		INR	international normalized ratio

INSS	international Neuroblastoma Staging System		PUJ	pelviureteric junction
IOUS	intraoperative ultrasonography		PUM	partial urogenital mobilization
IPPV	intermittent positive pressure ventilation		PUV	posterior urethral valves
IR	interventional radiology		PV	portal vein
ISSVA	International Society for the Study of Vascular Anomalies		PVT	portal vein thrombosis
			RICH	rapidly involuting congenital hemangioma
IUGR	intrauterine growth retardation		RIJV	right internal jugular vein
IVC	inferior vena cava		RSB	rectal suction biopsy
IVH	intraventricular hemorrhage		RUTI	recurrent urinary tract infections
LAARP	laparoscopic assisted anorectal pull-through		RWL	respiratory water loss
LACE	laparoscopic ACE		RYGBP	roux-en-Y gastric bypass
LDH	lactate dehydrogenase		SBS	short bowel syndrome
LG	long gap		SCM	sternocleidomastoid muscle
LHR	lung to head ratio		SCT	sacrococcygeal teratoma
LILT	longitudinal intestinal lengthening and tailoring		SG	sleeve gastrectomy
			SMV	superior mesenteric vein
LMA	laryngeal mask airway		SSEP	somatosensory evoked potential
LT	liver transplantation		STEP	serial transverse enteroplasty
LUQ	left upper quadrant		STEP	serial transverse enteroplasty procedure
MAGPI	meatal advancement and glanuloplasty		SVC	superior vena cava
MG	myasthenia gravis		TBSA	total body surface area
MGD	mixed gonadal dysgenesis		TBW	total body water
MIP	megameatus-intact prepuce		TDD	thoracoscopic debridement and decortication
MIS	Müllerian inhibiting substance		TEF	tracheoesophageal fistula
MMC	myelomeningocele		TEWL	transepithelial water loss
MOMS	Management of Myelomeningocele Study		TIP	tubularized incised plate
MRA	magnetic resonance angiography		TIPS	transjugular intrahepatic portosystemic shunts
MRCP	magnetic resonance cholangiopancreatography		TOF	tracheoesophageal fistula
MRI	magnetic resonance imaging		tPA	tissue plasminogen activator
MRU	magnetic resonance urography		TPN	total parenteral nutrition
NEC	necrotizing enterocolitis		TSH	thyroid stimulating hormone
NICH	non-involuting congenital hemangioma		TTTS	twin-to-twin transfusion syndrome
NIH	National Institutes of Health		TUM	total urogenital sinus mobilization
NPO	nil per os		UGI	upper gastrointestinal
NSAID	non-steroidal anti-inflammatory drugs		UGS	congenital adrenal hyperplasia
PAM	pulmonary airway malformation		UGS	urogenital sinus
PCNL	percutaneous nephrolithotomy		UNOS	United Network for Organ Sharing
PCR	polymerase chain reaction		UPJ	ureteropelvic junction
PD	peritoneal dialysis		URS	ureterorenoscopy
PDS	polydioxanone sutures		UTI	urinary tract infection
PEEP	positive end-expiratory pressure		UVJ	ureterovesical junction
PEG	percutaneous endoscopic gastrostomy		UVJ	uterovesical junction
PFIC	progressive familial intrahepatic cholestasis		UW	University of Wisconsin
PICC	percutaneously inserted central venous catheters		VA	venoarterial
			VATS	video-assisted thoracic surgery
PICC	peripheral intravenous central catheters		VATS	video-assisted thoracoscopy
PICC	peripherally inserted central catheter		VCUG	voiding cystourethrogram
PPD	primary peritoneal drainage		VMA	vanylmandelic acid
PSARP	posterior sagittal anorectoplasty		VP	ventriculoperitoneal
PSARVUP	posterior sagittal anorectovaginourethroplasty		VUR	vesicoureteric reflux
PTC	percutaneous transhepatic cholangiography		VV	venovenous
PTFE	polytetra-fluoroethylene		WHO	World Health Organization

SECTION I

General

Preoperative and postoperative management of the neonate and child

MATIAS BRUZONI and CRAIG T ALBANESE

INTRODUCTION

The physiology of the neonate, infant, child, and adolescent differ significantly from each other and from the adult. The most distinctive and rapidly changing physiologic characteristics occur during the neonatal period. This is due to the newborn infant's adaptation from complete placental support to the extrauterine environment, differences in the physiologic maturity of individual neonates, the small size of these patients, and the demands of growth and development. Advances in neonatal care have resulted in the survival of increasing numbers of extremely low birth weight infants. Extreme prematurity magnifies the already dynamic and relatively fragile physiology of the newborn period, predisposing these tiny infants to physiologic derangements in temperature regulation, fluid and electrolyte homeostasis, glucose metabolism, hematologic regulation, and immune function. In addition, physiologic and anatomic organ system immaturity make the preterm neonate vulnerable to specific problems such as intraventricular hemorrhage, hyaline membrane disease, and hyperbilirubinemia. From a surgical standpoint, these dynamic and fragile physiologic parameters are often the primary components that dictate the preoperative and postoperative management of the pediatric surgical patient. The first part of this chapter focuses on the physiology of the neonate, followed by general considerations on the perioperative care of the neonate, infant, and child.

LOW BIRTH WEIGHT INFANTS

Neonates may be classified according to their level of maturation (gestational age) and development (weight). This classification is important because the physiology of neonates may vary significantly depending on these parameters.

Under this classification system, a term, appropriate for gestational age infant is born between 37 and 42 weeks of gestation with a birth weight greater than 2500 g. However, approximately 7 percent of all babies do not meet these criteria. This may be due to prematurity or may be due to intrauterine growth retardation. From a clinical standpoint, neonates born under 2500 g are broadly classified as low birth weight (LBW) infants. Further subclassification into moderately low birth weight, very low birth weight, and extremely low birth weight infants has been used for epidemiologic and prognostic purposes (**Table 1.1**). Using this terminology, low birth weight infants may be preterm and appropriate for gestational age, term but small for gestational age (SGA), or both. The following sections will discuss several issues specific to the care of preterm and SGA infants.

Table 1.1 Newborn weight classification.

Classification	Birth weight	Premature births (%)
Low birth weight	Birth weight <2500 g	–
Moderately low birth weight	Birth weight between 2500 and 1501 g	82%
Very low birth weight	Birth weight between 1500 and 1001 g	12%
Extremely low birth weight	Birth weight <1000 g	6%

Preterm infant

By definition, preterm infants are born before 37 weeks' gestation. They generally have body weights appropriate for their age, though they may also be small for their gestational age. If the gestational age is not accurately known, the prematurity of an infant can be confirmed by physical examination. The principal features of preterm infants are a head circumference below the 50th percentile, thin, semi-transparent skin with an absence of plantar creases, soft and malleable ears with poorly developed cartilage, absence of breast buds, undescended testes (testicular descent begins around the 32nd week of gestation) with a flat scrotum in boys and relatively enlarged labia minora and small labia majora in girls.

In addition to these physical characteristics, several physiologic abnormalities exist in preterm infants. These abnormalities are often a result of unfinished fetal developmental tasks that normally enable an infant to successfully transition from intrauterine to extrauterine life. These tasks, which include renal, skin, pulmonary, immunologic, gastrointestinal, and vascular maturation, are usually completed during the final weeks of gestation. The more premature the infant, the more fetal tasks are left unfinished and the more vulnerable the infant to adverse sequelae of an early birth.

This physiologic and anatomic vulnerability sets the preterm infant up for several specific and clinically significant problems:

- Central nervous system immaturity leading to episodes of apnea and bradycardia and a weak suck reflex.
- Pulmonary immaturity leading to surfactant deficiency which can result in hyaline membrane disease (HMD).
- Cerebrovascular immaturity leading to fragile, unsupported cerebral vessels which lack the ability to autoregulate. This predisposes the preterm infant to intraventricular hemorrhage (IVH) – the most common acute brain injury of the neonate.
- Skin immaturity leading to an underdeveloped stratum corneum with significant transepithelial water loss (TEWL). This complicates the thermal regulation and fluid management of the infant.
- Gastrointestinal underdevelopment predisposing to necrotizing enterocolitis.
- Impaired bilirubin metabolism causing hyperbilirubinemia.
- Cardiovascular immaturity leading to a patent ductus arteriosus or patent foramen ovale. These retained elements of the fetal circulation can cause persistent left-to-right shunting, pulmonary hemorrhage and cardiac failure.
- Immature immune system which predisposes to a higher rate of infectious disorders in the preterm infant.

From a practical standpoint, the care of the preterm infant must be directed at preventing and/or treating these specific problems. Episodes of apnea and bradycardia are common and may occur spontaneously or as non-specific signs of problems, such as sepsis or hypothermia. Prolonged apnea with significant hypoxemia leads to bradycardia and ultimately to cardiac arrest. All preterm infants should therefore undergo apnea monitoring and electrocardiographic pulse monitoring, with the alarm set at a minimum pulse rate of 90 beats per minute. In the neonate with respiratory difficulties, chest radiography will help to detect hyaline membrane disease and cardiac failure. The lungs and retinas of preterm infants are very susceptible to high oxygen levels, and even relatively brief exposures may result in various degrees of hyaline membrane disease and retinopathy of prematurity. Infants receiving oxygen therefore require continuous pulse oximetry monitoring, with the alarm set between 85 and 92 percent. The preterm infant may also be unable to tolerate oral feeding because they have a weak suck reflex, necessitating intragastric tube feeding or parenteral nutrition. Finally, impaired bilirubin metabolism may necessitate serum bilirubin monitoring and phototherapy for rising levels of unconjugated bilirubin that can lead to kernicterus.

Small for gestational age infant

Infants whose birth weight is below the tenth percentile are considered to be small for gestational age. SGA newborns are thought to be a product of restricted intrauterine growth retardation (IUGR) due to placental, maternal, or fetal abnormalities. **Table 1.2** lists several conditions which may lead to intrauterine growth retardation in the neonate. However, it should be noted that not all infants in this group are truly growth retarded and therefore at higher risk. Some infants are simply born small as a result of a variety of factors including race, ethnicity, sex, and geography. It is important to differentiate these infants from those whose relatively low birth weight is a result of a genetic or an intrauterine abnormality.

Table 1.2 Common conditions associated with intrauterine growth retardation.

Age at delivery	Condition
Preterm	Placental insufficiency
	Discordant twin
	Chronic maternal hypertension
	Intrauterine infection
	Toxemia
Term	Congenital anomaly
	Microcephaly
Post-term	Placental insufficiency

The SGA infant can be divided into two broad categories: the symmetric SGA infant and the asymmetric SGA infant. This distinction is based primarily on when in the gestational period fetal growth was restricted. If fetal growth is restricted during the first half of pregnancy, when cellular hyperplasia and differentiation lead to tissue and organ formation, the neonate is generally a symmetric SGA infant. Fetal factors, such as genetic dwarfism, chromosomal abnormalities, congenital abnormalities, inborn errors of metabolism, and fetal infection, as well as maternal factors such as genetics, toxin ingestion, and substance abuse are all causative etiologies. While only 30 percent of SGA infants fall into this group, they have the highest morbidity and mortality rates. In contrast, asymmetric SGA infants are those who experience restriction in intrauterine growth during the last half of gestation, often during the third trimester. This is usually due to an inadequate nutrient supply. An example of this is twin gestations. Though both infants may be full term at birth, they generally have a low birth weight because placental function is inadequate to meet the growth demands of both fetuses. Other causes of asymmetric growth retardation include maternal conditions that reduce uteroplacental blood flow, such as hypertension, toxemia, cardiac disorders, and renovascular disorders.

In general, SGA infants have a body weight that is low for their gestational age, though their body length and head circumference are appropriate. The SGA infant is developmentally more mature than a preterm infant of equivalent weight. They therefore face significantly different physiologic problems. Because of the longer gestational period and resultant well-developed organ systems, the metabolic rate of the SGA infant is much higher in proportion to body weight than a preterm infant of similar overall weight. Fluid and caloric requirements are therefore increased. Intrauterine malnutrition results in a relative lack of body fat and decreased glycogen stores. In fact, body fat levels in SGA infants are often below 1 percent of their total body weight. This, coupled with their relatively large surface area greatly predisposes these infants to hypothermia and hypoglycemia. Close monitoring of blood sugar level is therefore essential. In addition, polycythemia is common in SGA infants due to increased red blood cell volumes. Occurring in 15–40 percent of asymmetric SGA babies, polycythemia may lead to the hyperviscosity syndrome characterized by respiratory distress, tachycardia, pleural effusions, and the risk of venous thrombosis. This may necessitate plasma exchange transfusions, as well as frequent monitoring of the infant's hematocrit level. Lastly, fetal asphyxia and distress due to inadequate placental support may lead to passage of meconium *in utero*. This results in an increased risk of meconium aspiration syndrome in SGA infants if the material is aspirated during labor and delivery. The perioperative management of these conditions will be detailed in the sections below. While the SGA infant is at a significant risk for morbidity and mortality associated with these problems, their adequate length of gestation puts them at a relatively lower risk for many of the conditions that affect preterm infants such as retinopathy of prematurity, intraventricular hemorrhage, and hyaline membrane disease.

PHYSIOLOGIC CONSIDERATIONS IN THE PERIOPERATIVE CARE OF THE NEONATE

As stated above, the dynamic physiologic changes that occur during the neonatal period significantly influence the perioperative care of the newborn surgical patient. In particular, physiologic derangements in temperature regulation, glucose metabolism, hematologic regulation, immune function, and fluid and electrolyte homeostasis often dictate perioperative management strategies.

Thermoregulation

Neonates are susceptible to heat loss because of their large surface area, low body fat to body weight ratio, and limited heat sink capacity due to their small size. In addition, neonates have a relatively high thermoneutral temperature zone. The optimal thermal environment (thermoneutrality) is defined as a range of ambient temperatures in which an infant, at a minimal metabolic rate, can maintain a constant normal body temperature by vasomotor control. The environmental temperature must be maintained near the appropriate thermoneutral zone for each individual. In adults, this critical temperature range is 26–28°C, while in the term infant it is 32–34°C. In the low birth weight infant, this critical range is even higher at 34–35°C.

In the neonate, heat loss may occur by evaporation, conduction, convection, and radiation. Evaporative heat loss occurs as a result of transepithelial water loss and depends on the gestational age of the infant, the relative humidity, and other environmental conditions. In addition, the presence of liquid in contact with an infant's skin also contributes to evaporative heat loss. Conductive heat loss occurs when an infant's skin is in contact with a solid object of lower temperature, causing heat to flow from the infant to the object at a rate dependent on the temperature difference between the two, as well as the insulating properties of the baby and the object. Similarly, convective heat loss occurs when the ambient air temperature is less than the infant's skin temperature. Convective heat loss depends on the temperature gradient between the infant's skin and the air, as well as the speed of the air current over the infant. Lastly, radiant heat loss occurs via the passage of infrared rays from the infant's skin to a cooler surface, such as the incubator or nursery wall. This type of heat loss is often the most difficult to control.

THERMOGENESIS IN THE NEONATE

Neonates generate heat by increasing metabolic activity. Unlike adults, neonates achieve this principally by non-shivering thermogenesis using brown fat. This has practical consequences because brown fat may be rendered inactive by pressors or anesthetic and neuromuscular blocking agents. Brown fat stores may also be depleted due to poor nutritional intake, such as in an SGA infant. When an infant is exposed to cold, metabolic work increases above basal levels and calories are consumed to maintain body temperature. If prolonged, this depletes the limited energy reserves of the neonate and predisposes to hypothermia and increased mortality.

Practical considerations

The environmental temperature of the neonate is best controlled in an incubator by monitoring the ambient temperature and maintaining it at thermoneutrality. Inside the incubator, clothing on the infant can increase insulation, reducing radiant and convective heat loss. In particular, covering the head with an insulated hat can reduce heat loss and total metabolic activity during cold stress by up to 15 percent. Similarly, conductive heat loss is minimized by the use of insulating padding. The incubators themselves are plastic walled containers that warm the infant by convection. The air in the incubator is heated by a heating element and then circulated by a fan. A servo system regulates incubator temperature according to the patient's skin temperature monitored by a skin probe. In this manner, the infant's skin temperature is maintained at a relatively constant value. Double-walled incubators minimize radiant heat loss by maintaining the inner wall of the incubator at the same temperature as the air temperature inside the incubator. Finally, humidity can be provided to the incubator environment, thereby reducing evaporative heat loss.

Optimal air temperatures for individual infants vary with the gestational age and condition of the infant, as well as with specific environmental factors, such as humidity and airflow. Standard nomograms are available that aid in determining the appropriate incubator temperature necessary to achieve thermoneutrality. Term infants usually require the incubator air temperature to be 32–34°C. Low birth weight infants may require temperatures at or above 35°C.

In contrast to incubators, radiant warmers provide open access and visibility to the infants. They are often used for surgical patients in whom frequent access to the patient and tubes/lines is necessary. Radiant warmers generate heat by means of an overhead panel that produces heat in the infrared range. However, their side rails are only minimally protective against convective heat loss and often lead to higher evaporative water and heat losses. This evaporative heat loss may be reduced by plastic sheets.

The feedback mechanisms of both incubators and radiant warmers are used to maintain an infant's skin temperature in the normal range. The normal skin temperature for a term infant is 36.2°C and for a low birth weight infant is 36.5°C. Increased metabolic activity can be detected by comparing skin and rectal temperatures, which normally differ by 1.5°C. A decreasing skin temperature with a constant rectal temperature suggests that the metabolic rate has increased to maintain the core temperature.

In a cold environment, such as the operating room or radiology suite, heat loss may be reduced by wrapping the head, extremities, and as much of the trunk as possible in clothing, plastic sheets, or aluminum foil. A variety of warming 'blankets' is available. A plastic sheet placed beneath the infant decreases the humidity of the microenvironment between it and the sheet. After draping, the infant is covered by a large adhesive plastic sheet which diminishes evaporative heat and water loss and prevents the infant from becoming wet during the operation. Any exposed intestine (e.g. gastroschisis) should be wrapped in plastic. An overhead infrared heating lamp should be focused on the infant during induction of anesthesia, preparation for operation, and at the termination of the operation. Solutions used for skin cleansing, as well as intracorporeal irrigation, should be warmed.

Glucose homeostasis

The fetus receives glucose from its mother by facilitated placental diffusion; very little is derived from fetal gluconeogenesis. The limited liver glycogen stores accumulated during the later stages of gestation are rapidly depleted within 2–3 hours after birth. The blood glucose level of the infant then depends on the neonate's capacity for gluconeogenesis, the adequacy of substrate stores, and the energy requirements of the infant. Of note, the neonate's ability to synthesize glucose from fat or protein substrates is severely limited, necessitating the intake of exogenous carbohydrates to maintain adequate blood glucose levels.

HYPOGLYCEMIA

The risk of developing hypoglycemia is high in low birth weight infants (especially SGA infants), those born to toxemic or diabetic mothers, and those requiring surgery who are unable to take oral nutrition and who have the additional metabolic stresses of their disease and the surgical procedure. The clinical features of hypoglycemia are non-specific and include a weak or high-pitched cry, cyanosis, apnea, jitteriness or trembling, apathy, and seizures. The differential diagnosis includes other metabolic disturbances or sepsis. Over 50 percent of infants with symptomatic hypoglycemia suffer significant neurologic damage. Neonatal hypoglycemia is defined as a serum glucose level less than 30 mg/dL in the full-term infant and less than 20 mg/dL in the low birth weight infant. However, neurologic abnormalities have been reported with higher blood glucose levels. Older children, particularly those with depleted stores and severe metabolic demands, are also at risk of hypoglycemia.

Practical considerations

All pediatric surgical patients, particularly neonates, are monitored for hypoglycemia. To avoid delay, blood glucose levels can be rapidly determined in the neonatal unit using blood glucose reagent strips. This may be correlated at intervals with serum glucose determinations, the frequency depending on the stability of the patient. Any intravenous fluids administered should contain at least 10 percent dextrose, and ready-made bags of parenteral nutrition should be initiated within the first few hours of life. If non-dextrose-containing solutions, such as blood or plasma, are being administered, close monitoring of the blood glucose level is essential. Hypoglycemia should be treated urgently with intravenous 50 percent dextrose, 1–2 mL/kg, and maintenance intravenous dextrose, 10–15 percent, 80–100 mL/kg for each 24 hours.

HYPERGLYCEMIA

Hyperglycemia is commonly a problem of very low birth weight infants on parenteral nutritional support since they have a low insulin response to glucose. Hyperglycemia may lead to intraventricular hemorrhage and renal water and electrolyte loss from glycosuria. Prevention of hyperglycemia is by small and gradual incremental changes in the glucose concentration and infusion rate.

Hematologic considerations

Total blood, plasma, and red cell volumes are higher during the first few hours after birth than at any other time in an individual's life. The levels may be further increased if a significant placental transfusion takes place at delivery (delayed umbilical cord clamping). Several hours after birth, plasma shifts out of the circulation and total blood and plasma volumes decrease. The high red blood cell volume persists, decreasing slowly to reach adult levels by the third postnatal month. Age-related estimations of blood volume are summarized in **Table 1.3**.

Table 1.3 Estimation of blood volume.

Age	Blood volume (mL/kg)
Preterm infants	85–100
Term infants	85
1–3 months	75
3 months to adult	70

POLYCYTHEMIA

In addition to SGA infants, neonatal polycythemia occurs in infants of diabetic mothers and infants of mothers with toxemia of pregnancy. In the neonate, polycythemia is defined as a central venous hematocrit greater than 65 percent or a hemoglobin level greater than 22 g/dL. Values at or above this threshold may be associated with high blood viscosity which is further increased by a fall in body temperature. Partial exchange transfusion may be indicated since hyperviscosity may be an etiologic factor for several disorders including central nervous system dysfunction or necrotizing enterocolitis.

ANEMIA

In the neonate, anemia is generally due to hemolysis, blood loss, or decreased erythrocyte production. Hemolytic anemia in the newborn is most often caused by placental transfer of maternal antibodies that destroy the infant's erythrocytes. Significant hemolytic anemia is most commonly due to Rh incompatibility producing jaundice,

pallor, hepatosplenomegaly, and in severe cases, hydrops fetalis. In addition, congenital infections, inherited hemoglobinopathies, and thalassemias may all manifest as hemolytic anemia in the newborn period. In severe cases, these conditions may require exchange transfusions.

In addition to hemolysis, severe anemia in the neonate may be secondary to acute hemorrhage. This can occur as a result of placental abruption or *in utero* bleeding into the intraventricular, intra-abdominal, subgaleal, or mediastinal spaces. Twin–twin transfusion syndrome may also result in severe anemia in the 'donor' co-twin. Lastly, anemia of prematurity due to decreased red blood cell production is another cause of significant neonatal anemia. This occurs in preterm infants born before a gestational age of 30–34 weeks, before erythropoietin release by the kidneys has occurred.

HEMOGLOBIN

Infant erythopoiesis does not occur until approximately two to three months of age. Until that time, fetal hemoglobin represents the vast majority of circulating hemoglobin in the neonate. In fact, approximately 80 percent of an infant's circulating hemoglobin is fetal at birth. This is significant in that the high proportion of fetal to adult hemoglobin in the neonate shifts their hemoglobin dissociation curve to the left. Since fetal hemoglobin has a higher affinity for retaining oxygen, lower peripheral oxygen levels are needed to release and deliver oxygen from fetal blood to the receiving end tissues. Thus, a high oxygen saturation percentage reading on a transcutaneous pulse oximeter may be associated with a relatively low blood pO_2 measurement. As fetal hemoglobin is broken down, a 'physiologic' anemia results with a nadir at about two to three months of age.

COAGULOPATHY

The routine administration of vitamin K to all neonates to prevent hypoprothrombinemia and hemorrhagic disease is established practice. This may be overlooked during the activities attendant on major congenital anomalies or conditions requiring urgent surgical evaluation. When in doubt, 1 mg of vitamin K should be administered by intramuscular or intravenous injection.

JAUNDICE

Heme pigments, notably hemoglobin, are catabolized in the spleen and liver to produce bilirubin. The bilirubin is conjugated with glucuronic acid in the liver, forming a water-soluble substance which is excreted via the biliary system into the intestine. In the fetus, the lipid-soluble, unconjugated (indirect) bilirubin is cleared across the placenta. In the fetal intestine beta-glucuronidase hydrolases conjugate bilirubin, which is then reabsorbed for transplacental clearance. Circulating unconjugated bilirubin is bound to albumin.

The neonate's capacity for conjugating bilirubin is not fully developed and may be exceeded by the bilirubin load, resulting in transient physiologic jaundice which reaches a maximum at the age of 4 days, but returns to normal levels by the sixth day. Usually, the maximum bilirubin level does not exceed 10 mg/dL. Physiologic jaundice is particularly likely to occur in SGA and preterm infants in whom a higher and more prolonged hyperbilirubinemia may be encountered.

High serum levels of unconjugated bilirubin may cross the immature blood–brain barrier in the neonate and can act as a neural poison leading to kernicterus. This condition, in its most severe form, is characterized by athetoid cerebral palsy and sensorineural hearing loss. Predisposing factors are hypoalbuminemia, acidosis, cold stress, Rh incompatibility, hypoglycemia, caloric deprivation, hypoxemia, and competition for bilirubin-binding sites by drugs (e.g. furosemide, digoxin, and gentamicin) or free acids.

Practical considerations

Clinical jaundice is apparent at serum bilirubin levels greater than 5 mg/dL. A rapid rise early in the neonatal period suggests hemolysis, secondary to inherited enzyme defects or to maternal–neonatal blood group incompatibilities. Prolonged (greater than 2 weeks postnatal) hyperbilirubinemia is often associated with an increase in conjugated bilirubin due to biliary obstruction or hepatocellular dysfunction. Breast milk jaundice commonly appears between 1 and 8 weeks of age. Mild indirect hyperbilirubinemia occurs with pyloric stenosis and quickly disappears after pyloromyotomy. Intestinal obstruction can intensify jaundice by increasing the enterohepatic circulation of bilirubin. Birth trauma with bleeding (e.g. caput medusae) can lead to jaundice as the blood is reabsorbed and hemolysed. Finally, jaundice is an early and important sign of septicemia.

If hemolysis is suspected, serial hematocrit estimations, reticulocyte counts, peripheral blood smears, and a Coomb's test are appropriate. Evaluation of neonatal sepsis includes hematocrit, white blood cell count and differential platelet count, chest radiography and cultures of blood, urine, and cerebrospinal fluid.

Phototherapy is widely used prophylactically in high-risk neonates to decrease the serum bilirubin levels by photodegradation of bilirubin in the skin to water-soluble products. It is continued until the total serum bilirubin level is less than 10 mg/dL and falling. The timing of phototherapy is based on the level of indirect bilirubin and the weight of the patient. Exchange transfusion is usually indicated if the indirect bilirubin level exceeds 25 mg/dL. The precise indications vary according to the individual patient, and in very low birth weight infants exchange transfusion is indicated at much lower serum bilirubin levels. Factors increasing the risk of kernicterus also influence the indications for exchange transfusion.

Immune function

As a group, neonates are particularly vulnerable to bacterial infections during the first 4 weeks of life. This may be due to maternal factors, as well as intrinsic deficiencies in their host defense system. Maternal factors independently associated with a higher incidence of neonatal sepsis include premature onset of labor, prolonged rupture of membranes (greater than 24 hours), chorioamnionitis, colonization of the genital tract with pathogenic bacteria such as group B Streptococci, and urinary tract infection. Neonatal factors include a diminished neutrophil storage pool, abnormal neutrophil and monocyte chemotaxis, decreased cytokine and complement production and diminished levels of type-specific immunoglobulins, including IgG, secretory IgA, and IgM. Overall, these factors lead to a significantly impaired host defense mechanism in the neonate with compromised anatomical barriers. These deficiencies are more severe in low birth weight infants.

Practical considerations

The impaired immune function and compromised anatomical barriers of neonates may contribute to postoperative infection. Specifically, wound infections, as well as infections precipitated by indwelling catheters may complicate the perioperative course of the neonate. For this reason, many surgeons advocate the use of prophylactic, broad-spectrum antimicrobials in neonatal surgical patients. While this practice may be common, it should be noted that the specific antibiotics used, as well as the duration of antibiotic therapy, are very site- and surgeon-specific parameters. At this time, there are no conclusive studies supporting the use of any particular regimen. Therefore, the prophylactic use of antibiotics in these patients must be determined on a case-by-case and surgeon-by-surgeon basis.

Fluid and electrolyte homeostasis

TOTAL BODY WATER

In the fetus, total body water (TBW) constitutes 94 percent of the body weight during early gestation. As the fetus grows, this percentage progressively diminishes to a value of 78 percent at term. This then decreases further by approximately 3–5 percent during the first 5 days of life, eventually reaching adult levels by nine months to one year of age. In addition to total body water, extracellular water (ECW) also declines until one to three years of age. In the term infant, ECW is often 40 percent of birth weight at 5 days. By three months of age, this value decreases to 33 percent, stabilizing at adult values of 20–25 percent by one to three years of age. Conversely, fetal intracellular water (ICW) slowly increases during gestation and the neonatal period. At 20 weeks' gestation, ICW is around 25 percent. This increases to 33 percent at the time of birth, finally reaching adult levels around 44 percent by three months of age.

The neonate must complete these water redistribution tasks to effectively transition from the intrauterine to the extrauterine environment. Under normal conditions, these changes in fetal body water progress in an orderly fashion *in utero* and after birth. If this process is interrupted by premature birth or intrauterine growth retardation, specific tasks may be left uncompleted predisposing the infant to increased risk for developing serious complications, such as patent ductus arteriosus and congestive heart failure.

RENAL FUNCTION

Compared to adults, the newborn infant has a relatively low renal blood flow and plasma flow and a high renovascular resistance. In fact, only 6 percent of the newborn's cardiac output is directed to the kidneys. This is in contrast to the 25 percent of cardiac output in adults. Overall, these factors lead to a relatively decreased glomerular filtration rate (GFR) in neonates. In term infants, the GFR rises rapidly during the first three months of life, nearing adult levels by 12–24 months of age. In premature infants, this process is delayed and GFR may lag behind the term infant.

In addition to GFR, the concentration capacity of the neonatal kidney is significantly lower than that of the adult kidney. While the adult kidney can concentrate urine up to 1200 mOsm/kg, the neonatal kidney is only able to achieve 500–600 mOsm/kg. Furthermore, newborn renal tubules are relatively insensitive to the effects of antidiuretic hormone (ADH) and aldosterone, compared to adults. These blunted responses are magnified in preterm infants. In addition, preterm infants are at a significant risk for salt wasting. This may lead to further growth retardation, as sodium appears to be a permissive factor for growth.

PRACTICAL CONSIDERATIONS FOR FLUID MANAGEMENT

Calculating maintenance needs

The neonate's basic maintenance requirement for water is the volume required for growth, renal excretion (renal water), and replacing losses from the skin, lungs, and stool. Stool water loss has been estimated at 5–10 mL per 420 J expended, the lower figure applying to those patients not being fed. In the surgical patient with postoperative ileus, stool water loss is usually insignificant. Growth is inhibited during periods of severe stress and is also not a major factor under these conditions. The basal fluid maintenance requirement is therefore renal water plus insensible loss. Requirements during the first day of life are unique because of the greatly expanded extracellular fluid volume in the neonate, which decreases after 24 hours. In addition, neonates with intestinal obstruction are not hypovolemic as a result of intrauterine adjustments across the placenta. During these first 24 hours, basic maintenance fluid should not exceed 90 mL/kg in preterm infants weighing less than 1000 g or less than 32 weeks' gestational age. In larger infants, maintenance fluid rates should not exceed 75 mL/kg.

The basic electrolyte and energy requirements are provided by NaCl (2–5 mEq/kg per day) in 5–10 percent dextrose with the addition of potassium (2–3 mEq/kg per day) once urine production has been established. Calcium gluconate (1–2 g/L fluid) may be added, especially in preterm infants.

RENAL WATER

The volume of water required for excretion by the kidney depends on the renal solute load and the child's renal concentrating ability. The solute load that the kidneys must excrete is derived from the endogenous tissue catabolism and exogenous protein and electrolyte intake. The osmolar load is thus reduced by growth and increased by tissue necrosis and high osmolar feeds/infusions. The volume of fluid administered should be sufficient to allow excretion of the solute load at an isotonic urine osmolality of 280 mOsm/dL. It is important to understand that there is no 'normal' urine output for neonates due to the fact that the osmolar load is highly variable in newborns. The calculated ideal urine output, representing the renal water required to excrete an osmolar load, is also therefore variable.

INSENSIBLE LOSSES

Invisible continuing loss of water occurs from the lungs (respiratory water loss, RWL) and through the skin (transepithelial water loss), and constitutes the insensible water loss (IWL). RWL accounts for approximately one-third of IWL in infants older than 32 weeks' gestation and is approximately 5 mL/kg body weight per 24 hours at a relative humidity of 50 percent. Transepithelial water loss for a full-term infant in a thermoneutral environment is approximately 7 mL/kg per 24 hours. The insensible water loss for a full-term infant in the thermoneutral environment at 50 percent humidity is therefore 12 mL/kg per 24 hours.

The main factors that affect IWL are the gestational age of the infant and the relative humidity of the environment. For infants 25–27 weeks' gestation, TEWL has been estimated at 128 mL/kg per 24 hours at 50 percent relative humidity. The relative humidity has a marked inverse effect on TEWL, which decreases to almost zero as the relative humidity approaches 100 percent. Plastic sheets may be used to increase the relative humidity around the infant and reduce TEWL by 50–70 percent. Conversely, radiant warmers and phototherapy increase IWL. This loss is magnified in the preterm infant.

MANAGEMENT PROGRAM

The most commonly used method of calculating fluid requirements is based on body weight. However, because of the many factors affecting maintenance requirements, there is no close or constant relationship between body weight and fluid and electrolyte needs. Thus, many surgeons advocate the use of a dynamic approach to fluid management. Such approaches generally begin with the administration of an initial fluid volume that is safe for the patient's status. This initial volume is essentially a 'best guess' volume. The effects of this volume on the patient's physiology are then monitored and appropriate changes are made.

CALCULATION OF ADDITIONAL LOSSES

External losses from stomas, fistulas, and drainage tubes are directly measured and replaced volume for volume with an appropriate electrolyte solution. In neonates, it is wise to measure the electrolytes in the fluid to guide replacement more accurately. Protein-rich losses (e.g. pleural fluid from chest tubes) can be replaced with 5–25 percent albumin solutions. Internal losses into body cavities or tissues (third space losses) cannot be measured, and adequate replacement of these losses depends on careful monitoring of the patient's response to fluid therapy.

CONSIDERING PRE-EXISTING FLUID DEFICITS OR EXCESSES

In addition to addressing maintenance requirements and additional losses, the fluid management of the neonate should include an assessment of any pre-existing fluid deficits or excesses. Pre-existing deficits may be due to *in utero* or intrapartum hemorrhage, as well as third space losses. Pre-existing excesses may be secondary to prematurity leading to a high total body water content. In all of these cases, the pre-existing condition should be considered when determining a fluid management plan.

MONITORING THE FLUID AND ELECTROLYTE PROGRAM

Once a fluid and electrolyte management program has been initiated, proper monitoring must occur to identify the newborn's response. In this manner, therapy may be adjusted dynamically to meet the specific needs of each neonate. The newborn's response to a fluid and electrolyte program may be monitored by the clinical examination, body weight measurements, and urine volume and composition measurements.

Clinical features

Severe isotonic and hypovolemic dehydration results in poor capillary filling and collapse of peripheral veins. The skin is cool and mottled, with reduced turgor; the mucous membranes are dry and the anterior fontanelle is sunken. These findings occur with 10 percent body fluid losses in an infant of more than 28 days of age and with 15 percent losses in a neonate. Hypertonic dehydration is more difficult to detect clinically because the decrease in circulating blood volume is considerably less than the total loss of body fluids. Signs of shock occur late and central nervous system signs, such as lethargy, stupor, and seizures, predominate.

BODY WEIGHT

Serial measurements of body weight are a useful guide to total body water in the neonate. Fluctuations over a 24-hour period are primarily related to loss or gain of fluid, 1 g body weight being approximately equal to 1 mL water. Errors will occur if changes in clothing, dressings, tubes, and standard intravenous boards are not accounted for, and if weighing scales are not regularly calibrated.

URINE VOLUME AND COMPOSITION

If the volume of fluid administered is inadequate, urine volume falls and its concentration increases. If excess fluid is administered, the opposite occurs. The authors aim to achieve a urine output which will maintain a urine osmolality of approximately 280 mOsmol/dL. In neonates, this usually results in a urine output of 2 mL/kg per hour. For infants and older children, hydration is adequate if the urine output is 1–2 mL/kg per hour with an osmolality of 280–300 mOsmol/kg. Serial hematocrit changes, in the absence of hemolysis or bleeding, also suggest a loss or gain of plasma water.

When the osmolar load is large, for example with extensive tissue destruction or with infusion of high osmolar solutions, urine flow may have to be increased to provide adequate renal clearance. Accurate measurements of urine flow and concentration are fundamental to the management of critically ill infants and children. In this situation, the insertion of an indwelling urinary catheter is recommended.

The specific gravity of the urine is a reliable indicator of hypertonicity (>1.012 specific gravity) and hypotonicity (<1.008 specific gravity), but is unreliable if urine is in the isotonic range (1.009–1.011 specific gravity). When fluid monitoring is critical, urine osmolality estimations provide more precise information than specific gravity. An increase in osmolality suggests that too little water or too much electrolyte has been given. A fall in osmolality suggests that sodium replacement is inadequate or that too much water has been administered. An unexpected change in osmolality, particularly an increase, requires immediate determination of serum levels of electrolytes, blood urea nitrogen, and glucose values, and a calculation of the osmolality. Serum osmolality can be measured directly or calculated by the formula:

$$\text{Osmolality} = \text{serum sodium} \times 1.86$$
$$+ \frac{\text{blood urea nitrogen}}{2.8} + \frac{\text{glucose}}{18} + 5$$

From this, it is possible to determine whether the rise in osmolality is due to an increase in serum sodium, the development of hyperglycemia or high blood urea nitrogen. Occasionally, the measured serum osmolality is higher than the calculated osmolality. This suggests that the increase in serum osmolality is due to some unidentified osmolar active substance, such as a metabolic byproduct resulting from sepsis, shock, or radio-opaque contrast material.

A rising blood urea nitrogen level and falling urine output may be due to acute renal failure or prerenal oliguria with azotemia resulting from hypovolemia. The distinction between these two states is important for appropriate treatment. Initially, the response to a fluid challenge of 20 mL/kg 5 percent dextrose and sodium chloride over 1 hour is monitored. If oliguria persists, the sodium, creatinine and osmolality levels in both the blood and urine are determined. The fractional excretion of sodium (Fe_{Na}) is calculated using the formula:

$$Fe_{Na} = \frac{\text{urine Na/serum Na}}{\text{urine creatinine/serum creatinine}} \times 100$$

A normal Fe_{Na} is 2–3 percent. A value below 2 percent implies prerenal azotemia and a value above 3 percent implies renal failure.

Calcium and magnesium homeostasis

In addition to fluid and sodium management, calcium and magnesium homeostasis are clinically significant challenges in the newborn surgical patient. The fetus receives calcium by active transport across the placenta, 75 percent of the total requirement being transferred after the 18th week of gestation. Hypocalcemia, defined as a serum level of ionized calcium below 1.0 mg/100 mL, is most likely to occur 24–48 hours after birth. Causes include decreased calcium stores, decreased renal phosphate excretion, and relative hypoparathyroidism secondary to suppression by high fetal calcium levels. Low birth weight infants are at a great risk (particularly if they are preterm), as are those born of a complicated pregnancy or delivery (e.g. diabetic mother), or those receiving bicarbonate infusions. Exchange transfusions or the rapid administration of citrated blood may also lead to hypocalcemia. The symptoms of hypocalcemia are non-specific and include jitteriness, high-pitched crying, cyanosis, vomiting, twitching, and seizures. Diagnosis is confirmed by determining the serum calcium level. However, the ionized fraction of the serum calcium may be low, resulting in clinical hypocalcemia without a great reduction in total serum calcium. Therefore, evaluation of the serum ionized calcium level is often useful.

Practical considerations

Hypocalcemia is prevented by adding calcium gluconate to daily maintenance therapy, 1–2 g per 24 hours intravenously or 2 g per 24 hours by mouth. Symptomatic hypocalcemia is treated by intravenous administration of 10 percent calcium gluconate in a dose of 1–2 mL/kg over 10 minutes; the rate should not exceed 1 mL/min.

Infants at high risk for hypocalcemia are also at risk for hypomagnesemia. In fact, the two conditions may coexist. If there is no response to attempted correction of a documented calcium deficiency, hypomagnesemia should be suspected and serum magnesium levels measured. Hypomagnesemia is corrected by administering 50 percent magnesium sulfate, 0.2 mEq/kg every 6 hours intravenously, followed by oral magnesium sulfate 30 mEq/day.

Although most seizures that occur in the neonatal period have a cerebral cause and are not secondary to hypoglycemia or hypocalcemia, hypocalcemia should be suspected in high-risk infants, particularly after surgery. Immediate blood glucose determination and serum glucose and calcium measurements should therefore be performed in a 'jittery' neonate. Treatment should be prompt, with intravenous glucose when hypoglycemia is suspected, followed by intravenous calcium if symptoms persist.

GENERAL CONSIDERATIONS IN THE PERIOPERATIVE CARE OF THE NEONATE AND CHILD

Preoperative care

The goals of appropriate preoperative care include:

1. Identifying and optimizing potential coexisting diseases
2. Preparing the patient and the family for the specific operation
3. Adequate patient identification: 'The time out'.

IDENTIFYING AND OPTIMIZING COEXISTING DISEASES

In a study performed on more than 90 000 pediatric non-cardiac and cardiac anesthesia cases, the incidence of perioperative cardiac arrest attributable to anesthesia was 0.65 per 10 000 anesthetics, suggesting that the large majority of perioperative cardiac arrests in children are caused by factors not related to anesthetic management. However, the preoperative evaluation performed by the anesthesia team is essential in identifying potential perioperative complications since neonates and infants continue to be at the highest risk for perioperative cardiac arrest and death during procedures requiring general anesthesia.

PREPARING THE PATIENT AND THE FAMILY FOR THE SPECIFIC PROCEDURE

Informed consent and family counseling

The American College of Surgeons has provided guidelines on the content of the information to be provided to patients to meet informed consent requirements. However, existing guidelines, although adequate for most adult patients, may not always satisfy the needs of the pediatric patient since by definition they lack decision-making capacity. The parents of the child can give informed 'permission' for the procedure, but it is very difficult to assess whether the child's best interests are being represented. Nevertheless, it is sufficient for ethical and legal purposes. The pediatric surgeon should spend quality time performing the informed consent because it helps gain the parent's trust and promotes a rewarding physician–patient/family relationship.

Informed consent should disclose, at the minimum:

- the surgeon's understanding of the problem;
- further measures to be taken to clarify the diagnosis, if indicated;
- the indication for emergency operation;
- a brief description of the procedure;
- alternatives to treatment, including the option to do nothing;
- the surgeon's recommendation as to the best alternative;
- the benefits and risks of the proposed operation, compared with alternatives;
- the anticipated outcome.

Surgical procedures instill a fair amount of preoperative fear for pediatric patients and their families. Separation anxiety, pain, disfigurement, loss of loved ones, and loss of control or autonomy all happen as the child is taken away from their parents and into the operating room. As a result, after undergoing surgery, children can feel betrayed by those whom they believed should protect them (e.g. parents). The entire health-care team is part of the surgical experience and should anticipate preoperative anxiety in both children and families since these factors may result in an overall negative surgical experience. Preoperative anxiety has been shown to delay the induction of anesthesia and provoke the release of stress hormones, which can hinder recovery.

The success of perioperative preparation programs in decreasing children's and families' anxiety, and in assisting families to deal with the stress of surgery has been widely documented. Child life services provide most of the preparation tools. A few examples include tours of the places they will see during the day of surgery, films about surgery or anesthesia, puppet shows, medical play, and photographs of previous children's experience. The anesthesia and preoperative team can also assist by the administration of anxiolytic medications.

Preoperative nil per os guidelines

NPO (nil per os) is the directive given to patients and their families concerning the timing of the fasting period before surgery. The preoperative fast is an attempt to avoid regurgitation and possibly aspiration of particulate matter and liquid from the child's stomach during induction of anesthesia. Each institution has its own NPO guidelines, however most will agree to a minimum of 6 hours of NPO for milk, formula, citrus juice, and solids; 4 hours for breast milk; and 2 hours for clear liquids.

'THE TIME OUT'

Adult data suggest that at least half of all surgical complications are avoidable. In 2008, the World Health Organization (WHO) published guidelines identifying multiple recommended practices to ensure the safety of surgical patients worldwide. Using these guidelines as a reference, the Safe Surgery Saves Lives Study Group implemented a prospective 19-point checklist and showed that the rate of any complication at all sites significantly decreased from 11 to 7 percent. A standard surgical checklist verifies the patient's identity, surgical site mark, introduction of all team members by name and role, review of the need for preoperative antibiotics and/or blood products, highlighting significant concerns or previous adverse reactions/allergies (including latex sensitization), need for any special equipment, and matching the operative procedure with the informed consent. The use of a preoperative checklist involves a radical change in the behavior of surgical teams since it introduces formal pauses in the usual flow of the operating room, as well as the implementation of briefings and postoperative debriefings. However, it sets a new bar in the care of surgical patients, and has the potential to prevent a large number of disabling complications and deaths in the perioperative period.

Monitoring

Due to the dynamic physiology of the neonatal period, most newborn surgical patients should be monitored postoperatively in the neonatal unit. In addition to providing continuous oxygen saturation readings, transcutaneous pulse oximetry is useful for monitoring episodes of apnea and bradycardia which can be common in the preterm infant. Transcutaneous CO_2 monitoring is gaining popularity for those on mechanical ventilators – it provides accurate trending data. Accurate monitoring of fluid status often requires an indwelling urinary catheter and frequent laboratory evaluations.

Invasive monitoring and access in the newborn can be achieved through the umbilical vessels, as they are relatively accessible in the first 24 hours of life in this population. Specifically, umbilical catheters provide quick central venous access and arterial pressure monitoring. A 3.5-Fr catheter is required for infants less than 1500 g, while infants 1500–3500 g can accommodate a 5-Fr catheter.

Nutrition

In pediatric surgical patients, proper nutrition must be delivered to meet their relatively large energy requirements. Specifically, neonates require a large energy intake because of their high basal metabolic rate, requirements for growth and development, energy needs to maintain body heat, and their limited energy reserves. These requirements vary according to age and environmental factors and are significantly increased by cold stress, surgical procedures, infections, and injuries. Energy requirements are increased 10–25 percent by surgery, greater than 50 percent by infections, and potentially more in children with burns. Energy reserves are limited in the neonate whose liver glycogen stores are usually consumed in the first 3 hours of life. These limited reserves are even more restricted in the preterm and SGA infant.

The energy needs of individual newborns can be calculated according to the requirements for basal metabolism plus growth. **Table 1.4** lists the energy requirements of children by age group. Consideration must also be given to the adequacy of energy reserves in the presence of stress factors such as cold, infection and trauma, and surgery. The average neonate should gain between 20 and 30 g/day, or 1–2 percent of the total body weight per day. Protein should be administered at a rate of 2–3 g/kg per 24 hours to achieve a normal weight gain and 30–40 percent of the total non-protein calories should be provided as fat.

Table 1.4 Energy requirements by age.

Age (years)	Energy required per 24 hours (cal/kg)
0–1	90–120
1–7	75–90
7–12	60–75
12–18	30–60
>18	25–30

The best means of providing calories is via the gastrointestinal tract either by mouth, nasogastric, or nasojejunal feeding tube, or through a surgically placed gastrostomy or jejunostomy tube. Enteral nutrition has a direct trophic effect on the bowel integrity and development. Furthermore, early enteral nutrition has been demonstrated to have a beneficial effect on maturing the intestinal tract of the very low birth weight and sick infant. It should be started right after birth unless otherwise contraindicated.

Some indications for parenteral nutrition in the pediatric surgical patient include: extremely low birth weight infant, gastrointestinal tract abnormalities with prolonged postoperative ileus (gastroschisis, necrotizing enterocolitis), short gut syndrome following extensive bowel resection, chronic diarrhea (malabsorption syndrome), inflammatory bowel disease, severe acute alimentary disorders (pancreatitis, necrotizing enterocolitis), chylothorax, intestinal fistulas, and persistent vomiting associated with cancer chemotherapy. The daily component requirements for total parenteral nutrition (TPN) are detailed in **Table 1.5**.

Table 1.5 Total parenteral nutrition requirements.

Component	Neonate	6 month–10 years	>10 years
Calories (kcal/kg/day)	90–120	60–105	40–75
Fluid (cc/kg/day)	120–180	120–150	50–75
Dextrose (mg/kg/min)	4–6	7–8	7–8
Protein (g/kg/day)	2–3	1.5–2.5	0.8–2.0
Fat (g/kg/day)	0.5–3.0	1.0–4.0	1.0–4.0
Sodium (mEq/kg/day)	3–4	3–4	3–4
Potassium (mEq/kg/day)	2–3	2–3	1–2
Calcium (mg/kg/day)	80–120	40–80	40–60
Phosphate (mg/kg/day)	25–40	25–40	25–40
Magnesium (mEq/kg/day)	0.25–1.0	0.5	0.5
Zinc (µg/kg/day)	300	100	3 mg/day
Copper (µg/kg/day)	20	20	1.2 mg/day
Chromium (µg/kg/day)	0.2	0.2	12 mg/day
Manganese (µg/kg/day)	6	6	0.3 mg/day
Selenium (µg/kg/day)	2	2	10–20/day

Pain management

Postoperative pain management in the newborn surgical patient may be challenging. In particular, the use of opioid analgesics in the neonate must be monitored carefully and may necessitate consultation with a pain management service. As a group, neonates have a narrower therapeutic window for postoperative opioid analgesia than older age groups. In addition, neonates treated with opioids exhibit variable pharmacokinetics and are at a high risk for respiratory depression. Despite these challenges, postoperative opiate analgesia can be effectively used to control pain in neonates.

The World Health Organization designed a three-step analgesic ladder, which is a reasonable way of approaching postoperative pain:

- Step 1: non-steroidal analgesics, such as acetaminophen, ketorolac, and ibuprofen;
- Step 2: mild opioids, such as codeine, oxycodone, and tramadol.
- Step 3: stronger opioids, such as morphine, fentanyl, and methadone.

FURTHER READING

Antonoff M, Marquez T, Saltzman D. Physiology of the newborn. In: Holcomb GW III, Murphy JP, Ostlie DJ (eds). A*shcraft's Pediatric Surgery*, 5th edn. Philadelphia, PA: WB Saunders, 2010: 3–18.

Flick RP, Sprung J, Harrison TE *et al.* Perioperative cardiac arrests in children between 1988 and 2005 at a tertiary referral center: a study of 92,881 patients. *Anesthesiology* 2007; **106**: 226–37; quiz 413–4.

Gawande AA, Thomas EJ, Zinner MJ, Brennan TA. The incidence and nature of surgical adverse events in Colorado and Utah in 1992. *Surgery* 1999; **126**: 66–75.

Haynes AB, Weiser TG, Berry WR *et al.* Safe Surgery Saves Lives Study Group. A surgical safety checklist to reduce morbidity and mortality in a global population. *New England Journal of Medicine* 2009; **360**: 491–9.

Pierro A, Eaton S, Ong E. Neonatal physiology and metabolic considerations. In: Grosfeld JL, O'Neill JA, Fonkalsrud EW, Coran AG (eds). *Pediatric Surgery*, 6th edn. Philadelphia, PA: Mosby Elsevier, 2006: 89–113.

Teitelbaum DH, Coran AG. Nutritional support. In: Grosfeld JL, O'Neill JA, Fonkalsrud EW, Coran AG (eds). *Pediatric Surgery*, 6th edn. Philadelphia, PA: Mosby Elsevier, 2006: 194–220.

2

Pediatric anesthesia

ROBERT BINGHAM and MARINA GEORGE

INTRODUCTION

Pediatric anesthesia is a recognized subspecialty of anesthesia, requiring different skills and knowledge from adult anesthesia. In different countries and institutions, the upper age limit for pediatric patients can vary, usually between 14 and 18 years, but it is generally accepted that it is most important for infants and younger children to receive the specialist care of pediatric anesthetists for both physiological and psychological reasons, and to reduce the incidence of adverse events.

The biochemical, physiological, and psychological needs peculiar to young children are best met in a children's environment, with all staff being trained and familiar with children and their needs. The recommended policy is to concentrate pediatric surgery and intensive care in children's departments and children's hospitals, so that each center for neonatal surgery serves a population of about 2 million. This is feasible because the transport of sick infants, even over very long distances, by surface or air, is now routine and safe, even for intubated and ventilated patients.

Many of the differences between adult and pediatric anesthesia are related to differences in anatomy and physiology – differences that are most marked in the very young. Surgical neonates with a gestational age as low as 24 weeks and a weight of 450 g are now surviving, so that the implications of the traditional neonatal period of 28 days of post-natal life is meaningless. From an anesthetic perspective, the neonatal period is better defined as up to 44 weeks after conception (**Figure 2.1**).

The age from birth is less important than the weight of the infant and the assessment of the function of its various organ systems. For a given gestational age, the morbidity and mortality are greater, the lower the birth weight. Therefore all children should be accurately weighed on admission to hospital. Many surgical procedures in children aged up to three years are for the correction of congenital defects, and it is important to remember that

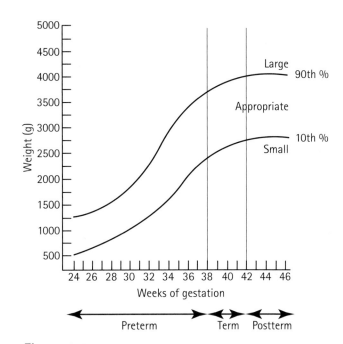

Figure 2.1 Percentile chart showing appropriate weight for gestational age.

such defects are often multiple. For example, a cardiac abnormality may be present in children with a cleft palate or esophageal atresia.

PHYSIOLOGIC DIFFERENCES BETWEEN NEONATES AND OLDER CHILDREN

Infants have poor respiratory reserves, and respiratory failure is a common sequel of pathology in any other system. Total pulmonary resistance, at 25 cmH_2O/L per second, is five times that of the adult. Lung compliance is very low (6 mL/cmH_2O compared with 160 mL/cmH_2O in the adult), but the infant chest wall is a very compliant structure, so that small infants have great difficulty in maintaining a normal functional residual capacity (FRC) in states in which pulmonary compliance is further reduced. The chest wall provides no counter-resistance to the collapsing forces of the lungs, as it will do later in life. Hence, the response to constant distending pressure in the form of positive end-expiratory pressure (PEEP) or continuous positive airway pressure (CPAP) is strikingly beneficial in this age group.

After birth, an eight-fold increase in the number of alveoli occurs and the adult number is reached by the age of six years. The resistance of the airways (and thus the work of breathing) remains high, until finally, the airways begin to enlarge; this occurs at the same time as the full complement of alveoli is present. Distal airway closure occurs within the tidal breathing range until six years of age, so there is an increase in physiologic right-to-left shunt during this period, with an even greater effect on oxygenation should the FRC fall, as it does with pulmonary disease or during anesthesia.

The resistance of the nasal passages in neonates is relatively great (45 percent of the total) and neonates are obligatory nose breathers, so respiratory obstruction may occur if the nares are blocked, for example by choanal atresia or by a large nasogastric tube. This dependence on nose breathing can be exploited with great effect in the use of nasal prongs or masks to apply distending pressure in the form of CPAP.

Alveolar ventilation and oxygen consumption per unit body weight are twice those of the adult, as manifest by the alarming rate at which hypoxemia occurs, if ventilatory problems arise.

Respiration during the early months of life is purely diaphragmatic (the bucket-handle effect of ribs becomes operational toward the end of the first year of life), so that respiratory failure may ensue if diaphragm movement is restricted, for example by abdominal distension or with phrenic nerve palsy. Attempts to increase alveolar ventilation can be made only by increasing the respiratory rate, which explains why a rising respiratory rate is a diagnostic sign of increased respiratory distress in infants. Phrenic nerve palsy may occur as part of a birth injury, but is also associated with damage to the phrenic nerve during thoracic or cardiac surgery.

The neonatal circulation is labile and may revert to the fetal pattern (with blood flowing from right to left through a patent ductus arteriosus and/or foramen ovale) if subject to conditions that promote pulmonary vasoconstriction: a state known as 'transitional circulation'. This state, previously known as persistent fetal circulation, is a transitional state between the fetal circulation, including the placenta, and that of the adult, when the right and left sides are quite separate (**Figure 2.2**).

The duct may reopen with exposure to hypoxia or fluid overload, until it is firmly closed by fibrosis after 3–4 weeks. Attempts can be made to close the duct pharmacologically, using small doses of a prostaglandin synthetase inhibitor, such as indomethacin. Conversely,

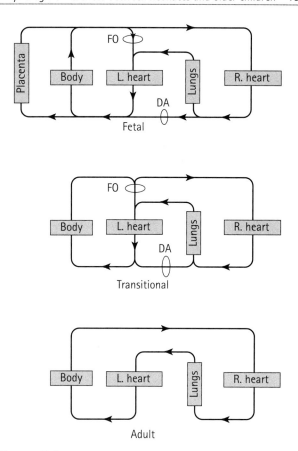

Figure 2.2 Transitional circulation. DA, ductus arteriosus; FO, foramen ovale.

prostaglandin E2 may be infused to maintain ductal patency where this is essential, for example in infants with pulmonary artery atresia, prior to surgical intervention.

The liability of the pulmonary vasculature is caused by abundant arteriolar smooth muscle, extending more peripherally than in later life (due to a failure of normal regression of the muscle in the first few hours of life). These arterioles constrict in response to hypoxia, hypercapnia, or acidosis via an adrenergic mechanism (this response is abolished after sympathectomy).

Infants with conditions such as respiratory distress syndrome of the premature infant, congenital diaphragmatic hernia, meconium aspiration or β-hemolytic streptococcal infections may develop the state of persistent pulmonary hypertension of the newborn and critical hypoxemia. If left untreated, these infants will die in a vicious cycle of cyanosis, acidosis, and falling cardiac output. Steps must be taken to reverse the high pulmonary vascular resistance: initially, a high inspired oxygen concentration (FiO_2), hyperventilation with a pH >7.4, and avoidance of painful or stress stimuli may be effective. If not, specific pulmonary vasodilators, such as inhaled nitric oxide or epoprostenol, can be employed. Extracorporeal membrane oxygenation (ECMO) may also be used for this condition at some specialist centers.

Neonates do attempt to maintain core temperature at 37°C, but may not succeed because of an initial low basal metabolic rate, a large surface-to-weight ratio, immature sweat function, and an inability to adapt to adverse conditions. Superficial thermoreceptors exist in the trigeminal area of the face; hence a cold stimulus causes an increase in metabolic heat production from hydrolysis of triglycerides in brown fat, causing a great increase in oxygen consumption, which may make existing hypoxia worse. Brown fat is distributed over the back and provides thermal lagging for the major intrathoracic vessels. The metabolic response to cold is inhibited by general anesthesia, hypoxia, hypoglycemia, and prematurity. Neonates are nursed in the neutral thermal environment at which their oxygen demands are minimal, as low as 31°C for a 3-kg term baby and up to 36°C for those with low birth weight (**Figure 2.3**). If preterm infants are allowed to cool, there is increased mortality and morbidity. They are more likely to develop respiratory disease, acidosis, hypoxia, coagulopathy, intraventricular hemorrhage, and a subsequent slower rate of brain growth.

The mean cord hemoglobin concentration is approximately 18 g/dL at birth and rises by 1–2 g/dL in the first days of life because of low fluid intake and a decrease in extracellular fluid volume. After that, the level declines (see **Figure 2.4**) and causes the physiologic anemia of infancy. Premature babies have a greater fall because of lower red cell production and survival. At birth, 70 percent of the hemoglobin is HbF, which has a greater affinity for oxygen, possibly because of a relative insensitivity to 2,3-diphosphoglycerate, which itself lowers the oxygen affinity of the hemoglobin molecule. The HbF is replaced by HbA by three months of age, at which time sickle tests become positive in children with sickle-cell disease, although most will have been diagnosed by electrophoresis in the newborn period. A hemoglobin concentration <10 g/dL is usually abnormal and severe anemias should be investigated prior to elective surgery.

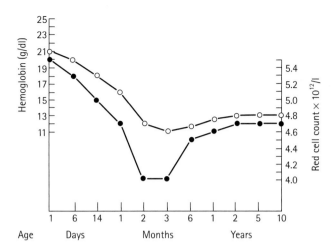

Figure 2.4 Changes in hemoglobin concentration and red cell count in the first ten years of life; ○, hemoglobin; ●, red cell count.

The blood volume of the neonate is more variable than that of the older infant and depends on the magnitude of the placental transfusion. Difficulties may arise if blood replacement is based on percentage of the estimated blood volume. The blood volume of an infant with normal hemoglobin is estimated to be 80–85 mL/kg, but in very premature infants it is greater, perhaps as much as 100 mL/kg.

Carbohydrate reserves of the normal neonate are relatively low and, as most glycogen is synthesized after 36 weeks' gestation, those of preterm infants may be very low. Blood sugar levels should average 2.7–3.3 mmol/L (50–60 mg/dL), and hypoglycemia of less than 1.6 mmol/L (30 mg/dL) is treated by infusion of 2–2.5 mL/kg of 10 percent dextrose. Frequent testing for blood sugar using point of care equipment gives improved control. There is no agreement as to the hypoglycemic effect of preoperative fasting, but 4 hours between the last clear drink and induction of anesthesia should be the very maximum, and small children should receive a drink of clear fluid containing sugar up to 2 hours preoperatively. The usual regimen for preoperative fasting at the major children's hospitals worldwide is 6 hours for food and formula feeds and 4 hours for breast milk, with 2 hours for clear fluids. Premature and very small babies receiving more frequent feeds may have shorter periods of fasting if this is discussed with the anesthetist. Children below 15 kg in weight are at greatest risk from perioperative hypoglycemia.

Maturity of liver enzyme systems is complete by two months of age. The synthesis of vitamin K-dependent clotting factors II, VII, IX, and X is suboptimal until then. Minimal levels of clotting factors occur on the second or third day of life, and this is partially prevented by routine oral administration of vitamin K to all neonates or by intramuscular injection if the oral route is not available. Hepatic immaturity also means that drugs metabolized in the liver, such as barbiturates and opiates, should be used with extreme caution. The conjugation of bilirubin is very inefficient, and uncoupling of at least one of the two

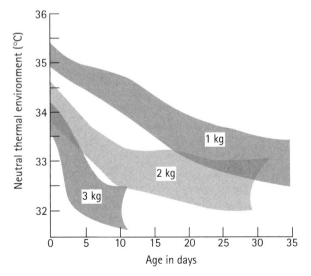

Figure 2.3 Neutral thermal environment for three groups of infants of differing birth weight.

molecules occurs at times of stress, such as during hypoxia or acidosis. After liver maturity is reached, most anesthetic drugs are well tolerated because of the high metabolic rate of the young child.

The neonate has no diuretic response to a water load for the first 48 hours of life. By the end of the first week, dilute urine can be produced, but the output falls before the full load has been excreted.

Fluid maintenance requirements for full-term infants start at 20–40 mL/kg per 24 hours on day 1, increasing by 20 mL/kg each day until the levels shown in **Table 2.1** are reached by the end of the first week of life.

Table 2.1 Basic fluid requirements of neonates 7 days after birth.

Birth weight (g)	Volume/24 hours (mL/kg)
<1000	180
1000–2500	150
>2500	120

There is usually marked fluid retention associated with the surgery, due to release of anti-diuretic hormone (ADH) and restriction to the requirements suggested for the neonatal period is necessary during and after operation. Pre- and postoperative maintenance fluids should contain glucose in newborns (depending on blood sugar), but abnormal losses must be replaced with an isotonic replacement fluid (0.9 per cent saline or buffered salt solution) separate to the maintenance solution. Added potassium chloride may be required. Due to the stress response, hyperglycemia may occur if glucose solutions are continued during the operation and glucose-free, balanced salt solutions are often used for both maintenance and replacement intraoperatively. Nevertheless, blood glucose levels must be measured frequently – hypoglycemia is likely in premature or small-for-dates babies and in those who have received preoperative glucose infusions.

ASSESSMENT OF THE PATIENT

Fitness for general anesthesia and surgery must be assessed in relation to the urgency of the surgery. Assessment often involves weighing up the risks related to an associated medical problem against the benefits of surgery. This requires cooperation between the anesthetist and the surgeon. Many centers run preoperative clinics in which medical problems can be identified, appropriate investigations performed, and treatment instituted in order to optimize the child's condition prior to surgery. The parents and patients may also be given the necessary instructions for admission to hospital, which is especially important for day-cases.

Elective surgery should not take place when the patient has an acute intercurrent illness. The operation should be deferred about one month after the last symptoms of respiratory tract infection, croup, or the acute exanthems have subsided, as related adverse events can occur for up to 6 weeks. However, some children requiring surgery, especially for ear, nose, and throat procedures, may suffer repeat upper respiratory infections, and the next episode may occur if the operation is postponed for too long a period.

After bronchiolitis, pulmonary abnormalities of increased resistance and reduced compliance may persist for as long as one year. In patients with chronic respiratory disease, lung function may be assessed by measuring airway resistance, compliance, and lung volumes, and by ventilation/perfusion scans. Baseline blood gas estimations are rarely indicated but may show metabolic alkalosis compensating for respiratory acidosis, or a raised $PaCO_2$ if there is incipient respiratory failure. Patients with values that are 50 percent of the predicted normal may be expected to develop respiratory problems after anesthesia and surgery, and in those with only 30 percent of predicted values with a resting $PaCO_2$ above 40 mmHg (5.3 kPa), postoperative respiratory support should be anticipated after major surgery and possibly even after apparently trivial procedures.

The history, including exercise tolerance and the physical examination of the child, should reveal any potential problems, such as respiratory obstruction or respiratory failure. The anesthetist is also alerted to possible problems, such as a difficult intubation due to a small jaw or limited mouth opening and neck movement, for example in patients with Pierre–Robin sequence or Still's disease.

A previously undiagnosed cardiac murmur needs preoperative investigation. Although a significant number of these murmurs are innocent, a thorough history and examination need to be performed in all cases. If the murmur is soft, or early systolic without a precordial thrill or electrocardiogram (ECG) changes, then surgery may proceed. However, if the child is less than one year of age, there is an associated syndrome or the features of the murmur are more pathological in nature, further investigation with echocardiography and a cardiology opinion should be sought preoperatively.

DAY–CASE SURGERY

Most minor surgery of all specialties is performed on a day-case basis as this arrangement is more cost-effective, more convenient for the parents, and has obvious psychological advantages for the child. Anesthetic techniques of premedication, intubation, inhalation, or intravenous anesthesia, local blocks, and postoperative analgesia need not differ significantly from those for hospitalized patients as both are geared to a rapid and pain-free return to normal function. Facilities must be available to admit a child overnight if the anesthesia or surgery has not been straightforward or if the parents feel they cannot manage at home. In general, babies of less than 46 weeks since conception should not be treated on a day-stay basis, even for minor surgery, as infants with a history of previous apneic attacks, or ex-premature babies of <46/40 post-conceptual age, have a risk of apnea for up to 24 hours after the operation.

Infants and small children are vulnerable to the psychological stress of being in hospital and undergoing surgery. They are totally dependent on their parents, and prolonged separation in the early months of life may cause problems with maternal bonding. Children between two and four years of age are especially vulnerable, as they may have unreasonable fears about hospitals and surgery, but may not yet have developed the intellectual mechanism to deal with these fears. Full preparation with a kindly and sympathetic approach is therefore required. Some children, despite this, will develop behavioral changes, which may last days or occasionally weeks.

PREMEDICATION

There is no ideal agent for premedication. The aim is to achieve mild sedation for most children, since a dose required to produce sleep in most, will cause over-sedation in a few. In recent years, preoperative medication has become less important, with parents usually present at induction and the universal use of topical anesthetic creams to allow painless intravenous induction of anesthesia. Opioid premedication is rarely used, as intramuscular injections are so disliked, and intraoperative and postoperative analgesia is usually managed by specific measures involving regional analgesia or intravenous opioid infusions.

Premedication drugs include midazolam 0.5 mg/kg, temazepam 0.50–1 mg/kg, and chloral hydrate 30–50 mg/kg – all administered orally. Other routes of administration, such as nasal or rectal, have been used, but no single method or agent has been shown to be superior. Clonidine 4 µg/kg orally may be used preinduction to reduce agitiation. Melatonin has few side effects and at a dose of 0.2 mg/kg orally has been shown to reduce the induction dose of propofol. The use of atropine as an anti-sialogogue used to be widespread, but since the development of non-irritant inhalational agents, it is now largely confined to specialist areas of practice, such as upper airway endoscopy.

EQUIPMENT

Specialized apparatus with low resistance to breathing (less than 30 cmH$_2$O/L per second during quiet breathing) and minimal dead space is necessary as infants already have a high airway resistance and a higher ratio of dead space to tidal volume than adults.

Jackson Rees' modification of Ayre's T-piece has almost universal approval for induction of anesthesia, particularly in infants and small children. With the advent of newer and more expensive volatile agents, such as sevoflurane and desflurane, circle systems are widely used during anesthetic maintenance for both spontaneous and intermittent positive pressure ventilation techniques.

Clear plastic, cuffed face masks provide a better fit to the face, and a firm fit also enables distending pressure to be applied to spontaneously breathing patients, which provides a 'pneumatic splint' to maintain upper airway patency and prevents reduction in FRC. The apparently larger dead space of some such masks is usually unimportant, as the fresh gas flow streamlines within the mask.

The infant larynx lies higher in the neck (opposite the fourth cervical vertebra) and more anterior than in the adult and, as the epiglottis is relatively large, laryngoscopy is best performed with a small, straight-bladed laryngoscope, the tip of which picks up the epiglottis. Perfect sizing, positioning, and fixation of the tracheal tube are central to pediatric anesthesia and intensive care.

The correct size of tube is that which allows a small air leak between it and the mucosa of the cricoid at a peak inspiratory pressure of 25 cmH$_2$O. The formula classically used to calculate the internal diameter (in mm) of the tube required (age over one year) is the age (in years) divided by 4 plus 4.5. The cricoid ring is the narrowest part of the upper airway in a child and is easily damaged by too large a tracheal tube, resulting in postoperative stridor or even subglottic stenosis (1 mm of mucosal edema in the infant cricoid will reduce the airway by 60 percent). Uncuffed tracheal tubes with a small leak have been traditionally used in both anesthesia and intensive care; however, the use of circle systems with low gas flow, and also the potential problems with a leak around the tube with non-compliant lungs, has popularized the use of cuffed tubes for both infants and children. Several studies have demonstrated that cuffed tubes are unlikely to cause damage provided they are properly positioned and that cuff pressure is monitored and maintained within the recommended limits. In certain circumstances, such as facial burns, cuffed tubes have significant advantages.

An oropharyngeal airway inserted alongside an oral tube can splint it and prevent lateral movement and kinking. An oral tube is usually fixed to the face by two pieces of adhesive strapping to prevent dislodgement. Nasal intubation is preferable for some head and intraoral surgery and is also a more secure route for long-term ventilation in infants and children, apart from very premature infants in whom the nasal cartilage is too soft and can erode due to the continuous pressure from the tube.

The laryngeal mask airway (LMA) designed by Sir Archie Brain, is routinely used in pediatric anesthesia and is suitable for all sizes of children, although there is an increase in the complication rate with diminishing LMA size. Modifications to the original design of the LMA have led to the development of airways specifically designed to increase flexibility of the connection point, allow intubation and allow the aspiration of gastric contents through a gastric port. Since the expiry of the patent on the original LMA, several new supraglottic airway devices have become available, some of which are available in pediatric sizes (iGel, Laryngeal Tube, Cobra Perilaryngeal Airway, air-Q Intubating Laryngeal Airway).

Intermittent positive pressure ventilation can be performed easily with the laryngeal mask in children, although many pediatric anesthetists would avoid this technique in smaller infants, as the potential to inflate the stomach and develop decreased compliance from diaphragmatic splinting may be significant. Use of disposable laryngeal masks will remove the theoretical risks of prion and other infective agent transfer.

Children with a potential for difficult laryngoscopy or intubation may require specific equipment. Devices which improve the glottic view using fiberoptics are particularly useful where the intubating difficulties are supraglottic. Equipment such as this are all available in pediatric sizes.

WARMING DEVICES

In addition to controlling the ambient temperature of the operating room environment, there are numerous heating devices available to help maintain normothermia in small children and infants during anesthesia. Many are either under-patient or over-patient hot air or water heaters with thermostatic servocontrols. The efficacy of most of these devices makes it mandatory that temperature measurement of the patient is closely monitored. In children receiving large volumes of intravenous fluids, especially blood, fluid warmers are essential. The most effective of these warm the fluid right up to the point where it enters the patient, such as the coaxial inline water heater. The use of heat and moisture exchange filters with a low dead space can prevent excessive heat loss through the breathing of cold inspired gases.

GENERAL PRINCIPLES OF ANESTHESIA

The principles of anesthesia in infants and children are similar to those for adults; however, infants weighing less than 5 kg are usually intubated for anesthesia, however minor the surgery, to allow controlled ventilation and avoid hypoxemia and hypercapnia. Metabolic studies clearly show that even neonates mount stress responses to surgery, and that these can be obtunded by opioid or regional anesthesia. Adverse responses may contribute to morbidity and mortality or the prolongation of recovery.

Induction and maintenance agents

Induction of anesthesia is usually achieved either by inhalation or intravenous administration. Halothane continues to be a popular agent worldwide as it is readily accepted by children, but in most developed countries it has been replaced by sevoflurane, which provides rapid and well-tolerated induction of anesthesia, with less myocardial depression and improved maintenance of cardiac output. Intravenous induction is usually with propofol (3 mg/kg), as it is very short acting and may be of advantage for day-case patients or where rapid recovery is desirable. Propofol also has antiemetic properties. Thiopentone sodium in doses of 4–5 mg/kg may be used as an alternative. Ketamine (1–2 mg/kg intravenously) is a useful agent for children with cardiovascular instability as it may enhance cardiac output by means of endogenous catecholamine release.

After induction, the depth of anesthesia can be controlled either intravenously or using inhalational gases. Isoflurane, sevoflurane and desflurane are commonly used for maintenance of anesthesia. The higher cost of sevoflurane and desflurane has been offset by the widespread use of circle systems with low fresh gas flow rates. Newer volatile agents have minimal toxicity, but all inhalational agents are known triggers of malignant hyperpyrexia in susceptible patients. There is also an association with emergence agitation, a phenomenon described as a disturbance in a child's awareness of their environment with disorientation and perceptual alterations.

Total intravenous anesthesia using target-controlled infusions of propofol in children is possible using enabled infusion devices, which use validated pharmacokinetic data to calculate the infusion rates required to achieve a preselected plasma level. Particular attention should be paid to minimizing the total dose of propofol infused for anesthesia to reduce the risk of propofol infusion syndrome.

Remifentanil, a selective μ-opioid receptor agonist, is particularly useful as part of a balanced anesthetic technique. Unlike other opioids, there is no increase in the context of sensitive half-life meaning a rapid recovery irrespective of the dose used or the duration of infusion.

Muscle relaxants

Sensitivity of the neuromuscular junction to non-depolarizing muscle relaxants exists during the first 2–3 weeks of life. This, together with wide individual variation, makes careful titration of dose with effect mandatory.

The progress of action of the relaxants can be monitored with a peripheral nerve stimulator. Atracurium besylate is the relaxant of choice for neonates as its metabolism is independent of hepatic and renal function, and it may be given by bolus (0.5 mg/kg) or continuous infusion (9 μg/kg per minute). The short-acting non-depolarizing relaxant mivacurium, inactivated by plasma cholinesterase, may also be given by infusion.

The reported resistance to succinylcholine (suxamethonium) in the neonate is caused by the dilution of a given dose in the relatively large extracellular fluid volume. Suxamethonium is hydrolyzed by butyrlcholinesterase and an inherited deficiency of this enzyme may result in a prolonged block requiring intubation and ventilation until recovery. Other side effects include hyperkalemia and the drug is a trigger for malignant hyperpyrexia. The indications for the use of this agent are significantly reduced with the introduction of newer agents; however, the rapid and optimal conditions produced for intubation are useful in rapid sequence inductions and critical airway management.

Any significant residual non-depolarizing neuro-muscular block at the conclusion of anesthesia should be antagonized using a reversal agent. Neostigmine (50 µg/kg) and edrophonium (1 mg/kg) are antagonists of acetylcholinesterase increasing the availability of acetylcholine at the neuromuscular junction. Atropine (20 µg/kg) or glycopyrrolate (10 µg/kg) should be administered before, or with the anticholinesterase to prevent muscarinic side effects. Sugamadex is a specific antagonist of rocuronium rendering it immediately inactive without the cardiovascular side effects seen with anticholinesterase drugs.

Prevention of aspiration

Cricoid pressure, used to prevent regurgitation of gastric contents, is as effective in infants as it is in adults if correctly applied and is used when there is a risk of pulmonary aspiration, for example in patients with intestinal obstruction. Cricoid pressure may distort the larynx and it should be removed if it compromises intubation of the airway.

ANALGESIA

Analgesia is balanced with anesthesia to provide stress-free conditions for surgery with improved outcomes. The technique used can either involve intravenous opioids, such as fentanyl (1–10 µg/kg) or morphine (0.05–0.2 mg/kg), or be regional, or a combination of the two. Great care must be taken when opioids are given to neonates unless postoperative mechanical ventilation is planned. Older infants and children tolerate up to 10 µg/kg fentanyl, in longer procedures (>1 hour), without the need for postoperative ventilation, and this provides excellent analgesia.

Regional anesthesia

Central or peripheral nerve blocks usually, but not necessarily, associated with light general anesthesia or sedation are routine in pediatric anesthesia. They obviate the need for opioid analgesia in high-risk groups, such as ex-premature infants. In day care, they result in good postoperative analgesia with a reduced incidence of side effects. Techniques such as spinal or extradural blocks with catheters are used even in neonates and have the advantage

that they can be continued into the postoperative period. Sacral lumbar and thoracic roots up to T10 may be blocked by caudal analgesia using 0.25 percent plain bupivacaine. Newer local anesthetic agents, such as ropivacaine and levo-bupivacaine, appear to be less cardiotoxic than the older agents.

Most pediatric surgery is suitable for the use of local anesthetic techniques of some type. Caudal epidural blocks are widely used, very safe, and easily performed in most children and are suitable for perineal, lower abdominal, and lower limb surgery in small children. In older ambulant children, the numb legs postoperatively may be a disadvantage, and ileoinguinal nerve block may be preferable for inguinal herniotomy or orchidopexy. The transversus abdominus plane block, which involves the placement of local anesthetic in the plane between the internal oblique and transversus abdominis muscles has gained recent favor for unilateral lower abdominal surgery. Penile blocks can be used for circumcisions and minor hypospadias repair, although caudal blocks are preferable for more extensive repairs. Axillary brachial plexus blocks are also easily and safely performed in children and are suitable for most upper limb surgery. The use of ultrasound imaging and nerve stimulation of peripheral nerves can improve the accuracy, quality and safety of nerve blocks. If a regional technique or nerve block is not possible, simple infiltration combined with either opiate intravenous analgesia or simple analgesics is also very effective, both for short procedures and for immediate postoperative analgesia.

Postoperative pain management

Since it was discovered that postoperative pain in children was being seriously under-treated, a great deal of attention has been given to the subject of acute pain relief in this patient group. Most children's hospitals and large centers have established acute pain services with physicians and nurses to treat, audit, and research this problem. Neonates present a unique problem of assessment and of treatment due to their sensitivity to the respiratory depressant effects of opioid analgesia. Regional techniques, as already described, including simple wound infiltration, are used whenever possible. Paracetamol is safe and effective in neonates in doses not exceeding 60 mg/kg per 24 hours. Non-steroidal anti-inflammatory drugs (NSAIDs) can be given to children over the age of three months provided they have normal renal function and are not wheezy, and are excellent in combination with paracetamol, especially for ambulatory care. Analgesia for neonates, infants, and children after major surgery is based on morphine intravenous infusions unless there is an epidural infusion. They obviate the need for painful intramuscular injections and avoid the peaks and troughs of bolus administration. A regimen appropriate to the patient, type of surgery, location of nursing (intensive care, high dependency, or ward), and the institution's protocols are essential, but most are based on infusions delivering 20–40 µg/kg per hour for older children and infants, with neonates receiving lower doses.

Patient-controlled microprocessor pumps can be used by children as young as five years, while younger children usually benefit from a higher background delivery supplemented by nurse-controlled boluses. Continuous epidural infusions of local anesthetics with or without opioids are widely used for pain relief after major abdominal and thoracic surgery in pediatric practice.

MONITORING

Suitable adaptations of standard techniques of monitoring used in adult practice are acceptable for all children, including neonates. Crucially, all monitors should be set up for the age of the child and the alarms set accordingly. Minimal standards of monitoring include electrocardiography (ECG), pulse oximetry, non-invasive blood pressure measurement, inspired and expired gas analysis, with CO_2 and O_2, and anesthetic agents. In addition, many anesthetists find the precordial or esophageal stethoscope a useful adjunct in pediatric practice. For all but the very briefest procedures, and for any in which a heating device is used, central temperature monitoring – usually nasopharyngeal – is mandatory. Peripheral temperature monitoring is useful in prolonged procedures and can help inform volume replacement. Direct measurement of arterial and central venous pressure is used routinely for much major pediatric surgery. Monitors designed to measure cardiac output and parameters to measure tissue perfusion, such as urine output base deficit and lactate, are useful to record. The use of near-patient blood testing of blood, allows close control of fluid therapy, blood replacement, and blood sugar monitoring. Cerebral function and depth of anesthesia can be monitored, but its use is yet to be validated in infants.

FLUID MAINTENANCE

Care is required with clear maintenance fluids during neonatal surgery, as fluids to flush drugs may be sufficient for requirements, particularly if the neonate has been receiving preoperative intravenous fluids. Neonates who have been on preoperative glucose infusions are prone to hypoglycemia if the glucose infusion is not continued. Frequent blood glucose monitoring is essential.

Older children may be given intraoperative fluids (as balanced electrolyte solution) at 6–10 mL/kg per hour. The routine use of the traditional 4 percent dextrose and 0.18 percent saline solution is no longer encouraged, as it is increasingly clear that hypoglycemia is rare outside the neonatal period and the injudicious use of functionally hypotonic solutions may be associated with severe hyponatremia.

Abnormal losses should be replaced with appropriate isotonic solutions such as 0.9 percent saline, human albumen solution, or artificial colloid solutions. The use of red cells is avoided unless absolutely necessary and should be guided by bedside testing of hematocrit. Much lower hemoglobin levels are now tolerated than in the past, and most anesthetists would not transfuse a fit older child without ongoing losses unless the hemoglobin fell below 7.0 g/dL. Techniques such as cell salvage and acute normovolemic hemodilution are increasingly used to avoid transfusion in major surgery.

RESPIRATORY SUPPORT AND POSITIVE PRESSURE VENTILATION

Many machines exist for the intraoperative mechanical ventilation of children. T-piece-occluding machines, such as the Penlon 200 series with the Newton valve, are satisfactory for simple cases in children with normal lungs, but most centers now use dedicated pediatric ventilators. Whatever ventilator is used, it is essential that it has a reliable alarm system.

Hand ventilation is still the 'gold standard' in situations of rapidly changing pulmonary compliance or if there is tracheal compression. Controlled ventilation should be used for all neonates because the respiratory depressant effect of inhalational anesthesia is so great at this age. Older infants may tolerate short periods of spontaneous ventilation via a tracheal tube, laryngeal mask, or facemask.

At the end of surgery, infants are extubated when fully awake, once spontaneous respiration is judged to be adequate. Because of the low respiratory reserve at this age, however, respiratory failure may ensue. Acute respiratory failure is a clinical diagnosis based on a rising respiratory rate, pulse rate, and oxygen dependence, and on an assessment of the work of breathing as shown by intercostal recession, tracheal tug, nasal flaring, restlessness, and grunting. Inability to clear secretions, or apneic attacks are further pointers. Blood gas levels may confirm the clinical impression, but if the need for postoperative blood gas analysis is anticipated, an arterial cannula should be left *in situ*, as intermittent sampling is painful and inaccurate.

Distending pressure in the form of CPAP can be used to avoid intubation, when an infant cannot maintain adequate saturations (>90 percent) in 60 percent oxygen. The CPAP may be administered via a tight-fitting facemask or nasal prong.

If postoperative ventilation is necessary, it is best provided via a nasotracheal tube, unless contraindicated. The complications of blockage, dislodgement, and subglottic stenosis can be avoided by meticulous care. Uncuffed tubes must be of a size to allow effective ventilation, but also some leakage of air around it, or damage to the cricoid mucosa may result. Cuff pressure must be carefully monitored if cuffed tubes are used.

TOXICITY OF ANESTHETIC AGENTS

Recent research has raised concerns over the potential toxicity of anesthetic agents on the developing brain. Both rats and Rhesus monkeys exhibit neuronal apoptosis when exposed to prolonged periods of anesthesia (>12 hours) with agents that antagonize NMDA receptors (e.g. ketamine) or potentiate the neurotransmission of gamma aminobutyric acid (e.g. isoflurane). There was no demonstrable effect with exposure to anesthetic agents for less than 3 hours. Although there have been no human studies of apoptosis, a large Danish cohort study compared academic performance in 2689 children who had an infant hernia repair with 14 575 children who had not received an anesthetic and found no significant differences in attainment. There is also an ongoing prospective, randomized international study comparing neurodevelopmental outcomes in children who had hernia repair under general anesthesia with those who had the surgery with local or spinal anesthesia (the GAS Study).

Clearly, if surgery is necessary, anesthesia must be administered and although there is no good evidence to suggest that any agent is better or worse than another in this respect, whichever agent is used, it is extremely unlikely that there will be any adverse consequence from a single exposure to less than 3 hours of anesthesia.

FURTHER READING

Association of Paediatric Anaesthetists of Great Britain and Ireland. *APA Consensus Guideline on Perioperative Fluid Management in Children*. London: APAGBI, 2007.

Bingham R, Lloyd-Thomas A, Sury M. *Hatch and Sumner's Textbook of Paediatric Anaesthesia*, 3rd edn. London: Hodder Arnold, 2008.

Lonnqvist PA. Regional anaesthesia and analgesia in the neonate. *Best Practice in Research Clinical Anesthesiology* 2010; **24**: 309–21.

McEwan AI, Birch M, Bingham R. The preoperative management of the child with a heart murmur. *Pediatric Anaesthesia* 2005; **5**: 151–6.

Stayer SA, Liu Y. Pulmonary hypertension of the newborn. *Best Practice in Clinical Research Anesthesiology* 2010; **24**: 375–86.

Operating room requirements and special consideration for laparoscopic surgery

HOCK LIM TAN and NICHOLAS SY CHAO

INTRODUCTION

Laparoscopic surgery has matured over the past decade to the extent that it is now routine in many centers to perform primary repairs of esophageal atresia, duodenal atresia, and other major reconstructive procedures which were thought impossible, or too challenging, not long ago. This is largely due to improvements in hand instruments, video technology, and new electrosurgical equipment, such as vessel-sealing devices which allow the pediatric surgeon to operate with a degree of precision and finesse previously impossible.

While open surgery can be performed with a minimum of equipment, the ability of a surgeon to perform delicate laparoscopic dissection and fine intracorporeal suturing is completely equipment dependent, and this chapter focuses on optimizing the operating room environment to perform complex laparoscopic operations with efficiency and safety. Ultimately, the goal is to improve the standard of surgical care and patient outcome.

ESSENTIAL SET-UP

The essential elements to optimize the ability to perform advanced laparoscopic procedures are:

- laparoscopic 'set-up';
- optimizing the operating room environment;
- choice and management of instruments.

OPTIMIZING VIDEO LAPAROSCOPIC EQUIPMENT SET-UP

The laparoscopic 'stack'

The laparoscopy stack evolved in the 1990s when the laparoscopic equipment required were simply 'stacked' on shelves mounted on a transportable cart and the video monitor placed on the topmost shelf because it was the heaviest and most cumbersome piece of equipment, and happened to sit best on the top of the stack.

1 While this served the needs of basic laparoscopic surgery, it is rarely possible to position a stack-mounted monitor in the most ergonomic position for advanced laparoscopic surgery without some compromise. The introduction of high definition flat screen monitors now allows them to be mounted on an adjustable side arm of a transportable laparoscopic stack thus allowing the monitor to be positioned in the most ergonomic position as illustrated.

While this allows greater flexibility, the moveable stack still occupies a significant 'footprint' and can be cumbersome especially if the stack has to be moved to reposition the video monitor because of the limited range of the side arm.

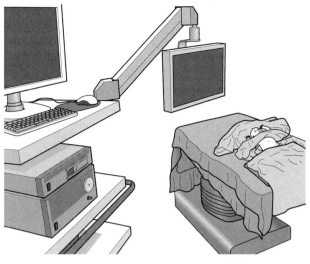

1a

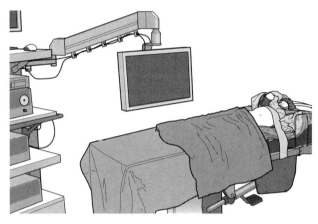

1b

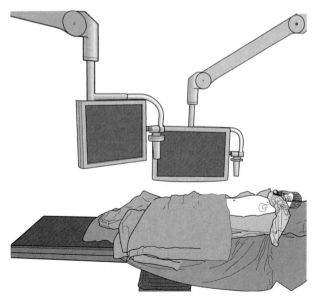

2 The most efficient option today is to mount the video monitor on a ceiling-mounted pendant, as this allows far greater flexibility of movement around the perimeter of table and provides for optimal height adjustment.

The increasing array of equipment required for contemporary laparoscopic surgery, robotic surgery, and the use of C arm severely challenges the physical constraints of the operating room, not only in terms of clutter but also safety, particularly if a wide assortment of cables and foot switches are strewn on the operating room floor.

2

3 The optimum environment for advanced laparoscopic surgery is to fully integrate the operating room control system. In a fully integrated operating room, much of the ancillary equipment can be located in an adjacent room, reducing the footprint in the operating room. The availability of voice or touch screen control in the sterile field also allows the surgeon to adjust electrosurgical equipment, such as insufflator and diathermy settings, operating room ambient lighting and environment, operating table height and pitch, teleconferencing and information servers, thus giving the surgeon full charge of the operating room, reducing the risk of errors, as can occur if the adjustment of equipment settings rests with a third party, in this environment of increasing complexity.

As an added feature, some integrated systems have a built-in electronic checklist and time-out system, in keeping with World Health Organization (WHO) requirements.

All these added features serve to reduce the incidence of adverse events in laparoscopic surgery which has been estimated to be around 10 percent of all laparoscopic procedures.

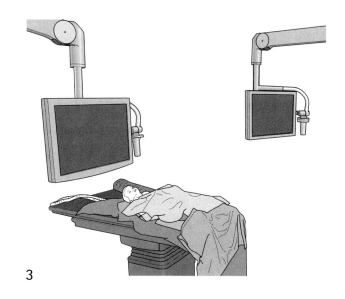

3

Video image quality

HIGH DEFINITION OR 3D CAMERA

The introduction of high definition (HD) video laparoscopic camera systems has resulted in a quantum leap in the clarity of the video image and allows the pediatric surgeon to identify with greater clarity the viscera in the operation field. Compared to a conventional DVD quality image with a resolution of 550 lines, HD images provide a resolution of 1080 lines, allowing far greater detail and clarity than was previously possible. This is now the gold standard. The superior image quality compensates for the lack of stereoscopic vision.

While there are many 3D or stereoscopic systems available capable of producing a stereoscopic image with the aid of special eye glasses, they are still in their infancy, and because the telescopes required to produce a stereoscopic image are 10 mm, they are generally unsuitable for use in infants and small children. A further disadvantage of 3D is the need for a shutter system to present alternating images to each eye, resulting in significant flicker and visual fatigue with extended use.

OPTIMIZING IMAGE QUALITY

While a high definition system is capable of producing an image of unsurpassed quality, it is important to appreciate that the image quality displayed depends on the source of the signal. It is important to ensure that the video signal for the monitor is sourced directly from the HDMI (high-definition multimedia interface) output in the camera control unit instead of taking the signal from the video recorder output which may lead to significant degradation of the image quality.

AMBIENT LIGHTING CONTROL

Many surgeons darken the room to improve image quality or brightness. This may be hazardous, especially if there are cables strewn across the floor. Newer operating rooms offer green ambient lighting which provides sufficient ambient lighting for operating room personnel to see and move around safely without interfering with the surgeon. Green ambient lighting also does not result in pupillary dilatation and has been shown to enhance the quality of the image on the flat screen.

Choice of laparoscopes

A wide range of laparoscopes are available today from 1.5-mm telescopes to 10-mm adult laparoscopes. In general, 4- and 5-mm rod lens telescopes provide sufficient illumination and image resolution for our requirements (except for bariatric surgery which may require a 10-mm adult telescope). Smaller telescopes (1.9-mm diameter) are available, but are only useful for simple diagnostic purposes as they are usually fiberscopes and will transmit a pixilated low resolution image.

Generally, it is best to have both 0° and 30° telescopes available.

PREPARATION OF HAND INSTRUMENTS

The key to providing an efficient service is to keep it simple. While there is a myriad of laparoscopic hand instruments available, in reality most surgeons use the same instruments for performing even complex procedures, and only need additional instruments when unexpected events occur. Around six hand instruments are required to perform a primary repair of duodenal or esophageal atresia, and the same applies to the entire range of complex reconstructive procedures.

In practice it is best to prepack selected instruments which are always used for the most common laparoscopic procedures performed in your institution, e.g. one pack for fundoplication, one for appendicectomy, and to have selected instruments you may need occasionally available in individually sterilized peel packs.

The most efficient set-up is to prepack instruments, and only open those instruments which are always required for a specific procedure, such as a duodenal grasper, pyloric knife, and spreader for laparoscopic pyloromyotomy. Other instruments, such as needle drivers which needed to repair a perforation, should be kept on standby and only opened if needed. This is efficient and will reduce the wear and tear of reusable instruments reducing the need to repack, clean and resterilize. Standardizing and keeping the entire instrument set-up as simple as possible will also increase the enthusiasm of the operating room personnel, especially scrub nurses, and will reduce the set-up and turnaround time.

OPTIMIZING WORK FLOW

Laparoscopic surgery inevitably involves increased workload for the operating room team. In addition to the usual documentation of patient details, checklist, and time out, the additional tasks required, such as setting up the equipment, ensuring correct insufflator settings, positioning of video monitors, and ensuring that the correct hand instruments are available adds significantly to the setting up and turnaround time. The complexity of these additional tasks also increases the risk of adverse events occurring.

Setting up of a laparoscopic service is challenging and has to involve team-building, but is also extremely rewarding once an efficient team has been established.

Special consideration has to be given to the care and maintenance of hand instruments and telescopes and it is best to assign a special member or team leaders to take specific charge of the cleaning, disassembly, and packaging of these delicate instruments, especially the telescopes, to avoid expensive breakages.

STORAGE FACILITIES

Most operating room suites have a common 'CSSD' to store for both laparoscopic and open surgery at sites often remote from the operating room itself. While this makes for ease of storage, consideration should be given to storing hand instruments, telescopes and other essential equipment, such as disposable staplers and clips in moveable trolleys which can be brought into the operating room. This will result in significant reduction in time wasted waiting for replacement instruments in case of malfunction or if instruments are accidentally dropped. In this age of economic prudency, such measures will result in significant cost saving, particularly as the operating room is one of the most expensive 'cost center'. It will also allow the OR team leader to manage stocktaking.

Unlike open surgery where much of the operation can continue in one form or another while waiting for replacement instruments, the complete dependence on equipment requires the development of a new paradigm shift in overall operating room management if we are to maximize our efficiency and reduce the incidence of untoward events.

FURTHER READING

Bharathan R, Aggarwal R, Darzi A. Operating room of the future. *Best Practice & Research Clinical Obstetrics & Gynaecology* Dec 2012; on line.

Endress A, Brucker S, Wallwiener D *et al.* Systems integration in the operating room: the challenge of the decade. *Gynecological Surgery* 2006; **3(1)**: 6–11.

Lingard L, Espin S, Whyte S *et al.* Communication failures in the operating room: an observational classification of recurrent types and effects. *Quality & Safety in Health Care* 2004; **13**: 330–4.

4

Vascular access

NIYI ADE-AJAYI and DEREK ROEBUCK

HISTORY

Secure vascular access is central to the delivery of many aspects of modern medical care. In 1628, William Harvey described the heart and circulation in detail. This provided the anatomical basis for subsequent vascular interventions. By the early 1900s, intravenous therapy was becoming established, replacing proctoclysis and cutaneoclysis as a means of delivering fluids and drugs to patients. Effective antimicrobials, chemotherapeutic agents, parenteral nutrition, and the evolution of a culture of intensive care are among the medical advances that have encouraged the development of innovative strategies for vascular access in children over the last 60 years. This group of procedures is now one of the most common performed by pediatric surgeons.

PRINCIPLES AND JUSTIFICATION

Venous and arterial access is a key part of the management of many children who require investigations, monitoring, and specific interventions. Access procedures may facilitate the monitoring of physiological, hematological, and biochemical indices. Therapeutic indications include the delivery of fluids, blood products, nutrition, and drugs, hemodialysis as well as miscellaneous interventions such as endovascular surgery and, increasingly, cellular transplantation.

Some children put forward for vascular access may be suitably managed by simpler, less invasive, and equally effective means. Despite improvements in devices, insertion techniques, and postoperative care, distress and complications related to catheter insertion are not infrequent and may be severe. In consultation with other members of the multidisciplinary team, it is the responsibility of the surgeon to ensure that the vascular access procedure proposed for each child can be justified.

OVERVIEW OF DEVICES AND TECHNIQUES

In most children, short-term venous access for sampling and the delivery of non-irritant infusions is achieved by the use of a short 14–26-gauge cannula inserted into a superficial vein in an upper or lower limb. In addition to easily visible veins, useful sites include the long saphenous vein anterior to the medial malleolus at the ankle, the cephalic vein at the wrist, the interdigital vein between the fourth and the fifth metacarpals on the dorsum of the hand, the external jugular vein, the superficial temporal vein of the scalp in small infants, and, occasionally, superficial veins on the trunk.

For children who require intravenous access for several days, the insertion of a 'short long line' early in the course of treatment, while superficial veins are well preserved, may reduce the frequency of recannulation. A number of suitable devices are available. Unless coincident with a general anesthetic for another reason, these procedures are generally performed in the awake child with the aid of topical anesthetic creams or sprays. Familiarity with peripheral venepuncture in children and maintenance of competence are recommended; however, the main role of the pediatric surgeon is related to central venous access.

The large number of central venous access devices fall into four broad categories: (1) percutaneously inserted central venous catheters (PICCs), (2) non-tunneled central venous catheters (CVCs), (3) tunneled CVCs (such as Hickman or hemodialysis catheters), and (4) venous port devices (Table 4.1). The type of central venous access device used will depend on the requirements of the individual child. The ideal position of the CVC tip is contentious. The options include the superior vena cava, the right atrium, and at the junction between the two. Individual patient requirements, government guidelines, manufacturer's recommendations along with institutional and personal experience and practice should be taken into consideration when deciding the final position. In general, our preference is for placement

Table 4.1 Types of central venous access device.

Device	Characteristics	Advantages	Disadvantages	Typical indications
Non-tunneled central venous catheter	Short, relatively stiff, usually multiple-lumen catheter	Ease of insertion	High infection rate	Short-term intravenous therapy, pressure monitoring, 'bridge access' before longer lasting line
Single-lumen Hickman catheter	Relatively soft catheter	Relatively low infection rate	No possibility of coadministration of incompatible infusions	Total parenteral nutrition, low intensity chemotherapy (e.g. nephroblastoma)
Multiple-lumen Hickman catheter	Relatively soft catheter with two or three lumens	Coadministration of blood products, parenteral nutrition, and drugs	Higher infection rate	Intensive chemotherapy protocols, bone marrow transplantation
Non-cuffed tunneled central venous catheter	Small-caliber soft catheter with one or two lumens	Ease of removal	Higher rate of inadvertent removal and infection	Short- to medium-term access with reliable blood sampling
Non-tunneled hemodialysis catheter	Large diameter catheter with offset lumens	Ease of insertion	Short lifespan, higher infection rate	Short-term hemodialysis, plasmapheresis, stem cell harvest
Tunneled (permanent) hemodialysis catheter	Large diameter catheter with offset lumens	Long lifespan, low infection rate	Higher incidence of damage to vein	Long-term hemodialysis
Central venous port device	Subcutaneous port with attached venous catheter	Even lower infection rate than Hickman catheter	Requires needle access, longer scar than Hickman catheter, visible 'port bump'	Chemotherapy, conditions requiring regular transfusions of blood products (e.g. hemophilia) or antibiotics (e.g. cystic fibrosis)
Peripherally inserted central venous catheter	Small-caliber soft catheter with one or two lumens	Safe insertion without general anesthetic, ease of removal	Higher rate of inadvertent removal and occlusion	Short- to medium-term access (e.g. for antibiotic therapy)

in the proximal right atrium. However, in line with UK government guidelines, stiff catheters inserted percutaneously are placed low in the superior vena cava, outside the pericardial reflection.

Emergency intraosseous access and arterial cannulation for monitoring are described below under **Emergency intraosseous venous access**, but other vascular procedures such as arterial access for diagnostic and therapeutic purposes, endovascular surgery, and extracorporeal membrane oxygenation are beyond the scope of this chapter.

PREOPERATIVE

Assessment and planning

A specific history and clinical examination are imperative, especially if there has been previous central venous cannulation. This should include the proposed site of insertion and exit site of the device and a search for stigmata that suggest potential venous access difficulty, such as multiple scars and dilated body wall veins. If such stigmata exist, preoperative vascular imaging may be indicated.

For the purposes of central venous access, the central veins may be defined as the superior vena cava (SVC), the right atrium, and the suprahepatic inferior vena

cava (IVC). The choice of vessels in order of preference should be determined in advance taking into account factors such as previous cannulation, the presence of other medical devices such as ventriculoperitoneal shunt and tracheostomy, and the child's skin condition. In general, the right internal jugular vein (RIJV) is the best site for central venous access. Other potential veins, in the usual order of preference, are the left internal jugular, external jugular, axillary, common femoral, and subclavian veins. If ultrasound-guided puncture is an option, this order may change and other veins, such as the brachiocephalics, considered. Less conventional methods, such as recanalization of occluded veins, the use of small collateral veins, and transhepatic or translumbar access to the inferior vena cava are occasionally required. These should be undertaken by personnel skilled in image-guided techniques and are outside the remit of this text.

Consent should be taken by the operating surgeon or a colleague with a clear understanding of the procedures and devices involved, as well as possible complications. Baseline blood tests should be performed and hemoglobin, platelet levels, and coagulation parameters optimized prior to surgery. With proper planning, most of these procedures can be carried out on planned lists, reducing risk to patients by a reduction of out-of-hours operating.

ANESTHESIA

Anesthetic experience should be appropriate to the complexity of the child undergoing surgery. Postoperative management may require intensive care facilities which should be arranged in advance.

Anesthetic strategies for vascular access procedures in children differ widely between centers. Intravenous sedation may be used with good results. Our institutional preference is for general anesthesia, but selected children will tolerate central venous catheter insertion under local anesthetic with or without an inhalational agent.

In the majority of cases, the airway is best secured by muscle paralysis and an endotracheal tube. A laryngeal mask may be appropriate for some patients if muscle relaxants are not used. Slight head down positioning and continuous positive airway pressure are advisable to reduce the risk of air embolus. Standard monitoring includes oxygen saturation, end-tidal carbon dioxide, temperature, blood pressure, and electrocardiography. The airway must be monitored closely, especially each time the position of the head is altered. Injection of local anesthetic at the site of all incisions is recommended. This should be done before incisions are made as it allows for a lighter general anesthetic and eliminates the risk of damaging the device following implantation.

PERCUTANEOUS CENTRAL VENOUS CATHETER INSERTION IN THE INFANT VIA A PERIPHERAL VEIN

1 In the small infant, percutaneous insertion of a fine Silastic central venous catheter can be performed awake (with oral sucrose) or with sedation. They are small, single or dual lumen catheters (outer diameter 0.6–1.0 mm, maximum crystalloid flow rate about 6 mL/min), and are particularly useful in neonates where the need for venous access is anticipated for a period of weeks. Blood sampling is possible but may be slow and shortens the lifespan of these catheters.

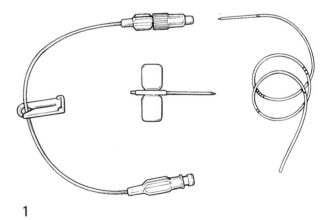

1

2a,b Popular insertion sites include the median cubital vein at the elbow, the long saphenous vein anterior to the medial malleolus, and the superficial temporal vein. For supracardiac veins, the distance from the chosen insertion site to the right nipple is measured as a guide to the length of the catheter that should be inserted. Good nursing assistance is essential. After antiseptic preparation of the skin, venepuncture is performed with a 19-gauge butterfly needle or other appropriate access device and the fine Silastic feeding line is inserted into the needle and threaded up the vein using fine non-toothed forceps. The progress of the catheter may be interrupted at venous junctions, but manipulating the limb will usually allow it to be advanced further. Once inserted to the desired distance, the butterfly needle is withdrawn and the line is connected to the infusion system via an inner blunt metal cannula and flushed with heparinized saline. Gentle suction on a 2-mL syringe should allow blood to be aspirated if the catheter tip lies in a large vein. The external catheter is firmly secured with a small piece of gauze covered by a transparent adhesive dressing. The position of the catheter tip should be confirmed radiologically. It is usually visible on a plain film with magnification, but it is easier to see if 0.5 mL of intravenous contrast material is injected prior to the chest radiograph.

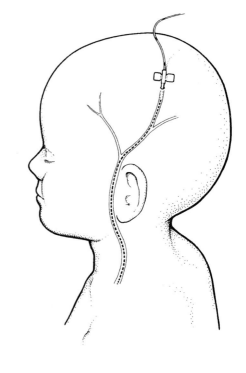

2a

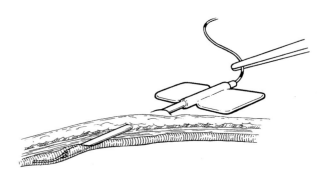

2b

Peripherally inserted central venous catheters

3a,b PICCs are single- or dual-lumen catheters typically made of silicone elastomer or polyurethane. They range in size from 2 Fr (0.67 mm) to 6 Fr (2.0 mm). Some PICCs have valves at the tip or hub, to prevent reflux of blood into the catheter. Although they are intended for short- to medium-term use (from 1 week to a few months), they are occasionally left in for much longer. Upper limb veins are generally used for PICCs, and many are inserted without image guidance. Imaging with ultrasound may, however, be required to gain access to a suitable vein, and the use of fluoroscopy significantly improves the chance of achieving a suitable final catheter tip position. The procedure is easier to perform in older children with larger cephalic and basilic veins. In certain circumstances when a short duration catheter is required, a device of this type may be used as a tunneled central venous catheter. The advantage over cuffed catheters is that it is easy to remove without sedation or anesthesia. For peripheral access, the arm is stabilized on a support board. Standard, sterile skin preparation is carried out and a local anesthetic injected after selection of an appropriate entry site to the basilic or cephalic vein, usually above the elbow. The vein is punctured with a 21-gauge needle or 22-gauge cannula. Aspiration of blood confirms successful puncture. A 0.018-inch (0.46-mm) guidewire is then advanced into the vein. If resistance is felt at this point, the needle or cannula should be repositioned (it is usually too far in). An appropriately sized PICC is selected. The needle or cannula is removed and a peel-away sheath of diameter just sufficient to accept the PICC is advanced over the guidewire. The guidewire should be fixed relative to the patient, and pressure applied over the puncture site as this is done. The guidewire and the dilator of the peel-away sheath are then removed, and the PICC inserted into the sheath. It is usually easier to advance the PICC to a central position if its stiffening wire is left in. In certain places, especially near the termination of the cephalic vein in the deltopectoral groove, it may be easier to fix the stiffening wire and advance the PICC over it, unsupported. When the tip lies in the low superior vena cava or upper right atrium, the peel-away sheath is split and removed, aspiration of blood is confirmed, and the catheter is flushed with normal saline. It is then sutured to the skin, and a transparent occlusive dressing applied. When no suitable superficial vein is available, ultrasound-guided puncture of a brachial vein (vena comitans of the brachial artery) is usually successful.

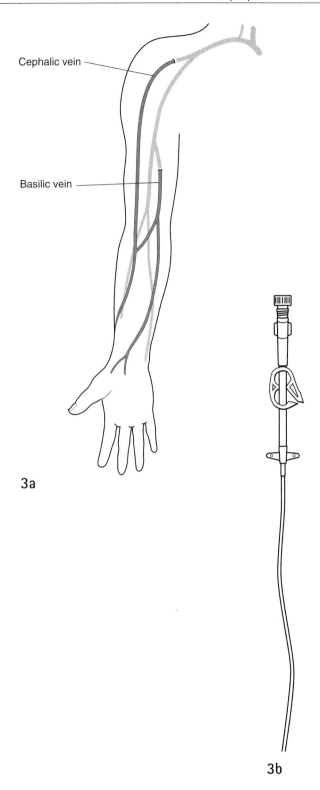

Cephalic vein

Basilic vein

3a

3b

Non-tunneled (percutaneous) CVC insertion

These short catheters, designed for insertion directly over a guidewire, include temporary hemodialysis catheters. Non-tunneled catheters are usually intended for short-term use (<10 days), because of the high rate of infection when they are left in for longer than this. Most of these lines are inserted using a percutaneous technique based on anatomical landmarks. Ultrasound guidance is recommended and increasingly being used for these and other CVC insertions.

Tunneled CVCs

4a,b These are intended for medium- to long-term venous access. There are two main types. Hickman and similar catheters have single or multiple lumens, a size range of 2.7–12 Fr, and a tissue in-growth cuff made of Dacron, which lies in the subcutaneous tunnel. The cuff is intended to reduce the risk of ascending infection and inadvertent removal. Hemodialysis catheters are similar, but have two lumens with offset openings at the tip, to prevent recirculation of blood during hemodialysis. The techniques for the insertion of these catheters are described below.

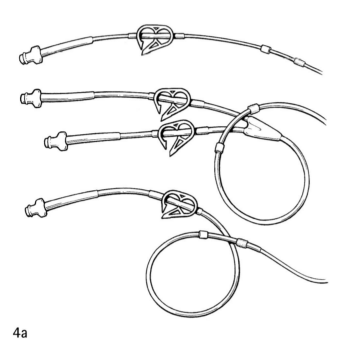

4a

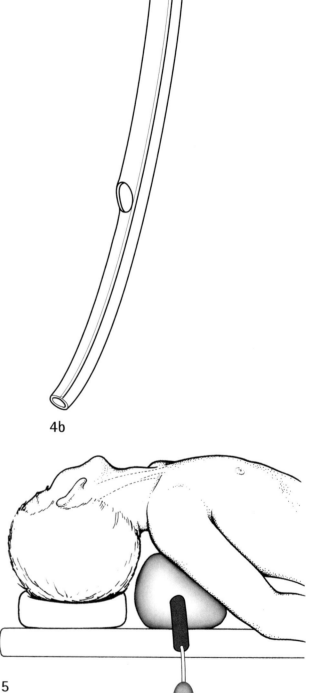

4b

OPEN INSERTION OF TUNNELED CVC
Internal jugular vein

5 The patient is positioned supine. A radiolucent pad (preferably inflatable) is placed under the scapulae and the head is turned slightly to the contralateral side. Alternatively, a soft roll may be utilized. Loupe magnification is an asset, particularly in infants and small children. After thorough skin preparation of the operative field, including the planned catheter exit site, the ipsilateral nipple and the neck, the drapes are secured with adhesive plastic or sutures.

5

6 A short skin crease incision is made 1–2 cm above the clavicle, overlying the diverging clavicular and sternal heads of the sternomastoid. The incision is deepened through platysma and the cervical fascia. The two heads of the sternomastoid are separated by blunt dissection. Small retractors are inserted to facilitate exposure of the internal jugular vein. Picking up and incising the fascia investing the internal jugular vein makes subsequent dissection easier. Using a Mixter, blunt right-angled forceps, a plane is developed on either side of the vein and the instrument is passed around the vein once a clear window has been established. A thin Silastic vessel loop is used to sling the vein. With this as a gentle retractor, a second vessel loop can be passed and a 1–2 cm length of vessel exposed between the slings. The retractors can be removed and the slings relaxed while the catheter tunnel is created.

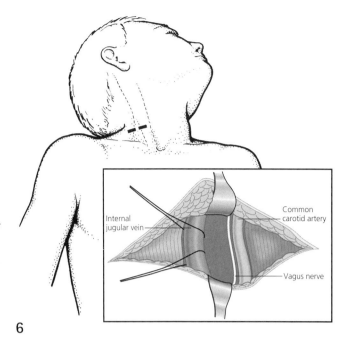

6

7 Various exit sites over the chest wall are possible but in girls, the developing breast and strap lines should be avoided. A small skin incision is made and a track of sufficient size to accommodate the catheter is developed using a hemostat. Local anesthetic from a syringe without a needle is injected into the track. Either a blunt tunneling rod to which the catheter is attached or a hollow tunneler is used to pass the catheter to the cervical wound. Soaking the Dacron cuff with aqueous antiseptic may be useful. It is then positioned about 2 cm from the exit site in order to facilitate future line removal. The distal catheter is cut to length with the tip beveled. On the right, the distance to the mid-right atrium is estimated by a point just above the nipple line and on the left, just below.

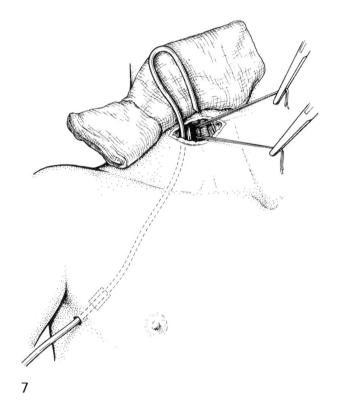

7

The prepared section of vein is elevated between the two slings by the assistant. Using fine non-toothed forceps and microvascular scissors, a short venotomy is made. This commences with the decisive use of the scissors to make a very small initial incision. This is followed by insertion of the closed scissor tips into the venotomy to widen it until it is equal to the external diameter of the catheter. The beveled catheter tip is now introduced into the vein with the aid of two non-toothed forceps. The assistant gently relaxes the lower sling to allow distal passage of the catheter and then tightens it to prevent back bleeding. The catheter should pass freely and, once inserted, free bidirectional flow should be confirmed. If required, the venotomy is closed around the catheter with 6/0 polypropylene vascular sutures, care being taken to avoid narrowing the vein. Hemostasis is checked with the slings relaxed. A purse-string suture around the catheter should be avoided as this may result in shearing of the vein upon removal.

8 The position of the catheter is checked using fluoroscopy. Allowance should be made for the radiolucent pad which when removed results in advancement of the catheter tip. Suboptimal positions resulting from anatomical variation or wrong catheter length should be corrected (e.g. left-sided SVC). The sternomastoid muscle is loosely approximated with an absorbable suture and the cervical wound is closed in two layers using a fine absorbable subcuticular suture. A topical biological skin glue and an adhesive dressing is an acceptable alternative. The catheter exit site incision is approximated around the catheter with a 4/0 monofilament suture and firmly tied without compression to the catheter to aid fixation. The catheter is flushed with heparinized saline (10 units/mL heparin). The exit site is dressed with gauze and a transparent adhesive plastic dressing. Adhesive tape is also used to secure the external part of the catheter, which should be looped to ensure that any pull on it does not result in direct traction to the line at the exit site. Unless soiled, the dressing is changed after 1 week.

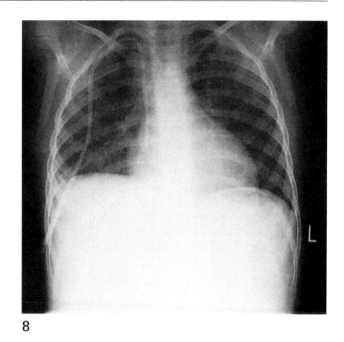

8

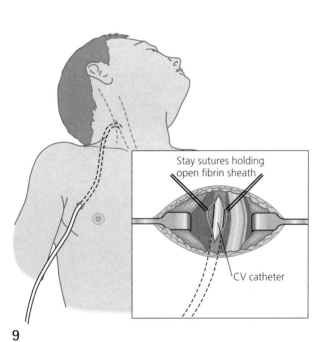

Stay sutures holding open fibrin sheath

CV catheter

9

VEIN REUSE

9 When indicated for mechanical failure in a tunneled central line that has been in place for weeks or more, the open exchange of a CVC provides very satisfactory results. The technique involves palpation of the old CVC just below the level of insertion into the RIJV, dissection onto the catheter, careful incision of the pericatheter fibrin sheath and control with fine stay sutures. At this stage, a new CVC (same size or smaller than the old), is tunneled via a fresh site, beside the old catheter in the neck and cut to length. With an assistant keeping the sheath open with gentle traction on the stay sutures, the surgeon removes the old line and immediately replaces it with the new. The final position is confirmed on screening and adjusted if required. The technique is simple and reliable. Its main drawback is that it cannot be used to increase the size of a catheter.

Alternative sites

Usually, the external jugular vein is easily visible and requires minimal dissection. It may provide a very useful alternative to the internal jugular vein; however, its use is limited by the caliber of the vein and the occasional difficulty of negotiating the junction with the subclavian vein.

10 The long saphenous vein is approached by a short transverse incision 1 cm below the groin skin crease, medial to the femoral artery. The vein is controlled with fine vessel loops. The catheter tip is positioned in the right atrium and the exit site, the lateral abdomen.

The femoral vein is especially useful for short-term access, but may also be used as a route for long-term catheters. The axillary vein is easily approached by an axillary incision and dissection, but size can be restricting. The common facial vein is a large anterior tributary of the internal jugular vein in infants that may be entered midway between the angle of the mandible and the clavicular head.

The cephalic vein is accessed in the deltopectoral groove, but tends to be small in young children. In some children who have required repeated, chronic venous access complicated by central vein thrombosis, other routes that can be used include the azygos, epigastric, iliac and renal veins, the inferior vena cava, and the right atrium. In these difficult cases, preoperative and intraoperative image guidance is advisable. Percutaneous techniques may avoid major dissection.

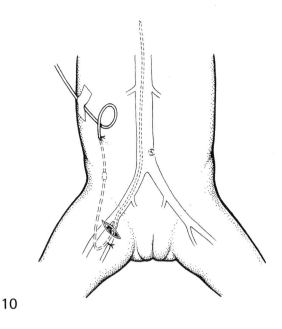

10

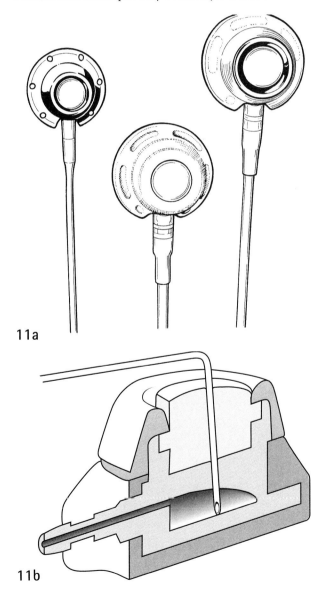

11a

11b

Ports

11a,b Totally implantable vascular access devices or 'ports' have a catheter connected to a small reservoir, which is implanted subcutaneously. A thick silicone membrane forming the roof of the port can be repeatedly injected percutaneously using a 22-gauge side-fenestrated, non-coring (Huber) needle. The ports are made from stainless steel, titanium, or hard plastic and are available in different shapes and sizes. Those with a preconnected catheter are easier to insert. One variety is designed to be implanted in the arm with central venous access through a peripherally inserted catheter. Because they have no external catheter, port devices have certain advantages over tunneled CVCs. In particular, they are less likely to require removal for infection, they cannot be accidentally removed, and they allow for activities such as swimming. They are therefore preferable for most children who require only intermittent (e.g. weekly) access, including those with hematological diseases and cystic fibrosis. They are less appropriate in children who cannot tolerate regular needle access, or who require continuous access, for example those who will need intensive chemotherapy or parenteral nutrition.

12 At the predetermined reservoir site, which must be easily accessible and rest on a firm surface, such as the anterolateral chest wall, the skin incision is deepened with diathermy. Hemostasis must be meticulous. A subcutaneous pocket is developed beneath the superficial fascia in such a way as to avoid placing the port directly under the skin incision. Placement of the port above rather than below the incision may reduce the impact of wound-related problems on port and line function. Before implanting the port, it is helpful to place non-absorbable sutures through the muscular fascia and the circumference of the port; when tied, these provide three-point fixation of the device. The catheter must be tunneled from the reservoir pocket to the site of venous access, such as the internal jugular vein in the neck. The port is flushed with saline, ensuring there are no kinks in the catheter. The distal catheter is cut to length (see above) and inserted by a cut-down or percutaneous technique. After confirming the catheter tip position by fluoroscopy, the port is flushed with heparinized saline and the skin incision is closed in two layers with an absorbable subcuticular skin suture.

Each injection must access the port vertically through the center of the silicone diaphragm such that the needle touches the base plate. As the needle is withdrawn, the port should be held in place and positive injection pressure applied to prevent reflux or blood into the catheter. A careful aseptic injection technique must always be used and the system flushed periodically.

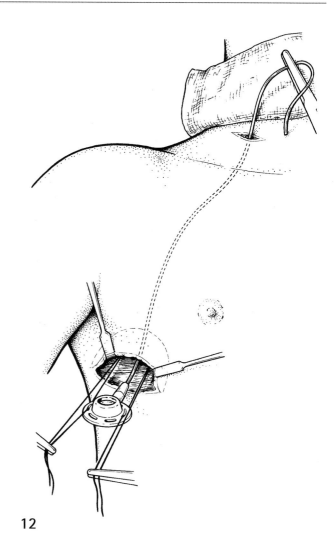

12

Removal

Most cuffed external catheters and all ports require a short general anesthetic for removal. With the former, the Dacron cuff can usually be dissected free with a hemostat and fine scissors via the exit site incision, which is then closed with absorbable sutures, skin tapes, or biological glue.

Ultrasound-guided insertion of central venous catheters

The use of real-time ultrasound guidance makes central venous access easy, quick, and safe in all but the most difficult cases. Potential advantages over surgical placement of central lines include a very high success rate at the first site attempted, a good cosmetic result because of the short puncture site incision, a short procedure time, and virtually no need for preoperative imaging in children who have had multiple central veins accessed in the past.

EQUIPMENT

13a,b A high-frequency (≥7 MHz) linear-array transducer is appropriate for the majority of punctures. In very small patients, a small 'hockey stick' transducer is a useful tool. The transducer is placed in a sterile probe cover for operative use.

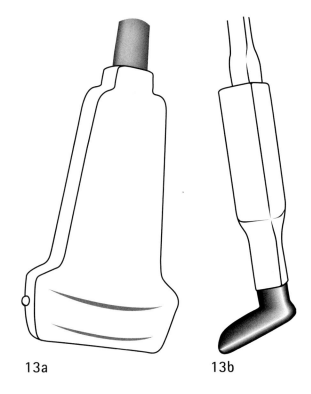

13a   13b

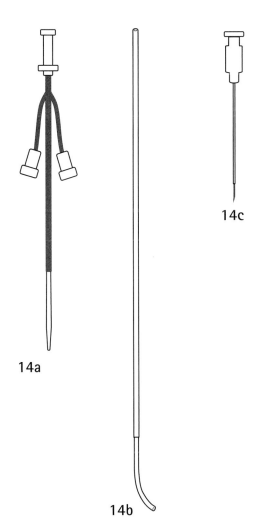

14c

14a

14b

14a–c In children weighing less than 10 kg, a 21-gauge one-part needle or 22-gauge cannula should be used for central venous puncture. These devices accept a 0.018-inch (0.46-mm) guidewire. The best guidewires have a stiff shaft and a short floppy tip. The stiff part of the wire is necessary to allow insertion of a peel-away sheath. In larger children, a wider (19- or 18-gauge) needle permits the use of a thicker guidewire, making insertion of the peel-away sheath easier. The percutaneous insertion of tunneled catheters requires the use of a peel-away sheath. These are available in a wide range of sizes. Although the stated size of a sheath is equal to the diameter of a catheter that can be introduced through it, this should be checked in advance, as it is sometimes necessary to use a sheath 0.5 Fr larger than the catheter.

INSERTION TECHNIQUE

15a–c Ultrasound is used to assess the available vessels and select one for access. The site of first choice is the right internal jugular vein. Skin preparation and draping is as described for open insertion. A trajectory for puncture is established using a 23-gauge needle attached to a syringe. The needle stops short of the vein wall. A small amount of local anesthetic is infiltrated as the needle is withdrawn and a skin crease stab incision made at the point of skin entry of the trajectory needle. This is widened slightly with a hemostat. We recommend tunneling the line (and when indicated, creation of a subcutaneous port pocket) at this stage. The line is introduced from the 'exit' site, along the track and out via the stab incision in the neck and wrapped in antiseptic-soaked gauze. The needle for vein puncture is attached to a syringe, and inserted at the medial end of the small cervical incision, taking care not to damage the catheter. There are two methods of puncturing the vein. In the first, the needle is advanced along the line of the vein, puncturing its anterior surface, with the probe held perpendicular to the needle and vein. The second method may be better for tunneled catheters and is our preferred technique: the anterolateral surface of the vein is punctured with the probe held in the same plane as the needle. In either case, it is important to puncture the vein with a sharp, stabbing motion to ensure that the tip of the needle enters the lumen of the vein with the bevel pointing downwards. The needle should be seen to move freely in the lumen, without a 'tent' of intima over the tip, and venous blood should aspirate freely. It is easy to create a subintimal hematoma if care is not taken at this stage. Inadvertent puncture of the opposite wall of the vein is usually not a problem, as the needle can be withdrawn into the lumen with ultrasound guidance. Once in the center of the vein, the angle of entry of the needle may be altered slightly so that it is pointing centrally. The guidewire is advanced into the vein, and its position confirmed by fluoroscopy. If it is easy to pass the guidewire through the right atrium and down the inferior vena cava, this should be done, as it makes insertion of the peel-away sheath easier and safer. Following removal of the needle, the peel-away sheath is advanced over the guidewire under fluoroscopic control. It is crucial to fix the guidewire (relative to the patient) at this stage. If this is not done, the dilator of the peel-away sheath may cause serious damage to the superior vena cava or heart. Catheter length can be determined as previously described by measurement against the nipple. Alternatively, fluoroscopy can be performed with the catheter on the anterior chest wall, projected over the peel-away sheath. If the catheter is cut at the T7 level,

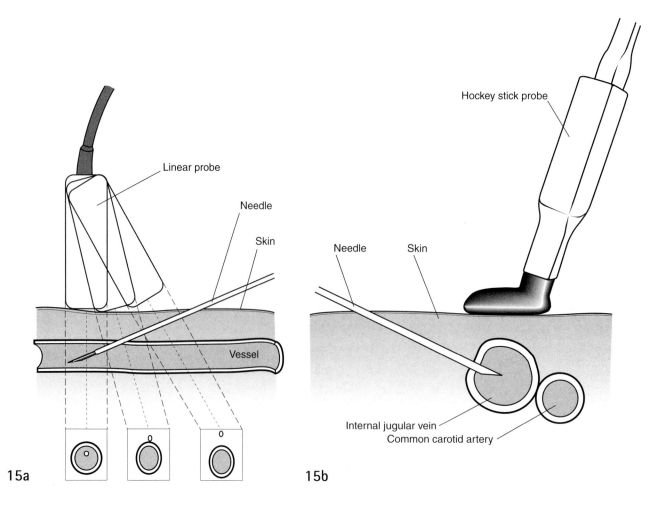

15a

15b

its tip will lie in the upper right atrium. The guidewire and the dilator of the peel-away sheath are removed. Mechanical ventilation with positive end-expiratory pressure effectively prevents air entering the peel-away sheath at this stage, but great care should be taken to avoid air embolism if the patient is breathing spontaneously. The catheter is advanced through the sheath, which is then split and removed. The position of the catheter tip is confirmed with fluoroscopy and adjusted if necessary. The catheter is flushed with heparin (10 units/mL) and sutured to the skin at the exit site. The cervical puncture can be closed with a subcuticular suture or tissue glue and adhesive tape. With minor modifications, this technique can be used at other sites or with other systems such as venous port devices.

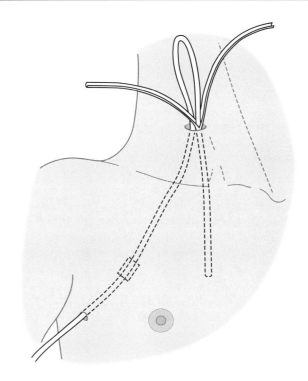

15c

EMERGENCY INTRAOSSEOUS VENOUS ACCESS

16 This route provides immediate vascular access during life-threatening emergencies in young children when rapid venous access cannot be achieved (cardiac arrest, shock, burns, and trauma). Contraindications include fracture or infection near the insertion site. After antiseptic preparation, the skin is punctured with a scalpel blade. The intraosseous needle is inserted into the medullary cavity of the proximal tibia through the middle of its flat anteromedial surface, 1–3 cm below the medial tuberosity (depending on the size of the child). The infusion needles (14- to 18-gauge) have an inner occluding stylet designed to facilitate bone penetration and should be inserted almost perpendicularly to the bone, but angled slightly away from the growth plate. Upon entering the marrow cavity, the resistance suddenly decreases. The needle should then stand firmly in the bone. It should be possible to aspirate bone marrow or flush the needle easily without extravasation. The needle flange is adjusted to skin level and taped in position. The patient's leg should be restrained with a support behind the knee. Crystalloids, blood products, and drugs can be infused, but blood sampling may occlude the needle.

The infusion needle should be removed once suitable conventional access has been obtained if potential complications (extravasation, compartment syndrome, fractures, osteomyelitis, fat embolism) are to be avoided. The distal femur and distal tibia are alternative sites.

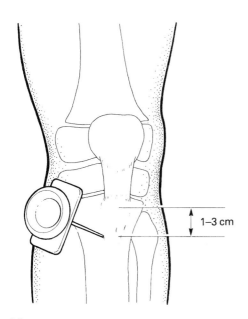

1–3 cm

16

ARTERIAL PUNCTURE AND CANNULATION

Intra-arterial access is used to provide continuous monitoring of systemic arterial blood pressure and to enable repeated arterial sampling for blood gas measurements.

17a–e The radial artery is the preferred site for both percutaneous and cut-down cannulation. The presence of adequate collateral flow must first be checked by the Allen test; both arteries are occluded at the wrist and after releasing the ulnar artery alone, the hand should flush pink (most hands have an ulnar dominant palmar arch). Alternatively, a Doppler ultrasound study may be performed. A small roll is placed under the supinated, extended wrist and the palm is taped to a padded surface, keeping the fingers exposed in order to assess the distal circulation. The skin is cleaned with antiseptic and a small quantity of local anesthetic is injected subcutaneously over the radial artery just proximal to the transverse crease at the wrist. The skin is punctured with a No. 11 scalpel blade and a 22- or 24-gauge Teflon cannula with a needle stylet is selected according to the size of the child. The artery position is verified by palpation. Two techniques are used. In the first, the needle and Teflon cannula are advanced at about 30° to the skin until a flashback of blood is seen. In the transfixion method, the artery is transfixed by the needle and cannula. The needle is then removed and the cannula is gently withdrawn until arterial blood appears when it is advanced up the artery lumen.

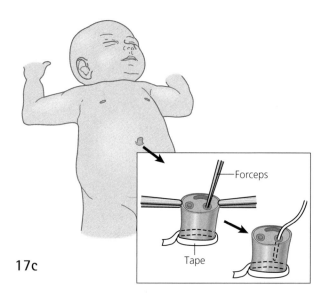

17c

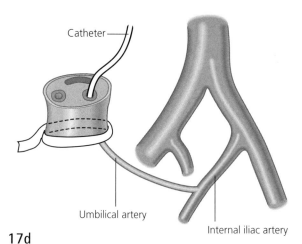

17d

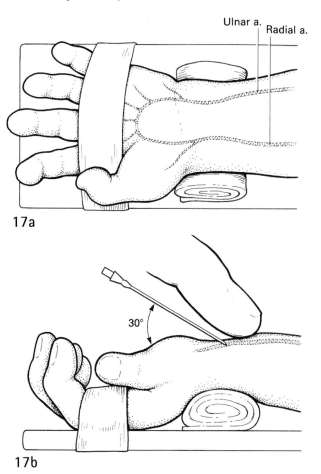

17a

17b

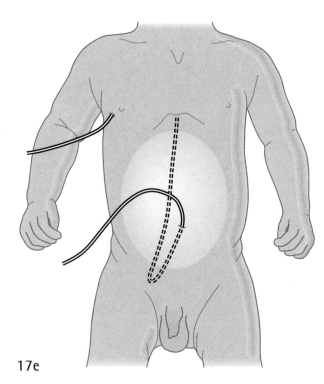

17e

In the cut-down technique, a small transverse incision over the artery allows the vessel to be punctured and cannulated under direct vision, with the option of proximal and distal vessel control. The catheter hub is sutured in place and the skin is sutured around the cannula.

Arterial cannulas require continuous perfusion with 0.5–1.0 mL/hour heparinized saline. Because of the risk of serious complications (ischemia, embolism, hemorrhage, sepsis), arterial access requires an even higher level of vigilance and should be used for the shortest possible time. The cannula should be removed if signs of digital ischemia develop. Alternative sites for arterial access include pedal, umbilical, femoral, brachial, and axillary arteries, but complications are more frequent than with radial artery cannulas.

Peripheral artery cannulation is not feasible in some sick infants who require intensive monitoring and umbilical artery cannulation may be required. If arterial and venous cannulation are necessary, it is recommended that arterial access (the more difficult) is carried out first. Arterial cannulation is described, but the principles are similar for venous access.

White tape under moderate tension is applied to control the cord at its base. The cord is cut with a No. 15 scalpel about 1 cm from skin level. The two thick-walled umbilical arteries and the one thin-walled vein are identified. A fine non-toothed forceps is introduced closed into the selected artery and opened gently to achieve dilatation. A preprepared and flushed catheter is grasped close to the tip using another pair of forceps and advanced into the umbilical artery, gently but firmly in a caudal direction. The catheter is thereby guided into the aorta via an internal iliac artery. Ready bleeding should be seen and a predetermined position aimed for and confirmed radiologically. In the 'low position', the catheter tip is just above the aortic bifurcation, while in the 'high position' it is just above the level of the diaphragm.

POSTOPERATIVE CARE

The postoperative care of CVCs is crucial to longevity and optimal function. Tunneled CVCs should be looped then secured with occlusive, transparent dressing. This ensures that distal traction is not directly transmitted to the line at the exit site. The development of dedicated teams and carefully defined protocols that cover aspects of management, such as frequency of flushing, line handling techniques for sampling and infusions, has also helped to reduce complications. If well cared for, the majority of catheters last the duration of the planned course of treatment. However, complications which may shorten this duration are well recognized and are summarized in **Table 4.2**.

Table 4.2 Complications of central venous access.

Timeline	Complication	Prevention	Management
Immediate	Pneumothorax	Avoid blind procedures	Chest drain
	Hemorrhage	Meticulous technique	Digital pressure, vein repair
	Air embolism	Positive pressure ventilation	Patient positioning, resuscitation
	Arterial puncture	Avoid blind procedures	Digital pressure
	Cardiac arrhythmia	Fix guidewire	Remove irritation, carotid massage, adenosine
	Malposition	Intraoperative fluoroscopy	Line revision
Early	Accidental removal	Secure exit site suture, loop catheter	Line replacement
	Catheter-related sepsis	Meticulous aseptic technique for insertion and subsequent line access	Antibiotic therapy, catheter removal
	Chest wall hematoma	Check and normalize coagulation parameters preoperatively	Pressure dressing
	Cardiac tamponade	Site stiff percutaneous catheters in low SVC	Pericardiocentesis, pericardiotomy
Delayed	Catheter-related thrombosis	Site catheter tip in upper right atrium, flush regularly	Conservative management, anticoagulation, thrombolysis
	Extravasation		
	Port-catheter separation	Use of preconnected catheter	Urgent exchange
	Catheter migration	Site catheter tip in upper right atrium	Catheter revision
	Catheter fracture	Gentle handling and careful removal	Fluoroscopic catheter retrieval of embolized fragments

SVC, superior vena cava.

FURTHER READING

Arul GS, Lewis N, Bromley P, Bennett J. Ultrasound-guided percutaneous insertion of Hickman lines in children. Prospective study of 500 consecutive procedures. *Journal of Pediatric Surgery* 2009; **44**: 1371–6.

Brevetti LS, Kalliainen L, Kimura K. A surgical technique that allows reuse of an existing venotomy site for multiple central venous catheterizations. *Journal of Pediatric Surgery* 1996; **31**: 939–40.

Donaldson JS, Morello FP, Junewick JJ *et al.* Peripherally inserted central venous catheters: US-guided vascular access in pediatric patients. *Radiology* 1995; **197**: 542–4.

National Institute for Health and Clinical Excellence, UK. Guidance on the use of ultrasound locating devices for placing central venous catheters. Technology Appraisal Guidance, No. 49. London: NICE, September 2002.

Stringer MD, Brereton RJ, Wright VM. Performance of percutaneous silastic central venous feeding catheters in surgical neonates. *Pediatric Surgery International* 1992; **7**: 79–81.

Vo JN, Hoffer FA, Shaw DW. Techniques in vascular and interventional radiology: pediatric central venous access. *Techniques in Vascular and Interventional Radiology* 2010; **13**: 250–7.

Head and neck

Ranula

MARCI M LESPERANCE

INTRODUCTION

1, 2 A ranula is a mucocele arising in the floor of the mouth, secondary to obstruction of the salivary ducts of the sublingual glands. The term 'ranula' is derived from the Latin roots *rana* (frog) and *ulus* (small). The simple ranula, confined to the sublingual space, is a true cyst with an epithelial lining. 'Plunging' ranulas present as masses involving the submandibular triangle or other neck spaces, resulting from extravasation of mucous and a consequent inflammatory response. The cervical component of a ranula is a pseudocyst lined by granulation or connective tissue without a true epithelial lining which may extend deeply into the soft tissues and fascial planes of the neck without respect for tissue planes. Ranulas may be congenital or acquired, and a simple ranula may develop into a plunging ranula after initial attempts at treatment. Ranulas are remarkable for the diversity of approaches to their treatment, which has led to some controversy in the literature.

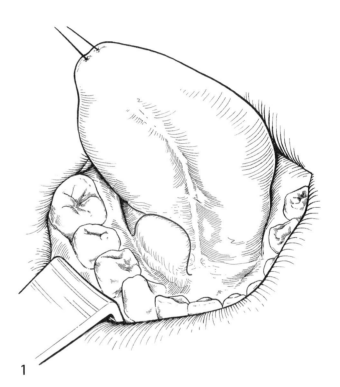

1

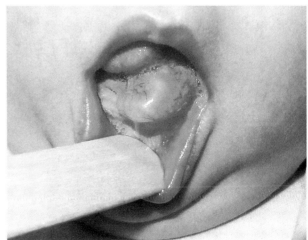

2

ANATOMY

The sublingual glands are almond-shaped structures located in the floor of the mouth, covered by mucosa in continuity with the mucosa of the ventral tongue and the gingiva of the mandible. The reflection of mucosa over the sublingual gland creates a fold known as the plica sublingualis on each side of the lingual frenulum. There may be several detached lobules of the sublingual gland, each with its own small duct that directly drains to the floor of the mouth. These small ducts are known as accessory ducts or ducts of Rivinus, some of which join to form the predominant sublingual duct (Bartholin's duct).

The floor of the mouth is supported by the mylohyoid muscle with contribution from the geniohyoid muscle. The submandibular duct, also known as the submaxillary or Wharton's duct, terminates into the sublingual caruncle, located on either side of the midline frenulum of the tongue. The sublingual ducts may drain into the submandibular duct, through the sublingual caruncle, or into the oral cavity at the plica sublingualis.

The main portion of the submandibular gland is located superficially in the submandibular triangle, the suprahyoid part of the anterior cervical triangle. A small deep or oral portion of the submandibular gland and its duct are found deep to the mylohyoid muscle, between the mylohyoid and the genioglossus and hyoglossus muscle. The oral portion of the submandibular gland is in close relationship to the sublingual gland, which may lead to the mistaken impression that a ranula is arising from the submandibular gland. Dehiscences in the mylohyoid muscle will allow the sublingual gland to herniate through into the submandibular space. Incisions through the floor of the mouth mucosa enter into the paralingual space, which contains the lingual nerve, the submandibular duct, and the sublingual glands, and is continuous with the submandibular space.

ETIOLOGY

As understood by contemporary authors, ranulas uniformly arise from the sublingual glands; the submandibular gland is not directly involved in their development. The sublingual gland produces saliva of high protein content, and secretion is constitutive; in contrast, the secretory activity of the submandibular gland increases in response to eating. The amount of fluid in a ranula reflects a balance between the continuous flow of mucous from the sublingual gland and the clearance of extravasated mucous by macrophages which are recruited in the inflammatory response and lymphatic drainage. Granulation tissue and fibrous tissue developing in response to inflammation may restrict the extravasation and seal the leak. Surgical treatment must address the primary pathology of impaired sublingual gland drainage; excision of the entire cervical pseudocyst portion is not necessary. Plunging ranulas may extend into other cervical triangles and mimic other lesions, such as macrocystic lymphangiomas. Ranulas may result from any type of traumatic or iatrogenic injury to the sublingual gland or its ducts, such as dental implants, sialoendoscopy procedures, frenulectomy, or submandibular duct rerouting procedures for the management of sialorrhea. Ranulas may be surgically induced in experimental animals by ligation of the sublingual duct. Finally, ranulas and oral mucoceles have been reported as the first presenting sign of HIV (human immunodeficiency virus) infection in patients from endemic regions.

EVALUATION

3 Imaging may be useful to diagnose the extent of a ranula and to confirm the diagnosis. Ranulas appear sonographically as hypoechoic (cystic) masses with internal echoes, and herniation of the sublingual gland through a dehiscence in the mylohoid muscle may also be seen. Computed tomography is chiefly useful for evaluation of plunging ranulas to rule out other etiologies, and will typically show extension into the sublingual and submandibular spaces. Magnetic resonance imaging will show high signal on T2-weighted images.

The presence of amylase in aspirated fluid contents will confirm the diagnosis of ranula, but is not typically necessary. Sialoendoscopy has recently been used to diagnose and treat salivary stones and other obstructive lesions of the parotid and submandibular glands; while ranula is a known complication of sialadenoscopy, a role for sialadenoscopy in the evaluation and management of ranula has not been established.

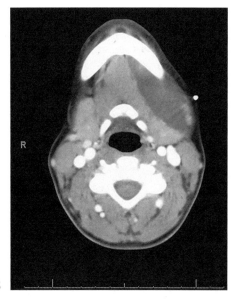

3

DIFFERENTIAL DIAGNOSIS

Lymphangiomas (cystic hygromas) of the neck may involve the floor of the mouth, extending from the submandibular space or tongue into the floor of the mouth region, characterized by a verrucous appearance of the oral mucosa. Other intraoral masses include congenital cysts unrelated to the sublingual gland or solid lesions such as dermoids. Neoplasms of the salivary glands, such as pleomorphic adenoma, are rare in children. Submandibular sialadenitis may result from stones in the submandibular duct and may require surgical excision of the gland. Thyroglossal duct cysts and branchial cleft cysts are usually readily distinguishable from ranulas, as neither typically involve the submandibular triangle.

TREATMENT

A wide variety of treatments have been reported for ranulas. With few exceptions, most reports consist of small case series. Simple incision and drainage is no longer advocated due to a very low success rate. Options include marsupialization, intraoral excision with or without sublingual sialadenectomy, or combined intraoral and cervical approaches.

Marsupialization involves unroofing the cyst, draining out the fluid, and either suturing the edges or using cautery to ensure that the cavity walls heal in an open fashion. Using a gauze pack to add positive pressure is thought to be more successful than simple marsupialization alone. Some authors advise packing with drainage for as long as 3 weeks, using antibiotics for 3 days, even for plunging ranulas. Lasers have also been used for marsupialization, with the goal of inciting sufficient fibrosis to prevent the edges from healing over and allowing reaccumulation of mucous. However, it is uncertain whether the laser provides sufficient advantages to justify the increased expense and risk.

The consensus in the current literature recommends excision of the sublingual gland to mitigate against recurrence. A prospective randomized clinical study of children with intraoral ranulas found a substantial recurrence rate after marsupialization with suturing of edges, compared to no recurrences in the sublingual sialadenectomy group. If the lesion arises from accessory lobes of salivary gland tissue distinct from the main sublingual gland, excising only the portion of the gland involved in the ranula may be sufficient. Simple intraoral excision of the cyst may be adequate for well-encapsulated, small lesions. Most authors would agree with removal of the sublingual gland at the time of salvage surgery if an initial conservative attempt fails.

For plunging ranulas, external approaches are still frequently used, although controversial. While most agree that the sublingual gland, rather than the submandibular gland, is the source of the ranula, the submandibular gland may develop post-obstructive sialadenitis if the function of its duct is compromised. Notably, ranula-like lesions involving the floor of the mouth, pterygomaxillary fossa and parapharyngeal space have been reported to occur after removal of an ipsilateral submandibular duct stone. Many authors suggest that it is not necessary to remove the entire pseudocyst wall of the ranula, because the wall consists of granulation tissue that will resolve once extravasation of mucous has ceased. Others advocate an external approach if the initial intraoral approach fails, as a cervical incision will provide excellent access to the submandibular triangle and facilitate identification of the lingual and hypoglossal nerves.

OK-432 (Picibanil) is a sclerosing agent which has been used for the treatment of ranulas in adults and children. OK-432 consists of a mixture of streptococcal antigen and benzylpenicillin, with demonstrated efficacy in the treatment of lymphangiomas. Using fluoroscopic guidance, the cyst is punctured, and its contents are aspirated. An equivalent volume of dilute OK-432 is injected into the cyst, which incites an inflammatory response, in some cases obviating the need for surgical excision. Success rates with OK-432 averaged 73 percent for oral ranulas and 59 percent for plunging ranulas. Postoperative fever, swelling, and odynophagia are common sequelae and up to five treatments may be necessary.

Spontaneous regression has been reported and some authors suggest deferring surgery until the lesion has been present for five months. Watchful waiting for up to six months may also be appropriate for ranulas occurring after surgical trauma or in cases of apparent recurrence. Postoperative imaging may demonstrate persistent subclinical accumulation of small amounts of extravasated mucous.

OPERATIVE PROCEDURE

4a–d In pediatric patients, general anesthesia with endotracheal intubation is advisable. Nasal intubation is an option but not strictly necessary, as an orotracheal tube may be taped off to the opposite side. If the endotracheal tube is uncuffed, a hypopharyngeal pack may be used. Either a mouth gag, such as a Jennings type, can be used, or retraction may be provided by an assistant using a Weider or Army–Navy retractors. It may be useful to place a silk suture through the tip of the tongue to aid in retraction, releasing tension intermittently to avoid tongue edema. Cannulation of the ipsilateral submandibular duct with a lacrimal probe is useful to identify and protect it.

Local anesthestic such as 1 percent lidocaine with 1:100000 epinephrine is infiltrated into the mucosa over the submandibular gland duct and the sublingual glands. The mucosa is incised with monopolar cautery along the anterior border of the submandibular duct. Placing stay sutures prior to incision may help to maintain visualization of the cyst itself, which is often very thin-walled. Excising a small ellipse of normal mucosa may be advisable rather than attempting to deliver the sublingual gland and the ranula through a mucosal incision. In revision cases with extensive scarring, an incision in the gingival sulcus with elevation of a full-thickness flap of mucoperiosteum from the lingual surface of the mandible to the floor of the mouth may be useful to avoid lingual nerve and hypoglossal nerve injury. The sublingual gland is dissected free from the submandibular duct, identifying the lingual nerve which is intimately associated with the duct. The intraoral incision is closed loosely with absorbable sutures.

The cervical fluid collection is drained from the intraoral approach without the need to excise the entire pseudocyst walls. Some authors describe placing a suction drain in a retrograde fashion, from the sublingual and submandibular space out through a small cervical incision, to provide postoperative drainage. For external approaches, a standard procedure for excision of the submandibular gland is utilized, identifying and preserving the lingual and hypoglossal nerves, and ligating the submandibular ganglion and the submandibular duct, while preserving the marginal mandibular nerve.

Postoperatively, the patient is allowed to resume a regular diet. Oral rinses after meals may be implemented in older children able to cooperate. Some authors recommend gavage feeds rather than feeding from a nipple in infants, and avoiding pacifier use. For external approaches or plunging ranulas, use of a suction drain through a cervical incision is recommended.

Antibiotics may be administered as a single perioperative dose; however, many authors use a short postoperative course of oral antibiotics, particularly if a drain or packing is in place. Some surgeons encourage the use of lemon drops or other sour candies and fruits to stimulate the secretion of saliva.

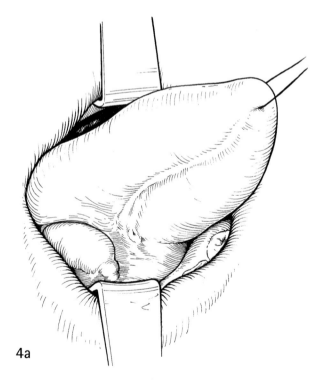

4a

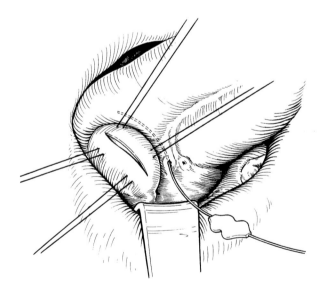

4b

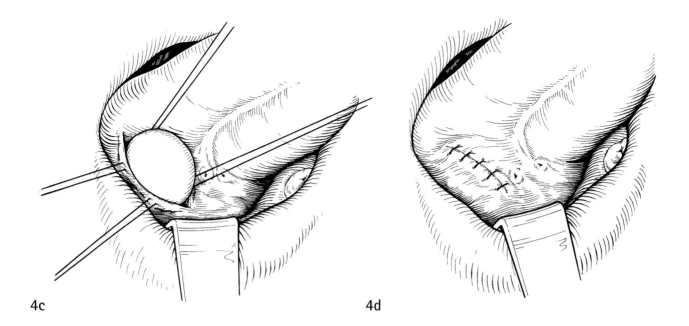

4c

4d

COMPLICATIONS

The most common complication is recurrence of the ranula with persistent or intermittent swelling. Surgical intervention may compromise the function of the submandibular duct or other sublingual ducts. Other risks of surgical intervention include lingual nerve injury resulting in tongue hypoesthesia, postoperative edema or hematoma, and infection. Less commonly, there is injury to the hypoglossal nerve or marginal mandibular nerve, which are more at risk from external cervical than intraoral approaches. However, traction injury to the marginal mandibular nerve may occur due to persistent intraoperative retraction.

CONCLUSION

Ranulas are benign lesions which may present challenges in treatment. Marsupialization with or without packing may be appropriate for small intraoral lesions. For both plunging and oral ranulas, excision of the ipsilateral sublingual gland and simple drainage is recommended. Complete excision of the pseudocyst wall is not necessary.

FURTHER READING

Baurmash HD. A case against sublingual gland removal as primary treatment of ranulas. *Journal of Oral and Maxillofacial Surgery* 2007; **65**: 117–21.

Harrison JD. Modern management and pathophysiology of ranula: literature review. *Head and Neck* 2010; **32**: 1310–20.

Jain P, Jain R, Morton RP, Ahmad Z. Plunging ranulas: high-resolution ultrasound for diagnosis and surgical management. *European Radiology* 2007; **20**: 1442–9.

Kim PD, Simental Jr A. Treatment of ranulas. *Operative Techniques in Otolaryngology–Head and Neck Surgery* 2008; **19**: 240–2.

Mahadevan M, Vasan N. Management of pediatric plunging ranula. *International Journal of Pediatric Otorhinolaryngology* 2006; **70**: 1049–54.

Patel MR, Deal AM, Shockley WW. Oral and plunging ranulas: what is the most effective treatment? *Laryngoscope* 2009; **119**: 1501–9.

Thyroglossal cyst and fistula

LEWIS SPITZ and PAOLO DE COPPI

HISTORY

The thyroglossal duct was first described in 1723 by Vater, who called it the 'lingual duct'. It was later referred to as the 'canal of His' following his descriptions in 1855 and 1891.

PRINCIPLES AND JUSTIFICATION

Development of thyroid gland and thyroglossal tract

The thyroid gland develops as a median thickening of the floor of the pharynx at the level of the second branchial arch (tuberculum impar), during the fourth week of gestation, and descends to its final position in the neck, leaving the thyroglossal duct extending caudally from the foramen cecum of the tongue to the pyramidal lobe of the gland, passing anterior through or posterior to the hyoid bone. The lateral lobes of the gland receive contributions from the fourth branchial clefts, which form the medullary C cells. Early in the fifth week of gestation, the attenuated duct loses its lumen and shortly afterwards breaks into fragments. Thyroid remnants may be found along the course of the thyroglossal duct.

Thyroglossal cysts

Thyroglossal cysts, the most common anterior cervical swelling in children, most frequently arise just inferior to the level of the hyoid bone. Occasionally, the duct deviates anterosuperiorly once it has passed the hyoid bone, giving rise to a thyroglossal cyst in the submental triangle, where it may be mistaken for a dermoid cyst. Although dermoid cysts may occur below the hyoid bone, they are more common in the submental triangle and can be distinguished from thyroglossal cysts by their softer, 'putty-like' consistency. Very occasionally, aberrant thyroid glandular tissue is found along the course of the thyroglossal duct.

Thyroglossal fistulas

A thyroglossal fistula usually results from rupture or incision of an inflamed thyroglossal cyst. The fistulous opening is usually at the level of the original cyst, but may appear lower down in the neck.

PREOPERATIVE

Assessment and preparation

In thyroid hypoplasia, a small central area of aberrant ectopic thyroid tissue may be mistaken for a thyroglossal cyst, and it is recommended that the precise location of the thyroid gland is determined, using isotope scanning or ultrasound examination, before undertaking surgery, as removal of the aberrant tissue may result in permanent hypothyroidism. The incidence of such aberrant tissue is, however, low (about 1 percent of all thyroglossal abnormalities) and it is easily recognizable when the lesion is exposed.

Occult staphylococcal infection is common in these cysts and perioperative antibiotic cover using a penicillinase-resistant agent, such as flucloxacillin or fusidic acid, is usually indicated.

Anesthesia

General anesthesia using an orotracheal or nasotracheal tube is recommended.

OPERATIONS

Excision of thyroglossal cyst

The aim of surgery is to remove the entire duct, including the central part of the body of the hyoid bone, to the level of the foramen cecum. Because side branches may arise from the duct within the muscles of the tongue, the intraglossal part of the duct should be removed with a surrounding cuff of muscle approximately 0.5 cm in diameter. Complete excision is essential to prevent recurrence and eliminate the risk of malignant degeneration. All thyroglossal cysts, however small, should be excised to avoid the risk of infection, which makes subsequent surgery more difficult, morbidity and recurrence rates higher, and cosmetic results less satisfactory. The operation may be performed on a day-case basis provided meticulous hemostasis has been achieved.

POSITION OF PATIENT

The patient is placed supine with the head extended and the shoulders elevated on a small sandbag.

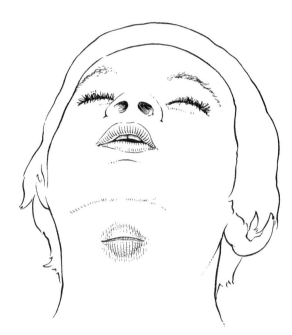

1

INCISION

1 A short (usually less than 3 cm) transverse incision is made in a skin crease over the main prominence of the cyst. Some authors recommend infiltration of the skin with epinephrine (adrenaline) to reduce bleeding.

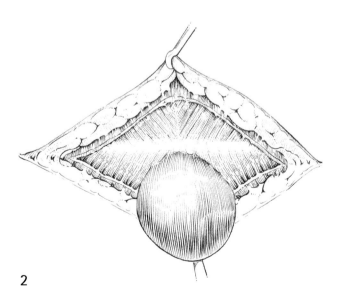

2

2 The subcutaneous fat, platysma, and deep cervical fascia are incised in the line of the incision with a diathermy needle and the cyst is freed from its superficial attachments by a combination of sharp and blunt dissection. Meticulous hemostasis is essential so that the operative field is not obscured.

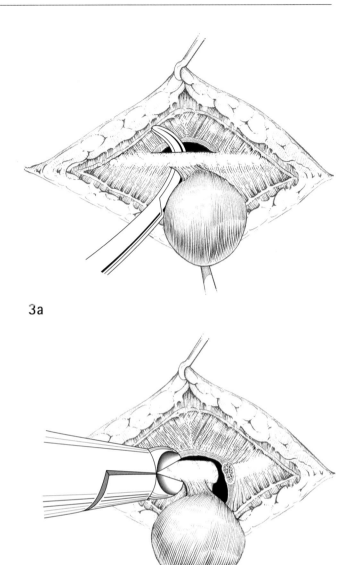

3a

3b

DISSECTION

3 The thyroglossal tract is identified at its deep attachment to the cyst and followed between the sternohyoid muscles to the hyoid bone. The centrum of the hyoid bone is freed from the sternohyoid muscles below and the mylohyoid and geniohyoid muscles above with a diathermy needle. The thyrohyoid membrane is separated from the posterior aspect of the centrum using artery forceps, a closed pair of scissors, or a McDonald dissector. Small bone-cutting forceps or strong Mayo scissors are then used to divide the body of the hyoid 5 mm to either side of the midline. This maneuver is facilitated by grasping and steadying the bone with Kocher artery forceps.

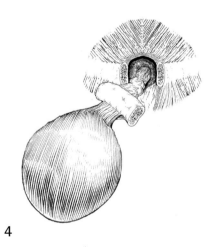

4

4 A cylinder of geniohyoid and genioglossus muscle 0.5 cm wide, including the duct, is excised to the foramen cecum; this is best performed using needle diathermy. It has been suggested that the dissection is made easier if the anesthetist uses a finger to depress the foramen cecum into the wound, but this is seldom of practical value and is a potential danger to the anesthetist. Meticulous hemostasis using diathermy will prevent postoperative respiratory obstruction due to hematoma formation.

WOUND CLOSURE

5 The muscles are approximated in the midline using sutures of 3/0 polyglycolic acid or chromic catgut to aid hemostasis. It is not necessary to reconstitute the hyoid bone because its cut ends tend to be approximated by the muscle sutures.

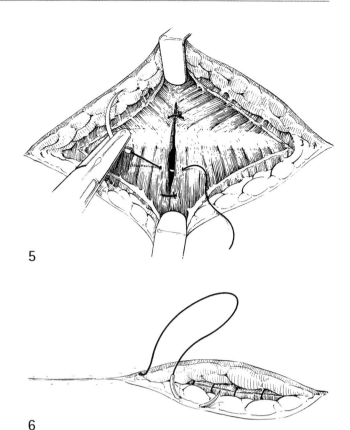

5

6 The fascia and platysma are closed with a continuous suture of 3/0 or 4/0 polyglycolic acid and the same suture is used in the subcutaneous layer to appose the skin edges. Alternatively, the skin edges may be approximated with self-adhesive wound tapes. The use of non-absorbable skin sutures or clips is not recommended as their removal causes anxiety and discomfort. If adequate hemostasis has been secured, no drains or dressings are required.

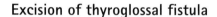

6

Excision of thyroglossal fistula

Treatment is similar to that for an uncomplicated thyroglossal cyst. All traces of the fistula must be excised to the foramen cecum.

POSITION OF PATIENT

The patient should be positioned as for excision of a thyroglossal cyst (see above under **Excision of thyroglossal cyst**).

INCISION

7 A small elliptical incision is made around the orifice of the fistula (sinus) in the neck.

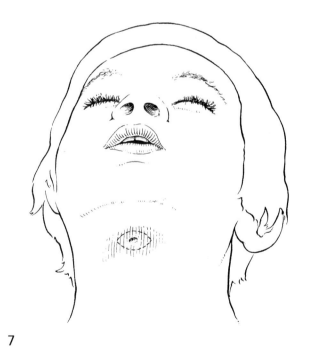

7

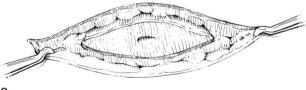

8

8 The ellipse of skin (including the sinus or fistulous tract) is traced through the subcutaneous tissues towards the hyoid bone.

RESECTION

9 The centrum of the hyoid bone is resected with the fistulous tract.

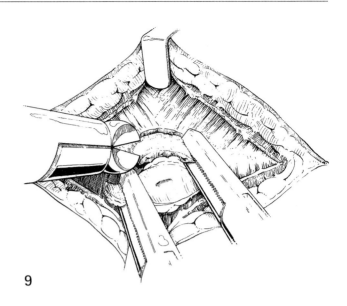

9

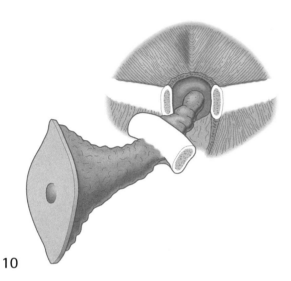

10

10 A core of geniohyoid and genioglossus muscles, including the tract, is excised up to the level of the foramen cecum.

WOUND CLOSURE

The wound is closed as for a thyroglossal cyst. It may be necessary to insert a drain if perfect hemostasis cannot be guaranteed or if there is florid inflammatory edema.

POSTOPERATIVE CARE

It is important to ensure that the airway does not become obstructed by reactionary hemorrhage. Infection is common, and spreading cellulitis may cause airway compression, so oral antibiotics should be continued for 2–3 days after the procedure. The child may be allowed home on the day after surgery.

OUTCOME

If the thyroglossal duct is excised with the cyst, recurrence is unlikely. Recurrence rates of 5–7 percent are reported. Cysts may recur, however, sometimes as much as ten years later, in more than 20 percent of patients treated by local excision only. This rate is reduced to 5 percent by removing the central part of the hyoid bone with the cyst. The recurrence rate of a thyroglossal fistula is higher than that for the uncomplicated cyst.

FURTHER READING

Brereton RJ, Symonds E. Thyroglossal cysts in children. *British Journal of Surgery* 1978; **65**: 507–8.

Brown BM, Judd ES. Thyroglossal duct cysts and sinuses. *American Journal of Surgery* 1961; **102**: 494–501.

Gallagher TQ, Hartnick CJ. Thyroglossal duct cist excision. *Advances in Oto-rhino-laryngology* 2012; **73**: 66–9.

Gupta P, Maddalozzo J. Preoperative sonography in presumed thyroglossal duct cysts. *Archives of Otolaryngology* 2001; **127**: 200–2.

Sistrunk WE. Technique of removal of cysts and sinuses of the thyroglossal duct. *Surgery, Gynecology and Obstetrics* 1928; **46**: 109–12.

Solomon J, Rangecroft L. Thyroglossal duct lesions in children. *Journal of Pediatric Surgery* 1984; **19**: 555.

Telander RL, Deane SA. Thyroglossal and branchial cleft cysts and sinuses. *Surgical Clinics of North America* 1977; **57**: 779.

Branchial cysts, sinuses, and fistulas

JOHN R WESLEY

PRINCIPLES AND JUSTIFICATION

Cysts, sinuses, and fistulas of the neck derived from branchial cleft remnants are common in the pediatric age group. Although all are present at birth, sinuses and fistulas are encountered more commonly in infants and children, while branchial cysts present more often in older children and young adults. Remnants of the first and second branchial apparatus are most common, accounting for 96 percent of all branchial anomalies with abnormalities of the second cleft outnumbering those of the first by 6:1. Abnormalities of the third and fourth branchial apparatus are rare, but recent case reports and reviews indicate that they may be more common than previously supposed.

1 A simple knowledge of head and neck embryology is helpful in understanding these abnormalities. The branchial arches appear by the 15th day of fetal life and present as bar-like ridges separated by grooves or clefts. Five paired ectodermal clefts and five endodermal pouches separate the six branchial arches. A closing membrane lies at the interface of the pouches and clefts. The four clinically significant arches and clefts are shown.

The pathogenesis of branchial cleft anomalies is controversial, and may occur as any combination of sinus, fistula, and cyst. Incomplete obliteration of the branchial apparatus, primarily the cleft, is accepted as the most likely etiology. Most branchial anomalies arise from the second branchial apparatus as the second branchial arch overgrows the second, third, and fourth branchial clefts, and finally fuses with the lateral branchial wall. As the arches coalesce during the growth of the embryo, part of the first branchial cleft remains open as the Eustachian tube and auditory canal. The second branchial cleft normally closes completely; however, either branchial cleft may form a sinus tract or cyst as it coalesces.

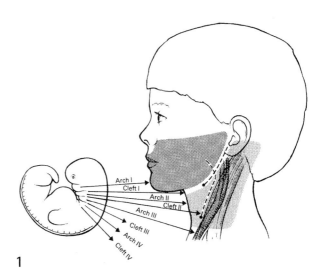

1

2 Remnants of the first branchial cleft, usually a short sinus track occasionally opening into the external auditory canal, occur along an imaginary line extending from the auditory canal behind and below the angle of the mandible to its midpoint. Second branchial cleft remnants are found anywhere along an imaginary line extending from the tonsillar fossa down to a point on the lower third of the anterior border of the sternocleidomastoid muscle.

Although branchial apparatus anomalies may present at any age, most branchial sinuses present clinically soon after birth or before the age of ten years.

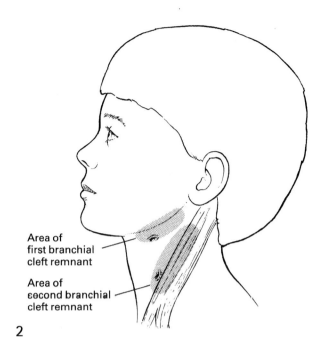

Area of first branchial cleft remnant

Area of second branchial cleft remnant

2

3 The more common second branchial cleft sinus presents as a pinpoint opening on the anterior border of the sternocleidomastoid muscle, one-quarter to one-third of its length cephalad from the sternal end. The defect is usually characterized by the appearance of small drops of clear fluid at the opening or by the occurrence of infection in the tract itself. The anomaly may be either unilateral or bilateral, and may be familial. Tracts that have an exterior opening occasionally become infected, although infection is a more common problem in sinuses and cysts in the older age group. Cysts of the first branchial cleft usually present as enlarging masses near the lower pole of the parotid gland and are more commonly seen in older children and young adults. Cysts of the second branchial cleft usually present in children and young adults as a mass at the mandibular angle along the anterior border of the sternocleidomastoid muscle, often associated with upper respiratory infection.

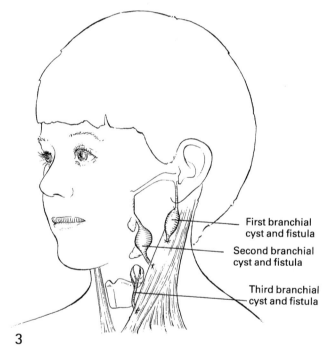

First branchial cyst and fistula

Second branchial cyst and fistula

Third branchial cyst and fistula

3

Case reports and recent reviews suggest that cysts or acute infections arising from a third or fourth branchial pouch sinus are rare but well-defined entities that offer diagnostic and therapeutic challenges not encountered with the anomalies of the first and second branchial remnants. These lesions present as an air-containing inflammatory lateral neck mass in the neonate or as acute suppurative thyroiditis in the infant or child. The etiology for both presentations is a fistulous track from the piriform sinus, most commonly on the left side, occurring as a result of a persistent remnant from the third or fourth branchial pouch. This condition should always be suspected in a neonate presenting with an inflammatory lesion containing air in the left side of the neck. Similarly, acute suppurative thyroiditis is rare and its presence should prompt consideration of a piriform sinus fistula as the etiology. Treatment of the acute infection should be followed by surgical extirpation in all cases.

PREOPERATIVE

Assessment and preparation

Cysts and sinuses of the first and second branchial clefts are diagnosed by their clinical appearance on careful physical examination. No special diagnostic imaging is indicated. The operation may be performed at any age, usually at the time of diagnosis, the main consideration in neonates being the availability of sophisticated pediatric anesthesia. The use of sclerosing solutions is contraindicated and may be dangerous. If infection is present, a course of antibiotics should be administered first. With respect to cysts or sinuses suspected to be of third or fourth branchial pouch origin, barium studies may demonstrate the presence of a piriform sinus fistula, particularly after a course of antibiotics and resolution of the surrounding inflammation. Computed axial tomography has also proved useful in diagnosing lesions of a third or fourth branchial pouch origin. If imaging techniques are not successful after resolution of the inflammation, then the next time the inflammation recurs, compression of the pus-filled cyst

Exposure of cyst

4 The most common branchial cyst is derived from the second branchial cleft. The skin incision is made over the cyst along Langer's lines or in a natural skin crease in order to obtain the best cosmetic result. The length of the incision will vary with the size of the cyst.

Infiltration of the overlying skin and adjacent tissues with dilute norepinephrine (noradrenaline) (1:1000 in isotonic saline) is optional, but generally unnecessary. A scalpel is used to incise the skin only, and subsequent dissection is accomplished by lifting the tissues off the underlying structures with Adson's tissue forceps and dissecting with a fine hemostat and electrocautery. The incision is carried through the subcutaneous tissues and platysma to the level of the cyst. The cyst is exposed by retracting the skin and muscle flaps, and is best accomplished with a self-retaining or ring retractor.

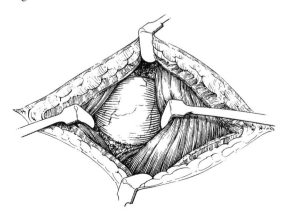

5

during endoscopy may reveal the origin of the fistula as pus exudes from the piriform sinus.

Anesthesia

Endotracheal inhalation general anesthesia, preferably by a pediatric anesthetist, is preferred.

OPERATIONS

Position of patient and preparation

The patient is placed in the supine position with a sandbag beneath the shoulders and a soft ring headrest beneath the cranium so that the neck is extended. The head of the table is raised slightly to diminish venous blood pressure in the head and neck. The chin is turned away from the side of the lesion, and the skin is prepared with 10 percent povidone-iodine solution. The field is draped with four towels held to the contours of the neck with plastic barrier drapes with one adhesive edge (Steridrape 1010). An electrocautery grounding plate is applied to the thigh.

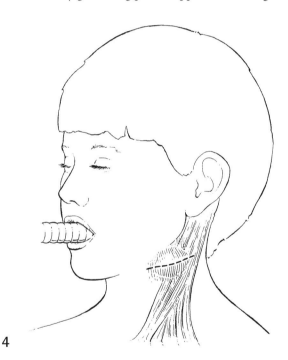

4

5 The deep cervical fascia is divided next to the anterior border of the sternocleidomastoid muscle, allowing the belly of the muscle to be retracted away from the cyst. Exposure is extended anteriorly and medially by retraction of the sternohyoid muscle. The fascia and soft tissue overlying the cyst are lifted and incised carefully to expose the superficial aspect of the cyst.

Dissection and removal of a second branchial cleft cyst

6 Great care is taken to avoid rupture of the cyst, as a tense cyst wall is easier to define and dissect than a collapsed cyst. Adjacent structures are separated from the cyst by blunt and electrocautery dissection along the cyst wall, special care being taken along the deep aspect of the cyst where the jugular vein and carotid arteries are in intimate relation. The pedicle of the cyst generally lies posterior to the jugular vein, usually coursing between the carotid artery bifurcation. It is then dissected cephalad towards the tonsillar pillar, where it is clamped and suture ligated with fine non-absorbable suture. Meticulous hemostasis is obtained and the wound irrigated with 1 percent povidone-iodine solution before closure.

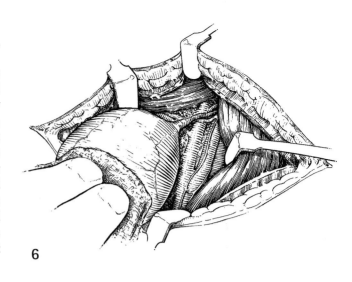

6

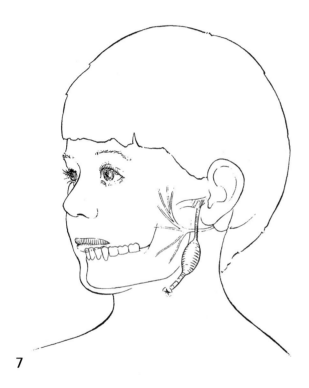

7

Dissection and removal of a first branchial cleft cyst

7 During dissection of the less common first branchial cleft cyst, care must be taken to avoid damage to the adjacent facial nerve in cases where there is a tract leading up to or into the external auditory meatus. Not uncommonly, the deep or superficial lobes of the parotid gland must be mobilized. A neurosurgical nerve stimulator is often helpful during the dissection.

Dissection and removal of a third or fourth branchial pouch cyst and sinus

Cysts and sinuses of the third and fourth branchial pouch are clinically similar because of their common origin in the piriform fossa and presentation as a neck or thyroid abscess. Common presentations include an air-containing inflammatory lateral neck mass requiring repeated incision and drainage. Preoperative resolution with antibiotics should be followed by a barium swallow or contrast computed tomography to allow visualization of the piriform sinus tract common to each of these anomalies. Exploration of the neck with excision of the entire tract to the level of the piriform sinus is necessary to prevent recurrence. Operative endoscopy at the start of the operation may enable cannulation of the tract from above, which greatly facilitates localization of the tract during resection. Once the cyst and tract are resected, the histological finding of squamous cell epithelial lining confirms the diagnosis of a branchial anomaly.

8 The thyroid gland is exposed through a standard collar incision, and the left lobe is mobilized. The recurrent and superior laryngeal nerves and parathyroid glands should be identified and protected. If no discrete cyst or tract is found, the fistula may be located at the laryngeal level near the cricothyroid membrane. The fibers of the inferior constrictor muscle are bluntly spread to expose the piriform recess. Extreme caution should be exercised in this region to preserve the external branch of the superior laryngeal nerve. The tract usually passes inferiorly, external to the recurrent laryngeal nerve along the trachea to the superior pole of the thyroid. It may end blindly near the gland or actually penetrate the capsule to terminate in the parenchyma of the left thyroid lobe. Thyroid lobectomy or resection of the superior pole is carried out as indicated by the extent of the cyst.

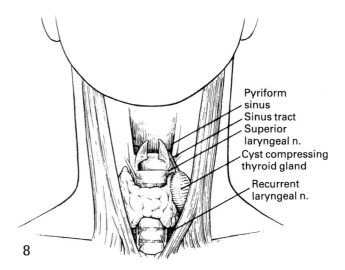

Pyriform sinus
Sinus tract
Superior laryngeal n.
Cyst compressing thyroid gland
Recurrent laryngeal n.

8

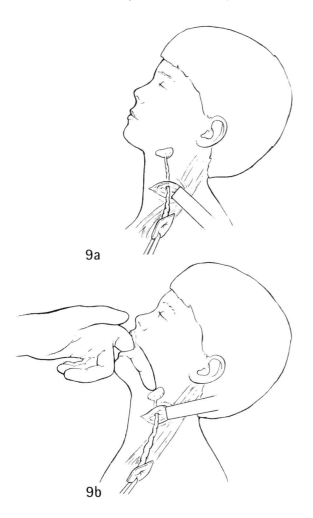

9a

9b

Excision of a second branchial cleft sinus

9a,b The operation to excise a second branchial cleft sinus begins with an elliptical transverse incision at the sinus opening, and cephalad dissection of the tract to its furthest extent, generally at the level of the tonsillar pillar. The dissection is kept directly on the tract to avoid injury to contiguous structures, e.g. the internal jugular vein, the bifurcation of the carotid artery, and the hypoglossal nerve. The operation can almost always be carried out through a single elliptical incision if the tract is kept under gentle traction and the anesthetist places a gloved finger in the tonsillar fossa and exerts downward pressure towards the field of dissection. In addition, the anesthetist's finger helps to localize the tonsillar fossa at the end point of dissection, where the sinus tract is suture ligated and divided. Dissection of the sinus tract may be facilitated by passing a fine silver probe or piece of heavy nylon suture the length of the tract and clamping this in position as the dissection progresses.

Minor branchial remnants

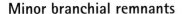

A branchial arch remnant may also occur along the lower anterior border of the sternocleidomastoid muscle near the sternoclavicular joint, and typically consists of a small cartilaginous mass presenting in the subcutaneous tissue. The lesion is usually visible and palpable, and bilateral occurrences are common. An accompanying sinus or cyst is seldom present, and infection is uncommon. Excision

may be carried out for cosmetic reasons or may be delayed indefinitely.

Preauricular sinuses or pits are common and have been attributed to vestiges of the first branchial cleft. These lesions probably relate to the infolding and fusion associated with formation of the ear. Asymptomatic lesions require no treatment; draining sinuses and infected cysts require antibiotic treatment, incision, and drainage if they fail to resolve, and later excision to prevent recurrence.

Wound closure

10 The cervical fascia and platysma are closed with interrupted sutures of 4/0 polyglycolic acid. When the dissection is carefully performed and the cyst or sinus is not infected, the incision may be closed without using a drain. The skin is closed with a running 5/0 subcuticular absorbable suture or pull-out nylon suture. Steristrips and a clear plastic dressing (Opsite) are applied as a wound dressing.

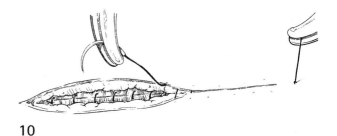

10

POSTOPERATIVE CARE

The operations described are carried out as outpatient procedures unless unusual difficulties are encountered or unless a drain is placed. Antibiotics (penicillin or a cephalosporin) are continued for 1–5 days after operation, depending on the presence of infection or degree of contamination. An occlusive dry sterile dressing is kept in place for 48 hours, after which the patient is permitted to bathe and shower normally. If a drain is placed, it is removed after 24 hours or whenever drainage has ceased. The patient is seen 7 days after operation for a wound check.

OUTCOME

The outcome for the procedures described is usually excellent, both functionally and cosmetically. Operative damage to related anatomical structures is rare and should not occur provided the surgeon has adequate knowledge of the anatomy and that meticulous hemostasis is obtained during dissection to ensure a clear field. Failure to excise the cyst or sinus completely may lead to its recurrence, in which case the patient should be treated with antibiotics and a thorough diagnostic re-evaluation initiated.

FURTHER READING

Makino S-I, Tsuchida Y, Yoshioka H, Saito S. The endoscopic and surgical management of pyriform fistulae in infants and children. *Journal of Pediatric Surgery* 1986; **21**: 398–401.

Mukherji SK, Fatterpekar G, Castillo M *et al.* Imaging of congenital anomalies of the branchial apparatus. *Neuroimaging Clinics of North America* 2000; **10**: 75–93.

Nicoucar K, Giger R, Jaecklin T *et al.* Management of congenital third branchial arch anomalies: a systematic review. *Otolaryngology, Head and Neck Surgery* 2010; **142**: 21–8.

Nicoucar K, Giger R, Pope HG Jr *et al.* Management of congenital fourth branchial arch anomalies: a review and analysis of published cases. *Journal of Pediatric Surgery* 2009; **44**: 1432–9.

Schroeder JW Jr, Mohyuddin N, Maddalozzo J. Branchial anomalies in the pediatric population. *Otolaryngology, Head and Neck Surgery* 2007; **137**: 289–95.

Waldhausen JHT. Branchial cleft and arch anomalies in children. *Seminars in Pediatric Surgery* 2006; **15**: 64–9.

External angular dermoid cyst

PAUL RV JOHNSON

PRINCIPLES AND JUSTIFICATION

Dermoid cysts are congenital cysts that result from sequestration of ectodermal and mesodermal elements. They occur along lines of embryologic closure, and the external angle of the supraorbital ridge is the most common site. External angular dermoid cysts are situated beneath the muscle and lie in a shallow depression in the outer table of the bone of the skull. A 'pit' within the bone is invariably present in the base of the bony depression through which the cyst receives its blood supply. Occasionally, these cysts have an intracranial extension in a 'dumb-bell' fashion, although this is far less common than with dermoid cysts situated at the internal angle of the eye or over the bridge of the nose.

External angular dermoids present as rounded, soft, semi-mobile swellings in the lateral part of the eyebrow. They are usually asymptomatic, although with time can enlarge and rupture or become infected. There are few conditions that cause diagnostic confusion in the infant or child. Treatment is by surgical excision of the cyst, which must be complete to prevent recurrence.

PREOPERATIVE ASSESSMENT AND PREPARATION

Radiology

The diagnosis is made on clinical grounds. If there is any suspicion of intracranial extension, magnetic resonance imaging should be performed preoperatively. However, unlike for dermoid cysts situated medially on the face, these are not indicated routinely. Skull x-rays are not helpful for excluding an intracranial extension as they may be misleading.

Consent

Informed consent must be obtained from one of the child's parents or the child's legal guardian. The complications of bleeding, infection, recurrence, and keloid scarring must be explained as part of this process.

Anesthesia

General anesthesia is administered via an endotracheal tube and the patient is placed supine on the operating table. The patient's head is positioned on a head ring.

OPERATION

Skin preparation and draping

There is no need to shave the eyebrow for this procedure. The eyelids are taped closed to prevent soiling of the eye. The skin is prepared with either aqueous betadine or aqueous chlorhexadine. A head towel is used to maintain the sterile field.

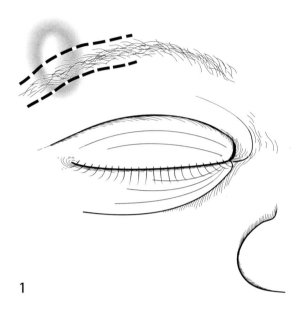

1

Incision

1 A 1–1.5-cm incision is made over the cyst in line with the upper or lower margin of the eyebrow. Care is taken not to cut the hair follicles of the eyebrow. Although this incision gives a good cosmetic result, an alternative approach is to make the incision in the palpebral crease itself.

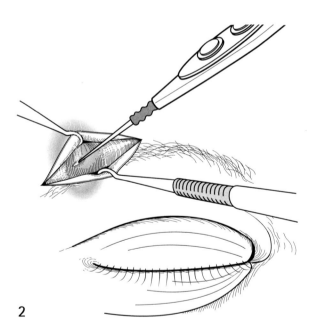

2

Dissection and excision

2 The incision is deepened using a fine monopolar diathermy point until the cyst becomes visible. Care is taken to avoid diathermy contact with the skin edges.

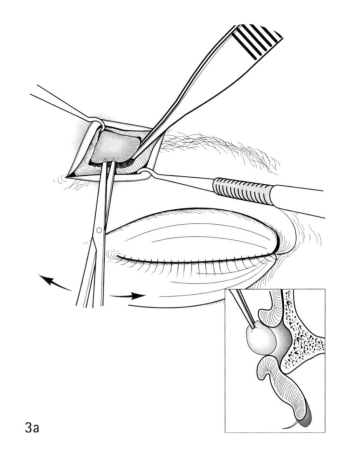

3a

3a,b The cyst is then mobilized using a mixture of blunt-scissor dissection and dissection with bipolar diathermy forceps. Meticulous hemostasis is ensured throughout. Instruments should not be applied directly to the cyst as this usually results in its rupture. The cyst is freed from its deep attachments, which often requires excising a circumferential rim of periosteum in continuity with the cyst. The feeding vessels passing through the pit of the bony depression are coagulated. Occasionally, this pit needs to be packed with bone wax to secure hemostasis. The cyst is removed and sent for routine histopathology to confirm the diagnosis. If rupture does occur during mobilization, the wound should be irrigated with saline and the contents and lining of the cyst completely removed to prevent recurrence.

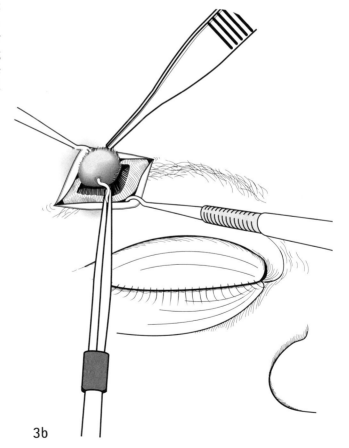

3b

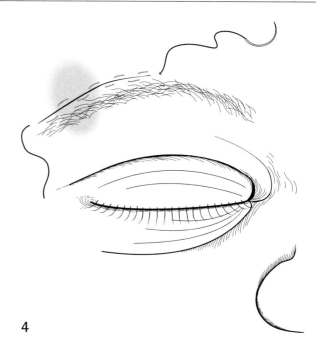

4

Closure

4 Once hemostasis has been confirmed, interrupted 4/0 polyglycolic sutures are placed in the muscle and fat layers, ensuring that the knots are buried. The skin is either closed using a subcuticular 5/0 undyed polyglycolic suture or a more predictable cosmetic result is achieved using interrupted 6/0 nylon sutures, although the latter can only be used in those infants in whom removal of sutures is practical. A Steristrip dressing is applied along the wound, followed by a small gauze/Mefix pressure dressing to prevent hematoma formation and thereby optimize the cosmetic result.

MINIMALLY INVASIVE APPROACHES

While both of the incisions described above usually give good cosmetic results, endoscopic-assisted procedures have recently been described that aim to make any scarring even less conspicuous. These include an endoscopic 'brow-lift' technique through a hairline incision within the scalp, as well as an endoscopic-assisted closed rhinoplasty approach. While several case series have been reported with good outcomes, these newer operations require more stringent evaluation before they become the 'gold standard'.

In the rare event of an intracranial extension, a formal craniotomy is required because the intracranial portion may be the larger of the two elements.

POSTOPERATIVE CARE

The majority of these procedures are performed as day cases. The pressure dressing is maintained for 48 hours after the operation and the wound kept dry during this time. If interrupted non-absorbable sutures have been used for skin closure, these should be removed 5 days postoperatively to prevent a tissue reaction to them.

OUTCOME

Complications are rare following this procedure. Postoperative hematoma and infection can occur, but are minimized by the techniques described above. Incomplete excision may result in recurrence of the cyst. The cosmetic result is usually good, although a keloid scar may result, especially if the wound becomes infected or the child is of Afro-Caribbean descent.

FURTHER READING

Cozzi DA, Mele E, d'Ambrosio G *et al.* The eyelid crease approach to angular dermoid cysts in pediatric general surgery. *Journal of Pediatric Surgery* 2008; **43**: 1502–6.

Dutta S, Lorenz HP, ALbanese CT. Endoscopic excision of benign forehead masses – a novel approach for pediatric general surgeons. *Journal of Pediatric Surgery* 2006; **41**: 1874–8.

Harris RL, Daya H. Closed rhinoplasty approach for excision of nasal dermoids. *Journal of Laryngology and Otology* 2010; **124**: 538–42.

9

Sternocleidomastoid torticollis

RONALD B HIRSCHL

HISTORY

Sternocleidomastoid torticollis is the term used to describe the presence of a shortened, fibrosed sternocleidomastoid muscle (SCM) which results in traction of the mastoid process toward the sternoclavicular joint. The head, therefore, is rotated away from and tilted toward the involved SCM.

The etiology of torticollis remains undefined. Light microscopic evaluation of the involved SCM demonstrates replacement of muscle bundles by dense fibrous tissue. Approximately 25–30 percent of patients presenting with SCM torticollis have a history of breech presentation at birth, with 62 percent involved in a complicated birth. Recent evidence suggests that SCM torticollis may be the manifestation of an *in-utero* positional disorder with development of an SCM compartment syndrome or related to prolonged intrauterine crowding or malposition. Bilateral SCM fibrosis is present in 2–3 percent of cases.

PRINCIPLES AND JUSTIFICATION

Approximately 30–40 percent of patients will present at age 1 to 8 weeks with a hard 1–3 cm, painless, discrete mass or pseudotumor, located within the substance of the middle or inferior portions of the SCM. This is often, but not always, accompanied by torticollis, with the face turned away from and the head tilted toward the side with the tumor. Such pseudotumors consist of fibrous tissue and mesenchyme-like cells, fibroblasts, and myoblasts at various stages of differentiation and degeneration. The remainder of patients will present with muscular torticollis (30 percent), in which there may be diffuse fibrosis of the SCM, or postural torticollis (22 percent). Passive neck range of motion exercises that emphasize rotation toward and side flexing away from the affected SCM should be performed by the parents, but also by a physical therapist. The parents should be encouraged to place toys and other desirable objects on the ipsilateral side in order to encourage turning toward that side. With physical therapy, resolution of the SCM pseudotumor and/or fibrosis is usually observed over the following three to four months. Therefore, operative intervention is not necessary in the majority (>90 percent) of newborns and young infants, but is required in 25 percent of the 3–6-month-old infants, 70 percent of the 6–18-month-old children, and 100 percent of those children older than 18 months. Torticollis will persist in approximately 7 percent of newborns, but this occurs usually in those with severe rotational limitations. In fact, large series have demonstrated that with the use of physiotherapy and manual stretching neck exercises, less than 8 percent of those with an SCM pseudotumor and 3 percent of those with muscular torticollis will require operative intervention. In general, operation is indicated in patients who are unresponsive after more than six months of manual stretching. Acquired plagiocephaly with flattening of both the frontal area on the ipsilateral side and the occipital region on the contralateral side may be noted in the first few months of life, but usually resolves spontaneously by one year of age after the infant begins to sit up.

Presentation in the child older than one or two years of age is more often refractory to conservative management, and operation is indicated if failure of physical therapy has been determined. Facial hemihypoplasia, which involves flattening and underdevelopment of the malar eminence and downward displacement of the eye, ear, and mouth on the affected side, may appear as early as six months of age, but most often appears after age 3–5 years. The development of facial hemihypoplasia is an indication for operative intervention, as potential resolution of skeletal abnormalities and subsequent normal growth and development of the facial skeleton will occur only after prompt operative correction of the torticollis.

PREOPERATIVE ASSESSMENT AND PREPARATION

Preoperative evaluation includes assessment to exclude other causes of abnormal head posture. Non-SCM causes for torticollis exist in 18 percent of patients and include neurologic disorders in 9 percent, such that the patient holds the head in a compensatory position most commonly due to the presence of ocular problems, such as nystagmus or strabismus, or vestibular disorders. Ocular examination is indicated in patients without a clear musculoskeletal cause of torticollis. Benign paroxysmal torticollis is an episodic functional disorder of unknown etiology that occurs in the early months of life in healthy individuals and resolves by the age of five years. It is thought that this disorder occurs as a migraine equivalent or due to a dystonic SCM. The child's head tilts to one side for a few hours or days, often without any associated symptoms, although vomiting, pallor, and ataxia may occur. Posterior fossa tumors may also present with torticollis, frequently accompanied by headache, nausea, and vomiting. Cervical spine radiologic evaluation may be necessary to exclude congenital osseous deformity of the cervical spine and the Klippel–Feil syndrome or C1–C2 cervical spine subluxation, which may rarely occur in patients presenting with torticollis. Usually the SCM is normal in these cases, but occasionally SCM fibrosis may coexist with other causes of torticollis. Atlantoaxial rotatory subluxation may be the cause of acute torticollis in children and also may be noted following head and neck procedures or infection. Imaging with computed tomography (CT) or magnetic resonance imaging (MRI) may be diagnostic and is indicated in children with torticollis without an SCM mass or evidence of muscular torticollis on examination.

The diagnosis of an SCM pseudotumor and torticollis in the newborn or infant presenting with an SCM mass can almost always be made based on physical examination, history, and clinical progression. Occasionally, ultrasound evaluation may help to differentiate such an SCM pseudotumor from a mass secondary to lymphadenopathy or neoplasm.

Photographic and/or CT evaluation for hemihypoplasia helps with the diagnosis and should be performed in any patient in whom torticollis persists beyond six months of age and as baseline before operative intervention. Radiologic evaluation of the hips and lower extremities should be performed because of the association (8–12 percent) with congenital dysplasia of the hip and abnormalities of the lower extremities in patients with torticollis. Hip dysplasia is observed in 7 percent of infants with a pseudotumor and is more commonly noted in infants with greater limitations in neck rotation. Preoperative open-mouth radiography of the odontoid process should be performed to look for tilt of the odontoid process to the side of the torticollis.

Anesthesia

General anesthesia with endotracheal intubation is required. The endotracheal tube should be secured sufficiently and placed appropriately to allow sterile preparation of the entire neck and full rotation of the neck in both directions.

OPERATION

The standard operation involves division of the SCM at the point where the sternal and clavicular heads converge. However, reports suggest that botulinum toxin injection into the SCM or lengthening of the SCM at its mastoid insertion may be effective. Selective peripheral denervation of the cervical muscles, including the spinal accessory branches to the SCM and C1–6 posterior nerve branches on the involved side, may also be effective, especially in those with an initial response to botulinum toxin injection. Early experience with a transaxillary and neck minimally invasive approach has also been effective.

Position of patient

The patient is placed in the supine position with a roll placed transversely under the shoulders in order to provide neck extension. The bed is flexed such that the head of the patient remains in a 30° upright position in order to decrease venous bleeding. The head is turned slightly to the side opposite the affected SCM. A sponge doughnut is placed under the head to maintain head position. The prepared field should include the entire neck extending up to just above the mandible, down to the areas of both shoulders, and to the infraclavicular regions bilaterally. Crumpled drapes are placed in the posterior aspect of the junction of the neck and shoulders bilaterally. Drapes are then placed along the inferior border of the mandible, at the level of the clavicle, and bilaterally along the posterolateral aspect of the neck.

1 An approximately 3 cm, transverse, curvilinear incision is made in a skin crease one to two fingerbreadths above the clavicle.

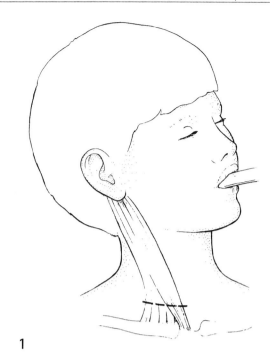

1

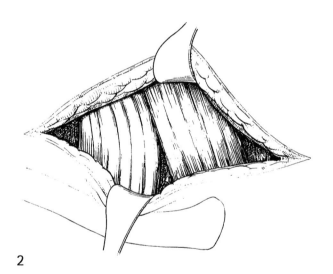

2

2 The platysma is divided. Subplatysmal flaps are developed along the SCM for 1–2 cm superiorly and to the level of the clavicle inferiorly. Division of the external jugular vein may be necessary. The posterior aspect of the SCM is then dissected free from the underlying carotid sheath structures at the point where the sternal and clavicular heads converge.

3 The sternal and clavicular heads, including the underlying investing cervical fascia, are divided at that level using electrocautery, with care taken to ensure hemostasis. The spinal accessory nerve is usually located superior to this region.

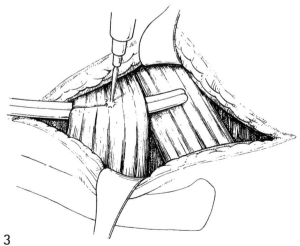

3

4 The ends of the transected SCM are then dissected free from the underlying carotid sheath structures. Limited dissection is performed superiorly while more extensive dissection is performed inferiorly down to the level of the sternum and clavicle.

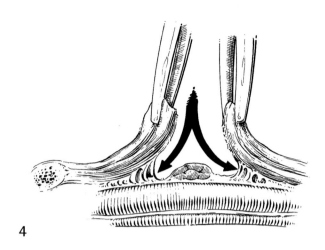

4

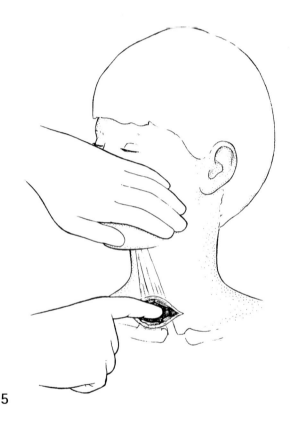

5

5 The head is then turned from side to side and the depths of the wound palpated to ensure that all contracted tissue is released. If tight lateral structures, such as the deep cervical fascia lateral to the SCM, are identified, these should be divided under direct vision. Although unusual, fascial tissue involved with the omohyoid muscle and the carotid sheath may occasionally require division.

6 The platysma muscle is then reapproximated with interrupted 3/0 vicryl sutures.

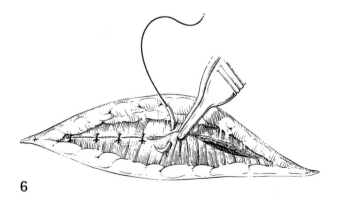

6

7 The skin is approximated with a running 5/0 vicryl subcuticular suture. Steristrips are placed perpendicular to the incision in overlying fashion such that a dressing is formed. The patient is maintained in a 30° head-up position during and after recovery.

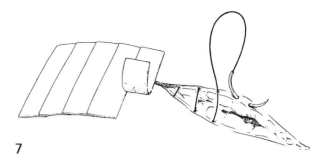

7

POSTOPERATIVE CARE

For the following 48 hours, the patient remains supine in the 30° head-up position without the use of a pillow. Careful assumption of the erect posture with initial assistance is then allowed. Some clinicians advise the use of a neck collar in the postoperative period. Physical therapy with resumption of passive neck range of motion exercises is then reinstituted and continued for the following six months. Full neck range of motion should be achieved by 7–10 days postoperatively. Older children must undergo retraining of the neck-righting reflexes in front of a mirror over the following months. Occasionally, a patient who is too young or not willing to cooperate with postoperative physical therapy will require placement of a Minerva cast for 6 weeks in order to maintain the head rotated toward the operatively treated side and tilted laterally toward the opposite side.

The most common complication is that of postoperative bleeding. Hematoma formation over the hours to days after the procedure may require evacuation. Specific attention to hemostasis during division of the muscular fascial tissues and to potential bleeding from tributaries of the internal jugular vein should prevent this complication. The risk of airway compromise secondary to postoperative bleeding is low. Injury to the spinal accessory or facial nerve is unusual.

OUTCOME

In the more than 90 percent of patients who are managed without operative intervention, follow up should include monitoring to ensure resolution of the SCM pseudotumor, residual SCM fibrosis, and torticollis. Specifically, close follow up should ensure the early detection of facial hemihypoplasia in those patients with persistent torticollis after six months of age. Overall, gross motor and cognitive function is normal by one year of age.

After operation, recurrent torticollis is observed in less than 3 percent of patients. Normal neck movement is observed with long-term follow up in 88 percent of patients. Follow up should include evaluation for facial hemihypoplasia and plagiocephaly, which, if present, will generally resolve. In addition, because of the high incidence of residual cervical and thoracolumbar scoliosis in patients with torticollis, radiologic spine evaluation is indicated to ensure identification and appropriate follow up of any spinal deformities.

FURTHER READING

Cheng JC, Tang SP, Chen TM *et al*. The clinical presentation and outcome of treatment of congenital muscular torticollis in infants – a study of 1,086 cases. *Journal of Pediatric Surgery* 2000; **35**: 1091–6.

Drigo P, Carli G, Laverda AM. Benign paroxysmal torticollis of infancy. *Brain and Development* 2000; **22**: 169–72.

Poungvarin N, Viriyavejakul A. Botulinum A toxin treatment in spasmodic torticollis: report of 56 patients. *Journal of the Medical Association of Thailand* 1994; **77**: 464–70.

Rogers GF, Oh AK, Mulliken JB. The role of congenital muscular torticollis in the development of deformational plagiocephaly. *Plastic and Reconstructive Surgery* 2009; **123**: 643–52.

Schertz M, Zuk L, Zin S *et al*. Motor and cognitive development at one-year follow-up in infants with torticollis. *Early Human Development* 2008; **84**: 9–14.

Tang ST, Yang Y, Mao YZ *et al*. Endoscopic transaxillary approach for congenital muscular torticollis. *Journal of Pediatric Surgery* 2010; **45**: 2191–4.

Tracheostomy

C MARTIN BAILEY and JOE GRAINGER

PRINCIPLES AND JUSTIFICATION

Tracheostomy should be performed as an elective procedure using the conventional dissection technique. Percutaneous dilatational tracheostomy, now widely used in adults, is not suitable for children because the airway is small and often precarious; the trachea is soft, flexible, and very mobile; landmarks can be difficult to palpate; and a displaced tube cannot be rapidly replaced.

INDICATIONS

- Airway obstruction:
  - Congenital anomalies, e.g. laryngeal web, subglottic stenosis.
  - Failed extubation with increasing subglottic edema and evidence of mucosal damage.
  - External trauma, e.g. hanging-type injuries.
  - Acute infection, e.g. acute epiglottitis or laryngotracheobronchitis, if endotracheal intubation is not available.
  - Tumors, e.g. hemangioma, lymphangioma.

- Functional obstruction, e.g. bilateral vocal cord palsy, cricoarytenoid joint fixation.
  - Tracheomalacia or extrinsic compression of the trachea.
- Long-term respiratory support, for example, for pulmonary pathology.
- Clearance of secretions, for example, in neurological injury or disease.
- As a covering procedure to secure the airway for subsequent surgery on the larynx, pharynx, or temporomandibular joints.

PREOPERATIVE

Anesthesia

The operation is performed under general anesthesia. Children are usually intubated, but in cases where intubation is deemed impossible a laryngeal mask airway (LMA) may be used, or even a facemask. Exceptionally, it might be necessary to undertake the procedure under local anesthesia, using lignocaine (lidocaine) 1 percent with epinephrine (adrenaline) 1:200 000.

OPERATION

Position of patient

1 The neck must be hyperextended. A jellyroll or sandbag is placed under the shoulders, and an adhesive tape 'chin strap' is applied and attached to the table on either side of the head to stabilize it. The occiput is supported by a head ring. The patient is tipped into a slightly head-up position. A fenestrated 'circumcision' drape is convenient and allows an anesthetic connector to be passed easily beneath it into the surgical field when the tracheostomy tube has been inserted. Bipolar diathermy should be available.

Incision

2 The neck is palpated carefully so that the hyoid bone, thyroid notch, and cricoid cartilage can be felt and marked. In neonates, the cricoid cartilage is not easily palpable. The skin midway between the cricoid and the suprasternal notch is marked and infiltrated using 1 percent lignocaine with 1:200 000 epinephrine. A horizontal skin incision approximately 2 cm in length is made through the infiltrated area, cutting through fat and platysma. In infants and young children, it is advantageous to defat the skin along the incision margins in order to improve access to the trachea, for which purpose microbipolar diathermy forceps are useful.

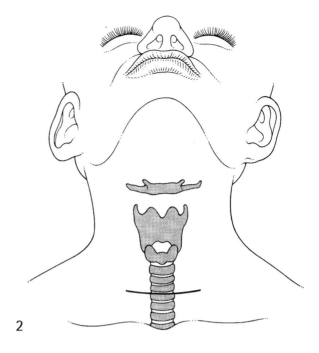

2

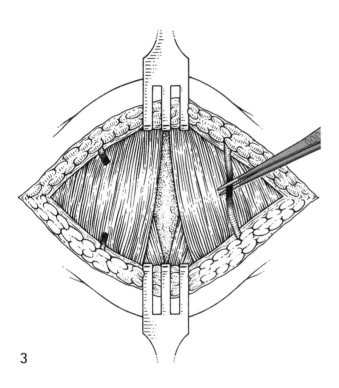

3 The incision is deepened in a horizontal plane until the deep cervical fascia investing the sternohyoid and sternothyroid strap muscles is encountered. Branches of the anterior jugular vein will be seen during this dissection; these should be coagulated and divided with the bipolar diathermy.

3

4 Having identified the strap muscles, a condensation of the investing layer of the deep cervical fascia will be seen running vertically between them in the midline. This interval is entered by blunt-scissor dissection and the strap muscles are separated and retracted laterally. Sprung self-retaining retractors of the Aberdeen pattern are very convenient for this purpose.

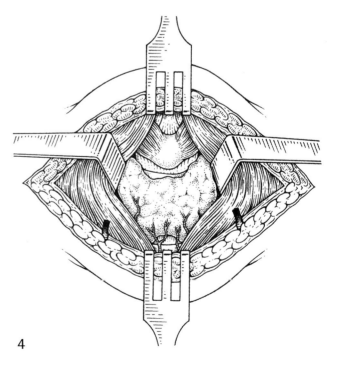

4

Exposure of the thyroid gland

Retraction of the strap muscles reveals the thyroid gland with the thyroid isthmus joining the two lobes of the gland. Above the isthmus, the cricoid is seen, although in the neonate it is easier to identify by palpation, feeling for its prominence with fine curved 'mosquito' artery forceps.

Dissection of the thyroid isthmus

5 The size and relationship of the thyroid isthmus to the trachea are variable, but in all cases the isthmus should be divided. A small incision is made through the condensation of the pretracheal fascia at the upper border of the isthmus, and the isthmus is then separated from the underlying trachea by blunt dissection using fine curved artery forceps. Branches of the inferior thyroid vein will be encountered at the lower border of the isthmus, and these should be coagulated with diathermy.

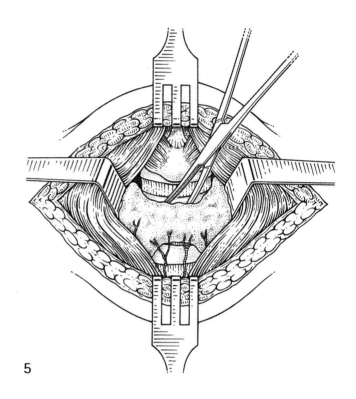

5

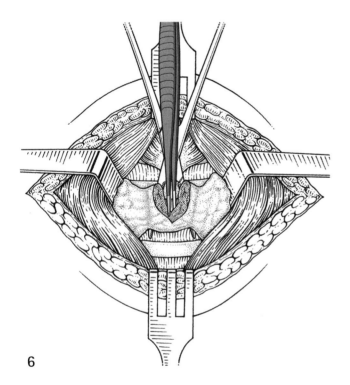

6

Division of the thyroid isthmus

6 The artery forceps are spread beneath the isthmus, and bipolar diathermy is used to divide it bloodlessly. In adolescents with a bulky, vascular isthmus it may be preferable to divide the isthmus between hemostats and secure the ends by suture transfixion and ligation.

Opening the trachea

Careful hemostasis is achieved, the cricoid is identified, and the tracheal rings counted. The first tracheal ring must not be included in the tracheostomy, and in neonates and infants, where distances are small, it is preferable to preserve the second ring as well.

7 Before making the incision, Prolene stay sutures are placed to help distract the tracheal opening: these are later taped to the skin and left in place until the first tracheostomy tube change. For routine tracheostomy in children, a vertical incision is made in the trachea through the third, fourth, and fifth tracheal rings. If a subsequent reconstructive operation on the larynx is planned, the incision in the trachea may be made through the fourth, fifth, and sixth tracheal rings. Care should be taken with a low tracheostomy that the end of the tracheostomy tube is clear of the carina, and in infants it is important to use a shorter 'neonatal'-length tube. A small sucker should be used to prevent blood from entering the trachea.

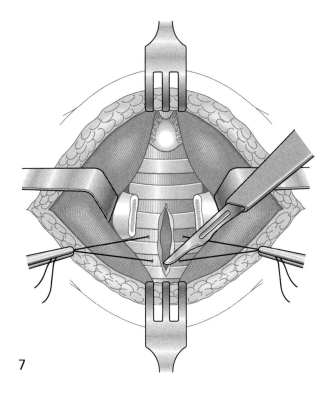

7

8a,b The stay sutures are now used to distract the cut edges of the trachea, if necessary, aided by fine skin hooks. The endotracheal tube will then be clearly seen.

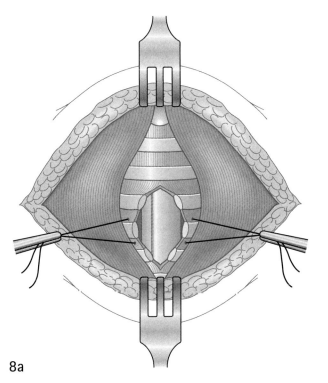

8a

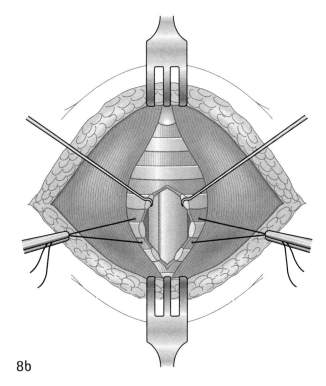

8b

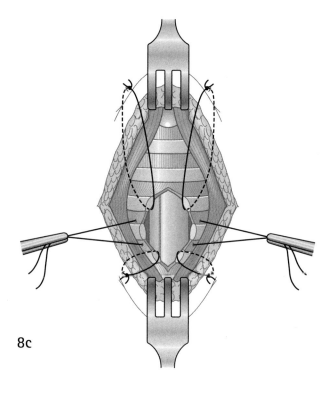

8c It is recommended that four Vicryl skin maturation sutures should be used to approximate the skin edges to the margins of the tracheal incision, thus creating a stoma and making it much easier to replace the tube should it become displaced.

8c

Insertion of tracheostomy tube

9a,b The anesthetist is asked to withdraw the endotracheal tube gently until its tip is just above the tracheostome. A plastic tracheostomy tube with a 15-mm termination is then inserted into the tracheal opening, a sterile anesthetic connector is fitted to it, and the end of the connector is passed out of the surgical field beneath the drape to the anesthetist. A sizing chart, such as that published by Tweedie *et al.* in 2008, reproduced in **Table 10.1**, should be used to select a tube of the correct diameter and length for the child's age.

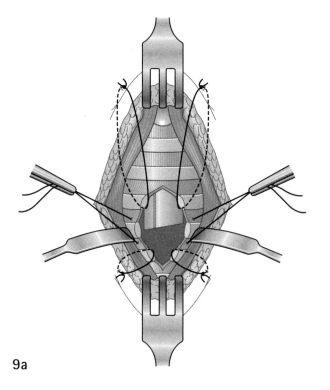

9a

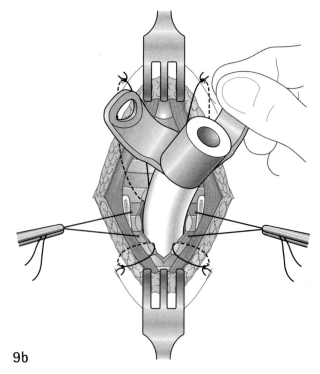

9b

Table 10.1 Great Ormond Street Hospital sizing chart for pediatric airways.

Material	Manufacturer	Measure	Preterm–1 month	1–6 months	6–18 months	18 mths – 3 yrs	3–6 years	6–9 years	9–12 years	12–14 years
	Trachea (Transverse Diameter mm)		5	5–6	6–7	7–8	8–9	9–10	10–13	13
PLASTIC	Great Ormond Street	ID (mm)	3.0	3.5	4.0	4.5	5.0	5.5	6.0	7.0
PLASTIC	Great Ormond Street	OD (mm)	4.5	5.0	6.0	6.7	7.5	8.0	8.7	10.7
PLASTIC	Shiley	Size	3.0	3.5	4.0	4.5	5.0	5.5	6.0	6.5
PLASTIC	Shiley	ID (mm)	3.0	3.5	4.0	4.5	5.0	5.5	6.0	6.5
PLASTIC	Shiley	OD (mm)	4.5	5.2	5.9	6.5	7.1	7.7	8.3	9.0
PLASTIC	Shiley	Length (mm) Neonatal	30	32	34	36				
PLASTIC	*Cuffed Tube Available	Paediatric		39	40	41*	42*	44*	46*	
PLASTIC		Long Paediatric					50*	52*	54*	56*
PLASTIC	Portex (Blue Line)	ID (mm)	3.0	3.5	4.0	4.5	5.0	5.0	6.0	7.0
PLASTIC	Portex (Blue Line)	OD (mm)	4.2	4.9	5.5	6.2	6.9	6.9	8.3	9.7
PLASTIC	Portex (555)	Size	2.5	3.0	3.5	4.0	4.5	5.0	5.5	
PLASTIC	Portex (555)	ID (mm)	2.5	3.0	3.5	4.0	4.5	5.0	5.5	
PLASTIC	Portex (555)	OD (mm)	4.5	5.2	5.8	6.5	7.1	7.7	8.3	
PLASTIC	Portex (555)	Length Neonatal	30	32	34	36				
PLASTIC	Portex (555)	Paediatric	30	36	40	44	48	50	52	
PLASTIC	Bivona	Size	2.5	3.0	3.5	4.0	4.5	5.0	5.5	
PLASTIC	Bivona	ID (mm)	2.5	3.0	3.5	4.0	4.5	5.0	5.5	
PLASTIC	Bivona	OD (mm)	4.0	4.7	5.3	6.0	6.7	7.3	8.0	
PLASTIC	Bivona — All sizes available with Fome Cuff, Aire Cuff & TTS Cuff	Length Neonatal	30	32	34	36				
PLASTIC		Paediatric	38	39	40	41	42	44	46	
PLASTIC	Bivona Hyperflex	ID (mm)	2.5	3.0	3.5	4.0	4.5	5.0	5.5	
PLASTIC	Bivona Hyperflex	Usable Length (mm)	55	60	65	70	75	80	85	
PLASTIC	Bivona Flextend	ID (mm)	2.5	3.0	3.5	4.0	4.5	5.0	5.5	
PLASTIC	Bivona Flextend	Shaft Length (mm)	38	39	40	41	42	44	46	
PLASTIC	Bivona Flextend	Flextend Length (mm)	10	10	15	15	17.5	20	20	
PLASTIC	TracoeMini	ID (mm)	2.5	3.0	3.5	4.0	4.5	5.0	5.5	6.0
PLASTIC	TracoeMini	OD (mm)	3.6	4.3	5.0	5.6	6.3	7.0	7.6	8.4
PLASTIC	TracoeMini	Length (mm) Neonatal (350)	30	32	34	36				
PLASTIC	TracoeMini	Paediatric (355)	32	36	40	44	48	50	55	62
SILVER	Alder Hey	FG		12–14	16	18	20	22	24	
SILVER	Negus	FG		16	18	20	22	24	26	28
SILVER	Chevalier Jackson	FG	14	16	18	20	22	24	26	28
SILVER	Sheffield	FG		12–14	16	18	20	22	24	26
SILVER	Sheffield	ID (mm)		2.9–3.6	4.2	4.9	6.0	6.3	7.0	7.6
	Cricoid (AP Diameter)	ID (mm)	3.6–4.8	4.8–5.8	5.8–6.5	6.5–7.4	7.4–8.2	8.2–9.0	9.0–10.7	10.7
	Bronchoscope (Storz)	Size	2.5	3.0	3.5	4.0	4.5	5.0	6.0	6.0
	Bronchoscope (Storz)	ID (mm)	3.5	4.3	5.0	6.0	6.6	7.1	7.5	7.5
	Bronchoscope (Storz)	OD (mm)	4.2	5.0	5.7	6.7	7.3	7.8	8.2	8.2
	Endotracheal Tube (Portex)	ID (mm)	2.5	3.0	3.5	4.0	4.5	5.0	6.0	8.0
	Endotracheal Tube (Portex)	OD (mm)	3.4	4.2	4.8	5.4	6.2	6.8	8.2	10.8

Table reproduced from 'Choosing a paediatric tracheostomy: an update on current practice'. Tweedie DJ, Skilbeck CJ, Cochrane LA, Cooke J, Wyatt ME. *Journal of Laryngology and Otology* 2008; **122**: 161–9.

Fixation of tracheostomy tube

When the tracheostomy tube is fully inserted it must be held by the assistant until it is properly secured. If necessary, the skin edges are approximated with a suture on each side of the tube. It is essential to leave a gap around the tube to avoid postoperative surgical emphysema. The Prolene stay sutures should be taped to the shoulders and the tapes clearly labeled 'Do Not Remove' as well as being marked 'left' and 'right'.

10 The jellyroll is then removed from beneath the patient's shoulders and the tracheostomy tube is secured by tying the tapes with a reef knot with the neck flexed. It is extremely important to remember this neck flexion and to tie the tapes fairly tightly; failure to do this may result in the tube becoming dislodged. Dislodgement of the tracheostomy tube must be avoided during the immediate postoperative period, as its subsequent reinsertion can be difficult in the first few postoperative days. A non-adherent dressing is applied to the wound, with a keyhole to accommodate the tracheostomy tube. This dressing should be kept clean and changed when necessary. At the end of the procedure, the surgeon should listen to the chest with a stethoscope to ensure that air entry is symmetrical; if it is reduced on the left, this suggests that the tracheostomy tube is too long and has intubated the right main bronchus. If necessary, a flexible fibreoptic laryngoscope or bronchoscope may be passed through the tracheostomy tube in order to confirm the position of the tube tip and establish that the tube is of the correct length.

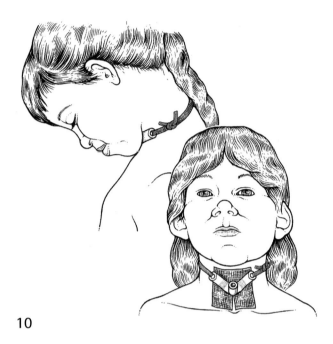

10

POSTOPERATIVE CARE

The following must be at the bedside:

- A spare tracheostomy tube of the same pattern and size as that in the patient, and a tube one size smaller (for use if difficulty is encountered replacing the tube with one of the same size); also scissors, spare tapes, and aqueous jelly to lubricate a replacement tube.
- Suction apparatus and sterile suction catheters with distal and lateral tip ports.
- A properly trained nurse.
- A supply of humidified air and an Ambu bag.

A portable chest radiograph should be arranged in the operating room recovery area or immediately on return to the ward, to check the length of the tracheostomy tube with regard to its proximity to the carina, and to ensure that there is no pneumothorax. The tracheostomy tube must be kept clear of secretions by the regular application of suction at hourly intervals for the first 12–24 hours, and thereafter as required. A sterile catheter is inserted into the tracheostomy tube gently but swiftly as far as the tube tip, and suction is applied only as the catheter is withdrawn.

If the tracheostomy tube is properly positioned and functioning satisfactorily, respiration should be virtually inaudible. If bubbling noises are heard, further suction is required.

Adequate humidification should be provided continuously for the first week, using a mechanical warm-air humidifier for infants and a room-temperature humidifier for older children. This will reduce the tenacity of the secretions and allow them to be cleared by suction more easily.

The tracheostomy tapes are changed daily, and the tracheostomy tube is changed routinely after 7 days, at which time the skin sutures and stay sutures are removed. However, if any difficulty is encountered during suction, or if breathing becomes noisy or obstructed despite suction, the tube must be changed immediately. This can sometimes be difficult with a new tracheostomy and should be done with adequate help: the child's neck must be extended with a rolled towel under the shoulders, good illumination is essential, and a headlight is desirable. As the tracheostomy tube is withdrawn, the stay sutures are pulled to distract the edges of the tracheal opening and bring them up to the surface of the neck. The tracheostome should thus be clearly visible (especially if the subcutaneous fat was reduced at the time of surgery and skin maturation sutures were placed) and a new tube is inserted under direct vision. If difficulty is encountered, a tracheal dilator is too large to be useful in small children; it is better to insert a suction catheter into the tracheal lumen and use the Seldinger technique to 'railroad' the new tube over it into the trachea (or use a smaller tube).

The most common cause of difficulty in suction is displacement of the tube into the pretracheal tissues, which may occur if the tapes are too loose, or if the tube is changed and the new tube is inserted incorrectly.

COMPLICATIONS

Intraoperative

- Bleeding may be encountered from an abnormally high left innominate vein. Careful controlled dissection of the structures in the lower part of the neck should avoid this.
- Damage to the cervical pleura may cause pneumothorax or possibly a pneumomediastinum; dissection lateral to the trachea should be avoided.
- Injury to the larynx, trachea, or esophagus should not occur when an elective tracheostomy is performed. Accidental decannulation may occur if the assistant does not hold the tube securely or if the tapes are tied too loosely.

Postoperative

- **Blocking and displacement of the tracheostomy tube.** These complications are preventable by careful nursing and attention to detail when tying the tracheostomy tube tapes.
- **Postoperative pneumonia.** This risk is small if a sterile technique is used for tracheal toilet and effective humidification is maintained. Adequate physiotherapy to encourage coughing is also desirable.
- **Surgical emphysema.** If this occurs, the wound should be opened fully. It is caused by suturing the wound too tightly around the tracheostomy tube.
- **Hemorrhage.** Reactionary hemorrhage from the wound may occur if hemostasis has been inadequate, a risk minimized by the use of bipolar diathermy dissection. Erosion of the anterior wall of the trachea may well occur if a metal tracheostomy tube of incorrect curvature is used. The overlying innominate artery may also be damaged, in which event a frequently fatal hemorrhage will result.

- **Stenosis.** This may occur at the tracheostome if cartilage is removed during the tracheostomy, or at the tip of the tube if suction is too vigorous or incorrectly applied. If the tracheostomy is placed too high and the cricoid cartilage is damaged by the tube, a subglottic stenosis may ensue.
- **Granuloma formation.** A suprastomal granuloma may form in the tracheal lumen at the upper margin of the tracheostome where it is irritated by the tube. If it becomes large enough to interfere with tube changes, phonation, or decannulation, it should be removed either with punch forceps via the stoma or endoscopically using the KTP laser through a bronchoscope. A tube-tip granuloma may arise as a result of irritation of the tracheal wall by either the tip of an ill-fitting tracheostomy tube or unskilled and over-vigorous suction.
- **Suprastomal collapse.** Some degree of suprastomal collapse of the anterior tracheal wall at the upper margin of the tracheostome is almost inevitable in long-term pediatric tracheostomies. Usually it is mild, but occasionally it is sufficiently severe to hinder eventual decannulation. When the suprastomal flap occludes up to 50 percent of the airway, it can be successfully vaporized using the KTP laser through a bronchoscope. If more than 50 percent of the airway is occluded, a formal surgical decannulation may be needed, with anterosuspension of the suprastomal flap or even stomal reconstruction using a cartilage graft.
- **Difficult decannulation.** In the absence of persisting pathology, decannulation is most safely undertaken by progressively downsizing the tube to one of 3.0 mm inner diameter, blocking it for 24 hours, and then removing it if the child can manage comfortably both awake and asleep with the blocked tube *in situ*.
- **Persistent tracheocutaneous fistula.** After prolonged tracheostomy, removal of the tube may result in a persistent fistula at the site of the tracheostomy in up to 50 percent of patients. If it fails to close spontaneously and continues to leak mucus, the tract may be excised and a formal closure performed.

CRICOTHYROTOMY

In an emergency, for example, in the case of acute epiglottitis when sudden airway obstruction may occur and peroral endotracheal intubation may not be possible, a cricothyrotomy should be considered in preference to a crash tracheostomy, which can be extremely difficult in the child whose trachea is soft and may not be easy to identify.

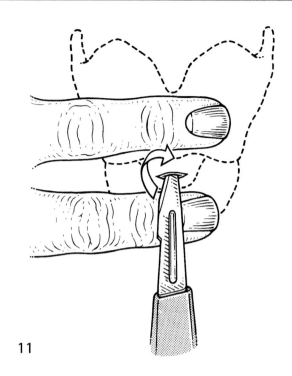

11 The child is held with the neck extended and the left hand is placed with the first finger over the cricoid cartilage and the second over the thyroid cartilage. A transverse stab incision is made through the cricothyroid membrane. The blade of the knife is then turned vertically, establishing the airway so that a tube of suitable size may be inserted to preserve the airway and to enable general anesthesia to be undertaken safely. Elective tracheostomy is then performed.

11

FURTHER READING

Hoeve HLJ. Tracheostomy: an ancient life saver due for retirement, or vital aid in modern airway surgery? In: Graham JM, Scadding GK, Bull PD (eds). *Pediatric ENT*. Berlin: Springer, 2007: 247–53.

McMurray JS, Prescott CAJ. Tracheotomy in the pediatric patient. In: Cotton RT, Myer CM (eds). *Practical Pediatric Otolaryngology*. Philadelphia, PA: Lippincott-Raven, 1999: 575–93.

Saunders M. Tracheostomy and home care. In: Gleeson M (ed.). *Scott-Brown's Otorhinolaryngology, Head and Neck Surgery*, vol. 1. Clarke R (ed.). Paediatric Otorhinolaryngology. London: Hodder, 2008: 1194–209.

Tweedie DJ, Skillbeck CJ, Cochrane LA *et al.* Choosing a paediatric tracheostomy tube: an update on current practice. *Journal of Laryngology and Otology* 2008; **122**: 161–9.

Wetmore RF. Tracheotomy. In: Bluestone CD, Stool SE, Alper CM *et al.* (eds). *Pediatric Otolaryngology*. Philadelphia, PA: Saunders, 2003: 1583–98.

Preauricular sinus

PAUL RV JOHNSON

PRINCIPLES AND JUSTIFICATION

The preauricular sinus is a congenital sinus whose opening is situated on the anterior aspect of the helix of the pinna. It results from ectodermal inclusions that arise during fusion of the six fetal tubercles that form the pinna. The course of the sinus is unpredictable and often consists of multiple branches. It passes anteriorly and inferiorly through the subcutaneous tissue to end in a racemose group of preauricular cysts and, contrary to some reports, frequently extends deep to the subcutaneous tissue to be attached to the cartilage of the pinna. The sinus is often familial, and may be unilateral or bilateral. In many cases, the preauricular sinus is completely asymptomatic and requires no treatment. However, it may present with an intermittent discharge or become infected, or as a preauricular abscess. Total excision of the sinus and the underlying group of preauricular cysts is essential for cure of the symptomatic sinus and this may also require excision of a small amount of underlying cartilage at the point of attachment. Incomplete excision results in a significant recurrence rate.

PREOPERATIVE ASSESSMENT AND PREPARATION

Definitive surgery should not be undertaken in the presence of active infection, which should be treated with anti-staphylococcal antibiotics. In the case of abscess formation, this requires either aspiration or excision and drainage. At the time of formal excision of the sinus, prophylactic antibiotics should be administered in those cases that have had previous episodes of infections.

Investigations

The decision about treatment is made on clinical grounds. No further investigations are routinely required preoperatively.

Consent

Informed consent must be obtained from one of the child's parents or the child's legal guardian. The complications of bleeding, infection, recurrence, and hypertrophic scarring must be outlined as part of this process.

Anesthesia

General anesthesia is administered by an endotracheal tube. Infiltration of the wound with local anesthetic agents often distorts the dissection plane if done preoperatively, and this is therefore best reserved for the end of the procedure. The patient is placed supine on the operating table and the patient's head positioned on a head ring.

OPERATION

Skin preparation and draping

Any hair anterior to the pinna should be shaved. The skin is prepared with either aqueous betadine or aqueous chlorhexidine. If bilateral sinuses are present, a head towel is used to maintain a sterile field. In the case of a unilateral sinus, a standard four-drape technique can be used. The injection of methylene blue has been advocated as a method for identifying the ramifications of the sinus. While some surgeons use this routinely, many find that in practice it does not prove helpful.

Incision

1 An elliptical incision is made around the punctum. The ellipse should also include any scarring that has resulted from previous infection. The incision is extended inferiorly in a vertical plane immediately in front of the pinna. An alternative incision is an inverted L-shape with an associated skin flap.

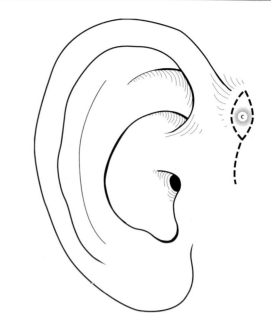

1

Dissection and excision

2 The incision is deepened using a fine monopolar diathermy point. The ellipse of skin containing the punctum and underlying sinus is then held using either toothed Adson forceps or a mosquito hemostat. Dissection is continued and the underlying group of preauricular cysts identified. Sometimes, insertion of a lacrimal probe is helpful to identify the course of the sinus.

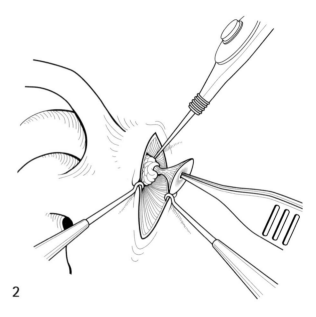

2

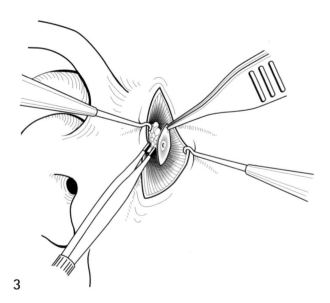

3

3 Further dissection is performed using bipolar diathermy forceps, ensuring that the skin ellipse, sinus, and cyst are dissected *en bloc*. As stated above, the deep attachment of the sinus is often lying on the cartilage, and excision of a small amount of cartilage at the point of attachment is often required to prevent recurrence. During deep dissection, particular care is taken to preserve the superficial temporal artery and the preauricular nerve. The sinus, together with the collection of cysts, is then removed and sent for routine histopathology. Meticulous hemostasis is ensured throughout.

Closure

Once hemostasis has been confirmed, interrupted 5/0 or 4/0 polyglycolic sutures are used to close any defect in the cartilage. Drainage of the wound is not routinely required. Bupivacaine 0.25 percent is infiltrated into the wound to ensure postoperative analgesia. Interrupted 4/0 polyglycolic sutures are then placed in the subcutaneous tissue, ensuring that the knots are buried.

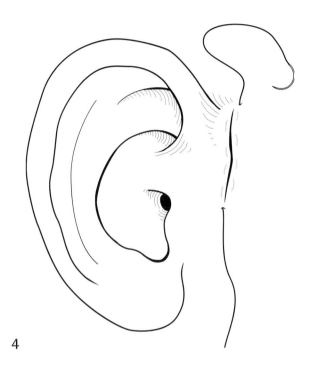

4 The skin is closed using either a subcuticular 5/0 undyed polyglycolic suture or, for a more predictable cosmetic result, interrupted 6/0 nylon sutures, although the latter can only be used in those infants for whom removal of sutures is practical. A Steristrip dressing is applied along the wound together with a small gauze/Mefix pressure dressing to prevent hematoma formation, and thereby optimize the cosmetic result.

4

POSTOPERATIVE CARE

Excision of a unilateral sinus is usually performed as a day case. The pressure dressing is maintained for 48 hours after the operation and the wound kept dry during this time. If interrupted non-absorbable sutures have been used for skin closure, these should be removed 5 days postoperatively to prevent a tissue reaction to them.

OUTCOME

Postoperative hematoma and infection can occur, but are minimized by the techniques described above. Incomplete excision may result in recurrence of the sinus. This risk is increased in those cases in which recurrent infection has preceded excision, as the dissection planes are often less clearly defined. Using the elliptical incision described above, the cosmetic result is usually good, although hypertrophic scarring may result, especially if the wound becomes infected or the child is of Afro-Caribbean descent.

FURTHER READING

Currie AR, King WW, Vlantis AC et al. Pitfalls in the management of preauricular sinuses. British Journal of Surgery 1996; 83: 1722–4.

Dickson JM, Riding KH, Ludemann JP. Utility and safety of methylene blue demarcation of preauricular sinuses and branchial sinuses and fistulae in children. Journal of Otolaryngology, Head and Neck Surgery 2009; 38: 302–10.

Scheinfeld NS, Silverberg NB, Weinberg JM, Nozad V. The preauricular sinus: a review of its clinical presentation, treatment, and associations. Pediatric Dermatology 2004; 21: 191–6.

Endoscopy

12

Bronchoscopy

JOE GRAINGER and BEN HARTLEY

PRINCIPLES AND JUSTIFICATION

Bronchoscopic examination of the pediatric airway may be performed electively for the diagnosis and/or management of airway disease. While flexible bronchoscopy may be regarded as less invasive, rigid bronchoscopy remains the most versatile method of airway assessment and is where this chapter will focus. Urgent rigid bronchoscopy may be required in the case of foreign body aspiration and, therefore, a good understanding of bronchoscopic technique is necessary for the pediatric surgeon. Rarely, the ventilating bronchoscope may be useful in securing the difficult airway.

INDICATIONS

- Diagnostic
  - airway assessment, e.g. for stridor
  - assessment of tracheomalacia
  - diagnosis of tracheo-esophageal fistula: H-type or recurrent
  - biopsy of tracheal/bronchial lesions
  - culture of secretions
- Therapeutic
  - removal of foreign bodies
  - dilatation of stenoses
  - laser destruction of lesions
  - management of severe upper airway obstruction
  - management of pulmonary/tracheal hemorrhage.

PREOPERATIVE

Investigations

Anteroposterior and lateral chest radiographs should be performed in the assessment of foreign body inhalation. Radio-opaque foreign bodies may be observed directly. In cases where the foreign body is radiolucent, air trapping, collapse, or consolidation may be seen.

Anesthesia

Rigid bronchoscopy is performed under general anesthesia using gaseous and/or intravenous anesthesia. Spontaneous ventilation is optimal, enabling a dynamic assessment of airway lesions and is preferred in cases of severe airway obstruction.

Children should be premedicated with atropine in order to reduce airway secretions and facilitate the effective application of topical anesthesia to the larynx. Following the application of topical anesthesia to the larynx to prevent laryngospasm, a nasopharyngeal airway is passed in order to deliver inhalational anesthesia and/or oxygen until the bronchoscope is in place.

OPERATION

Preparation

The ventilating bronchoscope and any associated ancillary equipment should be prepared prior to the induction of general anaesthesia (**Figures 12.1** and **12.2**) (**Table 12.1**). For diagnostic evaluation in the spontaneously ventilating patient, a rigid Hopkins rod endoscope may be used alone, reducing equipment diameter and, therefore, reducing mucosal trauma. A defogging solution is used to prevent condensation forming on the lens.

Table 12.1 Storz bronchoscope sizes relative to the child's age and airway diameter.

		Preterm–1 month	1–6 months	6–18 months	18 months–3 years	3–6 years	6–9 years	9–12 years	12–14 years
Cricoid (AP diameter)	ID (mm)	3.6–4.8	4.8–5.8	5.8–6.5	6.5–7.4	7.4–8.2	8.2–9.0	9.0–10.7	10.7
Endotracheal tube size	ID (mm)	3.0	3.5	4.0	4.5	5.0	6.0	7.0	8.0
Bronchoscope size (Storz)	Size	2.5	3.0	3.5	4.0	4.5	5.0	6.0	6.0
	ID (mm)	3.5	4.3	5.0	6.0	6.6	7.1	7.5	7.5
	OD (mm)	4.2	5.0	5.7	6.7	7.3	7.8	8.2	0.2

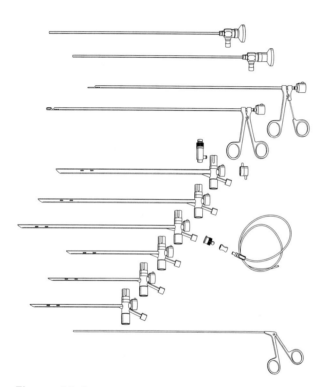

Figure 12.1 Storz ventilating bronchoscopes and ancillary parts, Hopkins rod endoscopes, and selection of grasping forceps.

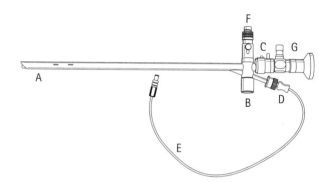

Figure 12.2 An assembled Storz ventilating bronchoscope: (A) ventilating bronchoscope; (B) 15-mm anesthesia port; (C) bridge; (D) suction post with bung; (E) flexible suction tubing; (F) prismatic light deflector; (G) 0° Hopkins rod endoscope with fiberoptic light port.

Position of the patient

1 The child should be placed supine on the operating table. The neck should be extended with a shoulder roll and the head supported by a head ring.

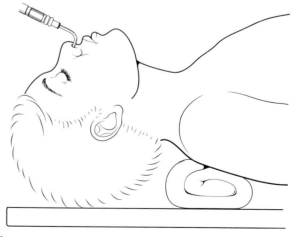

1

Direct laryngoscopy

2 A moistened swab may be used to protect the upper alveolar ridge in infants. In older children, a silastic gum guard may be preferred. Direct laryngoscopy is performed using an appropriate sized open laryngoscope with a lateral slot. Once the tip of the laryngoscope is in the vallecula, the larynx is exposed by pulling the epiglottis forward. Using the upper alveolus or dentition as a fulcrum should be avoided.

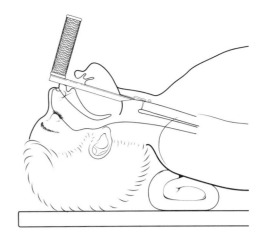

2

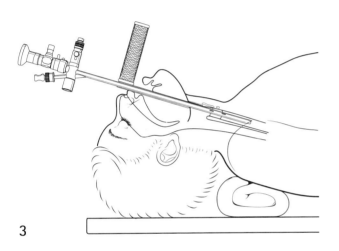

3

Diagnostic bronchoscopy

Diagnostic evaluation is performed in a systematic fashion. The bronchoscope is passed distally identifying the carina, which may appear rather broad in the neonate. From the carina, to enter the right main bronchus, the child's head is rotated to the left and simultaneously the bronchoscope is angled to the right. The opposite procedure is followed to enter the left main bronchus.

A fine flexible suction tube may be passed through the suction port of the bronchoscope to clear secretions.

Introducing the bronchoscope

3 The bronchoscope is inserted through the laryngoscope lumen. It is sometimes helpful to unlock the Hopkins rod from the bronchoscope during insertion and withdraw it slightly into the lumen of the bronchoscope. As the vocal cords are approached, the bronchoscope is rotated 90° so that its leading edge is in an anteroposterior direction. As the bronchoscope enters the trachea, it is rotated back 90° and the laryngoscope is withdrawn. The fingers of the left hand may be used to support the bronchoscope at the mouth and protect the lips and alveolus. While the bronchoscope is in place, the anesthetic circuit should be connected to the side port of the bronchoscope.

Foreign body removal

Having identified the foreign body, an assessment is made as to whether the foreign body can be safely removed endoscopically. Dilute epinephrine solution (1–2 mL of 1:10 000) may be instilled around the foreign body using the flexible suction catheter, provided there is no contraindication. This reduces mucosal edema and facilitates foreign body removal.

The bronchoscope is left in place and the Hopkins rod endoscope removed from its lumen. An appropriate optical forceps is selected according to the nature of the foreign body. A variety of types of forceps are available, but optical forceps are preferred over flexible side arm forceps where possible.

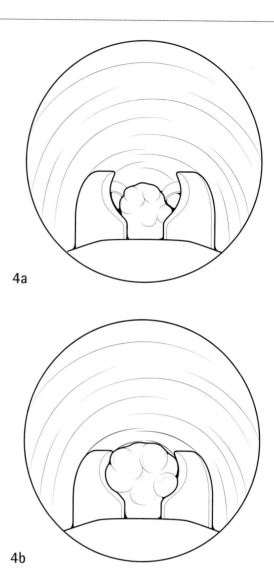

4a

4b

4   The optical forceps are inserted through the bronchoscope, which should be positioned just proximal to the foreign body. The foreign body is grasped and drawn into the bronchoscope lumen. Larger foreign bodies should be withdrawn to the leading edge of the bronchoscope and then the entire apparatus withdrawn.

Following removal, a further endoscopic examination should be performed in case of multiple foreign bodies being present.

POSTOPERATIVE CARE

Following recovery from anesthesia, children should be observed for at least 24 hours. Where bronchoscopy has been performed in the presence of significant airway narrowing, or where there has been significant mucosal trauma, dexamethasone may be administered in the immediate postoperative period to reduce edema.

Respiratory distress following rigid bronchoscopy may be helped by dexamethasone and nebulised epinephrine. However, increasing airway obstruction may necessitate intubation.

After foreign body removal, most children recover rapidly with no long-term sequelae. In cases where a foreign body has been present for some time or where there are radiographic changes suggesting infection, a course of antibiotics may be indicated.

COMPLICATIONS

Intraoperative

- Dental injury or damage to the alveolar margin may occur, especially where there is micrognathia. Protection of the teeth and gingivae during the procedure with the operator's fingers and gauze swabs can avoid this.
- Bleeding may be encountered if granulation tissue is removed or mucosal injury occurs. This usually resolves spontaneously, but topical epinephrine may be helpful.
- Hypercarbia occurs with prolonged use of the ventilating bronchoscope, especially when smaller sized bronchoscopes (<4.0) are used. Removal of the Hopkins rod endoscope from the lumen every 5 minutes or so can prevent this.

Postoperative

- Laryngospasm: this may be minimized by good anesthetic technique, use of topical local anesthetic to the larynx, minimal mucosal contact and ensuring there is no active bleeding at the end of the procedure.
- Airway obstruction may occur as a result of trauma to an already compromised airway along with the effects of anesthesia. Nebulized epinephrine and oral or intravenous dexamethasone may provide time for edema to settle, but in severe cases intubation or tracheostomy may be necessary.
- Aspiration: sufficient time should elapse following the application of topical anesthesia to the larynx before feeding in order to prevent aspiration.

OTHER THERAPEUTIC OPTIONS

A full description of other therapeutic airway techniques is beyond the scope of this chapter. However, the ventilating bronchoscope has many other roles including the management of tracheal stenosis, tracheal and suprastomal granulations, and indwelling stent removal.

In addition to foreign body forceps, balloon catheters and laser fibers may be used down the bronchoscope alongside a Hopkins rod endoscope.

The bronchoscope may also be a valuable adjunct in the management of the difficult pediatric airway where other intubation methods have failed. A far lateral approach to the glottis through the glossotonsillar sulcus can often be successful, provided the operator is familiar with the ventilating bronchoscope.

FLEXIBLE BRONCHOSCOPY

In some cases, particularly where therapeutic intervention is not required and the child's airway not significantly compromised, flexible bronchoscopy may provide a 'less invasive' alternative to rigid endoscopy. However, in contrast to adult flexible bronchoscopy, general anesthesia is still required for flexible bronchoscopy in children, reducing some of the benefits seen in adult flexible bronchoscopy.

Flexible bronchoscopy may be used instead of rigid endoscopy for the assessment of tracheobronchial lesions, biopsy of lesions, and bronchoalveolar lavage. Flexible bronchoscopy may be performed in the spontaneously ventilating patient in a similar fashion to rigid endoscopy or through an endotracheal tube or laryngeal mask airway. Performing flexible bronchoscopy through an endotracheal tube ensures a secure airway and enables mechanical ventilation. However, a distally placed endotracheal tube may obscure proximal tracheal lesions or stent malacic tracheal segments.

FURTHER READING

Ayari-Khalfallah S, Froehlich S. Airway endoscopy and assessment in children. In: Graham JM, Scadding GK, Bull PD (eds). *Pediatric ENT*. Berlin: Springer, 2007: 177–82.

Casselbrant ML, Alper CM. Methods of examination. In: Bluestone CD, Stool SE, Alper CM *et al.* (eds). *Pediatric Otolaryngology*. Philadelphia, PA: Saunders, 2003, 1379–94.

Green CG, Holinger LD, Gartlan MG. Technique. In: Holinger LD, Lusk RP, Green CG (eds). *Pediatric Laryngology and Bronchoesophagology*. Philadelphia, PA: Lippincott-Raven, 1997: 97–116.

Kuo M, Rothera M. Emergency management of the pediatric airway. In: Graham JM, Scadding GK, Bull PD (eds). *Pediatric ENT*. Berlin: Springer, 2007, 183–8.

Mani N, Soam M, Massey S *et al.* Removal of foreign bodies – middle of the night or the next morning? *International Journal of Pediatric Otorhinolaryngology* 2009; **73**: 1085–9.

13

Esophageal dilatation

NIYI ADE-AJAYI

HISTORY

Dilatation is indicated when the esophagus is obstructed with resultant dysphagia, drooling, and aspiration. Interventions for esophageal strictures date back to the sixteenth century. Readily available materials such as wax were initially used as tools for blind dilatation. Pioneers such as Ambrose Pare (1510–90) carried out disimpaction of the esophagus. Later, Thomas Willis (1621–75) used whale bone with a sponge on the tip for regular dilatation of achalasia. Other early materials included leather and swan feathers. The introduction of rigid esophagoscopy in the mid-nineteenth century facilitated more accurate dilatation. Lead dilators were the precursors of a range of carefully considered and manufactured dilators. Chevalier Jackson developed a range of practical instruments, including bougies, for dealing with strictures and esophageal foreign bodies.

Radiology was a very useful adjunct added to the armamentarium in the early twentieth century. While the principles of esophageal dilatation have remained unchanged over the years, the available tools for this group of interventions have evolved considerably. There are now several options available to the pediatric surgeon who manages esophageal strictures.

PRINCIPLES AND JUSTIFICATION

The conditions that result in occlusion of the esophagus in childhood are virtually all benign and include relatively common conditions such as gastroesophageal reflux, corrosive narrowing, and anastomotic strictures following surgery for esophageal atresia, as well as less common problems such as cartilaginous rings and dystrophic epidermolysis bullosa (**Table 13.1** and **Figure 13.1**).

Table 13.1 Clinical conditions resulting in esophageal stricture.

Category	Condition	Types/characteristics
Congenital	Muscular hypertrophy	
	Esophageal web	
	Cartilaginous ring	
Acquired	Gastroesophageal reflux disease	Peptic, short, few dilatations if early, recalcitrant if long-standing and fixed
	Corrosive ingestion with narrowing	Caustic, irregular, often long, tend to be recalcitrant
	Schatzi's ring	Predominantly adolescents, disruption of ring at dilatation. Important to prevent recurrence of symptoms
	Dystrophic epidermolysis bullosa	Shearing forces should be avoided during dilatation, balloon superior to bougie
	Postoperative	Anastomotic stricture postesophageal atresia, tight Nissen fundoplication, sclerotherapy
	Achalasia	Large balloon to dilate
	Eosinophilic esophagitis	
	Foreign body	Fixed if long-standing, beware tracheoesophageal fistula
	Drug ingestion	
	Infective	

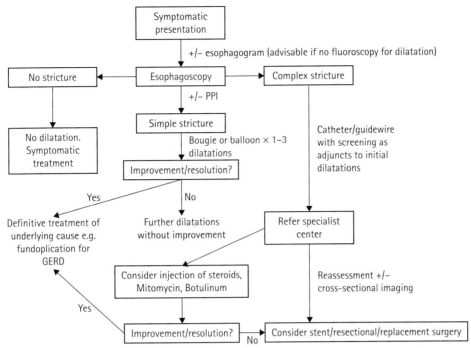

Figure 13.1 Algorithm for esophageal dilatation. PPI, proton pump inhibitor; GERD, gastroesophageal reflux disease.

Children at risk of developing strictures should be closely monitored clinically and with the judicious use of radiology and endoscopy so that, when indicated, intervention is timely. Esophageal dilatation may play a key role in management. However, some children put forward for esophageal dilatation are more appropriately managed conservatively with, for example, proton pump inhibitors. Some children are more suited to bypass by way of gastrostomy while others may require stricture resection or esophageal replacement surgery. Careful consideration should be given to patient selection, type of stricture, and timing of intervention in addition to the specific technique used.

It is useful to consider strictures in terms of complexity. Simple strictures are short and straight while complex ones are tight, long, and irregular. The majority of strictures are amenable to dilatation using one or more of the methods described below. However, recent perforation is a contraindication. The key goals of intervention are the relief of dysphagia, oral nutrition, and airway protection. At the commencement of intervention, an estimate of the number of dilatations likely to result in cure is helpful. This helps to avoid children having large numbers of dilatations without commensurate clinical benefit. Those with complex esophageal strictures and, in particular, the recalcitrant ones who have undergone numerous dilatations with little improvement in dysphagia and limited oral nutritional intake, are best managed in the context of a multidisciplinary team, including surgeon with esophageal replacement expertise, gastroenterologist, interventional radiologist, and dietician. When the multidisciplinary expertise is not locally available, referral to an appropriate center is advisable for complex and recalcitrant strictures.

OVERVIEW OF DEVICES AND TECHNIQUES

The range of available procedures has increased over the past few decades. The choice of device and specific technique is dependent on the condition being treated and characteristics of the stricture. While a specific plan for dilating should be made preoperatively, a wide range of tools should be available. An esophageal contrast study may be helpful at the outset, particularly if fluoroscopy is not available for dilatation. Flexible endoscopic assessment is recommended, although rigid endoscopy also allows for direct visualization and remains a suitable alternative. At the outset, detailed information regarding the stricture should be documented and include site, degree of tightness, length, and mucosal inflammation.

Devices for dilatation may be put into three broad categories: (1) bougies, (2) balloon dilators, and (3) stents. Bougies can be subdivided into those that are passed over a guidewire or not. They come with a range of different tips: blunt, conical, olive-tipped, and tapered. Stents are divided depending on material (metal or plastic) and whether or not they are covered (**Table 13.2**).

The rigid endoscope allows direct assessment of the stricture and facilitates the passage of smaller bougies. Flexible endoscopy enables direct visualization and in addition allows the targeted introduction of a guidewire or balloon. The endoscope can then be withdrawn and be replaced with an appropriate bougie or balloon dilator. If a guidewire is used, insertion can be achieved fluoroscopically using a catheter. A number of catheter types and guidewires may be suitable, but typically for a tight stricture, a floppy tipped, hydrophilic guidewire (0.035 inch) is passed via a 5 Fr catheter with curved tip. Screening contrast after

Table 13.2 Types of esophageal dilators, stents, and related equipment.

Main type of dilator	Subtype of dilator	Material	Characteristics/method
Bougie	Savary–Gilliard	Polyvinyl chloride	Central hollow for guidewire, tapered tip, radio-opaque marker at maximum diameter
	Eder–Puestow	Metal	Graduated olive shape on flexible shaft, central hollow for guidewire
	Chevalier–Jackson	Polythene, gum elastic	Passed via rigid esophagoscope, best when warmed up, 'memory' when curved
	Filiform	Polythene, gum elastic	Fine filiform is inserted via stricture then a 'follower' is attached and used to achieve dilatation
	Tuckers	Silicone	Frequent dilatation of long-standing stricture, loop each end to tie to string
	Maloney	Rubber – mercury or tungsten filled	Tapered tip. May be used blindly, but fluoroscopic control recommended
Balloon	Single or multiple diameter	Non-latex	Accurate fluoroscopic positioning across stricture possible, disposable, higher cost. May be passed via an endoscope, over a guidewire or without. Variety with radiolucent marks recommended. Expanded by liquid pressure with or without pressure monitor
	Special achalasia balloons		Wire-guided, large diameter
Stent	Covered and uncovered	Metal, plastic or biodegradable, e.g. polydioxanone	Simple deployment, tissue ingrowth, stent migration, traumatic removal. Biodegradable variety do not require removal

dilatation need not be routine, particularly for simple strictures. However, the threshold for carrying this out immediately post-dilatation or subsequently should be low for early diagnosis of a perforation and reduced morbidity. If early dilatation of a tight stricture is planned, a nasogastric tube may be left in place to facilitate the next procedure.

PREOPERATIVE

Assessment and planning

Detailed history and clinical examination are important. Any underlying clinical conditions should be carefully evaluated and related anomalies taken into account. For example, if there has been aspiration secondary to the stricture, this should be treated by chest physiotherapy and appropriate antibiotics prior to the procedure. In the case of reflux-related strictures, therapy with prokinetics and proton pump inhibitors should be optimized. An esophageal contrast study as a road map may be helpful before embarking on intervention(s). Stricture position, regularity, length, and evidence of external compression are established, and associated conditions such as reflux and hiatus hernia identified. The objective should be clear for the individual patient and type of stricture, taking natural history into account. For example, with a long-standing postanastomotic stricture, small incremental dilatations may be ideal, whereas for achalasia a more forceful dilatation with the aim of disrupting the fibers of the distal esophageal sphincter is appropriate. For those who require multiple dilatations, frequency between dilatations should be carefully considered. Early on in the series of interventions, the intervals may necessarily be of short duration. This can then be lengthened as a pattern is established. Dilatation of simple strictures or

those that have previously been dilated without difficulty can be planned on a day-case basis. The procedures can be carried out in a general operating room, radiology department, or in a specially designed combined interventional radiology and surgery suite. Appropriate team support should include an anesthetic team experienced at managing the pediatric airway, nursing staff and surgical assistant. Informed consent is mandatory and should be obtained by the surgeon performing the intervention or a colleague in the team with an understanding of the subtle differences in the devices and techniques employed. The process should include a discussion regarding management options and complications, particularly esophageal perforation. Lead suits with thyroid protectors should be provided for all staff present in the operating room during radiation exposure. Efficient routines will help reduce the burden of ionizing radiation (particularly important for those who require multiple dilatations). Routine antibiotics are recommended for infants and small children and should be used selectively for those with long established strictures.

ANESTHESIA

For the majority of patients, a general endotracheal anesthetic is used. Sedation is an option for selected children with simple strictures or where the dilatation routine has been established. It is not recommended for complex strictures at the start of interventions. For the duration of the procedure, oxygen saturation, end-tidal carbon dioxide, and cardiac function are monitored. The endotracheal tube should be securely strapped down and the anesthetic team vigilant about maintaining its position and preventing inadvertent dislodgment particularly with withdrawal of scopes and dilators.

Bouginage of esophageal stricture without guidewire

1 This is preceded by rigid esophagoscopy with the child in the supine position with the neck extended on a head ring. The index finger of the operator's non-dominant hand is used to pull back the upper teeth and the thumb used to protect the teeth from damage by the esophagoscope. With the esophagoscope advanced to immediately proximal to the stricture, the selected bougie is prepared with hydrophilic gel and gently passed. The ideal grip involves thumb and index finger, supported behind by the middle finger; a gentle rather than a 'fist' grip. This is preferred in order to reduce the amount of force applied and thus lessen the risk of perforation. The choice of initial dilator size is based on radiological/endoscopic assessment. Bouginage without the rigid endoscopy is not recommended.

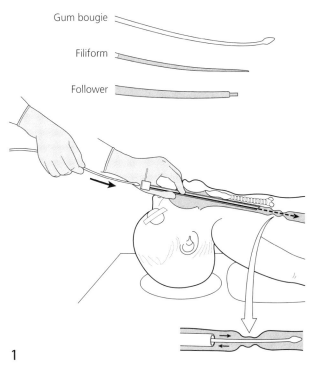

Gum bougie

Filiform

Follower

1

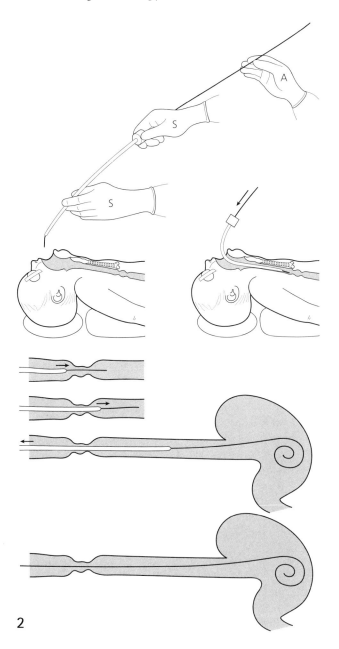

2

Bouginage of esophageal stricture with guidewire

2 The flexible endoscope is passed as outlined elsewhere in this text until it is just proximal to the stricture. The instrument channel should be irrigated with saline. A suitable stiff and wet guidewire with a floppy tip (typically 0.035 inch and 260 cm) is advanced via the instrument channel under direct vision. Redundant guidewire in the stomach should be confirmed fluoroscopically. The endoscope is then slowly withdrawn ensuring that as this takes place, commensurate insertion of the guidewire occurs to maintain the original position in the stomach. As the endoscope is removed, the guidewire is controlled at the level of the lips to allow complete disengagement of the endoscope from the guidewire without dislodgment. The guidewire channel of a suitably sized and shaped bougie (such as the Savary–Gilliard) is irrigated and advanced over the guidewire. Dilatation is carried out progressively as appropriate.

Balloon dilatation fluoroscopic

3 For practical purposes, fluoroscopic and endoscopic balloon techniques are often interchanged to achieve optimum outcomes. Balloon size is determined by the estimated size of the normal esophagus of the child, tightness and duration of stricture, and the underlying condition. An early peptic stricture, even when tight, should dilate up readily and balloon size could be taken from the size of the child's thumb. On the other hand, a caustic stricture should be dilated in small increments. If the underlying condition is achalasia, the aim is to dilate by rupturing and a large balloon size should be chosen.

A suitably shaped catheter is inserted into the upper esophagus with fluoroscopic guidance and a contrast study is performed (illustration shows a stricture of the cervical esophagus outlined by contrast). The stricture is then crossed with a guidewire (b, shorter than required when used with an endoscope), which is then advanced to the stomach. The combination of a curved (steerable) tip of the catheter and fine floppy guidewire ensures that the majority of even very tight strictures can be traversed. The catheter is removed and replaced with a balloon of appropriate diameter. The angioplasty catheter is advanced over the guidewire until the radio-opaque markers indicating the position of the balloon straddle the stricture. The balloon is then inflated with dilute radiographic contrast (c). Fluoroscopy is essential at this stage to confirm that the stricture has been successfully dilated, as shown by abolition of the waist on the balloon. There is no general agreement on the optimum duration of dilatation, but prolonged maintenance of pressure does not appear to improve the results. Our practice is to maintain pressure for 30–60 seconds once the maximum diameter has been reached. The balloon is then deflated and the catheter and guidewire are removed. There is often a small volume of blood on the dilator. In the main, this does not pose a clinical problem. Stricture position and the starting and completion diameter should all be carefully recorded, including relationship with bony and soft tissue landmarks.

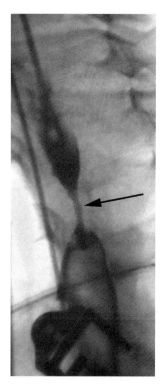

3a

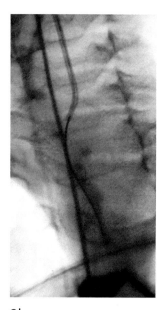

3b

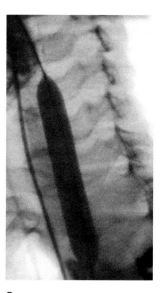

3c

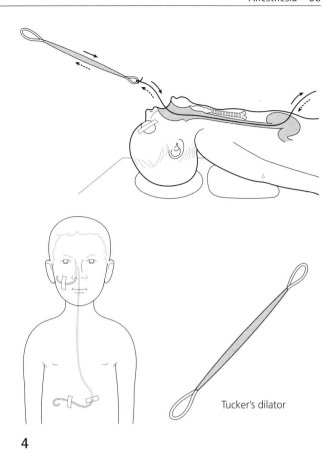

Retrograde dilatation

4 If antegrade cannulation of a tight stricture proves impossible, it can be approached from below. This is usually carried out via an established gastrostomy and can be facilitated by flexible endoscopy, or fluoroscopy and guidewire. Once the stricture has been traversed, every effort should be made to keep the lumen open and a channel for future rapid dilatation. A nasogastric tube between dilatations usually achieves this. The tip should be cut off in order to be able to pass the guidewire and retrieve the nasogastric tube during the next dilatation.

Tucker's dilator

4

Alternative strategies for recalcitrant strictures

INJECTIONS AND STENTS

5 When multiple conventional dilatations have failed to achieve sustained luminal opening and relief of symptoms, alternative methods, usually in the context of a specialist center are appropriate. These include direct endoscopic injection into the stricture using a sclerotherapy needle. Agents that can be injected include steroids, mitomycin, and botulinum toxin. A four-quadrant technique is used, with the overall dose divided into four and administered into each quadrant.

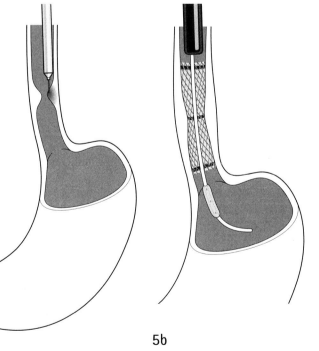

5a   5b

Plastic or metal stents have been a medium-term option for recalcitrant strictures for over two decades. Conventional dilatation of the stricture precedes stent insertion. A guidewire is left in place. Deployment is carried out aided by fluoroscopy. A push or pull technique is employed; the stent is loaded onto a delivery system which is advanced over the previously placed guidewire. Within the delivery system, the stent is positioned so it is above and below the stricture (making allowance for shortening). When the correct position has been confirmed, the stent is deployed. The final position is confirmed endoscopically. The biodegradable versions which have recently come onto the market do not require retrieval. This is an attractive option and may result in increased use of this tool for conditions such as stricture secondary to caustic ingestion.

POSTOPERATIVE CARE

If a nasogastric tube has been left in place, this should be secured with occlusive, transparent dressing. Monitoring following dilatation should be carried out in a designated recovery area immediately following dilatation and should include regular measurements of pulse, heart rate, temperature, and blood pressure. If an adequate luminal diameter has been achieved, clear fluids may be permitted by mouth when the child is fully awake. If this is tolerated, then progression to milk is allowed followed by a soft diet if appropriate. A dietician should liaise with the carers to ensure adequate nutrition between dilatations.

OUTCOME

With appropriate adjunctive treatment, the majority of children with an esophageal stricture have a satisfactory and sustained response to a few dilatations. Complication rates are low in experienced hands. They occur most often during dilatation of corrosive strictures followed by those associated with gastroesophageal reflux. Other at-risk patients include those with dystrophic epidermolysis bullosa. Careful postoperative monitoring and a low threshold for chest x-ray and upper gastrointestinal contrast study facilitate early diagnosis. Three types of esophageal injury occur. Guidewire perforation of the esophagus can be recognized at fluoroscopy and treated conservatively. Submucosal tears of the esophagus are seen as contained extravasation of contrast. These also seem to do well with conservative treatment. Full thickness perforation of the esophagus is uncommon. Small perforations require nasogastric or parenteral feeding and broad-spectrum antibiotic therapy. Large perforations, if recognized early, may be managed best by surgical repair.

FURTHER READING

Earlam R, Cunha-Melo JR. Benign oesophageal strictures: historical and technical aspects of dilatation. *British Journal of Surgery* 1981; **68**: 829–36.

Lan LCL, Wong KKY, Lin SCL *et al.* Endoscopic balloon dilatation of esophageal strictures in infants and children: 17 years' experience and a literature review. *Journal of Pediatric Surgery* 2003; **38**: 1712–15.

Lew RJ, Kochman ML. A review of endoscopic methods of esophageal dilation. *Journal of Clinical Gastroenterology* 2002; **35**: 117–26.

Taitelbaum G, Petersen BT, Barkun AN *et al.* Tools for endoscopic stricture dilation. *Gastrointestinal Endoscopy* 2004; **59**: 753–60.

14

Esophagogastroduodenoscopy

ROBERT E CILLEY and PETER W DILLON

HISTORY

Endoscopists in the nineteenth century used open, rigid tubes to visualize the upper gastrointestinal tract. The characteristics of rigid endoscopies were improved by the addition of conventional lenses that provided magnification and some increase in the viewing angle. When miniaturized for pediatric applications, the narrow viewing angle and the poor light transmission inherent in these devices limited their usefulness. A major advance in the field of endoscopy was the development of the rod-lens telescope, which first became available in 1966. Flexible fiberoptic endoscopes were first developed in 1958. Technical improvements combined with the development of specialized equipment have expanded the diagnostic and therapeutic potential of this technique. Flexible endoscopes for upper gastrointestinal endoscopy are now available in small sizes ideally suited to pediatric applications.

PRINCIPLES AND JUSTIFICATION

Indications

Endoscopy of the upper gastrointestinal tract is performed for both diagnostic and therapeutic reasons. The most common diagnoses requiring esophagogastroscopy in children include esophageal foreign bodies and reflux disease. Other diagnoses include caustic ingestion, food impaction, and tracheoesophageal fistula evaluation. The most common symptoms requiring endoscopy include dysphagia, pain, bleeding, and food refusal. Additional procedures performed in conjunction with esophagogastroscopy include stricture dilatation and percutaneous gastrostomy insertion.

UPPER GASTROINTESTINAL TRACT BLEEDING

Flexible esophagogastroduodenoscopy causes most upper gastrointestinal tract bleeding. Definitive or palliative treatment may be provided for specific lesions. Esophageal varices may be treated by endoscopic sclerotherapy or variceal banding. Ulcer bleeding may be controlled by the injection of sclerosants or coagulation using electric current, heat, or laser energy.

ESOPHAGEAL FOREIGN BODIES

Either flexible or rigid esophagoscopy is mandatory in the evaluation and treatment of suspected esophageal foreign bodies. When encountered, foreign bodies may be removed or advanced into the stomach. Most gastric foreign bodies will pass spontaneously. Those that fail to pass after a period of observation require extraction with a flexible scope.

ESOPHAGEAL STRICTURE

Endoscopy is beneficial in the diagnosis and treatment of strictures and achalasia. Dilatation of either process may be made easier and safer using endoscopy to visualize and assist in the passage of guidewires, strings, and dilators. Fluoroscopy to confirm proper guidewire position and to monitor the passage of each dilator is a useful adjunct to minimize the risk of esophageal perforation or damage. Traditionally, dilators of progressively larger size are passed to the point of maximal dilation. Clear end-points for dilation are difficult to determine (e.g. blood on dilator, subjective increase in difficulty). Balloon dilators are now available in multiple sizes that can be used in all patients. Balloon dilators apply force to the stricture in a radial fashion and may be safer than traditional dilators. Esophageal injury and perforation can occur with any technique.

CAUSTIC INGESTION/ESOPHAGEAL INJURY

Esophagogastroscopy is useful in the evaluation of infants following suspected ingestion of caustic substances. The degree of esophageal injury and likelihood of subsequent stricture formation is difficult to determine from the appearance of the mucosa. Follow-up evaluations can assess mucosal healing and early stricture formation. As most children have mild injury after caustic ingestion, the role of mandatory esophagoscopy in all caustic injury patients is debated.

ADJUNCTS TO FEEDING

Endoscopic techniques may be used to place gastrostomy tubes (percutaneous endoscopic gastrostomy) and transpyloric feeding tubes.

CHOICE OF ENDOSCOPE

The choice of rigid or flexible endoscopes depends on the procedure planned and the experience and training of the surgeon. The safety and ease of flexible endoscopy make it the procedure of choice for most pediatric upper gastrointestinal endoscopic procedures. The ability to insufflate air and thus distend the esophagus and allow complete visualization ahead of the advancing esophagoscope is the principal advantage of the fiberoptic endoscope. Removal of an impacted foreign body may be easier with the rigid esophagoscope. Endoscopists should be familiar with both techniques. Image processing systems that allow the endoscopic image to be viewed on a video monitor and recorded for documentation are used routinely.

Rigid esophagoscopes

The Storz–Hopkins rod-lens telescope is utilized almost exclusively in rigid esophagoscopy. Unlike a conventional telescope that uses small lenses with long intervening air spaces, this system uses long glass rods with their ends shaped in the form of a lens and small intervening air space. The lens system allows transmission of a brilliant magnified image through a small-diameter tube. A wide variety of endoscopic instruments is available to perform

such tasks as foreign body retrieval and sclerotherapy. General anesthesia with endotracheal intubation is required.

Flexible endoscopes

Flexible adult endoscopes are typically 11–12.6 mm in diameter. Although they may be passed into the esophagus of children, they are too large for maneuvers such as intragastric retroflexion for fundic visualization or transduodenal passage. Large endoscopes with two channels may have some advantages in emergency sclerotherapy for bleeding, as one channel can be used for suction and irrigation while the other is used to direct the sclerotherapy needle. Endoscopes of intermediate size, 9–10 mm, are versatile and may be used in both adults and older children. High-resolution 5-mm instruments are now available, allowing complete upper gastrointestinal endoscopy to be performed on the smallest of infants.

PREOPERATIVE AND ANESTHESIA

Patients should be 'nil by mouth' for an appropriate period of time before sedation or anesthesia (e.g. 4 hours for infants and 6 hours for toddlers and young children). The mouth should be examined for loose and potentially dislodgable teeth. Explanations appropriate to the age of the child should be given. Gastrointestinal endoscopy should be performed either in the operating room or in an appropriately equipped, dedicated endoscopy suite, ideally under the care of a pediatric anesthesiologist.

OPERATION

The following endoscopic techniques are commonly used in pediatrics.

Rigid esophagoscopy

1 For this procedure, the child is anesthetized and endotracheally intubated. The endotracheal tube has been omitted from the figure for clarity. Supporting towels are placed under the shoulders to maintain the head in full extension. The oropharynx is suctioned. Although the esophagoscope may be passed into the cervical esophagus by direct visualization, this maneuver is facilitated by lifting the tongue and epiglottis with a laryngoscope and directly visualizing the entry into the esophagus. It is critically important that the oroesophageal axis is straight (sword-swallower's position) during rigid esophagoscopy. The teeth, if present, are protected by a gauze pad or plastic guard.

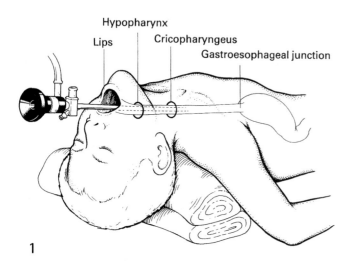

Hypopharynx
Lips   Cricopharyngeus
        Gastroesophageal junction

1

2 The esophagoscope is grasped with the supporting hand much as one would grasp a pencil, while the remaining fingers of that hand rest against the maxilla or upper teeth. The esophagoscope is then advanced – in the words of Chevalier Jackson, '... the word insinuate is better than introduce, since it implies to introduce slowly, as through a winding and narrow passage ... the esophagoscope is advanced ... watching the folds as they unfold and recede'. If any difficulty is encountered in negotiating the lumen of the esophagus, a small soft catheter may be used as a lumen finder. Again, Jackson advises, 'When no lumen is visible a search for a lumen is made by gentle palpation with the lumen finder. When the lumen is found, the esophagoscope may be gently and safely advanced. The lumen finder is not, in any sense, a mandril for blind introduction ... when it has found and entered deeply into the lumen, the esophagoscope is advanced'. The narrowest points along the way are the cricopharyngeus and the gastroesophageal junction. Once the stomach has been entered, the esophagoscope is slowly withdrawn. It is during the removal of the esophagoscope that the best examination of both the stomach and the esophagus can be obtained.

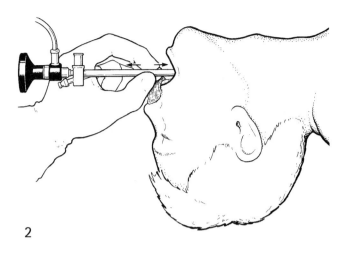

2

Flexible esophagoscopy

Though conscious, sedation can be used in children undergoing flexible esophagoscopy. General anesthesia with endotracheal control of the airway is preferred, especially if procedures such as foreign body removal or dilation are to be performed. The patient can be supine or positioned laterally with the left side down. The instrument is introduced by directly visualizing the oropharynx and the entry into the esophagus through the cricopharyngeus. The primary advantage of the flexible endoscope during advancement through the esophagus is the ability to insufflate air easily through the endoscope and with precise control in order to distend the esophageal lumen. Controlled air insufflation not only lessens the danger of esophageal injury during insertion of the endoscope, but also provides a valuable tool for examining the esophageal lumen since the distensibility of the esophageal wall may be altered in pathologic conditions. It must be emphasized that the same dangers found in using rigid instruments are present during flexible esophagoscopy. The esophagoscope should never be forcibly or blindly advanced. The esophagus may be injured just as easily during manipulations with flexible instruments.

Air insufflation, although invaluable in visualizing the esophagus, must be controlled, especially in infants and small children. Gaseous distension of the abdomen can compromise ventilation. The lowest adjustment possible of the air insufflation rate is used, and the abdomen is left uncovered so that it may be continuously inspected. The child's temperature may need to be supported by elevating the room temperature, external warming lights, or a warming mattress.

After the stomach is entered, insufflation is used to allow a panoramic view. Excessive fluid is suctioned to allow complete visualization of the mucosa. A gastrostomy, if present, must be occluded to allow the stomach to fill. Orientation and endoscopic maneuvers are similar in the lateral and supine positions. Once the stomach is filled with air, the endoscope can be retroflexed, and the gastroesophageal junction visualized. The endoscope is straightened, and the remainder of the stomach is visualized. With the pylorus in view, the endoscope is advanced. Entering the pylorus may be facilitated by rotation of the endoscope. The best visualization of the pyloric channel may be obtained during the slow removal of the endoscope. In a patient with a pronounced angulation at the incisura (the 'J-shaped' stomach), a considerable length of the endoscope may need to be advanced before the tip will enter the pylorus. Changing the patient's position from supine to lateral or from lateral to supine may also be helpful. The ampulla of Vater is recognized by the drainage of bile. Cannulation of the ampulla for retrograde cholangiopancreatography is beyond the scope of this discussion. The duodenum, including the bulb and pylorus, is carefully inspected as the endoscope is slowly withdrawn.

Biopsy techniques

Small cup biopsy forceps that pass easily through the suction channel of the flexible endoscope or alongside the telescope within the rigid endoscope allow precisely directed biopsies to be performed.

Grading of esophagitis

Endoscopic grading of esophagitis is not uniform and is subject to both inter-user and intra-user variability. Nevertheless, description of the mucosal appearance should be part of the language of the endoscopist. The severity of esophagitis can be roughly graded on the basis of the visual appearance alone. Mild esophagitis is indicated by abnormal erythema and friability of the mucosa; moderate esophagitis describes linear erosions and superficial ulcers; and severe esophagitis refers to confluent erosions, deep ulcers, and diffusely hemorrhagic mucosa.

Esophageal mucosal biopsies through the endoscope may help diagnose and manage such pathologic entities as gastroesophageal reflux, eosinophilic esophagitis, and Crohn's disease.

Esophageal sclerotherapy and banding for variceal bleeding

Esophageal variceal bleeding usually stops spontaneously in children with conservative treatment and correction of coagulopathy. Emergency endoscopy to control bleeding is rarely required. Endoscopic variceal ligation has been proven to be safe and effective in children.

Under most circumstances, varices are present circumferentially in the distal esophagus and extend a variable distance proximally. Each sclerotherapy session is limited to 0.5 mL of sclerosant/kg body weight. Sodium morrhuate, 50 percent dextrose, and absolute alcohol have all been used for this purpose. The authors use a combination of perivariceal and intravariceal injection and preferentially obliterate an entire column of varices using injections at multiple levels rather than injecting circumferentially at one level. After injection of the varix, the endoscope is advanced and used to tamponade bleeding at the injection site.

With variceal banding, the varix is drawn into the end of the band applicator using suction. The band is released around the base of the varix, resulting in its thrombosis and subsequent obliteration. As many as six bands have been applied in one procedure.

Esophageal foreign body removal

The most common esophageal foreign bodies in children are coins. Other objects include toy parts, hair beads, small bones, and food impaction. Although some advocate fluoroscopically guided balloon extraction of coins as a safe and cost-effective alternative to endoscopic removal, the authors have not adopted this technique. The controlled environment of the operating room is preferred, where adjunctive equipment is readily available to provide airway control. In addition, when the foreign body is removed endoscopically, the esophagus can be directly assessed for damage. The most important technical consideration in foreign body removal is the availability of the proper grasping forceps. A 'coin forceps' with small teeth at its distal end, allowing it to grasp the edge of a coin or small solid object firmly, is essential. Removal of an irregular object, such as impacted food material, may be facilitated by the passage of a balloon catheter beyond the material, which is then withdrawn under direct vision while the airway is controlled by endotracheal intubation.

Food impactions in previously healthy children without known esophageal disease should prompt investigation for eosinophilic esophagitis.

Esophageal stricture

Stricture dilatation can be facilitated by the passage of a guidewire through the side channel of the endoscope and across the stricture. Proper position can then be confirmed with fluoroscopy before attempted passage of a dilator or a pneumatic dilating device. Very tight strictures can be initially dilated with sequential ureteral dilators before advancing to larger sizes.

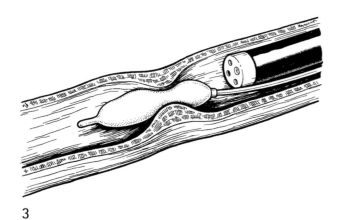

3

3 When balloon dilatation is performed for esophageal strictures, the flexible endoscope is essential to position the balloon properly. It is worth noting that, since the operating channel of pediatric gastroscopes is small and passage of the larger dilating balloons may be difficult, the balloon may be directly inserted into the esophagus alongside the gastroscope and still be precisely positioned under direct vision. The dilating balloon is inflated to a preset pressure according to its diameter, as recommended by the manufacturer, and held at that pressure for 2 minutes. The application of radial forces using a balloon results in much less shear force to the esophageal lining than an equivalent dilatation using prograde or retrograde techniques.

Percutaneous endoscopic gastrostomy

Percutaneous gastrostomy placement may be performed using either conscious sedation or general anesthesia in the endoscopy suite, intensive care unit, or operating room.

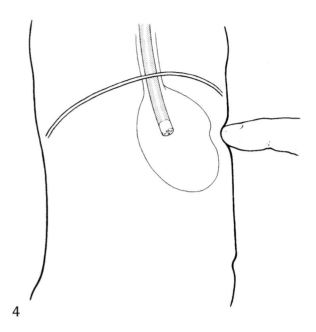

4 The gastroscope is passed and used to identify the anterior stomach in contact with the anterior abdominal wall. Orientation is provided endoscopically visualizing the deformation of the anterior wall of the stomach caused by indenting the proposed gastrostomy site with a probe or finger.

4

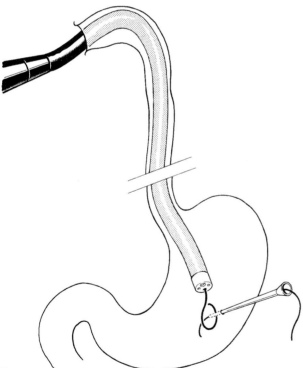

5

5 A small incision is made at the proposed site and a needle is introduced through the gastrostomy site, through the full thickness of abdominal wall, and into the stomach, where its entry is visualized endoscopically. A wire passed through this needle is grasped with the endoscopic forceps or in a snare and withdrawn with the gastroscope out of the mouth.

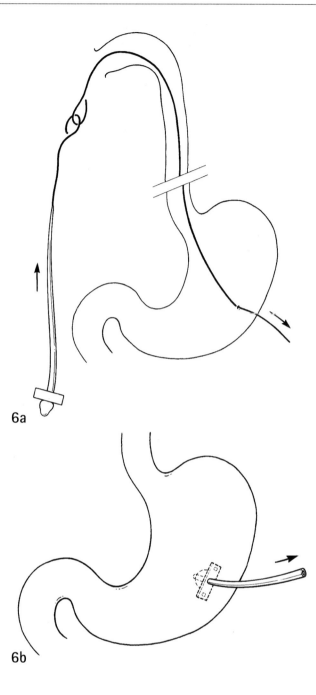

6a,b This wire is used to guide a dilator, on the end of which is a flanged feeding tube that will seat the stomach securely against the anterior abdominal wall when it is drawn out of the gastrostomy exit site.

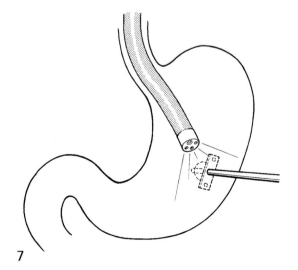

7 The gastroscope is again passed into the stomach and the proper positioning of the feeding tube is confirmed.

POSTOPERATIVE CARE

The endoscopic procedure itself may be performed on an outpatient basis. Concurrent or underlying disease may necessitate hospitalization. A chest radiograph is obtained whenever significant manipulation of the esophagus has occurred, such as during a dilatation procedure. The finding of mediastinal air or pneumothorax mandates esophagography with a water-soluble contrast medium to assess the degree of injury. Minor, self-contained perforations may be treated conservatively with antibiotics and hospitalization and possibly pleural drainage. Large perforations with significant pleural or mediastinal communication should be primarily repaired and drained.

Sclerotherapy may result in significant chest pain requiring narcotic analgesia. Esophageal ulceration and stricture may also result. Strictures following sclerotherapy usually respond to dilatation.

Percutaneously placed gastrostomy tubes may be used for feeding almost immediately. Percutaneous gastrostomies require immediate operation for early tube dislodgment.

Abdominal wall cellulitis will usually respond to antibiotic therapy. Failure to secure the gastric wall to the abdominal wall with resultant intraperitoneal leakage requires operative correction. Gastrocolic fistula may result from inclusion of a portion of the transverse colon in the path of the tube.

FURTHER READING

Baskin D, Urganci N, Abbosoglu L et al. A standardized protocol for the acute management of corrosive ingestion in children. *Pediatric Surgery International* 2004; **20**: 824–8.

Celinska-Cedro D, Teisseyre M, Woynarowski M et al. Endoscopic ligation of esophageal varices for prophylaxis of first bleeding in children and adolescents with portal hypertension: preliminary results of a prospective study. *Journal of Pediatric Surgery* 2003; **38**: 1008–11.

Gans SL. Principles of optics and illumination. In: Gans SL (ed.). *Pediatric Endoscopy*. New York: Grune and Stratton, 1983: 1–8.

Jackson C. Difficulties and pitfalls in the insinuation of the esophagoscope. *Annals of Otology, Rhinology and Laryngology* 1936; **45**: 1109–13.

Putnam PE, Rothenberg ME. Eosinophilic esophagitis: concepts, controversies and evidence. *Current Gastroenterology Reports* 2009; **11**: 220–5.

Schwesinger WH. Endoscopic diagnosis and treatment of mucosal lesions of the esophagus. *Surgical Clinics of North America* 1989; **69**: 1185–203.

15

Colonoscopy

IAN SUGARMAN and JONATHAN SUTCLIFFE

PRINCIPLES AND JUSTIFICATION

Indication

The indications for colonoscopy can be divided into diagnostic, screening, surveillance, and therapeutic. In diagnostic cases, the most common indication is to investigate symptoms suggestive of inflammatory bowel disease (IBD). These include failure to thrive or weight loss, chronic diarrhea, anemia, bleeding, passage of mucous per rectum, or when there is radiologic abnormality (e.g. narrowed terminal ileal abnormality on ultrasound, small bowel follow-through or magnetic resonance imaging (MRI)). The second most common is to look for rectal/colonic polyps in children presenting with rectal bleeding.

Colonoscopy is preferable to a contrast enema since it allows visualization of the bowel wall, histological assessment, and can be performed without irradiation. When indicated, it is feasible to perform both colonoscopy to the terminal ileum and gastroscopy to the duodenum (esophagogastroduodenoscopy (EGD)) at a single exam-ination. A large proportion of the gastrointestinal tract is thus rendered accessible to inspection, biopsy, or instrumentation in one procedure. Performing EGD at the same sitting as colonoscopy is particularly useful for children with potential IBD for whom evidence of Crohn's disease may exist in the upper gastrointestinal (GI) tract before it appears in the lower GI tract.

Contraindications

There are few contraindications to colonoscopy in experienced hands with appropriate instrumentation. Examination is unlikely to be helpful in constipation and the diagnostic yield is extremely low in abdominal pain unaccompanied by features to suggest systemic illness.

There is a risk of translocation leading to septicemia in marasmic, immunodepressed, or immunosuppressed subjects, who should receive appropriate antibiotics. A risk of bacterial peritonitis contraindicates colonoscopy in the presence of ascites.

PREOPERATIVE

Bowel preparation

A variety of bowel preparation regimens for children are now available that will produce a clean colon. In our institution we use Picolax® in doses dependent on the child's age, or Senna® in children aged less than one year (see Table 15.1).

Table 15.1 Bowel preparation used at our institution.

Age (years)	Medication	First dose (24 hours preoperatively)	Second dose (18 hours preoperatively)
<1	Senna	5–10 mL	5–10 mL
1–2	Picolax	Quarter of a sachet	Quarter of a sachet
2–5	Picolax	Half a sachet	Half a sachet
5–10	Picolax	1 sachet	Half a sachet
>10	Picolax	1 sachet	1 sachet

Sedation or anesthesia?

Premedication may be useful for apprehensive children, for whom reassurance and explanation are often ineffective. Colonoscopic examination is, however, often uncomfortable or painful for a short period, as the instrument stretches the sigmoid colon mesentery or the visceral peritoneum, and anesthesia is therefore recommended.

Choice of instrument

There is an increasing array of colonoscopes available in terms of size, length, variable stiffness, definition, and narrow band imaging; however, a summary of what is used at our institution is given in **Table 15.2**, with their characteristics.

Is radiographic control needed?

Most examinations do not require radiographic screening control and the majority of colonoscopists never use it. It has been shown that magnetic endoscopic imaging (which involves passing a magnetic probe through the biopsy channel, such that loops can be seen and hand pressure to prevent the loops is more controlled) is a useful tool for training and dealing with the more difficult loops that may occur.

OPERATIONS

Colonoscopy

POSITION OF PATIENT

Infants are usually examined supine, while in older patients the left lateral position is the norm, and it is often possible to complete the examination without a position change. If there are mechanical difficulties at any stage of the procedure, a change in position may alter the configuration of the bowel and facilitate examination. Such movement under general anesthesia may require a number of people to be present in a larger child. Changing to the right lateral position will make the splenic flexure less acute and can also help to drain fluid from the descending colon and facilitate air distension within it if the view is poor. Soft padding is used to protect pressure areas at all times.

INSERTION AND PASSAGE THROUGH THE RECTOSIGMOID

An important component of the examination is an examination under anesthetic to exclude abdominal masses and perineal inspection; the presence of tags, deep fissures, and induration makes the diagnosis of Crohn's disease more likely. Prior to intubation of the anus, a rectal examination should be performed to exclude a distal polyp. Proctoscopy not only allows visualization of the distal rectum, but also will allow liquid stool to be drained from within the rectum which in turn improves examination of the rectal ampulla.

The tip of the colonoscope and the perianal region are lubricated with jelly. On insertion, initially there may be no view because the tip is against the wall of the rectum. The instrument must be withdrawn slightly and air insufflated before a view is obtained, the tip then being angled and the instrument shaft rotated as necessary to follow along the lumen of the rectosigmoid. In passing the many bends of the rectosigmoid, the object is to avoid distending or stretching the bowel so as to keep it short and pass almost straight to the descending colon. This is easier to suggest than to achieve, but is made more likely by observing the points set out below:

- As little air as possible should be insufflated; excess air should be aspirated from time to time.
- The bowel lumen should be followed accurately.
- If the view is lost, even for a few seconds, the control knobs must be released and the colonoscope withdrawn a short distance – the lumen will automatically reappear. Blind pushing should be avoided, but on acute bends this may be necessary for a few seconds providing the mucosa continues to move and the general direction is known.
- If the tip will not negotiate round a bend, an attempt should be made to 'corkscrew' the instrument by pulling the shaft back straight and twisting it one way or the other.
- The colonoscope should be pulled back repeatedly after passing a bend and before starting each inward push. A straight colonoscope and a shortened colon will result.
- The instrument shaft should be held in the fingertips as far as possible – gripping in a clenched fist causes clumsiness.

Table 15.2 Endoscopes used and their characteristics (review of over 600 patients).

Name	Make	Age (years)	Weight (kg)	Outside diameter (mm)	Working channel diameter (mm)	Length (mm)	Variable stiffness	Bend up/down (°)	Bend left/right (°)	Field of view (°)
EG450PE	Fujinon	2 or under	Less than 10	8.2	2.2	1100	No	210/90	100/100	120
PCF240I	Olympus	8 or under	10 and over	10.3	3.2	1330	No	180/180	160/160	140
CF240AL	Olympus	6 and over	17 and over	12.2	3.2	1680	Yes	180/180	160/160	140
CFQ260AL	Olympus	8 and over	22 and over	13.2	3.7	1680	Yes	180/180	160/160	140

SIGMOID N-LOOP: HOOK AND TWIST MANEUVER

1a–c The most common situation on reaching the junction of the sigmoid and descending colon, in spite of all care, is for there to be an N-loop forming an acute tip angle which makes direct passage difficult or impossible. If the tip can be passed a short way around the bend, looking into the retroperitoneal part of the descending colon, it can be held there without consciously hooking while the instrument is withdrawn 10–40 cm to reduce and straighten out the loop. Putting a clockwise twisting force or torque onto the shaft of the colonoscope while it is withdrawn will help to straighten out this loop and keep the tip in the descending colon.

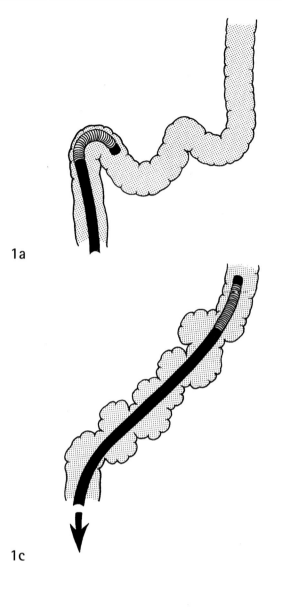

1a

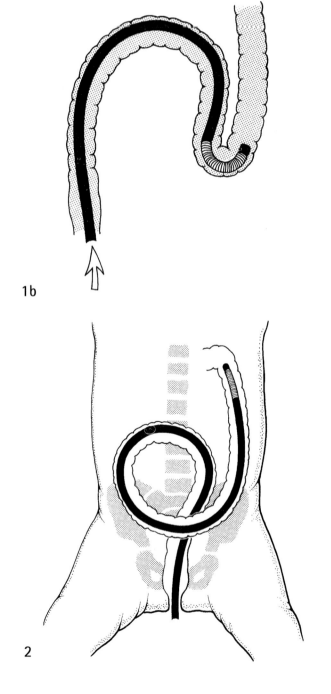

1b

1c

2

SIGMOID 'ALPHA' LOOP

2 Often, if there is a redundant colon, a loop is obviously forming but the tip runs in easily without discomfort to the patient. This suggests that a spiral 'alpha' loop is forming. The correct thing to do is to continue pushing (in as far as is comfortable for the patient if awake), at least to the proximal descending colon and preferably to the splenic flexure. Once around the splenic flexure, the instrument can be 'hooked' over the flexure while attempting to withdraw and straighten it out to remove the loop as described below.

STRAIGHTENING OUT LOOPS

3 Having reached the transverse colon, the sigmoid colon loop should be straightened, since loops create friction in the control wires and stress the instrument just as much as they stress the patient. To straighten a loop, the instrument shaft should be withdrawn until the tip begins to slide past the mucosa or resistance to withdrawal is felt. While pulling back, twisting the colonoscope, usually in a clockwise direction, will prevent the tip slipping back excessively and facilitate the straightening of the instrument. Once 1:1 movement is obtained, i.e. for each centimeter of movement of the scope by the operator there is a commensurate centimeter of movement at the tip of the scope, the scope can be readvanced. Leaving the same direction of torque on the scope as it is advanced is likely to allow reinsertion without reforming a loop. It is sometimes possible to ask an assistant to apply external pressure to the apex of a loop (often higher than might be expected) which in turn reduces the likelihood of a loop progressing.

In the young child, it is very likely that the colon will prove to be hypermobile, without conventional fixation of the descending colon and splenic flexure. In the 20–30 percent of patients who have a mobile colon, unpredictable and sometimes uncontrollable loops may form.

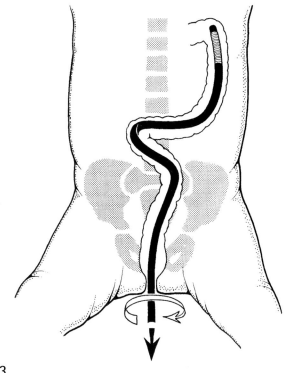

3

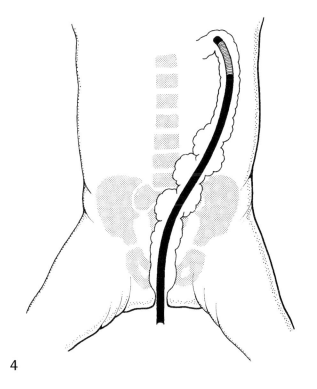

4

SPLENIC FLEXURE: KEEPING THE SIGMOID COLON STRAIGHT

4 With the colonoscope straightened in the proximal descending colon or splenic flexure, some care may be needed to prevent the sigmoid loop reforming. Continued clockwise (or sometimes anticlockwise) twist on the shaft during reinsertion is often enough to keep it straight. It is at this point that the variable stiffness colonoscopes come into their own. Once the loop is removed, by placing the instrument on maximum stiffness, the chance of the loop recurring is diminished. Shaft insertion without tip movement, or losing the 1:1 relationship between shaft and tip, indicates looping. The instrument is immediately pulled back again and the assistant pushes into the left iliac fossa to resist the tendency for the sigmoid loop to rise up from the pelvis. In the splenic flexure, this tendency to reloop in the sigmoid colon results because the hooked instrument tip impacts in the splenic flexure.

A combination of the following small corrective measures will usually overcome this:

- The instrument shaft should be pulled back straight.
- As described above, if possible, the scope should be stiffened.
- Hand/finger pressure should be applied by the assistant over the left iliac fossa.
- The instrument shaft should be twisted clockwise.
- If necessary, the instrument should be re-aimed toward the lumen, avoiding over-angulation.
- It should be pushed slowly inwards, continuing the clockwise twist.

Sometimes, it is easier to reposition the child in the right lateral position to cause the splenic flexure to drop down and flatten out.

REDUNDANT TRANSVERSE COLON

The transverse colon may sometimes be pushed down by the instrument into a deep loop, which makes it difficult and painful to reach the hepatic flexure. Once again, the correct procedure is to withdraw the instrument to shorten this loop. If necessary, withdrawal may need to be repeated several times, the instrument advancing a few centimeters on each withdrawal ('paradoxical movement') until the loop is straightened. Keeping the colon deflated also helps to shorten the hepatic flexure region, making it easier both to reach and to pass. In addition, an assistant pushing the transverse colon upwards and straightening this loop out is often helpful.

Difficulty in the transverse colon is often due to recurrent looping in the sigmoid colon, and the best corrective measures are abdominal pressure in the left iliac fossa and gentle clockwise twisting during reinsertion.

PASSING THE HEPATIC FLEXURE

Do not mistake the hepatic flexure for the cecum; the presence of the liver often produces a blue discoloration visible through the wall of the colon, but if doubt remains, briefly increasing the intensity of the scope light will allow the tip of the scope to be located in the right upper quadrant.

Having reached and deflated the hepatic flexure, and angled acutely around it into the ascending colon, the transverse loop may remain and make it difficult to pass the rest of the instrument into the ascending colon. By once again withdrawing the colonoscope and straightening out this loop, it becomes easier to pass. Deflating the ascending colon by aspiration and simultaneously steering carefully to avoid haustral folds will often cause the colonoscope to descend spontaneously towards the cecum.

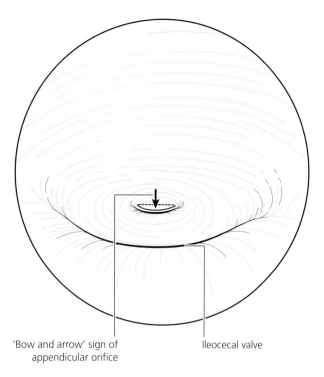

'Bow and arrow' sign of   Ileocecal valve
  appendicular orifice

REACHING THE CECUM

5 Reaching the cecal pole can be facilitated by change of position, deflation, abdominal pressure, and clockwise twist on the straightened instrument; aggressive pushing usually only results in looping. The colonoscope is seen to have reached the cecum when the bulge of the ileocecal valve is seen or, 2–5 cm beyond it, the appendix orifice is identified. The ileocecal valve is the largest fold lying close to the cecal pole and can often be identified by following the arrow, in the 'bow and arrow' sign of the appendix orifice.

5

Brilliant transillumination in the right iliac fossa is usually apparent at this point. The depth of insertion of the straightened instrument is variable according to the age of the patient: 70–80 cm in a teenager, down to 25 cm in a small infant. During withdrawal, the splenic flexure or descending colon is found at appropriately shorter distances. During insertion, in mobile colons or if any loops have been formed, these distance rules may not apply, but if the room is darkened, transillumination will show the position of the instrument tip.

To enter the terminal ileum, it is necessary first to identify the bulge of the ileocecal valve, which may bubble or gush on deflation. The instrument tip is then pushed in just proximal to the bulge, angled in towards it, and slowly withdrawn until a 'red-out' indicates embedding into the valve region, at which point air is insufflated to attempt to distend the ileum.

Alternatively, the biopsy forceps are advanced through the end of the scope which is placed such that the ileocecal valve lies adjacent to its 6 o'clock position (and therefore closest to the scope's biopsy forceps channel). The tip of the scope is positioned just over the ileocecal valve, the biopsy forceps advanced 1 cm and then the tip angulated down slightly. As the scope is gently withdrawn, the biopsy forceps will often enter the ileocecal valve. If the forceps are then advanced by 1–2 cm, the scope itself can then be advanced over the forceps thus entering the ileum.

Ileal mucosa is characteristically granular or nodulated by lymphoid hyperplasia, in contrast to the shiny surface and vascular pattern of the colon.

In infants under one year of age, entry into the ileum may be impossible, either because the orifice is too narrow or because the dimensions of the cecum are too small to allow the instrument to make the necessary right-angle turn.

EXAMINATION

The colon is visualized to some extent during insertion of the instrument, but active examination, biopsy, or polypectomies are normally undertaken during withdrawal because the instrument is then straight and easy to maneuver, the view is better, and the patient is more comfortable. At all stages during the examination, but particularly during withdrawal, it is best for the endoscopist to control the instrument, using a one-handed technique. Very active maneuvering of the controls, with rotation and to-and-fro movements of the shaft, allow a good view to be obtained of nearly all areas, although around acute bends and convoluted folds there may be some blind spots. Ensure representative photographs are taken throughout this phase of the examination.

BIOPSIES

Most colonoscopies are diagnostic and the diagnosis is made both on the macroscopic and microscopic findings. It is recommended that two specimens are taken from any segment as this helps to assess the histological patchiness of inflammation and may help in distinguishing between Crohn's and ulcerative colitis. Our standard practice is to take biopsies from the terminal ileum, cecum, ascending colon, transverse colon, sigmoid, and rectum. If localized pathology is seen in a segment, abnormal and adjacent macroscopically normal colon should be biopsied.

COLONOSCOPIC POLYPECTOMY

The principles of colonoscopic polypectomy are identical to those for proctosigmoidoscopic polypectomy, but it is particularly important that full coagulation of polyp stalk vessels is achieved before transection, as any hemorrhage is difficult to control endoscopically. Most polyps in pediatric practice are hamartomatous, thin-stalked, and easy to coagulate. If a thick stalk (1 cm or more) is to be snared, it may be wise to inject it with epinephrine (adrenaline) (1 mL of 1:100 000 solution), using a long Teflon sclerotherapy needle before applying the polypectomy snare. Alternately, a ligating loop can be placed on the proximal stalk before the more distal stalk is divided with diathermy snare.

6a–e Endoscopic snare wires are characteristically thick, to guard against cutting too fast, but care should be taken not to apply excessive mechanical pressure before adequate electrocoagulation has occurred, otherwise 'cheese-wiring' of an uncoagulated stalk may occur with consequent hemorrhage. A low-power coagulating current (15–25 W) is employed until local whitening or swelling of the stalk indicates adequate coagulation, at which point tight strangulation should result in severance of the head. If bleeding does occur, the stalk remnant can be quickly regrasped with the loop and strangulated for 15 minutes, after which bleeding will not normally recur. The correct position of the snare is shown in panel (a). Care must be taken to avoid contact of the polyp surface with the opposite wall leading to burns from dissipation of the current (b). Burns may also result if the active electrode or metal components of the colonoscope tip are in contact with the local tissue (c,d) or if the electrode is in contact with a pool of fluid (e).

Rarely, sessile polyps are found. These may be removed by endomucosal resection (EMR), but this is an advanced technique and beyond the scope of this chapter.

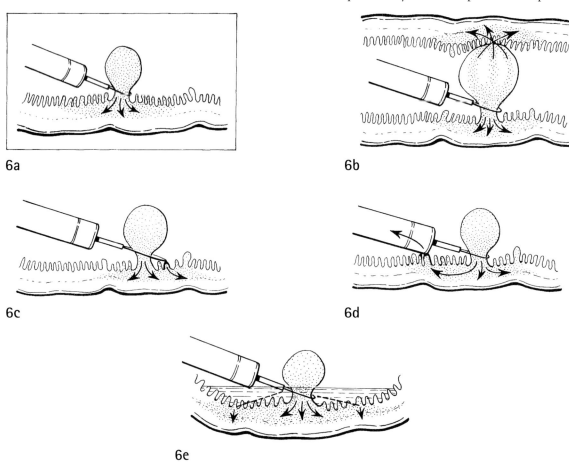

6a

6b

6c

6d

6e

Other therapeutic maneuvers

Electrocoagulation of a telangiectasia or cavernous hemangioma (blue rubber-bleb nevus syndrome) is easy through the colonoscope. The use of laser photocoagulation for this purpose has been described but is probably unnecessary, since careful local electrocoagulation with hot biopsy forceps or judicious scleropathy of raised lesions, repeated as necessary, gives excellent results. Strictures, particularly anastomotic strictures after resection of Crohn's disease, can be successfully dilated with transendoscopic balloon dilators. The colonoscope can be used to introduce guidewires, tubes, and other devices to any point in the colon, although this is rarely indicated in pediatric practice. The use of submucosally injected Indian ink can be useful as a long-lasting marker. Surface irrigation with colorant (1:4 dilution of washable blue fountain pen ink is convenient) can be helpful in demonstrating the smallest lesions in conditions such as familial adenomatous polyposis.

A final therapeutic use of the colonoscope is that of insertion of an ACE button to allow colonic irrigation. The button can be placed in the cecum (ACE) or sigmoid (DACE) and is performed in two stages. First, inserting a tube and then, 6 weeks later, changing the tube for a button. The first stage is performed exactly as per insertion of a PEG tube (**Chapter 44, Gastrostomy**) and in the cecum is a relatively easy and quick procedure. It is more challenging in the sigmoid as it is difficult to keep the sigmoid insufflated compared to the cecum (or stomach).

The authors first place a 15 Fr Freka tube® so that when it is changed to a 14 Fr MicKey® or Mini button®, the button slips in with no resistance.

POSTOPERATIVE CARE

In most cases, no special care is needed after colonoscopy, apart from a short period of rest until the after-effects of sedation or anesthesia wear off. Food and drink can be taken immediately. When the patient appears and feels well, normal activities can be resumed, with many examinations being performed on a day-case basis.

Follow up is probably unnecessary after colonoscopic polypectomy if only between one and three juvenile polyps are present in the colon; larger numbers may suggest the possibility of juvenile polyposis, which mandates follow up because of the association with dysplastic foci. The other most common group undergoing surveillance is children with familial adenomatous polyposis prior to corrective surgery.

Complications

The main risk is that of perforation. The risk is about 1:1000. The presence of severe acute inflammatory bowel disease with peritonism or deep ulceration, however, increases the possibility of perforation. Even in a normal colon, if the procedure proves technically difficult, common sense may nonetheless recommend abandonment of an examination. It is expected that successful cecal intubation is greater than 90 percent and ileal intubation is greater than 85 percent. Neonatal examination is the most difficult. The highest percentage of complications occurs following therapeutic maneuvers, such as snare polypectomy, when both perforation and bleeding have been reported. It is recognized that delayed perforation after polypectomy may occur, and this may also be seen after a 'hot biopsy' which is why EMR is now preferable to hot biopsies in adult practice.

FURTHER READING

Cotton PB, Williams CB. *Practical Gastrointestinal Endoscopy: The Fundamentals*, 6th edn. Oxford: Wiley-Blackwell, 2008.

Hassall E, Ament M. Total colonoscopy in children. *Archives of Disease in Childhood* 1983; **58**: 76–7.

Wyllie R, Kay MH. Colonoscopy and therapeutic interventions in infants and children. *Gastrointestinal Endoscopy Clinics of North America* 1994; **4**: 143–60.

SECTION IV

Thoracic

Thoracic surgery: general principles of access

SHAUN M KUNISAKI and JAMES D GEIGER

PRINCIPLES AND JUSTIFICATION

This chapter describes the basic operative approaches to the chest in pediatric thoracic surgery. These approaches include traditional posterolateral thoracotomy, muscle-sparing thoracotomy, axillary thoracotomy, median sternotomy, and more recently, thoracoscopy. The skilled pediatric surgeon should be comfortable with all of these modes of access. Based on the underlying pathology, a properly chosen incision can provide optimal exposure of the structure of interest. Conversely, the wrong thoracic approach can lead to poor visualization of the operative field with unnecessary intraoperative and postoperative morbidity.

ANESTHESIA

General endotracheal anesthesia is required for most intrathoracic operations. The notable exception to this rule would be a biopsy in a child with tracheal compression from a giant anterior mediastinal mass. In this case, local anesthesia would be advised because of the risk of complete airway loss associated with using muscle relaxants upon induction.

Following the administration of general anesthesia, tracheal intubation can be sufficient for many open and minimally invasive procedures, such as thoracoscopic pulmonary decortication, because of the relatively easy visualization of the pleural space following collapse of the ipsilateral lung with carbon dioxide insufflation. In these situations, asking the anesthesiologist to ventilate with smaller tidal volumes, lower peak pressures, and high respiratory rates can sometimes further enhance exposure.

However, there are many cases, such as in thoracoscopic pulmonary lobectomy, in which selective intubation to better isolate the lung is essential. These techniques require an experienced anesthesiologist. Intubation of the contralateral mainstem bronchus with an uncuffed tube is one relatively easy option for selective intubation in all age groups. However, one drawback is that mainstem intubation does not always give complete lung isolation unless there is a good seal and no overflow ventilation.

Another well-described technique is the bronchial blocker, which is a 5-Fr catheter that is deployed to occlude the ipsilateral mainstem bronchus. Bronchial blockers have a high-volume, low-pressure balloon to isolate the lung, but require at least a 4.5-sized endotracheal tube for deployment. Therefore, bronchial blockers are generally restricted to children who are at least 6–12 months of age. A 3- or 4-Fr Fogarty balloon can similarly act as a useful bronchial blocker in smaller infants but is discouraged because the low-volume, high-pressure properties of the balloon can theoretically damage the airways with prolonged occlusion. In our experience, bronchial blockers can be difficult to properly position within the mainstem bronchus, can often become displaced, and thus are not an ideal option for lung isolation.

Double lumen tubes can be an excellent choice for lung isolation since they provide contralateral ventilation and ipsilateral balloon occlusion. Unfortunately, these devices generally cannot be used in children of less than eight to ten years of age (about 25 kg) since the smallest tubes require a 26-Fr airway.

The management of postoperative pain after a thoracotomy incision should be discussed with the anesthesiologist prior to the operation. The options include patient/nurse-controlled anesthesia, thoracic epidural catheters, pleural catheters, and intermittent intravenous dosing of pain medications, depending on the type of incision and the age of the patient.

OPEN APPROACHES

Posterolateral thoracotomy

Because children have more compliant ribs and are relatively short along their longitudinal axis compared to their adult counterparts, visualization of the pediatric hemithorax through a traditional posterolateral thoracotomy incision is generally excellent.

POSITION OF PATIENT AND INCISION

1 The child lies in the full lateral decubitus position. In older children, exposure of the intercostal spaces can be enhanced by positioning the patient's iliac spine over the point of flexion on the table. The ipsilateral arm is rotated anterior and cephalad above the nipple. An axillary roll may reduce iatrogenic injury to the brachial plexus, particularly in longer cases. The child is firmly stabilized in position with towel rolls, gel padding, or a vacuum-type bean bag at the front and back of the chest and abdomen. Care is taken not to create any obstruction or impedance of the incision on range of motion during thoracoscopic approaches. Adhesive strapping is attached across the hips to the operating table and similarly across the uppermost arm and shoulder. The lower leg is well padded and should be flexed at the knee. The upper leg should be straight.

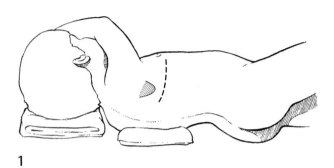

1

The skin is widely cleansed with antiseptic solution. Sterile towels are placed to keep the nipple, lower scapula, spine, and costal margin visible as landmarks. The position of the scapula tip, as well as the nipple, should be marked. A large adhesive plastic sheet can be applied to stabilize the towels and reduce heat loss. The lower chest wall is included in the operative field for later chest drain placement, if required.

The transverse skin incision starts around the mid-axillary line just below the level of the nipple. In prepubertal girls, the skin incision should be kept well away from the nipple to avoid scarring of the underlying mammary tissue. The incision extends posteriorly about 1 cm below the inferior tip of the scapula. In teenagers and young adults, an adult-type posterolateral thoracotomy incision that extends posterior to the latissimus dorsi may be required. Rarely, the incision may have to be gently curved further along a line that bisects between the vertebral column and the posterior aspect of the scapula. The subcutaneous tissues are divided.

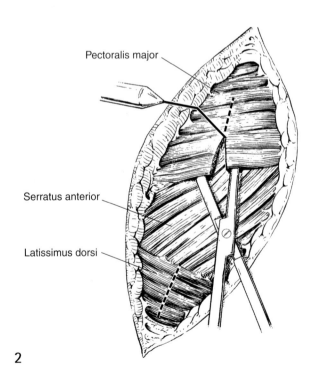

Pectoralis major

Serratus anterior

Latissimus dorsi

2

2 In the traditional posterolateral thoracotomy, the latissimus dorsi muscles and the serratus anterior muscle are divided. Artery forceps are used to elevate each muscle while it is incised with diathermy. Posteriorly, the latissimus dorsi muscle can be transected as far as the erector spinae muscle without concern for causing iatrogenic scoliosis. Bleeding vessels are accurately coagulated using fine-toothed forceps. The long thoracic nerve runs near the anterior border of the serratus anterior muscle and must be protected. Should it be necessary to divide the nerve, this can be done as far caudally as possible to minimize the effect of a winged scapula. If necessary, the pectoralis major may be incised.

Once the intercostal muscles are identified, the scapula is elevated with a retractor. The ribs are palpated and counted. In an older child, the highest rib that can be palpated is usually the second rib, on which the posterior scalene muscle inserts laterally. In an infant, the first rib can usually be palpated. The target rib is marked with the diathermy. The fifth intercostal space provides adequate exposure for most pediatric thoracic procedures, including those involving the diaphragm. A key exception is esophageal atresia in which the fourth intercostal space is optimal.

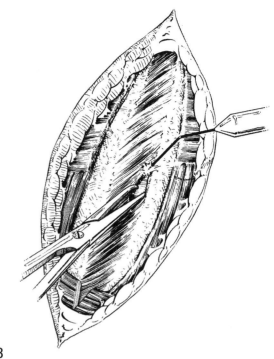

OPENING THE CHEST: INTERCOSTAL TRANSPLEURAL APPROACH

3 The fifth intercostal space is entered by dividing the intercostal muscle and pleura along the superior aspect of the sixth rib with diathermy. This avoids injury to the neurovascular bundle that lies just inferior to the rib in a recessed groove. A short incision is made initially, using artery forceps to spread the muscle and with the ipsilateral lung deflated by the anesthesiologist. The remaining intercostal muscles and pleura are divided, using a peanut swab or similar retractor to protect the lung.

3

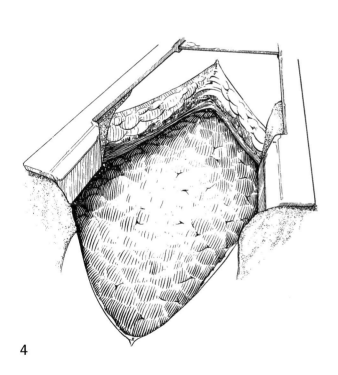

4 The rib retractor (such as the Finochietto retractor) is inserted and opened slowly while dividing the intercostal muscles anteriorly and posteriorly until there is visualization of the longitudinal fibers of the sacrospinus muscles. Care must be taken to avoid excessive pressure from the retractor as this may fracture the ribs posteriorly, particularly in infants. Because the ribs are more compliant in children, excision of a subperiosteal segment of the rib, often referred to as shingling, is not necessary. The chest wall muscles and subcutaneous tissues may also need to be incised further to ease the tension on the ribs.

4

OPENING THE CHEST: INTERCOSTAL EXTRAPLEURAL APPROACH

5 Division of the intercostal muscles begins as above using artery forceps to enter the extrapleural space in the posterior half of the incision and diathermy to incise the muscle. Great care must be taken not to open the parietal pleura.

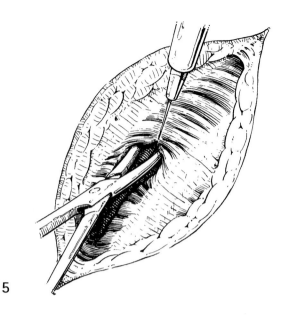

5

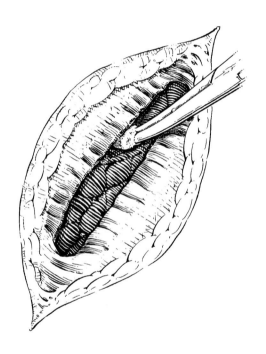

6

6 A moist cotton tip applicator is used carefully to extend the dissection in the extrapleural plane. The initial dissection should proceed in a posterior direction. Anteriorly, the parietal pleura is adherent to the ribs and can be easily torn.

7 A cotton tip applicator is used to further develop the extrapleural space posteriorly and superiorly in order to further strip the pleura from the chest wall. The rib retractor is readjusted and the extrapleural dissection to the posterior mediastinum is completed under direct vision. A moistened gauze sponge can also be used to facilitate this dissection.

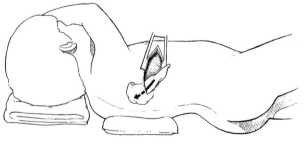

7

WOUND CLOSURE

8 Before closing the chest, posterior rib blocks with bupivicaine above and below the level of the thoracotomy should be performed. Between two and four pericostal sutures are passed around the ribs above and below the incision, taking care to avoid the intercostal vessels. In infants, an absorbable suture is used and the ribs are loosely approximated such that the normal intercostal space is preserved. Tight apposition of the ribs is to be avoided to prevent rib fusion that may lead to increased pain and other morbidities. Repair of the intercostal muscles is not essential.

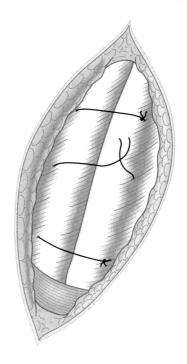

8

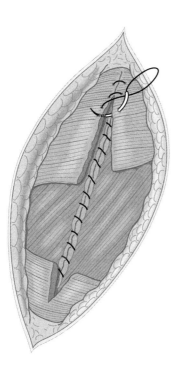

9

9 Any divided chest wall muscles are accurately realigned and approximated in anatomic layers using continuous absorbable sutures. The subcutaneous tissues and skin are closed in layers to provide a watertight seal. Additional local anesthetic can be infiltrated into the subcutaneous tissues.

POSTOPERATIVE CARE

Effective systemic analgesia is essential for the patient's comfort and to facilitate early postoperative physiotherapy and mobilization, which will reduce the risk of atelectasis and pulmonary infections. The use of intravenous and/ or oral non-steroidal inflammatory medications can be effective adjuncts in pain management.

COMPLICATIONS

Early complications include intercostal vessel bleeding and wound infection. Damage to the long thoracic nerve results in winging of the scapula. If the incision is too close to the inferior angle of the scapula, adhesions to the scapula may develop, leading to limited shoulder abduction and elevation. Overzealous reapproximation on the ribs can lead to chest wall deformities and scoliosis. In infants, all follow-up evaluations should include an examination of the spine to screen for scoliosis.

Muscle-sparing thoracotomy

10 The muscle-sparing thoracotomy approach is an excellent alternative to the traditional posterolateral thoracotomy in children. Preservation of the chest wall muscles may reduce postoperative pain and other morbidities. The same skin incision is utilized, and the dissection is carried down through the subcutaneous tissues. Following this, superior and inferior skin flaps are raised, leaving the fascia intact on the muscle. The thin fascial attachments along the anterior border of the latissimus dorsi are incised with diathermy to facilitate retraction of the muscle posteriorly. The fascia along the inferior border of the serratus anterior is incised. The serratus anterior is retracted both anteriorly and superiorly to expose the intercostal muscles. Occasionally, the lowermost origins of the serratus anterior limit the exposure and can be divided with diathermy. The thoracic cavity is entered through the fifth intercostal space, and the dissection proceeds as described above.

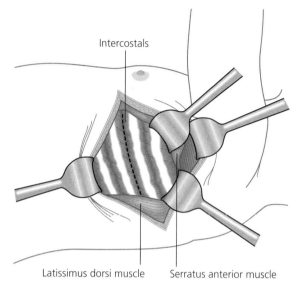

Intercostals

Latissimus dorsi muscle   Serratus anterior muscle

10

Axillary thoracotomy

Axillary thoracotomy is another approach to thoracic access, particularly when visualization of the upper mediastinum is desired. This incision gives excellent exposure of the lung apex, ductus arteriosus, sympathetic chain, and upper esophagus through either the third or fourth intercostal spaces. Axillary thoracotomy can be performed without dividing any major muscle groups and leaves a less conspicuous scar when compared to posterolateral thoracotomy.

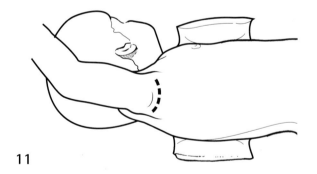

11

11 With the infant in the lateral decubitus position and the arm abducted at least 90° above the head, a curvilinear incision is made in a natural axillary skin crease, extending from the lateral border of the pectoralis muscles to the posterior axillary fold formed by the latissimus dorsi muscle. A vertical incision in the mid-axillary line down to the ninth intercostal space has also been advocated, but tends to leave a less cosmetically appealing scar.

12 The axillary fat pad and lymphoid tissues are then swept superiorly. The pectoralis and latissimus dorsi muscles are left intact. The serratus anterior is split transversely along the line of its fibers, taking care to avoid injury to the long thoracic nerve. Alternatively, the serratus anterior can be mobilized posteriorly and retracted anteriorly to preserve the long thoracic nerve. The thoracic cavity is entered through the third or fourth intercostal space, and the dissection proceeds as described above.

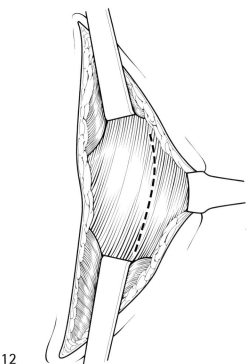

12

Median sternotomy

Although median sternotomy is widely popular in cardiac surgery, this mode of access has a limited role in non-cardiac, thoracic operations because visualization of the carina, lower lobes, and diaphragm is generally unsatisfactory. However, a median sternotomy can occasionally be useful when simultaneous access to the bilateral upper/middle lobes or anterior mediastinum (e.g. thymus, upper trachea) is desirable.

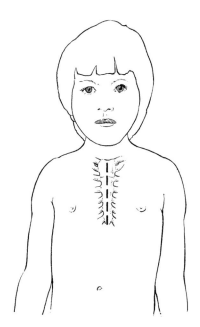

13

POSITION OF THE PATIENT AND INCISION

13 The child lies supine with the arms tucked and a shoulder roll placed to hyperextend the thoracic spine and bring the sternum forward. Slight elevation of the head of the operating table reduces venous congestion. The skin is incised from just below the suprasternal notch to the xiphoid cartilage. To minimize blood loss, diathermy is used to incise the subcutaneous tissues and decussating fibers of the pectoralis major muscle down to the periosteum.

14 In the suprasternal notch the soft tissues are dissected off the superior and posterior aspects of the manubrium with sharp and blunt dissection, taking care to avoid the innominate vein which runs transversely just underneath the sternal notch. Inferiorly, the xiphoid is mobilized and divided vertically with heavy scissors or diathermy. The retrosternal plane can be entered cranially and caudally using a peanut swab or index finger to free the mediastinal structures from the back of the sternum.

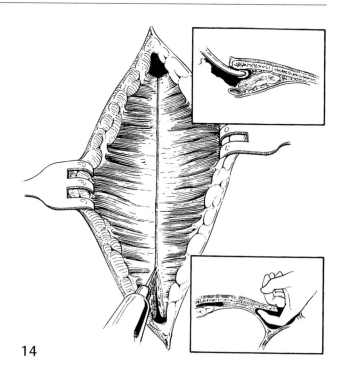

14

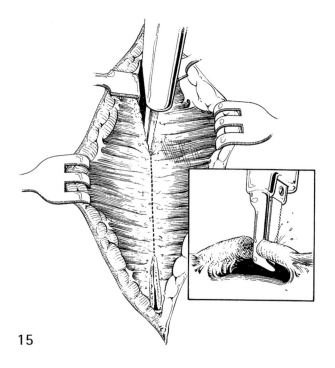

15

DIVIDING THE STERNUM

15 The sternum is divided vertically in infants using heavy shears. In older children, a bone saw is required. Ventilation should be suspended while this is done to avoid opening the pleura. Bleeding, which is usually from the periosteum or bone marrow, is controlled with diathermy and bone wax.

A self-retraining retractor is inserted and opened slowly while dissecting the soft tissues off the inner aspect of the ribs on either side, taking care not to tear the pleura. In the infant, it may be necessary to mobilize and retract or partially excise the thymus gland. This is done by sharp and blunt dissection from below cranially, ligating larger vessels as needed. Laterally, care must be taken not to damage the phrenic nerves.

WOUND CLOSURE

Regardless of whether the pleural cavity has been opened or not, one or two closed suction drainage catheters should be placed in the retrosternal space and brought out through stab incisions below and lateral to the xiphoid process. The drains are sutured to the skin with non-absorbable sutures.

16 The two halves of the sternum are apposed with No. 2 steel wires. Heavy sutures (e.g. polydioxanone sutures (PDS), polypropylene) can alternatively be used in infants. In older children, closure with No. 4 or No. 5 wires may be necessary. Wires should be driven through the sternum or taken around the edge of the sternum between sternocostal junctions.

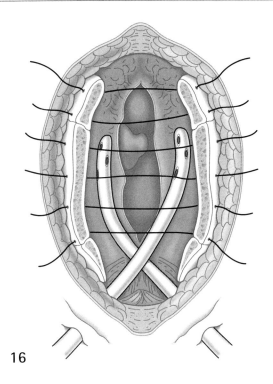

16

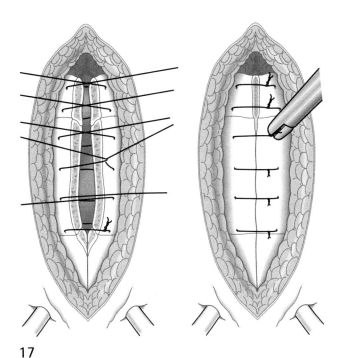

17

17 The ends of the wires are crossed, pulled, and twisted together between five and seven times. The surplus wire is then cut short and buried into the sternal tissues. The subcutaneous tissues are closed with continuous absorbable suture. The margins of the incision are infiltrated with local anesthetic, and the skin is approximated with fine absorbable subcuticular sutures.

POSTOPERATIVE CARE

Systemic analgesia is essential to ensure early mobilization. The drains are removed after 24 hours if no drainage or clinically significant pneumomediastinum is present.

THORACOSCOPIC SURGERY

Minimally invasive techniques have become the preferred operative approach for many thoracic operations, including lung biopsy, pulmonary decortication, and pleurodesis. In the hands of an advanced thoracoscopic surgeon, additional procedures, including diaphragmatic hernia repair, pulmonary lobectomy, and esophageal atresia/tracheoesophageal fistula repair can also be routinely performed in this manner.

Thoracoscopy offers a number of advantages compared to traditional thoracotomy including less pain and better cosmesis. Moreover, the current resolution of high definition optical systems gives better magnification and therefore superior visualization of the thoracic mediastinum, particularly in the apex. Another potential advantage of minimally invasive techniques is the avoidance of some of the long-term, postoperative morbidity associated with thoracotomy, including limitations in shoulder abduction, chest wall deformities, and scoliosis. Relative contraindications to thoracoscopy include hemodynamic instability requiring pressors, non-conventional ventilation, weight less than 2 kg, and concurrent support on extracorporeal membrane oxygenation (ECMO).

POSITION OF PATIENT AND INCISION

Proper positioning is especially critical for successful thoracoscopy in children. For lobectomy, lung biopsy, and pulmonary decortication, the patient should be in the lateral decubitus position. The same is true for diaphragmatic hernia repair, although the infant should be placed crosswise on the operating table to allow the surgeon to stand above the infant's head and preserve appropriate ergonomic alignment between the surgeon, diaphragm defect, and video monitor.

18 A modified supine position with the ipsilateral thorax elevated about 30° is preferred for biopsy of anterior mediastinal masses, aortopexy, and thymectomy. This position allows the lung to retract posteriorly to optimize visualization.

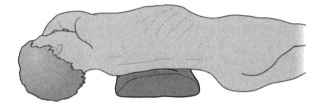

18

19 Conversely, a modified prone position is useful for posterior mediastinal masses, such as foregut duplications and neuroblastoma, and for esophageal atresia/tracheo-esophageal fistula repair.

19

Once appropriate padding of the child is ensured, the skin is widely cleansed with antiseptic solution and draped since emergent conversion to a thoracotomy is always a consideration. Careful planning of trocar placement is imperative because of the small intrathoracic working space and the potential to damage the thin and delicate thoracoscopic instruments against the rigid chest wall. Common regions for initial entry into the chest cavity are over a rib either posterior to the scapula tip in the 'triangle of auscultation' or inferiorly at a proposed chest tube site. After the skin incision is made, the pleural space is accessed with a Veress needle or artery forceps. A 5-mm trocar is gently inserted, and the thorax is insufflated with carbon dioxide to 4 mmHg at a flow rate of 0.1–5 L/second. Higher flow rates can lead to desiccation of the tissues. A 5-mm 30° thoracoscope is used to inspect the chest cavity. For all these positions, the use of gravity by rotation of the bed can be helpful to keep the uninvolved lung and other structures out of the field. If necessary, insufflation pressures of up to 12 mmHg can be tolerated for short periods of time if initial operative visualization is poor.

20 Many chest procedures require dissection in a focused area within the mediastinum. In these situations, a triangular arrangement of the trocars works best with the camera port placed slightly above and between the two working ports. This allows the surgeon to look down on the field of view and to minimize instrument dueling. The use of 3- or 5-mm ports/instruments is standard in children, depending on the size of the patient. Larger children have wider intercostal spaces that can usually accommodate 12-mm trocars for endoscopic linear stapling. Larger trocars are ideally placed through a lower interspace to maximize working space for the staple head. If the anesthesiologist can effectively establish lung isolation, some surgeons prefer to insert and remove instruments through stab incisions since maintaining positive insufflation pressures within the mediastinum may not be necessary. Upon completion of the procedure, all incisions are infiltrated with local anesthetic and closed in one or two layers using non-absorbable sutures.

Lesion

Port sites

20

CHEST TUBES

Any thoracotomy or thoracoscopic procedure in which an air leak or accumulation of pleural fluid is anticipated postoperatively requires placement of an intercostal chest tube at the end of the procedure. Typical tube sizes range from 12 to 28 Fr, depending on the size of the patient and type of pleural drainage anticipated.

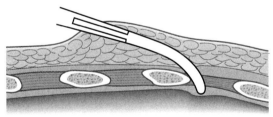

21

21 Under direct visualization, the chest tube is positioned posteriorly and towards the apex to facilitate drainage and re-expansion of the lung. The skin incision is ideally placed well away from the thoracotomy incision or through one of the existing trocar sites. An incision adjacent to the costodiaphragmatic recess at least one intercostal space below the site of intercostal entry is preferred to minimize postoperative leakage, particularly in children who have a thin chest wall. The tube should always exit the body anterior to the mid-axillary line extending down to the anterior superior iliac spine. Chest tubes placed posterior to this are more painful and prone to kink. Many chest tubes placed in infants may need to be cut in length to avoiding kinking. Heavy non-absorbable suture is used to secure the tube to the skin followed by application of an occlusive, adherent dressing.

Depending on the level of concern for a parenchymal air leak, the chest tube should immediately be connected to low-pressure suction (5–15 cm water) or water seal. A chest radiograph to confirm adequate chest tube positioning is mandatory. The use of antibiotic prophylaxis while the chest tube is in place remains controversial. The chest tube should be removed if the lung stays fully expanded on water seal, air leaks have resolved for 24–48 hours, and fluid drainage is minimal, typically defined as less than 2.5 mL/kg per day.

FURTHER READING

Bianchi A, Sowande O, Alizai NK *et al.* Aesthetics and lateral thoracotomy in the neonate. *Journal of Pediatric Surgery* 1998; **33**: 1798–800.

Jaureguizar E, Vazquez J, Murcia J *et al.* Morbid musculoskeletal sequelae of thoracotomy for tracheoesophageal fistula. *Journal of Pediatric Surgery* 1985; **20**: 511–14.

Rodgers BM. The role of thoracoscopy in pediatric surgical practice. *Seminars in Pediatric Surgery* 2003; **12**: 62–70.

Rothenberg SS, Pokorny WJ. Experience with a total muscle-sparing approach for thoracotomies in neonates, infants, and children. *Journal of Pediatric Surgery* 1992; **27**: 1157–9.

Singh SJ, Kapila L. Denis Browne's thoracotomy revised. *Pediatric Surgery International* 2002; **18**: 90–2.

Soucy P, Bass J, Evans M. The muscle-sparing thoracotomy in infants and children. *Journal of Pediatric Surgery* 1991; **26**: 1323–5.

Esophageal atresia with and without tracheoesophageal fistula

LEWIS SPITZ and AGOSTINO PIERRO

HISTORY

The first description of esophageal atresia is credited to Durston who, in 1670, described esophageal atresia in one of a pair of conjoined twins. Thomas Gibson in 1697 accurately described the clinical features of esophageal atresia. In 1913, Richter proposed a plan of management, which comprised dividing the tracheoesophageal fistula (TEF) and feeding the infant by gastrostomy until the 'technical difficulties of an esophageal anastomosis' had been overcome. Ladd and Leven were independently the first to achieve long-term survival in 1939, but only by a staged approach. Haight in 1941 is credited with the first successful primary anastomosis.

PRINCIPLES AND JUSTIFICATION

Embryology

The respiratory primordium first appears as a ventral diverticulum of the foregut at day 22–23 of gestation. This is followed by a period of rapid growth when the ventrally placed trachea separates from the dorsally placed esophagus. One theory postulates that the trachea becomes a separate organ as a result of rapid longitudinal growth of the respiratory primordium away from the foregut. An alternative theory is that the trachea initially grows as part of an undivided foregut and then becomes a separate structure as a result of a separation process that starts at the level of the lung buds and proceeds in a cranial direction. This process is associated with a precise temporospatial pattern of expression of the developmental gene sonic hedgehog (*Shh*). The primary defect resulting in esophageal atresia is persistence of an undivided foregut either as a result of failure of tracheal growth or of failure of the already specified trachea to separate physically from the esophagus.

Classification of esophageal atresia

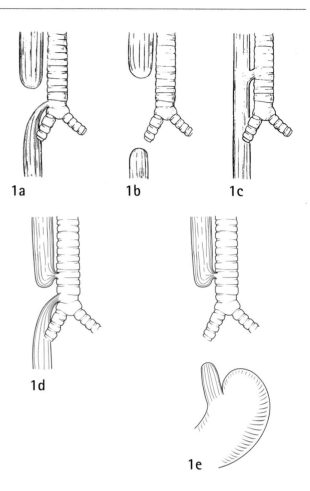

1a–e The various types of esophageal atresia are: (a) esophageal atresia with distal fistula (85 percent), Gross C; (b) esophageal atresia without fistula (6 percent), Gross A; (c) H-type TEF (4 percent), Gross E; (d) esophageal atresia with proximal and distal fistula (1 percent), Gross D; (e) esophageal atresia with proximal fistula (4 percent), Gross B.

Associated anomalies

At least 50 percent of infants with esophageal atresia have one or more associated anomalies (**Table 17.1**). Most common are cardiac malformations, particularly ventricular septal defects and tetralogy of Fallot, and these are responsible for the majority of deaths. Next most common are gastrointestinal and anorectal anomalies, followed by genitourinary tract abnormalities. The VACTERL association (V, vertebral; A, anorectal; C, cardiac; T, trachea; E, esophageal; R, renal; L, limb) is a well-known combination of defects.

Table 17.1 Anomalies associated with esophageal atresia.

	%
Cardiovascular	29
Anorectal	14
Genitourinary	14
Gastrointestinal	13
Vertebral/skeletal	10
Respiratory	6
Genetic	4
Other	11

A full clinical examination should be made at the outset for associated anomalies, and special investigations, including echocardiography and renal ultrasonography, are carried out as indicated.

Prognosis

In 1962, Waterston proposed a risk classification for infants with esophageal atresia based on his experience in the management of 218 infants as follows:

- **Group A** (95 percent survival): birth weight over 5.5 lb (2.5 kg) and well.
- **Group B** (68 percent survival):
  - birth weight 4–5.5 lb (1.8–2.5 kg) and well;
  - higher birth weight, moderate pneumonia, and congenital anomaly.
- **Group C** (6 percent survival):
  - birth weight under 4 lb (1.8 kg);
  - higher birth weight, severe pneumonia, and severe congenital anomaly.

An amended classification more relevant to modern pediatric surgical practice is shown in **Table 17.2**.

Table 17.2 Spitz prognostic classification.

Group		Survival (%)
I	Birth weight >1500 g and no major cardiac anomaly	98
II	Birth weight <1500 g or major cardiac anomaly	82
III	Birth weight <1500 g plus major cardiac anomaly	50

Diagnosis

ANTENATAL

Polyhydramnios is present in 95 percent of patients with isolated atresia without fistula and in 35 percent of cases with a distal fistula.

With expert fetal ultrasonography, it is possible to visualize the blind upper esophageal pouch filling and emptying, and an inability to detect the stomach would suggest atresia without fistula. The combination of polyhydramnios with a small or absent fetal stomach has a 56 percent positive predictive value for esophageal atresia.

POSTNATAL

A nasogastric tube (8–10 gauge) should be passed at birth in all cases where polyhydramnios was present during pregnancy. Failure to advance the tube beyond 10 cm from the nose or mouth indicates esophageal atresia.

Symptoms that develop in the neonatal period include inability to clear secretions from the mouth, cyanotic episodes with or without attempting to feed the infant, inability to swallow, and respiratory distress.

PREOPERATIVE

Investigations

2 Plain radiography of chest and abdomen demonstrates a radio-opaque nasogastric tube (Replogle type) arrested in the upper mediastinum, and air in the stomach and intestine confirms the presence of a distal TEF.

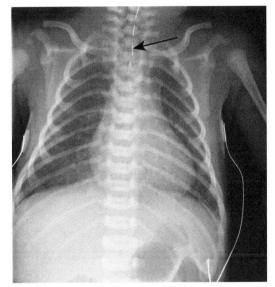

2

3 The absence of intestinal air suggests the diagnosis of pure esophageal atresia. Contrast studies of the upper pouch are seldom indicated. Endoscopic examination of the upper esophagus and/or bronchoscopy immediately before surgery will detect an upper pouch fistula if present (10 percent of cases with distal atresia). If contrast medium is used, the examination should be performed with extreme care by an experienced radiologist.

3

Initial management

Immediate surgery for esophageal atresia is seldom necessary. Scheduling the operation 12–24 hours after admission allows for full assessment for associated anomalies and resolution of pulmonary atelectasis if aspiration has occurred prior to referral. Neonates with respiratory distress requiring assisted ventilation, particularly if associated with gastric distension, should undergo emergency transpleural ligation of the distal fistula. This will immediately improve the respiratory status, and gas exchange in the lungs will improve as the escape of gas through the fistula is halted. In some infants, the improvement is so dramatic as to allow primary repair of the atresia to proceed. In others, the procedure is terminated pending improvement in the infant's condition. The repair can be safely postponed for up to 7 days; further delay increases the risk of the fistula reopening. Gastrostomy as a primary procedure in these high-risk neonates is to be avoided.

While awaiting surgery, the upper pouch is continuously aspirated using a Replogle tube attached to low-pressure suction. Intravenous fluids (10 percent dextrose in 0.18 percent saline) will maintain fluid and electrolyte balance and prevent hypoglycemia. Preoperatively, a vitamin K analog should be routinely administered intramuscularly. An echocardiogram prior to surgery is highly recommended to diagnose cardiac defects and to determine the position of the aortic arch.

Choice of operation

In most neonates with esophageal atresia and a distal TEF, division of the fistula and primary anastomosis of the esophagus are possible. The anastomosis should be attempted, even if performed under extreme tension. The presence of a right-sided aortic arch, best identified on an echocardiogram, would indicate a left-sided thoracotomy to provide easier access to the mediastinum.

A short upper pouch on the preliminary plain x-ray may also indicate that a primary anastomosis may be difficult. The presence of a distal TEF requiring division dictates the necessity for right thoracotomy, and the possibility of obtaining a satisfactory primary anastomosis should not be ruled out until the anatomy has been inspected at the time of the thoracotomy.

The absence of a lower pouch fistula is usually associated with a long gap between the upper and lower esophagus. This situation is usually managed by a preliminary feeding gastrostomy. If esophageal replacement is the procedure of choice, a cervical esophagostomy is necessary, unless a primary replacement in the neonatal period is proposed. The alternative is a delayed primary anastomosis after several weeks of gastrostomy feeding and upper pouch suction. The decision about when to attempt the delayed primary anastomosis is based on radiological assessment of the intervening gap. With a Replogle tube in the proximal esophagus and a urethral dilator introduced into the distal esophagus through the gastrostomy stoma under fluoroscopic control, the size of the gap between the upper and lower esophagus is measured. If the gap measures less than the width of two vertebral bodies, primary anastomosis should be attempted. A gap greater than six vertebrae may indicate the need for an esophageal replacement. In general, it is not profitable to wait longer than 8–12 weeks before deciding how to proceed.

PREOPERATIVE

The Replogle tube or a similar large-bore tube should be in position in the upper pouch. Careful attention is paid to maintaining body temperature with a heating blanket, and to preventing heat loss by covering the infant with foil. Broad-spectrum antibiotics should be administered either preoperatively or at the time of induction.

Anesthesia

Premedication is with atropine alone. The endotracheal tube requires careful positioning to permit adequate ventilation with minimal gas flow through the fistula. The majority of pediatric anesthetists will control ventilation

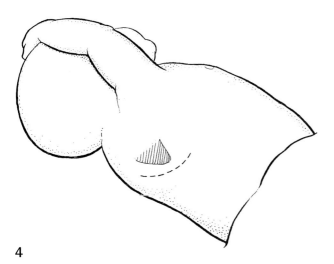

4

from an early stage following intubation. An intravenous infusion is sited in a limb other than the right upper limb.

Preliminary endoscopy

Many surgeons advocate preliminary bronchoscopy to define the site of entry of the distal TEF, to exclude the presence of a proximal fistula, and to assess the degree of tracheomalacia. A distal TEF entering the trachea at the level of the carina may indicate a 'wide-gap' atresia. Esophagoscopy will define the length of the upper pouch and exclude an upper pouch fistula (more common in isolated atresia) that enters the side of the proximal pouch at some distance from its distal end (see **Figure 17.1** which shows the steps to consider in the treatment of isolated esophageal atresia).

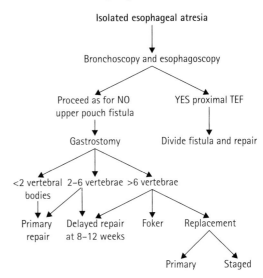

Figure 17.1 Steps to consider in the treatment of isolated esophageal atresia.

OPERATION

Classic repair

INCISION

4 The infant is positioned on the left side and stabilized with jelly bags. The right arm is extended above the head and fixed. Care must be taken to ensure that the neck is flexed. A curved incision is made 1 cm below the inferior angle of the scapula extending from the mid-axillary line to the paravertebral region posteriorly. Division of the subcutaneous tissues and muscles is carried out with diathermy to minimize blood loss. The latissimus dorsi muscle is divided along the length of the incision. Serratus anterior is retracted forwards, but if additional exposure is required, the lowermost fibers only are divided in order to preserve its nerve supply. Alternatively, access to the intercostal spaces may be via the angle of auscultation whose borders are trapezius above, latissimus dorsi below, and the medial border of the scapula laterally. Following division of the muscles, the scapula is elevated and the rib spaces are counted by palpation.

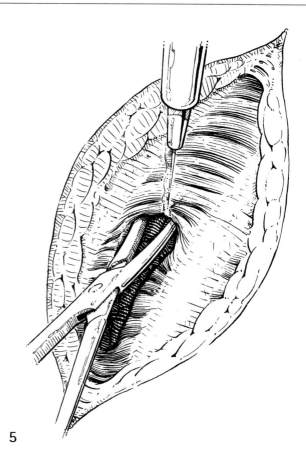

5 The thorax is entered through the fourth or fifth intercostal space by carefully dividing the external and then the internal intercostal muscles. The muscle fibers are gently elevated from the underlying parietal pleura and divided using diathermy.

5

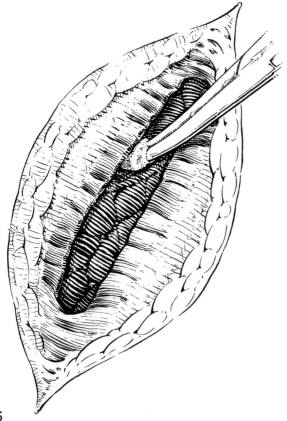

6

6 Having exposed the pleura through the intercostal space, stripping of the pleura from the chest wall is best carried out by the gentle insertion of a gauze swab into the extrapleural space. On withdrawing the swab, an extensive area of dissection will have resulted; a rib spreader can then be inserted and the ribs gently separated. Further posterior dissection of the pleura is achieved by using moist pledgets; a pair of pledgets used simultaneously is most satisfactory.

7 The azygos vein and the posterior mediastinum should be exposed, enabling the lower pouch, upper pouch, and fistula to be seen. Anterior dissection of the pleura should be sufficient only to allow the ribs to be adequately spread. Very occasionally, the size or position of the fistula may make it impossible for the anesthetist to ventilate the lungs adequately. In that situation, the more rapid transpleural approach to the fistula may be necessary. In order to expose the posterior mediastinum effectively, lung retraction is essential, but care must be taken to ensure that the retractor does not compress the mediastinal structures.

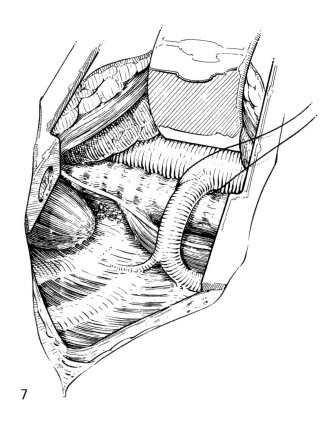

7

MOBILIZATION OF LOWER ESOPHAGUS AND DIVISION OF FISTULA

The azygos vein is ligated and divided. The lower esophagus may be obvious, distending with each inspiration as it lies in the lower posterior mediastinum. The close proximity of the vagus nerve to the lower esophagus aids in its identification.

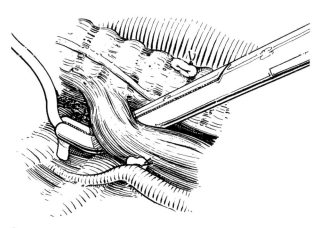

8

8 Every attempt must be made during dissection to preserve the fibers of the vagus nerve supplying the lower esophagus. The lower esophagus is dissected circumferentially to just distal to the fistula and a loop is placed around it. Traction on this loop controls the fistula and enables the junction of the lower esophagus and trachea to be accurately defined and dissected. In addition, occlusion of the fistula by traction on the loop or applying a soft clamp across the fistula while inflating the lungs will eliminate the possibility of mistaking the right main bronchus for the distal esophagus.

9a,b After carefully defining the junction between the trachea and esophagus, two 5/0 polypropylene (Prolene) sutures are placed in the trachea at the extremities of the fistula and the fistula is divided a few millimeters distal to its entry into the trachea. The trachea is closed with interrupted sutures. The air-tightness of the closure should be tested by instilling a few milliliters of saline into the mediastinum and watching for bubbles on ventilation. An alternative means of closing the fistula is to transfix it close to the trachea with a 5/0 suture. A small tube is passed through the open end of the distal esophagus into the stomach to ensure that an adequate lumen exists and to enable air distending the stomach to be aspirated. Dissection of the lower esophagus needs care to preserve the vagal attachments and prevent damage to the adjacent thoracic duct and left pleura. A 5/0 stay suture allows traction to be exerted on the lower esophagus without handling with forceps. Dissection should be the minimum required to achieve an anastomosis.

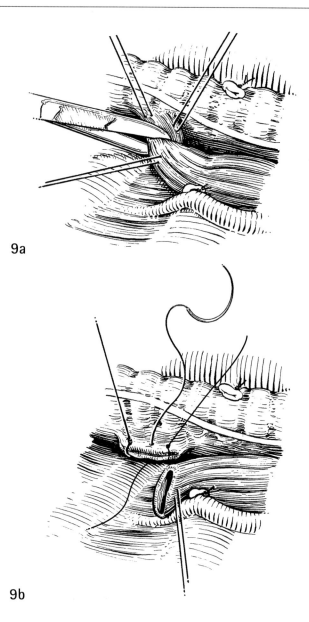

9a

9b

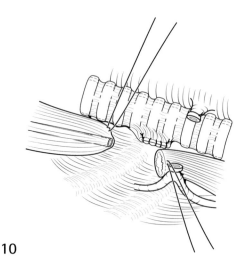

10

IDENTIFICATION OF UPPER POUCH

10 If the upper pouch is not immediately visible, pressure on the Replogle tube by the anesthetist will usually advance it into the mediastinum. Dissection of the upper pouch should be sufficient to allow an opening to be made in the distal end for an anastomosis to be performed. As with the lower esophagus, branches of the vagus supplying the upper esophagus should not be disturbed. Dissection in the plane between the esophagus and trachea should be carried out with extreme care to avoid inadvertently opening either structure. A stay suture can be placed in the muscular wall of the esophagus to facilitate its exposure and minimize the need for forceps traction. When opening the upper esophagus, care should be taken to ensure that the opening is at the lowermost point; this is most reliably recognized by pushing the Replogle tube down and incising the esophagus over the tip of the tube. The size of the opening in the upper esophagus should correspond to the diameter of the lower esophagus.

ANASTOMOSIS

11 This is achieved using interrupted 5/0 or 6/0 sutures positioned along the posterior aspect of the anastomosis, particular care being taken to ensure that both mucosa and muscle are included in each suture. It is seldom necessary to insert more than four or five sutures. Unless the two ends of the esophagus are very close together, all the sutures are placed in position in the posterior layer before they are tied in sequence.

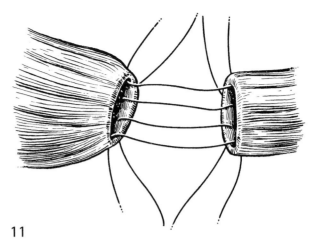

11

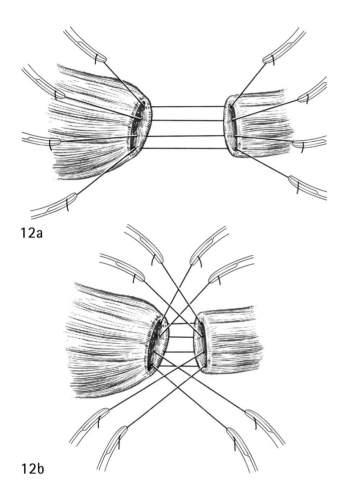

12a

12b

ANASTOMOSIS UNDER TENSION

12a,b The posterior layer of sutures is inserted and the ends of each suture are held separately in artery forceps. The sutures with the attached forceps are crossed over and gradual tension applied, bringing the proximal and distal halves of the posterior esophagus toward each other. While maintaining tension on the sutures, each one is tied in turn, thereby distributing the tension on the suture line over a wider area.

13 Following completion of the posterior layer of the anastomosis, a fine-bore feeding tube may replace the Replogle tube and it is then advanced across the anastomosis into the stomach. The anterior layer of the anastomosis is then completed over the tube. The use of a nerve hook avoids the need to use forceps on the open ends of the esophagus when placing the sutures. Once the anastomosis is complete, the intraesophageal tube may be withdrawn; if it is to be left *in situ* for feeding, its mobility should be checked to ensure that a suture has not inadvertently passed through or around it.

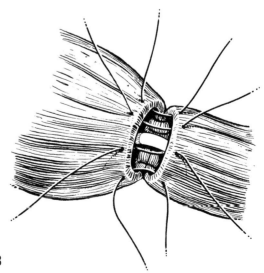

13

WOUND CLOSURE

14 The lung is expanded following the placement of two pericostal 3/0 sutures. The muscles and subcutaneous tissues are closed with a 4/0 suture and the skin with a subcuticular suture.

A chest drain is only used in specific circumstances, e.g. trauma to the underlying pleura and lung, or occasionally in a very tight anastomosis. The tip of the drain should be sutured to the lateral chest wall away from the anastomotic site with 4/0 chromic catgut.

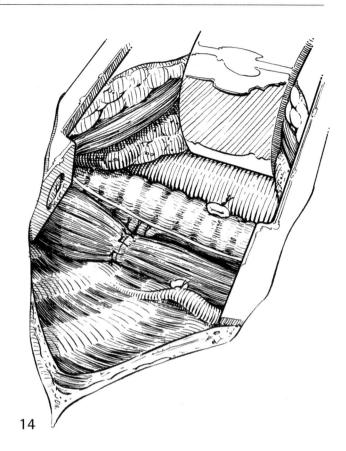

14

Thoracoscopic repair

THORACOSCOPIC REPAIR OF ESOPHAGEAL ATRESIA WITH TRACHEOESOPHAGEAL FISTULA

The main advantage of the thoracoscopic repair is the reduction in the musculoskeletal sequelae that may develop following thoracotomy in the newborn. Musculoskeletal deformities, including 'winged' scapula, asymmetry of the thoracic wall secondary to atrophy of the serratus anterior muscle, and thoracic scoliosis, have been reported in 33 percent of neonates who have had a thoracotomy for esophageal atresia. Mammary maldevelopment has also been reported. Theoretical advantages also include improved anatomical visualization and less extensive dissection of the esophageal pouches. Conversely, the incidence of anastomotic stricture and the recurrence of TEF may be higher after thoracoscopic repair.

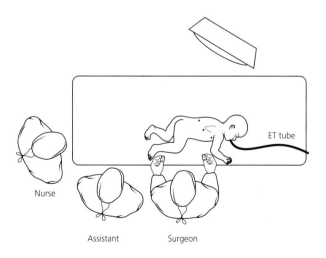

Nurse

Assistant   Surgeon

Position

15 Under general endotracheal anesthesia, the infant is placed in a three-quarter left prone position. This will allow the right lung to deflate and fall away from the operation site by natural gravity to expose the operative field without the need for retraction. The surgeon stands on the left side of the table with the screen opposite at the right upper end of the table. The assistant is at the surgeon's left side, and the scrub nurse at the bottom end of the table.

15

Insertion of cannula

16 Three cannulae are inserted in the right chest in a V-shape. The first cannula (5 mm) is inserted just anterior to the angle of the scapula. A 30° telescope is inserted and the chest insufflated with CO_2 at 5 mmHg and flow of 2 L/min until the lung is collapsed. Following this, the CO_2 insufflation pressure can be reduced. A 3-mm port is inserted posterior to the scapula for the use of 3-mm working instruments. A further 3- or 5-mm port is inserted in the axilla. A transpleural approach is made and the lung collapses or is retracted anteriorly to visualize the posterior mediastinum. This transpleural approach provides an excellent visualization of the posterior mediastinum. Occasionally, if the lung does not collapse completely, it may be necessary to introduce a further 3-mm port posterior to the other two working ports to retract the lung anteriorly using an atraumatic forceps.

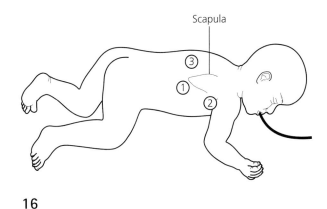

16

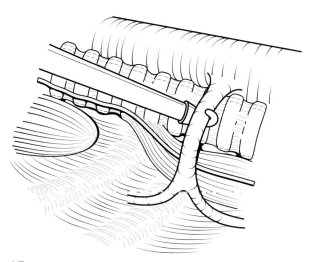

17

Operation

17 The vagus nerve is seen clearly and used as a guide to identify the esophagus. The azygos vein is freed and transected after coagulation of the vessel using a hook diathermy (the authors' preferred technique). Alternatively, the azygos vein is divided between 4/0 ligatures. The mediastinal pleura covering the proximal esophageal blind pouch is opened and the pouch mobilized. For guidance, the anesthetist pushes on the Replogle tube in the proximal esophagus. Grasping of either esophageal pouches is to be avoided.

Division of the tracheoesophageal fistula

18a,b The TEF is visualized during ventilation. If the dissection is carried out too posteriorly, the aorta could come into view mimicking the esophagus distal to the TEF. A Kelly clamp is used to dissect completely the TEF from the trachea and the posterior mediastinum. Before ligating and dividing the fistula, an atraumatic clamp is used to occlude the fistula and ascertain that the right lung is still ventilating. The fistula is suture ligated close to the posterior tracheal wall using a single 4/0 or 5/0 Prolene suture. The fistula is now transected and air leak from the trachea is excluded by Valsalva maneuver. A 4- or 6-Fr nasogastric tube is inserted via the axillary port and passed through the distal esophagus into the stomach to exclude distal obstruction.

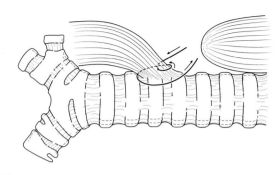

18a

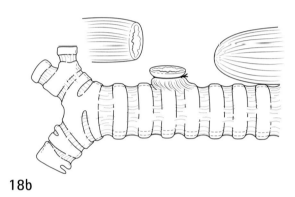

18b

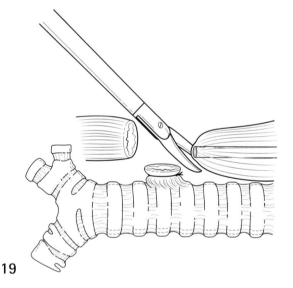

19

Mobilization of the proximal esophageal pouch

19 The proximal esophageal pouch is visualized again by asking the anesthetist to push on the Replogle tube. To mobilize the upper pouch, it is useful to insert a traction suture of Vicryl 4/0 in the pouch and dissect it from the trachea. The cleavage plane between the proximal esophagus and trachea is developed using scissors to avoid damage to the esophagus and trachea. Hook diathermy is only used when the dissecting is not close to the tracheal wall. The distal end of the upper pouch is opened using dissecting scissors.

Anastomosis

20 The end-to-end esophageal anastomosis is performed using interrupted full thickness sutures of 4/0 or 5/0 Prolene and intracorporeal knots. Sutures are initially placed in the posterior wall. The anesthetist then passes a transanastomotic tube (4 or 6 Fr) and the anterolateral part of the anastomosis is completed using the same suture material. By leaving the end of a suture a little longer, traction can be applied so that the next suture can be placed more easily.

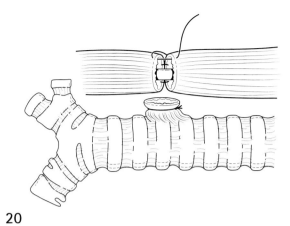

20

Closure

The 5-mm port site used for the camera is closed by inserting a suture for the muscle layer and skin glue or Steristrips for the skin. The 3-mm port sites are closed only at skin level as indicated above.

The authors prefer to leave a chest drainage tube for 24 hours to avoid a postoperative tension pneumothorax usually caused by inadvertent lung lesion during the introduction of the working instruments.

The postoperative care is as for the open repair.

OUTCOME

There has been no randomized controlled trial comparing the thoracoscopic and open approach for the repair of this anomaly. Preliminary data indicate that arterial pCO_2 rises during the operation and the arterial pH decreases. It is imperative to monitor arterial gases regularly during the operation. To avoid a prolonged intraoperative acidosis and hypercapnia, consideration should be given to (1) reducing the insufflation pressure or totally avoiding insufflation; (2) pausing the operation and allowing the acidosis to correct; or (3) converting the operation to the open procedure.

Published series show comparable results from thoracoscopic repair versus previous historic reports of neonates undergoing repair by thoracotomy. A retrospective study of 104 infants reported that 12 percent of infants developed an early leak or stricture at the anastomosis and 32 percent required at least one esophageal dilatation. A recurrent fistula developed in two infants (2 percent).

To minimize serious complications related to surgery, it is important that the thoracoscopic approach is restricted to surgeons fully trained in minimally invasive surgery and capable of performing the repair through a very limited space.

POSTOPERATIVE CARE

The infant is nursed in the neonatal intensive care unit. Intravenous fluids are administered and antibiotic prophylaxis is continued. Feeds via the transanastomotic nasogastric tube may be commenced on the second or third day after the operation. Oral feeding is gradually introduced. Regular chest physiotherapy, with nasopharyngeal suction, as required, is carried out to avoid respiratory infection.

If the esophageal anastomosis has been performed under extreme tension, it is recommended that the infant is electively paralyzed and mechanically ventilated for an arbitrary period of 5 days.

COMPLICATIONS

- Early:
  - anastomotic leakage
  - anastomotic stricture
  - recurrence of fistula.
- Late:
  - gastroesophageal reflux
  - tracheomalacia
  - dysmotility.

Anastomotic leaks occur in 15–20 percent of cases, but major disruption is rare. Minor leaks are generally detected on 'routine' contrast studies and can be managed conservatively. Major leaks present in the first 48 hours postoperatively with a tension pneumothorax. Emergency treatment is by insertion of an intercostal drain. Consideration should be given to re-exploration of the anastomosis with the intention of repairing the leak.

Anastomotic strictures develop in 30–40 percent of cases, most responding to one or two dilatations. Risk factors include anastomotic tension, anastomotic leakage, and gastroesophageal reflux.

Recurrent TEFs develop in 5–14 percent of cases and present with choking or cyanotic attacks with feeding or with recurrent episodes of pneumonia.

FURTHER READING

Bax KM, van der Zee DC. Feasibility of thoracoscopic repair of esophageal atresia with distal fistula. *Journal of Pediatric Surgery* 2002; **37**: 192–6.

Beasley SW, Myers NA, Auldist AW. *Oesophageal Atresia.* London: Chapman & Hall, 1991.

Holcomb GW III, Rothenberg SS, Bax KM *et al.* Thoracoscopic repair of esophageal atresia and tracheoesophageal fistula: a multi-institutional analysis. *Annals of Surgery* 2005; **242**: 422–8.

Lopez PJ, Keys C, Pierro A *et al.* Oesophageal atresia: improved outcome in high-risk groups? *Journal of Pediatric Surgery* 2006; **41**: 331–4.

Myers NA. The history of oesophageal atresia and tracheo-oesophageal fistula 1670–1984. *Progress in Pediatric Surgery* 1986; **20**: 106–57.

Rothenberg SS. Thoracoscopic repair of a tracheoesophageal fistula in a newborn infant. *Pediatric Endosurgical Innovative Techniques* 2000; **4**: 289–94.

Rothenberg SS. Thoracoscopic repair of esophageal atresia and tracheo-esophageal fistula. *Seminars in Pediatric Surgery* 2005; **14**: 2–7.

Spitz L. Esophageal atresia: past, present and future. *Journal of Pediatric Surgery* 1996; **31**: 19–25.

Spitz L, Kiely EM, Morecroft JA, Drake DP. Oesophageal atresia: At-risk groups for the 1990s. *Journal of Pediatric Surgery* 1994; **29**: 723–5.

van der Zee DC, Bax KN. Thoracoscopic treatment of esophageal atresia with distal fistula and of tracheomalacia. *Seminars in Pediatric Surgery* 2007; **16**: 224–30.

18

Cervical esophagostomy

LEWIS SPITZ

PRINCIPLES AND JUSTIFICATION

Although this procedure is relatively seldom performed, it should still form part of the repertoire of the pediatric surgeon.

Indications

The principal indication is long-gap esophageal atresia, where the atretic segment extends beyond six or eight thoracic vertebral bodies or when attempts at delayed primary anastomosis have failed. Other indications include disruption of a previous primary repair of esophageal atresia, extensive stricture of the esophagus – caustic ingestion or peptic esophagitis – with chronic aspiration, and foreign-body perforation of the esophagus.

In general, performing a cervical esophagostomy commits the surgeon to carrying out an eventual esophageal replacement.

OPERATION

Position of patient and incision

1 The patient is positioned supine on the operating table under general endotracheal anesthesia. A large-bore nasogastric tube is placed as far distally as possible in the esophagus. A jelly bag is placed under the shoulders, and the neck is moderately extended.

The esophagostomy may be sited on either side of the neck, but the left side is preferred, as it is more suited to the anastomotic site following esophageal replacement. A transverse incision is made on the left side of the neck 1 cm above and parallel to the medial third of the clavicle.

Using diathermy, the incision is deepened through the subcutaneous fat and platysma muscle, ligating and dividing the anterior jugular vein.

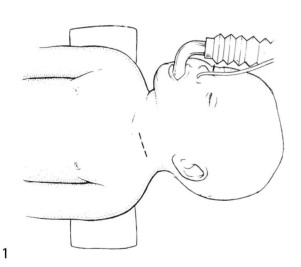

1

2 The clavicular head of the sternocleidomastoid muscle is divided in the line of the incision using electrocoagulation to provide hemostasis. The sternothyroid muscle is similarly divided or retracted posteriorly to reveal the carotid sheath and its contents. The common carotid artery lies medial to the internal jugular vein.

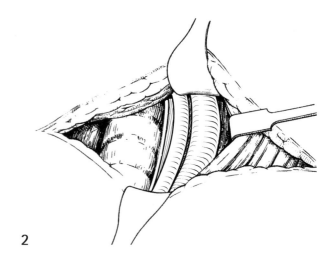

2

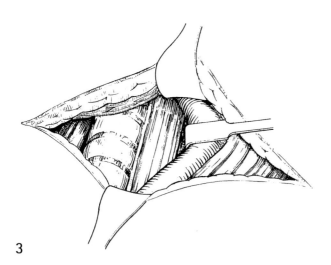

3

Preservation of recurrent laryngeal nerve

3 The carotid sheath containing the carotid artery, vagal nerve, and internal jugular vein is retracted laterally. This exposes the cartilaginous rings of the trachea anteromedially and the closely applied esophagus lying on its posterior surface. It is important to identify and preserve the left recurrent laryngeal nerve, which runs in the groove between the trachea and esophagus.

The esophagus is clearly identified by palpating the nasogastric tube within its lumen. It may also be helpful to leave a flexible gastroscope in the esophagus. By gradually withdrawing the gastroscope, the esophagus can be accurately identified by viewing the light at the end of the gastroscope as it passes through the neck.

Mobilization of the esophagus

4 The esophagus is carefully separated from the posterior surface of the trachea by blunt dissection, and, remaining close to the esophageal wall, the dissection is continued posteriorly and to the opposite side until the esophagus has been encircled. By keeping the dissection close to the esophageal wall, the risk of traumatizing the right recurrent laryngeal nerve will be minimized.

It is important to mobilize the full thickness of the esophagus. It is easy to enter the submucosal plane and to mobilize a mucosal cuff only. A soft rubber sling is placed around the esophagus, and the dissection continued distally, remaining on the muscle wall.

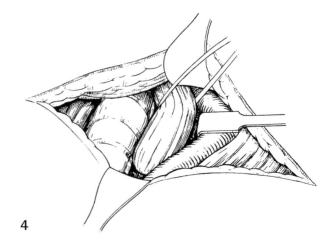

4

5 In isolated esophageal atresia, the proximal esophageal segment is usually short and the blind end soon comes into view. In other cases, e.g. strictures, it is necessary to divide the esophagus at a convenient place, leaving sufficient proximal esophagus to reach the skin incision without tension while permitting accurate closure of the distal esophagus.

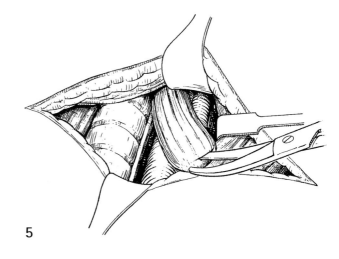

5

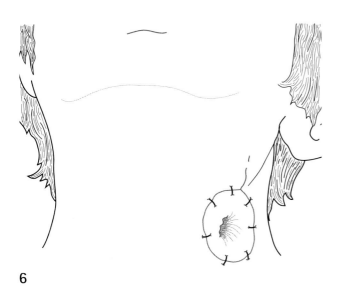

6

Fashioning the esophagostomy

6 The end of the esophagus is brought out of the lateral end of the incision and sutured to the skin edges with interrupted, full-thickness, fine, absorbable sutures. There should be no tension on the suture line, and a nasogastric tube should be able to exit the stoma unimpeded.

Wound closure

The remainder of the wound is closed with interrupted sutures to the platysma muscle and subcuticular sutures to skin.

POSTOPERATIVE CARE

The esophagostomy should be covered initially with paraffin gauze and ultimately left open to drain freely onto the surface.

An adhesive plastic bag may be applied to the skin around the esophagostomy site to collect saliva. In infants with esophageal atresia, it is vitally important to practice sham feeding pending the esophageal replacement. Failure to do this will result in tremendous difficulty in establishing oral feeds when the esophageal replacement is performed.

COMPLICATIONS

Stricture of the cervical esophagostomy occurs as a consequence of impaired vascularity. Kinking of the esophagus occurs when mobilization has been inadequate and will result in inefficient drainage of saliva.

19

H-type tracheoesophageal fistula

LEWIS SPITZ and STEVEN S ROTHENBERG

HISTORY

Described by Lamb in 1873, the first operative success was reported in 1939 by Imperatori.

PRINCIPLES AND JUSTIFICATION

An isolated or H-type tracheoesophageal fistula most commonly presents during the first few days of life, when the neonate chokes on attempting to feed and/or has unexplained cyanotic episodes. The associated gaseous distension of the gastrointestinal tract may be sufficiently severe to mimic that of intestinal obstruction. Older infants and children are likely to present with recurrent chest infections, particularly involving the right upper lobe.

H-type tracheoesophageal fistula constitutes about 4 percent of tracheoesophageal anomalies.

Investigations

The most reliable method of establishing the diagnosis of an H-type fistula is by a prone tube video esophagogram. A small-caliber nasogastric tube is passed into the distal esophagus and contrast medium is gradually injected while the tube is slowly withdrawn. The escape of contrast from the esophagus into the trachea may only show up in one or two frames. Caution must be taken to avoid spillover from the larynx into the trachea. The presence of an H-fistula may be missed in over 50 percent of routine contrast swallows.

Bronchoscopy with esophagoscopy will confirm the presence of a fistula. If performed immediately before ligation of the fistula, it should be possible to pass a fine tube, e.g. a ureteric catheter, through the fistula to aid in its subsequent identification at surgical exploration.

Having accurately identified the position of the fistula, a decision can be made on the most suitable approach. Some fistulas, including a recurrent fistula associated with a previous repair for esophageal atresia, will be best approached through the thorax, but the majority of isolated tracheoesophageal fistulas can be divided through a cervical approach with moderate neck extension. Another alternative is to address these lesions using thoracoscopy. While it is difficult to approach H-type fistulas through a standard thoracotomy because of their position high in the thoracic inlet, the exposure and access afforded by thoracoscopy is excellent.

The thoracic approach to a tracheoesophageal fistula is similar to that previously described for esophageal atresia and tracheoesophageal fistula (see **Chapter 17**).

OPERATION

Position of patient

1 The child is placed supine on the operating table with the head turned to the left. Before extending the neck, the site of the incision is drawn with a marker pen in a suitable skin crease 1 cm above and parallel to the clavicle. Failure to mark the site of the incision before extending the neck may result in a cosmetically unsatisfactory incision.

A jelly bag of appropriate size placed under the shoulders ensures adequate neck extension. An approach through the right side is usually preferred. A nasogastric tube of adequate size should be passed after induction of anesthesia.

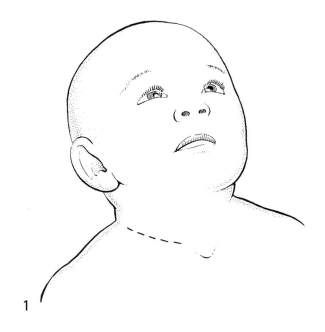

1

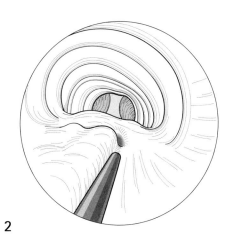

2

2 In ideal circumstances, a ureteric catheter will have been passed through the fistula under bronchoscopic control. This is invaluable in identifying the fistula site during exploration.

Operative approach

3 Having incised the skin and subcutaneous tissues, the sternocleidomastoid muscle is retracted posteriorly, dividing the sternal head of this muscle if necessary to allow adequate exposure. The plane medial to the carotid sheath is identified, and dissection allows the sheath to be retracted posteriorly. The thyroid gland, trachea, and esophagus lie medially. Palpation of the endotracheal and nasogastric tubes facilitates identification of these structures. The inferior thyroid artery and middle thyroid vein are identified crossing the space between the retracted carotid sheath and the thyroid, and division of these vessels may be necessary. The plane between the trachea and esophagus is gently dissected, care being taken to identify and preserve the right recurrent laryngeal nerve.

3

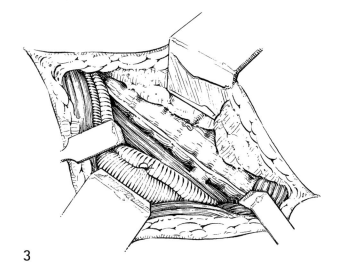

Dissection of fistula

4 Identification of the fistula requires careful dissection, and it is usually rather higher than anticipated because of the extension of the neck. Slings positioned around the esophagus above and below the fistula will facilitate dissection, but extreme care is required to preserve the left recurrent laryngeal nerve, which lies on the opposite side of the neck and is difficult to visualize.

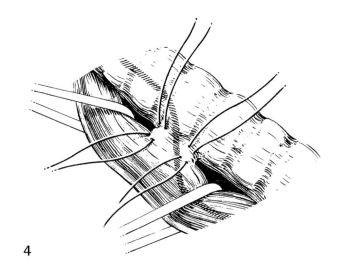

4

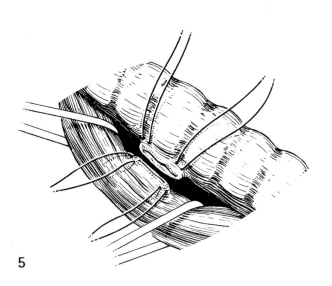

5

5 Having isolated the fistula, stay sutures are placed on the esophageal side to mark its position because, following division of the fistula, rotation and retraction of the esophageal end may make it difficult to identify. On the tracheal side, a 5/0 polypropylene suture is placed at both limits of the fistula.

6 Following division of the fistula, the tracheal defect is closed with interrupted sutures. The esophageal end of the fistula is closed with one or two interrupted fine polyglycolic acid sutures.

The retracted tissues will now assume a more normal position. Some surgeons advocate interposing tissue, e.g. fascia or muscle, between the two opposing suture lines in order to reduce the likelihood of recurrence of the fistula. The wound is closed in layers with absorbable sutures and with a subcuticular suture for the skin.

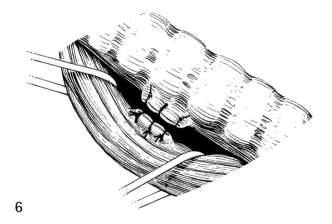

6

7 Three ports are used for the procedure, similar to that for repair of a type 3 tracheoesophageal fistula (TOF). The camera port is placed just posterior to the tip of the scapula in the fourth or fifth interspace. The right and left operating ports are placed one interspace below and are anterior and posterior to the camera port. A 30° optic should be used for the procedure.

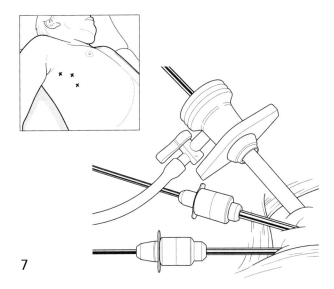

7

Thoracoscopic approach

The patient should be placed in a left lateral decubitus position. A selective left mainstem intubation is helpful, but not necessary. Adequate exposure of the thoracic apex can be obtained from the use of CO_2 insufflation alone, usually at a pressure of 4–6 mmHg.

The pleura in the posterior apex of the chest is incised longitudinally exposing the esophagus and trachea. The membranous wall of the trachea is identified and it is gently separated from the esophagus near the thoracic inlet. The membranous wall of the trachea is then followed superiorly until the bottom of the fistula is encountered. This is facilitated by having a small catheter across the fistula as previously mentioned. The magnified view afforded by the thoracoscope allows for easy identification of the fistula, as well as visualization of the vagus and laryngeal nerves. This fact should decrease the risk of injury to these structures.

8 Once the lower edge of the fistula is identified a more distinct plane between the esophagus and trachea is developed. Dissection is then carried out at the upper limit of the fistula to complete the mobilization. A Maryland dissector or right angle dissector should be easily passed behind the fistula prior to division to ensure that no inadvertent injury to the trachea, esophagus, or recurrent laryngeal nerve is caused. Once the fistula is dissected out, the internal catheter is removed.

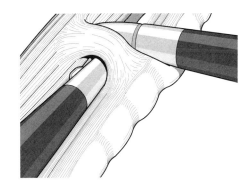

8

Depending on the size of the patient, there are two options for division of the fistula. Endoscopic 5-mm clips can be placed across the fistula on the esophageal and tracheal side and then the fistula is divided; or the fistula can be divided and oversewn using 4/0 PDS suture. Both of these techniques have been used successfully.

Some of the fatty tissue lying in the adjacent thoracic inlet can be interposed between the two ends if desired. The pleura is then sutured closed with a running absorbable suture to prevent contamination of the pleural space should a leak occur. No chest drain is necessary. The pneumothorax is simply eliminated with positive pressure ventilation prior to removal of the last trocar.

POSTOPERATIVE CARE

Extensive dissection of the trachea and esophagus is often required during this operation. Invariably this produces some tracheal edema, which may be minimal immediately after operation, but progresses in severity for up to 24 hours. It is reasonable, particularly in premature infants or in those with pre-existing lung disease, to leave an endotracheal tube in position.

Following extubation, the movement of the vocal cords should be assessed. A proportion of these neonates will require intubation for some considerable time and may have a tendency to stridor, particularly when crying or coughing, for weeks or months afterwards. Feeds can be given through a nasogastric tube.

Recurrence of an H-type fistula is rare.

FURTHER READING

Benjamin B, Pham T. Diagnosis of H-type tracheoeso-phageal fistula. *Journal of Pediatric Surgery* 1991; **26**: 66–71.

Gans SL, Johnson RO. Diagnosis and management of 'H' type tracheo-esophageal fistula in infants and children. *Journal of Pediatric Surgery* 1977; **12**: 233–6.

Rothenberg SS. Experience with thoracoscopic tracheal surgery in infants and children. *Journal of Laparoendoscopic and Advanced Surgical Techniques* 2009; **19**: 671–4.

Rothenberg SS. Thoracoscopic repair of esophageal atresia and tracheo-esophageal fistula in neonates: evolution of a technique. *Journal of Laparoendoscopic and Advanced Surgical Techniques A.* 2012; **22(2)**: 195–9.

Recurrent tracheoesophageal fistula

LEWIS SPITZ

PRINCIPLES AND JUSTIFICATION

The incidence of recurrent tracheoesophageal fistula ranges from 5 to 10 percent. Infants who develop respiratory symptoms following repair of an esophageal atresia, e.g. gagging, coughing, apneic or cyanotic spells during feeding, or suffer from recurrent chest infections should be suspected of having a recurrent fistula.

1 Cine tube esophagography performed in the prone position is the most reliable method of establishing the diagnosis.

Bronchoscopy with cannulation of the fistula is also a reliable diagnostic method and is invaluable in locating the fistula during the operative procedure.

PREOPERATIVE

Diagnosis

Radiographs of the chest and abdomen may show an air esophagogram or an excessive amount of gas in the gastrointestinal tract. Routine contrast swallows will only detect about 50 percent of recurrent fistulas. Esophagoscopy carries a low diagnostic rate.

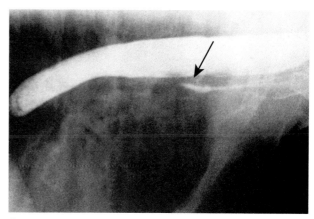

1

Anesthesia

Anesthesia for repair of recurrent fistula is fraught with danger. Lung function may be compromised by chronic aspiration, and vascular access may have been compromised by previous surgery or the use of parenteral nutrition. Intraoperative ventilation may be difficult because of gaseous escape through a large fistula. Meticulous intraoperative monitoring is mandatory, including continuous oxygen saturation measurements. Hand ventilation with high gas flow rates may be necessary because of changes in pulmonary compliance. Because of pleural adhesions following previous surgery, blood loss may be excessive and should be replaced – volume for volume. Postoperative ventilation and intensive care are often necessary, particularly in young infants because of respiratory stridor.

OPERATION

Bronchoscopy and cannulation of fistula

2 A rigid Storz bronchoscope of suitable size for the child's age (2.5–3 Fr for infants) is passed and the fistulous opening in the posterior wall of the trachea at or just above the carina is identified. A fine (4–6 Fr) ureteric catheter is passed through the suction channel of the bronchoscope, through the fistula into the esophagus, advanced well down into the esophagus and left *in situ*.

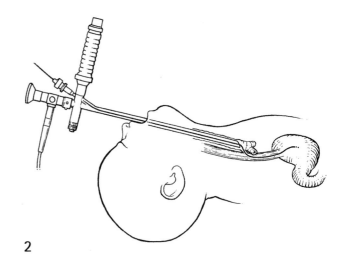

2

Incision

A posterolateral thoracotomy via the previous incision is the preferred approach. The fourth or fifth intercostal space is opened in the length of the incision and a small rib spreader is used to widen the thoracotomy. Access to the mediastinum is via a transpleural route as the extrapleural approach is not an option, having been used in the repair of the esophageal atresia.

Mediastinal dissection and mobilization of esophagus

3 The mediastinal pleura is opened longitudinally over the esophagus, exposing its lateral wall proximal and distal to the fistulous site. The esophagus proximal and distal to the fistula (identified by palpating the ureteric catheter within its lumen) is carefully mobilized from the surrounding tissue and rubber slings are passed around it above and below the fistula.

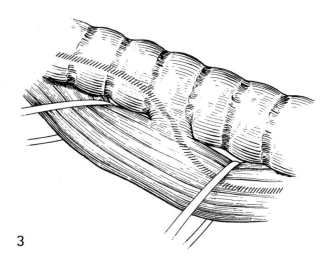

3

Dissection of fistula

4 Having identified and isolated the fistula, stay sutures of 5/0 polypropylene (Prolene) are inserted in the upper and lower walls of the fistula on both the tracheal and esophageal ends. These sutures are invaluable in facilitating accurate closure of the defects following division of the fistula.

4

Division of fistula

5 The fistula is now opened. The ureteric catheter should be positively visualized traversing the fistula before being withdrawn through the mouth to allow complete division of the fistula.

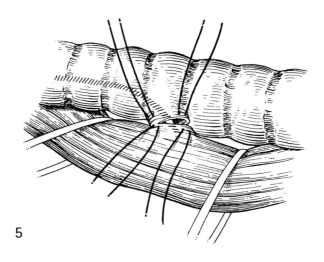

5

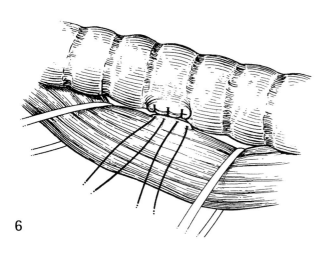

6

Closure of fistulous openings

6 The tracheal and esophageal orifices of the fistula are securely closed with interrupted 5/0 polypropylene sutures. In experienced hands, the procedure can be performed thoracoscopically.

Separation of the suture lines

To prevent the two contiguous suture lines becoming adherent and to prevent refistulization, mediastinal pleura, intercostal muscle, or a flap of pericardium may be interposed between the esophagus and trachea. In the author's experience, once the fistula has been divided and the defects in the trachea and esophagus repaired, the two suture lines tend to rotate away from each other so that interposing tissue between is unnecessary. An intercostal drain is inserted with the tip some distance away from the area of repair.

Wound closure

The thoracotomy wound is closed with pericostal 3/0 polyglycolic acid sutures and the muscles of the chest wall are approximated with continuous 4/0 polyglycolic acid sutures. The skin is closed with a subcuticular suture.

Endoscopic treatment

A variety of endoscopic methods to promote closure of recurrent tracheoesophageal fistulas have been described. The agents used include tissue glues (Histoacryl), fibrin sealant (Tisseel), and lasers. Reported series are small, with variable success rates and short-term follow up.

POSTOPERATIVE CARE

Endotracheal intubation and elective mechanical ventilation are usually required for 48–72 hours after operation due to tracheal edema. A contrast swallow may be performed on the seventh day after operation and the chest drain removed following confirmation that there is no leak from the esophageal repair.

COMPLICATIONS

These include pneumothorax and esophageal leak with consequent empyema. There is a 10–20 percent risk of fistula recurrence.

FURTHER READING

Bruch SW, Hirschl RB, Coran AG. The diagnosis and management of recurrent tracheoesophageal fistulas. *Journal of Pediatric Surgery* 2010; **45**: 337–40

Ein SH, Stringer DA, Stephens CA *et al*. Recurrent tracheoesophageal fistulas: seventeen-year review. *Journal of Pediatric Surgery* 1983; **18**: 436–41.

Filston HC, Rankin JC, Kirks DR. The diagnosis of primary and recurrent tracheoesophageal fistulas: value of selective catheterization. *Journal of Pediatric Surgery* 1982; **17**: 144–8.

Ghandour KE, Spitz L, Brereton RJ, Kiely EM. Recurrent tracheoesophageal fistula: experience with 24 patients. *Journal of Paediatrics and Child Health* 1990; **26**: 89–91.

Willetts IE, Dudley NE, Tam PKH. Endoscopic treatment of recurrent tracheoesophageal fistulae: long-term results. *Pediatric Surgery International* 1998; **13**: 256–8.

21

Aortopexy

EDWARD KIELY

HISTORICAL BACKGROUND

In 1948, Gross and Neuhauser were the first to recognize and successfully treat innominate artery compression of the trachea by suturing the innominate artery to the sternum. Some 20 years later, Mustard and colleagues reported on 285 patients with innominate artery compression of whom 39 underwent surgery. The operation was performed through a right thoracotomy and the ascending aorta and origin of the innominate artery were sutured to the sternum.

The association of tracheomalacia with tracheoesophageal anomalies and its subsequent management by aortopexy was first reported in 1976 by Benjamin *et al.* More recently in 2000, DeCou *et al.* described thoracoscopic aortopexy.

Diagnosis

1a,b The diagnosis is confirmed endoscopically when expiratory collapse of the trachea is seen during quiet respiration. Complete obliteration of the lumen is common under these circumstances. The tracheal collapse in infants previously treated for esophageal atresia and/or tracheoesophageal fistula is usually proximal to the site of entry of the original fistula.

Severe symptoms are unusual when more than 20 percent of the lumen remains open.

PRINCIPLES AND JUSTIFICATION

Tracheomalacia is suspected when an infant develops expiratory stridor on exertion – feeding and crying. Increasing difficulty with expiration leads to difficulty with feeding, cyanotic spells, and, in extreme cases, apnea and collapse (death attacks). In infants with tracheoesophageal anomalies, symptoms often become pronounced with increasing body mass over the age of about three months. Expiratory stridor at rest or biphasic stridor is an ominous sign of severe airway compromise.

The symptoms are similar to features of severe gastro-esophageal reflux and recurrent tracheoesophageal fistula, and the three conditions may coexist.

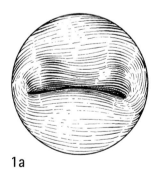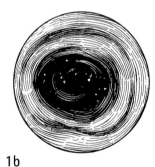

1a   1b

OPERATION

Position of patient

The patient is positioned supine with a small roll beneath the shoulders and the left arm abducted.

Incision

2 The procedure may be performed open or thoracoscopically. Conventionally, the chest is entered anteriorly through the bed of the third rib. Alternatively, an upper median sternotomy extending to a level just below the manubrium may be utilized.

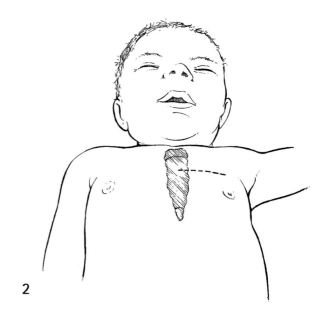

2

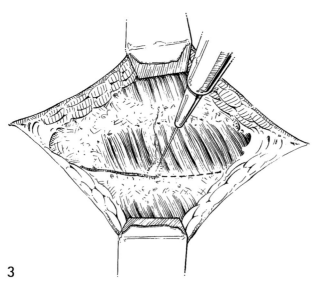

3

3 The perichondrium and periosteum are incised with diathermy and separated from cartilage and bone, respectively. The chest is entered through the bed of the rib and the internal mammary vessels are divided at the medial end of the incision.

4 The thoracotomy is widened by means of an infant-sized chest retractor. The left lung is retracted and held out of the operation field by a moist gauze swab.

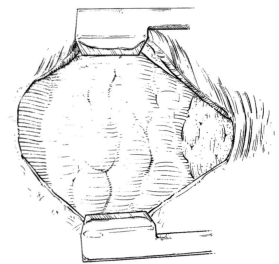

4

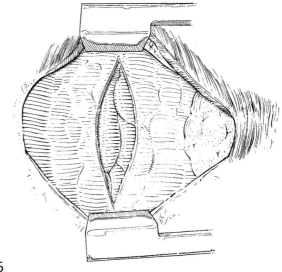

5 The pleura is incised longitudinally over the left lobe of the thymus gland.

5

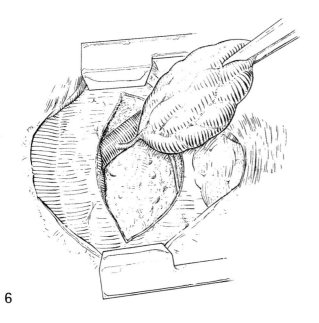

6

6 The left lobe of the thymus gland is excised with care to protect the phrenic nerve. The thymic vein, which enters the innominate vein, is identified, coagulated, and divided. The great vessels are then in view.

7 The roots of the great vessels are within the pericardium, which is incised transversely just below its reflection on the aorta. Meticulous attention to hemostasis is required.

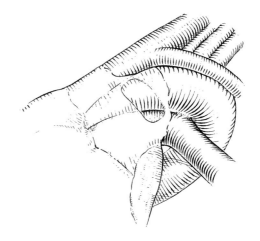

7

8 Three 4/0 polypropylene sutures are sufficient to perform the aortopexy. The pericardial reflection and aortic adventitia are picked up with two or three bites of each suture. Care is taken to remain superficial to the tunica media of the aorta. The sutures are then inserted into the posterior aspect of the sternum and are left untied until all three are in place.

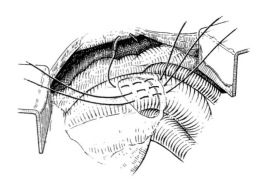

8

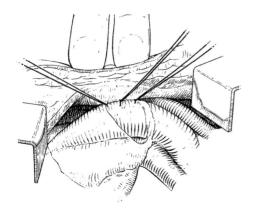

9

9 The assistant then depresses the sternum firmly and holds this position until all three sutures have been tied. The sternum is then released and the aorta moves forward with it. The anterior tracheal wall also moves anteriorly to fill the potential space between the aorta and trachea. There are no connections between the aorta and trachea.

Thorascopic procedure

10 The camera port is inserted in the left anterior axillary line in the fourth interspace. A 0° telescope is used. Two other ports are inserted in the second and fifth spaces, the upper posterior to the pectoralis major and the lower slightly posterior to the telescope position. At least one 5-mm port should be used for removal of the thymus.

11 The pleura is incised over the thymus in the manner described for the open operation. Excision of the left lobe of the thymus is accomplished piecemeal with every effort to minimize bleeding. It is necessary to do this in order to see the great vessels clearly.

12 The pericardium is incised to expose the root of the aorta. The internal mammary vessels are coagulated to avoid bleeding from needle puncture. The sutures are passed from outside through an intercostal space. For each suture, a short stab incision is used over the sternum, intercostal space, or costal cartilage, depending on the level of the pericardial reflection. The needle is inserted through the stab incision and the suture retrieved using a large bore needle inserted through the same incision.

13 Three sutures are placed as before and left untied. The assistant then depresses the sternum and the sutures are tied. Aftercare is as described for the open operation.

Wound closure

The wound is closed in the normal manner. If the operative field is dry, a chest drain is unnecessary.

POSTOPERATIVE CARE

Oral feeding may be commenced the same day and early discharge is possible if symptoms are alleviated.

FURTHER READING

Benjamin B, Cohen D, Glasson M. Tracheomalacia in association with congenital tracheoesophageal fistula. *Surgery* 1976; **79**: 504–8.

Calkoen EE, Gabra HO, Roebuck DJ *et al.* Aortopexy as treatment for tracheo-bronchomalacia in children: an 18-year single-centre experience. *Pediatric Critical Care Medicine* 2011; **12**: 545–51.

Corbally MT, Spitz L, Kiely E *et al.* Aortopexy for tracheomalacia in oesophageal anomalies. *European Journal of Pediatric Surgery* 1993; **3**: 264–6.

DeCou JM, Parsons DS, Gauderer MWL. Thoracoscopic aortopexy for tracheomalacia. *Pediatric Endosurgical Innovative Techniques* 2000; **4**: 92.

Schaarschmidt K, Kolberg-Schwerdt A, Pietsch L, Bunke KJ. Thoracoscopic aortopericardiosternopexy for severe tracheomalacia in toddlers. *Pediatric Surgery* 2002; **37**: 1476.

Schwartz MZ, Filler RM. Tracheal compression as a cause of apnea following repair of tracheoesophageal fistula: treatment by aortopexy. *Journal of Pediatric Surgery* 1980; **15**: 842–8.

22

Esophageal replacement with colon

YANN RÉVILLON and NAZIHA KHEN-DUNLOP

HISTORY

The first description of the anatomic details of esophageal replacement with colon is credited to Vuillet and Kelling in 1911. Von Hacker was the first to perform the procedure three years later. For many years, the colon was the primary substitute for a damaged or atretic esophagus but has recently been superseded by the newer techniques transposing the stomach. Many of the pitfalls using the transposed colon in adults stem from problems with vascular supply to the graft. These problems are less commonly seen in the pediatric population.

PRINCIPLES AND JUSTIFICATION

Even though preservation of the patient's own esophagus should always be attempted, the motility of repaired esophagus may not allow normal oral feeding and esophageal replacement may be required. In the pediatric population, long-gap esophageal atresia or failed primary anastomosis and extensive caustic injury are the main indications for graft interpositions. Colon and stomach are the most commonly used, depending more on local preference and experience than on objective data, both producing good functional outcome, but are also associated with a high morbidity and specific complications. The ideal replacement is yet to be found and tissue engineering may be the next advance. The normal esophagus contracts with forceful peristaltic contractions in response to initiation of a swallow, while the normal colon contracts in a more complex pattern as a result of distension mediated by hormonal and neurogenic stimuli. The colon interposed into the esophageal bed needs large volume distension before emptying. Animal studies of isolated segments of colon have shown more rapid emptying in isoperistaltic compared with antiperistaltic loops.

There are a number of advantages with colon interposition. It has an excellent, mobile vascular supply via the marginal artery, it always provides adequate length to reach up into the chest or the neck and it is the appropriate caliber for anastomosis. In addition, it avoids problems of acid production in the conduit that can lead to Barrett's esophagus.

The minimal age for replacement with colon is still debatable. Some authors advocate waiting until the child starts to walk, others prefer to carry out the procedure at five to six months. Before this age, the small size of colonic vessels could lead to graft vascular compromise.

The laparoscopic approach has been recommended for the mediastinal dissection and esophagectomy as it achieves more precise hemostasis and reduces trauma to the trachea and nerves compared with conventional blunt dissection.

BOWEL PREPARATION

During gastrostomy (for esophageal atresia or caustic injury), the middle colonic artery may be ligated to increase the vascularity of the colon by increasing blood flow through the marginal vessels.

Prior to esophageal replacement, the child is admitted and clear liquids are given for 24 hours preoperatively. Polyethylene glycol electrolyte solution is given at a rate of 25–40 mL/kg per hour until stools are clear.

Intestinal antiseptics are given orally 3 days before surgery with neomycin and erythromycin. On the day of surgery, intravenous cephalosporin and metronidazole are added.

ANESTHESIA

The procedure is carried out under general endotracheal anesthesia. An epidural catheter can facilitate the intraoperative anesthesia and postoperative pain control.

OPERATION

Position of the patient

The patient is placed in a 45° left lateral decubitus position with the right arm prepped into the operative field. The table is rolled laterally to afford greater exposure for the abdominal portion of the procedure.

1a,b A midline incision is made and the colon is examined. Vascular supply to the colon dictates the segments to be transposed into the chest. Right, transverse, or left colon can be mobilized and brought up to the neck in most children without compromise of the blood supply to the graft. Most surgeons use the left colon and a small section of the left transverse colon based on the marginal artery of Drummond (the ascending branches of the left colic vessel). Small vascular clamps are placed on the middle colic artery, if not previously ligated, to evaluate the graft perfusion before dividing the vessels. At the same time, intestinal clamps are placed at the two extremities of the graft to stop the transmural vascularization. The perfusion of the proposed graft by the residual blood supply is assessed after 10 minutes and if adequate, the clamped vessels are divided centrally at their origin, preserving

Abdominal incision

Starting the surgical procedure via the abdominal approach has two advantages: it confirms the technical feasibility of a well-vascularized colonic graft before the thoracic incision and it may avoid a thoracotomy completely if the esophagectomy can be performed via transhiatal dissection.

collaterals in the marginal artery system of the colon segment.

Where possible, mediastinal blunt dissection is performed. An umbilical tape is passed from the colonic mesentery through the diaphragmatic hiatus to the level of the proximal esophageal segment in the neck. This tape helps determine the length of colon necessary for replacement. Accurate measurement of the distance between the site of the upper and lower anastomosis is necessary to avoid graft tension (if too short) and prevents secondary colon redundancy (if too long). The colon is then divided at the appropriate length. An alternative, where the left colon is not available, is to use the right colon, cecum and a section of the distal ileum, based on the ileocolic vessels, passed retrosternally isoperistaltically into the neck, with the ileum anastomosed to the cervical esophagus.

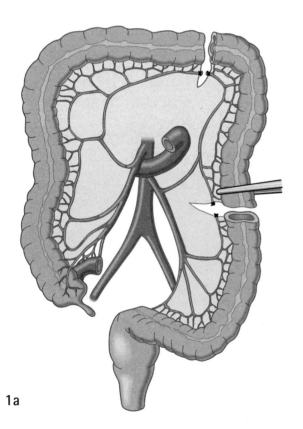

1a

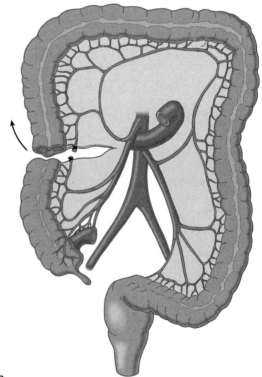

1b

Thoracic incision

2a,b The table is rolled laterally to expose the thoracic region and the right arm is raised.

In the case of a mid-esophagus stricture, a posterolateral thoracotomy incision is made in the sixth intercostal space. The latissimus dorsi is retracted laterally. If there had been no prior thoracotomy, an extrapleural approach can be used via the sixth intercostal space or via subperiosteal resection of the sixth rib with incision into the extrapleural space through the posterior periosteum to facilitate the approach. A transpleural approach is made in the case of previous thoracotomy. The lung is retracted anteromedially and the proximal esophagus identified with the aid of the manipulation of a nasoesophageal tube by the anesthesiologist. The proximal esophagus is mobilized to the thoracic inlet followed by the esophagectomy. The distal esophageal segment is mobilized to the esophageal hiatus. In children with minimal scarring of the esophageal bed, transhiatal dissection and esophagectomy without thoracotomy is possible.

In cases of previous esophagostomy, minimal dissection of the proximal esophagus is carried out to prevent recurrent laryngeal nerve injury and to preserve the blood supply to the esophagus. Alternatively, the cervical esophagus is approached via an oblique or transverse right neck incision. The neck vessels are retracted and the proximal esophagus is mobilized within the thoracic inlet.

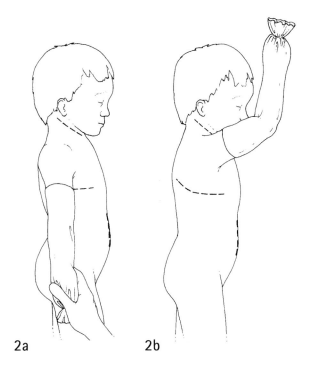

2a   2b

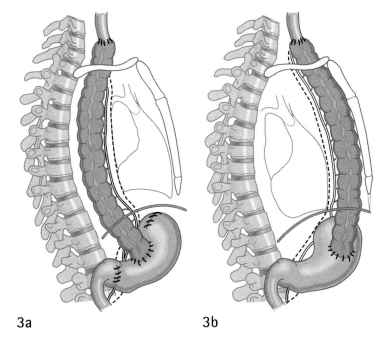

3a   3b

Colonic interposition

3a,b Once the colon graft is mobilized, the distal esophageal stump is resected, if possible, at the stomach with a linear stapling device to avoid reflux in the stump. In some cases, a normal gastroesophageal junction may be preserved, anastomosing distal esophagus to colonic interposition.

Colonic interposition is passed behind the stomach and pulled through the chest. The graft is placed in the posterior mediastinum in the esophageal bed. This is the preferred route as it is the shortest distance to the cervical region and results in less dysphagia and reflux and improved graft function. In cases with severe scarring in the native esophageal bed, the graft is placed retrosternally.

Anastomosis

4 The proximal anastomosis between esophagus and colon is created in the neck with a single layer of absorbable sutures and colon is fixated to the neck muscle. While the anastomosis can be created in the neck or the chest, a cervical anastomosis avoids the potential disaster of an intrathoracic leak, which carries high morbidity.

The gastrocolic anastomosis is performed at the anterior gastric wall which limits gastrocolonic reflux compared with cardiac positioning. The anastomosis is partially wrapped with stomach. Pyloroplasty is created and temporary gastrostomy is left for gastric decompression and transition to oral feeds.

Colocolic anastomosis ends the procedure, anterior to the vascular pedicle, to re-establish colonic continuity. The thoracic dissection is drained before abdominal closure. A nasocolonic tube is also placed in the interposed colon for postoperative graft decompression to prevent distension and hypoperfusion of the colon graft.

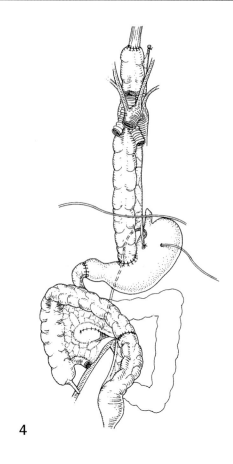

4

Colonic patch esophagoplasty

Although not commonly used, this procedure can be helpful in selected cases. The technique was proposed for the correction of persistent, isolated, short strictures of the esophagus as an alternative to esophageal replacement.

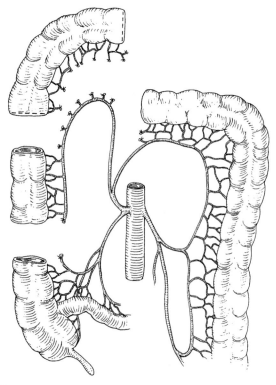

5a

5a–d A thoracic approach is made exposing the area of stricture. Via an abdominal incision, the colon is measured and pedicle created as if performing an esophageal replacement procedure. A segment based on the right colic artery is preferred. The esophageal stricture is then opened and the length of stricture to be patched is determined. A segment of colon equal to the length of the esophageal defect is measured. The segment of colon distal to the patch segment, but adjacent to the mobilized vascular pedicle, is removed. The marginal artery is carefully preserved by dividing vessels close to the wall of the segment of bowel to be discarded. The colon patch segment is opened along its antimesenteric border and the patch is created from a template of the esophageal defect. The patch is then passed behind the stomach through the esophageal hiatus. If the patch is too large, a pseudodiverticulum may develop. A single layer of interrupted or continuous absorbable suture is used to secure the patch in place.

The anastomotic site is drained and gastrostomy performed as in esophageal replacement.

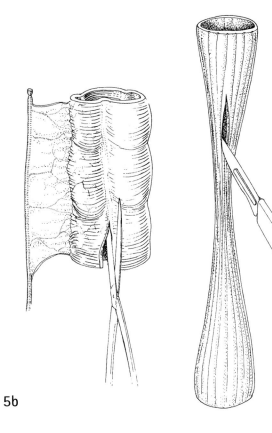

5b

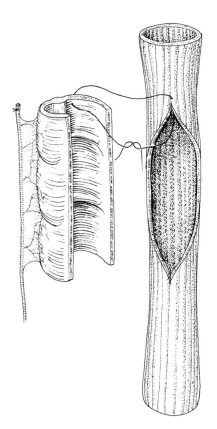

5c

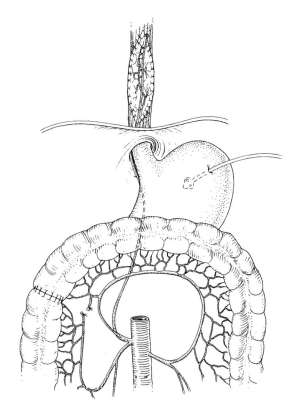

5d

POSTOPERATIVE CARE

The nasocolonic tube is removed on postoperative day 3, if no graft distension is seen on chest radiograph.

A contrast swallow is performed on postoperative day 7. If no leak is detected, oral feeding may be initiated and thoracic drainage catheters subsequently removed. As the child recovers, clinical evidence of dysphagia or obstruction should prompt a contrast swallow or endoscopy to detect anastomotic stricture. Identified strictures are usually amenable to dilatation.

OUTCOME

The 'colon patch' avoids many of the functional disadvantages of the segmental colon interposition, and problems related with redundancy and difficulty with emptying are not seen. Endoscopic evaluations of patients with colon patch have also demonstrated re-epithelialization and scar regression of the esophagus. However, it includes a long intrathoracic suture line, thereby increasing the potential for perioperative leakage and secondary pseudodiverticulum are observed.

In the pediatric population, ischemic anastomotic strictures are not a common problem occurring in 5–10 percent of cases. Anastomotic leaks develop in about 10–20 percent. With respiratory problems and local infections, postoperative complications are observed in 50 percent of cases, but mortality remains low (1–5 percent).

Most patients who have undergone esophageal replacement with colon lead a relatively normal life. Their quality of life is deemed acceptable despite frequent late complications: scoliosis is reported in 25 percent of cases and reflux in 40 percent.

The main disadvantage of esophageal replacement with colon is that the segment does not establish peristaltic contractions coordinated with swallowing as in the native esophagus. Contractions can be measured in the interposed colon in response to distension thus emptying is primarily by gravity, and transit of solids is slow. Consequently, the colon interposition becomes redundant over time, leading to obstruction.

Despite a high morbidity, colon interposition is a proven, satisfactory, durable replacement for the esophagus in children that allows normal swallowing. Because of the risks of late strictures and excessive tortuosity of the neo-esophagus, long-term follow up is necessary.

FURTHER READING

Burgos L, Barrena S, Andrés AM et al. Colonic interposition for esophageal replacement in children remains a good choice: 33-year median follow-up of 65 patients. *Journal of Pediatric Surgery* 2010; **45**: 341–5.

Esteves E, Sousa-Filho HB, Watanabe S et al. Laparoscopically assisted esophagectomy and colon interposition for esophageal replacement in children: preliminary results of a novel technique. *Journal of Pediatric Surgery* 2010; **45**: 1053–60.

Hadidi AT. A technique to improve vascularity in colon replacement of the esophagus. *European Journal of Pediatric Surgery* 2006; **16**: 39–44.

Hamza AF, Abdelhay S, Sherif H et al. Caustic esophageal strictures in children: 30 years' experience. *Journal of Pediatric Surgery* 2003; **38**: 828–33.

Othersen HB Jr, Parker EF, Chandler J et al. Save the child's esophagus. Part II: Colic patch repair. *Journal of Pediatric Surgery* 1997; **32**: 328–33.

Zani A, Pierro A, Elvassore N, De Coppi P. Tissue engineering: an option for esophageal replacement? *Seminars in Pediatric Surgery* 2009; **18**: 57–62.

23

Gastric replacement of the esophagus

LEWIS SPITZ and AGOSTINO PIERRO

INTRODUCTION

One of the alternatives for replacing the esophagus is gastric transposition involving the whole stomach. This method has the advantage of involving only one anastomosis, which is well vascularized and is associated with a low incidence of leakage.

HISTORY

In 1922, Kummell described the technique of gastric transposition via the mediastinal route in two patients, both of whom died. In 1945, Sweet recorded 12 esophageal resections with esophagogastric anastomosis above the aortic arch. In 1980, Atwell reported on six children who underwent gastric transposition, with good long-term results in four. Gastric transposition is currently the procedure of choice for esophageal replacement in adults with esophageal carcinoma.

OPERATION

The procedure may be performed either by a thoracoabdominal approach or transhiatally via the posterior mediastinum without having to resort to a thoracotomy. This latter method will be described in detail. If the posterior mediastinum is severely scarred from previous surgery, the left pleural or retrosternal route may be preferred.

The importance of sham feeds in infants with long-gap esophageal atresia who have undergone a cervical esophagostomy in simplifying the initiation of oral nutrition following the interposition should not be underestimated.

Initial gastrostomy

The initial feeding gastrostomy should ideally have been sited on the anterior surface of the body of the stomach, well away from the greater curvature, in order to preserve the vascular arcades of the gastroepiploic vessels.

INCISION

1 The preferred approach is via a midline upper abdominal incision extending from the xiphisternum to the umbilicus. Alternatively, a left upper abdominal transverse muscle-cutting incision may be used.

The gastrostomy is carefully mobilized from the anterior abdominal wall and the defect in the stomach closed in two layers with interrupted 4/0 polyglycolic acid sutures.

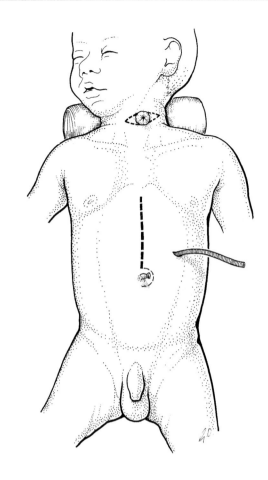

1

MOBILIZING THE STOMACH

Adhesions between the stomach and the left lobe of the liver are released, taking care not to damage any of the major blood vessels.

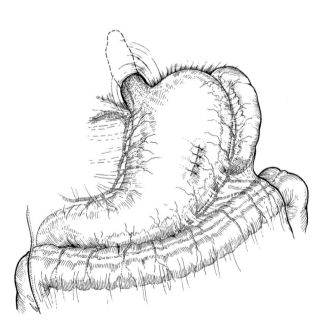

2 The greater curvature of the stomach is mobilized by ligating and dividing the vessels in the gastrocolic omentum and the short gastric vessels. These vessels should be ligated well away from the stomach wall in order to preserve the vascular arcades of the right gastroepiploic vessels. Meticulous care must be exercised to avoid damaging the spleen.

The lesser curvature of the stomach is freed by dividing the lesser omentum from the pylorus to the diaphragmatic hiatus. The right gastric artery is carefully identified and preserved, while the left gastric vessels are ligated and divided close to the stomach. The lower esophagus is exposed by dividing the phrenoesophageal membrane, and the margins of the esophageal hiatus in the diaphragm are defined.

2

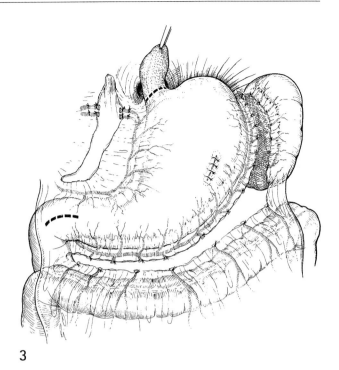

RESECTION OF THE DISTAL ESOPHAGUS

3 The inevitably short, blind-ending lower esophageal stump is dissected out of the posterior mediastinum by a combination of blunt and sharp dissection through the diaphragmatic hiatus. The anterior and posterior vagal nerves are divided during this part of the procedure. The body and fundus of the stomach are now free from all attachments and can be delivered into the wound.

The esophagus is transected at the gastroesophageal junction and the defect closed in two layers with 4/0 polyglycolic acid sutures.

The second part of the duodenum may be Kocherized to obtain maximum mobility of the pylorus.

3

PREPARING FOR GASTROESOPHAGEAL ANASTOMOSIS

4a,b The highest part of the fundus of the stomach is identified and stay sutures of different material are inserted to the left and the right of the area selected for

the anastomosis. These sutures help to avoid torsion of the stomach occurring as it is pulled up through the posterior mediastinum into the neck.

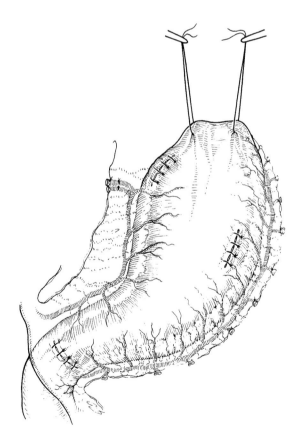

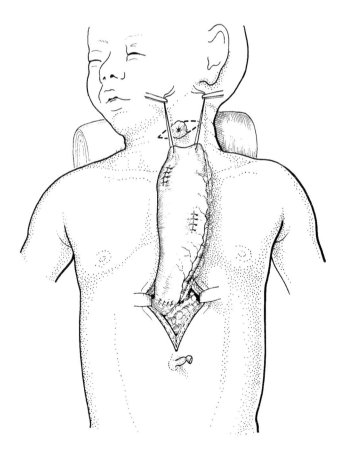

4a   **4b**

PYLOROPLASTY

A short Heinecke–Mikulicz pyloroplasty is performed, the transverse incision being closed horizontally with interrupted fine polyglycolic acid sutures. An alternative is to perform a short pyloromyotomy.

The stomach is now ready for its transposition into the neck.

MOBILIZATION OF THE CERVICAL ESOPHAGUS

5 Attention is now turned to the neck, where the previously constructed cervical esophagostomy (preferably performed on the left side) is mobilized via a 3–4 cm transverse incision, taking care not to damage the muscular coat of the esophagus. The recurrent laryngeal nerve coursing upwards on the posterolateral surface of the trachea is identified and preserved. It is important to mobilize at least 1–1.5 cm full-thickness esophagus to allow a satisfactory anastomosis to take place. If a cervical esophagostomy had not previously been constructed, then the cervical esophagus is exposed as shown in Chapter 18 on cervical esophagostomy.

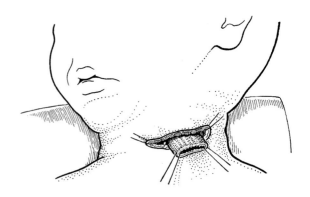

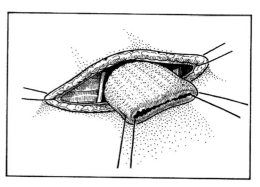

5

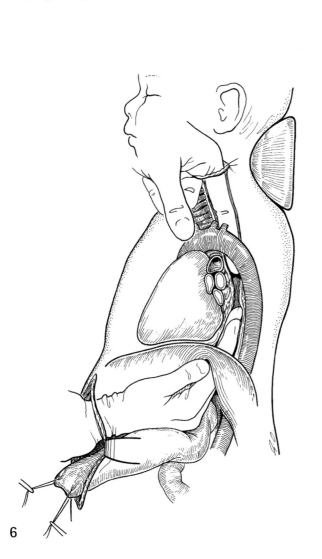

6

PREPARING THE POSTERIOR MEDIASTINAL TUNNEL

6 A plane of dissection between the membranous posterior surface of the trachea and the prevertebral fascia is established, and a tunnel is created into the superior mediastinum by blunt dissection immediately in the midline.

A similar tunnel is fashioned from below in the line of the normal esophageal route, by means of blunt dissection through the esophageal hiatus in the posterior mediastinal space posterior to the heart and anterior to the prevertebral fascia.

When continuity of the superior and inferior posterior mediastinal tunnels has been established, the space to be occupied by the stomach is developed into a tunnel of two to three fingers' breadth.

There will be occasions when fashioning of the posterior mediastinal tunnel by blind dissection is impossible or hazardous due to inflammation, fibrosis from previous surgery, or adhesions following previous perforation or caustic ingestion. Under these circumstances, it is necessary to perform a lateral thoracotomy and for the dissection to be carried out under direction vision.

TRANSPOSING THE STOMACH

7a,b A wide-caliber nasogastric tube is passed through the posterior mediastinal tunnel from the cervical incision to appear via the esophageal hiatus into the abdominal wound. The two stay sutures on the fundus of the stomach are tied to the tube, which is then gently withdrawn, pulling the stomach up through the esophageal hiatus and the posterior mediastinal tunnel into the cervical incision. Orientation of the fundus is checked by realigning the stay sutures in their correct position to avoid torsion of the stomach in the mediastinum.

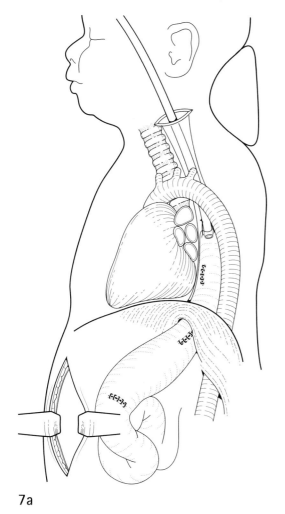

7a

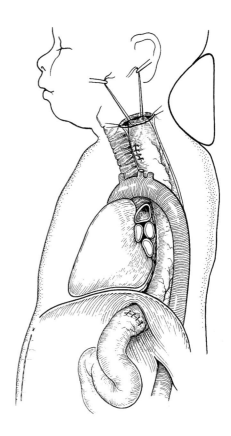

7b

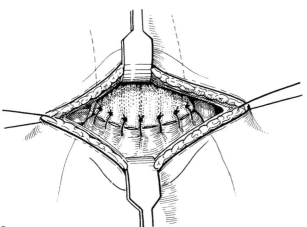

8

GASTROESOPHAGEAL ANASTOMOSIS

8 The transected end of the cervical esophagus is now anastomosed to the highest part of the stomach using a full-thickness single layer of interrupted 4/0 polyglycolic acid sutures.

A 10–12 Fr transanastomotic nasogastric tube is inserted into the intrathoracic stomach before completing the anterior layer of the anastomosis. This is left on free drainage and aspirated at regular intervals to prevent acute gastric dilatation in the early postoperative period.

WOUND CLOSURE

A soft rubber drain may be placed at the site of the anastomosis in the neck and the wound is closed in layers.

The margins of the diaphragmatic hiatus are sutured to the antrum of the stomach with a few interrupted sutures – 4/0 polyglycolic acid or braided polyamide (Nurolon) – so that the pylorus lies just below the diaphragm.

A fine-bore feeding jejunostomy has been found to be of considerable value in providing enteral nutrition in the first few weeks following gastric transposition, before full oral nutrition is established.

The abdominal incision is closed en masse or in layers.

Final anatomy

9 The gastroesophageal anastomosis is shown in the cervical region with the nasogastric tube passing into the intrathoracic stomach. The pyloroplasty is below the diaphragm and a feeding jejunostomy tube is inserted for postoperative feeding. This is particularly important for infants with esophageal atresia who have previously not acquired the skill of oral feeding. The jejunostomy is a source of potential complications and it is probably wise to omit it in older children who have previously taken full oral nutrition, e.g. caustic strictures.

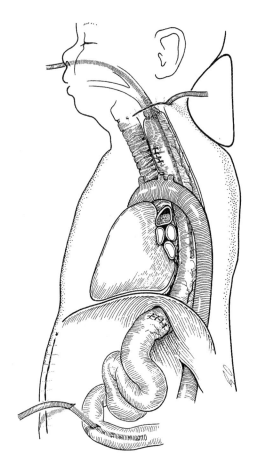

9

Laparoscopic–assisted gastric replacement of the esophagus

The open method of gastric transposition has been the procedure of choice in our institution for almost three decades. During the past few years, we have performed the laparoscopic-assisted gastric transposition. Few reports have been published on this technique due to the challenging nature of this procedure and the steep learning curve required.

The preoperative preparation of the patient and the details of the anesthesia are discussed above.

The following approaches are considered for the laparoscopic-assisted gastric interposition:

- No previous thoracic surgery or corrosive esophagitis (patient with or without cervical esophagostomy):
  - laparoscopic mobilization of the stomach and distal esophagus;
  - mobilization of esophagus in the neck;
  - esophagectomy via laparoscopic and neck approach (no thoracotomy or thoracoscopy);

  - transposition of the stomach;
  - esophagogastric anastomosis in the neck.
- Previous thoracic surgery or corrosive esophagitis (patient without cervical esophagostomy):
  - laparoscopic mobilization of the stomach;
  - laparoscopic mobilization of distal esophagus;
  - thoracoscopic or open thoracotomy for esophagectomy;
  - transposition of the stomach;
  - esophagogastric anastomosis in the neck or upper mediastinum.
- Previous thoracic surgery or corrosive esophagitis and esophagostomy (patient with cervical esophagostomy):
  - thoracoscopic mobilization of the esophagus;
  - laparoscopic mobilization of the stomach and distal esophagus;
  - mobilization of esophagus in the neck;
  - esophagectomy via laparoscopic and neck approach;
  - transposition of the stomach;
  - esophagogastric anastomosis in the neck.

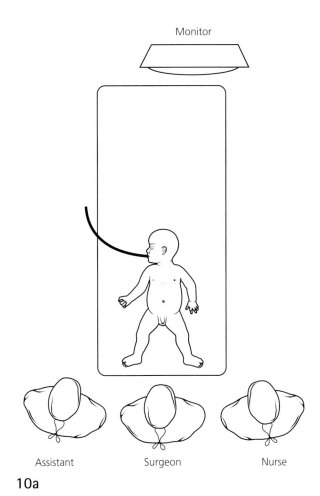

Monitor

Assistant   Surgeon   Nurse

10a

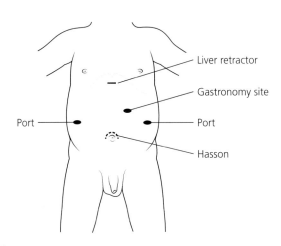

Liver retractor

Gastronomy site

Port

Port

Hasson

11

APPROACH 1: NO PREVIOUS THORACIC SURGERY OR CORROSIVE ESOPHAGITIS (PATIENT WITH OR WITHOUT CERVICAL ESOPHAGOSTOMY)

Patient positioning

10a,b The child is positioned at the foot of the operating table accordingly to the floor plan and the video monitor is placed at the head of the table. The table should be tilted head up about 20–30°. In older children, the legs are abducted using a special split table and the operator works between the legs at the bottom of the table; the position of the video monitor is as above.

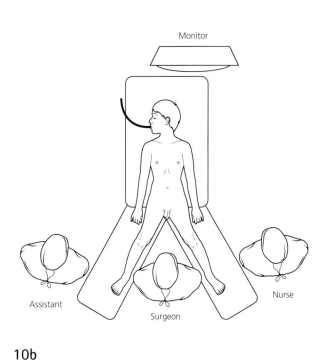

Monitor

Assistant   Surgeon   Nurse

10b

Port placements

11 The operation is performed with three ports. A primary port for the telescope (5-mm Hasson) is usually placed above the umbilicus. Two ports for insertion of instruments are placed in the right and left upper quadrants of the abdomen; it is important to insert these ports laterally, placed so that a wide angle is created that facilitates the intracorporeal suturing. The port on the right upper quadrant can be 3 or 5 mm depending on the size of the patient. The authors prefer a 5-mm disposable port in the left quadrant since it allows the introduction of needles for suturing and accommodates both 3- and 5-mm laparoscopic instruments. In the midline of the epigastrium, a small incision is made for the introduction of a Nathanson liver retractor without insertion of a port. The liver retractor size is decided on the basis of the liver and child size. The liver retractor is kept in position with the help of a fast clamp.

Laparoscopy

During the following operative steps a 30° camera is used.

- **Mobilization of the stomach.** The gastrostomy is mobilized from the anterior abdominal wall using a hook diathermy. To facilitate closure, the gastrostomy tube is left in place until the first suture is inserted on the stomach; the remaining part of the gastrostomy is closed using intracorporeal sutures of 3/0 or 4/0 Prolene. Using the Nathanson liver retractor, the liver can be easily retracted upwards, allowing mobilization of the stomach. When a failed open or laparoscopic fundoplication and/or a gastrostomy had been previously performed, adhesions will be present between the stomach and the liver. These adhesions are carefully divided using hook diathermy and the liver retractor is moved in the desired position. Mobilization of the greater and lesser curve of the stomach is performed following the same principles described in the open technique (see Figure 23.3). The right gastric artery is identified and preserved and the left gastric vessels are divided using hook diathermy or Harmonic scalpel.

- **Resection of the distal esophagus.** The distal esophageal pouch is resected as described above and the esophagogastric junction is closed with intracorporeal sutures of 3/0 or 4/0 Prolene.

- **Pyloroplasty or pyloromyotomy.** A short Heinecke–Mikulicz pyloroplasty is performed, the transverse incision being closed horizontally with interrupted 3/0 or 4/0 Prolene. Alternatively, a short pyloromyotomy is performed.

Mobilization of the cervical esophagus

The cervical esophagus is mobilized as described above and a posterior mediastinal tunnel is developed from above, using digital dissection (see Fig. 5).

Tunnel in posterior mediastinum

12 The posterior mediastinum is visualized from below using a 0° camera inserted via the Hasson cannula. Space is created in the posterior mediastinum using a 'two-stick' triangulation maneuver with blunt dissection by two laparoscopic graspers advanced through the esophageal hiatus or by monopolar hook diathermy. Occasionally, if previous thoracic surgery has been performed, it may be necessary to mobilize the esophagus in the mediastinum via a thoracoscopic approach.

The mediastinal tunnel is further dilated using a long blunt-ended forceps and, then, increasing sizes of a Hegar dilator (Seward Thackray, Gwent, UK) to accommodate the transposed stomach. The laparoscopic camera is advanced above the hiatus and the Hegar dilators are introduced through the cervical approach and are seen emerging into the upper mediastinum.

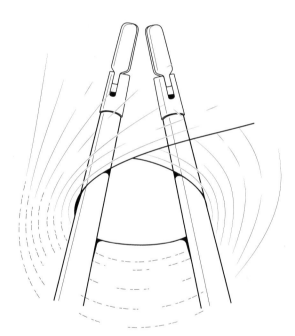

12

Transposition of the stomach

An intercostal drain is inserted via the neck and advanced in the posterior mediastinum. It is retrieved in the abdomen and secured to two sutures positioned in the most proximal part of the fundus of the stomach.

Eesophagogastric anastomosis

The stomach is drawn into the neck and sutured to the cervical esophagus in a single-layer anastomosis, using interrupted sutures.

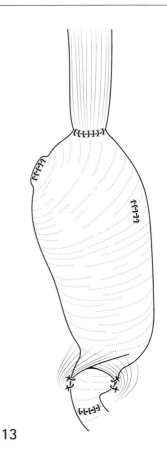

Hiatal defect

13 To prevent herniation of intestine through the esophageal hiatus, the authors recommend: (1) a meticulous reapproximation of the diaphragmatic crura once the stomach has been pulled up and (2) suturing of the antrum of the stomach to the diaphragmatic crura.

The wounds are closed with interrupted sutures, and the port sites are closed with tissue glue. A nasogastric tube is used, with the tip positioned in the middle of the mediastinum. If the chest is not opened, a chest drain is not required.

A feeding jejunostomy is performed when appropriate.

13

APPROACH 2: PREVIOUS THORACIC SURGERY OR CORROSIVE ESOPHAGITIS (PATIENT WITHOUT CERVICAL ESOPHAGOSTOMY)

The laparoscopic procedure is performed first as described in Approach 1. The position of the patient for laparoscopy is illustrated above.

The thoracoscopy (or if necessary, thoracotomy) approach is performed.

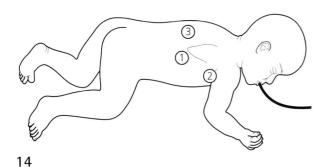

14 The child is placed in a three-quarters left prone position. The surgeon is at the left side of the table with the screen opposite at the right upper end of the table. The assistant is at the surgeon's left side, and the scrub nurse at the bottom end of the table.

14

15 Three cannulae are inserted in the right chest in a V-shape. The first cannula, a 5-mm one is inserted just anterior to the angle of the scapula. A 30° telescope is inserted and the chest insufflated with CO_2 at 5 mmHg and flow of 2 L/min until the lung is collapsed. Following this, the CO_2 insufflation pressure can be reduced. A 5-mm port is inserted posterior to the scapula for the use of working instruments. A further 5-mm port is inserted in the axilla. The lung collapses or is retracted anteriorly to visualize the posterior mediastinum. Occasionally, if the lung does not collapse completely, it is necessary to introduce another 5-mm port posteriorly to the other two working ports to retract the lung anteriorly by using an atraumatic forceps. Meticulous dissection is performed due to the adhesions in the mediastinum.

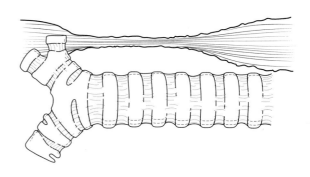

15

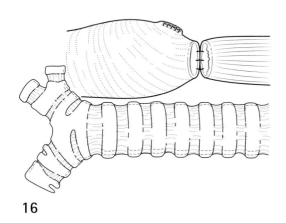

16

16 The esophagus is fully mobilized and the stomach pull-through is in the chest. The esophagectomy is performed and the esophagogastric junction is closed using the technique described above. The esophagogastric anastomosis is performed in the upper mediastinum using a single layer of interrupted stiches of Prolene 4/0 or 3/0. A chest drain is left through one of the ports.

APPROACH 3: PREVIOUS THORACIC SURGERY OR CORROSIVE ESOPHAGITIS (PATIENT WITH CERVICAL ESOPHAGOSTOMY)

The thoracoscopic (or thoracotomic) approach is performed first. The position of the patient and the port placement is described in Approach 2. The esophagus is fully mobilized.

The patient is positioned supine, and the remainder of the operation is as described in Approach 1.

The postoperative management after the laparoscopic-assisted operation does not differ from the open operation.

There are few reports on the laparoscopic-assisted gastric replacement of the esophagus in children. In 2007, Shalaby and colleagues published a series of 27 cases of post-corrosive esophageal stricture that were treated with laparoscopic-assisted transhiatal esophagectomy and gastric transposition. They reported an anastomotic leakage rate of 11 percent and a stricture rate of 15 percent. Recently, we noticed that the development of a large hiatus hernia appears to be more frequent in the laparoscopic approach compared to the more established open operation.

The minimally invasive procedure described above is challenging and should be performed by surgeons with experience in performing advanced laparoscopy and thoracoscopy.

POSTOPERATIVE CARE

Careful monitoring of vital functions is essential in the early postoperative period. There has been a fairly extensive dissection in the tissues posterior to the trachea, and edema may produce respiratory embarrassment. Elective nasotracheal intubation with assisted ventilation for a few days will simplify the postoperative course and reduce the incidence of respiratory problems.

Jejunal feeds are instituted on the second or third day after operation. The safest method of delivery of these feeds is by a slow continuous infusion rather than as a bolus, which can provoke a 'dumping' effect. A contrast swallow is performed 5–7 days after surgery, and if no leak is identified at the anastomosis, oral feeding may be commenced. The cervical drain is removed when the integrity of the anastomosis has been demonstrated.

COMPLICATIONS

In the period 1981–2005, 192 gastric transpositions were performed at Great Ormond Street Hospital, London, UK. Fifty-two percent were via the posterior mediastinal route without thoracotomy. The mortality rate was 5.2 percent. Anastomotic leakage occurred at the esophagogastric connection in 12 percent and strictures developed in 19 percent. All leaks except one closed spontaneously and all strictures except three responded to endoscopic dilatation. Strictures were more common (38 percent) after caustic ingestion.

Delayed gastric emptying and dumping syndrome also occurred in some patients, but usually resolved spontaneously within a few months. Feeding problems and recurrent vomiting are commonly encountered in the early postoperative period, but are generally transient.

OUTCOME

Good to excellent results are achieved in 90 percent of patients. Growth and development do not appear to be affected, and respiratory function is not impaired.

FURTHER READING

Hirschl RB, Yardeni D, Oldham K *et al*. Gastric transposition for esophageal replacement in children: experience with 41 consecutive cases with special emphasis on esophageal atresia. *Annals of Surgery* 2002; **236**: 531–9.

Orringer HB, Sloan H. Esophagectomy without thoracotomy. *Journal of Thoracic and Cardiovascular Surgery* 1978; **76**: 643–54.

Shalaby R, Shams A, Soliman SM *et al*. Laparoscopically assisted transhiatal esophagectomy with esophagogastroplasty for post-corrosive esophageal stricture treatment in children. *Pediatric Surgery International* 2007; **23**: 545–9.

Spitz L. Gastric transposition via the mediastinal route for infants with long-gap esophageal atresia. *Journal of Pediatric Surgery* 1984; **19**: 149–54.

Spitz L. Gastric transposition for esophageal substitution in children. *Journal of Pediatric Surgery* 1992; **27**: 252–9.

Spitz L, Kiely E, Pierro A. Gastric transposition in children – a 21-year experience. *Journal of Pediatric Surgery* 2004; **39**: 276–81.

Spitz L, Kiely E, Sparnon T. Gastric transposition for esophageal replacement in children. *Annals of Surgery* 1987; **206**: 69–73.

Stanwell J, Drake D, Pierro A *et al*. Paediatric laparoscopic assisted gastric transposition. Early experience and outcomes. *Journal of Laparoendoscopic and Advanced Surgical Techniques* 2010; **20**: 177–81.

Ure BM, Jesch NK, Sümpelmann R, Nustede R. Laparoscopically assisted gastric pull-up for long gap esophageal atresia. *Journal of Pediatric Surgery* 2003; **38**: 1661–2.

24

Jejunal interposition

DAVID C VAN DER ZEE

HISTORY

Reconstruction of the esophagus in long gap esophageal atresia (type A) has always been a challenge. The fact that many different techniques have been developed over the years indicates that reconstruction is not an easy procedure. In 1946, Reinhoff performed an intrathoracic jejunal replacement of the esophagus. Jejunal interposition for long gap esophageal atresia was first described by Akiyama *et al.* in 1971, and was later adopted by Bax *et al.* The technique is demanding, but the results are encouraging, even in the long term.

PRINCIPLES AND JUSTIFICATION

The jejunum is ideally suited for esophageal replacement, because it maintains good isoperistalsis and has a growth rate similar to that of the normal esophagus. In contrast to other techniques, there is little or no reflux and there are no pulmonary sequelae.

With good nursing care and a sump drain in place, the proximal esophagus can be drained adequately in the period before the reconstruction and a cervical esophagostomy is not always necessary. A prior esophagostomy necessitates that a cervical proximal anastomosis will be performed when a reconstruction is undertaken. The crucial part of the procedure is meticulous dissection of the jejunal pedicle graft. Ideally, the proximal anastomosis is placed in the thorax.

The procedure commences with a right-sided thoracotomy or thoracoscopy to obtain an accurate assessment of the proximal and distal esophagus and to determine whether a primary anastomosis is possible. If it is decided that a jejunal interposition is needed, the thoracic procedure is terminated and the patient is repositioned into a supine position for a midline laparotomy and preparation of the jejunal pedicle graft. If the graft is judged to be of adequate length, a path is created retrocolic through the lesser omentum and esophageal hiatus. It is vitally important to ensure that the pedicle is not twisted when bringing it up into the thorax. After the abdominal wound has been closed again, the thoracotomy is performed/reopened, and the graft is tailored to its proper size. Both the proximal and distal anastomosis is preferably made intrathoracically.

PREOPERATIVE ASSESSMENT AND PREPARATION

The first step in a neonate with a long gap esophageal atresia usually is the placement of a gastrostomy for feeding. During this procedure, a tracheobronchoscopy is carried out to exclude a proximal fistula. A proximal fistula usually prevents the proximal esophagus from increasing in length. Through the gastrostomy, the length of the distal esophagus can be determined, either with bougies or by contrast study. An intestinal contrast study to determine the length of the small intestine is performed just prior to the interposition procedure.

No specific preoperative bowel management measures are necessary.

ANESTHESIA

Jejunal interposition is accomplished under general anesthesia. An epidural catheter for intra- and postoperative pain management is inserted. An arterial line is placed for sampling during the procedure and postoperatively. Because of the length of the procedure, a urine catheter is introduced.

OPERATION

1, 2 The patient is positioned either in a left lateral decubitus position for thoracotomy or in a three-quarter left prone position for thoracoscopy.

The proximal esophagus in the superior mediastinum is mobilized. It is important to confirm that there is no proximal fistula present to prevent full mobilization of the proximal esophagus.

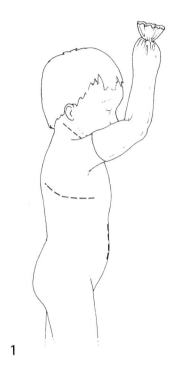

1

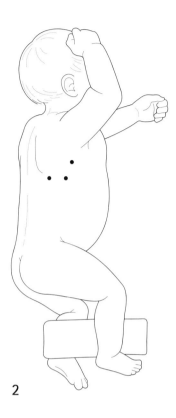

2

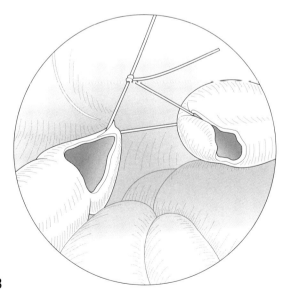

3

3 The distal esophagus is now assessed. If the surgeon has the impression that the distal esophagus may have sufficient length for a primary anastomosis, the distal esophagus is fully mobilized towards the hiatus. If the remaining gap is less than 1–2 cm under maximal traction, an attempt may be undertaken to approximate the two ends of the esophagus. Two or three full-thickness sutures are inserted in the proximal and distal ends of the esophagus, and with a sliding knot, they are slowly advanced bringing the two ends together. This can either be undertaken thoracoscopically or open. If this is successful an anastomosis can still be made.

When this option is unsuccessful, or the primary situation is such that an attempt to anastomosis is not possible, the distance between the two ends is measured, in order to prepare the jejunal pedicle graft. The thorax is closed provisionally, the patient is positioned in a supine position and a midline laparotomy is undertaken. When in place, the gastrostomy is taken down. The proximal jejunal loops are inspected for anomalies in their anatomy that might preclude the dissection.

The next step is to prepare everything for transposition of the graft into the thorax. This entails mobilization of the esophageal hiatus to allow the passage of the graft into the thorax. Usually the short gastric vessels are taken down in order to facilitate the entrance to the lesser omentum and hiatus. The hiatus is dilated using Hegar dilators up to H14.

The proximal jejunum is transected approximately 3–5 cm from the ligament of Treitz and two mesenteric branches are severed centrally to gain length of the pedicle. The length of the pedicle is measured to determine if sufficient length has been obtained before the distal jejunal end is transected just proximal to the third mesenteric branch. The two ends of proximal and distal jejunum are anastomosed.

4a–c Only the most proximal 3–5 cm of jejunum will be used for the interposition and the rest of the mobilized jejunal is carefully dissected from its vasculature at the level of the jejunal serosa and resected. Initially the distal portion of jejunum may appear somewhat bluish due to the 'steal' of circulation in the proximal part of the jejunum, but as dissection progresses the circulation improves and the final 3–5 cm of jejunum remaining on the pedicle resumes good vascularity. It is import to keep an eye on the position of the vasculature at all times to avoid twisting or strangulation of the vascular stalk.

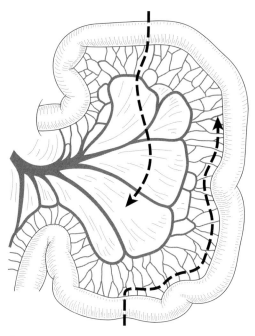

4a

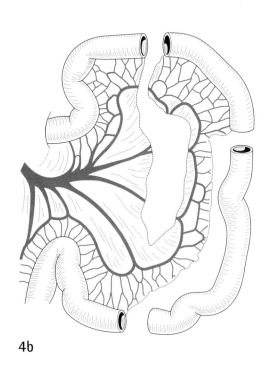

4b

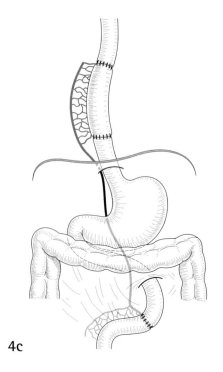

4c

An opening is now made in the mesentery of the transverse colon somewhat on the left side to pass the jejunal graft with its pedicle through in a comfortable way. The graft and its blood supply are closely observed at all times while it is passed through the lesser omentum and through the esophageal hiatus. The jejunal graft is carefully placed in the lower thorax.

Because time now plays an important role, the abdomen is closed provisionally.

The patient is repositioned in a left lateral decubitus position and the thorax is opened again. After retraction of the lung, the pedicled graft is located and carefully stretched into the thorax carefully maintaining the vasculature. The definitive length of the graft is determined and if necessary adjusted. First the proximal end of the jejunal graft is anastomosed to the proximal esophagus using Vicryl® 5 × 0 and only after that anastomosis has been completed, can the distal portion be adjusted for anastomosis to the distal esophagus. As the distal esophagus in many instances is hypoplastic, the distal esophagus is opened obliquely to obtain an adequate diameter for the anastomosis. The anastomosis is made using Vicryl 5 × 0 interrupted sutures.

A transanastomotic tube is passed into the stomach. A thoracic drain is left *in situ* for the first few postoperative days.

After closure of the thorax, the patient is turned back into the supine position for refashioning of a gastrostomy and final closure of the laparotomy wound.

POSTOPERATIVE CARE

A contrast swallow is performed on postoperative day 5. If there is no leakage, oral feeding can be initiated.

If the child returns with feeding difficulties, a contrast study can exclude anastomotic strictures. Sometimes when the distal esophagus is but a small bud there may be dysphagia, requiring dilatation, but usually swallowing problems resolve in due course.

OUTCOME

Although the procedure is demanding, there has been no graft loss in our series. Twenty-seven children received a jejunum interposition between 1988 and 2009, of whom 22 had long gap esophageal atresia (eight had a proximal fistula), three had caustic burns, and two severe peptic strictures. Five patients developed an anastomotic leak – four thoracic and one abdominal. On follow up, four children had complaints of reflux for which they were treated with antireflux medication. Five children occasionally experience functional stenosis at the distal anastomosis that responds well to domperidon. Two children are treated for upper airway complaints.

The major advantage of jejunal pedicle grafts is that they grow at the same speed as the native esophagus, redundancy does not occur, and the grafts display peristalsis facilitating good passage of solid food.

FURTHER READING

Akiyama H, Ishii K, Kodaira Y *et al*. Esophageal reconstruction with a pedicled jejunum in esophageal atresia (type A). *Shujutsu* 1971; **25**: 711–19.

Bax KN. Jejunum for bridging long-gap esophageal atresia. *Seminars in Pediatric Surgery* 2009; **18**: 34–9.

Bax KN, Roskott AM, van der Zee DC. Esophageal atresia without distal tracheoesophageal fistula: high incidence of proximal fistula. *Journal of Pediatric Surgery* 2008; **43**: 522–5.

Bax NM, van der Zee DC. Jejunal pedicle grafts for reconstruction of the esophagus in children. *Journal of Pediatric Surgery* 2007; **42**: 363–9.

25

Foker technique

JOHN FOKER

INTRODUCTION

1 The difficulty of a primary repair in esophageal atresia (EA) is directly related to the distance or gap between the two atretic segments (see illustration 1). The majority of patients have a short gap between segments because of a lower tracheoesophageal fistula (TEF) (type C). Longer gaps are found in patients with pure esophageal atresia with the lower segment ending above the diaphragm (type A2) or those with an upper pouch TEF (type B). The most difficult cases include pure EAs where the lower end might not even reach the diaphragm (type A_1) and patients in whom the initial attempt at repair has failed and a long gap (LG) has resulted. A true primary repair requires that the gastroesophageal (GE) junction remains below the diaphragm and no circular myotomies are done.

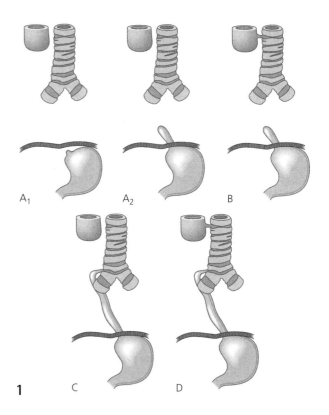

1

HISTORY

Many approaches have been used to solve the problem of long gap EA (LG-EA). Delayed repair, with or without bougienage, may be successful, but if not, other procedures such as circular myotomies, gastric pull ups, and interposition grafts have been used to close the gap. Unfortunately, these are frequently attended by a variety of short- and long-term problems.

Time and bougienage, when successful, result in a true primary esophageal repair and support the belief that growth of the segments is possible. A reliable and relatively rapid method to achieve a true primary esophageal repair across the entire EA spectrum, however, has been missing. Recently, growth induction by axial tension on the segments has been shown to reliably provide the signal to accomplish this goal.

PRINCIPLES AND JUSTIFICATION

The esophageal segments are clearly capable of growth, making EA a developmental rather than a primary genetic defect. Tension is common among the physiological signals for tissue growth. Esophageal growth can be relatively rapidly induced by traction sutures.

PREOPERATIVE ASSESSMENT AND PREPARATION

Evaluation and imaging

Beyond the usual patient evaluation for other anomalies, an estimation of gap length is useful in preoperative planning and can be achieved in several ways.

2, 3 The author favors an unstressed 'gapogram' achieved by contrast material in the gastrostomy tube to define the lower esophageal segment and a radio-opaque catheter or injection of air into the upper pouch. For the infant with a gasless abdomen (isolated atresia), placement of a gastrostomy tube aids in the estimation of gap length and provides a route for feeding until EA repair. This method provides a reasonable assessment of the difficulty of the cases, although it does not provide information on the gap length after dissection and pulling the ends together. The judgment about the feasibility of a primary repair, however, should be made in the operating room before opening the segments. When there is doubt, a period of, traction-induced growth will usually solve the problem.

When instruments, such as Hegar dilators are used to push the ends together as closely as possible for the preoperative gap evaluation, a false impression may result that a relatively short gap exists. In the operating room, the last centimeter or two of gap may be very difficult to bridge.

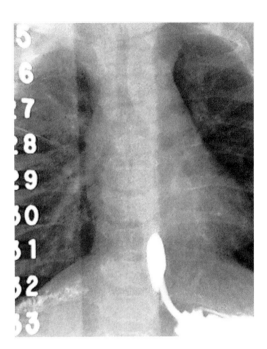

2

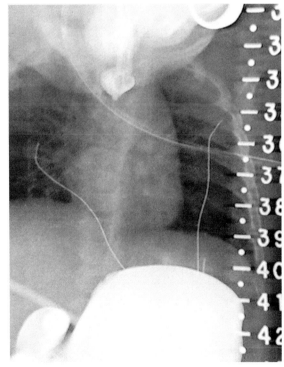

3

Timing

Growth induction requires tissue strength during traction. The aim should be to allow the infant to attain the weight of 3–3.5 kg, at which stage the tissues will be sufficiently sturdy for traction in order to produce a strong growth response and achieve a relatively prompt repair.

OPERATION

Position for the thoracotomy incision

A right posterior-lateral thoracotomy incision is used. For a baby 3–6 kg in weight, a 3-cm incision will suffice. An

4 This incision allows any part of the thoracic cavity to be accessed by varying which interspace is entered. When there is considerable separation between the segments and both will be put on traction, two intercostal incisions through the single skin incision are desirable. For assessing the gap length, a thorascope can be used.

When traction sutures will be used, a transpleural approach allows the esophageal segments to move as freely as possible. Otherwise, the pleura will drape over the esophageal segments, adhere, and shut down growth.

easily removed plastic tape such as Micropore (R) holds the patient firmly in a straight lateral position as shown.

The incision and exposure

The esophagus resides in the posterior mediastinum, therefore the incision is begun below the tip of the scapula and carried posteriorly until the paraspinal ligaments are reached. The incision meets the requirements of location, exposure, flexibility and, with care in closing, minimal long-term consequences for the chest wall and shoulder girdle.

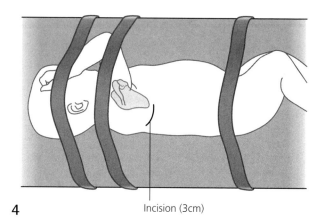

4   Incision (3cm)

Location and mobilization of the segments

For the experienced surgeon, the upper and lower esophageal segments can be reliably found. When the segments are very small or there have been previous operations in the area, they can be more difficult to identify.

Effective dissection of the upper pouch begins with a

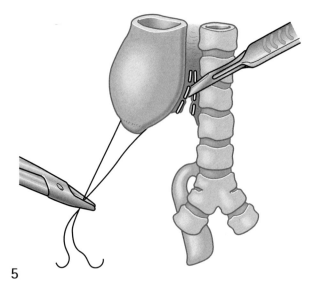

5

longitudinal incision in the parietal pleura posterior to the trachea to open up the space in which the upper pouch will be found. A tube placed down from the mouth will elongate and make the upper pouch more easily visible. A 5/0 prolene suture doubly placed superficially in the end of the pouch will aid in the dissection and minimize tissue injury from grasping it with instruments.

5 The main difficulty in dissecting free the upper pouch may come from a variable degree of tissue fusion with the membranous portion of the trachea. When considerable fusion is present, the dissection can be aided as shown. By first doubly clipping the tissue, it can be sharply divided with little risk of bleeding.

6 In more extreme cases of LG-EA, the lower segment may be at or below the diaphragm. If the lumen is over 10 mm in length by contrast study and/or endoscopy, it should be found through a low intercostal opening. For purposes of illustration, the intercostal opening is shown much longer than in life and the anterior extension illustrated contributes nothing to the operation. At the level of the diaphragm posteriorly, the vagus nerve is found and the parietal pleura close to the nerve incised. The tissue near the vagus nerve is grasped and pulled upward (the nerve is not grasped). Dissection is carried into the posterior mediastinum crossing over to the left side where the esophageal hiatus and the small lower segment will be.

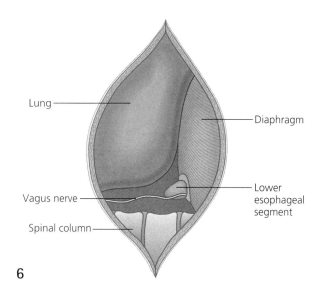

6

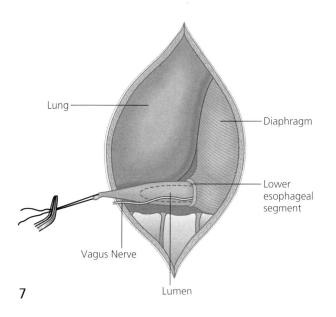

7

7 In order to minimize damage to the segment, a 5/0 prolene suture doubly placed at the tip is helpful during the dissection. The dissection continues down to the diaphragmatic hiatus, but not into it to ensure the GE junction remains below the diaphragm and stomach does not herniate into the chest.

Even a small nubbin (3–4 mm) of esophagus can be grown into a very adequate lower esophageal segment (see illustration 3). In these cases, the primordial esophageal segment must be found through an abdominal incision and will require very careful placement of 7/0 prolene sutures anchored to the diaphragm to provide the stimulus of internal traction to begin the growth process. Several reconfigurations of the traction sutures may be needed for sufficient growth to allow the lower segment to be pulled through the diaphragm so that external traction can begin.

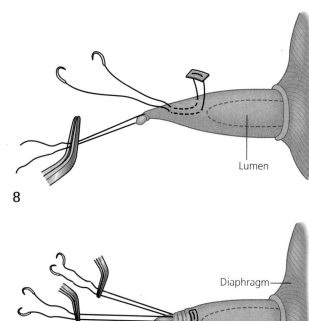

8

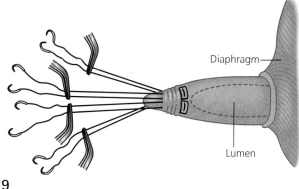

9

The traction sutures

8, 9 The tendency of the sutures to pull out can be reduced by using pledgeted (either autologous fascia or bovine pericardium) horizontal mattress sutures of 5/0 prolene. Prolene suture is suitable because it slides easily, is non-reactive and relatively sturdy but it does stretch. Because the sutures themselves lengthen with stretching, they may have to be re-tied to shorten them during the period of external traction.

The traction sutures should be carefully placed to both maximize the holding power and minimize the chance of a leak developing from either esophageal pouch. The sutures are placed to incorporate as much tissue as possible for holding power without entering the lumen. Four sutures are placed in each segment for external traction. For internal traction to the prevertebral fascia, three sutures seem better.

From time to time, sutures will pull out and if two or more sutures do pull out before adequate growth has been obtained, the sutures should be replaced and traction continued. Similarly, if a leak develops, the hole should be repaired.

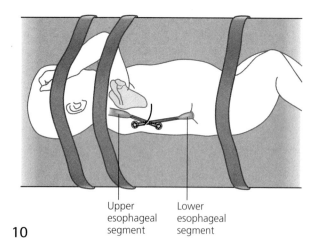

10

The traction apparatus

10 To maximize the slipperiness of the system, the esophageal segments are loosely wrapped in a cylinder of very thin Silastic sheeting (not shown).

The lower segment sutures are brought out of the chest wall above the incision and the upper pouch sutures below it.

11 The four pairs of eight sutures are brought out in a simple square of about 1 cm on the side. A thick piece of Silastic sheeting is cut into a circle and four holes placed in it resembling a button. Each suture pair is passed through the holes on one side and tagged. Because the tension that will be placed on the esophageal segment will be significant, the presence of the Silastic button will help dissipate the force and prevent the sutures from pulling through the skin. Tension can be increased daily to keep the growth signal active. A method which gives a feel for the tension consists of tying the suture pairs over short lengths of 2.5-mm diameter Silastic tubing with additional pieces of tubing inserted underneath the sutures at least daily to increase the tension.

When the number of tubing pieces becomes unwieldy, it is helpful to shorten the loop and start again. Once a familiarity is gained with the technique of the growth method, remarkable growth responses can be expected.

Growth induction necessarily means that at least two operations will be required for a primary esophageal repair. The first procedure will be to place the traction sutures which will induce growth. The second operation will be a primary repair of the grown esophageal segments. Between the two operations, tension is increased at least daily to ensure a good response.

The anastomosis

When growth is adequate, as assessed radiologically by introducing contrast medium into each segment, the original thoracotomy incision is reopened. Whatever the gap between the segments initially, the anastomosis tends to be located at the usual mid-thoracic level.

The segments are pulled together using the traction

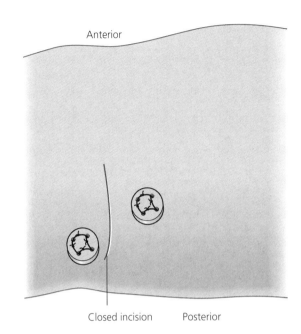

Anterior

Closed incision   Posterior

11

sutures to allow a final assessment as to whether or not the anastomosis can be readily achieved. If the two ends cannot be made to touch, an additional period of external traction should be used. If the ends can be brought together but with significant tension, internal traction will produce additional growth in 4–5 days. Although this may seem complicated, a true primary repair makes it worthwhile.

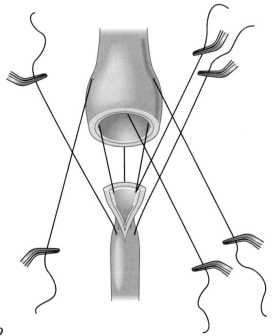

12 With the two ends open, the corner sutures are placed. Tagging the sutures will hold open the ends. The back row of sutures is placed with very generous full thickness bites and so they will be tied on the inside. The sutures are tagged individually as shown. Even after apparent adequate growth, it may take significant tension to bring the ends together. After the back row is placed, the sutures are crossed and with increasing traction over 5–10 minutes, the ends will slowly meet and can be held together. The individual sutures can be tied free of tension. Tension will gradually shift to the tied sutures.

12

13 The anterior row is placed in a similar fashion.

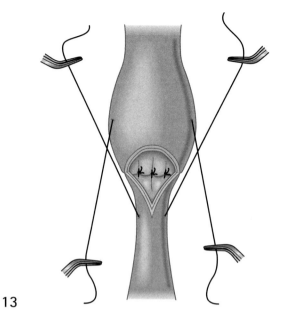

13

Closure

Late chest wall deformities from a thoracotomy incision depend mainly on two factors: (1) incision through the serratus anterior which can easily be avoided and (2) fusion of the ribs following an intercostal opening. There is little distractive force on the chest wall and the ribs should not be pulled together. To inhibit fusion further, we place a folded piece of thin Silastic sheeting between the ribs which is left behind.

Postoperative issues

For the first 3–5 days post-anastomosis, the patient is kept in a head elevated position (>20°) and on ventilatory support with moderate paralysis.

It has been found that LG-EA has a high incidence of GE reflux. The very small lower segment often appears not to have a narrowing at the area of the GE junction and external traction, despite keeping the GE junction below the diaphragm, may be detrimental to the sphincter. Whatever the causes, GE reflux is very common and our approach has been to treat it actively.

After about 2–3 weeks, a contrast study is done to assess the anastomosis and evaluate for GE reflux. If reflux is significant, a Nissen fundoplication within the next week or two is recommended.

The external traction will pull the GE junction and the fundus of the stomach up against the diaphragm making a laparoscopic Nissen more difficult. Consequently, our usual approach has been through a short left subcostal incision. An effective wrap will require about 2 cm of intra-abdominal esophagus. To ensure this, we place a 3/0 prolene suture around the esophagus at the level of the GE junction with superficial bites of tissue. Pulling down on this suture will ensure the wrap is around the esophagus.

Outcome

The longer-term results have been very encouraging. We believe that these patients, if the postoperative issues of GE reflux and stricture formation are effectively treated, will have an outcome indistinguishable from the best repairs of esophageal atresia/tracheoesophageal fistula (it should be noted that there is a significant incidence of GE reflux and stricture symptoms in EA/TEF patients).

Without effective postoperative treatment, however, the overall result will be compromised and these children will require significant medications, frequent clinic visits, and intermittent esophageal dilations.

FURTHER READING

Boyle EM, Irwin ED, Foker JE. Primary repair of ultra long gap esophageal atresia: results without a lengthening procedure. *Annals of Thoracic Surgery* 1997; **57**: 576–9.

Foker JE, Linden BC, Boyle EM, Marquardt C. Development of a true primary repair for the full spectrum of esophageal atresia. *Annals of Surgery* 1997; **226**: 533–43.

Foker JE, Kendall TC, Catton K, Khan KM. A flexible approach to achieve a true primary repair for all infants with esophageal atresia. *Seminars in Pediatric Surgery* 2005; **14**: 8–15.

Foker JE, Kendall Krosch TC, Catton K *et al.* Long gap esophageal atresia treated by growth induction: the biological potential and early follow-up results. *Seminars in Pediatric Surgery* 2009; **18**: 23–9.

Khan K, Foker JE. Use of high-resolution endoscopic ultrasound to examine the effect of tension of the esophagus during primary repair of long-gap esophageal atresia. *Pediatric Radiology* 2007; **37**: 41–5.

Khan KM, Krosch TC, Eickhoff JC *et al.* Achievement of feeding milestones after primary repair of long-gap esophageal atresia. *Early Human Development* 2009; **85**: 387–92.

Rintala RJ, Sistonen S, Pakarinen MP. Outcome of esophageal atresia beyond childhood. *Seminars in Pediatric Surgery* 2009; **18**: 50–6.

26

Congenital diaphragmatic hernia

ERICA R GROSS and CHARLES JH STOLAR

BACKGROUND

Although Paré was the first to describe diaphragmatic hernia in the sixteenth century, Bochdalek did not discuss the concept of an embryologic etiology until 1848, erroneously believing that the diaphragm ruptured after formation.

1 Congenital diaphragmatic hernia (CDH) is a field defect, involving the lungs, foregut, and chest wall, resulting from failure of the diaphragm to separate the pleuroperitoneal canal into the thorax and abdomen before the midgut returns through the umbilicus. Consequently, the abdominal viscera translocate into the chest in the first trimester when the lungs are at a vulnerable lung bud or glandular stage.

Both lungs are involved, the ipsilateral greater than the contralateral lung. Affected infants are born with a complex interface of pulmonary hypoplasia and pulmonary hypertension. There is decreased surface area available for gas exchange, compromised bronchiolar and pulmonary vascular beds and muscular hypertrophy of the intra-acinar arterioles. These anatomical changes are most severe in term neonates. Severe pulmonary hypoplasia can preclude extrauterine life, whereas successful management of pulmonary hypertension can lead to survival. Despite significant advances in neonatal intensive care and pediatric surgery, a cohort of affected infants does not survive.

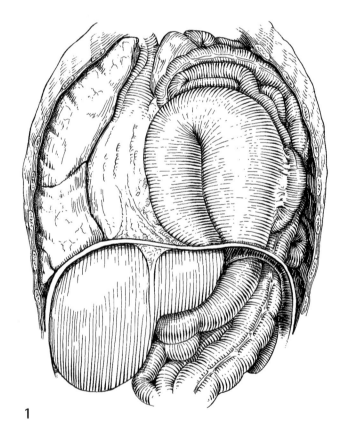

1

DIAGNOSIS

2a–c Most infants with CDH are diagnosed antenatally. Ultrasound may show bowel and/or liver in the chest, the heart and stomach in the same plane, or mediastinal shift. Magnetic resonance imaging (MRI) has also become a useful adjunct to differentiate CDH from lung bud anomalies. With right-sided CDH, MRI can identify eventration, hepatopulmonary fusion, and right atrial drainage of the hepatic veins, all of which have important

surgical implications. MRI can also estimate fetal lung volume or lung-to-head ratio (LHR), predictors of survival, but neither measurement is universally accepted.

CDH infants are typically near-term and present immediately with respiratory distress, tachypnea, grunting, and cyanosis. Physical examination reveals a scaphoid abdomen, asymmetric respiration and a barrel chest. Chest radiography confirms the diagnosis, showing multiple gas-filled bowel loops above the diaphragm, contralateral mediastinal shift, and a paucity of abdominal bowel gas.

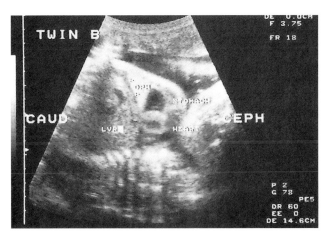

2a

2b

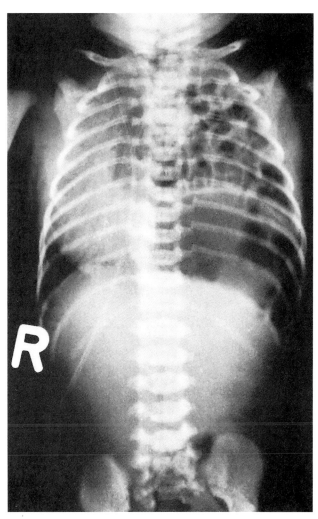

2c

PREOPERATIVE

Resuscitation

With antenatal diagnosis, the mother and fetus require transfer to an experienced center capable of appropriate neonatal, surgical, and extracorporeal membrane oxygenation (ECMO) care. If diagnosed postnatally, the infant is stabilized and transferred to the same type of specialized center prior to operation. Surgical intervention

is not an emergency. Recent experience demonstrates that infants can be medically stabilized over several days and then undergo elective repair. Infants with pulmonary hypoplasia incompatible with life are not candidates for ECMO. Infants with overwhelming pulmonary hypertension and some degree of pulmonary hypoplasia refractory to conventional therapy should be considered for resuscitation with ECMO.

Initial treatment starts with prompt intubation, nasogastric decompression, and vascular access. Bag-mask ventilation should be avoided to limit distention of the stomach in the chest. Umbilical artery catheterization allows accurate blood pressure monitoring and blood sampling. Because of right-to-left shunting at the ductus arteriosis, blood gas monitoring from the umbilical artery is misleading. A preductal arterial catheter or pulse oximetry is essential in guiding therapeutic interventions and evaluating gas exchange potential.

Respiratory care must avoid muscle paralysis and allow spontaneous respiration to minimize barotrauma. Ventilator settings range from low rates and modest peak airway pressures to high frequency oscillatory ventilation. The prevention of secondary lung injury cannot be over-emphasized.

Pharmacologic support consists of nitric oxide, which reduces right ventricular afterload by decreasing pulmonary vascular resistance, and ionotropes, to prevent hypotension and worsening acidosis. Milrinone, dopamine, and dobutamine are commonly used in this setting. Sildenafil, an agent that relaxes smooth muscle, may also be useful in decreasing the level of pulmonary hypertension.

ECMO is useful in the preoperative infant who has already demonstrated evidence of adequate lung function, based on preductal oxygenation, but who then deteriorates because of pulmonary hypertension. Such an infant is unlikely to tolerate surgery prior to respiratory stabilization.

Diaphragmatic repair is performed electively on infants who are hemodynamically stable with a physiologic acid-base status and are able to tolerate conventional ventilation. A follow-up echocardiogram should show resolution of pulmonary hypertension. For infants requiring ECMO, the same parameters demonstrating improvement of pulmonary vascular resistance are used prior to surgical repair.

Anesthesia

The airway should be controlled with an appropriately sized nasotracheal tube, preferred to orotracheal intubation because of decreased incidence of airway complications. Single lung ventilation is unnecessary. Intravenous anesthesia is administered as needed and complemented by muscle paralysis and narcotics. Mechanical ventilation is controlled throughout surgery with a pressure-cycled infant ventilator rather than the conventional anesthesia machine. Continuous oxygen saturation monitoring, both preductal and postductal, is critical. An arterial line should already be placed and accessible for intraoperative blood gases. A heating mattress is used, and the head and extremities are wrapped to minimize heat loss. Prophylactic antibiotics should be given perioperatively and can be continued postoperatively if any contamination is encountered.

SURGERY

Traditional open repair is accomplished transabdominally. Thoracoscopic techniques are also being advocated.

Transabdominal

POSITION OF PATIENT

The infant is positioned supine, elevating the thoracolumbar spine. Both the upper abdomen and chest are prepared as the operating fields.

INCISION

3 An ipsilateral subcostal incision is made 1 cm below the costal margin. To create a muscle flap with the transversalis abdominis muscle, make the incision 2 cm below the costal margin.

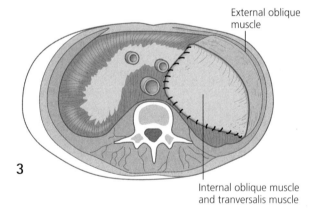

External oblique muscle

3

Internal oblique muscle and tranversalis muscle

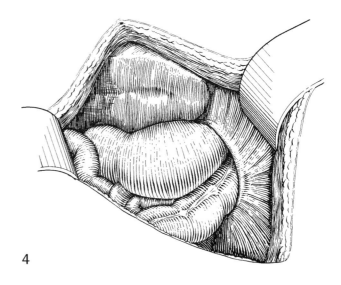

4

STEPS

4 The defect is exposed after the stomach is decompressed, and the viscera are reduced from the chest. The unfixed spleen and its attachments to the colon and pancreas are especially vulnerable. Reduction of the liver and spleen may be challenging, but can be accomplished by careful manual reduction using downward pressure from above.

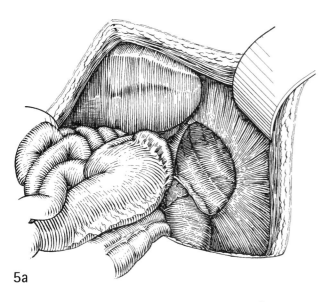

5a

5a–c If a true hernia sac exists, it must be excised to ensure proper healing of the defect. The posterior rim can be identified by tracing the anterior rim medially. Its mesothelial covering is sharply incised and carefully mobilized. Primary repair is accomplished with interrupted, simple, non-absorbable sutures.

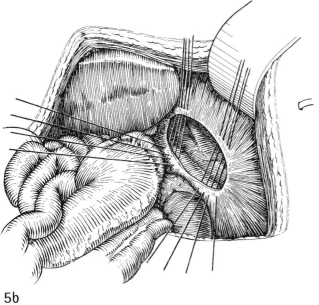

5b

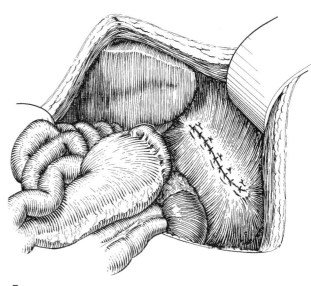

5c

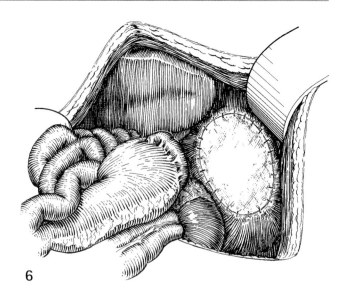

6 If a prosthetic patch is required, 1-mm polytetra-fluoroethylene (PTFE; Gore-tex™) is preferred. Laterally, the patch can be anchored to the ribs. An ipsilateral thoracostomy tube is unnecessary unless there is concern for bleeding or an air leak.

6

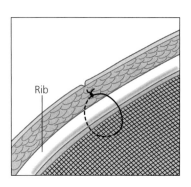

7

7 In cases of true diaphragmatic agenesis, the posterior and medial rim of diaphragm usually used to anchor mesh for a patch repair are absent. A larger prosthetic patch should be used for these defects and can be placed using pericostal sutures to bring the patch to the posterior wall, through the chest wall, through the diaphragm, and back out of the chest. Secure the knot in the subcutaneous tissue. Recurrent diapharagmatic hernias are very common in these patients.

Correction of malrotated midgut or an appendectomy is not indicated. Postoperative volvulus is rare, but significant bleeding after heparinization may be a major problem. Electrocautery is used as much as possible to perform the operation because of the potential need for ECMO and heparin postoperatively.

WOUND CLOSURE

Loss of abdominal domain challenges abdominal closure. Vigorous stretching of the abdominal wall should be avoided. If the abdomen cannot be closed safely, without compromising venous return, a 1-mm PTFE patch can augment the abdominal wall temporarily. A silo can be employed if bleeding or compromise to bowel circulation is a concern.

Transthoracic

While a thoracotomy may be used for CDH repair, it is generally avoided due to its morbidity. Thoracotomy for left CDH repair can be challenging because loss of abdominal domain makes reduction of thoracic contents difficult. Diaphragmatic repair through a right thoracotomy may be of value in cases of hepatopulmonary fusion or other anatomical variations that make reduction of the liver complicated. However, thorascoscopic repair is an option in a stable infant. Thoracoscopy should not be performed on infants on ECMO due to the high risk of bleeding.

Thorascopic repair

POSITION OF PATIENT

8 The infant is placed in a near-lateral decubitus position with a small raised support placed beneath. The chest is prepared from sternum to spine, including the abdomen, in anticipation of conversion to a transabdominal approach. Anesthesia should be positioned at the side of the operative table, and the operating surgeon stands at the head of the bed with a monitor by the patient's feet.

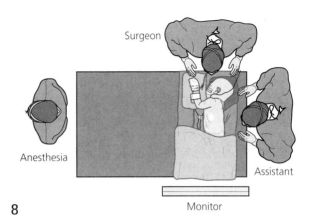

8

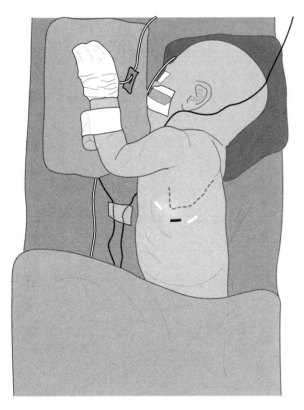

9

INCISION/ACCESS

9 A Veress needle is placed below the scapular tip in the midaxillary line while holding respiration. Carbon dioxide is insufflated, achieving an intrathoracic pressure of 3–5 mmHg. The Veress needle is then exchanged for a 4-mm trocar, and a 4-mm, 30° scope is inserted. Two additional 3- or 4-mm trocars are placed under direct visualization in the anterior and posterior axillary lines, cephalad to the camera port.

STEPS

Herniated abdominal contents are reduced into the abdominal cavity using cotton-tipped Kittners.

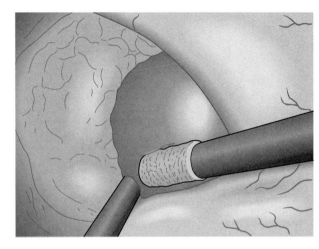

10 If the diaphragmatic defect can be easily approximated, primary repair is performed using interrupted, non-absorbable suture.

10

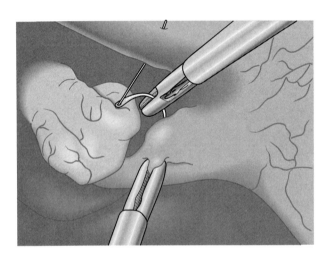

11

11 Pledgets should be used in areas of attenuated diaphragm. Silk or braided nylon is best for intracorporeal knot tying. Pericostal sutures can facilitate lateral closure of the defect as well.

12 External pressure on the chest wall aids approximation of diaphragmatic edges. When the defect cannot be closed primarily, a PTFE patch can be cut to size. Total diaphragmatic agenesis usually warrants conversion to an open, transabdominal approach.

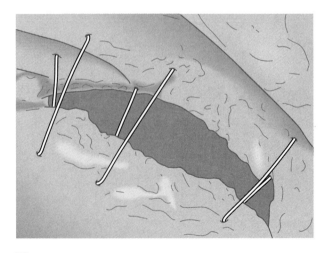

12

WOUND CLOSURE

The muscle is approximated with 4/0 Vicryl, and skin is closed with 5/0 Vicryl. Evacuation of the pneumothorax is accomplished by inserting a catheter into the chest before closure of the final port incision. A thoracostomy tube should only be used in cases with a concern for bleeding.

POSTOPERATIVE MANAGEMENT

The therapeutic strategy used in the preoperative period is reinstituted in the postoperative period. Muscle paralysis is discontinued to allow spontaneous respiration. Adequate analgesia with narcotics is mandatory. Sufficient intravenous fluids are given to maintain adequate circulating blood volume and hemoglobin for oxygen delivery.

OUTCOME

These patients require acute and long-term follow-up care by a multidisciplinary team consisting of pediatric surgeons, pulmonologists, cardiologists, and gastroenterologists. These children are not only at risk for hernia recurrence, but for chronic pulmonary hypertension and gastroesophageal reflux disease.

The risk of recurrent herniation after open, trans-abdominal repair has been reported to be as high as 10 percent, especially in the setting of ECMO and use of a prosthetic patch. Experience with thoracoscopic CDH repair has been well reported. We have observed outcomes of thoracoscopic and open repairs simultaneously and found a statistically higher recurrence rate in the infants repaired thoracoscopically (23 versus 0 percent). Therefore, we cannot support thoracoscopic repair as the standard of care for surgical management of CDH at this stage in its development.

ECMO

Although this therapy is discussed in detail in a separate chapter (**Chapter 27**), there are some special considerations for ECMO in these patients. Because ECMO may be appropriate both before and after operation, these infants should be transferred to an ECMO center as soon as possible after diagnosis and the infant (or fetus) is stable enough for transport. For patients repaired on ECMO, the use of Amicar should be considered.

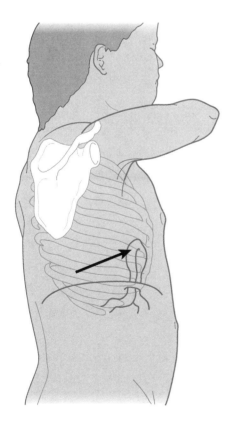

13

MORGAGNI HERNIA

13 A much less common type of diaphragmatic hernia, referred to as Morgagni hernia, occurs anteromedially on either side of the junction of the septum transversum and the thoracic wall. Morgagni hernias differ significantly from Bochdalek hernias in incidence, severity, presentation, and treatment.

Anterior diaphragmatic hernias account for less than 5 percent of all congenital diaphragmatic defects. Right-sided Morgagni hernias (90 percent) are significantly more common than left, due to the additional strength of the pericardial attachment to the diaphragm on the left. Bilateral Morgagni hernias are not an uncommon finding, and occasionally, communicate in the midline, constituting a large anterior diaphragmatic defect. Hernia sacs are much more common in patients with Morgagni hernia (95 percent) compared to Bochdalek hernia. The transverse colon and small bowel herniate most commonly.

Unlike Bochdalek hernia, Morgagni hernias rarely present in the neonatal period. When this defect is seen in the pediatric age group, recurrent pulmonary infection is the most common complaint, while gastrointestinal symptoms are much less frequent. Diagnosis can be made with a combination of posterior–anterior and lateral chest radiographs and upper gastrointestinal fluoroscopy.

Treatment of Morgagni hernias in asymptomatic patients is considered by some to be controversial. Repair can be performed transthoracically or transabdominally, however, transabdominal repair is advocated because it allows for repair of bilateral hernias, which are often only diagnosed intraoperatively. Repair consists of suturing the diaphragm to the underside of the posterior rectus sheath at the costal margin after reduction of the hernia. Most surgeons also advocate for resection of the sac, however this may increase the risk of pneumopericardiam or pneumothorax. Patients with Morgagni hernias are typically more stable preoperatively than patients with Bochdalek hernia and are better candidates for minimally invasive approaches to repair.

FURTHER READING

Al-Salem AH. Congenital hernia of Morgagni in infants and children. *Journal of Pediatric Surgery* 2007; **42**: 1539–43.

Boloker J, Wung J-T, Stolar CJH. Congenital diaphragmatic hernia in IZO infants treated consecutively with permissive hypercapnea, spontaneous respiration, elective surgery. *Journal of Pediatric Surgery* 2002; **37**: 357–66.

Gander JW, Fisher JC, Gross ER *et al.* Early recurrence of congenital diaphragmatic hernia is higher after thoracoscopic than open repair: a single institution study. *Journal of Pediatric Surgery* 2011; **46**: 1303–8.

Geggel RL, Murphy JD, Langleben D *et al.* Congenital diaphragmatic hernia: arterial structural changes and persistent pulmonary hypertension after surgical repair. *Journal of Pediatrics* 1985; **107**: 457–64.

Lansdale N, Alam S, Losty PD, Jesudason EC. Neonatal endosurgical congenital diaphragmatic hernia repair: a systematic review and meta-analysis. *Annals of Surgery* 2010; **252**: 1–7.

Reid L. Embryology of the lung. In: de Reuck AVS, Porter R (eds). *Development of the Lung*. London: Churchill, 1967: 109–30.

Silen ML, Canvasser DA, Kurkchubasche AG *et al.* Video-assisted thoracic surgical repair of a foramen of Bochdalek hernia. *Annals of Thoracic Surgery* 1995; **60**: 448–50.

Simpson JS, Gossage JD. Use of abdominal wall muscle flap in repair of large congenital diaphragmatic hernia. *Journal of Pediatric Surgery* 1971; **6**: 42–4.

27

Extracorporeal membrane oxygenation

THOMAS PRANIKOFF and RONALD B HIRSCHL

HISTORY

Extracorporeal membrane oxygenation (ECMO) has been used to describe a method of extracorporeal life support (ECLS) using extrathoracic cannulation for cardiopulmonary support. ECLS is a supportive rather than a therapeutic intervention. It provides adequate perfusion and gas exchange (venoarterial bypass) or gas exchange alone (venovenous support), and so avoids deleterious effects from high oxygen concentration and positive pressure ventilation, while allowing resolution of reversible heart and lung pathology.

PRINCIPLES AND JUSTIFICATION

Vascular access for ECLS in the neonate is particularly challenging due to the small vessel size. The route of access depends on the method used. Venoarterial (VA) bypass is indicated if both cardiac and pulmonary support are required, and in neonates where access for venovenous (VV) support cannot be obtained.

VV support is the method of choice for pulmonary failure and can adequately support most infants, including those with depressed cardiac function from high pressure ventilation used to manage their severe respiratory failure prior to ECMO. VV support is more physiologic than VA and provides well-oxygenated blood to the pulmonary circulation which acts as a potent vasodilator to reduce right to left shunting. It also obviates the need for arterial cannulation and thereby lowers risk of arterial embolization and from carotid ligation or repair. Various access sites, including the umbilical, femoral, and carotid/jugular vessels, have been used.

For VA access, the preferred site is the right atrium via the right internal jugular vein for venous drainage and the aortic arch via the right common carotid artery for arterial infusion. The internal jugular vein and carotid artery are relatively large in the neonate and may be distally ligated without major sequelae.

For VV access, a double-lumen cannula is placed into the right atrium via the right internal jugular vein. This technique is limited by the size of the vein, because the smallest cannula currently available is 12 Fr.

Technique selection

VA bypass requires arterial ligation to prevent distal embolization from flow past the cannula. VV support can be performed either using this technique or without vessel ligation via a percutaneous or semi-open technique. Percutaneous access utilizes the Seldinger technique to place the cannula. Because the size of the vessel in relation to the cannula is unknown, vessel disruption is a risk. For this reason, our preferred method is the semi-open technique. This technique requires a small incision to visualize the size of the vein as an aid to select the correct cannula size (usually 12 F or 15 F in a newborn). Cannula insertion can also be visualized through this incision. With this technique, vessel ligation is not utilized. This has several advantages: cephalad flow into the cannula increases the amount of deoxygenated blood available to enter the bypass circuit, the vessel may remain patent after decannulation, and kinking of the cannula at the vessel is reduced.

ECMO circuit

1 Blood is drained from the right atrium via the venous cannula into a small bladder by siphon/gravity. As long as venous drainage is adequate to fill the bladder, blood enters the raceway (tubing within the pump head) where it is actively pumped into the membrane lung. Here, blood travels in a countercurrent fashion to the sweep gas, separated by a thin silicone membrane. Oxygen enters the blood and carbon dioxide enters the sweep gas by simple diffusion along a concentration gradient. Blood then enters the heat exchanger where it is warmed to body temperature before entering the arterial cannula. This blood may either enter the arterial (VA bypass) or venous system (VV support).

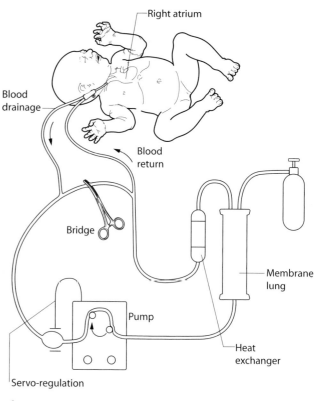

1

PREOPERATIVE

Vascular cannulation and decannulation are performed in the neonatal intensive care unit under adequate sedation and neuromuscular blockade. Neuromuscular blockade is especially important in preventing the potentially lethal complication of an air embolus during introduction of the venous cannula. The instruments and sterile procedures used are identical to those used in the operating room. Heparin sodium (100 units/kg) is drawn up for subsequent administration.

Anesthesia

Local anesthesia is administered by infiltration of 1 percent lidocaine.

OPERATION

Position of patient

The patient is placed supine with the head turned to the left. A roll is placed transversely beneath the shoulders. Special attention is paid to assuring that the endotracheal tube is positioned to prevent kinking under the drapes during the procedure. This can be accomplished by using a piece of suction tubing split lengthwise and placed over the tube at the connector to prevent kinking. The chest, neck, and right side of the face are aseptically prepared and draped.

Venoarterial/venovenous cannulation: open technique

INCISION

2 A transverse cervical incision, approximately 2–3 cm in length, is made one finger's breadth above the clavicle over the lower aspect of the right sternocleidomastoid muscle.

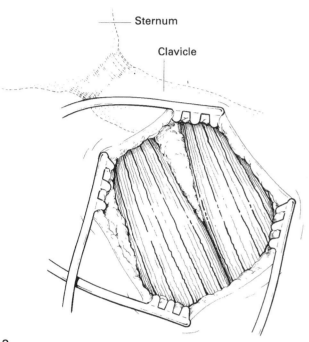

2

Sternum

Clavicle

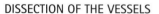

3

EXPOSURE OF THE CAROTID SHEATH

3 The platysma muscle and subcutaneous tissues are divided with electrocautery and the sternocleidomastoid muscle exposed. Dissection is continued bluntly between the sternal and clavicular heads of the muscle. The omohyoid muscle will be seen superiorly. It may be necessary to divide the omohyoid muscle tendon to expose the carotid sheath. Two alternating self-retaining retractors (e.g. Weitlanders) are placed.

DISSECTION OF THE VESSELS

4 The carotid sheath is opened and the internal jugular vein, common carotid artery, and vagus nerve are identified and isolated. Dissection is progressed proximally and distally along the vessels, dissecting the vein first. Special care should be taken while dissecting the vein to avoid induction of spasm, which makes subsequent introduction of a large venous cannula difficult. Manipulation of the vein therefore should be minimized. There is often a branch on the medial aspect of the internal jugular vein which must be ligated. Ligatures of 2/0 silk are placed proximally and distally around the internal jugular vein. The common carotid artery lies medial and posterior and has no branches, which makes its dissection proximally and distally safe. Ligatures of 2/0 silk are also placed around the carotid artery. The vagus nerve should be identified.

Once vessel dissection is completed, heparin (100 units/kg) is administered intravenously and 3 minutes allowed for circulation. During this waiting period, papaverine is instilled into the wound to enhance venous dilatation.

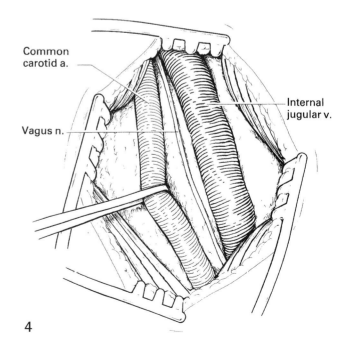

Common carotid a.

Vagus n.

Internal jugular v.

4

ARTERIOTOMY/VENOTOMY

5 For venoarterial bypass, the arterial cannula is chosen (usually 10 Fr, but will vary depending on the size of the infant) and marked with a 2/0 silk ligature, left uncut, at a point that will allow the tip of the cannula to lie at the ostium of the brachiocephalic artery (about 2.5 cm). The venous cannula (usually 12–14 Fr) is similarly marked at a point equal to the distance from the venotomy to the right atrium (roughly 6 cm). An obturator is placed into the venous cannula to prevent blood from flowing out through the side holes during introduction into the vessel. The common carotid artery is ligated distally. Proximal control is obtained with the use of an angled ductus clamp. A transverse arteriotomy is made near the distal ligature. The arteriotomy may be 'fish mouthed' by angling the incision. Care should be taken to make the arteriotomy and venotomy only as large as needed for the cannula selected to prevent weakness that might cause the vessel to tear more easily with traction during cannula insertion. Full thickness stay sutures of 6/0 polypropylene are placed on the proximal edge of the artery to prevent subintimal dissection during cannula insertion. Following arterial cannulation, a venotomy is performed in a similar fashion. Gentle retraction of the caudal ligature around the vein precludes the need for a ductus clamp during venotomy and venous cannulation. Stay sutures are also not routinely necessary for venous cannulation.

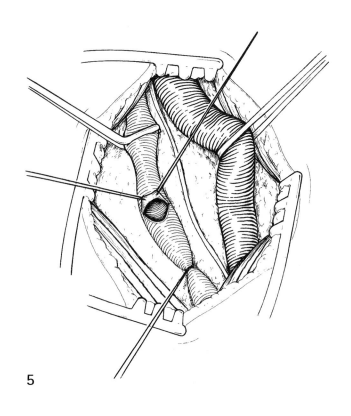

5

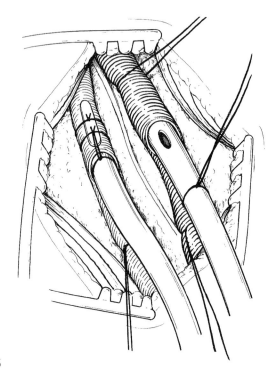

6

CANNULA PLACEMENT

6 The cannulas are carefully placed into the artery and vein and secured using two circumferential 2/0 silk ligatures, with a small piece of silastic vessel loop inside the ligatures to protect the vessels from injury during decannulation when the ligatures are sharply divided. The ends of the marking ligatures are tied to the most distal circumferential ligature for extra security. Immediately after each cannula is secured, it is carefully debubbled via back-bleeding and filling with heparinized saline. If the infant is hypovolemic, back-bleeding can be increased by compressing over the liver. During connection of the tubing to the cannula, it is helpful to gently squeeze the tubing to prevent air from entering the connection. Saline may also be simultaneously squirted over the connection.

For venovenous support, the double-lumen cannula is placed into the venotomy and advanced 5.5 cm. It is crucial to maintain the arterial reinfusion (red) port anteriorly, while securing for proper orientation to minimize recirculation of reinfused blood.

WOUND CLOSURE

7 The wound is irrigated with saline and hemostasis obtained. The skin is closed with continuous monofilament suture. The wound is dressed with gauze. The cannula is sutured to the skin with several 2/0 silk sutures. Special attention should be directed to affixing the cannulas securely to the bed.

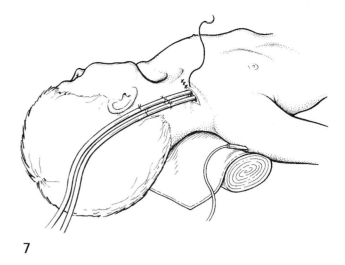

7

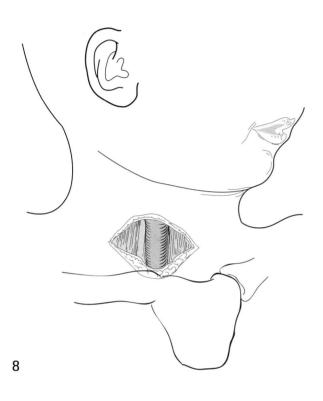

8

Venovenous cannulation: semi-open technique

INCISION AND VEIN EXPOSURE

8 A transverse cervical incision approximately 1.5–2 cm in length is made 2 cm above the right clavicle between the heads of the sternocleidomastoid muscle. The platysma is divided with electrocautery and the anterior surface of the internal jugular vein is exposed with minimal dissection. The vessel is observed and either a 12 F or 15 F Origen venovenous ECMO cannula (Origen Biomedical Inc, Austin, TX, USA) is selected.

GUIDEWIRE PLACEMENT

9 The cannula skin exit position is selected so that the cannula will lie behind the right ear when the head is returned to the midline. The needle/catheter is placed through the skin 2 cm superior to the incision and into the internal jugular vein to enter either under the skin flap or just inside the incision. The needle is removed and a 0.035-inch diameter guidewire is advanced and the catheter is withdrawn. A Teflon guiding obturator is placed over the guidewire into the vessel and right atrium. The use of fluoroscopy, if available, is helpful. Alternatively, single or multiple radiographs may be used. The skin exit is slightly enlarged with a scalpel.

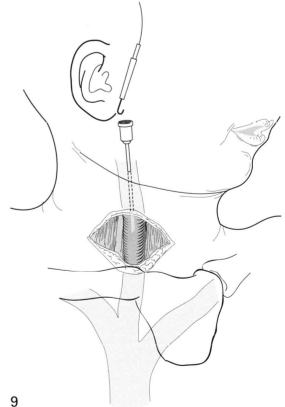

9

CANNULA PLACEMENT

10 Heparin (100 units/kg) is administered and 3 minutes allowed for circulation. The selected cannula is advanced over the Teflon obturator into the vein under direct vision to confirm entrance into the vein. The arterial (red) port of the cannula must be directed anteriorly to allow the arterial blood to cross the tricuspid valve and minimize recirculation of circuit blood. The tip of the cannula is placed at 6–9 cm from the skin.

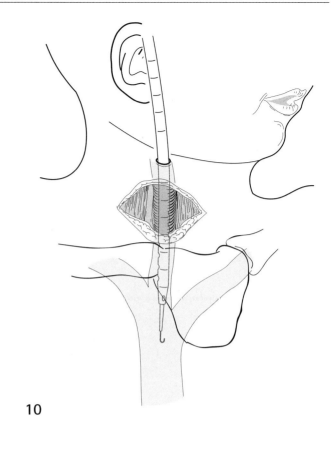

10

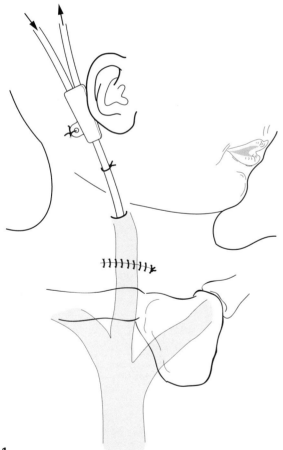

11

WOUND CLOSURE AND CANNULA FIXATION

11 The relatively low venous pressure allows adequate hemostasis around the venotomy site without any ligature. This prevents kinking of the thin-walled cannula which often occurs at the area of a ligature if used around the vessel. Repositioning of the cannula only requires removing the skin sutures, repositioning the cannula, and replacing skin sutures. The cannula is fixed to the skin with several 2/0 silk sutures. The incision is closed with a monofilament suture.

DECANNULATION

After respiratory failure has resolved to allow ventilation without extracorporeal support, cannulation can be performed by removing the skin sutures, pulling the cannula, and holding pressure on the catheter exit site for 5 minutes or until bleeding stops. Care must be taken to rapidly remove the entire cannula to prevent air from entering the side holes while the end of the cannula remains in the vessel.

POSTOPERATIVE CARE

The cannulas are connected to the extracorporeal bypass circuit, ensuring that no air bubbles are present, and bypass is initiated. Dopamine infusion into the ECLS circuit reinfusion connector is often necessary for inotropic support with the initiation of venovenous support if the patient required this type of support prior to ECLS initiation. A chest radiograph should be obtained following the procedure to verify optimal cannula placement distal to the aortic arch (arterial cannula) and inferior aspect of the right atrium (venous cannula). If flow is poor due to limited venous return, several maneuvers may help. Elevation of the bed and infusion of volume into the circuit may help. Cannula position can be checked with chest radiograph or echocardiogram. The venous cannula should be marked at its tip by a barium dot if not radio-opaque to the tip. The tip should be well into the right atrium. Occasionally, cardiac echography may be helpful to guide the catheter into the correct position.

Bleeding from the wound is controlled by lowering activated clotting times, platelet transfusions, admin-istration of fresh frozen plasma, and local instillation of fibrin glue. Bleeding not controlled by these maneuvers should be investigated and controlled by operative exploration after the open technique. Placement of a purse-string suture around the catheter exit site controls bleeding after the semi-open technique.

OUTCOME

More than 24 000 neonates have been treated since 1972, with an overall survival rate of 85 percent. The four most common diagnoses requiring ECLS in neonatal patients are meconium aspiration syndrome, congenital diaphragmatic hernia, pneumonia/sepsis, and persistent pulmonary hypertension. Survival rates of 94, 51, 57, and 78 percent, respectively, have been achieved.

FURTHER READING

Hogan MJ. Neonatal vascular catheters and their complications. *Radiological Clinics of North America* 1999; **37**: 1109–25.

Peek GJ, Firmin RK, Moore HM, Sosnowski AW. Cannulation of neonates for venovenous extracorporeal life support. *Annals of Thoracic Surgery* 1996; **61**: 1851–2.

Pranikoff T, Hines MH. Vascular access for extracorporeal support. In: Van Meurs K, Lally KP, Peek G, Zwischenberger JB (eds). *ECMO: Extracorporeal Cardiopulmonary Support in Critical Care.* Ann Arbor, MI: Extracorporeal Life Support Organization, 2005.

28

Eventration of the diaphragm

ROBERT E CILLEY

HISTORY

Eventration of the diaphragm refers to the radiographic finding of an abnormally elevated hemidiaphragm. The physiologic consequences of the loss of diaphragm function may result in respiratory insufficiency made worse in infants due to the mobility of the mediastinum. When the normal hemidiaphragm descends during inspiration, the mediastinum shifts to the normal side, while the eventration side paradoxically elevates. Acquired eventration (paralytic eventration) is understood on the basis of injury to the phrenic nerve, most commonly occurring at the time of intrathoracic surgery. Congenital eventration of the diaphragm is less well understood and probably includes a number of different entities. Phrenic nerve injury from birth trauma is similar to operative injury in that the diaphragm is developmentally normal. Other congenital eventrations (nonparalytic eventration) of the diaphragm are associated with anatomic abnormalities of the diaphragm. The diaphragm muscle is thinned and may be entirely absent from a portion that is normally muscular. In its most extreme forms, eventration is indistinguishable from a congenital diaphragmatic hernia with a hernia sac. Surgical treatment is based on removing the laxity of the abnormal diaphragm leaf to prevent paradoxical motion.

PRINCIPLES AND JUSTIFICATION

Diaphragm eventration may be discovered incidentally as an elevated hemidiaphragm on a chest radiograph obtained for other reasons, or it may be the cause of severe symptoms such as respiratory failure or pneumonia. The most common presentation of diaphragm eventration is postoperative respiratory failure as a result of phrenic nerve injury following an intrathoracic operation. Small eventrations with minimal compromise of lung volume may be monitored by serial radiographs. Recurrent symptoms or respiratory distress that requires mechanical ventilation are indications for surgical correction. When the possibility of reversible phrenic nerve injury exists, such as that due to birth trauma or operative injury, a period of observation is indicated. If there is no improvement in diaphragm function after a reasonable period of observation (2–4 weeks), diaphragm plication is performed. Some function may eventually return to the previously paralyzed diaphragm, but this may require many months. Operative plication does not preclude some recovery of diaphragm function.

Transabdominal–transthoracic techniques have been used for the correction of eventration. The abnormally lax diaphragm may be removed by excision and closure of the resultant defect, suture of a portion of the diaphragm to the chest wall, or various methods of 'gathering' or 'pleating' the excess tissue with sutures. All of these procedures have in common the creation of a taut diaphragm that is mechanically resistant to elevation when negative intrathoracic pressure is created during spontaneous breathing. Specific abnormalities lend themselves to repair by the different methods.

Video-endoscopic techniques may also be used to perform diaphragm plication. Thoracoscopic techniques are preferred. Cases of robotic repair in infants and children have also been described. When concurrent abdominal pathology that requires operative correction is present, the transabdominal/laparoscopic approach is used. The transthoracic/thoracoscopic approach is used for isolated unilateral eventration. It allows better visualization of the course of the phrenic nerve.

No portion of the diaphragm needs to be excised in cases of acquired eventration. The muscular diaphragm may ultimately regain some function, and excision only increases the risk of additional injury to the intradiaphragmatic portion of the phrenic nerve. In congenital eventrations with muscular aplasia or atrophy, the thinned portion of the diaphragm may be excised when the thoracic approach is used and the course of the phrenic nerve is visualized. This allows the edges that will be brought together to be visualized precisely. Sutures may be placed with less risk of injury to intra-abdominal organs. Pledgets and non-absorbable sutures provide the most secure closure. Since diaphragmatic defects come in all shapes and sizes, the precise orientation of the plication procedure and the decision to excise some or all of the eventration must be made on an individual basis.

The descriptions of thoracoscopic repairs have not involved excision of the thinned out diaphragm. Both interrupted and continuous suture techniques are described. Reinforcing pledgets have not been used. Reduced postoperative pain and quicker recovery compared to open repairs are reported.

PREOPERATIVE

Assessment and preparation

Unilateral eventration is suspected when the right hemidiaphragm is greater than two rib levels higher than the left, or the left hemidiaphragm is more than one rib level higher than the right. A rare bilateral eventration is suspected when respiratory failure is present in association with radiographic demonstration of bilateral diaphragm elevation. Chest radiographs may be misleading in the patient on positive pressure mechanical ventilation. The most convincing diagnostic tests are those that allow dynamic visualization of diaphragm function during spontaneous respiration. These include fluoroscopy and ultrasonographic imaging. Ultrasonography has the advantage that it can be performed easily at the patient's bedside in the intensive care unit. Absent or paradoxic elevation of the hemidiaphragm during spontaneous inspiratory effort is diagnostic.

An echocardiogram should be performed in the presence of congenital eventration to rule out associated structural cardiac abnormalities. Diaphragm eventration has been associated with intestinal rotational abnormalities and gastric volvulus. It is noted in rare genetic conditions. Upper gastrointestinal contrast studies or computed tomography (CT) scanning may be indicated if associated malformations are suspected.

Anesthesia

General endotracheal anesthesia is used. Unilateral intubation improves exposure, but, if difficult to perform or not well tolerated, it is not mandatory because the lung is easily retracted. Unilateral ventilation and low pressure insufflation facilitate the thoracoscopic approach. Intraoperative orogastric intubation with regular gastric aspiration is important since a dilated stomach is at risk of injury when diaphragmatic sutures are passed.

OPERATIONS

Whatever technique is chosen for repair, it is imperative that a taut diaphragm is created and that adjacent organs are not injured. A taut diaphragm is necessary to provide mechanical stability to the mediastinum during inspiration. The stomach, colon, and spleen are at particular risk during transthoracic procedures.

For illustrative purposes, the diagrams below refer to the open repair of a left-sided acquired eventration with a structurally normal, but non-functioning hemidiaphragm.

In the case of a congenital eventration, the central portion of the diaphragm is 'thinned out'. Although the diaphragm may be 'gathered' (see below) in a fashion similar to the repair of an acquired eventration, excising the thin central portion of the diaphragm allows the edges to be visualized clearly so that sutures may be placed in normal muscularized tissue and the abdominal viscera avoided. If excessive tension is required to bring the tissues together, a prosthetic patch may be used to close the defect. This is rarely necessary.

In the open repair, a transverse upper abdominal incision is used for bilateral eventration or in cases of unilateral eventration with malrotation. A lateral muscle-sparing seventh intercostal space thoracotomy is used for the open repair of an isolated left or right eventration.

Thoracoscopic procedures use three or four ports. Patients are placed in the lateral position, with the camera port entering superiorly. Two working ports are then triangulated to typically allow an anterior–posterior orientation of the repair. A fourth port is placed to assist with the reduction of the abdominal viscera if needed. Low pressure pneumothorax facilitates visualization and reduction of the abdominal contents. In congenital eventration, the central thinned portion of the diaphragm is not excised. Pledgets and 'gathering' techniques have also not been used in thoracoscopic procedures.

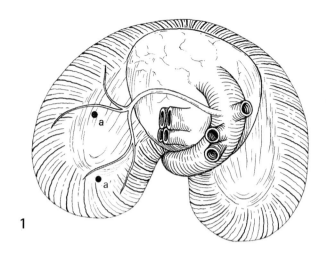

1

Transthoracic repair of diaphragm eventration

1 The main phrenic nerve on each side divides into an anterior and posterior division. Subsequent divisions usually include a sternal branch immediately off the anterior division and a bifurcation of the posterior division. The branches run in a medial to lateral orientation, allowing sutures to be placed to minimize the risk of injury to the muscular branches of the nerve. Viewed from above in this figure, the points *a* and *a'* represent the portions of the diaphragm that will be brought together by the plication.

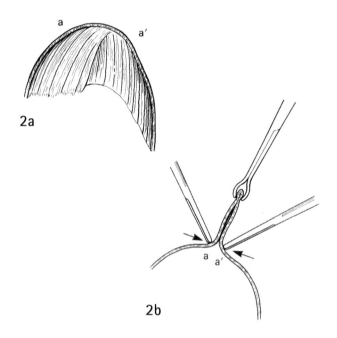

2a

2b

2a,b The diaphragm is grasped and manipulated to determine the amount that must be included in the plication to create a taut closure. This is conveniently performed by grasping the center of the diaphragm with a non-crushing clamp. The extent of the plication, determined by manipulations with the two forceps, is marked with a surgical marker.

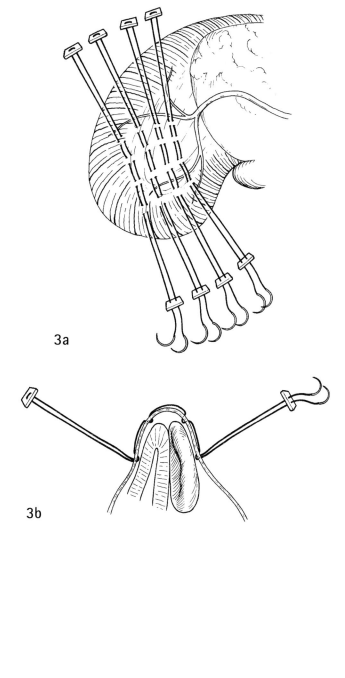

3a

3b

3a,b Several non-absorbable sutures are placed to bring the marked portions of the diaphragm together. The sutures are passed through the intervening diaphragm muscle three or four times. This maneuver is referred to as 'gathering', 'reefing', or 'pleating'. Pledgeted mattress sutures are shown. Care must be taken that the sutures are passed adequately through muscle, but not deeply enough to penetrate adjacent abdominal viscera.

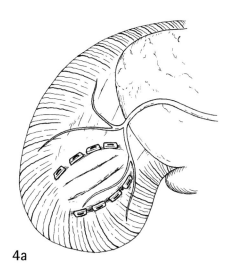

4a

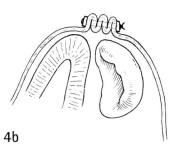

4b

4a,b The final result of the plication creates a taut diaphragm.

Transabdominal repair of bilateral eventration

Rotational abnormalities of the intestine are addressed if present.

5 The undersurface of the diaphragm is exposed on the left by mobilizing the liver as necessary. The stomach and spleen are retracted and mobilized to give complete exposure. The right lobe of the liver is mobilized if needed. Plicating sutures are arranged to avoid the phrenic nerve based on its expected location. The plication is oriented anteromedial to posterolateral, identical to the transthoracic approach.

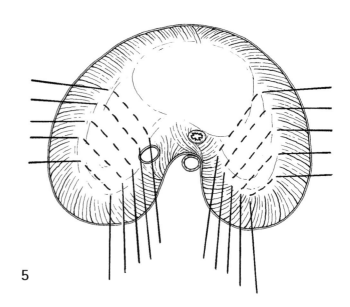

5

POSTOPERATIVE CARE

Response to operation may be immediate, allowing prompt weaning and extubation. In patients who have required prolonged mechanical ventilation prior to operation, slower ventilator weaning is performed. Intrapleural drainage may be used briefly after surgery and the drainage tube is usually removed within a few days.

OUTCOME

Although death may result from chronic respiratory failure and pneumonia, outcome is largely dependent on the presence of associated conditions, such as pulmonary hypoplasia or congenital heart disease. Long-term survival is variably reported as 69–100 percent. Children with bilateral eventration fare less well.

Surgical correction is durable and recurrence requiring repeat plication rare. Inadequate plication may result if the diaphragm is not made taut at the initial operation, and the plication process will need to be repeated.

Transdiaphragmatic injury may occur with either open or throacoscopic techniques. Intra-abdominal injuries, such as gastric or colon perforation, require immediate operative attention. Herniation into the site of the repair can occur.

Many patients examined years after diaphragm plication have evidence of appropriate, although diminished, movement of the involved side.

There is no long-term follow up that compares risks and outcome of video-endoscopic and open techniques of diaphragm plication. Small technical differences, such as the use of pledgets, and the ability to assess the completeness of the plication ('tautness') must be considered. In a condition that is relatively rare, surgeons should be cautious to make sure that the video-endoscopic procedure they perform is as safe and effective as the open approach.

FURTHER READING

Becmeur F, Talon I, Schaarschmidt K *et al.* Thoracoscopic diaphragmatic eventration repair in children: about 10 cases. *Journal of Pediatric Surgery* 2005; **40:** 1712–15.

Cherian A, Stewart RJ. Thoracoscopic repair of diaphragmatic eventration. *Pediatric Surgery International* 2004; **20:** 872–4.

Flageole H. Central hypoventilation and diaphragmatic eventration: diagnosis and management. *Seminars in Pediatric Surgery* 2003; **12:** 38–45.

Groth SS, Andrade RS. Diaphragmatic eventration (review). *Thoracic Surgery Clinics* 2009; **19:** 511–19.

Yazici M, Karaca I, Arikan A *et al.* Congenital eventration of the diaphragm in children: 25 years' experience in three pediatric surgery centers. *European Journal of Pediatric Surgery* 2003; **13:** 298–301.

29

Lung surgery

SALEEM ISLAM and JAMES D GEIGER

PRINCIPLES AND JUSTIFICATION

Lung surgery is a relatively rare event in childhood, since acquired lesions such as carcinoma or chronic infections, are much less common than in adults. Many operations are performed for congenital problems, and less commonly for infectious etiologies. **Table 29.1** lists the indications for pulmonary resection in children.

In general, the principles of lung surgery are similar in adults and children. Children usually have a greater physiologic reserve and withstand resections better than older patients. In the first seven years of life, there is ongoing alveolar development, which may diminish the impact of resection. Depending on the indications and the anatomic location for pulmonary resection, the approach and operative principles have to be adjusted. Minimally invasive techniques are being used more frequently in children and there is growing experience in thoracoscopic

pulmonary resections in this age group. However, in cases of severely altered anatomy, such as inflammatory conditions, an open procedure is usually performed.

Complications of lung surgery in children are typically less than in adults. Major bronchial stump air leaks are rare in healthy pediatric patients. Scoliosis and/or the development of chest wall deformities are potential long-term complications unique to children who have undergone open thoracotomy, but are actually quite rare. Children with inflammatory conditions such as lung abscess, pneumonia, cystic fibrosis, and bronchiectasis are at greater risk for postoperative complications such as prolonged air leak.

We will first discuss the major conditions that result in the need for pulmonary resections in infants and children. These mainly consist of congenital problems, such as lobar over-expansion, pulmonary airway malformations, and sequestrations.

Table 29.1 Pediatric lung conditions requiring surgery.

Congenital	Acquired
Sequestration	Acquired lobar emphysema
Cystic adenomatoid malformation	Bronchiectasis
Lobar over-expansion	Apical (or other) blebs
Lung cysts (single, multiple)	Metastatic lesions
Hamartomas	Fungal infections (lobar)
Congenital pulmonary insufficiency (needing biopsy for diagnosis)	Diffuse pulmonary disease

CONGENITAL LOBAR OVER–EXPANSION (EMPHYSEMA)

1a,b Lobar over-expansion can be found in neonates and infants. These may be acquired from mucous plugs or structural abnormalities obstructing a portion of the airway. Congenital lobar over-expansion is caused by absence of the bronchial cartilage in 35 percent of cases, leading to ball valve-type air trapping. Occasionally, extrinsic compression (e.g. congenital heart anomalies) can lead to distal air trapping and over-expansion. Bronchogenic cysts are also seen in association with this condition. A number of cases result from alveolar hyperplasia in a specific lobe of the lung leading to an emphysematous appearance. The symptoms arise from compression of other thoracic and mediastinal structures, which may occur acutely or chronically. Some infants do not require surgical intervention and remain stable without removing the lesion. Of those who need an operation, 50 percent will develop symptoms within a few days of birth, while the remaining present a few months later. Chest radiograph will show a hyperlucent area in the affected chest with a variable degree of compression of the mediastinal structures. The diaphragm is flattened on the affected side. Involvement is usually restricted to the upper lobes (42 percent left upper, 21 percent right upper, 35 percent right middle), with less than 1 percent involving the lower lobes. Differential diagnosis includes pneumothorax, pulmonary airway malformation, pneumatocele, and atelectasis.

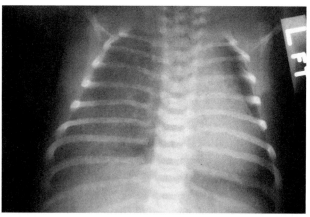

1a

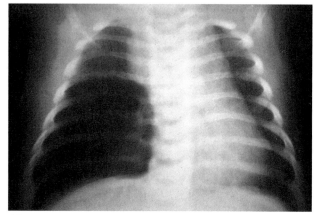

1b

Additional studies are usually unnecessary, but ventilation perfusion scans are occasionally used and show delayed uptake and poor vascular supply to the affected lobe. In some instances, it is necessary to perform an emergency thoracotomy for life-threatening compression. The lobe will usually herniate out as soon as the chest is opened, with immediate clinical improvement. Importantly, the anesthesia team should not over-ventilate the patient, but should use rapid small tidal volumes; and the surgeon must be prepared to rapidly open the chest, as deterioration may occur with positive pressure ventilation.

Resection usually involves a lobectomy. If possible, bronchoscopy should be performed before resection to rule out a mucous plug or another obstructing lesion.

CONGENITAL PULMONARY AIRWAY MALFORMATIONS

Pulmonary airway malformations (PAM, previously known as cystic adenomatoid malformations (CAM)) are lesions that are mostly diagnosed with prenatal ultrasound. They form 25 percent of all congenital lung malformations, but are still rare. Some become large enough that they cause lung hypoplasia and can also impede caval blood return, thus causing polyhydramnios and hydrops fetalis. Some of the affected fetuses will be stillborn. In selected centers, fetal thoracotomy and lung resection are performed in those who develop hydrops, with resultant improved survival. PAMs are found in the left lower lobe in 25 percent, left upper lobe in 20 percent, right lower lobe in 19 percent, and right upper lobe in 10 percent.

2a,b Some neonates have respiratory distress at birth, and can present with severe pulmonary hypertension requiring extracorporeal membrane oxygenation (ECMO) for stabilization prior to resection. Chest x-ray will often reveal an irregular cystic mass in the affected lung, which may involve the entire chest and have mediastinal shift. In most cases, however, postnatal chest x-ray is normal, and a subsequent chest computed tomography (CT) (generally performed at one to two months of age) confirms the prenatal diagnosis. In patients who are in no distress after birth, resection is usually delayed until the child is between six and 18 months of age. Operation at a younger age may be easier due to the lack of inflammation. The risks of infection and cancer remain the major indications for elective resection. Bronchoalveolar carcinoma, pleuropulmonary blastoma, and rhabdomyosarcoma have been reported to arise in these lesions, but the incidence is considered very low.

In symptomatic patients, resection is performed in the early neonatal period. The most common procedure is a lobectomy, although segmentectomy has been reported as well. It is considered vital to resect the entire PAM due to recurrence or prolonged air leak. In some cases the PAM may involve multiple lobes, and in very rare cases pneumonectomy may be considered, although most would perform segmental resections in order to spare lung tissue.

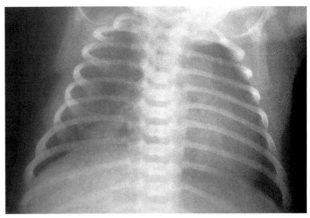

2a

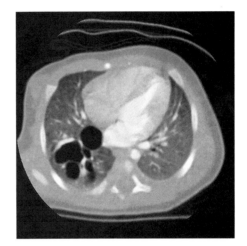

2b

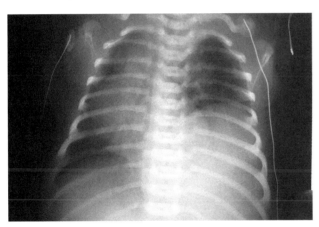

3a

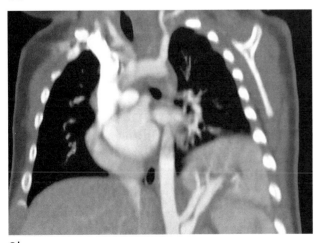

3b

SEQUESTRATION

3a,b A bronchopulmonary sequestration is a congenital malformation in which a portion of the lung receives systemic arterial supply and has no bronchial communication. There are two types, intralobar and extralobar sequestrations. Most large series describe a preponderance of extralobar lesions. These may coexist with other malformations such as bronchogenic cysts, PAM, and congenital heart lesions. Extralobar sequestrations are also associated with diaphragmatic hernias and eventrations. They may also occur in the abdomen, usually in the vicinity of the left adrenal gland. Most intralobar sequestrations are found in the lower lobes, with only 15 percent in the upper lobes. Presentation of intralobar lesions may be in the form of recurrent pneumonias, although increasingly they are being diagnosed by prenatal ultrasound. Extralobar sequestrations are usually discovered during repair of a congenital diaphragmatic hernia or eventration. They also may be found incidentally as a posterior mediastinal mass. It is important to remember that there may be a communication of the sequestration with the foregut (esophagus or stomach). During resection, these communications should be sought and repaired if present.

The vascular supply arises from the abdominal aorta in 85 percent and needs to be carefully ligated at the outset. It is usually found in the inferior pulmonary ligament, and care must be taken when mobilizing the structure. There is no bronchial attachment, which makes the resection easier. Intralobar sequestrations usually have a clear demarcation from the normal lung parenchyma and this forms a good plane of dissection. Lobectomy for intralobar lesions is the procedure of choice.

PREOPERATIVE ASSESSMENT AND PREPARATION

If the patient meets the indications for lung surgery, pulmonary function should be optimized and infections should be controlled as much as possible with preoperative antibiotics, especially in the patient with cystic fibrosis (CF). Lobectomy and non-anatomic resections less than a lobectomy are well tolerated in healthy children. In patients with CF or other generalized pulmonary diseases in which lung reserve is reduced, resections, especially lobectomy, may not be tolerated. Preoperative work up in older children may include measurement of forced expiratory volume in the first second (FEV_1) and forced vital capacity (FVC) to assess potential effects of resection, although this is not done in most otherwise healthy children. Most patients should have a minimum baseline measurement of hemoglobin, and a type and screen with blood readily available in complex resections (see **Chapter 12, Bronchoscopy**, for additional discussion).

ANESTHESIA CONSIDERATIONS

Many lung operations in children can be successfully performed using a standard endotracheal tube without single lung ventilation. If required, single lung ventilation can be accomplished in infants and young children by either selective main stem intubation or the use of bronchial blockers, which make the main stem intubation usually technically easier and more reliable. In the older child, the use of double-lumen tubes (when at least a 7-mm endotracheal tube can be utilized) will allow for selective ventilation. For many simple thoracoscopic procedures, gentle insufflation at pressures of 5–10 mmHg will be enough to collapse the lung sufficiently, and selective ventilation may not be needed. However, for lobectomies, it is preferable to have the ipsilateral lung decompressed.

Postoperative pain relief after a thoracotomy is another important consideration, and the use of thoracic epidurals should be liberally considered. Epidurals facilitate anesthetic delivery intraoperatively and decrease postoperative narcotic requirements. Intercostal nerve blocks can also be performed or, alternatively, a pleural catheter can be placed for delivery of local anesthetic.

Monitoring of children undergoing major lung surgery intraoperatively may involve the placement of an arterial line and a central venous line, but these are dependent on the patient's preoperative condition, and on surgeon and anesthesiologist preference, and are not considered mandatory.

OPERATIONS

These are discussed in two broad categories: (1) the general principles of pulmonary resection and specific approaches to various lobectomies, and (2) the indications and operations needed for specific conditions.

Principles of pulmonary resection

ACCESS TO THE LUNG

Operations on the lung can be performed in two ways, via thoracotomy or thoracoscopy. Thoracotomy can be performed by one of three approaches. The first is an anterolateral approach mostly used for open lung biopsies, or wedge resections. The second is a posterolateral thoracotomy, which is the most common method used for open lung resections. A third approach through a prone position is employed to reduce spillover of infected secretions into the contralateral lung. However, with modern anesthesia techniques allowing single lung ventilation, as well as more effective antimicrobial therapy, this approach is less common. A median sternotomy is used by some surgeons when bilateral wedge resections are required, such as in osteosarcoma metastases.

The anterolateral thoracotomy is performed by elevating the patient with a roll 30–45° from the table. The incision is performed below the level of the nipple in the fourth, fifth, or sixth interspace, taking care not to injure the breast bud in a prepubertal female. The incision may be extended along the ribs toward the axilla as required. The pectoralis and intercostal muscles are then divided to enter the pleural cavity. After performing the desired resection or biopsy, a chest tube may be placed a couple of interspaces below the incision. The ribs are approximated loosely with an absorbable pericostal stitch (polygalactin). The muscle fascia is approximated with a running absorbable suture, followed by subcutaneous closure with either a running or interrupted suture and subcuticular closure of the skin (both with absorbable suture).

4 Posterolateral thoracotomy is performed with the patient in the lateral decubitus position. An axillary roll is used and appropriate padding of the legs is placed. The upper arm is allowed to lie on the same side with support to prevent excessive stretching of the arm as well as the brachial plexus. A wide preparation is done from the vertebral column posteriorly to the sternum anteriorly. The nipple and areola are marked, as is the tip of the scapula, to help guide the incision. A gently curved thoracotomy incision is performed in the interspace chosen. In most cases, a muscle-sparing approach can be employed (see **Chapter 16, Thoracic Surgery: general principles** for details), in which the serratus anterior is retracted anteriorly or detached from the rib cage and the latissimus dorsi is reflected posteriorly. These muscles may be partially or completely divided as needed to gain wider access during the operation. Care is taken not to divide the paraspinal muscles, but to free them up longitudinally. This move, as well as avoiding division of the trapezius and rhomboids, may help in reducing the development of scoliosis. The ribs are held apart with a self-retaining metal retractor (Finochietto). After the resection is performed, a chest tube may be placed a couple of interspaces below the incision. Pericostal sutures are placed in an interrupted fashion and appropriately secured avoiding excessive approximation of the ribs. Fascia and skin are closed as described previously.

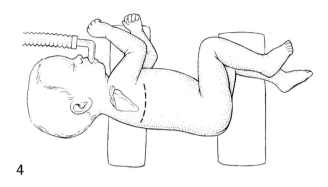

4

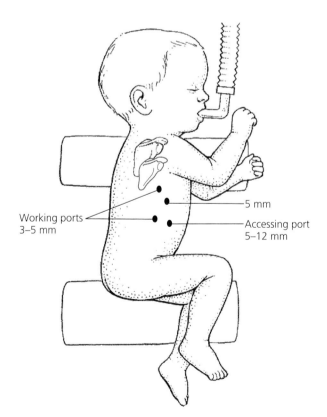

Working ports 3–5 mm

5 mm

Accessing port 5–12 mm

5 Thoracoscopic approaches are now being increasingly employed. Lung biopsies, wedge resections, and lobectomies can be performed using this approach. Improved optics with high-definition cameras and brighter light sources have made visualization excellent, and the development of energy devices such as the Ligasure (Covidien, Mansfield, MA, USA) electrocoagulator for dissection and control of vessels up to 7 mm in diameter has allowed these resections to be performed safely. The clear benefits in cosmesis, decreased pain and length of stay, and potentially less scoliosis have been the driving forces, but have yet to be proven. For thoracoscopic resections of any kind, the patient is placed in a decubitus position, as described previously. The table may be rotated to the right or left as needed for exposure. Some surgeons prefer to have the patient in the position described for the anterolateral thoracotomy. It is important to extensively use gravity as a retractor and the surgeon should vary the position accordingly. Single lung ventilation should be used to facilitate exposure for lobectomy, although CO_2 insufflation suffices for other procedures. The chest is prepared as for a thoracotomy and a 5-mm incision made in the mid-axillary line in the fourth to sixth interspace. A Veress needle is placed into the chest carefully just above a rib to avoid the neurovascular bundle.

5

Insufflation with CO_2 to a pressure of 3–7 mmHg, at least initially, facilitates exposure and creates a functional working space. A 5-mm port is placed and the 4- or 5-mm 30° telescope is introduced. The remaining port sites are then chosen based on the specific anatomy and which lobe is to be operated upon. Usually, two additional ports are placed to facilitate triangulation and dissection of the fissure and lobe. These positions are variable and can move one or two interspaces up or down as needed, and for lobectomy are typically located in the anterior axillary line. A fourth access site may be used for retraction if necessary. If an endoscopic stapling device is to be used, a 12-mm port will be required. One of the port sites may need to be enlarged slightly to remove the specimen. Upon completion of the procedure, a chest tube may be placed through one of the dependent port sites and secured. The fascia may be closed with an absorbable stitch and the skin approximated by suture or other means.

LUNG BIOPSY AND WEDGE RESECTION

This procedure is performed for diagnostic or therapeutic purposes. Indications for biopsy include infectious processes, diffuse parenchymal diseases, and presence of lung nodules where a diagnosis of an inflammatory or malignant process is being considered. Those patients who have diffuse disease may not tolerate single lung ventilation, and in these cases the procedure will have to be performed with the lung expanded. Thoracoscopic procedures allow visualization of the entire lung making a small wedge resection easy to perform with a stapling device. An open operation with a small anterolateral thoracotomy is also a reasonable technique for a wedge biopsy with a stapling device. A persistent air leak after a non-anatomic resection can be controlled by a second firing of the stapling device after removing the knife blade, or by over-sewing the suture line. Buttressed staplers or fibrin sealant may also decrease the risk of air leaks. Chest closure is performed in the same way as described previously.

Non-anatomic wedge resections may also be performed for metastatic disease of the lung. In general, an open thoracotomy is preferred for osteosarcoma metastatic disease, to allow palpation of the lung parenchyma and to remove as many lesions as possible, which is thought to improve survival. Usually both lungs are evaluated in this fashion for metastatectomy.

In other tumors, it may be reasonable to utilize a thoracoscopic approach. Smaller or deep parenchymal lesions may not be accessible via thoracoscopy. Some authors have described using CT-guided marking of the lesions with methylene blue ink immediately preoperatively to facilitate localization and resection with thoracoscopy.

Apical bleb disease leading to recurrent or persistent pneumothorax can also be treated thoracoscopically. The apex is visualized and wedges of parenchyma with blebs are removed using an endoscopic stapling device. In most cases, it is best to use these devices with the vascular load, which has smaller staples and thus results in less bleeding. Again, if there is an air leak from the staple line, a further firing of the device after removing the blade or using a stapler that has been reinforced with bovine pericardium may be helpful. Fibrin glue can be applied over the staple line as an adjuvant to help control air leaks.

LOBECTOMY

The principles of lobectomy are similar in children and adults. The most important considerations are adequate visualization and exposure of the hilar structures, namely, the blood vessels and bronchus. In most instances, it is better to dissect out and control the pulmonary arterial branches first, venous drainage second, and the bronchus last. Occasionally, as in the case of a severe, purulent infectious process, it is better to divide the bronchus first.

The anatomic considerations involved in the removal of different lobes will now be discussed in detail. The surgeon must have a complete understanding not only of the normal anatomy but also of the variations in anatomy that are frequently encountered during lung resections.

Right upper lobectomy

6a,b The patient is positioned for either a posterolateral thoracotomy via the fifth interspace or a thoracoscopic approach. The lung is retracted posteriorly and the pleura covering the hilum of the right lung is opened anteriorly and posteriorly to a level below the right mainstem bronchus. Care is taken to avoid injury to the right phrenic nerve. It should be noted that considerable variation in vascular anatomy occurs, but the usual pattern is shown in the illustration. The first vessel to be encountered will be the superior pulmonary vein which will have the upper and middle lobar branches. The main pulmonary artery is identified behind the superior pulmonary vein, and dissection is carried out peripherally to expose the superior and inferior pulmonary arterial trunks. The superior pulmonary arterial trunk, with its branches to the anterior, posterior, and apical segments, is exposed and then branches individually ligated. The ligation of the vessels is aided by dissecting into the parenchyma to gain length. This technique also allows one to ligate arteries of smaller caliber more effectively using clips or energy devices. The superior lobe vein is identified and dissected laterally, usually exposing three segmental pulmonary veins. The middle lobe veins entering the superior pulmonary vein must be identified and preserved. It is often easier and safer to ligate the individual venous branches peripherally and in the lung parenchyma. The oblique fissure is then opened and completed between the upper and lower lobes. This permits the dissection of the posterior ascending segmental pulmonary arterial branch, which ordinarily comes off the pulmonary artery after the middle lobe branches. All the vessels are best managed by ligation with non-absorbable suture, as well as suture ligation proximally.

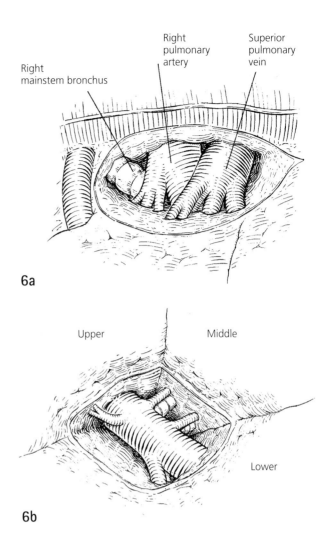

After division of the arterial and venous branches of the right upper lobe, adventitial tissue surrounding the bronchus is cleared away. The bronchus only needs to be cleared to show its origin, as further dissection may compromise the blood supply and delay healing of the bronchial stump. Stay sutures of non-absorbable material are placed on either side of the bronchus and it is divided about 1 or 2 cm from the mainstem in order to avoid a long stump, which may accumulate secretions. After division of the bronchus, the stump is closed with interrupted sutures of 3/0 or 4/0 monofilament or braided non-absorbable material, or with a stapling device.

When performing the operation with video-assisted thoracic surgery (VATS), the Ligasure or similar bipolar device is used to coagulate a portion of the vessel and divide it. Of note, the right upper lobe is probably the technically most difficult one to perform thoracoscopically. Most of the electrosurgical devices are approved to control vessels up to 7 mm in diameter. The dissection begins similarly, with the exposure of the superior vein and branches; it is easier to ligate and divide these branches before the arterial branches. Teasing the lung off the vessels is a good technique to use in these cases to gain length and ensure no compromise to the main vessel. This maneuver also allows for thermoligation of smaller vessels which may be somewhat safer. Completion of the fissure can be performed with the Ligasure, again without air leak.

Thoracoscopically, the same choices exist for handling the bronchus, with most surgeons preferring interrupted sutures, especially in small children. The use of non-absorbable Hem-O-Lock® clips (Teleflex Medical, Reading, PA, USA) for the bronchus as well as hilar vessels has also been described. Torsion of the right middle lobe has occurred after an upper lobectomy, and the right middle lobe should be sutured to the right lower lobe if the major fissure is complete after a right upper lobectomy is performed. After closure, warm saline is poured into the chest and the stump is tested for a leak by applying a pressure of 30–40 cmH$_2$O with the ventilator. Surrounding pleura may be used to reinforce the stump and possibly promote healing. A chest tube is placed and secured as described previously.

Right middle lobectomy

7 The arteries to the right middle lobe are best exposed through the oblique fissure between the upper and middle lobes. After development of the interlobar fissure, one or two middle lobe vessels are usually encountered; these are ligated as described by creating length. The lung is retracted posteriorly to expose the anterior hilum, and one or two right middle lobe veins are found in the area mentioned previously, joining the superior pulmonary vein. Once the middle lobe has been separated from the upper lobe and both arterial and venous branches divided, the lobe is retracted anteriorly and the bronchus is dissected and divided. The stump is controlled in the fashion described previously. The potential for injury to the ascending posterior segmental artery of the upper lobe makes this operation somewhat more technically demanding than upper and lower lobectomies.

The working ports are shifted one or two interspaces up in the anterior axillary line for the middle lobectomy when done with VATS. The minor fissure is dissected and the arteries are encountered near the confluence of the major and minor fissures. The vein is located after posterior retraction of the lobe and dissection of the anterior pleura. The bronchus is easily identified near the apex of the lobe. It is considered safer to divide this sharply and close it with interrupted sutures using a stapler due to the risk of compromising the other lobar bronchi.

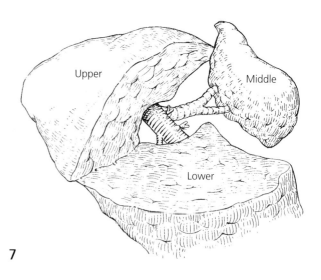

7

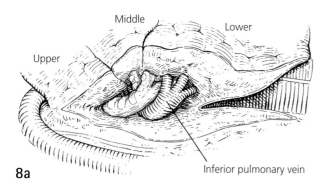

8a

Inferior pulmonary vein

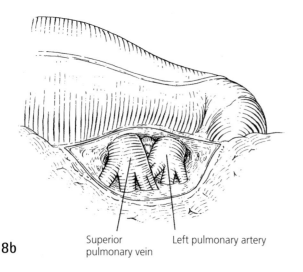

8b   Superior pulmonary vein   Left pulmonary artery

Right lower lobectomy

8a,b For performing a right lower lobectomy, a lower intercostal space may be used. The interlobar fissure is exposed by retraction of the upper and middle lobes superiorly and the lower lobe inferiorly. The branches of the interlobar portion of the right pulmonary artery are exposed and carefully identified. Just beyond the middle lobe arteries and opposite them, one or two superior segmental arteries supplying the superior segment of the lower lobe are encountered. These are divided after ligation. There is a remaining vessel to the basilar segments, which should be identified and similarly ligated. The lobe is then retracted anteriorly to expose the posterior hilum. The inferior pulmonary vein is exposed by opening the inferior pulmonary ligament and carrying the pleural dissection upwards to isolate and facilitate ligation of the inferior pulmonary vein. After this, the right lower lobe bronchus can be easily identified by posterior retraction. Care is taken to keep the bronchial stump length short.

When doing this resection using the thoracoscope, the first move is typically dissection of the inferior pulmonary ligament to expose the inferior pulmonary vein. During this dissection, it is prudent to look for an aberrant systemic vessel as occurs in a sequestration. The vein is not ligated until after the arterial dissection to avoid congestion of the lobe. The upper and middle lobes are then retracted superiorly to expose the fissure which is completed and the vessels are dissected as described for the open approach. Each vessel is divided after the Ligasure has been used and dissected in the parenchyma to create length. The vein is then similarly ligated at the branch level. The bronchus can be visualized and divided as previously described.

Left upper lobectomy

9a,b After positioning the patient in the appropriate right lateral decubitus position, a posterolateral thoracotomy is performed. As for the right lung, the pleura overlying the hilum of the lung anteriorly is incised and carried superiorly and posteriorly below the level of the left mainstem bronchus. The left pulmonary artery is best identified anteriorly first, and then found as it courses superiorly and posteriorly to the upper lobe bronchus. Four to six branches of the left pulmonary artery to the upper lobe can be noted. Anteriorly, the anterior, apical, and posterior segmental arteries are seen. The apical segmental artery may be encountered superiorly, and anterior segmental and lingular segmental branches are usually seen in the interlobar fissure. After ligation of all these branches, the lung is retracted posteriorly and the left superior pulmonary vein is ligated just before it divides. Occasionally, the left superior and inferior pulmonary veins form a common vein, so before ligating the superior vein on the left side, the inferior vein should be identified separately. With anterior retraction, it is possible to see the bronchus to the upper lobe and lingula and divide these close to the origin as described.

The thoracoscopic approach is similar to that mentioned for the right upper lobe, with exposure of the pulmonary vein and then the arterial branches, as discussed in the open technique.

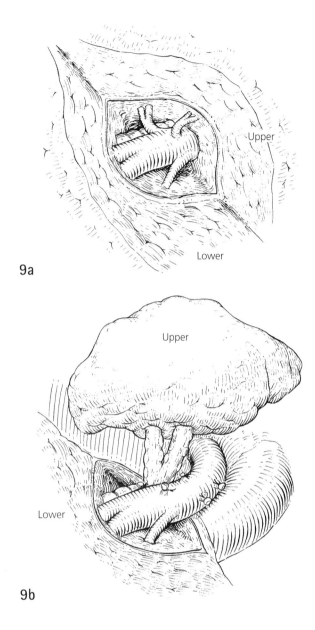

9a

9b

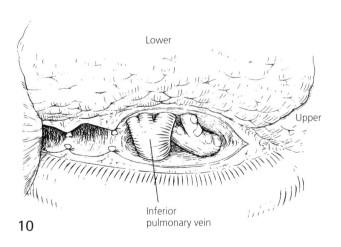

10

Left lower lobectomy

10 After gaining access to the chest, the interlobar fissure is exposed to identify the arteries. One or two arteries supply the superior segment, but care must be taken as the superior segmental artery may arise proximal to the lingular vessels. Thus, the lingular arteries must be identified in the course of this dissection. Following ligation of these vessels, the basilar portion of the left pulmonary artery may be divided just distal to the lingular arteries. After this, the lung is retracted anteriorly to expose the posterior hilum. The inferior pulmonary ligament is divided to expose the inferior pulmonary vein. The vein is then divided as described, taking care to be sure the superior lobe has good venous drainage. After vascular division, the lobe is retracted posteriorly and the bronchus isolated and divided as described previously.

Thoracoscopic left lower lobectomy is very similar to the right one, as described previously. The vein is isolated first by taking down the inferior pulmonary ligament; however, the vein is not ligated until after pulmonary artery ligation. The pulmonary arterial branches are then dissected in the fissure and ligated using the Ligasure device taking care to identify the lingular vessels. The vein branches previously isolated are then ligated at this point. The bronchus is divided using a stapler or by sharp division and suture closure.

POSTOPERATIVE CARE

Important principles of postoperative care after lung surgery involve ensuring adequate pulmonary toilet. Pain control is critical to optimizing postoperative pulmonary lung function and may be provided by a thoracic epidural. The epidural, if used, is usually maintained for 48–72 hours postoperatively. A Foley catheter for bladder drainage may be needed with epidural pain relief. Pain may not be a prominent feature following thoracoscopic procedures, but often the chest tube is a major cause of postoperative pain and should be removed as soon as possible. The chest tube is maintained for 1–3 days, initially on suction and then on underwater seal. The tube is removed once there is no air leak and the drainage is minimal.

Antibiotics may be given for 24 hours. Some surgeons continue antibiotics until the chest tube is removed, although there are no good data to support this practice. Narcotics should be used judiciously and non-narcotic analgesia incorporated into the algorithms for pain control. Feeding is usually resumed the day after surgery.

Intensive care is required for patients with significant underlying lung disease and reduced pulmonary function. Most patients are able to go home within 3–4 days, although older children may need to stay longer because of pain issues. After thoracoscopic procedures, the hospital stays are usually shorter.

OUTCOMES

Mortality following lung resection, including lobectomy or bilobectomy should be minimal with modern surgical techniques and postoperative care. The only group at increased risk is those with significant other comorbidities, such as congenital heart disease, or those with additional pulmonary disease.

Mortality and morbidity after lung biopsy are mainly dependent on the underlying disease process. The risk of prolonged air leak with diffuse parenchymal disease also exists and can add significantly to morbidity.

Infectious complications are not common following lung resection for congenital lobar over-expansion, uncomplicated CAM, or sequestrations. When there is a pre-existing infection or abscess, the risk is higher. Bronchial stump leaks are very rare compared to adults.

FURTHER READING

Aziz D, Langer JC, Tuuha SE et al. Perinatally diagnosed asymptomatic congenital cystic adenomatoid malformation: to resect or not? Journal of Pediatric Surgery 2004; **39**: 329–34.

Azizkhan RG, Crombleholme TM. Congenital cystic lung disease: contemporary antenatal and postnatal management. Pediatric Surgery International 2008; **24**: 643–57.

Puligandla PS, Laberge JM. Infections and diseases of the lungs, pleura and mediastinum. In: O'Neill JA, Rowe MI, Grosfeld JL et al. (eds). Pediatric Surgery, 6th edn. Boston, MA: Mosby, 2006: 1001–37.

Rothenberg SS. First decade's experience with thoracoscopic lobectomy in infants and children. Journal of Pediatric Surgery 2008; **43**: 40–4.

Rothenberg SS. Thoracoscopic lobectomy. In: Holcomb GW, Georgeson KE, Rothenberg SS (eds). Atlas of Pediatric Laparoscopy and Thoracoscopy. Philadelphia, PA: Saunders Elsevier, 2008: 253–60.

Su WT, Chewning J, Abramson S et al. Surgical management and outcome of osteosarcoma patients with unilateral pulmonary metastases. Journal of Pediatric Surgery 2004; **39**: 418–23.

30

Empyema

CASEY M CALKINS, SHAWN D ST PETER, and GEORGE W HOLCOMB III

HISTORY

The accumulation of purulent material in the pleural space is termed 'empyema or empyema thoracis'. Usually a complication of inflammation or an infection within or adjacent to the pleural space, empyema rarely resolves spontaneously because host defenses are limited by the anatomy and physiology of the pleural space. In children, the majority of cases occur as a result of pneumonia. However, infection of the chest wall or a subphrenic abscess can also lead to empyema. In the United States, among children less than 18 years of age, the annual empyema-associated hospitalization rate increased nearly 70 percent between 1997 and 2006, despite decreases in the rates of bacterial pneumonia and invasive pneumococcal disease, and the utilization of the conjugate pneumococcal vaccine.

Empyema develops by progression through three well-recognized stages. Initially, sterile pleural fluid accumulates in the pleural space as an inflammatory response to neighboring infection. In this stage, known as the acute or exudative stage (stage I), a parapneumonic effusion develops that is characterized by clear, low viscosity pleural fluid with normal pH and glucose levels, and a low level of lactate dehydrogenase (LDH). The visceral and parietal pleura in this stage are not fused. Thereafter, the transitional or fibropurulent stage (stage II) is characterized by turbid pleural fluid with an increasing accumulation of leukocytes and decreasing pH and glucose. The LDH of the fluid begins to increase and a fibrinous peel develops along both pleural surfaces that may limit full expansion of the lung. Finally, the chronic or organizing stage (stage III) is characterized by ingrowth of capillaries and fibroblasts into the fibrinous peel along with fusion of the visceral and parietal pleural surfaces. This typically occurs 4–6 weeks following the onset of the process. At the end stage of disease, the pleural fluid has a pH of less than 7 and a glucose level of less than 40 mg/dL.

Since the last iteration of this chapter, much has been written about the use of fibrinolysis in the treatment of empyema thoracis in children. Also, two prospective randomized trials compared fibrinolytic therapy to thoracoscopic debridement and decortication (TDD) as the initial therapy for empyema. A prospective, randomized trial was conducted at Children's Mercy Hospital comparing TDD with intrapleural fibrinolysis using tPA (tissue plasminogen activator). We (authors SDS and GWH) concluded that there are no therapeutic or recovery advantages between TDD and fibrinolysis. Also, initial TDD resulted in significantly greater charges. In addition, we concluded that fibrinolysis may pose less risk of acute clinical deterioration and recommend that it be the initial therapy for children with empyema. These findings were confirmed in another prospective, randomized trial comparing fibrinolytic therapy (urokinase) to primary TDD. These authors also found no difference in clinical outcome between intrapleural urokinase and TDD for the treatment of childhood empyema. Urokinase was again found to be a less costly treatment option compared with TDD and this group similarly concluded that initial fibrinolytic therapy should be the primary treatment of choice. The failure rate for fibrinolysis was 16 percent in both studies demonstrating that the majority of patients with loculated pleural space disease can avoid an operation.

Despite these findings, the pediatric surgery community remains divided on best practice as it pertains to the initial treatment for the child with empyema. Today, the initial treatment remains largely governed by personal experience and training, hospital historical norms, and data from retrospective case series. Although there is no clear gold-standard approach to the treatment of empyema, we advocate that surgeons charged with the care of children utilize the data from these prospective, randomized controlled trials to develop a rational management strategy to approach this disease. We present one evidence-based approach based on level 1 evidence for the treatment of the child with empyema, and will review the available operative techniques to carry out operative treatment when necessary.

PRINCIPLES AND JUSTIFICATION

Stage I

Traditionally, parapneumonic effusions associated with stage I empyema are treated by tube thoracostomy and intravenous antibiotic therapy. This approach is reserved for children with simple effusions that are not loculated. In our experience, the effusion can be adequately assessed by either plain chest x-ray with decubiti films, or more effectively, by ultrasonography or chest computed tomography (CT). We do not advocate simple aspiration of the fluid in these cases as high rates of subsequent reintervention have been reported. Instillation of fibrinolytic agents into the pleural space for management of a parapneumonic effusion is recommended when the white blood cell count in the pleural fluid is greater than 10 000/μL.

Stage II

Progression to the second stage of empyema with the development of fibrinous adhesions and loculations is best treated by clearing the pleural space with chemical or mechanical debridement. Continued conservative therapy with intravenous antibiotics and tube thoracostomy risks the development of stage III empyema and subsequent lung trapping with respiratory dysfunction.

1a–c To prevent the development of end-stage empyema, we advocate initial therapy with fibrinolysis, we wait several days before deciding that the patient has failed non-operative therapy. Illustrations 1a and 1b demonstrate pre- and post-therapy (one month post-therapy) plain radiographs of a patient treated successfully with fibrinolysis alone. It should be noted that radiographic improvement often lags behind physiologic recovery. If fever and/or oxygen requirement persist after fibrinolysis and chest tube removal, then the pleural space should be assessed for residual stage II empyema using ultrasound or CT scan. Although these studies often demonstrate residual parenchymal disease, they can serve to allow the clinician evidence to suggest that pleural debridement is indicated. This CT scan (1c) demonstrates residual parenchymal and pleural-based disease following fibrinolysis. Pleural space disease is debrided thoracoscopically(TDD), and a soft suction drain (19F round Blake drain; Ethicon, Piscataway, NJ, USA) is inserted under direct vision at that time.

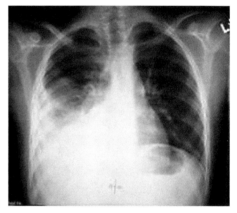

1a

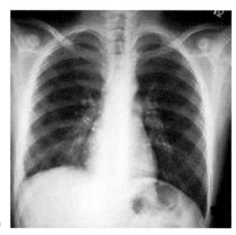

1b

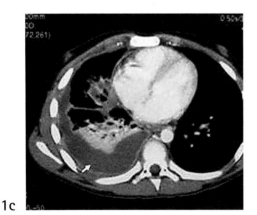

1c

Stage III

A minimally invasive approach may be difficult when the visceral and parietal pleural surfaces have fused in stage III empyema because there is minimal, if any, pleural space to work. Patients with entrapped lung and persistent pulmonary dysfunction often benefit from open decortication to liberate the lung from the thickened visceral pleural peel and allow for re-expansion of the underlying pulmonary parenchyma, although the thoracoscopic approach may be used by experienced surgeons.

PREOPERATIVE ASSESSMENT AND PREPARATION

2 An algorithmic approach to patients with empyema is employed. Children are begun on intravenous antibiotic therapy consisting of a third-generation cephalosporin (e.g. ceftriaxone) and a macrolide (e.g. clindamycin). For the rare pediatric patient with a hospital-acquired pneumonia, gram-negative coverage should be added.

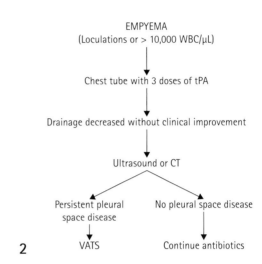

2

SURGICAL MANAGEMENT

Tube thoracostomy and pleural fibrinolysis

Patients are sedated with midazolam and intravenous narcotics are used for pain control. Cardiorespiratory monitors are placed. The skin and soft tissues about the fifth intercostal space in the mid-axillary are infiltrated with either ¼ percent marcaine or 1 percent lidocaine (1 cc/kg maximum). For instillation of fibrinolytics, we prefer to use a 12 Fr chest tube (Thal-Quick Chest Tubes; Cook Critical Care, Bloomington, IN, USA) introduced using the Seldinger technique. The authors have not felt it necessary to use image guidance in the majority of patients. Once the tube is inserted, the effluent is sent for culture, and the tube is secured to a $-20\,\mathrm{cmH_2O}$ suction collection device. Fibrinolysis is performed by mixing 4 mg of tPA in 40 mL of normal saline. (Other fibrinolytics such as urokinase or reteplase can also be used.) The prepared tPA solution is instilled directly into the thoracic cavity via tube, which is immediately clamped for 1 hour. After the dwell time, the tube is unclamped and left on to continuous suction. Two additional doses are subsequently given at 24-hour intervals utilizing the same technique. The tube is removed once there is no evidence of an air leak and the output is less than 1 mL/kg per day.

3a–c Although the authors no longer place traditional chest tubes for the treatment of empyema prior to surgical intervention, for the sake of completeness, the technique for tube thoracostomy has been included. A transverse skin incision is made in the intercostal space below which the tube will pass. Blunt dissection is then carried subcutaneously over the rib and into the pleural space cephalad to the rib. Another well-tolerated technique is to use a 10-mm expandable sleeve and cannula (Step™; Covidien, Mansfield, MA, USA) as an avenue for insertion of a soft suction drain (19 Fr round Blake drain) The cannula with its blunt trocar is inserted over a rib and into the pleural space directing it posterior and cephalad. The soft suction drain is subsequently inserted through the cannula. The cannula is then removed and the tube is secured to the skin. Soft, flexible tubes have been shown to be equally safe compared with the traditional stiff chest tubes in pediatric thoracic surgery, with the added benefit of being less painful when studied in adults. These tubes have been utilized effectively following TDD for the surgical treatment of empyema, and we have found that they can also be successfully used in providing effective drainage of the pleural space prior to TDD. If these step cannulas or soft flexible tubes are not available, an appropriate size chest tube is chosen, and then loaded on the end of a hemostat which is used to insert the tube into the pleural space directing it posterior and cephalad. The tube is secured to the skin with a nonabsorbable suture, and a sterile occlusive dressing with hydrophobic gauze is applied. The tube is then connected to a pleurovac-type system to −20 cmH$_2$O suction. A post-procedure chest radiograph is obtained to confirm the position of the tube.

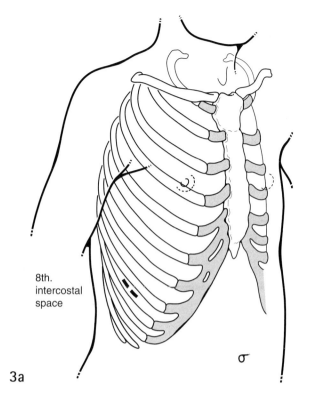

8th. intercostal space

3a

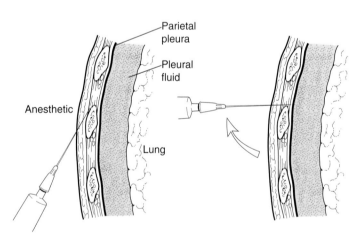

Parietal pleura

Pleural fluid

Anesthetic

Lung

3b

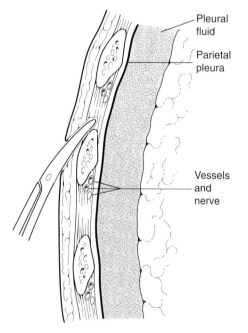

Pleural fluid

Parietal pleura

Vessels and nerve

3c

OPERATIONS

Anesthesia

For each of the following operative techniques, the procedure is performed under general anesthesia with tracheal intubation, yet is facilitated by selective, single lung ventilation. To this end, we employ either double lumen endotracheal intubation or tracheal intubation with bronchial blockade.

4 The patient is positioned in the lateral decubitus position with the affected side up, and an axillary roll is placed. One should aim to position the patient with the level of the iliac crest rests at the break in the table to allow for increased opening of the intercostal spaces. Raising the kidney rest, if available, can also assist in this goal.

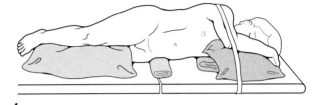

4

Thoracoscopic debridement and decortication

5 For TDD, an initial incision is placed in an area deemed advantageous for accessing the majority of disease after review of the ultrasound or CT scan. Typically, this initial 10-mm port is best placed directly overlying the empyema. Usually, placement of the cannula in the fifth intercostal space at the mid-axillary line is a good starting point. A 10-mm angled telescope is used to create a working space by sweeping the adhesions and lung away from the chest wall with the end of the telescope. Once the underlying lung is freed adequately, a second incision is placed in a location to maximize the ease with which the majority of pleural disease can be removed. When two incisions are not sufficient, a small third incision for a 5-mm cannula can be placed to provide a second working port. A low pressure (4 mmHg), low flow (1 L/min) CO_2 pneumothorax facilitates lung collapse. Pleural debridement is then undertaken using a ring forceps or Yankauer suction to remove the pleural peel and debris. Alternatively, an atraumatic grasping forceps can be used. Samples for gram stain and culture are routinely sent by attaching a Lukens trap to the suction device. Once all pockets of fluid have been drained and the majority of the pleural debris is removed, a single chest drain/tube (preferably a 19 Fr round Blake drain, if available) is inserted into the pleural space under direct vision.

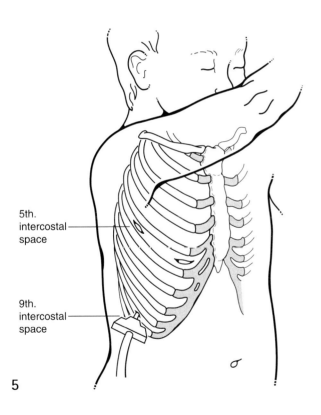

5th. intercostal space

9th. intercostal space

5

6 To lessen the possibility for pneumothorax when the tube is removed, the drain/tube is tunneled over the rib space cephalad to the port site through which it is going to exit. Incisions are closed with absorbable suture and sterile dressings are applied.

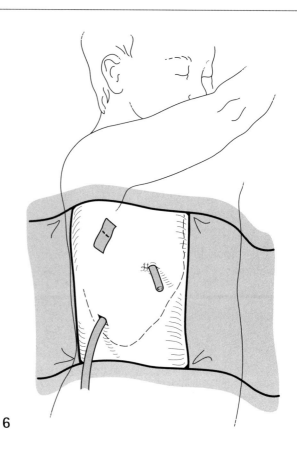

6

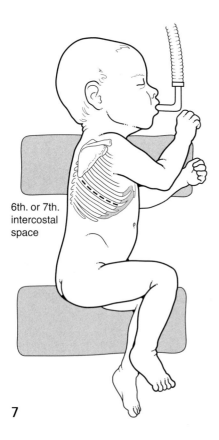

6th. or 7th. intercostal space

7

Mini-thoracotomy pleural debridement

7 When videoscopic equipment is not available, pleural debridement through a small thoracotomy incision can be easily performed. In addition, thoracoscopic debridement in small children can be accomplished via mini-thoracotomy with equivalent results. A small (3 cm) incision is situated in the mid-axillary line at the level of the fifth intercostal space.

8 Use of an appropriately sized mediastinoscope with a good light source facilitates visualization of the pleural space. Debridement ensues under direct vision. A suction device can be inserted through the mini-thoracotomy whereby loculations and debris are bluntly removed and lysed. An appropriate sized chest drain is tunneled over the ribs caudal to the incision. The intercostal muscles are reapproximated with polygalactin suture and the chest drain is secured to the skin with nonabsorbable suture.

Thoracotomy

Pleural debridement via a posterolateral thoracotomy is reserved for patients in whom thoracoscopy or mini-thoracotomy is unsafe or has proven ineffective. However, this is rarely needed. Open decortication is reserved for patients with persistent pleural thickening (>3 months) and persistent abnormalities in pulmonary function or evidence of entrapped lung on radiographic evaluation (CT scan).

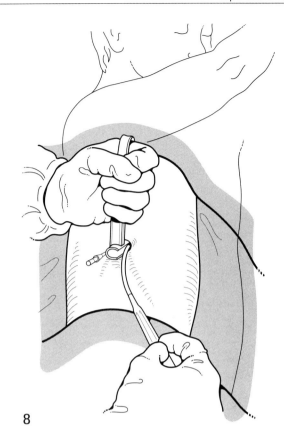

8

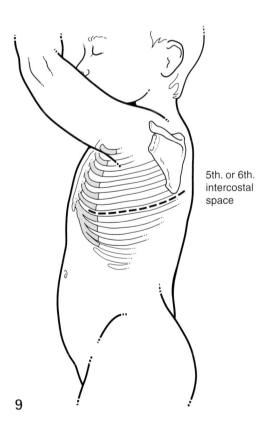

5th. or 6th.
intercostal
space

9

9 Through a posterolateral thoracotomy, the pleural space is developed, and the visceral pleural peel is dissected away from the underlying pulmonary parenchyma. This tedious and meticulous dissection is facilitated by incising the peel in its thickest portion, and teasing the peel away from the lung with a Kitner or peanut type of instrument. The dissection proceeds until most of the peel has been removed and the lung can be expanded. The lung parenchyma is then observed for an air leak. Large areas of air leak can be controlled with a suture ligature (chromic or polygalactin) or alternatively, with fibrin sealant. Small areas can be covered with either fibrin sealant or observed as most will resolve spontaneously. A tunneled thoracostomy tube is placed, and the ribs are approximated with large polygalactin suture. The lung is observed for full re-expansion prior to final closure of the chest.

Complicated empyema cavities in critically ill patients who may not tolerate thoracoscopy or a lengthy open debridement may be drained by rib excision and tube drainage of the cavity. This is accomplished by excising a small segment of one to three ribs at the most dependent portion of the cavity, and inserting a large bore thoracostomy tube which is secured to the skin and connected to suction initially. Thereafter, it is gradually withdrawn after the tube is trimmed and drainage is controlled with an ostomy appliance. Fortunately, in children, this technique is seldom necessary.

POSTOPERATIVE CARE

The chest drain/tube is initially connected to a pleurovac with 20 cm H_2O suction. A postoperative chest radiograph is obtained in the recovery room to ensure that the lung has expanded completely, and the chest drain/tube is in the appropriate position. The chest drain/tube is maintained on suction until drainage is less than 1 mL/kg per day in a 24-hour period. Thereafter, it is connected to an underwater seal, and removed when there is no evidence of air leak, the lung is completely expanded, and there is no significant reaccumulation of pleural fluid on the chest film. Antibiotics are continued postoperatively for 10–14 days, and tailored to the microbiologic evaluation of the cultured pleural fluid. Patients are discharged when the chest drain/tube has been removed, and pain control and nutritional issues are optimized. A follow-up visit and chest radiograph is recommended 3–4 weeks following discharge.

OUTCOME

Single institution retrospective case-series reports (level 4 data) on primary thoracoscopic intervention have shown that primary TDD results in a short hospitalization, less hospital cost, and fewer instances of patients proceeding to stage III disease. However, these conclusions are typically based on comparison to historical controls, at best. The results from the aforementioned prospective randomized, controlled trials from The Children's Mercy Hospital and Great Ormond Street Hospital demonstrate no significant difference in several important outcome variables (including length of stay, cost, and resolution of fever) between initial TDD and intrapleural fibrinolytic therapy. Although we advocate an initial attempt at fibrinolytic therapy in patients with empyema, we recognize that primary TDD is likely to be equally as effective, given the circumstances of one's practice. Despite the availability of level I evidence to guide therapy, these decisions will continue to be governed by historical and practice-specific algorithms.

FURTHER READING

Kurt BA, Winterhalter KM, Connors RH *et al.* Therapy of parapneumonic effusions in children: video-assisted thoracoscopic surgery versus conventional thoracostomy drainage. *Pediatrics* 2006; **118**: e547–53.

Singh M, Mathew JL, Chandra S *et al.* Randomized controlled trial of intrapleural streptokinase in empyema thoracis in children. *Acta Paediatrica* 2004; **93**: 1443–5.

Sonnappa S, Cohen G, Owens CM *et al.* Comparison of urokinase and video-assisted thoracoscopic surgery for treatment of childhood empyema. *American Journal of Respiratory and Critical Care Medicine* 2006; **174**: 221–7.

St Peter SD, Tsao K, Spilde TL *et al.* Thoracoscopic decortication vs tube thoracostomy with fibrinolysis for empyema in children: a prospective, randomized trial. *Journal of Pediatric Surgery* 2009; **44**: 106–11.

Valusek TA, Tsao K, St Peter SD *et al.* A comparison of chest tubes versus bulb-suction drains in pediatric thoracic surgery. *Journal of Pediatric Surgery* 2007; **42**: 812–14.

Velaiutham S, Pathmanathan S, Whitehead B, Kumar R. Video-assisted thoracoscopic surgery of childhood empyema: early referral improves outcome. *Pediatric Surgery International* 2010; **26**: 1031–5.

31

Chylothorax

SHAUN M KUNISAKI, ARNOLD G CORAN, and DANIEL H TEITELBAUM

INTRODUCTION

A chylothorax is a pleural effusion composed of lymphatic fluid. In children, the most common etiology is iatrogenic following an operation within the posterior mediastinum. Procedures on the esophagus and thoracic aorta, such as ligation of a patent ductus arteriosus, coarctation repair, and Fontan procedure, are at highest risk for this complication. Ten percent of chylothoraces in the pediatric population are congenital. Other important causes of chylothoraces in children include superior vena cava obstruction, blunt and penetrating trauma, lymphatic malformations, malignancy, and following diaphragmatic hernia repair, particularly in the setting of right heart failure.

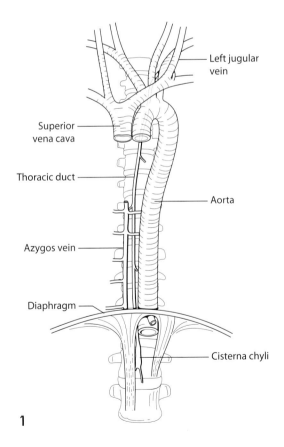

PRINCIPLES AND JUSTIFICATION

1 The thoracic duct, which carries between 70 and 90 percent of all fats absorbed by the gut into the venous circulation, originates within the abdomen at the cisterna chili located over the second lumbar vertebral body. The duct extends into the thorax through the aortic hiatus and then passes upward into the posterior mediastinum on the right before shifting toward the left at the level of the fourth or fifth thoracic vertebra. It then ascends behind the aortic arch and into the posterior neck to the junction of the left subclavian and internal jugular veins. Therefore, disruption of the thoracic duct below the fifth thoracic vertebra produces a right chylothorax. Disruption of the thoracic duct above the fifth thoracic vertebra produces a left chylothorax.

Any child with the suspicion of having a chylothorax mandates an analysis of the pleural fluid obtained by thoracentesis or tube thoracostomy. Chylous fluid appears straw colored in chronically fasted patients, but turns milky with enteral feeding. A pleural fluid cell count greater than 1000 cells per microliter with more than 70–90 percent lymphocytes is diagnostic for a chylothorax. In older non-fasted children, a triglyceride level of more than 110 mg/dL supports the diagnosis.

A trial of medical management is always indicated before operative management for a chylothorax is attempted. All patients require an indwelling transthoracic chest tube to drain the fluid and to promote pulmonary re-expansion. Apart from the obvious respiratory embarrassment from the accumulation of chyle in the pleural space, a chylothorax, even in infants, can produce several hundred milliliters of fluid per day, resulting in hyponatremia, hypoalbuminemia, and immunologic derangements secondary to the loss of lymphocytes. The latter can lead to an overwhelming bacterial and/or fungal sepsis and death. Electrolyte derangements and intravascular volume losses should be corrected. The routine use of antibiotics has not been shown to be effective.

A major cornerstone in the initial treatment of any chylothorax is complete restriction of enteral intake with the administration of intravenous alimentation. If no clinical effect is seen after several days, continuous intravenous somatostatin therapy may also be useful as an adjunct to facilitate closure of the leak. Somatostatin is thought to act on gastric, pancreatic, and biliary secretions to decrease the overall volume and protein content of fluid going to the thoracic duct. Serum glucose levels need to be monitored during somatostatin therapy. Finally, high clinical suspicion for central venous obstruction as an underlying cause for the chylothorax should be evaluated by magnetic resonance venography since such cases may be amenable to intravenous thrombolysis and/or intravascular balloon dilation. If the chest tube output improves on medical management, the child can be advanced to a medium-chain triglyceride enteral diet for several weeks before transitioning to a regular diet.

If medical management fails after 1–4 weeks of therapy, operative management is indicated. The exact timing of surgical intervention depends on the etiology, volume of output, severity of nutritional/immunologic depletion, and clinical stability of the patient. Preoperative lymphoangiograms or nuclear scintigraphy can be performed, but these studies are technically difficult to obtain and are seldom helpful in operative planning.

ANESTHESIA

General anesthesia is desirable, although pleuroperitoneal shunts can be placed under local anesthesia, if desired. Lung isolation is ideal in thoracoscopy and thoracotomy because of the need to clearly visualize the medial aspect of the posterior mediastinum. This can usually be accomplished by selective intubation of the contralateral mainstem bronchus. In toddlers and school-age children, a bronchial blocker is another good option. Adolescents should receive a double-lumen endotracheal tube.

The management of postoperative pain should be discussed with the anesthesiologist prior to the operation. Options include patient-/nurse-controlled anesthesia, thoracic epidural catheters, and intermittent intravenous dosing, depending on whether a thoracotomy is planned and the age of the patient.

OPERATIONS

The surgical armamentarium for the management of refractory chylothoraces includes thoracic duct ligation, pleurectomy, pleurodesis, and pleuroperitoneal shunts. Each of these procedures can be performed as a stand-alone procedure or in combination, depending on surgeon preference and the clinical scenario.

Thoracic duct ligation

Thoracic duct ligation is the preferred operation in suspected cases of localized, iatrogenic injury. The thoracic duct should be approached from the ipsilateral side, whereas in cases of bilateral effusion, the right chest should be chosen initially. Thoracoscopic duct ligation has become the current standard given its superior view of the posterior mediastinum at the level of the diaphragm, even in neonates and small infants. However, some children, such as those with significant pulmonary adhesions or severe congenital diaphragmatic hernia, should be approached via a posterolateral thoracotomy, typically through the sixth or seventh interspace.

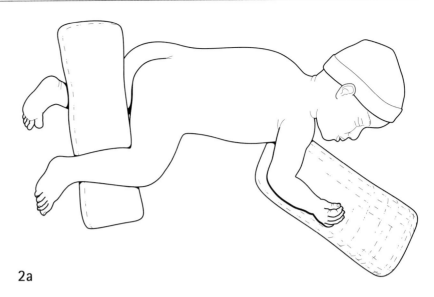

2a

2 One hour prior to operative incision, approximately 60 mL of heavy cream is administered through a post-pyloric feeding tube. This maneuver can occasionally be helpful in identifying the chyle leak intraoperatively. Because of the post-pyloric position, infusion may continue during the procedure itself and this may increase the likelihood of detection of a thoracic duct leak. The child is positioned in a modified prone position with 45° of elevation of the ipsilateral thorax with padded rolls or a beanbag. An axillary roll is placed to minimize the risk of brachial plexus injury. The ipsilateral arm is elevated anteriorly out of the way or alternatively prepped in its entirety into the sterile field.

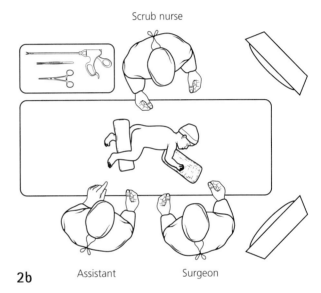

Scrub nurse

2b   Assistant   Surgeon

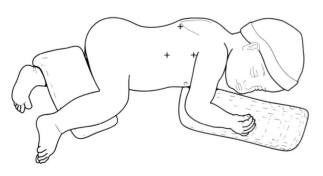

3

3 A 5-mm incision is made in the sixth intercostal space midway between the nipple and scapula tip along the mid-axillary line. The pleural space is entered with a Veress needle or artery forceps. A 5-mm port is placed, and the hemi-thorax is insufflated with carbon dioxide to 4 mmHg. The posterior mediastinum is visualized using a 5-mm 30° thoracoscope. Two additional ports are placed in a triangular configuration along the mid-axillary and posterior axillary lines. This orientation of the ports allows for optimal visualization of the posterior mediastinum at the level of the diaphragm.

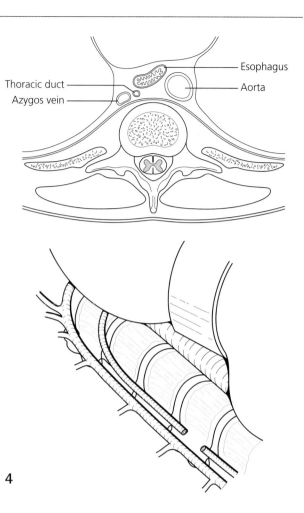

4 Depending on the size of the patient, either 3- or 5-mm instruments are used to mobilize the lung and take down any adhesions. The inferior pulmonary ligament can be divided with diathermy, if necessary, to optimize exposure. The esophagus is visualized with the assistance of an orogastric tube placed by the anesthesiologist at induction. On the right side, the thoracic duct is located between the azygous vein and the aorta.

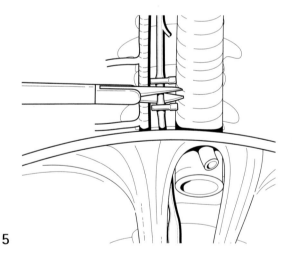

5 Once the duct is identified, it should be carefully ligated as it enters the chest through the aortic hiatus with small metallic endoscopic clips. This should be performed regardless of whether a specific area of leakage is identified. The duct can similarly be ligated cephalad to the area of leak site if one is identified. If no definitive duct is visualized, mass ligature of the adjacent tissues with fine absorbable sutures should be performed, and this may require conversion to an open thoracotomy. After ligation, it is often advantageous to cover the area of the thoracic duct with fibrin glue or a pleural flap. At the conclusion of the procedure, a chest tube is placed through the inferior port site.

Pleurodesis

Although pleurodesis can be performed as a stand-alone operation to treat a refractory chylothorax, the procedure is more commonly employed in combination with thoracic duct ligation, particularly if no focal leak is identified. Once access to the parietal pleura is obtained either by thoracotomy or thoracoscopy, the entire parietal pleura of the lower thorax adjacent to the thoracic duct is mechanically abraded with a surgical sponge, peanut, or cautery scratch pad. An alternative approach to pleurodesis is to instill a chemical agent, such as bleomycin, doxycycline, or talc, all of which are known to facilitate significant pleural inflammation. Chemical pleurodesis is generally reserved for treatment in older children and in patients with congenital lymphangiomatosis. A chest tube should be left in place after pleurodesis.

Parietal pleurectomy

Pleurectomy, which involves manual stripping of full thickness parietal pleural, is a preferred first-line technique in the setting of chylothorax secondary to central venous obstruction or diffuse lymphatic leak.

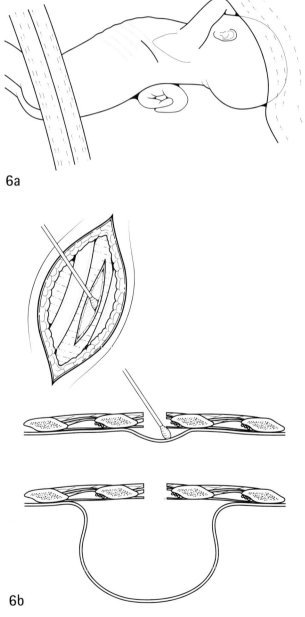

6a

6a,b Pleurectomy is routinely performed through a fifth or sixth interspace posterolateral thoracotomy. The posterior mediastinum is accessed using an extrapleural dissection with the aid of cotton-tipped applicators or Freer elevator. Once the thoracic duct is exposed, the entire parietal pleura adjacent to the diaphragm and lung hilum is mobilized and excised from the chest wall with diathermy. Special attention is paid towards avoiding injury to the phrenic nerve medially and the recurrent nerve superiorly. Although the procedure is rarely associated with significant blood loss, diffuse oozing from the chest wall surfaces may occur in cases where a previous thoracotomy has been performed. Therefore, a relatively large bore chest tube should be left *in situ*. Pleurectomy may be particularly useful in cases where the leak is diffuse, or is poorly identified (e.g. superior vena caval occlusion).

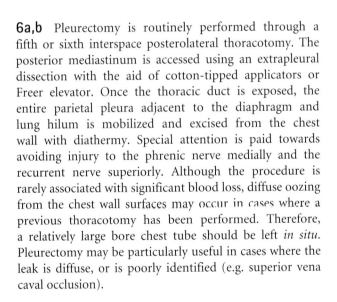

6b

Pleuroperitoneal shunts

The placement of a shunt is another potential option in the treatment of chylothorax. These shunts are less invasive, making them ideal for high operative risk patients. However, shunts are associated with relatively high failure rates, particularly in infants, and are therefore reserved as a last resort in those who have failed other operative interventions. The one-way pumping chamber can be positioned either externally or internally in the subcutaneous tissues depending on the size of the patient.

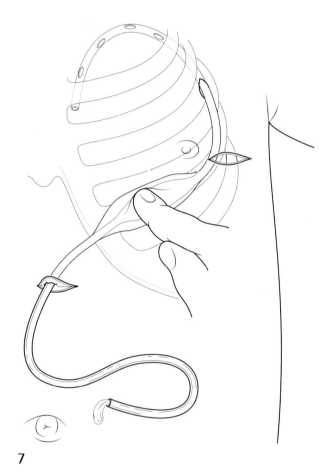

7

7 A small transverse skin incision is made along the mid-axillary line caudal to the proposed intercostal space for pleural catheter insertion. A second small skin incision is made over the anterior rectus sheath midway between the umbilicus and xiphoid. The fibers of the rectus sheath are separated longitudinally. Two concentric purse-string absorbable sutures are placed through the posterior rectus sheath and peritoneum. A subcutaneous tunnel between the two incisions is created.

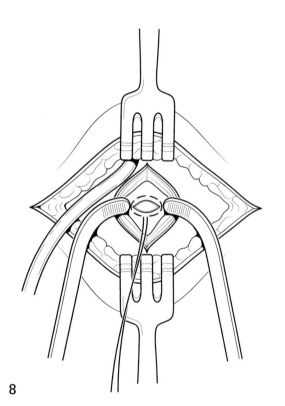

8

8 The shunt system is composed of two segments of ventriculoperitoneal shunt tubing connected together by a one-way pumping chamber. The system is primed with saline. Special attention is paid toward orienting the pumping chamber towards the abdomen. The pleural end of the catheter is trimmed to the appropriate length and tunneled into the pleural space as far posterior as possible to allow for optimal dependent drainage. Care must be taken to not kink the catheter as it enters the pleural space. A long atraumatic clamp is then passed from the lower incision to the upper incision through the subcutaneous pocket. In small infants, a low-profile ventriculoperitoneal shunt device works well. As the device may require active pumping, the pump/reservoir chamber should be placed over the thoracic cage to allow for ease of pumping.

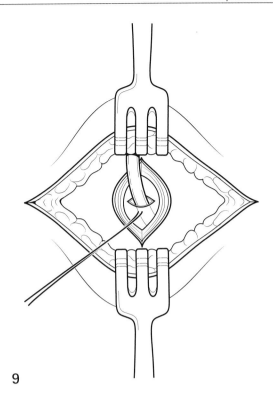

9 For the internal reservoir/chamber system, the peritoneal catheter and pumping chamber are drawn into the pocket by traction.

9

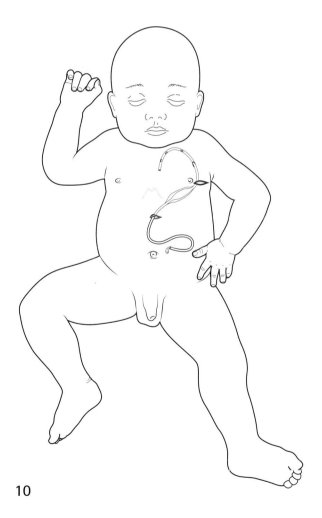

10

10 For the external chamber system, an additional stab incision is made near the xiphoid to create a long subcutaneous tunnel for the catheter prior to entry into abdominal cavity. The catheter entry and exit sites are secured to the skin with non-absorbable sutures.

The peritoneal catheter is trimmed to the appropriate length and inserted into the abdominal cavity. The purse-string sutures are tied securely. The incisions are closed in layers using fine absorbable sutures. The chamber should be manually pumped five to ten times every 6–8 hours to ensure catheter patency and removal of fluid. Over the ensuing weeks, the pumping sessions can be weaned accordingly. Pleuroperitoneal shunts can remain in place for months, if necessary, until pleural drainage ceases.

In some cases drainage into the peritoneal cavity may be unsuccessful or not possible. In these cases, one could consider drainage into the central venous system, via the internal jugular vein. This would use a similar operative approach, with the pumping chamber oriented to permit unidirectional flow toward the vein.

OUTCOME

The majority of chylothoraces, particularly those that are congenital in etiology, cease spontaneously under proper medical management. An operative strategy that includes thoracic duct ligation, often in conjunction with pleurectomy and pleurodesis, is effective in most of the remaining medically refractory cases. Chest tubes can be safely removed after the initiation of regular feeds with minimal output.

FURTHER READING

Beghetti M, La Scala G, Belli D et al. Etiology and management of pediatric chylothorax. *Journal of Pediatrics* 2000; **136**: 653–8.

Gonzalez R, Bryner BS, Teitelbaum DH et al. Chylothorax after congenital diaphragmatic hernia repair. *Journal of Pediatric Surgery* 2009; **44**: 1181–5.

Helin RD, Angeles ST, Bhat R. Octreotide therapy for chylothorax in infants and children: a brief review. *Pediatric Critical Care Medicine* 2006; **7**: 576–9.

Katanyuwong P, Dearani J, Driscoll D. The role of pleurodesis in the management of chylous pleural effusion after surgery for congenital heart disease. *Pediatric Cardiology* 2009; **30**: 1112–16.

Murphy MC, Newman BM, Rodgers BM. Pleuroperitoneal shunts in the management of persistent chylothorax. *Annals of Thoracic Surgery* 1989; **48**: 195–200.

Teitelbaum DH, Teich S, Hirschl RB. Successful management of a chylothorax in infancy using a pleurectomy. *Pediatric Surgery International* 1996; **11**: 166–8.

32

Mediastinal masses

ROBERT C SHAMBERGER

PRINCIPLES AND JUSTIFICATION

Mass lesions of the mediastinum have multiple origins and may appear at any age throughout infancy, childhood, and adolescence. The mass may be cystic or solid, and of either congenital or neoplastic origin. The symptoms produced by a mediastinal mass are almost as diverse as the underlying pathology of these lesions, but most symptoms are due to the 'mass effect' of the lesion which may compress the airway, vasculature, esophagus, or the lung. Occasionally, they present with pain resulting from inflammation produced by infection or perforation of a cyst. Invasion of the chest wall by a malignant tumor will also produce pain. Many mediastinal lesions, in fact, are found as a radiographic abnormality on a study obtained for symptoms unrelated to the mass. Respiratory symptoms of expiratory stridor, cough, dyspnea, or tachypnea require urgent investigation. Cystic or solid lesions located at the carina may produce major airway obstruction. Lesions at this site are often 'hidden' in the normal mediastinal shadow and may not be apparent on the anterior–posterior or lateral chest radiographs. Orthopnea and venous engorgement from superior vena caval syndrome occur with extensive involvement of the anterior mediastinum and are harbingers for respiratory obstruction upon induction of a general anesthetic. Less frequently, dysphagia from pressure on the esophagus is the presenting symptom. Neurologic symptoms from spinal cord compression or Horner's syndrome may occur with neurogenic tumors arising in the posterior mediastinum.

INDICATIONS FOR RESECTION

Management of mediastinal masses is determined by the presumed diagnosis. Cystic lesions in the anterior mediastinum are generally resected. Acute enlargement in thymic cysts has been noted following viral respiratory illnesses. Teratomas, because of their possible malignant degeneration, are also resected. Lymphatic malformations may secondarily involve the mediastinum with their predominant component in the cervical–facial area. Isolated mediastinal involvement is seen in less than 5 percent of cases. Pericardial cysts are the most innocent of these lesions and if well demonstrated on scans and radiographs often are simply followed because they rarely increase in size and are unlikely to compress any vital structures.

The solid lesions require establishment of a histopathologic diagnosis. The most common solid tumor in the anterior mediastinum is Hodgkin's disease followed by non-Hodgkin's lymphoma. Primary treatment of these tumors is by chemotherapy often in conjunction with radiotherapy; the surgeon's role is to establish the diagnosis. The primary treatment of the malignant germ cell tumors is also chemotherapy, with surgical resection of residual masses after treatment. Teratomas or dermoids are the only neoplastic lesions which require resection as they may become secondarily infected or undergo malignant degeneration. Retrosternal thyroid goiters are generally resected through the neck. These latter tumors and substernal extension of cystic hygromas can often be quite readily removed from a suprasternal incision; with progressive retraction and dissection one can remove quite sizable retrosternal masses originating in the neck.

Bronchogenic cysts and esophageal duplications arise in the middle and posterior mediastinum. They develop in the embryo during separation of the aerodigestive systems. Bronchogenic cysts are generally lined by respiratory epithelium and esophageal duplications by intestinal mucosa, but ectopic mucosa may be present in both lesions. These should be resected because of their potential for growth with accumulation of secretions. They can also become secondarily infected or develop malignancy. Lesions with gastric mucosa can erode into the bronchus, esophagus, or pleural cavity.

Solid tumors in the posterior mediastinum should be resected. For thoracic neuroblastoma, this is a major component of its treatment. The requirement for radiation therapy or chemotherapy will depend on the age of the child, the presence of metastatic disease, and the cytogenetic findings of the tumor, particularly amplification of the *MYCN* oncogene or normal ploidy, both of which predict an aggressive tumor. Ganglioneuroma, while a benign tumor, may grow locally, may erode the ribs, and may extend into the spinal canal producing neurologic symptoms. While these benign lesions are often identified when asymptomatic, resection generally is recommended to establish diagnosis and prevent local extension. A paraganglioma (extra-adrenal pheochromocytoma) should be removed to control the systemic manifestations of neuropeptide production. The patient should be well prepared for surgery with alpha- and beta-blocking agents and volume repletion. Pulmonary sequestrations are generally resected to obtain a definitive pathologic diagnosis, to treat the arteriovenous shunt which may be present, and to avoid infection in the intralobar sequestrations.

DIAGNOSIS

The preoperative diagnosis of a mediastinal mass can be established quickly with only a few diagnostic studies. Anterior–posterior and lateral chest radiographs will demonstrate the area of the mediastinum in which the mass arises. The location and knowledge of whether the mass is cystic or solid and the age of the patient will often allow an accurate diagnosis to be made.

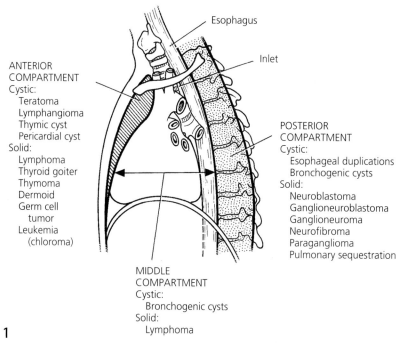

1 Lesions occurring in each of the three compartments of the mediastinum are shown, grouped by their cystic or solid nature. Further investigation is determined by the location of the lesion.

ANTERIOR COMPARTMENT
Cystic:
 Teratoma
 Lymphangioma
 Thymic cyst
 Pericardial cyst
Solid:
 Lymphoma
 Thyroid goiter
 Thymoma
 Dermoid
 Germ cell
  tumor
 Leukemia
  (chloroma)

Esophagus

Inlet

POSTERIOR COMPARTMENT
Cystic:
 Esophageal duplications
 Bronchogenic cysts
Solid:
 Neuroblastoma
 Ganglioneuroblastoma
 Ganglioneuroma
 Neurofibroma
 Paraganglioma
 Pulmonary sequestration

MIDDLE COMPARTMENT
Cystic:
 Bronchogenic cysts
Solid:
 Lymphoma

1

Masses in the anterior compartment

Masses in the anterior mediastinum may produce respiratory symptoms and cause compression of the trachea. Computed tomography (CT) scan is generally best for evaluation of masses in this area; it defines the cystic or solid nature of the lesion and most accurately demonstrates the extent of tracheal compression. The extent to which the trachea is compressed will determine the safety of anesthesia required for further diagnosis or resection.

Cystic lesions may be differentiated by their structure and location. A teratoma generally has both cystic and solid components with areas of varying density that are well demonstrated on the CT scan. Most lymphatic malformations have multiple cysts with very thin walls which often extend up into the neck. Only a small proportion is limited entirely to the anterior mediastinum. Thymic cysts are often single, thin-walled, and contiguous with the thymus. Pericardial cysts arise in the inferior portion of the chest adjacent to the pericardium.

Solid anterior mediastinal lesions are also easily assessed on a CT scan. A dermoid or entirely solid teratoma has areas of varying fat and water density and often calcification. A substernal thyroid goiter arises from the thyroid gland and extends into the retrosternal space. Thymomas are extremely rare in children. Lymphomas involve multiple nodal sites. The CT scan also defines lymph node enlargement in the pulmonary hilum and pulmonary parenchymal lesions. Germ cell tumors are uncommon, arising primarily in teenagers or young adults. They are usually diagnosed with serum markers.

Masses in the middle compartment

A bronchogenic cyst at the carina may be 'hidden' in the mediastinal shadow on the chest x-ray despite it being large enough to produce significant respiratory distress. Fluoroscopy of the infant will demonstrate compression and anterior displacement of the airway, and ingestion of barium into the esophagus will demonstrate posterior displacement of the esophagus and confirm the presence of a space-occupying lesion. While CT scan and magnetic resonance imaging (MRI) will demonstrate these lesions more definitively, the sedation required for these studies in infants may be dangerous if respiratory compromise is significant.

Masses in the posterior compartment

The main cystic lesions in this area are bronchogenic cysts and esophageal duplications which are typically ovoid in shape and may be suspected on routine x-rays.

The solid neural tumors have a fusiform shape and are based in the posterior sulcus between the vertebral bodies and the ribs. The age of the patient will give some hint of the diagnosis: neuroblastomas and ganglioneuroblastomas arise more often in infants. Ganglioneuromas occur in older children and are generally asymptomatic, but they can extend into the spinal canal and produce neurologic symptoms. Neurofibromas arise primarily in conjunction with neurofibromatosis (von Recklinghausen's disease) and are often associated with scoliosis. Paragangliomas may arise in the posterior mediastinum, although they are rare. They often present with symptoms related to catecholamine secretion particularly paroxysmal hypertension, diaphoresis, and palpitations. Extralobar pulmonary sequestrations arise in the posterior mediastinum with arterial supply from the aorta. They generally can be distinguished by a triangular shape.

MRI is often used to evaluate patients with masses in the posterior mediastinum, because it provides a better definition of possible extension of the tumor into the spinal canal than does a CT scan. It is important to identify this extension prior to surgical resection. In infants and young children in whom neuroblastoma is a major diagnostic concern, evaluation for metastatic disease is also important. This should include a bone marrow biopsy, bone scan, and urine should be collected to measure catecholamines which are elevated in 95 percent of infants and children with neuroblastoma. The majority of esophageal and bronchogenic cysts are not associated with vertebral anomalies, but some rare cases in which large duplication cysts originate from the stomach, pancreas, or duodenum and extend into the thoracic cavity will demonstrate abnormalities of the vertebrae.

PREOPERATIVE

Solid lesions require further histopathologic diagnosis. The most common solid tumor in the anterior mediastinum is Hodgkin's disease followed by non-Hodgkin's lymphoma. Other areas of lymph node involvement besides the mediastinum, particularly the neck, should be sought where biopsy could be more easily performed. In those rare instances where only the mediastinum is involved, a germ cell tumor should be suspected and serum alpha-fetoprotein and human chorionic gonadotrophin (hCG) levels should be obtained. In cases where there is no extrathoracic tumor, either a needle biopsy with radiographic guidance or a limited anterior thoracotomy may be required to establish a tissue diagnosis. The rare chloroma of leukemia presenting as a mediastinal mass can be diagnosed with the initial complete blood count and bone marrow biopsy.

Preparation for surgery

The child should be prepared for surgery after completion of diagnostic studies. If a bronchogenic cyst is compressing the airway sufficiently to produce pneumonia or respiratory distress, no undue delay should occur. Appropriate antibiotic coverage and physiotherapy should be instituted for pneumonia. Preliminary bronchoscopy should be avoided in these patients, because a tenuous airway in an infant or child will be further compromised by manipulation. Catecholamine-secreting tumors, primarily paragangliomas, require institution of alpha- and beta-blocking agents and volume repletion. Direct involvement of the bronchus is very rare and compression of the airway can be defined most safely radiographically. In the occasional case of a thymoma and associated myasthenia gravis, the neuromuscular deficit should be minimized as much as possible prior to surgical intervention.

Anesthesia

Anesthesia is of major concern primarily for solid lesions of the anterior compartment which often compress the airway. A cross-sectional tracheal area of less than 50 percent of that expected for age or a peak expiratory flow rate of less than 50 percent of predicted suggests that a child is at significant risk for respiratory collapse upon induction of anesthesia. Children with either of these two findings must be limited to local anesthesia with sedation; general anesthesia (particularly paralytic agents) must be avoided at all costs. Bronchogenic cysts in the area of the carina may also cause significant airway obstruction in infants, but the endobronchial tube can generally be passed down one of the main stem bronchi to provide adequate ventilation until the pressure is relieved. This maneuver may not be feasible in children with a solid mass compressing the airway.

Appropriate monitoring of these patients requires transcutaneous oximetry and, in those children requiring extensive resections, a central venous line, as well as arterial pressure monitoring, are utilized. Uncuffed endotracheal tubes are routinely used in younger children to avoid any injury to the airway from pressure. An 'air leak' should be present around the endotracheal tube to confirm that pressure on the subglottic mucosa, the narrowest segment of an infant's upper airway, is not excessive.

For thoracoscopic procedures, single lung ventilation will often facilitate the resection. Double lumen endotracheal tubes are available down to 26 Fr caliber which may be used on children of over 25 kg. In smaller children or infants, main stem intubation of the contralateral bronchus or placement of a balloon catheter (bronchial blocker) will allow deflation of the lung to facilitate exposure.

CHOICE OF APPROACH AND APPLIED ANATOMY

The approaches to these masses are based primarily on their location and nature; most may be resected through a posterolateral thoracotomy or by video-assisted thoracic surgery (VATS). The robotic approach has been reported as well, but no true comparison between the robotic and video-assisted thoracoscopy has been completed. If a teratoma or a dermoid is primarily located in the midline, it may be most easily resected through a median sternotomy. These lesions are often asymmetric and prolapse into one of the hemithoraces allowing them to be resected from that side. This is also true of a thymic cyst. Extensive lymphatic malformations, if they extend into the thoracic cavity, are also best dealt with through a thoracotomy. Sternotomy should be avoided for suspected lymphomas because compression of the airway can occur when the sternum is closed after biopsy of the mass. Posterolateral thoracotomy and video-assisted approaches are appropriate for lesions of the posterior compartment depending on the size of the lesion and experience of the surgeon. Extension into the spinal canal from benign tumors requires a preliminary laminectomy with resection of the tumor or a combined laminectomy and thoracotomy. Swelling of the residual segment of tumor in the canal after resection of the thoracic component could produce neurologic sequelae. The anatomic considerations and steps of the procedures are identical for open or thoracoscopic resections.

2 The major structures of concern on the right side of the mediastinum are shown. Particular care should be taken to preserve the phrenic nerve, avoiding loss of diaphragmatic function. The upper mediastinum and carina are most readily approached from the right side because of the aortic arch and its branches on the left.

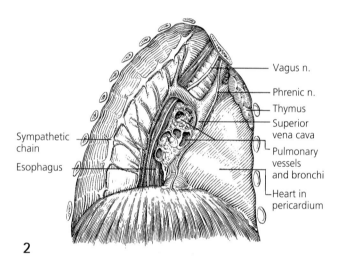

Vagus n.
Phrenic n.
Thymus
Superior vena cava
Pulmonary vessels and bronchi
Heart in pericardium
Sympathetic chain
Esophagus

2

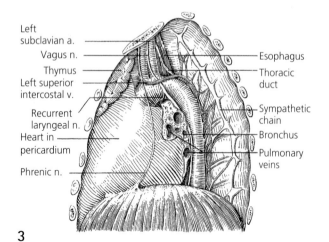

Left subclavian a.
Vagus n.
Thymus
Left superior intercostal v.
Recurrent laryngeal n.
Heart in pericardium
Phrenic n.
Esophagus
Thoracic duct
Sympathetic chain
Bronchus
Pulmonary veins

3

3 On the left side, in addition to the phrenic nerve, attention must be paid in the upper mediastinum to the course of the vagus nerve and the recurrent laryngeal nerve which loops around the aortic arch before it ascends to the larynx.

OPERATION

Posterolateral thoracotomy and thoracoscopy

POSITION OF THE PATIENT

4 The patient's back should be perpendicular to the ground. For thoracoscopy to resect a posterior mediastinal mass, allowing the chest to come around more anteriorly toward a prone position will allow the lung to fall away from the mass without retraction. The lower leg should be flexed, the upper leg straight with a pillow placed between them. The axilla should be padded. The uppermost arm should be angled at 90° and brought anterior to the chest. Greater extension should be avoided as traction injury to the brachial plexus may occur. Adequate padding of all weight-bearing areas on the table is critical, particularly for extended procedures. For a midline sternotomy, the child is placed supine. The head must be adequately extended to provide ready access to the sternal notch without dislodging the endotracheal tube.

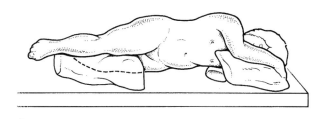

4

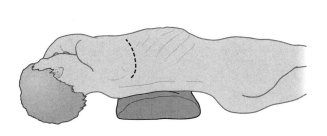

5

INCISION

5 The incision curves from below the nipple in the estimated inframammary crease to a point two finger breadths below the tip of the scapula, traveling superiorly to a point midway between the scapula and the spinous processes. This incision does not have to extend very far superiorly in children because of the mobility of the scapula. The latissimus dorsi muscle is divided with electrocautery. The serratus muscles can generally be mobilized adequately anteriorly and are not divided.

The intercostal space is then entered; if the mass is in the superior mediastinum, the chest is best entered in the fourth intercostal space; if the mass is lower, the fifth intercostal space is used. Neurogenic tumors with an inferior location near the diaphragm are approached through the sixth or seventh intercostal space. A thoracoabdominal incision is occasionally required for extensive neurogenic tumors with abdominal and thoracic components. The surgeon should take care not to be 'trapped' through an incision that is too low and does not allow access to the apex of the mass. It is rarely necessary to remove a rib in children for adequate exposure. The pleura is opened and the chest is entered.

For thoracoscopic approaches, at least three and occasionally four port sites are required: one for the camera, one or two sites for the retraction instruments, and one for the dissection instrument. They are often placed along the potential line for the incision should conversion to an open procedure be required. Often the middle of these sites is placed below the line for the incision for use with the camera and for a postoperative chest tube if one is required. The sites can be shifted anteriorly, posteriorly, or superiorly based on the location of the lesion, but adequate distance must be maintained to triangulate the sites to provide working space between the instruments.

Bronchogenic cysts

6 The thoracic cavity is explored to identify the extent of the mass to be resected and its relationship with the vital intrathoracic structures. The lung is retracted anteriorly to expose the mass. During the resection of cystic lesions, aspiration is unnecessary unless the airway is compressed or the lesion is too large for safe dissection. Keeping the cyst filled with secretions often actually facilitates its dissection. These lesions can be resected by either open or thoracoscopic methods.

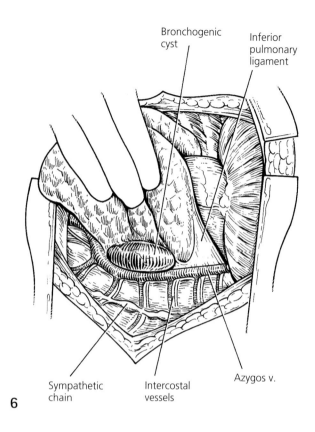

6

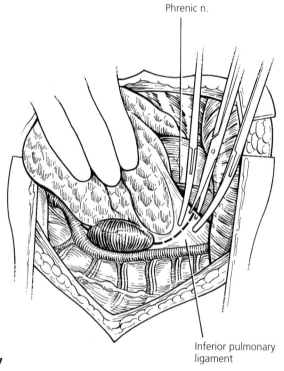

7 The pleura around a cystic lesion is incised first.

7

8 Bronchogenic cysts generally lie adjacent and posterior or lateral to the bronchus or trachea, but direct communication is extremely rare. They can be easily dissected away from surrounding structures and removed intact. Extreme caution must be taken to avoid injury from dissection or cautery to the membranous part of the trachea and bronchus. Delayed recognition of this injury has been reported after thoracoscopic resections.

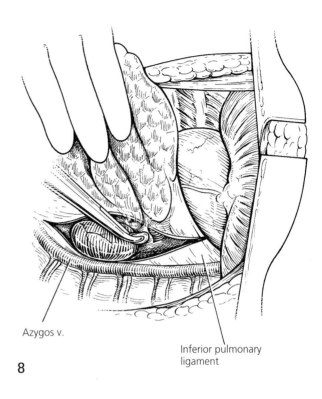

Azygos v.

Inferior pulmonary ligament

8

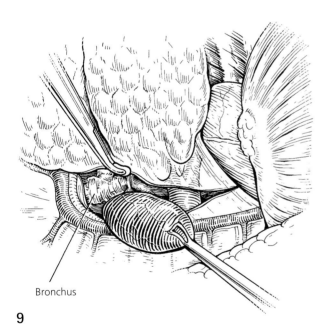

Bronchus

9

9 Cysts associated with the right bronchus, carina, and central left bronchus are best approached through the right chest; only more peripheral lesions of the left bronchus lateral to the aortic arch are resected through the left chest.

An inflammatory reaction around the cyst suggests ectopic gastric mucosa within the cyst or secondary infection of the cyst. Only rarely, when acid produced by the gastric mucosa has eroded through the cyst wall, will it be densely adherent to either the bronchus or esophagus. Significant hemorrhage or pulmonary reaction can occur in this situation. Cysts with gastric mucosa eroding into the bronchus or the esophagus may present with hemoptysis, hematemesis, or pain.

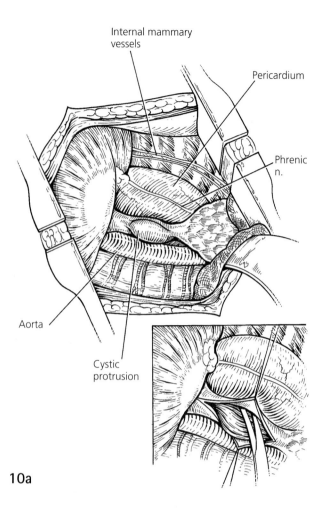

Internal mammary vessels

Pericardium

Phrenic n.

Aorta

Cystic protrusion

10a

Esophageal duplications

10a,b Esophageal duplications are generally surrounded by esophageal muscle. They are best approached through the side of the thorax into which they protrude. These can also be resected by either open or thoracoscopic methods. The pleura is incised first over the esophagus and then the muscle overlying the cystic lesion is opened longitudinally. It is particularly helpful to keep the cyst intact during this dissection.

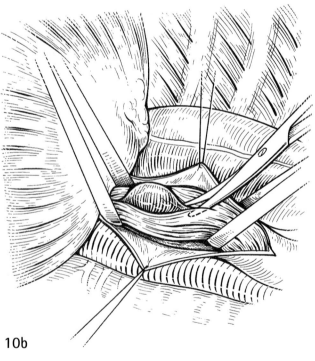

10b

11a,b Submucosal resection is the safest plane of dissection of the cyst from the esophagus to avoid an untoward entrance into the esophageal lumen. A single muscular layer comprises the common wall between the esophagus and the duplication. After completion of the resection, a nasogastric tube or bougie can be passed to confirm that the mucosa is intact. Reapproximation of the muscular wall may prevent the formation of a diverticulum which occurs following resection of the cyst in some cases.

Bronchogenic cysts and esophageal duplications should have their mucosa removed in its entirety. Any remaining mucosa may cause the cyst to recur. Aspiration or sclerosis of these lesions is not recommended because the mucosal surface will regenerate and produce a recurrent mass. The risk of development of malignancy in the mucosa must always be considered.

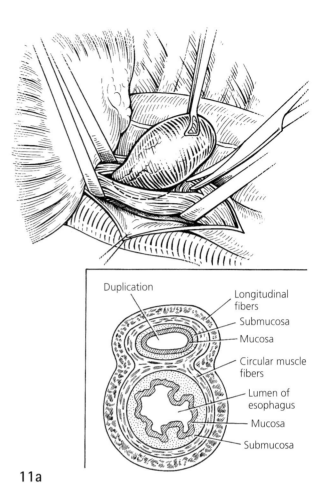

11a

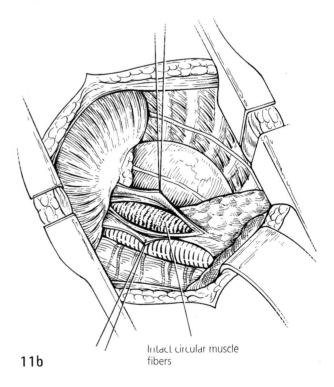

11b

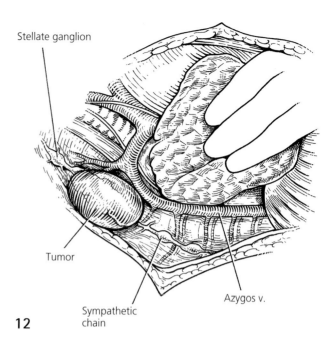

Stellate ganglion

Tumor

Sympathetic chain

Azygos v.

12

Solid posterior masses

12 Solid posterior mediastinal lesions are most frequently neurogenic in origin. They generally are broad based and adhere to the ribs, intercostal muscles, and the lateral surface of the vertebral bodies. They commonly arise from the sympathetic chain and may involve the stellate ganglion. Resection of this ganglion with an apical tumor will produce Horner's syndrome with apparent ptosis, miosis, and anhidrosis. The family and child should be forewarned of this possibility.

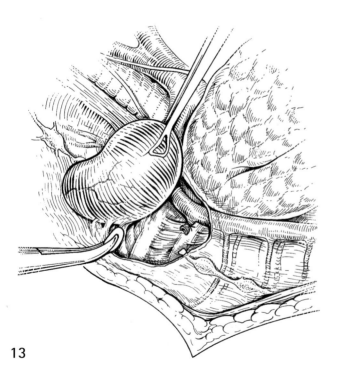

13 After incision of the pleura around the periphery, blunt dissection is used to elevate the tumor off the ribs. This will facilitate identification of the plane between the tumor and the intercostal muscles. These lesions may be densely adherent to the chest wall making thoracoscopic resection challenging.

13

14 The most difficult part of this dissection occurs at the sulcus, where the tumor may extend into the neural foramina. An artery and vein accompany the nerve from each foramen. The use of bipolar cautery in this area avoids the risk of conduction of the current to the spinal cord. The aorta and esophagus, when involved, can generally be dissected from the anterior aspect of the tumor easily as direct involvement of the tumor is rare. As the aorta or azygos vein are dissected forward, each of the intercostal arteries should be controlled and ligated or clipped or cauterized for thoracoscopic resections. The tumor rarely extends through the periosteum of the vertebral bodies. A combination of blunt and cautery dissection is utilized to mobilize the tumor off each of the vertebral bodies.

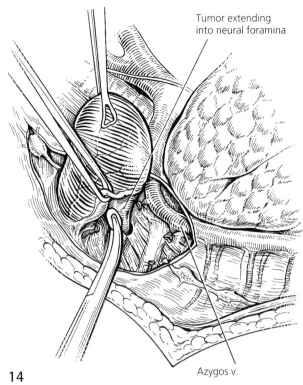

Tumor extending into neural foramina

14

Azygos v.

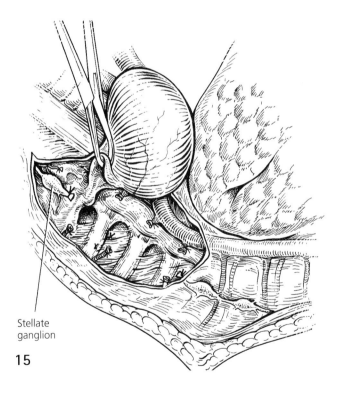

Stellate ganglion

15

15 Dissection proceeds around the mass, working where progress can most readily be achieved. The sympathetic chain is divided superior and inferior to the tumor. The stellate ganglion should be preserved if it is distinct from the mass to avoid Horner's syndrome. Ganglioneuromas and neurofibromas do not have an extensive blood supply and are firm and fibrous and easy to keep intact during the dissection. Neuroblastomas are much softer and more vascular and rupture should be avoided. If preliminary chemotherapy is administered, the neuroblastoma becomes much firmer and also less vascular. A nasogastric tube in the esophagus will facilitate its identification and dissection from a large tumor.

Once the mass, whether cystic or solid, has been completely resected, the area should be inspected for any ongoing bleeding or evidence of lymphatic leak. These should be controlled and an intercostal chest tube inserted. While oxidized regenerated cellulose (Surgicel) may be used to help control bleeding in the chest cavity or foramina, it should not be left in the pleural space when the neural foramina have been dissected during the resection as it has been reported to migrate into the spinal canal and produce compression of the cord as the material expands.

The bed of a resected neuroblastoma should be marked with radio-opaque titanium clips to facilitate radiation therapy planning if it is required, particularly if gross residual tumor is present, which should be rare in the mediastinum, except for tumor extending through the neural foramina.

WOUND CLOSURE

It is rarely possible to cover the defect with pleura, particularly following resection of a solid tumor, where a significant amount of pleura is removed. A chest tube is placed in the mid-axillary line two intercostal spaces below the incision so it can be brought up through the muscle in a superior trajectory. It can also be brought out at an appropriately positioned port site. It is secured with non-absorbable sutures. The ribs are then approximated with pericostal sutures and each of the musculofascial layers is reapproximated with absorbable sutures. Subcuticular polyglycolic acid absorbable sutures are used to reapproximate the skin edges. For the thoracoscopic port sites, absorbable sutures are used to approximate the musculofascial layer and the dermis.

POSTOPERATIVE CARE

Management of the airway

Most children can be extubated following surgery unless the procedure has been particularly long or required significant volume replacement. In infants and children, a humidified oxygen tent will often be better tolerated than a face mask. In very small infants, a short period of postoperative ventilation will allow equilibration and progressive withdrawal of respiratory support. If a child is to remain intubated an 'air leak' must exist around the endotracheal tube; this confirms that the uncuffed tube is not producing undue pressure on the tracheal or subglottic mucosa with a risk of developing a postoperative stricture.

Intercostal drainage

Suction is employed for 24–48 hours and if drainage is insignificant, the tube can then be removed. An air leak is rare following these resections. The intercostal tube is removed once it is confirmed that there is full expansion of the lung with no air leak. Serous drainage is common, but does not usually require extended intercostal drainage. A chest x-ray should be obtained once the drain is removed to document continued full expansion of the lung.

Analgesia and sedation

Young children and adolescents require analgesia for the first several days after surgery. For major resections through a full posterolateral thoracotomy, an epidural catheter may provide optimum pain relief, particularly in adolescents. Infants require a shorter duration of analgesia. Sedation is also necessary in all infants and children during mechanical ventilation.

FURTHER READING

Hammer GB. Single-lung ventilation in infants and children. *Pediatric Anesthesia* 2004; **14**: 98–102.

Hirose S, Clifton MS, Bratton B *et al.* Thoracoscopic resection of foregut duplication cysts. *Journal of Laparoendoscopic Advanced Surgical Techniques* 2006; **16**: 526–9.

Lacreause I, Valla JS, de Lagausie P *et al.* Thoracoscopic resection of neurogenic tumors in children. *Journal of Pediatric Surgery* 2007; **42**: 1725–8.

Meehan JJ, Sandler AD. Robotic resection of mediastinal masses in children. *Journal of Laparoendoscopic Advanced Surgical Techniques* 2008; **18**: 114–19.

Petty JK, Bensard DD, Partrick DA *et al.* Resection of neurogenic tumors in children: is thoracoscopy superior to thoracotomy? *Journal of the American College of Surgeons* 2006; **203**: 699–703.

Saenz NC, Schnitzer JJ, Eraklis AE *et al.* Posterior mediastinal masses. *Journal of Pediatric Surgery* 1993; **28**: 172–6.

Shamberger RC. Preanesthetic evaluation of children with anterior mediastinal masses. *Seminars in Pediatric Surgery* 1999; **8**: 61–8.

Tolg C, Abelin K, Laudenbach V *et al.* Open vs thorascopic surgical management of bronchogenic cysts. *Surgical Endoscopy* 2003; **19**: 77–80.

33

Surgical treatment of chest wall deformities in children

ROBERT C SHAMBERGER, MICHAEL J GORETSKY, and DONALD NUSS

PECTUS EXCAVATUM

Principles and justification

Pectus excavatum is the most common chest wall deformity in infants, children, and adolescents. Its incidence is estimated at between 1 and 400 live births and 7.9 per 1000 births and has a male to female ratio of 3:1. The exact etiology of pectus excavatum is unknown. It has a genetic predisposition with patients having a family history of chest wall deformities in 37 percent of cases. Patients may have a family history of a carinate or protrusion deformity. The pectus excavatum depression is created by two components. First, is a posterior angulation of the sternum generally at the level of the insertion of the second or third costal cartilages. The second component is posterior angulation of the costal cartilages to meet the sternum. In older teenagers, the posterior angulation may involve the most medial portion of the osseous rib, as well as the cartilaginous component. The pectus excavatum depression may be symmetric or asymmetric. In the asymmetric deformities, the more acute and severe depression is primarily on the right side. The rarest configuration of pectus excavatum is a combination of ipsilateral depression and a contralateral carinate protrusion. In approximately 90 percent of cases, the excavatum deformity is noted within the first year of life. This is in marked contrast with a carinate deformity where almost half the patients have the protrusion noted after they enter the pubertal growth spurt.

INDICATIONS

Children with pectus excavatum may present with symptoms of shortness of breath during strenuous exercise and rapid development of fatigue. Symptomatic improvement after repair is frequently noted. Multiple studies have demonstrated a 'restrictive' defect with a decrease in the vital capacity, total lung capacity, and maximum breathing capacity. Despite the symptomatic relief often seen in patients and improvement in their exercise tolerance, the pulmonary function tests are not consistently improved after repair. Several recent studies have suggested that the symptomatic improvement results from enhanced cardiac function with increased stroke volume achieved by resolution of the anterior compression of the right ventricle following surgical repair. It has also been demonstrated that the chest wall deformity, as well as the physiologic components, can have a significant adverse psychologic impact on patients. Therefore, consideration for surgical repair must include both the physiologic and psychologic aspects of this congenital deformity. Children and their parents must be apprised of the risks and benefits of the surgery prior to proceeding with repair.

OPERATIONS

Multiple repairs have been developed for correction of pectus excavatum, but none has been uniformly accepted as the optimal procedure, although the Nuss repair is increasingly utilized. This would suggest that none of the alternatives provide perfect results. The current standard open repair is frequently attributed to Ravitch. His initial description included resection of the costal cartilage and the perichondrium with anterior fixation of the sternum with Kirschner wires. Welch and Baronofsky subsequently stressed the vital importance of preservation of the perichondrium to achieve optimal regeneration of the cartilage after repair.

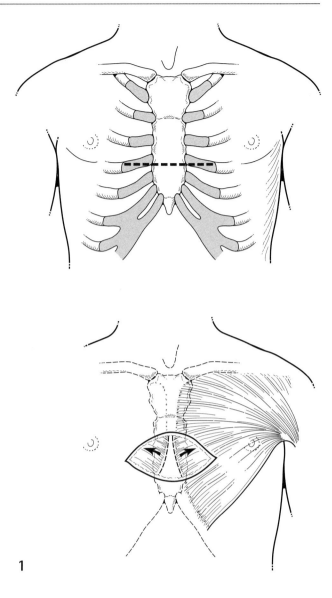

1

OPEN REPAIR

1 In the standard open procedure, a transverse incision is made below and well within the nipple lines and, in females, at the inframammary crease. The pectoralis major muscle is elevated from the sternum along with portions of the pectoralis minor and serratus anterior bundles.

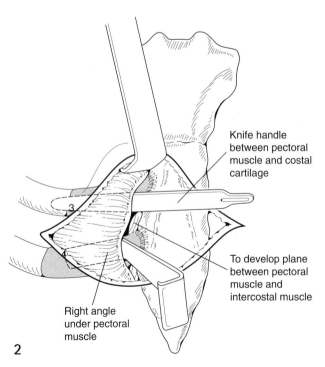

Knife handle between pectoral muscle and costal cartilage

To develop plane between pectoral muscle and intercostal muscle

Right angle under pectoral muscle

2

2 The correct plane of dissection of the pectoral muscle flap is defined by passing an empty knife handle directly anterior to a costal cartilage after the medial aspect of the muscle has been elevated with electrocautery. The knife handle is then replaced with a right-angle retractor, which is pulled anteriorly. The process is then repeated anterior to an adjoining costal cartilage. Anterior distraction of the muscles during the dissection facilitates identification of the avascular areolar plane and avoids entry into the intercostal muscle bundles. Elevation of the pectoral muscle flaps is extended bilaterally to the costochondral junctions of the third to fifth ribs and a comparable distance for ribs 6 and 7 or to the lateral extent of the deformity.

3 Subperichondrial resection of the costal cartilages is achieved by incising the perichondrium anteriorly. The perichondrium is then dissected away from the costal cartilages in the bloodless plane between perichondrium and costal cartilage. Cutting back the perichondrium 90° in each direction at its junction with the sternum (inset) facilitates visualization of the back wall of the costal cartilage.

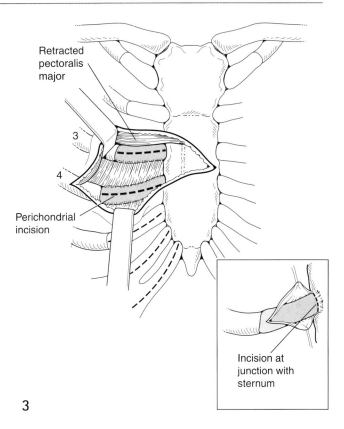

Retracted pectoralis major

Perichondrial incision

Incision at junction with sternum

3

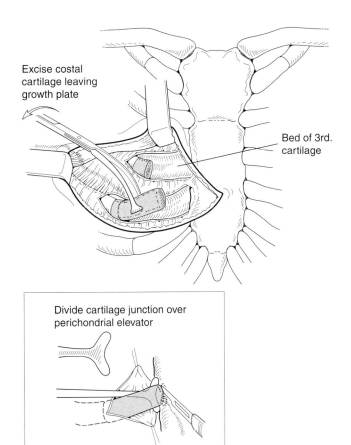

Excise costal cartilage leaving growth plate

Bed of 3rd. cartilage

Divide cartilage junction over perichondrial elevator

4

4 The cartilages are divided with a knife at their junction with the sternum as a Welch perichondrial elevator is held posterior to the costal cartilage to elevate the cartilage and protect the mediastinum (inset). The divided cartilage can then be held with an Allis clamp and elevated. The costochondral junction is preserved by leaving a segment of costal cartilage on the osseous ribs by incising the cartilage with a scalpel. Fonkalsrud has described resection of segments of the deformed portion of the costal cartilage rather than the entire segment suggesting that regeneration is improved with this modification. Costal cartilages three to seven are generally resected, but occasionally the second costal cartilages must be removed if posterior displacement of the sternum extends to this level. Segments of the sixth and seventh costal cartilages are resected to the point where they flatten to join the costal arch. Familiarity with the cross-sectional shape of the medial ends of the costal cartilages facilitates their removal. The second and third cartilages are broad and flat, the fourth and fifth are circular, and the sixth and seventh are narrow and deep.

5 The sternal osteotomy is created at the level of the posterior angulation of the sternum, generally at the level of the insertion of the third cartilage, but occasionally the second. Two transverse sternal osteotomies are created through the anterior cortex with a Hall air drill 3–5 mm apart, and the wedge of bone is partially mobilized. The base of the sternum and the rectus muscle are elevated with two towel clips, and the posterior plate of the sternum at the osteotomy is fractured. The xiphoid can be divided from the sternum if its anterior angulation produces an unsightly bump below the sternum when it is elevated in its corrected position. The insertion of the rectus muscle into the sternum can generally be preserved by dividing the xiphoid with electrocautery by a lateral approach. Preservation of the attachment of the perichondrial sheaths and xiphoid to the sternum avoids an unsightly depression that can occur below it. When a strut is not used, the osteotomy is closed with several heavy silk sutures as the sternum is elevated by the assistant.

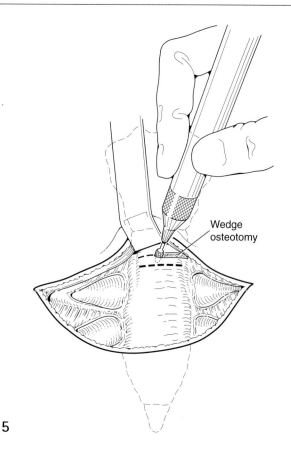

Wedge osteotomy

5

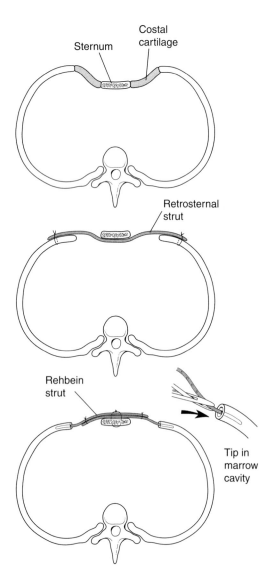

Sternum

Costal cartilage

Retrosternal strut

Rehbein strut

Tip in marrow cavity

6

6 This figure demonstrates the use of both retrosternal struts and Rehbein struts. Rehbein struts are inserted into the marrow cavity (insert) of the third or fourth ribs, and the struts are then joined medially with stainless steel wire to create an arch anterior to the sternum. The sternum is sewn to the arch to secure it in its corrected position. The retrosternal strut is placed behind the sternum and is secured to the rib ends laterally to prevent migration.

7 Anterior depiction of the retrosternal strut. The perichondrial sheath to either the third or fourth rib is divided from its junction with the sternum, and the retrosternal space is bluntly dissected to allow passage of the strut behind the sternum. It is secured with two pericostal sutures at each end to prevent lateral migration. The wound is then flooded with warm saline and cefazolin solution to remove clots and inspect for a pleural entry. A single-limb medium Hemovac drain is brought through the inferior skin flap and placed in a parasternal position.

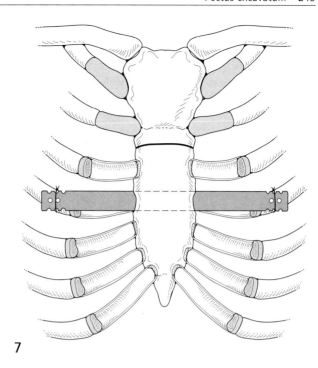

7

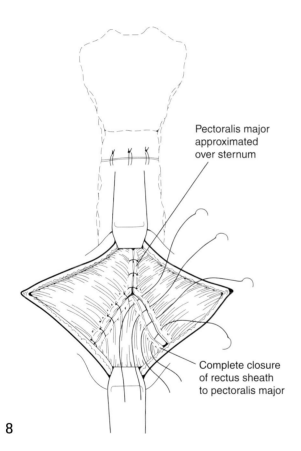

Pectoralis major approximated over sternum

Complete closure of rectus sheath to pectoralis major

8

8 The pectoral muscle flaps are secured to the midline of the sternum advancing the flaps inferiorly to obtain coverage of the entire sternum. The rectus muscle fascia is then joined to the pectoral muscle flaps, closing the mediastinum.

Postoperative care

Perioperative antibiotics are utilized by most surgeons. Pain control is managed by either an epidural catheter or intravenous narcotics in the immediate perioperative period. Most surgeons utilize closed drainage early after repair to minimize the risk of hematoma or seroma development under the flaps. Children are encouraged to ambulate early after repair. Contact sports are generally avoided during the first six months of repair with either suture or strut elevation of the sternum.

Outcome

Generally successful repair of pectus excavatum is reported. It is critical that children are followed until they reach their full stature for it is during the period of rapid growth during puberty that recurrences may occur. No randomized studies between sternal fixation with struts and suture fixation have been performed. Comparable outcomes are reported in large series using both techniques. One long-term series from a single institution, however, reports improved outcome in those patients with retrosternal strut fixation.

STERNAL TURNOVER

The 'sternal turnover' approach for repair of pectus excavatum was first proposed by Judet and Judet and Jung in the French literature. It has been utilized primarily in Japan with a large series reported by Wada and colleagues.

9 This technique involves use of a free graft of the sternum and costal cartilages which is divided en bloc and rotated 180° and secured to the costal cartilages and sternum from which it has been divided. This technique can result in major complications including wound infection, dehiscence, and necrosis of the sternum. Because of these complications, Taguchi proposed a modification which preserves the internal mammary artery in an effort to avoid ischemic osteonecrosis and its sequelae. Other authors have suggested revascularization of the turnover by microvascular reconstruction of the internal mammary arteries. The sternal turnover is generally considered a radical approach for children with pectus excavatum given the acceptable alternative methods.

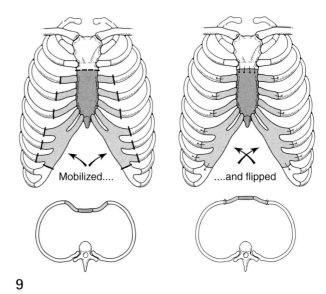

9

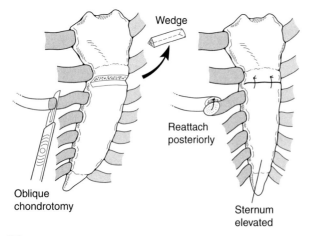

10

TRIPOD FIXATION

Haller developed a technique known as 'tripod fixation'.

10 The subperichondrial resection of the abnormal cartilages is performed followed by a posterior sternal osteotomy. The lowest normal cartilages are then divided obliquely in a posterior/lateral direction. Elevation of the sternum rests the sternal ends of the cartilage on the costal ends to which they are secured providing further anterior support of the sternum.

NUSS TECHNIQUE OR MINIMALLY INVASIVE REPAIR OF PECTUS EXCAVATUM

Indications

A complete history and physical examination is performed on all patients and includes documenting photographs. Patients who have a mild to moderate pectus excavatum are treated with an exercise and posture program in an attempt to halt progression of the deformity. The exercises are designed to improve posture, strengthen the chest and back muscles, and improve exercise tolerance. These patients are followed at 6–12-month intervals.

Patients who have a severe deformity or who have documented progression are also treated with the exercise and posture program, but, in addition, they undergo objective studies to see whether their condition is severe enough to warrant surgical correction. These studies include a thoracic computed tomography (CT) scan, pulmonary function tests, and a cardiac evaluation that includes an electrocardiogram (EKG) and an echocardiogram. The use of magnetic resonance imaging (MRI) can easily be substituted for a CT scan. The authors are currently evaluating the use of cardiac MRI to replace CT and echocardiograms.

Determination of a severe pectus excavatum and the need for repair requires two or more of the following criteria: (1) a Haller CT index greater than 3.25; (2) pulmonary function studies that indicate restrictive and/or obstructive airway disease; (3) a cardiology evaluation demonstrating the compression is causing murmurs, mitral valve prolapse, cardiac displacement, or conduction abnormalities on the echocardiogram or EKG tracings; (4) documentation of progression of the deformity with associated physical symptoms other than isolated concerns of body image. When utilizing these criteria, less than 50 percent of patients are found to have a deformity severe enough to warrant surgery.

Our experience has shown that the optimal age for repair is 10–14 years, as the patients' chests are still soft and malleable and they show rapid recovery and return to normal activities, and have excellent structural results. After puberty, the flexibility of the chest wall is decreased, which often necessitates the insertion of two bars. It also takes the patients longer to recover when they are older. However, we have performed the procedure in patients up to age 31 years with equally good long-term results.

Technique

A first-generation cephalosporin is used for antibiotic coverage and continued for 24 hours. The arms are abducted at the shoulders and care is taken to pad all pressure points and keep the upper extremities extended without tension on the brachial plexus.

11 The length of the pectus bar is determined by measuring the distance from the right mid-axillary line to the left mid-axillary line and subtracting 2 cm (or 1 inch), because the bar takes a shorter course than the tape measure. The measurement is done over the area of the deepest depression that is still part of the sternum. The bar is bent to the desired convex configuration, bearing in mind that the center of the bar should be flat for 2–4 cm to provide greater stability.

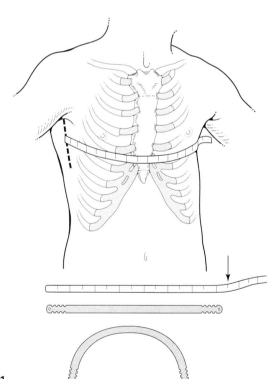

11

12 A thoracoscope is inserted into the right chest two intercostal spaces below the site of planned bar placement to confirm that the internal anatomy corresponds with the external markings and to look for unexpected pathology. If all is well, then transverse lateral thoracic incisions are made between the mid- and anterior axillary lines and subcutaneous tunnels are created to the greatest apex of the pectus deformity which is marked with an 'X'. These Xs represent the entrance and exit sites of the bar from the chest. They are in the intercostal space that is in the same horizontal plane as the deepest depression marked with a circle and care should be taken that they are placed medial to the greatest apex of the chest.

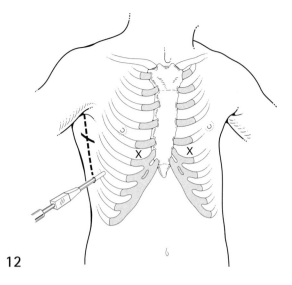

12

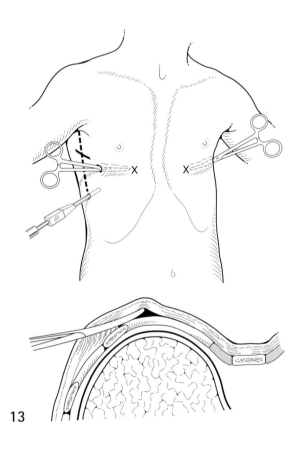

13

13 Skin tunnels are created above the muscle starting from each of the lateral thoracic incisions to the top of the pectus ridge on each side. The tunnel can also be created between the pectoralis major and minor muscles to minimize skin retraction. The tunnels should be created so that the entry and exit sites of the bar from inside the chest are medial to the top of the pectus ridge on each side. With the thoracoscope in place, a tonsil clamp is inserted into the subcutaneous tunnel on the right and a blunt thoracostomy is created at the site marked 'X', taking care not to injure the intercostal vessels, lung, or pericardium.

14 Under continuous thoracoscopic visualization, a Biomet™ (Biomet Microfixation, Jacksonville, FL, USA) introducer is inserted into the chest through the right tunnel and thoracostomy site at the top of the pectus ridge. With great care and thoracoscopic guidance, the pleura and pericardium are dissected off the undersurface of the sternum creating a substernal tunnel. The introducer tip is kept in view at all times and slowly advanced across the mediastinum and brought out through the corresponding intercostal space on the left and advanced out of the incision on the contralateral side. Again, this exit site is medial to the top of the pectus ridge.

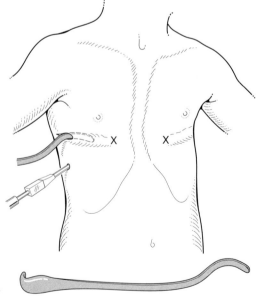

14

15 A 30° scope facilitates visualization during the substernal dissection and care is taken to keep the point of the dissector adjacent to the undersurface of the sternum at all times to push the heart out of the way of the dissection plane. There should be a clear plane between the pericardium and the sternum. During the dissection, the EKG monitor should be turned to maximum volume to listen for ectopy or arrhythmias. A subxiphoid incision and manual elevation of the sternum can be used as an adjunct for those patients with very severe deep depressions where adequate visualization cannot be achieved. In severe deep depressions, it is usually necessary to create two tunnels. By creating the first tunnel more superiorly and leaving the introducer in place, the sternum remains elevated making tunneling under the deepest point of the depression much easier, as well as more safe.

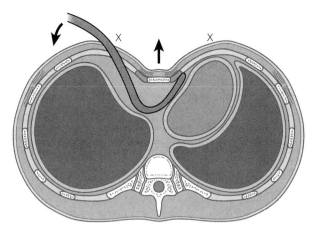

15

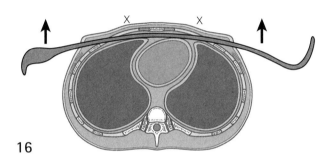

16

16 The introducer is pushed out of the thorax through the previously marked intercostal space 'X' on the left and advanced out through the corresponding tunnel and incision. When the introducer is fully in place, the sternum is elevated by lifting the introducer on each side, thus correcting the pectus excavatum. The sternum is lifted out of its depressed position with the introducer numerous times, as well as pressing down on the lower chest wall while lifting the introducer.

17 Once the sternal depression has been corrected, an umbilical tape is attached to the introducer and the introducer is slowly withdrawn from the chest cavity with the umbilical tape attached.

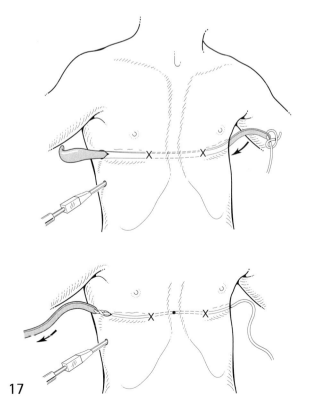

17

18 The pectus bar that was previously bent into a convex shape is then attached to the umbilical tape and slowly guided through the right subcutaneous tunnel under thoracoscopic visualization and guided through the substernal tunnel with its convexity facing posteriorly until it emerges on the contralateral side.

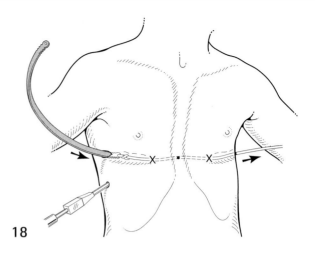

18

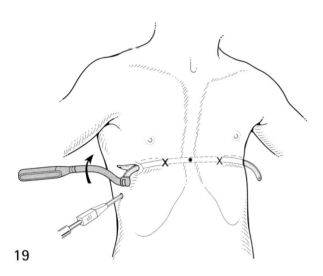

19

19 The pectus bar is positioned inside the chest with its convexity facing posteriorly with an equal amount of bar protruding on each side. Using the specially designed Biomet bar flippers, the bar is rotated 180° achieving an immediate correction to the pectus deformity. The sides of the bar should be resting comfortably against the musculature and should not be too tight or too loose. If the bar does not fit snugly on each side because of pressure on the middle, the bar can be reflipped and molded as necessary while still in place in the chest.

20 Bar stabilization is essential for a successful outcome. The bar is stabilized first by attaching a stabilizer to the left end of the bar and wiring the bar and stabilizer together with No. 3 surgical steel wire, or alternatively FiberWire™ (Arthrex, Naples, FL, USA) can be used. If two bars are placed, a stabilizer is placed on each bar on alternating sides. An additional stabilizing technique utilizes a laparoscopic 'autosuture' needle to place multiple '0' polidioxanone sutures (PDS) or Vicryl sutures around the bar and underlying ribs with thoracoscopic guidance. Ideally, these sutures should be placed around separate ribs for each bar. Since thoracoscopy is usually performed on the right, we place these pericostal sutures on the right and the metal stabilizer on the left. The stabilizer and bar are also secured by placing numerous interrupted absorbable sutures through the holes in the bar and adjacent fascia.

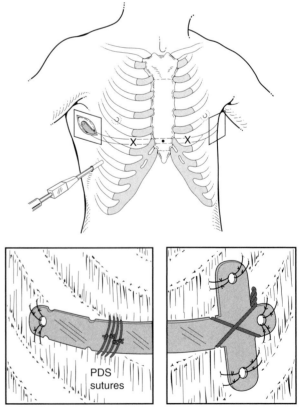

20

21a–c Bars are removed electively between two and four years after placement. Bar removal is performed under general anesthesia, using positive end-expiratory pressure (PEEP) to minimize the risk of a pneumothorax. We recommend opening all incisions and mobilizing both ends of the bar (a). It is not uncommon to encounter significant calcifications that require a rongeur and/or chisel to remove. Once the stabilizer is removed, the bars are unbent using Biomet bar flippers or alternatively Biomet Multi-Benders. (b) The bars are then removed from the right side gently under positive pressure ventilation using an orthopedic bone hook (c). We routinely perform bar removals as an outpatient procedure and the use of postoperative narcotics is minimal.

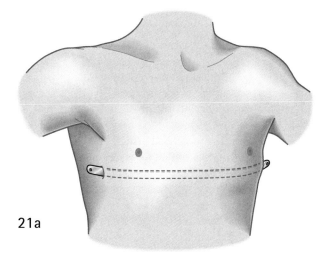

21a

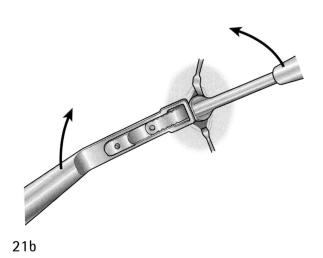

21b

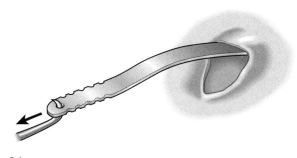

21c

Postoperative care

Perioperative antibiotics are continued for 24 hours. We use patient-controlled analgesia pumps for all patients and transition to oral pain medications on postoperative day 2–3. The patients are discharged on a combination of narcotic, anti-inflammatory, and muscle relaxant medications usually on postoperative day 4 or 5. The use of bilateral ON-Q® Pain Buster® (I-Flow Corporation, Lake Forest, CA, USA) recently have been a beneficial adjunct to the perioperative pain management to minimize use of narcotics. These are placed at the time of operation and usually pulled on postoperative day 4.

For the first 6 weeks, patients are prohibited from playing sports, but are encouraged to do deep breathing exercises and to ambulate. At 6 weeks post-repair, they are encouraged to resume normal activities, and at three months they may resume competitive sports. Heavy contact sports, such as American football, boxing, and ice hockey, are prohibited until the bar has been removed, but other aerobic sports are encouraged.

Outcome

In 1997 we published our initial ten-year experience with 42 patients utilizing the minimally invasive technique

for pectus repair. In 2010, we published our 21-year experience performing the Nuss repair on 1215 patients. Of those patients, 92 were redo operations, and only 11 of those patients had their primary repair performed at our institution yielding a less than 1 percent rate of recurrence overall.

There have been no deaths at our institution and minimal postoperative morbidity. The most common early complication is a pneumothorax, which usually resolves spontaneously and rarely requires a chest tube. The infection rate is less than 2.5 percent. Bar displacement has been decreased to 1 percent with the advent of wiring the stabilizers to the bar on the left side, using PDS sutures around the bar and underlying rib on the right side, and the liberal use of two bars on stiff and older patients.

SILASTIC IMPLANTS

A technique for superficial correction of the depression utilizes implantation of silastic molds into the subcutaneous space to fill the deformity. Although this approach may improve the contour of the chest, it fails to increase the intrathoracic volume with its potential benefit for both pulmonary and cardiac function.

PECTUS CARINATUM

The carinate deformity is much less common than the depression deformity with approximately a 1:5 ratio of occurrence. It is more common in boys than in girls (4:1), as is pectus excavatum. As noted previously, the deformity frequently appears after the 11th birthday. In those children in whom a protrusion is noted at birth or in childhood, it often worsens during the period of rapid pubertal growth. The etiology of this deformity is no better understood than is that of pectus excavatum. A family history is identified in 26 percent of patients suggesting a genetic predisposition. Scoliosis occurs in conjunction with pectus carinatum in 15 percent of children which implies a diffuse abnormality in connective tissue development. Consideration for repair of this deformity is based entirely upon the severity of the anterior protrusion. Cardiopulmonary abnormalities are rarely identified. Correction of the deformity by bracing has been reported and is now the first approach for correction, particularly of the symmetric abnormalities. Compliance with the compression regimen may be an issue.

Operation

Repair of pectus carinatum has had a colorful past. Early attempts at repair included such maneuvers as tangential resection of the anterior table of the sternum and removal of the distal half of the sternum with reattachment of the rectus muscle higher up on the body of the sternum. Current techniques stress the need for preservation of the perichondrial sheath with sternal osteotomies tailored to the specific deformity of the sternum. Pectus carinatum presents in three primary configurations. The most common is protrusion of the body of the sternum (gladiolous) and costal cartilages and is termed the 'chondrogladiolar protrusion'. This protrusion can be asymmetric producing a keel-like protrusion along one side of the sternum. As mentioned previously, some children can have a 'mixed' deformity with ipsilateral carinate and contralateral depression components. The sternum is often rotated to one side in these cases. The rarest configuration is the chondromanubrial protrusion, also referred to as a 'pouter pigeon breast'. In this deformity, the manubrium and the first and second costal cartilages protrude, and there is relative depression of the body of the sternum.

The exposure of the sternum and costal cartilages is identical with that of the open repair for pectus excavatum. The protruding costal cartilages are resected with attention to maximum preservation of the perichondrial sheaths.

22 A single or double transverse osteotomy with fracture of the posterior plate after resection of the costal cartilages allows posterior displacement of the sternum to an orthotopic position.

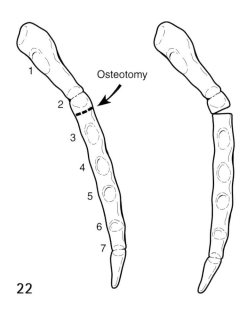

22

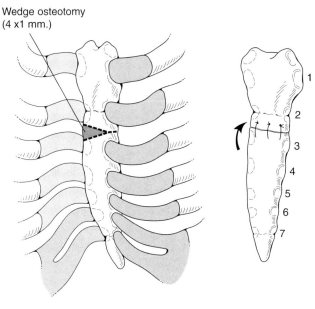

23 The mixed pectus deformity is corrected by full and symmetric resection of the involved costal cartilages, followed by a transverse offset (0–10° wedge-shaped sternal osteotomy). Closure of this defect achieves both anterior displacement and rotation of the sternum

Mixed deformity (anterior view) 9.2%

23

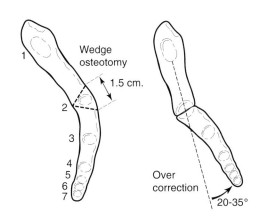

24

24 In the chondromanubrial deformity, both the protrusion of the manubrium and depression of the body of the sternum must be corrected. A broad, wedge-shaped sternal osteotomy is placed through the anterior cortex of the obliterated sternomanubrial junction. Closure of the osteotomy after fracture of the posterior cortex achieves posterior displacement of the superior portion of the sternum, which is attached only by its junction with the first rib. The lower portion of the sternum is overcorrected 20–35° and is secured in position by strut or suture fixation correcting both components of the abnormality.

Outcome

Generally, excellent results are achieved with repair of pectus carinatum. Repair at a young age may result in development of a protrusion of cartilages which have not been resected, or in cases of a unilateral abnormality, contralateral protrusion may occur. For this reason, correction of pectus carinatum is generally deferred until children have completed the majority of their pubertal growth.

STERNAL CLEFT

The sternal cleft deformity is the least severe of the sternal abnormalities which also include thoracic and thoracoabdominal ectopia cordis. A sternal cleft results from incomplete fusion of the sternal bars in the fetus. The heart is in an orthotopic position. While intrinsic cardiac anomalies are common in thoracoabdominal and thoracic ectopia cordis, they are rare in infants with a sternal cleft. Repair of the sternal cleft relieves the paradoxical motion often seen in this anomaly. The sternal cleft may be complete, but in most cases the inferior base of the sternum is fused. Repair is best achieved in the newborn period or within the first several months of life when the chest wall is most flexible and primary repair is tolerated by the infant.

Operation

25a–d (a) Repair of the bifid sternum is best performed through a longitudinal incision extending the length of the defect. (b) Directly beneath the subcutaneous tissues, the sternal bars are encountered. The pectoral muscles insert lateral to the bars. (c) The endothoracic fascia is mobilized off the sternal bars posteriorly with blunt dissection to allow safe placement of the sutures. In many cases, excision of a wedge of cartilage from the most inferior portion of the defect will facilitate approximation of the two sternal halves during suture closure. (d) Closure of the defect is achieved with 2-0 Tevdek or PDS sutures.

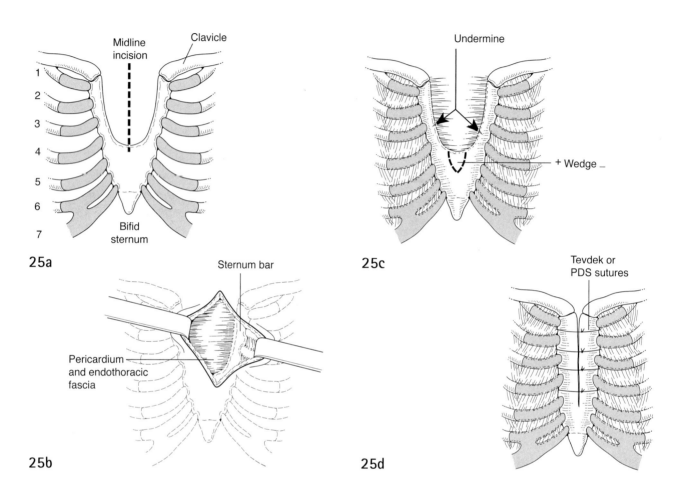

25a

25b

25c

25d

More complex repairs are required in older children including bilateral oblique incisions through the costal cartilages to increase their length allowing midline approximation of the sternal halves or by division of the cartilages allowing them to be swung medially to cover the defect.

Outcome

Repair at an early age is most satisfactory. Closure with cartilage or rib grafts often leads to instability of the chest with progressive growth.

POLAND'S SYNDROME

Poland's syndrome is a constellation of anomalies including absence of the pectoralis minor muscle, absence of the costal portion of the pectoralis major muscle, hypoplasia of the breast and nipple or complete absence of the breast and nipple, and brachysyndactyly of the digits. A variable deformity of the chest wall occurs ranging from hypoplasia to a severe excavatum deformity to aplasia of several ribs.

26a–d These figures depict the spectrum of thoracic abnormality seen in Poland's syndrome. (a) Usually, an entirely normal thorax is present, and only the pectoral muscles are absent. (b) Depression of the involved side of the chest wall, with rotation and often depression of the sternum. A carinate protrusion of the contralateral side is frequently present. (c) Hypoplasia of ribs on the involved side, but without significant depression may be seen. It usually does not require surgical correction. (d) Aplasia of one or more ribs is usually associated with depression of adjacent ribs on the involved side and rotation of the sternum.

This deformity has its gravest implication in females in whom significant abnormality of the breast is seen. In females, repair of the underlying chest wall depression facilitates correction of the absence or hypoplasia of the breast with a prosthetic implant. Often simultaneous rotation of the latissimus dorsi muscle is performed to create a more natural texture to the breast. In males, repair of the aplastic segment is undertaken in adolescence to avoid impairment of growth resulting from surgery at an early age.

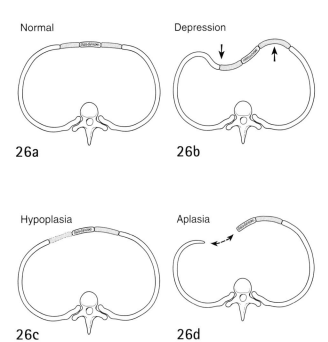

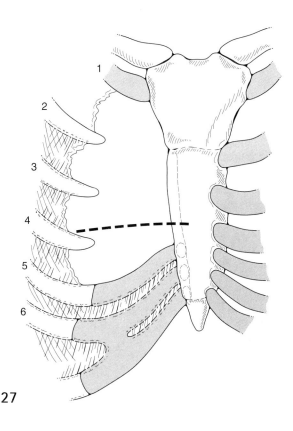

27 Schematic depiction of a severe deformity with rotation of the sternum and aplasia of three ribs. Ironically, the contralateral side of the chest may have a carinate protrusion which accentuates the depression on the ipsilateral side. The rotation of the latissimus dorsi muscle that is occasionally utilized in males has the potential drawback of decreasing strength of the shoulder.

Operation

The incision for repair is similar to that in pectus excavatum and carinatum. A transverse incision is placed below the nipples and, in females, in the inframammary crease.

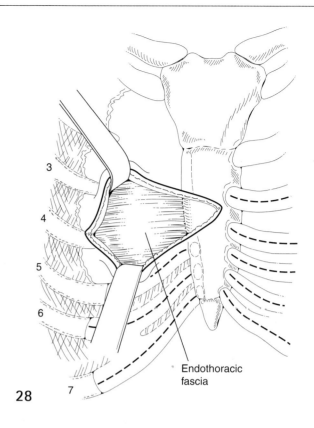

28 In patients with aplasia of the ribs, the endothoracic fascia is encountered directly below the attenuated subcutaneous tissue and pectoral fascia. The pectoral muscle flap is elevated on the contralateral side and the pectoral fascia, if present, on the involved side. Subperichondrial resection of the costal cartilages is then carried out, as shown by the bold dashed lines. Rarely, this must be carried to the level of the second costal cartilages.

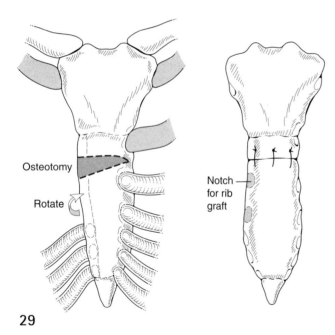

29 A transverse, offset, wedge-shaped sternal osteotomy is created below the second costal cartilage. Closure of this defect with heavy silk sutures or elevation with a retrosternal strut corrects both the posterior displacement and the rotation of the sternum.

30 In patients with rib aplasia, split rib grafts are harvested from the contralateral fifth or sixth rib and then secured medially with wire sutures into previously created sternal notches and with wire to the native ribs laterally. Ribs are split as shown along their short axis to maintain maximum mechanical strength.

Outcome

A broad spectrum of chest wall abnormalities is seen in Poland's syndrome, and surgical intervention must be appropriately tailored to the severity of the deformity. Hypoplasia of the chest without a localized posterior depression does not require repair. A significant posterior depression, particularly in females, warrants repair in adolescence.

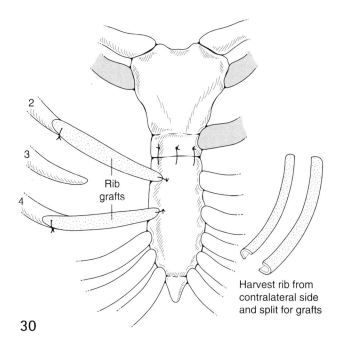

30

ACKNOWLEDGMENTS

Step figures 1–5 and 8 from Shamberger RC, Welch KJ. Surgical repair of pectus excavatum. *Journal of Pediatric Surgery* 1988; **23**: 615, with permission. Step figure 4 adapted from original figure. Step figures 6 and 7 from Shamberger RC. Chest wall deformities. In: Shields TW (ed.). *General Thoracic Surgery*, 5th edn, 2005, with permission Lippincott, Williams & Wilkins.

Step figures 9 and 10 are reproduced from Shamberger RC. Depression deformities: pectus excavatum. In: *Pediatric Surgery and Urology: Long-Term Outcomes*, 1998, with permission from WB Saunders.

Step figures 22 and 23 are reproduced with permission from Shamberger RC, Welch KJ. Surgical correction of pectus carinatum. *Journal of Pediatric Surgery* 1987; **22**: 48–53.

Step figure 24 is reproduced with permission from Shamberger RC, Welch KJ. Surgical correction of chondromanubrial deformity. *Journal of Pediatric Surgery* 1988; **23**: 319.

Step figure 25 is reproduced with permission from Shamberger RC, Welch KJ. Sternal defects. *Pediatric Surgery International* 1990; **5**: 156.

Step figures 26 and 30 are reproduced with permission from Shamberger RC, Welch KJ, Upton J III. Surgical treatment of thoracic deformity in Poland's syndrome. *Journal of Pediatric Surgery* 1989; **24**: 760.

FURTHER READING

Croitoru DP, Kelly RE Jr, Nuss D *et al.* Experience and modifications update for the minimally invasive Nuss technique for pectus excavatum repair in 303 patients. *Journal of Pediatric Surgery* 2002; **37**: 437–45.

Kelly RE, Shamberger RC, Mellins RB *et al.* Prospective multicenter study of surgical correction of pectus excavatum: design, perioperative complications, pain, and baseline pulmonary function facilitated by internet-based data collection. *Journal of the American College of Surgeons* 2007; **205**: 205–16.

Kelly RE, Goretsky MJ, Obermeyer R *et al.* Twenty-one years of experience with minimally invasive repair of pectus excavatum by the Nuss procedure in 1215 patients. *Annals of Surgery* 2010; **252**: 1072–81.

Nuss D, Croitoru DP, Kelly RE Jr *et al.* Review and discussion of the complications of minimally invasive pectus excavatum repair. *European Journal of Pediatric Surgery* 2002; **12**: 230–4.

Nuss D, Kelly RE Jr, Croitoru DP *et al.* A 10-year review of a minimally invasive technique for the correction of pectus excavatum. *Journal of Pediatric Surgery* 1998; **33**: 545–52.

Shamberger R. Surgical treatment of thoracic deformity in Poland's syndrome. *Journal of Pediatric Surgery* 1989; **24**: 760–6.

Shamberger R. Congenital chest wall deformities. *Current Problems in Surgery* 1996; **33**: 471–542.

Shamberger R, Welch KJ. Sternal defects. *Pediatric Surgery International* 1990; **5**: 156–64.

34

Patent ductus arteriosus

NEIL J SHERMAN and JAMES E STEIN

PRINCIPLES AND JUSTIFICATION

The ductus arteriosus of many preterm infants remains patent at birth. Patency approaches 90 percent under 28 weeks' gestation, 75 percent at 28–31 weeks, 45 percent at 31–33 weeks, and 21 percent at 34–36 weeks. When correlated with weight, there is 83 percent patency under 1000 g; this falls to 47 percent in those weighing 1000–1500 g at birth and 27 percent in neonates weighing more than 1500 g. While spontaneous closure is directly related to arterial oxygen tension, there are many additional factors that affect functional and anatomic closure, and reopening, in both the premature and full-term infant.

Indications

Approximately 70 percent of infants delivered before 28 weeks' gestation will need the ductus closed, medically or surgically. A patent ductus arteriosus (PDA) results in increased blood flow to the lungs, exposing them to systemic blood pressures. The left-to-right shunt decreases organ perfusion, which correlates with such clinical problems as necrotizing enterocolitis and lower glomerular filtration rates.

Clinical findings of a left-to-right shunt include collapsing pulses (widened pulse pressure), cardiomegaly, and a continuous murmur. Practically, this produces a continuing dependence on mechanical ventilation and an increasingly or persistently high oxygen requirement. Traditional therapy includes restricting intravenous fluids, administering digitalis, diuretics, and dopamine, and adding positive end-expiratory pressure. All of these may influence the degree of shunting, but do not directly promote closure.

Diagnosis is confirmed by two-dimensional echocardiography, which is invaluable in assessing both patency and pressures. The hemodynamic significance of a patent ductus arteriosus, rather than its patency, determines the course of treatment. The decision about when to close a patent ductus arteriosus by medical or surgical means remains a clinical one.

NON-SURGICAL CLOSURE

The treatment of choice for non-surgical closure of a patent ductus arteriosus in most neonatal intensive care units is indomethacin. Two or three courses are usually required to promote closure, and further administration beyond this rarely improves the success rate. Indomethacin tends to be less effective as the infant grows older. Contraindications to giving indomethacin include sepsis, necrotizing enterocolitis, azotemia, and prolonged coagulation. When these conditions exist, surgical intervention is necessary.

OPERATION

1 The infant is placed in the lateral decubitus position with the right side down. The surgeon stands on the right side, facing the infant's abdomen. A headlight provides valuable illumination of the small operative field. A lateral incision is made and the subcutaneous layer is mobilized from the underlying muscles. The flimsy attachment of the anterior margin of the latissimus dorsi, which overlies the inferior edge of the serratus anterior, is incised. The latissimus is elevated and retracted posteriorly, and the serratus is freed and retracted anteriorly. It is unnecessary to divide any muscle to achieve exposure.

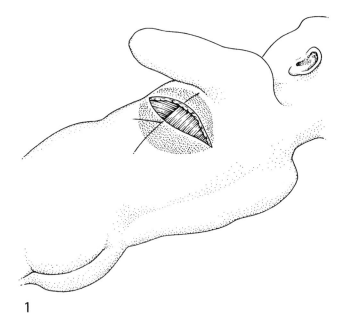

1

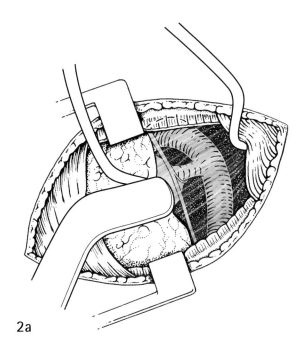

2a

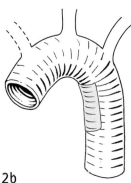

2b

2 The third or fourth intercostal space is entered and a small self-retaining retractor (Finochetto) is placed. A second retractor (Gelpi) retracts the muscles in an anterior–posterior direction (2a). The ductus arteriosus may be as large as, or larger than, the aorta. Its exact position is variable; as it arises from the ventral side of the aorta, it may be located just inferior to or more distal from the aortic arch (2b). When mediastinal edema exists, and in the tiniest babies, the usual landmarks can be obscure. Identification of the vagus nerve and its recurrent branch always leads to the ductus arteriosus (photo). (VN, vagus nerve; PDA, patent ductus arteriosus; AO, aorta; RLN, recurrent laryngeal nerve.)

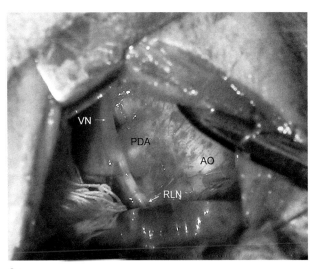

2c

3 The mediastinal pleura overlying the aorta is opened; a large superior intercostal vein often overlies the ductus, and if present must be divided. A malleable retractor over a moist sponge holds the lung anteriorly and inferiorly for exposure, but in unstable patients it is often necessary to allow intermittent lung expansion during surgery. The vagus nerve and recurrent branch are visible and are reflected anteriorly with the pleura.

Adequate exposure of the ductus is achieved by incising and spreading the tissue just above and below the ductus. This delicate areolar tissue can be grasped with forceps, but care should be taken to avoid direct handling of the ductus, which is extremely friable. The use of tenotomy scissors enhances the accuracy of this dissection. The superior angle between the aorta and the ductus arteriosus (*) is particularly vulnerable, and dissection here must be performed with great care.

It is not necessary to completely dissect and encircle the ductus unless it is too large for a metallic clip and requires ligation. The dissection is complete once most of the circumference can be visualized; the posterior shaded area (inset) remains undissected.

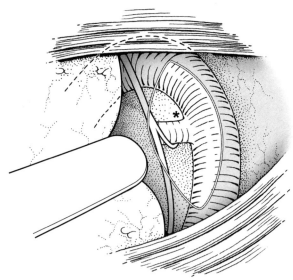

3a

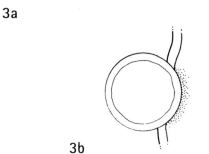

3b

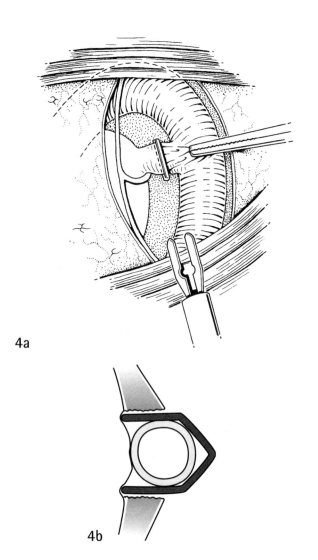

4a

4b

4 The adventitia of the aorta can be grasped and pulled away from the surgeon when necessary to provide enough length to place the clip. The tip of the metallic clip must extend beyond the margin of the ductal wall to ensure complete occlusion. The appropriate-sized metallic clip is placed closer to the aortic end of the ductus arteriosus (but not flush against the aorta). When ligation is necessary, a heavy ligature is safest, as it decreases the likelihood of cutting through the wall. It should be passed around the ductus arteriosus using a right-angled clamp.

Several absorbable pericostal sutures are placed to appose the ribs and close the intercostal space gently. Since a muscle-sparing incision is used, no muscular sutures are needed. The lung is gently re-expanded with the ventilator and, although rarely needed, a small rubber catheter or thoracostomy may be placed into the pleural cavity and gentle suction applied. The catheter may be removed once the pericostal sutures have been tied, unless there is an obvious air leak. The intercostal muscle is not sutured, and a very fine skin closure is performed.

Thoracoscopic ductal ligation

5 Thoracoscopic patent ductus arteriosus ligation is an alternative to open thoracotomy. It offers the theoretical advantages of better chest wall compliance, decreased risk of scoliosis, and cosmetic improvement. In this approach, three small skin sites in the fourth intercostal space are used. A 3-mm port can be placed in the mid-axillary line for the scope. An additional site anterior to this is used for lung retraction with a cotton-tip applicator and a posterior 5-mm site is used to introduce a dissector and then the clip applier. Lung compliance and reduced visualization due to bleeding are the main reasons for conversion to an open approach.

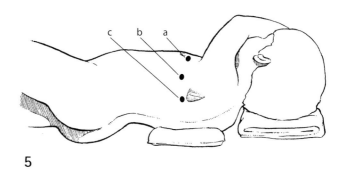

5

POSTOPERATIVE CARE

In many centers, the operation is performed in the neonatal intensive care unit, as transportation of these tiny, unstable infants can be challenging. The operation should be completed in less than 30 minutes. After surgery, lung re-expansion is confirmed by chest radiography. The infant should recover quickly from the short-acting intravenous agents. The hemodynamic response of interrupting a large left-to-right shunt is immediate, but the gratifying increase in blood pressure may require prompt treatment to avoid central nervous system hemorrhage.

COMPLICATIONS

Postoperative complications are uncommon, but chylothorax, transient vocal cord paralysis, and incomplete occlusion have been reported, in addition to the usual sequelae of any thoracic surgical operation. If the ductus is torn, or there is inadvertent ligation of the left pulmonary artery or aorta, the baby is unlikely to survive.

OUTCOME

Improvement in cardiopulmonary function starts immediately, depending on the volume of flow through the left-to-right shunt and the preoperative status of the heart and lungs. Many studies have tried to compare the results of indomethacin versus surgical ligation but fail to be convincing because the patient groups are different, and many babies undergo surgery only because medical therapy has failed. Because the method of ductal closure appears to have little influence on overall survival, accurate comparison of these modalities is difficult.

VIDEO-ASSISTED THORACOSCOPIC APPROACH

Video-assisted thoracoscopic PDA ligation has been shown to be feasible. Large series of patients undergoing this technique report similar outcomes with the standard advantages of thoracoscopy over thoracotomy being noted. These include improved cosmesis, reduced pain, shorter recovery time, and better visualization. While there have been reports of successful treatment of premature neonates, this procedure generally is reserved for the pediatric population and is often compared to percutaneous techniques, such as coil occlusion. The application of thoracoscopic ligation in small premature neonates is limited due to clinical stability of the patient, operative mechanics such as instrument size, and visualization on high frequency ventilation, as well as the risk and impact of injury to the ductus, aorta, and pulmonary artery.

FURTHER READING

Hines MH, Raines KH, Payne RM *et al*. Video-assisted ductal ligation in premature infants. *Annals of Thoracic Surgery* 2003; **76**: 1417–20.

Little DC, Pratt TC. Patent ductus arteriosus in micropreemies and full-term infants: the relative merits of surgical ligation versus indomethacin treatment. *Journal of Pediatric Surgery* 2003; **38**: 492–6.

Malviya M, Ohlsson A, Shah S. Surgical versus medical treatment with cyclooxygenase inhibitors for symptomatic patent ductus arteriosus in pre-term infants. *Cochrane Database of Systematic Reviews* 2003; (**3**): CD003951.

35

Thoracoscopic sympathectomy

EDWARD KIELY

BACKGROUND

Hyperhidrosis is a condition of unknown etiology whereby excess sweating occurs from the eccrine glands in the palms, axillae, and soles of the feet. Excess axillary sweating does not occur in prepubertal children.

Onset may be as early as infancy and a family history of the condition is not unusual.

Severe palmar sweating may render schoolwork almost impossible. As a general rule, the condition worsens during adolescence. The only permanent cure is by interruption of the sympathetic supply to the eccrine glands by sympathectomy. At the present time, plantar hyperhidrosis is not treated, and treatment is confined to the management of palmar and axillary sweating.

Topical medication is ineffective in those who are severely affected. Injection of botulinum toxin provides temporary relief in axillary hyperhidrosis.

Endoscopic thoracic sympathectomy was first performed in 1942 and has since become the standard treatment for the condition.

OPERATION

Position of patient

The patient lies supine on the operating table with the thorax elevated about 20°. Both arms are abducted to 90°.

Single-tube endotracheal anesthesia is employed. The aim is to deal with both sides at one operation.

We have employed a two-port technique, using one port for the camera and the second for the diathermy probe.

Incision

Two incisions are made, both in the mid-axillary line. The initial incision is 1 cm in length in about the sixth or seventh interspace. Local anesthesia is employed initially, followed by blunt dissection with an artery forceps until the pleura is entered. Subsequently, a Veress needle is utilized to achieve a pneumothorax. Pressure greater than 10 mmHg is unnecessary.

A blunt Hasson trocar and cannula is inserted and subsequently a 5-mm telescope (0° or 30°).

Procedure

1 Once lung collapse had been achieved, a stab incision is made about three intercostal spaces above the initial incision. A 3- or 5-mm diathermy probe is then introduced under vision. The sympathetic trunk is identified either overlying the necks of the ribs or medial to the heads of the ribs. The first rib and stellate ganglion are covered by Sibson's fascia and are not seen. The most proximal rib seen is the second rib.

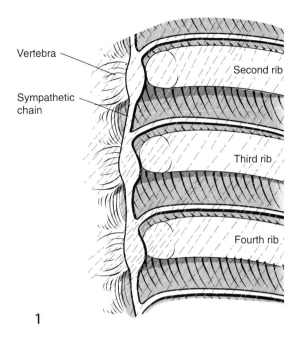

1

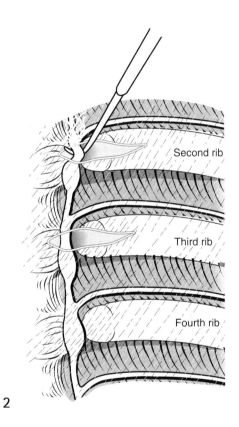

2

2 The trunk is divided with diathermy. This is most easily done by pressing the diathermy hook down onto the bone beneath. The incision through trunk and periosteum is about 1.5 cm in length. For palmar sweating in prepubertal children, the trunk is divided over the second and third ribs. For axillary sweating in adolescents, an additional level is added.

3 Once the sympathectomy is complete, the lung is inflated under vision and the procedure is repeated on the contralateral side. Chest drains are not used routinely. Skin closure is achieved with tissue glue.

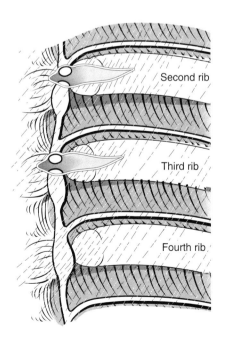

3

Side effects

Horner's syndrome has been reported and occurs in perhaps 1–2 percent of cases.

Compensatory trunk sweating is very common in adult practice (>80 percent), but seems much less problematic in prepubertal children. Occasionally, this symptom is disabling in adults.

No adverse long-term consequences have been reported in children who have undergone this procedure.

FURTHER READING

Cerfolio RJ, De Campos JR, Bryant AS *et al.* The Society of Thoracic Surgeons expert consensus for the surgical treatment of hyperhidrosis. *Annals of Thoracic Surgery* 2011; **91**: 1642–8.

Lin T-S. Transthoracic endoscopic sympathectomy for palmar and axillary hyperhidrosis in children and adolescents. *Pediatric Surgery International* 1999; **15**: 475–8.

Ojimba TA, Cameron AEP. Drawbacks of endoscopic thoracic sympathectomy. *British Journal of Surgery* 2004; **91**: 264–9.

Steiner Z, Cohen Z, Kleiner O *et al.* Do children tolerate thoracoscopic sympathectomy better than adults? *Pediatric Surgery International* 2008; **24**: 343–7.

36

Thymectomy

STEVEN S ROTHENBERG

HISTORY

The first thymectomy was performed by Sauerbrunchin in 1911 in a woman with hyperthyroidism and myasthenia gravis. The thymectomy was performed to treat her hyperthyroidism, but both conditions improved temporarily. Further understanding of the surgical approach to the thymus and its relationship to systemic disease was documented by Blalock and his colleagues when they successfully removed the thymus in a young woman with a thymic cyst and myasthenia gravis (MG). She eventually underwent complete remission. They later reported the removal of an anatomically normal thymus with clinical improvement of the disease and this became the basis for the surgical management of myasthenia.

PRINCIPLES AND JUSTIFICATIONS

It is well known that the thymus is necessary for the development of cellular immunity and T lymphocytes. However, once past infancy the thymus seems to have little function and removal causes no alterations in immune function of normal individuals. The role of the thymus in MG is now clearly recognized and thymectomy is an established and accepted therapy as part of the overall treatment plan. Myasthenia is an autoimmune disorder of the postsynaptic nicotinic acetylcholine receptor and manifests as weakness and fatigue of skeletal muscles. Ptosis, diplopia, dystonia, and loss of facial expression are often common early findings. More severe symptoms include severe weakness and even respiratory compromise. Initial medical therapy consists of drugs aimed at blocking the effect of antibodies at the neuromuscular junction. First-line drugs are anticholinesterases, such as pyridostigmine and mestinon. Steroids and other immunosuppressants are used in more severe cases. Plasmapheresis has also been used to filter out antibodies to the acetylcholine receptors.

Thymectomy is an established therapy in the management of generalized MG and can be implemented as a supplement to medical therapy, or in cases where medical therapy has failed to improve symptoms. The course of the disease is highly variable and the severity of the disease often changes. The timing of thymectomy is controversial, but most agree that pediatric patients who present with the disease do better with thymectomy.

The other indication for thymectomy is thymic tumors, and these are often associated with immunodeficiency syndromes as well. Nearly 50 percent of patients with thymic tumors present with symptoms of MG. The majority of others are asymptomatic, but may present with chest pain, dyspnea, cough, fatigue, and weight loss. These tumors can include benign thymic cysts (10 percent), and thymomas.

INVESTIGATIONS

The work up for patients with a thymic mass is relatively straightforward. In the case of large masses, the patient may present with symptoms of respiratory compromise or distress from tracheal compression. A routine chest x-ray may show evidence of mediastinal widening or shift.

A computed tomography (CT) scan or, in some cases, a magnetic resonance imaging (MRI) are usually obtained to determine the extent of the mass and to plan the best surgical approach. No specific investigations are required preoperatively in cases of MG, however the preoperative and postoperative management are more critical.

Most patients with MG are on anticholinesterase therapy and may be on steroids as well. These medications need to be maximized and monitored closely both pre- and postoperatively. Depending on the severity of muscle weakness and respiratory compromise, plasmapheresis may be indicated preoperatively to try and diminish postoperative respiratory issues. Intravenous immunoglobulin therapy can also be instituted to diminish the necessity for postoperative ventilation.

OPERATION

There are a number of different surgical approaches to thymectomy and the decision of which one to use depends on the disease process and surgeon preference. However, with perhaps the exception of a giant anterior mediastinal mass, a thoracoscopic approach is generally the most preferable in terms of overall surgical exposure of the gland and the significantly decreased morbidity for the patient. Other approaches include a full median sternotomy, a partial sternal split, or a transverse cervical incision. The anatomy of the thymus often plays a role in surgeon bias when contemplating the surgical approach, especially in cases of MG where a complete resection of all thymic tissue is required.

1 The thymus lays in the anterior mediastinum and overlies the pericardium and the great vessels. The thymus is a bilobed structure with upper and lower poles resembling an H. The upper poles extend up into the neck and are attached to the thyroid gland by the thyrothymic ligament. The lower poles extend down over the pericardium. The hilum of the thymus lies over the left innominate vein. The venous drainage of the thymus is usually through one or two small branches to this vein. The arterial supply comes in laterally off the internal mammary or thyroid arteries.

The extensive length of the thymus both above and below the thoracic inlet is what caused many surgeons to advocate a median sternotomy, as there is concern that a more limited incision made complete resection difficult if not impossible. A thoracoscopic approach eliminates this concern as visualization of the entire anterior mediastinum, including up into the neck, is facilitated by use of the thoracoscope.

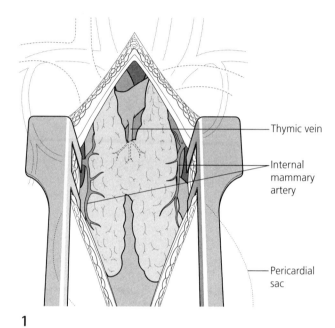

Thymic vein

Internal mammary artery

Pericardial sac

1

ANESTHESIA

The keys to anesthesia are really the preoperative preparation as already mentioned. The greatest concern is being able to extubate the patient postoperatively because of the weakness of the respiratory muscles.

If a median sternotomy is used, this is a significant concern. A cervical or a thoracoscopic approach is associated with significantly less pain and these patients are usually more easily extubated.

Some advocate single lung ventilation during a thoracoscopic thymectomy and this does ease access and improve exposure. The authors prefer to approach the thymus through the left chest so generally use a mainstem intubation of the right bronchus to achieve this. Other options include the use of a double lumen endotracheal tube or bronchial blocker.

Adequate exposure can also be obtained by insufflation with CO_2 alone. Generally, a pressure of 4 to 6 is adequate to collapse the lung sufficiently to allow safe dissection of the thymus.

STERNOTOMY

2a A sternotomy is a relatively standard and straightforward approach. The patient is in the supine position with the arms at the side. The incision runs in the midline from the sternal notch to the xiphoid. The sternum is split using an oscillating sternal saw and exposure of the thymus is obtained by use of a sternal retractor. The dissection is relatively easy and can begin with either the lower or upper horns. The thymus is relatively easily dissected off the pericardium and great vessels. Care must be taken to protect the phrenic nerve, which runs along the lateral border of the thymus, down the pericardium. Care should also be taken to avoid entering the pleural cavity if possible.

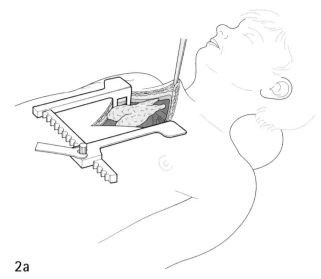

2a

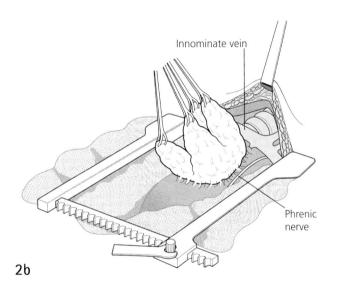

Innominate vein

Phrenic nerve

2b

2b The vascular supply is easily addressed as the arterial branches come in anteriorly and laterally off the internal mammary, and the veins are easily exposed by rolling the thymus medially off the left brachiocephalic vein once the upper and lower pole are mobilized. Complete excision of the thymus should be guaranteed with this approach as the entire gland is exposed.

TRANSVERSE CERVICAL INCISION

This approach has been advocated to avoid the morbidity of a sternotomy, especially the respiratory compromise. With the advent of thoracoscopy, there is probably little advantage to this technique, although it should avoid any disruption of the pleural space.

A transverse incision is made just above the sternal notch extending from the anterior border of the sternocleidomastoid muscle on one side to the other. Dissection is carried down in the midline to the trachea. The thymic isthmus and the upper horns of the right and left lobe should be easily identified. Dissection of the upper poles is under direct vision and straightforward. Once the upper poles are mobilized, gentle cranial traction is placed on the gland, and the body and lower poles are teased up

into the incision. The thymic and brachiocephalic veins must be carefully looked for and the thymic vein ligated as it is easy to avulse the vein through this approach. If this happens, it is extremely difficult to regain vascular control through this limited incision. The key is constant gentle traction without tearing the gland. The major criticism of this approach is that adequate exposure of the lower horns cannot be obtained and that there will be retained thymic tissue left in the lower anterior mediastinum. The phrenic nerves are also not visualized using this approach.

THORACOSCOPIC THYMECTOMY

This is by far the most common approach today and avoids the pitfalls of the other techniques.

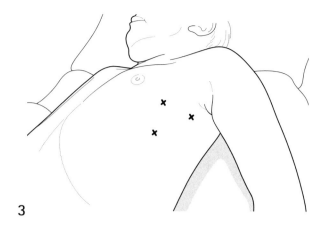

3 The patient is in a modified supine position with the left side elevated 20–30° to allow access to the lateral chest for trocar insertion.

3

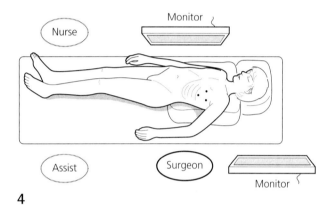

4

4 This position allows gravity to retract the lung posteriorly, exposing the anterior mediastinum. The arm is placed at the side, slightly hyperextended or can be draped across the upper chest. The surgeon and assistant stand on the patient's left with the monitor directly across from them.

5 The chest is first insufflated with CO_2 using a Veress needle to ensure adequate collapse. This is done in the anterior axillary line in the fourth or fifth inner space. A 5-mm trocar is then inserted in this site and a 5-mm 30° scope is used for the procedure. Two other 5-mm ports are then placed superiorly and inferiorly to the camera port as shown.

The thymus can easily be visualized lying on the pericardium.

With a Maryland in the left hand and a scissor or tissue sealer/divider in the right, the pleura overlying the lateral border of the lower pole of the thymus, is incised. Prior to this, the left phrenic nerve needs to be identified and care taken to avoid injury to this structure during the entire dissection.

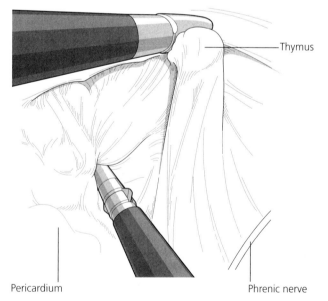

Thymus

Pericardium

Phrenic nerve

5

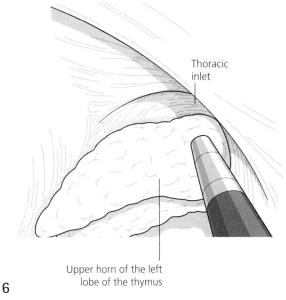

6 Once the parietal pleura is open, the lower pole is freed by gently dissecting it off the pericardium and retracting it anteriorly and medially. Dissection is continued superiorly along the lateral border of the thymus up toward the upper pole. Small arterial branches may be encountered, but these are easily taken with the tissue sealer or cautery. Gentle traction is placed on the upper pole and blunt dissection is used to free it from the thyrothymic ligament. The thoracoscope provides for direct vision high into the neck through the thoracic inlet, allowing for complete dissection of the upper pole.

Thoracic inlet

Upper horn of the left lobe of the thymus

6

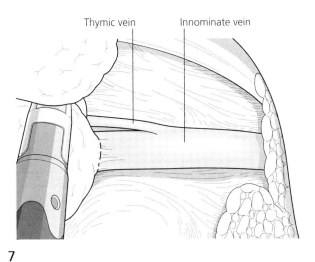

Thymic vein   Innominate vein

7 With the upper and lower poles mobilized, the isthmus is retracted medially exposing the back of the thymus gland and the left innominate vein. The thymic vein(s) is usually easily identified and it is further dissected out with gentle blunt dissection.

7

8 Once mobilized, the vein can be clipped and divided or sealed with the tissue sealer and divided.

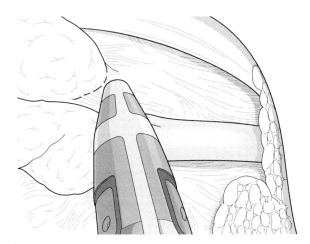

8

With this maneuver completed, the left lobe is now retracted into the left chest pulling the right lobe of the thymus medially. The right upper and lower horns are gently dissected off their fascial attachments by blunt and sharp dissection. The thymus should be able to be dissected out of the right side of the mediastinum without entering the right pleural space.

The only danger to this part of the dissection is possible injury to the right phrenic nerve, as it cannot be easily visualized. The key to avoiding injury to this nerve is to maintain steady traction on the thymus pulling it into the left chest, and using mostly blunt dissection for this part of the procedure. This pulls the gland away from the nerve and protects it.

Once the thymus is completely free, it is placed in an endoscopic specimen bag and brought out through a slightly enlarged trocar site.

The CO_2 insufflation is stopped and the right lung reinflated using the trocar to evacuate the pneumothorax. The last trocar is then withdrawn under positive pressure and an occlusive dressing is applied. No chest tube is necessary.

9 In cases of tumors, the same approach is used although the side of chest entry may vary depending on where the tumor lies.

The ability to resect the tumor thoracoscopically depends on the size of the mass and the surgeon's experience.

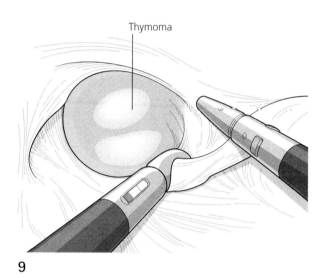

Thymoma

9

POSTOPERATIVE CARE

The patient should be extubated at the end of the procedure and simply requires aggressive chest physiotherapy. No chest tube is left in place and there will likely be a small residual pneumothorax on the chest x-ray, but this will resolve spontaneously over the next 24–48 hours.

Most patients are discharged on the first postoperative day. In cases of MG, the patient's medications are tapered over the next several weeks.

FURTHER READING

DeFilippi VJ, Richman DP, Ferguson MK. Transcervical thymectomy for myasthenia gravis. *Annals of Thoracic Surgery* 1994; **45**: 242–7.

Kogut KA, Bufo AJ, Rothenberg SS *et al*. Thoracoscopic thymectomy for myasthenia gravis in children. *Journal of Pediatric Surgery* 2000; **35**: 1576–7.

Seguier-Lipszyc E, Bonnard A, Evrard P *et al*. Left thoracoscopic thymectomy for myasthenia gravis in children. *Surgical Endoscopy* 2005; **19**: 140–2.

SECTION V

Abdominal

37

Hernias in children

JAY L GROSFELD, SCOTT A ENGUM, and PAUL KH TAM

INGUINAL HERNIA AND HYDROCELE

History

The first reference to hernia repair in children is credited to Celsus who in AD25 recommended removal of the hernia sac and testes through a scrotal incision. Pare recommended treatment of childhood hernia; however, the first accurate description was made by Pott in 1756. Czerny performed high ligation of the hernia sac through the external ring in 1877, and in 1899, Ferguson recommended that the spermatic cord should remain undisturbed during inguinal hernia repair. In 1912, Turner documented that high ligation of the sac was the only procedure necessary in most children. Herzfeld later advocated for outpatient surgical repair in 1938, followed by early repair in infancy being recommended by Ladd and Gross in 1941. The concept of bilateral inguinal exploration was promoted by Duckett, Rothenberg, and Barnett, among others. Advances in neonatal intensive care have resulted in improved survival of premature infants who have a high incidence of hernia and an increased risk of complications. These cases have stimulated great interest into considerations regarding the timing of operation and choice of anesthesia. With the advent of laparoscopy, surgeons now have the choice of open or laparoscopic repair of inguinal hernias.

There is no consensus on how to approach the contralateral groin in an infant or child who presents with unilateral inguinal hernia. Many would advocate exploration in those who are under the age of two years based on the concepts that bilateral involvement was most frequent in the first six months of life, and then the incidence dropped gradually. The controversy of contralateral groin exploration has further been fueled by advances in laparoscopy, which allows a more accurate evaluation of whether a contralateral patent processus vaginalis is present.

Principles and justification

1 The occurrence of congenital inguinal hernia is related to descent of the testis which follows the gubernaculums testis as it descends from an intra-abdominal retroperitoneal position to the scrotum. Those factors affecting descent (androgenic hormonal influences for the abdominal descent phase and local hormonal influences, such as GFRH release from the genitofemoral nerve for the scrotal descent phase) are beyond the scope of this chapter. However, as the testis passes through the internal ring it drags with it a diverticulum of peritoneum on its anteromedial surface referred to as the 'processus vaginalis'. In girls, this pouch was described by Anton Nuck in 1691 and is referred to as the canal of Nuck. It is an abnormal patent pouch of peritoneum extending into the labia majora and is analogous to the processus vaginalis in males. The layers of the processus vaginalis normally fuse in >90 percent of full-term infants, obliterating the entrance to the inguinal canal from the peritoneal cavity. Failure of obliteration may result in a variety of inguinal–scrotal anomalies, including complete persistence resulting in a scrotal hernia, distal processus obliteration, and proximal hernial patency, complete patency with a narrow opening at the internal ring referred to as a communicating hydrocele, hydrocele of the canal of Nuck in girls or inguinal canal in boys, and a hydrocele of the tunica vaginalis.

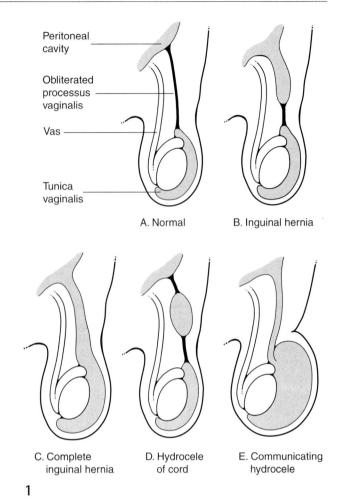

A. Normal   B. Inguinal hernia

C. Complete inguinal hernia   D. Hydrocele of cord   E. Communicating hydrocele

1

CLINICAL PRESENTATION

The majority of inguinal hernias in infants and children are indirect hernias. Boys are more commonly affected than girls in a ratio of 9:1; 60 percent present on the right side due to later testicular descent and obliteration of the processus vaginalis on the right, 25 percent occur on the left side, and 15 percent are bilateral. The diagnosis is often visually as a bulge and can be observed in the groin with crying, straining, or standing. Scrotal enlargement and frequent change in scrotal size may be noted and are the result of fluid transfer (or bowel) between the peritoneal cavity and the sac. Physical examination will often confirm these observations: however, not uncommonly, the diagnosis may depend on visualization of these events by the referring pediatrician or parents; this may be aided by having a photograph taken by the parent when the hernia appears. The distinction between a hernia and a hydrocele is the history and/or physical sign of reducibility of the swelling in the former.

Inguinal hernia is a high-risk hernia, particularly in early infancy, as it is frequently complicated by incarceration, occasionally leading to intestinal obstruction and strangulation. In young infants with undescended testes and associated hernia, the testis is sometimes at risk of torsion or atrophy caused by compression of the vascular supply by a hernia sac filled with bowel at the level of the internal inguinal ring. The incidence of incarceration is highest in the youngest patients, particularly premature infants and infants under the age of one year where an incarceration rate of 31 percent has been reported. The incarceration rate in children up to 18 years of age is 12–15 percent.

INDICATIONS

Because of the high rate of complications associated with inguinal hernia, there is no place for conservative management except in instances of an isolated hydrocele of the tunica vaginalis. The natural history of this particular abnormality is often associated with spontaneous involution at 6–12 months of age. As long as the hydrocele does not change in size, this can be observed. All other inguinal scrotal anomalies require surgical intervention. In addition to instances of incarceration seen in boys, girls can present with a mass in the labia majora due to a sliding hernia of the ovary and Fallopian tube. This may be associated with a risk of torsion of the ovary in the hernia sac.

Preoperative assessment and preparation

The operation is usually performed shortly after the diagnosis is made. Attempts to reduce an incarcerated hernia using sedation and manual reduction are successful in more than 80 percent of cases. An elective operation is then typically carried out within 24 hours of the reduction as the recurrence rate for incarceration is noted to be as high as 15 percent if repair is delayed beyond 5 days. In instances of symptomatic hernias in small premature infants already hospitalized in the neonatal intensive care unit because of other illnesses, elective repair is carried out just before discharge and/or a weight greater than 2.0 kg. For infants diagnosed after discharge from the hospital who required ventilatory support or experience episodes of apnea and/or bradycardia in the neonatal period, elective repair may be delayed until 50 weeks of corrected conceptional age to optimize their clinical status. Although most infants and children can be managed in an ambulatory setting, infants with bronchopulmonary dysplasia, anemia, prematurity (less than 50 weeks of corrected conceptional age), or those who required ventilator support at the time of birth should be observed after operative repair in an extended observation (23 hours) center and monitored for episodes of apnea and/or bradycardia.

Anesthesia

Mild sedation may be administered preoperatively (midazolam 0.5–1.0 mg/kg orally 15–20 minutes prior to going to the operating room) to minimize patient anxiety. The operation is usually performed under general anesthesia, however, regional analgesia methods for inguinal hernia repair have attracted increasing interest. Caudal block, lumbar epidural block, ilioinguinal nerve block, and wound infiltration have all been used with varying success. Spinal anesthesia has become a popular technique, but some studies report intraoperative restlessness and pain during the repair which may be due to peritoneal sac traction. The lower abdomen (umbilicus included), inguinal scrotal area, perineum, and thighs are prepared with a sterilizing solution of choice and then draped appropriately for herniotomy.

Operation: open approach

2 A transverse incision is made in the lowest inguinal skin crease above the external inguinal ring on the affected side. One must be aware of the superficial epigastric vein to avoid bleeding and subsequent ecchymoses in the superficial wound in the postoperative period. Scarpa's fascia is incised and the external oblique fascia identified. The external oblique fascia exposed and traced laterally to the inguinal ligament. The inguinal ligament is traced inferiorly to expose the external inguinal ring. This minimizes the risk of opening the inguinal canal too medially.

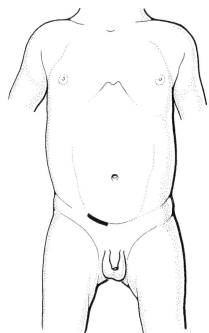

2

3 Once the superficial inguinal ring is identified, the external oblique fascia is opened superiorly in the long axis of its fibers, perpendicular to the ring, for a distance of 1.0–2.0 cm (near the deep inguinal ring). Care is taken during this maneuver to minimize accidental injury to the ilioinguinal nerve.

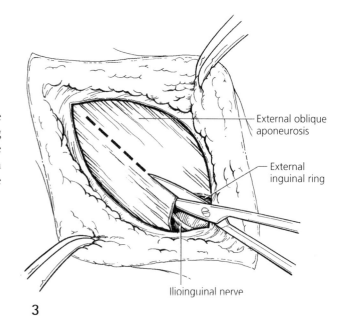

External oblique aponeurosis

External inguinal ring

Ilioinguinal nerve

3

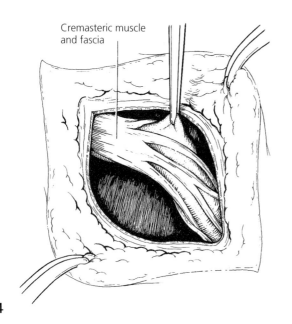

Cremasteric muscle and fascia

4

4 The undersurface of the superior leaflet of the external oblique is gently dissected free from the internal oblique and abdomen's transverse muscle. The inferior leaflet is mobilized down to the inguinal ligament. During this mobilization, the iliohypogastric and ilioinguinal nerves are located. The ilioinguinal nerve can be seen on the outer vestment of the spermatic fascia. The cremasteric muscle is teased open by blunt dissection on the anteromedial surface of the cord and spread to expose the glistening peritoneum of the indirect hernia sac.

5 The sac is elevated anteromedially and the spermatic vessels are identified and carefully dissected free from the diverticular structure of the inguinal hernia sac. Once the spermatic vessels are mobilized away from the sac, the vas deferens is visualized. The vas deferens is often intricately adherent to the sac and should never be grasped directly with a forceps or a clamp during the dissection as this can result in an injury. The hernia sac often extends to the testicular area. Once the vital structures (vessels and vas deferens) are identified and cleared laterally, the hernia sac can be divided between clamps and the upper end dissected superiorly to the level of the internal (deep) inguinal ring. The proper extent of the superior dissection is identified by the presence of retroperitoneal fat at the neck of the sac.

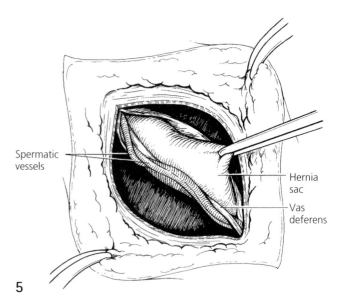

Spermatic vessels

Hernia sac

Vas deferens

5

6 At this point, the sac can be opened on the most distal end and a 2- or 3-mm trocar is advanced into the abdomen and secured with a tie to minimize insufflation leak. The abdomen is insufflated with CO_2 to 8–10 mmHg pressure and a 70° laparoscope is advanced through the trocar into the abdomen to view the opposite internal ring. It may be of advantage to have the patient in some degree of Trendelenburg position to aid the bowel in moving out of the pelvis and away from the contralateral internal ring.

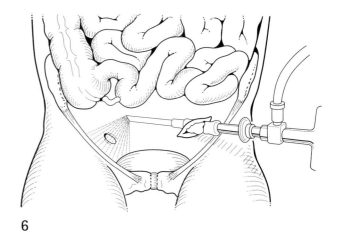

6

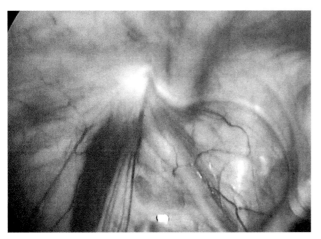

7a

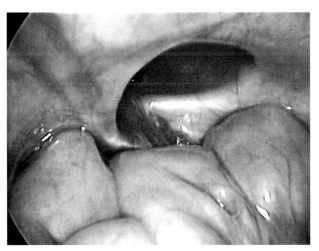

7b

7 Viewing the left internal ring via the right inguinal hernia sac, one can see in Step figure 7a a normal internal ring with the vas deferens medially and the spermatic cord vessels located laterally. There is no inguinal hernia evident. In Step figure 7b, while viewing the right internal ring via the left inguinal hernia sac, a large indirect inguinal hernia is noted with weakening of the inguinal floor. When a contralateral hernia is noted, a similar repair can be performed on the opposite groin during the same anesthetic with limited morbidity. This technique avoids unnecessary routine contralateral exploration for all patients without a recognizable bulge on the opposite side and limits repair to those babies that have a demonstrable hernia on laparoscopy. Alternatively, laparoscopic hernia repair (see below under Operation: laparoscopic approach) allows concomitant examination of the contralateral internal inguinal ring.

8 Following laparoscopy, the trocar is removed and any contents in the sac should be reduced into the peritoneal cavity. The base of the sac may be twisted to ensure that all the contents are fully reduced. If contents seem to remain within the sac, one should suspect a sliding component within the posterior wall of the sac. Sliding hernias often present as a more chronic hernia with the bulge often noted for a prolonged period of time prior to referral. In these instances, a viscus is usually a component of the sac. The sac may contain bowel – partly intraperitoneal and partly extraperitoneal. The bladder can occasionally be found medially and on the right lateral side a slider of the cecum might be noted. The pelvic colon may be part of the sac on the left lateral side. In girls, the Fallopian tube, ovary, and occasionally the uterus can be part of the sliding component. Unwise dissection may result in an accidental injury to any of these structures. Similarly, failure to recognize the sliding component may result in injury if the surgeon attempts to perform high suture ligation of the sac and includes the viscus in the suture.

The best treatment usually involves the separation of the spermatic vessels and vas deferens from the sac, opening the sac, and delicately dissecting the intra-abdominal structures off the sac. Following reduction of the sliding component into the abdomen, a high ligation of the sac at the internal ring can then be safely carried out. A forceps (or slotted spoon) may then be placed at the base of the sac to protect the cord structures. The neck of the sac is transfixed twice with a non-absorbable 4/0 (or 3/0 in older children) suture ligature. A free tie is avoided because of the risk of postoperative abdominal distension and the possibility of dislodgment of the free-tie from the peritoneum.

If the dissection has been sufficient, retraction of the sutured hernia sac stump into the preperitoneal space will occur. The distal end of the hernia sac is then opened on its anterior surface and excess tissue excised. If a separate hydrocele is present, this should be excised at the same time. If the internal ring is excessively large, this can be made smaller inferior to the cord vessels with an interrupted 4/0 non-absorbable suture placed across the transversalis fascia. The floor of the inguinal canal is usually normal and requires no specific repair, and during the procedure, the surgeon should avoid any injury to the transversalis fascia as high ligation of an infant hernia is usually all that is required.

In rare cases where there is an associated direct inguinal hernia, or the internal ring is excessively large, this can be repaired by inserting a few non-absorbable sutures between the conjoined tendon and Poupart's ligament. If the direct component comprises a majority of floor of the canal, a Cooper's ligament repair may rarely be necessary. The testis should be returned to a normal intrascrotal location at the end of the procedure. Administration of a local anesthetic (e.g. bipivacaine 0.25 percent, use 0.25 mL/kg per hernia repair side for a maximum of 3 mg/kg dose) along the ilioinguinal and iliohypogastric nerves will reduce postoperative pain.

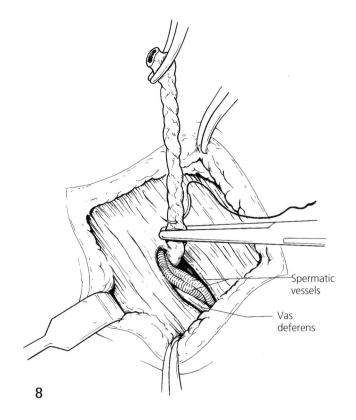

Spermatic vessels

Vas deferens

8

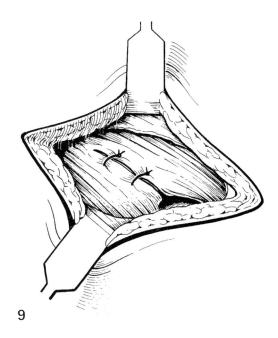

9 Wound closure is accomplished with an interrupted or running absorbable 4/0 suture approximating the external oblique fascia leaflets to the external ring.

9

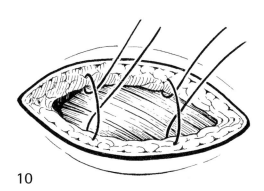

10

10 Scarpa's fascia is closed with one or two interrupted 4/0 absorbable sutures. The skin edges are opposed with either interrupted or running subcuticular 4/0 or 5/0 absorbable sutures. The skin edges are approximated with a Dermabond dressing in infants if they are not toilet-trained. Alternatively, Mastisol and sterile skin closure strips (e.g. Steristrips) and a semipermeable adhesive film dressing (e.g. Opsite) is applied in older children.

Operation: laparoscopic approach

11 Laparoscopic hernia repair is an effective and increasingly popular alternative to open herniotomy. After the induction of general endotracheal anesthesia, the patient is placed in the Trendelenburg position. The abdomen, groin, and scrotal areas are prepped with a sterile solution and draped with linens. Hernia contents, if still present, are reduced manually. The surgeon and assistant stand at the head of the operating table, and the television monitor is placed at the foot of the table. A 3-mm trocar is placed through an umbilical incision and the abdomen is insufflated with CO_2 to 5–8 mmHg pressure. Under telescopic vision, two 2-mm ports are placed superior and medial to the anterior superior iliac spine.

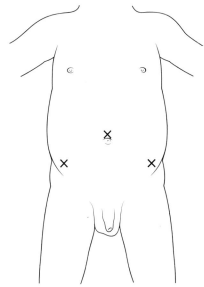

11

12 The internal opening of the hernia is confirmed, and the contralateral side is examined – contralateral patent processus vaginalis is found in 30–40 percent of cases and can be repaired at the same operation.

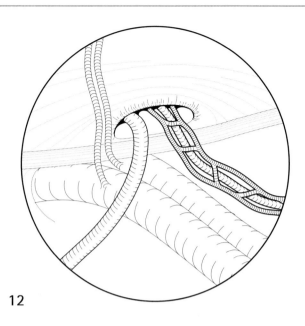

12

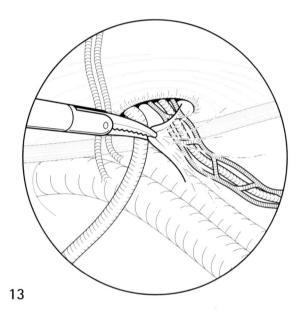

13

INTRAPERITONEAL PURSE-STRING CLOSURE

13 For boys, subperitoneal injection of normal saline to separate the vas deferens and testicular vessels from the peritoneum allows the safe application of a purse-string stitch. The peritoneum overlying the testicular vessels and vas deferens is picked up with a laparoscopic grasper.

14 An injector (6 F, 155-mm NM-3K injector, Olympus, Tokyo, Japan) is introduced and the needle enters the space beneath the 'tented' peritoneum under vision; 2 mL of normal saline are injected to elevate the peritoneum away from the vas and testicular vessels – the position of the tip of the needle may need to be adjusted during the injection and, if necessary, another 2 mL of normal saline can be introduced to achieve adequate separation of the vas and testicular vessels from the peritoneum. The injector is then withdrawn. Some surgeons also diathermize or incise the neck of the hernia sac with a diathermy hook.

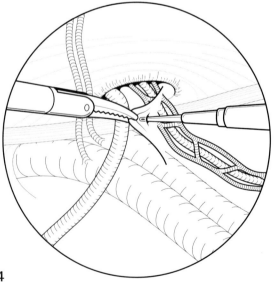

14

15 A 10- to 15-cm 4/0 non-absorbable monofilament (Prolene) suture is passed into the peritoneal cavity through the abdominal wall next to the lateral port under vision. The purse-string stitch commences at the 2 o'clock position of the internal hernia opening; the needle should be seen to traverse the subperitoneal space free of the vas and testicular vessels at each successive 'bite' of the peritoneum around the hernia ring.

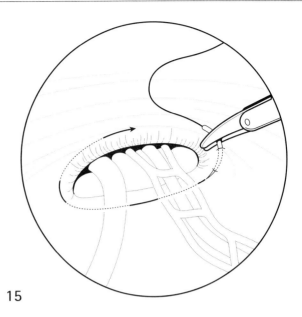

15

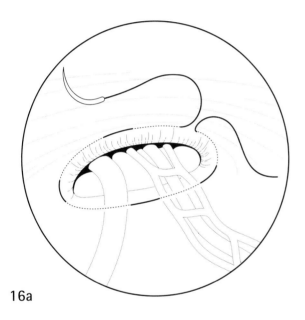

16a

16a–c Care is taken to ensure that a 'complete ring' of peritoneum has been included in the purse-string stitch without significant gaps (the exit and entry sites of successive 'bites' of peritoneum should be as close as possible). For the anterior aspect of the internal hernia ring, sometimes it may be easier to pick up the peritoneum at the rim and apply 'over and over' suturing until the 2 o'clock position is reached.

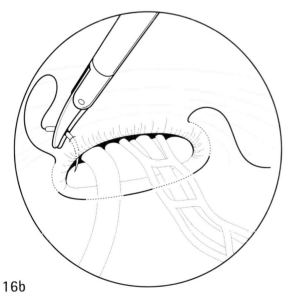

16b

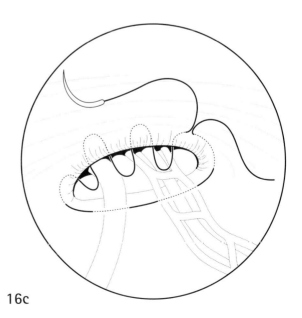

16c

17 Before the stitch is tied, the intraperitoneal pressure is lowered to 2–4 mmHg, and gas in the hernia sac is expelled by compression of the groin/scrotum. The purse-string suture is tied tightly with several intraperitoneal knots. Airtightness of the hernia closure is tested by increasing the intraperitoneal pressure transiently to 15 mmHg. There should be no gas leakage into the groin/scrotal hernia sac and the intraperitoneal pressure can be returned to 5–8 mmHg; if there is gas leakage, a second purse-string stitch can be added proximal to the first one. The ends of the stitch are cut, and the needle is retrieved through the abdominal wall. The ports are removed after release of the pneumoperitoneum. The umbilical wound is repaired in layers using absorbable sutures for fascia and skin, respectively. The lateral wounds are closed simply with Steristrips.

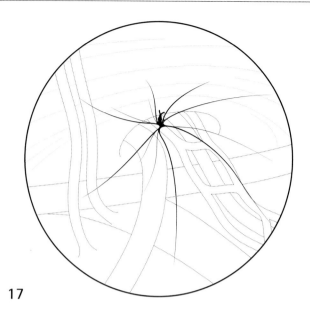

17

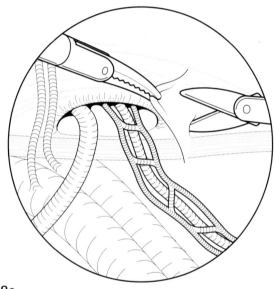

18a

18a–c An alternative method of intraperitoneal hernia repair is the 'flip-flap' technique. Briefly, a cut is made on the peritoneum 1 cm lateral to the internal inguinal ring. A flap of peritoneum is raised and 'flipped' across to the internal inguinal ring to cover the hernia opening in the manner of a trap door. Closure of the hernia ring is secured with a continuous suture between the free edge of the peritoneal flap and the adjacent hernia ring. The use of a peritoneal flap avoids tension in the closure of large hernias.

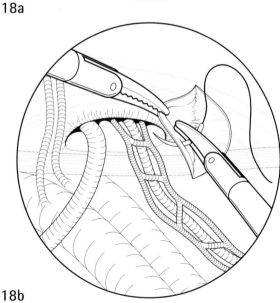

18b

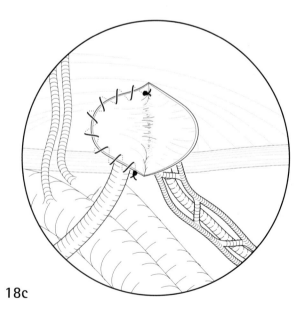

18c

EXTRAPERITONEAL CLOSURE

19a,b Laparoscopic closure of inguinal hernia can also be achieved by an extraperitoneal encircling suture. A 3-mm telescope is introduced into the peritoneal cavity via an umbilical incision and pneumoperitoneum is established. A 2- or 3-mm grasper is inserted midway between the umbilicus and suprapubic tubercle under telescopic guidance. A small stab wound is made just lateral to the internal inguinal ring. The incision is deepened to the preperitoneal space. A hernia hook (Karl Storz, 26167HH, Tuttlingen, Germany; or its equivalent) carrying a 3/0 non-absorbable suture is passed through the tract into the preperitoneal space and the deep ring is dissected from the lateral to medial aspect posteriorly, avoiding the vas and testicular vessels. The tip of the hook then pierces the peritoneum half-way around the internal ring and the suture is pulled free of the hook into the peritoneal cavity with the laparoscopic grasper.

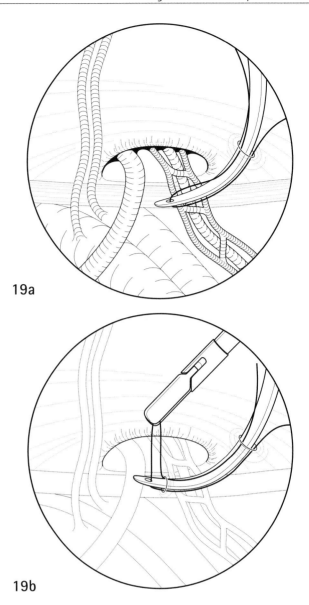

19a

19b

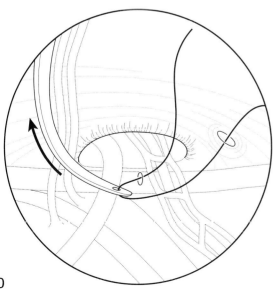

20

20 The hook is withdrawn and reinserted into the anteromedial aspect of the preperitoneal space; the medial semicircle of the internal inguinal ring is similarly dissected as before until the previous hook entry site in the peritoneum is reached. The hook re-enters the peritoneal cavity. The suture is threaded through the eye of the hook. On withdrawal of the hook, the suture which it carries will completely encircle the internal inguinal ring. The distal hernia sac is compressed and pneumoperitoneum is released. The encircling suture is tied extracorporally and airtightness of the hernia closure is tested by reintroduction of pneumoperitoneum. Wounds are closed as described in the previous section.

Postoperative care

With the exception of infants who require extended observation, most patients are discharged from the day surgery room within 2 hours of operative repair. Oral intake may be resumed when the child awakens. Tylenol with codeine is used for analgesia for approximately 48 hours following the procedure. Baths can be resumed on postoperative day 3. There are no activity restrictions for infants, but older children should refrain from bicycle riding or other vigorous physical activity until their pain has subsided. Treatment of routine inguinal hernias usually includes a postoperative clinic visit. Prospective assessment of the necessity for the traditional approach has shown that there is no difference in overall satisfaction with the care received when given a follow-up clinic visit or no follow up and a detailed instruction sheet. Accurate postoperative instructions and an open access to follow up, when required, is as effective as the traditional postoperative clinic visit, especially with individual families traveling great distances.

Outcome

Injury to the spermatic vessels or vas deferens is unusual but may occur in approximately 3 per 1000 cases. If the vas deferens is divided, it should be repaired with interrupted 7/0 or 8/0 monofilament sutures. The use of magnifying loupes or an operating microscope will make the repair more precise.

Intraoperative bleeding is also an unusual complication unless the floor of the canal is weakened and requires repair. Needle-hole injury to the epigastric vessels or the femoral vein can usually be controlled by withdrawal of the suture and direct pressure.

Postoperative complications include wound infection, scrotal hematoma, postoperative hydrocele, and recurrent inguinal hernia. The wound infection rate at most major pediatric centers is quite low (1–2 percent). An increased incidence of infection might be expected in patients presenting with an incarcerated hernia.

Recurrent inguinal hernia is a relatively uncommon complication in children with recurrence rates of less than 1 percent having been reported by experienced pediatric surgeons. Of these, 80 percent are noted within the first postoperative year. The major causes of recurrent inguinal hernia in children include: (1) a missed hernial sac or unrecognized peritoneal tear; (2) a broken suture ligature at the neck of the sac; (3) failure to repair (snug) a large internal inguinal ring; (4) injury to the floor of the inguinal canal, resulting in a direct inguinal hernia; (5) severe infection; (6) increased intra-abdominal pressure (patients with ventricular–peritoneal shunts and continuous ambulatory peritoneal dialysis); (7) in patients with cystic fibrosis and chronic cough; and (8) connective tissue disorders (i.e. Ehlers–Danlos syndrome). Most

surgeons would approach a first time recurrent inguinal hernia repair through the previous inguinal site. However, a preperitoneal repair (Cheatle-Henry type) or traditional laparoscopic repair should be considered in selected cases with multiple recurrences.

Postoperative hydrocele may rarely occur after high ligation of the proximal hernial sac and incomplete excision of the distal portion. To avoid this complication, the anterior and lateral aspects of the sac are partially resected. The postoperative hydrocele often resolves spontaneously. Rarely, long-term persistence of the hydrocele may require a hydrocele aspiration and possible formal hydrocelectomy.

Testicular atrophy has been observed after repair of incarcerated hernias and in instances of large, acute tense hydroceles in young infants, but is very rare after a typical hernia repair. There continues to be debate on the pros and cons of open versus laparoscopic inguinal hernia repair, as well as to the superiority of which method of laparoscopic repair. Several studies, including a prospective randomized controlled study, suggest that laparoscopic repair is associated with less pain, faster recovery, and better wound cosmesis; in addition, laparoscopic hernioplasty allows detection and concomitant repair of contralateral hernia. With technical refinements of laparoscopic hernioplasty, the recurrence rate which was high in some early series is no longer a concern. While data on long-term outcome of laparoscopic hernioplasty remain scarce, we have observed satisfactory results on patients with laparoscopic repair with more than ten years' follow up.

FEMORAL HERNIAS

Principles and justification

A femoral hernia is a protrusion of preperitoneal fat or viscus through a defect in the femoral canal. It is the least common hernia occurring in the inguinal region in infants and children. The diagnosis, however, must be considered when examining a swelling in the inguinal region, especially if the bulge or mass presents inferior to the inguinal ligament. Femoral hernia may occasionally be confused with an enlarged swollen infected lymph node near the saphenofemoral junction (lymph node of Cloquet) just inferior to the inguinal ligament. Femoral hernias are often misdiagnosed and treated as inguinal hernias. Careful examination for a lower extremity focus of infection should be performed. Femoral hernias are most common in girls aged between five and ten years. Occasionally, a femoral hernia may be noted shortly after an ipsilateral inguinal hernia repair. This may represent either a missed femoral hernia or operative damage involving the femoral canal. Some individuals advocate the use of laparoscopy in the child with presumed recurrent inguinal hernias because of the concern for a missed diagnosis. The anatomic boundaries of the femoral canal can be divided into anterior, posterior, lateral, and medial.

The anterior border involves the iliopubic tract and/or the inguinal ligament. Posterior includes the pectineal ligament (Cooper's) and iliac fascia. The lateral boundary involves a connective tissue septum and the femoral vein. Medially, the canal is bordered by the aponeurotic insertion of the transversus abdominis muscle and tranversalis fascia.

INDICATIONS

The presence of a femoral hernia is an indication for operation. Conservative management is contraindicated because of the risk of incarceration and strangulation. The fixed margins of the femoral ring result in early compression of swollen tissues and increase the risk of visceral compromise when incarceration occurs.

CHOICE OF PROCEDURE

There are four possible methods to repair a femoral hernia: (1) the lower infrainguinal ligament procedure of Langenbeck; (2) transinguinal Cooper's ligament repair (McVay procedure); (3) abdominal extraperitoneal repair (Cheatle-Henry); and (4) laparoscopic repair. Although femoral hernia repair has also been performed using endoscopic techniques through the laparoscope in adults and there are limited reports in children, the authors have not used this technique. It may have a role in instances of recurrent hernias.

An inguinal or extraperitoneal approach should be used in instances of strangulated obstruction; however, since this is rarely seen in infants and young children, the low infrainguinal repair is preferred. If a concomitant inguinal hernia is present, an inguinal incision and McVay repair are recommended.

Preoperative assessment and preparation

In elective cases, the infant or child is kept without oral intake for 4–6 hours before the anticipated procedure.

Anesthesia

In elective cases, an outpatient operation may safely be carried out. Mild sedation is administered preoperatively (midazolam 0.5–1.0 mg/kg orally 15–20 minutes prior to going to the operating room) and general endotracheal anesthesia is employed. Following appropriate skin cleansing of the lower abdomen, inguinoscrotal (or labial) area, thigh, and perineum, sterile drapes are applied.

Operation

The infrainguinal (Langenbeck) repair will be described as the other approaches are dealt with in the section on inguinal hernia.

INFRAINGUINAL (LANGENBECK) REPAIR

21 A transverse incision is made in a skin crease over the mass from a point just inferior to the pubic tubercle medially, extending laterally just past the palpable pulsation of the femoral artery.

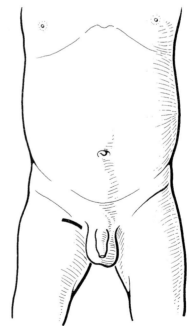

21

22 Hemostasis is effected with an electrocoagulator and the wound is deepened to expose the hernia sac bulge. The sac is covered by cribriform fascia and groin fat, and may overlie the femoral vein and extend upwards over the inguinal ligament.

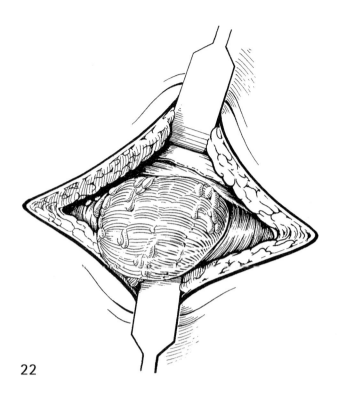

22

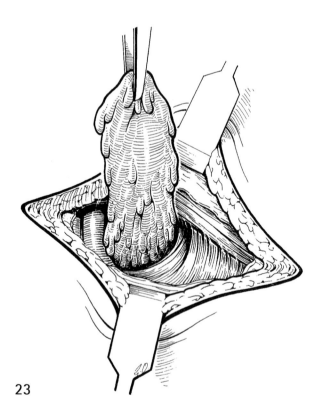

23

23 The cribriform fascia and fat layers are incised, exposing the femoral hernia sac. Note that the femoral sac protrudes into the femoral canal medial to the femoral vein, inferior to the iliopubic tract, above the Cooper's ligament, and lateral to the reflected fibers of the iliopubic tract. The sac should be carefully palpated for visceral contents which should be gently reduced through the defect. In the event that the sac is challenging to identify, an umbilical laparoscopic trocar can be placed and visualization of the femoral hernia can be noted and with insufflation and guidance of the telescope, clear delineation of the sac can be accomplished. Occasionally, when incarceration is present and reduction is difficult, the sac is released by carefully incising the insertion of the iliopubic tract into the Cooper's ligament at the medial margin of the femoral ring.

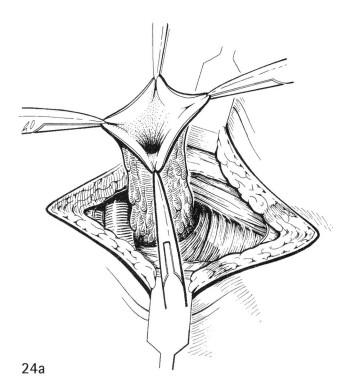

24a,b The peritoneal sac is small; however, it may have a considerable amount of retroperitoneal fatty tissue at its base. The sac can be opened (to ensure reduction of contents) if there is any question of a complete reduction. Hernial repair is initiated with high ligation of the sac similar to an inguinal hernia. This is accomplished with 3/0 non-absorbable suture ligatures. The sac may be bulky, however, and an alternative method of sac closure is inversion and reduction of the intact sac, placing one or two 3/0 non-absorbable purse-string sutures at a level just above the femoral defect.

24a

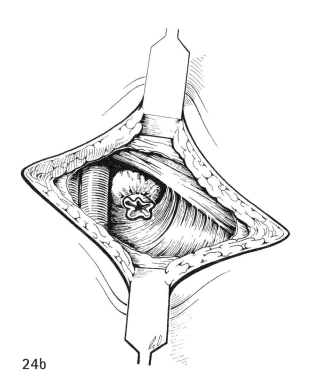

24b

25 Repair of the femoral defect is facilitated by placing a small retractor to raise the inguinal ligament superiorly in order to expose the pectineus fascia and Cooper's ligament. If this is not performed, the femoral vessels may be traumatized with suture placement. The hernia repair is completed by suturing these two structures together, thereby obliterating the femoral canal medial to the femoral vein. All sutures are placed between Cooper's ligament and the inguinal ligament under direct vision before tying. The authors use interrupted 3/0 non-absorbable suture material in older children and 2/0 suture in adolescents. Special attention is given to avoid either injury to the femoral vein by the needle or its compression when the sutures are tied. Gentle lateral retraction of the vein during suture insertion is useful. In the posterior approach, the external iliac–femoral vein is easily seen and can be maintained out of the line of suturing. In addition, one can maximize the degree of closure of the femoral canal without compressing the vein.

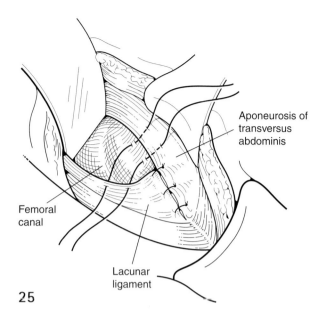

Aponeurosis of transversus abdominis

Femoral canal

Lacunar ligament

25

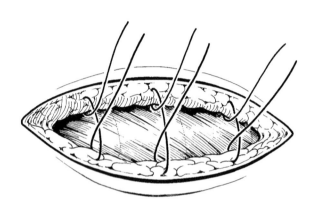

26 Prior to closing, it is important to evaluate the rest of the groin to ensure there is no evidence of another hernia, as a missed hernia may present as a recurrent femoral hernia. Wound closure is accomplished with a few interrupted inverting 4/0 absorbable sutures. The wound edges are approximated with 5/0 subcuticular absorbable suture material and the skin sealed with Steristrips and a semipermeable adhesive film dressing (e.g. Opsite) in children or with Dermabond in infants who are not toilet trained.

Postoperative care

Oral intake may be resumed when the infant is alert. Acetaminophen with codeine may be used for pain control for 24–48 hours. Most young children return to normal activity within a few days. The family is instructed to keep the wound dry for the first few days to minimize wound complications. In older children or teenagers, avoidance of competitive athletics and bicycle riding is advised until the pain has subsided.

Outcome

In most cases, recovery from elective femoral hernia repair is uncomplicated. A superficial wound infection may develop in 1 percent of cases and should be recognized promptly and the wound opened or administration of oral antibiotics should be initiated early to avoid possible extension of a closed infection to the deeper tissues. A wound hematoma is rarely observed and may be caused by an unrecognized tear in a saphenous/femoral venous branch.

Pain and ipsilateral leg swelling may be the result of compression of the iliac or femoral vein which can be obviated or minimized with meticulous attention, while placing the hernia repair sutures as previously described.

Since a femoral hernia is relatively rare in children, data concerning recurrence are not available and a recurrence rate of 1–2 percent in children might be expected. In the event of a recurrence, one must rule out an associated inguinal hernia. Some have adopted the preperitoneal approach for recurrent repair due to the higher rate of secondary recurrences. Since recurrences may be the result of a localized collagen defect and direct reapproximation of the weakened tissue may not be appropriate, the use of a prosthetic buttress may be indicated. The posterior approach will avoid reoperation through a previous surgical site, allow evaluation and exclusion of all groin-related hernia defects, facilitate the repair by easy visualization of Cooper's ligament and the iliopubic tract, and if a prosthetic buttress is chosen, the principles of distributing even intra-abdominal pressure to the prosthetic patch are employed.

UMBILICAL HERNIA

Principles and justification

An umbilical hernia is commonly encountered in infants and young children. The hernia sac protrudes through a defect in the umbilical ring due to a failure of complete obliteration at the site where the fetal umbilical vessels (umbilical vein and the two umbilical arteries) are joined to the placenta during gestation.

Approximately 20 percent of full-term neonates may have an incomplete closure of the umbilical ring at birth. However, 75–80 percent of premature infants weighing between 1.0 and 1.5 kg may show evidence of an umbilical hernia at birth. Umbilical hernia is more common in girls than boys. Black children have a higher incidence than white children.

The umbilical bulge becomes more apparent during episodes of crying, straining, or even during defecation, and may result in considerable protrusion of the sac and, at times, visceral contents through the ring. The hernial protrusion is composed of peritoneum adherent to the undersurface of the umbilical skin. The hernia often causes considerable parental anxiety and frequent requests for operative repair in early infancy.

Although rupture or incarceration of an umbilical hernia occurs, this is an exceptionally rare event in the authors' experience. The hernia is rarely a cause of pain or other symptoms. Almost 80 percent of umbilical hernias will decrease in size and close spontaneously by four or five years of age. Careful counseling will usually allay unnecessary parental anxiety and fear.

INDICATIONS

As the majority of these very low-risk hernias will close spontaneously, it is safe to wait until the child is four years of age (particularly if the umbilical ring is less than 1.5 cm in diameter) before attempting repair. In contrast, defects of more than 1.5–2.0 cm diameter rarely close spontaneously. Since there is a significant risk of complications including incarceration and strangulation in adults with umbilical hernia, those hernia defects that do not close by four years of age should be electively repaired. The umbilical defect can also be repaired in children less than four years of age when the ring is more than 1.5 cm, or they have symptoms related to the hernia.

Preoperative assessment and preparation

The child is kept without oral intake for 6 hours before the anticipated time of the procedure. The operation can safely be carried out on an outpatient basis. Careful preparation of the skin is essential as the umbilicus is often a repository of surface debris, lint, etc., and is not always kept immaculate. Preoperative cleansing with cotton applicator sticks may be useful.

Anesthesia

After administration of mild preoperative sedation (oral midazolam), the procedure is carried out under general anesthesia via endotracheal intubation or laryngeal mask airway. Some facilities will advocate regional anesthesia, such as a rectus sheath block, to improve pain management following the hernia repair. Interest in the block has been renewed following favorable reports in adult series comparing the block with opioids alone for analgesia. These continue to be limited to small case series in children; however, with the more frequent availability of ultrasound in the operating room, ultrasound-guided umbilical nerve block is becoming more common.

Operation

27 After appropriate skin preparation and application of sterile linen drapes, a curved ('smile') incision is made in a natural skin crease immediately below the umbilicus. A supraumbilical incision is also acceptable, especially if a supraumbilical defect is encountered. Placement of four-quadrant traction by the assistant on the abdominal wall and slight upward traction of the defect allows selection of the site of the incision. The curved incision should typically not extend beyond 180°.

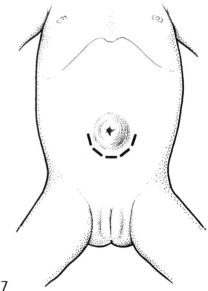

27

28a,b The subcutaneous tissue is incised and bleeding points controlled with a fine tip electrocoagulator. With upward traction on the inner margin of the upper lip of the incision, dissection is carried out down along the sac to the level of the anterior abdominal wall fascia. By blunt dissection with a mosquito clamp, a plane is developed on either side of the sac, extending superiorly to gain control of the entire circumference of the sac. Any contents in the sac should be reduced into the peritoneal cavity. If the sac is large, the surgeon or assistant places an index finger in the skin defect to evert the sac where it is attached to the skin. The sac is dissected free from its skin attachments, preserving the umbilical skin for an umbilicoplasty. Separation of the sac may require its transection near the skin to preserve the umbilicus for cosmetic purposes.

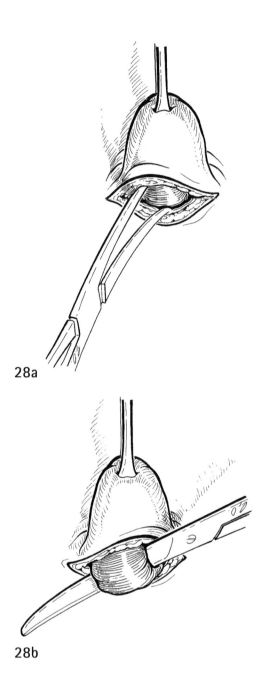

28a

28b

29a,b The entire sac is elevated by mosquito clamps to maintain control of the edge of the defect and to have direct visualization during placement of sutures to avoid visceral injury. The sac is opened and any contents reduced. The rim of the defect is identified and the sac incised to allow placement of sutures starting at the corner farthest from the surgeon. Continuous or interrupted 3/0 (infants and young children) or 2/0 (older children and teenagers) sutures are placed. The sutures are elevated to maintain upward traction on the abdominal wall. The sac is partially excised at the level of the abdominal wall as more sutures are placed. A traction suture may also be placed at the corner of the transverse wound closest to the operating surgeon to offer exposure as the remaining sac is excised and sutures placed. If considerable redundant tissue is present or the initial tissue layer seems sparse, a layer of fascia can be imbricated over the initial line of repair with interrupted or continuous absorbable suture.

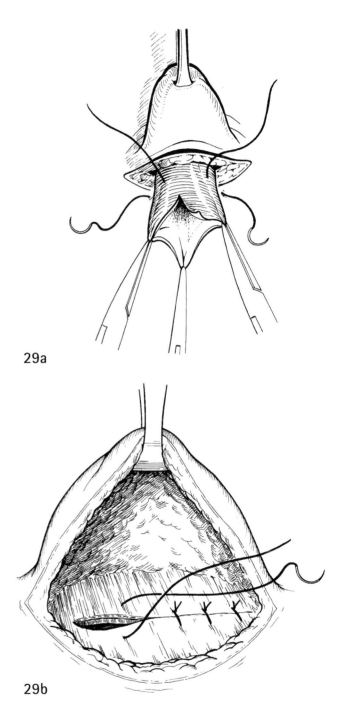

29a

29b

30a,b An umbilicoplasty is performed for cosmetic purposes by inverting the undersurface of the redundant umbilical skin to the anterior abdominal wall fascia with one or two interrupted 4/0 absorbable sutures. Any remnant of the peritoneum on the umbilical sac that is adherent to the skin may be safely left behind, excised, or cauterized. In children with a very large protuberant hernia with redundant skin, following the removal of the sac and fascial closure, the umbilicoplasty can sometimes be frustrating to the surgeon and patient. The volume and variety of literary material on the repair of umbilical defects attest to the fact that there exists no single ideal approach. The management of the excess umbilical skin can be completed using numerous methods, such as a purse-string suture, complicated V–Y advancement procedures, four equilateral triangular skin flaps, or the Mercedes-Benz umbilicoplasty.

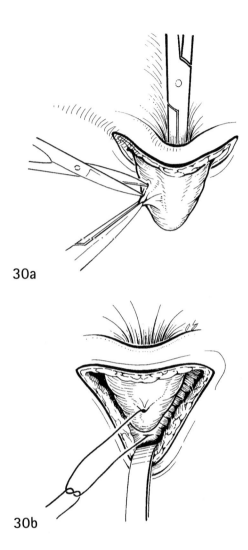

30a

30b

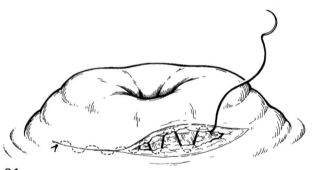

31

31 The wound is closed by a few interrupted inverted 4/0 absorbable sutures in the subcutaneous fascia. The skin edges are opposed with a running subcuticular suture. A Dermabond dressing may be applied or one may use Steristrips and an Opsite dressing in older patients. There is no benefit to minimizing the rate of wound complications by the use of a pressure dressing.

Postoperative care

Oral fluids can be offered when the infant or child is alert. Acetaminophen with codeine may be used for pain control for 24–48 hours. Postoperative activity restrictions are similar to those for an inguinal hernia repair.

Outcome

Complications are unusual and are limited to a wound infection (1 percent) or an occasional wound hematoma. Bowel injury is the rarest of complications. Recurrence is rare as well, and those that do recur are typically in children with associated comorbidities, such as long-term continuous ambulatory peritoneal dialysis, ventricular peritoneal shunts, or a connective tissue disorder.

SUPRAUMBILICAL AND EPIGASTRIC HERNIAS

Principles and justification

A number of defects may be observed along the linea alba between the xiphoid process and the umbilicus. Failure of fixation of the medial borders of the rectus abdominis muscles at the linea alba in infants, results in a large,

bulging defect (a diastasis recti) which is virtually of no consequence and resolves spontaneously as the baby grows and the linea alba becomes a firm structure.

Epigastric hernias usually occur in the mid-epigastrium. The actual defect may be small; however, it is often symptomatic. Fat from the falciform ligament or the omentum can incarcerate and cause pain. In some cases, a tender mass of incarcerated fatty tissue can be palpated in the defect. Since epigastric hernias do not spontaneously close and are often symptomatic, they should be repaired on an elective basis. As the hernial defect may be small, it is wise to mark the skin over the exact site before surgery with the child awake in a standing position prior to the procedure.

Preoperative assessment and preparation

Repair can be performed on an outpatient basis. It is critical to mark the patient's hernia in the preoperative holding area to assure easy operative recognition.

Anesthesia

General anesthesia is typically required. The abdomen is prepared with a cleansing solution and sterile drapes applied.

Operation

32 A transverse incision is made directly over the premarked area identifying the site of the hernia defect, or in the case of a supraumbilical defect, a supraumbilical frown incision may be made to maximize cosmesis.

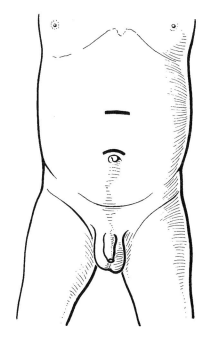

32

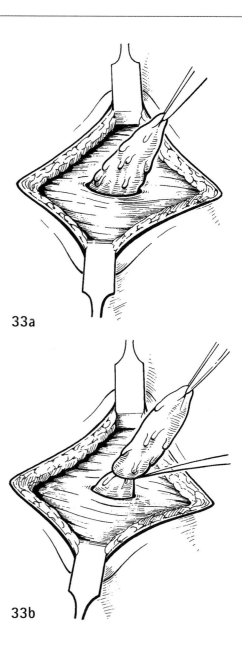

33a

33b

33a,b Hemostasis is controlled with an electrocoagulator. There is often no peritoneal sac identified in instances of epigastric hernia. A fatty mass protruding through the defect in the linea alba is observed and may be suture ligated and excised or inverted and reduced into the peritoneal cavity.

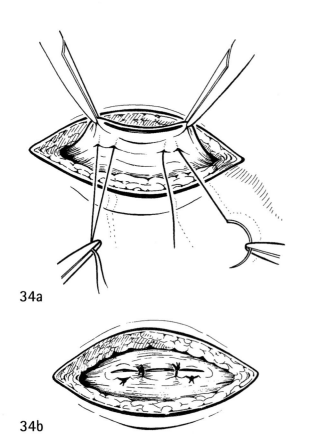

34a

34b

34a,b The small defect (not uncommonly the size of a pencil tip) is repaired with interrupted 3/0 absorbable sutures. Wound closure is accomplished with a running subcuticular 5-0 absorbable suture and the skin edges approximated with either Steristrips or Dermabond dressing.

Postoperative care

Postoperative care is similar to that described for umbilical hernias.

FURTHER READING

Chan KL, Hui WC, Tam PKH. Prospective, randomized, single-center, single-blind comparison of laparoscopic vs open repair of pediatric inguinal hernia. *Surgical Endoscopy* 2005; **19**: 927–32.

Chan KL, Chan HY, Tam PKH. Towards a near-zero recurrence rate in laparoscopic inguinal hernia repair for pediatric patients of all ages. *Journal of Pediatric Surgery* 2007; **42**: 1993–7.

Maria BDJ, Gotzens V, Mabrok M. Ultrasound-guided umbilical nerve block in children: a brief description of a new approach. *Pediatric Anesthesia* 2007; **17**: 44–50.

Melone JH, Schwartz MZ, Tyson DR *et al.* Outpatient inguinal herniorrhaphy in premature infants: is it safe? *Journal of Pediatric Surgery* 1992; **27**: 203–8.

Niyogi A, Tahim AS, Sherwood WJ *et al.* A comparative study examining open inguinal herniotomy with and without hernioscopy to laparoscopic inguinal hernia repair in a pediatric population. *Pediatric Surgery International* 2010; **26**: 387–92.

Parelkar SV, Oak S, Gupta R *et al.* Laparoscopic inguinal hernia repair in the pediatric age group – experience with 437 children. *Journal of Pediatric Surgery* 2010; **45**: 789–92.

Rescorla FJ, West KW, Engum SA *et al.* The 'other side' of pediatric hernias: the role of laparoscopy. *American Surgeon* 1997; **63**: 690–3.

Reyna TM, Hollis HW, Smith SB. Surgical management of proboscoid herniae. *Journal of Pediatric Surgery* 1987; **22**: 911–12.

Scherer LR, Grosfeld JL. Inguinal hernia and umbilical anomalies. *Pediatric Clinics of North America* 1993; **40**: 1121–31.

Schier F, Montupet P, Esposito C. Laparoscopic inguinal herniorrhaphy in children: a three-center experience with 933 repairs. *Journal of Pediatric Surgery* 2002; **37**: 395–7.

Skinner MA, Grosfeld JL. Inguinal and umbilical hernia repair in infants and children. *Surgical Clinics of North America* 1993; **73**: 439–49.

Treef W, Schier F. Characteristics of laparoscopic inguinal hernia recurrences. *Pediatric Surgery International* 2009; **25**: 149–52.

Willschke H, Senberg AB, Marhofer P *et al.* Ultrasonography-guided rectus sheath block in paediatric anaesthesia – a new approach to an old technique. *British Journal of Anaesthesia* 2006; **97**: 244–9.

Yip KF, Tam PKH, Li MKW. Laparoscopic flip-flap hernioplasty: an innovative technique for pediatric hernia surgery. *Surgical Endoscopy* 2004; **18**: 1126–9.

38

Omphalocele/exomphalos

THOMAS R WEBER

HISTORY

Ambrose Paré, the famous French surgeon, first described an infant with omphalocele in 1634. Although small omphaloceles were subsequently successfully repaired, there were few reported survivors of larger abdominal wall defects until the 1940s, when Gross described a two-stage closure of an omphalocele using skin flaps followed by ventral hernia repair. Further advancement in the treatment of massive omphalocele defects occurred when Schuster devised an extracelomic 'pouch' to house eviscerated bowel temporarily. This was later modified by Allen and Wrenn, who devised the additional innovation of staged reduction of abdominal contents to allow gradual enlargement of the abdominal cavity. The development of total parenteral nutrition in the 1960s allowed vigorous nutritional support of infants with abdominal wall defects, in whom a period of 1–3 weeks of intestinal dysfunction is expected after the operation. The basic principles of occasional non-operative therapy, primary closure when possible, and staged reduction with a temporary Silastic 'pouch', remain the mainstays of contemporary therapy for these congenital defects.

EMBRYOLOGY

Although controversy continues regarding the similarities, relationships, and embryological events surrounding omphalocele and gastroschisis, it is probably most reasonable to consider these as separate entities. Omphalocele is basically a persistence of the body stalk in the midline, where somatopleure normally develops. Failure of return of the normally herniated midgut at fetal week 12 either causes or aggravates the condition. Unless ruptured, omphaloceles are covered with a sac consisting of inner peritoneum and outer amnion. Infants with omphalocele frequently have associated anomalies (cardiac, renal), chromosome abnormalities (trisomy 13–15, 16–18), or recognizable syndrome associations (Beckwith–Wiedemann, Cantrell's pentalogy, caudal regression).

PRINCIPLES AND JUSTIFICATION

Because of the possibility of serious, life-threatening, or even lethal associated anomalies, infants with omphalocele are occasionally treated non-operatively. Painting the sac with agents designed to induce eschar formation, followed by gradual epithelialization from the base of the defect upwards, will eventually produce a covered ventral hernia. Early use of alcohol, iodine, and mercury-containing compounds produced toxicity due to systemic absorption of these compounds, and they have therefore been largely replaced by silver nitrate solutions or silver sulfadiazine cream.

The operative treatment of choice for small- to medium-sized omphaloceles is excision of the sac, with primary closure of fascia and skin. If fascia closure increases intra-abdominal pressure sufficiently to cause respiratory embarrassment, skin closure alone, with later repair of the ventral hernia, is advisable. For giant omphaloceles, frequently containing liver as well as bowel, attaching a Silastic 'pouch' to the fascia allows gradual (10–14 days) reduction of the contents into the abdominal cavity, with eventual skin flap closure. Occasionally, a prosthetic patch is needed to close the fascial defect in this setting, but skin must be mobilized sufficiently to cover the prosthesis.

PREOPERATIVE ASSESSMENT AND PREPARATION

Newborn infants with omphalocele must be placed immediately in a warm, aseptic environment to prevent evaporative fluid loss, hypothermia, and infection. A non-adherent sterile gauze can be placed on the defect, covered by transparent plastic wrap. Alternatively, a transparent plastic drawstring 'bowel bag' may be used, which can be kept sterile in the delivery room. The lower two-thirds (to the axillae) of the neonate can be placed within the bag. Safe transport of the infant to a center that is experienced in the management of these complex infants can then be accomplished.

Infants with large omphaloceles, especially when the liver is in the sac, should be positioned on their side to prevent twisting of the inferior vena cava from the sac 'tipping' to one side. Alternatively, rolls can be used to support the sac if the infant is placed supine.

Intravenous access must be established soon after birth to replace evaporative fluid loss and administer broad-spectrum antibiotics. Placement of the intravenous line above the diaphragm is preferable because of the possibility of inferior cava compression and partial obstruction as the eviscerated bowel and/or liver are reduced. An oral gastric or nasogastric tube should be placed to prevent gastric distension. Preoperative endotracheal intubation is reserved for premature infants or those with significant respiratory distress. The latter is occasionally encountered because pulmonary hypoplasia can be associated with omphalocele. All infants with omphalocele should undergo complete cardiac and renal evaluation before they are subjected to operative repair.

Anesthesia

General, endotracheal anesthesia, with complete muscle paralysis, is recommended for all infants with omphalocele. As stated above, infants with omphalocele who have serious or life-threatening associated anomalies, especially cardiac, should probably be treated non-operatively with application of escharotic agents to the sac.

OPERATIONS

Small- to moderate-sized omphalocele

1 A small ('hernia into cord') or moderate omphalocele, which may contain a small portion of liver, has the umbilical cord inserted into the top of the sac.

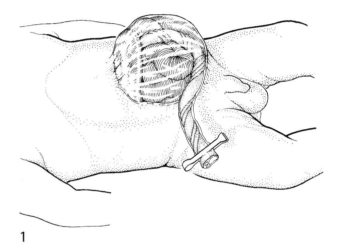

1

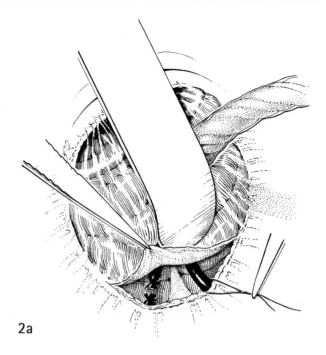

2a

2a,b Although some surgeons advocate leaving the sac intact and repairing the fascia and skin over it, most surgeons favor excision of the sac to allow complete intra-abdominal exploration. The sac is sharply removed at the skin/fascia edge, with careful identification and ligation of the umbilical vessels.

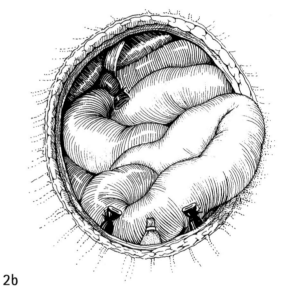

2b

3 The abdominal cavity can be enlarged by manual stretching.

3

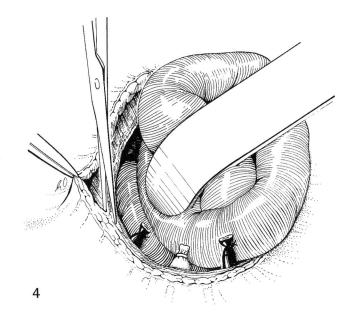

4 The skin is carefully 'undermined', separating it from the deep fascia layers.

4

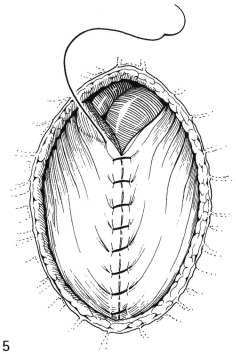

5

5 The fascia is closed with running or interrupted absorbable sutures (polyglactin or polydioxanone) and the umbilicus reconstructed.

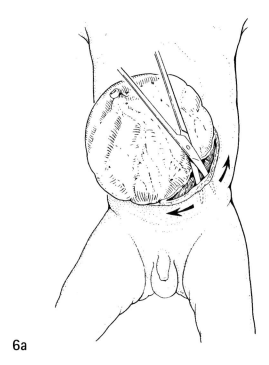

6a

Large omphalocele: staged repair

6a–c Large omphaloceles, frequently containing most of the liver, are usually not fully reducible at the first operation, and staged repair is necessary. After undermining the skin, the skin is closed over the abdominal viscera, producing a ventral hernia that can be repaired 6–12 months later.

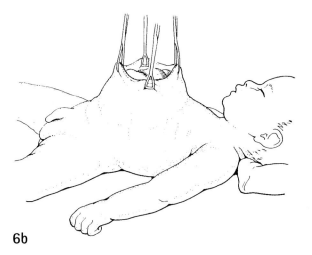

6b

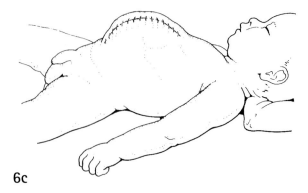

6c

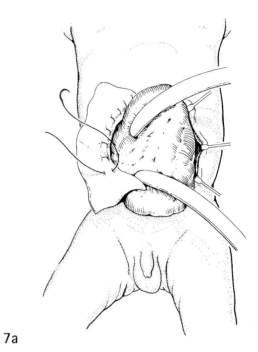

7a,b An alternative approach utilizes prosthetic closure of the fascia defect over polyethylene or Silastic sheeting to prevent adhesion of the viscera to the prosthetic material. The skin is closed over the fascia prosthesis.

7a

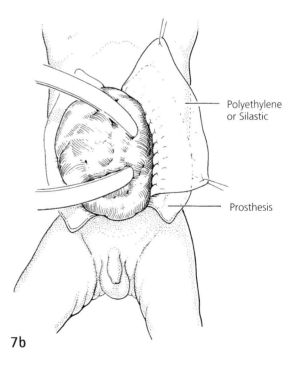

Polyethylene or Silastic

Prosthesis

7b

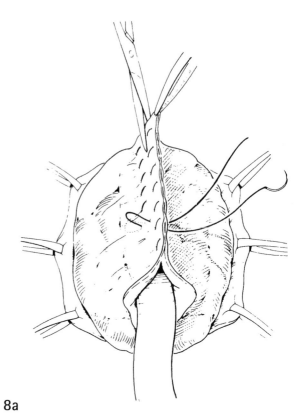

8a

8a,b At 4–6-week intervals, the wound can be reopened and the skin dissected from the prosthesis. The central portion of the prosthesis and sheeting are resected and resutured to pull the fascia together. Eventually, the fascia can be closed without the prosthesis.

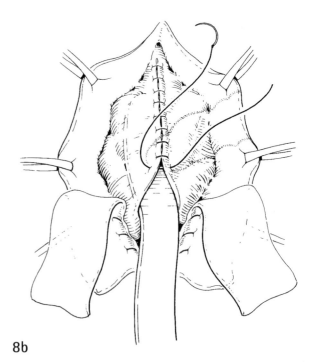

8b

9a–d In cases of ruptured omphalocele, an alternative method of management is necessary if the viscera cannot be reduced primarily and there is insufficient skin for coverage. A Dacron-reinforced Silastic sheet is attached to the abdominal wall with a running, non-absorbable suture and fashioned into a 'pouch' using the same suture. A preformed 'pouch', with a spring-loaded base that fits into the abdominal cavity to hold the 'pouch' in place and therefore does not require suturing, is also commercially available.

The viscera are gradually reduced into the abdominal cavity, using gentle squeezing pressure on top of the 'pouch', which is then occluded by umbilical tape tie or suture to maintain reduction. This is usually performed without anesthesia every other day, over a 7–10-day period, until the gut is fully reduced.

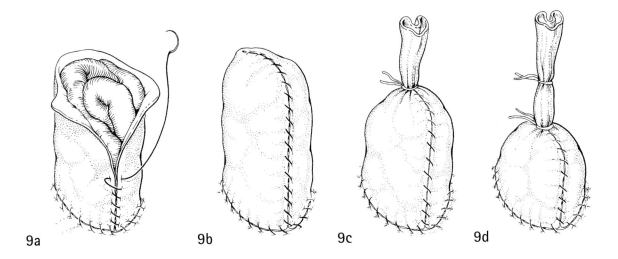

9a 9b 9c 9d

10 The infant is then returned to the operating room for removal of the 'pouch', with fascia and/or skin closure. A newer approach to infants with large omphalocele is the use of progressive wrapping of the defect. By this method, the amnion is left intact. The surgeon applies an antibacterial ointment to the amnion, and then wraps the defect first with gauze, and then an elastic wrap. By gradually applying more pressure in downward and lateral directions, the herniated organs gradually return to the abdominal cavity, and the cavity, itself, grows in size. While this process may take several months to fully reduce the herniation, the gradual process often avoids respiratory embarrassment, and greatly facilitates the eventual closure. Great care must be take to avoid trauma to the amnion early on, as excessive shear forces could tear the sac, resulting in a significantly more complicated form of reduction.

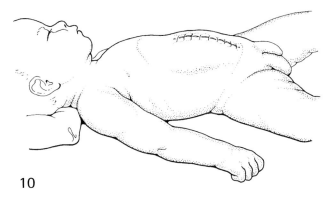

10

POSTOPERATIVE CARE

All infants should be maintained on systemic antibiotics for 5–7 days or until the prostheses are removed. Intravenous nutrition should be initiated as soon as possible and continued until bowel function returns. In infants with omphalocele, this may be a period of several days.

Respiratory compromise is common after primary repair, or during staged reduction of omphalocele, and endotracheal intubation, ventilators, sedation, and, occasionally, muscle relaxants are common interventions in these infants in the early postoperative period.

OUTCOME

The outcome in these infants depends on the presence and degree of prematurity, associated anomalies, and the loss of bowel length due to atresia or gut infarction from mesenteric vascular compromise.

Neonates with omphalocele have a high (50–60 percent) incidence of associated anomalies and chromosome abnormalities that precludes long-term survival in 20–30 percent of cases. Severe cardiac defects are particularly troublesome in these infants. Modern neonatal intensive care, improved ventilator management, and intravenous nutrition have undoubtedly been responsible for the continued improvement in survival for these critically ill infants.

FURTHER READING

Christisan-Lagay ER, Kelleher CM, Langer JC. Neonatal abdominal wall defects. *Seminars in Fetal and Neonatal Medicine* 2011; **16**: 164–72.

Grosfeld JL, Dawes L, Weber TR. Congenital abdominal wall defects; current management and survival. *Surgical Clinics of North America* 1981; **61**: 1037–49.

Grosfeld JL, Weber TR. Congenital abdominal wall defects: gastroschisis and omphalocele. *Current Problems in Surgery* 1982; **19**: 159–213.

Schuster SR. A new method for the staged repair of large omphaloceles. *Surgery, Gynecology and Obstetrics* 1967; **125**: 837–50.

Van Ejick FC, Aronson DA, Hoogeveen YL, Wijnen RM. Past and current surgical treatment of giant omphalocele. *Journal of Pediatric Surgery* 2011; **46**: 482–8.

Weber TR, Au-Fliegner M, Downard C, Fishman S. Abdominal wall defects. *Current Opinion in Pediatrics* 2002; **14**: 491–7.

39

Gastroschisis

MARSHALL Z SCHWARTZ and SHAHEEN J TIMMAPURI

HISTORY

The first successful surgical repair of gastroschisis was performed by Watkins in 1943. Although there were improvements in the perioperative management and surgical procedures for gastroschisis, the mortality remained significant and was reported to be as high as 90 percent. Two major advances occurred in the late 1960s that led to a dramatic improvement in the survival of infants with gastroschisis. In 1967, Schuster et al. described a technique of staged reduction of the herniated bowel and abdominal closure for patients in whom primary closure was not possible. The second major advance was the evolution of intravenous nutrition, which, remarkably, allowed for growth and development during the prolonged period that these infants would not tolerate enteral feeding.

Over the past three decades, the outcome for infants with gastroschisis has dramatically improved. The survival rate is now greater than 90 percent.

PRINCIPLES AND JUSTIFICATION

1 Gastroschisis is an anterior abdominal wall defect that occurs *in utero*, through which there is herniation of intra-abdominal viscera into the amniotic sac. It is thought to result from a defect at the site of involution of the second (right) umbilical vein. This anomaly is accompanied by non-rotation of the bowel and an increased incidence of intestinal abnormalities, including atresia, perforation, and infarction, resulting from midgut volvulus or vascular thrombosis. The incidence of gastroschisis is approximately 1 in 4000–6000 live births.

Most infants with gastroschisis are born prematurely (35–37 weeks' gestation), weighing 2000–2500 g. The defect is almost always to the right of the umbilicus and generally measures 2–3 cm in diameter. All or a portion of the midgut is usually herniated through the defect. In addition, the stomach, urinary bladder, and, in females, the Fallopian tubes and ovaries may also be extracelomic.

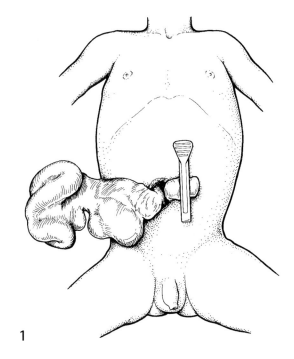

1

2 The intestine is foreshortened, edematous, and generally has a fibrin coating. Atresia of the small and large intestine occurs more often (approximately 14 percent) than in patients with omphalocele (1 percent). The most striking difference in appearance between omphalocele and gastroschisis is the absence of a sac or membrane covering the herniated contents in gastroschisis. Continuous contact of the herniated contents with amniotic fluid has been proposed as the reason for the thickened, foreshortened, and edematous bowel. There is also increasing evidence that the fascial defect begins to decrease in diameter near the end of the third trimester, which could lead to venous congestion of the midgut and contribute to the abnormal appearance of the bowel at birth. Therefore, serial fetal ultrasonography in the third trimester is warranted to follow the appearance of the bowel. Bowel dilatation and echogenic bowel have been described as possible predictors of postnatal morbidity. Progressive worsening of these findings could lead to future complications and may be an indication for early delivery. Routine Cesarean section is not recommended for infants with gastroschisis.

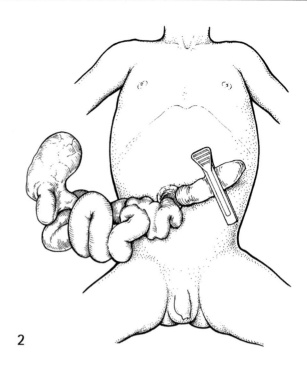

2

Preoperative assessment and preparation

Gastroschisis requires prompt surgical intervention. Delays in surgical management should only be incurred as a result of transport of the infant to a pediatric surgical center or the need for prolonged preoperative stabilization. The evaluation of other life-threatening anomalies, which are rare, may delay surgery. Appropriate preoperative preparation is essential to ensure a good outcome.

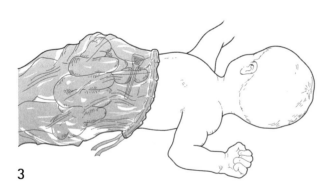

3

3 Maintenance of the infant's temperature within the normal range is critical because heat loss from the exposed herniated contents can be significant. There are numerous methods to minimize this heat loss depending on what supplies are available in the delivery room or intensive care nursery. Damp, warm gauze sponges or a damp, warm roll of gauze is wrapped around the intestine. Next, a plastic bag containing the baby from the chest to the feet may be used to maintain normal body temperature and diminish evaporative fluid loss. Alternatively, dry rolls of gauze may be wrapped around the patient's abdomen and the damp gauze-covered bowel to create an appropriate environment. It is imperative to stabilize the bowel and, therefore, diminish the risk of compromising its blood supply at the fascial ring. The infant should be in a warming isolette or under an overhead radiant warmer to help maintain normothermia.

Most infants with gastroschisis are dehydrated at birth and require at least 125 percent of normal maintenance fluids to regain normovolemia. Eventually, almost all infants with gastroschisis will require central venous access. However, attempts are made to delay the placement of a tunneled central venous catheter until 2–3 days after surgery to decrease the risk of catheter contamination by bacterial translocation or other sources. It is appropriate to give broad-spectrum antibiotics during the perioperative period because of exposure of the bowel and peritoneal cavity to bacterial contamination at the time of birth. A nasogastric tube placed at the time of birth is necessary for gastrointestinal decompression because of the bowel inflammation and resulting ileus.

Thus, before surgery, the infant with gastroschisis should be normothermic, hemodynamically stable, and have normal serum electrolytes following adequate fluid resuscitation.

ANESTHESIA

General anesthesia is required for appropriate operative management of gastroschisis. The choice of anesthetic agents should be made by the anesthetist, but two points should be emphasized: first, muscle paralysis is useful in optimizing the chances for complete reduction of the herniated bowel and primary abdominal wall closure, and second, nitrous oxide should not be used as it diffuses into the lumen of the bowel causing distension and

compromising the likely success of primary abdominal wall repair.

OPERATION

The operation should be performed under conditions that maintain normothermia. Several methods exist to accomplish this goal. An overhead radiant warmer, warming lights, or a warming blanket should be used to maintain the infant's temperature in the normal range during the procedure. Raising the temperature in the operating room may also be necessary. After the induction of general anesthesia, the dressing previously placed over the herniated contents should be removed. The bowel should be handled with sterile gloves. The umbilical cord, which has usually been left long, should be clamped 2–3 cm above the abdominal wall and the excess cord then removed. Holding the bowel and clamp on the umbilical cord in one hand, the bowel should be prepared using gauze sponges soaked in a 50:50 mixture of povidone-iodine solution and saline. The antiseptic solution must be warm to the touch in an effort to minimize heat loss. After gently washing the bowel and the anterior and lateral abdominal wall, drapes are appropriately placed and the herniated contents are laid on the drapes. The surgeon should then scrub and put on gown and gloves. Next, the herniated intestine should be carefully inspected for areas of perforation or sites of atresia, although no effort should be made to dissect matted loops of intestine.

4 It is sometimes necessary to extend the abdominal wall defect to facilitate reduction of the herniated bowel. This is generally done by extending the defect superiorly in the midline by 1–3 cm. Extending the incision caudally is not recommended because the urinary bladder is in close proximity to the inferior aspect of the abdominal wall defect. The length of this incision depends on the size of the original defect and the bulkiness of the herniated bowel.

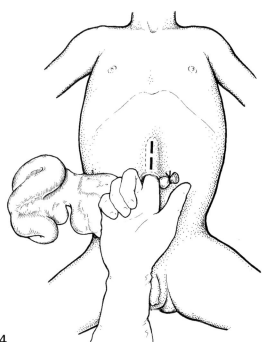

4

The herniated intestine is reduced as much as possible, distributing the bowel to all quadrants of the peritoneal cavity. Two techniques have been described to facilitate complete bowel reduction and abdominal wall closure: (1) stretching of the anterior abdominal wall and (2) 'milking' the intestinal contents into the stomach where they can be aspirated through the nasogastric tube. Some surgeons also find milking out the colonic contents to be an effective maneuver for decompressing and reducing the bowel. Although gentle stretching of the anterior abdominal wall can be useful, the authors are opposed to vigorous stretching. This maneuver can lead to rectus muscle hemorrhage and abdominal wall edema, producing a non-compliant, firm anterior abdominal wall, resulting in ventilation difficulties and wound-related problems. Nor do the authors advocate manipulating the intestine to 'milk' the intestinal contents into the stomach, believing that this can cause further damage to the bowel wall resulting in increased bowel wall thickening and additional delay in bowel recovery.

5 If reduction of the herniated intestine is successful, the abdominal wall is assessed for primary closure. If it can be closed without undue tension, 3/0 absorbable, monofilament sutures are used. These sutures are placed in a figure-of-eight, as this results in fewer knots. When all the sutures have been placed, they are tied in sequence with a thin, malleable retractor initially underneath the fascia to prevent a loop of intestine from becoming entrapped under the sutures. The umbilical stalk is retained to create a more natural umbilical appearance when the wound is fully closed.

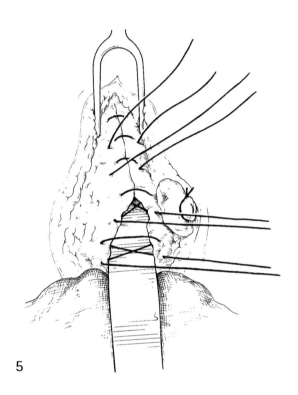

5

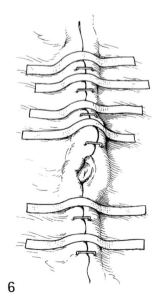

6

6 When the fascia has been closed, the skin edges are approximated using interrupted absorbable sutures or a few skin staples and sufficient sterile skin closure strips, allowing distribution of skin tension over a wider surface area and thus reducing the likelihood of skin disruption.

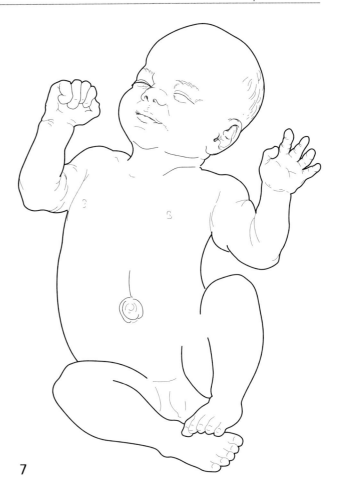

7 Appearance 1 week after primary closure. Note the umbilicus was retained.

7

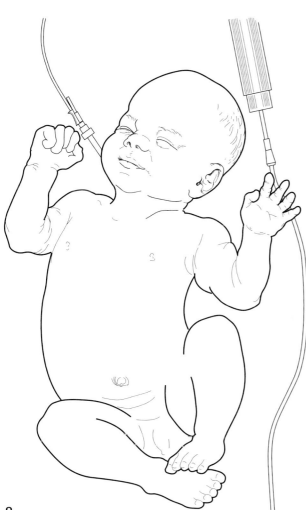

8

8 Appearance 3 weeks after primary closure.

About 60–70 percent of infants with gastroschisis can be operatively treated in this way without creating undue intra-abdominal pressure or tension in the abdominal wall closure. It is best to avoid high intra-abdominal pressure and excessive suture line tension. This can result in abdominal compartment syndrome, possibly leading to intestinal necrosis, renal hypoperfusion, and difficulty in ventilation, as well as wound disruption. Intragastric and bladder pressure monitoring has been used by some pediatric surgeons to determine intra-abdominal pressure. These two measurements are used as a guide to monitor intra-abdominal pressure during primary or staged closure of gastroschisis. The goal of therapy, to maintain intra-abdominal pressure below 20 mmHg, is based on prior studies showing that higher pressures compromise intra-abdominal organ perfusion.

9 For patients in whom complete reduction of the herniated bowel and abdominal wall closure are not possible or appropriate, the staged reduction technique described by Schuster in 1967 has proved to be very useful. Reinforced Silastic sheeting (0.8–1.0 mm thick) is sutured to the fascial edges. This is accomplished with interrupted 3/0 silk mattress sutures. It is generally necessary to enlarge the fascial defect prior to suturing the Silastic sheet. However, extending the fascial opening too far inferiorly should be avoided as bladder injury may occur.

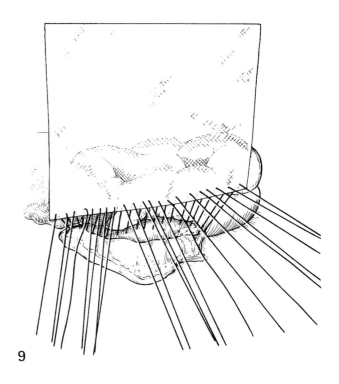

9

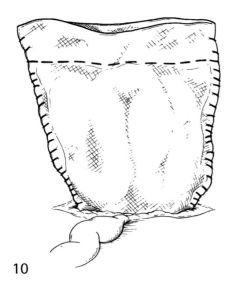

10

10 The cephalad and caudad vertical edges of the silo are constructed with running 3/0 monofilament sutures. Before closing the top of the silo, as much of the bowel as possible is reduced into the peritoneal cavity by manual compression within the sac while avoiding excessive intra-abdominal pressure. The top of the sac is oversewn with a 3/0 monofilament suture placed in a running horizontal mattress fashion. Suture is also placed through the skin and looped over the Silastic sac (illustration 11) in order to pull the skin edges together and minimize skin retraction.

The Silastic sac is covered with povidone-iodine ointment followed by dry roll gauze to act as a protective dressing and provide support to the Silastic sac at the fascial level.

11 The staged reduction technique requires daily reduction of the herniated intestine within the silo. The target for completely reducing the bowel, removing the Silastic sac, and closing the abdominal wall is within 1 week of age. Any delay beyond 1 week substantially increases the risk of fascial infection, tearing away of the Silastic sheeting from the anterior abdominal wall, and failure of the technique. This is also true when using the spring-loaded, preformed silo. Daily reduction of the intestinal contents within the sac can be accomplished in the neonatal intensive care unit using sedation and sterile technique. Each time the procedure is performed, the sac and anterior abdominal wall are prepared with warm povidone-iodine solution before the reduction, and povidone-iodine ointment is applied followed by roll gauze after the procedure. Some pediatric surgeons do not use this approach when using the spring-loaded silo, but simply leave it exposed. General anesthesia is not necessary. When the herniated bowel has been successfully reduced into the peritoneal cavity and the fascial edges brought to within 1 cm of each other, the infant is ready for removal of the sac and primary abdominal wall closure in the operating room under general anesthesia. An alternative 'gentle touch' technique has been described. This method involves bedside placement of a spring-loaded silo, followed by passive reduction of the herniated contents into the abdomen via gravity. The infant is kept paralyzed or sedated and intubated with assisted ventilation during the passive reduction. The author states that this process typically takes 4–5 days. Subsequently, closure of the abdominal wall defect is performed.

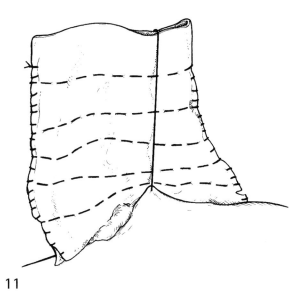

11

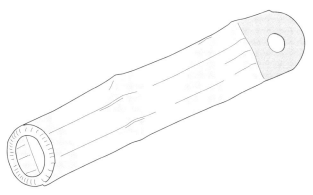

12

12 An alternative method is the placement of a preformed, spring-loaded silo at the bedside. This can be accomplished without general anesthesia. The preformed silo comes in different diameters and should be selected appropriately to accommodate the size of the defect and bulkiness of the herniated contents.

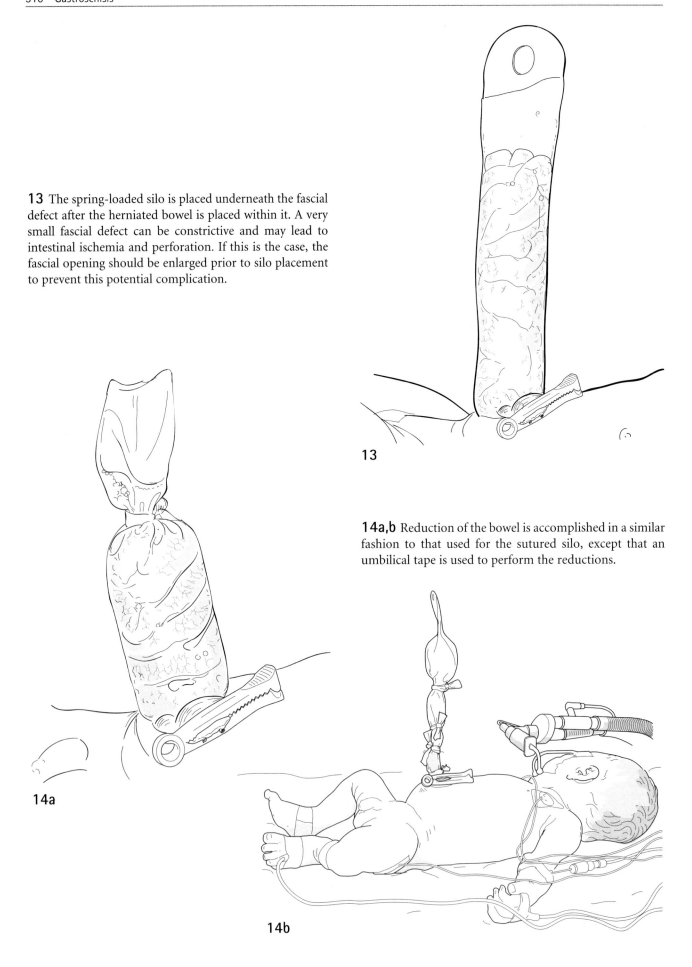

13 The spring-loaded silo is placed underneath the fascial defect after the herniated bowel is placed within it. A very small fascial defect can be constrictive and may lead to intestinal ischemia and perforation. If this is the case, the fascial opening should be enlarged prior to silo placement to prevent this potential complication.

13

14a,b Reduction of the bowel is accomplished in a similar fashion to that used for the sutured silo, except that an umbilical tape is used to perform the reductions.

14a

14b

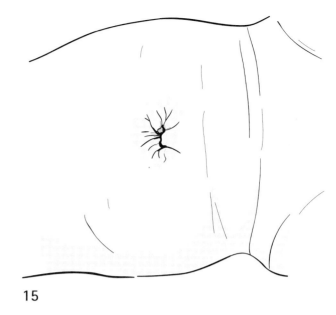

15 Appearance after fascial closure and purse-string technique of skin closure. Umbilicus was removed.

15

POSTOPERATIVE CARE

Most patients with gastroschisis require parenteral nutrition to provide the necessary calories intravenously while awaiting bowel reduction and recovery of bowel function. Until recently, this was accomplished via a cuffed Silastic central venous catheter. An alternative is the placement of a small Silastic catheter inserted via a peripheral vein and threaded centrally (commonly referred to as a PICC (peripherally inserted central catheter) line). Parenteral nutrition is typically required for 2–6 weeks after the operation while awaiting the return of intestinal function. Nasogastric decompression is necessary until there is evidence of bowel function. Broad-spectrum antibiotics are generally continued for a minimum of 5 days. Those infants who undergo the staged approach require a longer period of antibiotic treatment (usually until 1–2 days after the sac has been removed).

Once there is evidence of gastrointestinal function, enteral feeding can be introduced and gradually progressed using breast milk or a low-residue elemental-type formula with appropriate caloric intake. In the past, enteral feeding in these patients was generally delayed for at least 4–6 weeks after surgery, as it was thought that early feeding could lead to an increased risk of developing complications. However, this approach has not been supported with clinical evidence and, more recently, enteral feedings have been started as early as 10–14 days postoperatively, with no increase in adverse outcomes.

COMPLICATIONS

It is generally not recommended to attempt a bowel resection or anastomosis because of the marked thickening and inflammation of the intestinal wall. Intestinal atresia can be managed by the creation of a stoma if primary abdominal wall closure is possible or by leaving the atresia *in situ* if staged reduction is undertaken. A stoma can be created at the time of removal of the Silastic sac and primary abdominal wall closure. A devastating complication can be partial or complete necrosis of the midgut as a result of excessive intra-abdominal pressure or kinking of the blood supply to the bowel at the time of reduction of the herniated bowel. This complication may lead to the death of the patient or to short bowel syndrome.

Additional complications associated with the abdominal wall closure are wound dehiscence and intestinal–cutaneous fistula formation. These complications are also often associated with excessive intra-abdominal pressure. It is preferable to use the staged reduction approach when primary abdominal wall closure might result in excessive intra-abdominal pressure.

A delayed complication is the development of necrotizing enterocolitis. The incidence of necrotizing enterocolitis in patients with gastroschisis has been reported to be as high as 20 percent. It generally has a delayed onset, usually 3–6 weeks after birth. The causes remain unknown, but associations have been made with total parenteral nutrition (TPN)-induced cholestasis and delay in feeding. Necrotizing enterocolitis associated with gastroschisis can be mild or severe and can involve a significant portion of the bowel resulting in a high mortality.

Finally, sepsis, resulting from intra-abdominal or wound infections, and central line infections are additional causes of morbidity in the patient with gastroschisis.

16a,b Complications in infants with gastroschisis are generally related to the gastrointestinal tract or the abdominal wall closure. As noted earlier, *in utero* complications from intestinal atresia or perforation can occur. Intestinal perforation can be managed in one of several ways, depending on the specific circumstances. The options at the time of birth include suture closure, resection of the site of perforation with oversewing of the two ends of the bowel (i.e. creating 'intestinal atresia'), or creation of a stoma if primary abdominal wall closure can be accomplished.

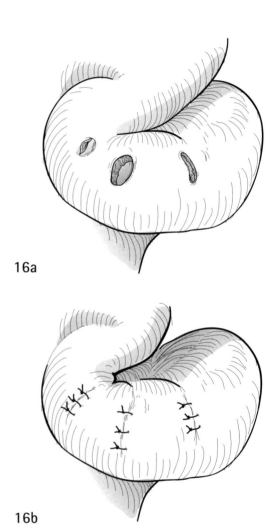

16a

16b

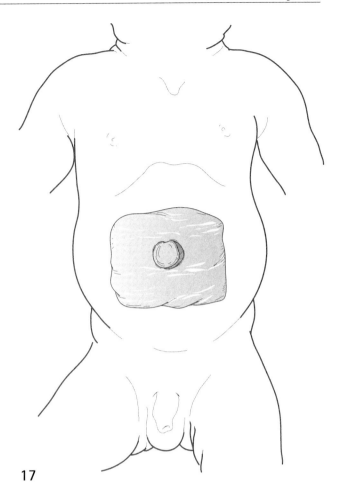

17 Recently, a new method for 'sutureless' gastroschisis closure has been described. In this technique, the bowel is reduced in the usual fashion either primarily or after placement in a silo. However, instead of placing sutures to approximate the fascia, the defect is covered with the umbilical stump or a non-adherent dressing. Occlusive dressings are then placed over the site and the wound is allowed to granulate. Once granulation tissue covers the wound bed, the area is covered with dry dressings. Proposed advantages of this technique include insignificant changes in intra-abdominal pressure and decreased narcotic and sedation requirements. Nearly all infants have an umbilical hernia following this method of repair, but many of these resolve spontaneously, similar to isolated umbilical hernias.

17

OUTCOME

The availability of neonatal intensive care units, parenteral nutrition, and the technique of staged reduction have resulted in significant improvement in the outcome for infants with gastroschisis over the past four decades. The survival of infants with gastroschisis has exceeded 90 percent. Morbidity should be relatively low if attention is paid to the details of the surgical correction. In the authors' experience, infants successfully treated for gastroschisis do not have significant complications during later infancy and childhood.

In addition to the marked improvement in survival, the length of time to initiation of feedings and hospital discharge have been significantly shortened. Whereas hospitalization usually averaged approximately 6 weeks, the average is now around 4 weeks.

FURTHER READING

Badillo A, Hedrick H, Wilson R *et al.* Prenatal ultrasonographic gastrointestinal abnormalities in fetuses with gastroschisis do not correlate with postnatal outcomes. *Journal of Pediatric Surgery* 2007; **43**: 647–53.

Jona JZ. The 'gentle touch' technique in the treatment of gastroschisis. *Journal of Pediatric Surgery* 2003; **38**: 1036–8.

Lacey SR, Carris LA, Beyer J *et al.* Bladder pressure monitoring significantly enhances care of infants with abdominal wall defects: a prospective clinical study. *Journal of Pediatric Surgery* 1993; **28**: 1370–5.

Oldham KT, Coran AG, Drongowski RA *et al.* The development of necrotizing enterocolitis following repair of gastroschisis: a surprisingly high incidence. *Journal of Pediatric Surgery* 1988; **23**: 945–9.

Riboh J, Abrajano C, Garber K *et al.* Outcomes of sutureless gastroschisis closure. *Journal of Pediatric Surgery* 2009; **44**: 1947–51.

Schlatter M, Norris K, Uitvlugt N *et al.* Improved outcomes in the treatment of gastroschisis using a preformed silo and delayed repair approach. *Journal of Pediatric Surgery* 2003; **38**: 459–64.

Schuster SR. A new method for the staged repair of large omphaloceles. *Surgery, Gynecology and Obstetrics* 1967; **125**: 837–50.

Schwartz MZ, Tyson KR, Milliorn K *et al.* Staged reduction using a Silastic sac is the treatment of choice for large congenital abdominal wall defects. *Journal of Pediatric Surgery* 1983; **18**: 713–19.

40

Ergonomics, heuristics, and cognition in laparoscopic surgery

HOCK LIM TAN

INTRODUCTION

Ergonomics is the study of people at work or in structured activities.

Laparoscopic surgery is not intuitive. Unlike open surgery, where there is very little need to interact with sophisticated surgical equipment, even the simplest diagnostic laparoscopy requires the surgeon to interact with laparoscopic equipment without which it is impossible for them to visualize the operative field, and to manipulate the instruments.

ERGONOMICS OF LAPAROSCOPIC SURGERY

The basic premise in laparoscopic surgery is that all instruments have to work around a fulcrum, which is the point of entry of the instrument or telescope into the body cavity. There is no exception to this, and because of the fulcrum, all internal movements are paradoxical. Moving an instrument to the right will result in the opposite movement inside the body. This is a first-order paradox and is similar to rowing a boat.

Working in first-order paradox is easily mastered provided one follows the simple rule that the telescope must be pointed directly away from the surgeon towards the video monitor which should be sited directly in front of the surgeon (**Figure 40.1**). The further the surgeon deviates from this, the further removed they are from first-order paradox, to the extent that if the telescope is pointed towards the surgeon, horizontal movements seen on the video monitor are no longer paradoxical, but the vertical movements will remain so (**Figure 40.2**).

This is second-order paradox and even the simplest manipulation becomes challenging if the surgeon has to manipulate hand instruments under a second-order second paradox environment. While most surgeons intuitively place themselves in the optimum position for

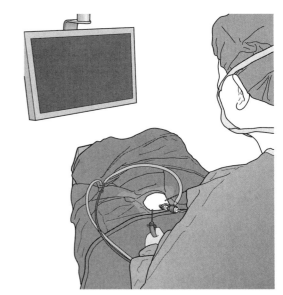

Figure 40.1 Optimum working optimum position for first-order paradox.

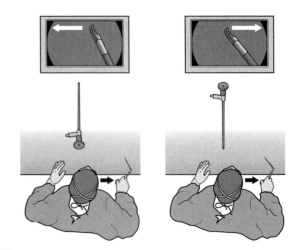

Figure 40.2 Horizontal movements are not paradoxical if the camera is pointed towards the surgeon.

manipulating instruments in first-order paradox, this is not necessarily the case when it comes to positioning the assistant surgeons or nurses. While it is logical in open surgery to position the assistant and nurse opposite the operating surgeon, and is the rule of thumb for most open surgical procedures, it is not ergonomic for laparoscopy. If the assistant and operating room nurse are positioned opposite the surgeon, the camera will be pointing towards them and they will be working under second-order paradox, even if they have an extra video monitor placed in front of them. This makes even the simplest task arduous (**Figure 40.3**).

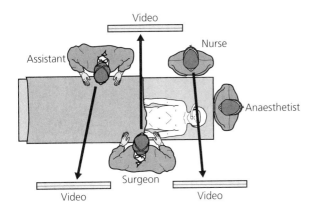

Figure 40.3 Example of how placing the assistant and operating room nurse opposite the surgeon creates a second-order paradox.

To overcome the problem with second-order paradox, the optimum position for the operating team is one which allows everyone to work with the camera pointed away. This usually requires that they stand on the same side for most operations, with few exceptions (**Figure 40.4**).

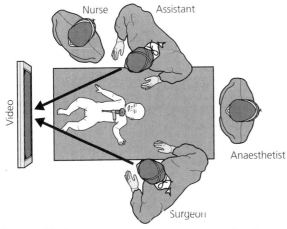

Figure 40.4 In-line position for the surgeon and assistant.

THE ERGONOMICS OF PORT PLACEMENT

Surgeons intuitively place open surgical incisions close to the operative field to gain maximum extensile exposure to the surgical field. This is not applicable in laparoscopic surgery, because the amount of internal space available to manipulate instruments is determined by the volume of the cone formed from the point of entry of your surgical instrument to the operation site (**Figure 40.5**).

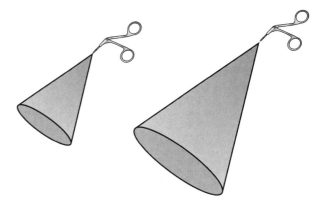

Figure 40.5 The amount of internal space available is determined by the volume of the cone formed from the point of entry of the instrument to the operation site.

The closer the port is to the operation site, the less room there will be to maneuver. The optimum port position for laparoscopic surgery is one which provides direct access to the target organ, optimizing the volume of the internal space to allow the manipulation of instruments with minimal exaggerated movements. Ports should be positioned so that the surgeon is able to manipulate hand instruments with minimum strain and maximal comfort.

PRINCIPLES OF PORT PLACEMENT

The principles of port placement are:

1. Place the instrument ports to allow for direct access to the organ. Do not forget that some 'unimportant' structures which are easily retracted at open surgery e.g. such as the falciform ligament, can form a curtain which may obstruct direct access to the contralateral subdiaphragmatic area if the instrument ports are positioned too high in the contralateral upper quadrant.
2. Maximize the internal volume available to manipulate instruments. When operating in an extremely confined space, such as when repairing a duodenal atresia, it will be necessary to break some ergonomic rules in order to maximize the internal space available to allow for accurate suturing.

3. Minimize exaggeration of external movements. The optimum port position is to have approximately the same length of instrument on the inside as you would on the outside.
4. Position ports to allow you to manipulate instruments with your arms completely adducted by the side of your body, with shoulders in resting position, i.e. a comfortable position (**Figure 40.6**).
5. Position the suturing port in line with the intended anastomosis. It is impossible to perform an anastomosis if the suturing port is not parallel to the intended line of the anastomosis because of restricted freedom of movement (**Figure 40.7**).

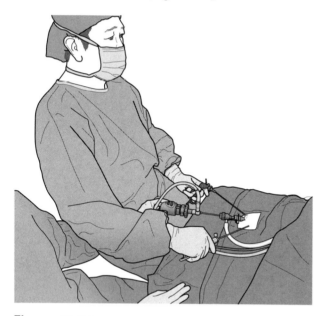

Figure 40.6 The ports should be positioned so that instruments can be manipulated comfortably.

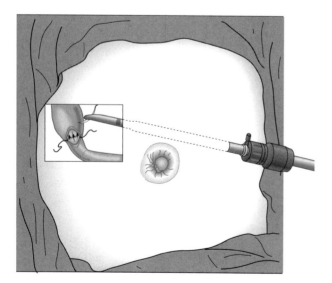

Figure 40.7 The suturing port should be in line with the intended anastomosis e.g. duodenal atresia.

POSITIONAL REQUIREMENTS

The best and most stable position for a surgeon to work is in the most comfortable position possible and this usually means the position of rest.

In practice, the optimum position is for the surgeon to be sitting down, and for both arms to be adducted and resting comfortably by the side of the body without elevating the shoulders. This requires that the operating table be lowered to a much lower position than conventional surgery to avoid 'chicken winging'. Operating with the table at the same height for open surgery will result in unnecessary neuromuscular strain if the surgeon has to work with arms extended or abducted for prolonged periods (**Figure 40.8**).

The same applies with the positioning of the video monitor. Before the advent of pendant-mounted video monitors, it was necessary to position the monitor on the top of the 'stack', resulting in suboptimal operating conditions for the surgeon, making it necessary to turn the head to view the monitor mounted on top of the 'stack'.

Contemporary laparoscopic operating rooms with pendant-mounted video monitors allow the video monitor to be positioned at eye level or even lower to approximate conditions found in open surgery, creating a virtual window to look into the celomic cavity (**Figure 40.9**).

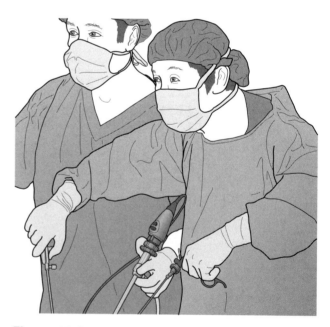

Figure 40.8 The operating table should be lower than in conventional surgery to avoid 'chicken winging'.

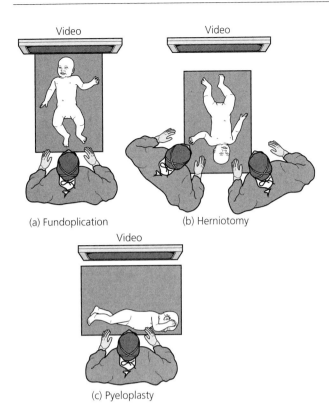

Figure 40.9 Examples of ergonomic positions for video monitors: (a) fundoplication; (b) herniotomy; (c) pyeloplasty.

MANIPULATING INSTRUMENTS

A common problem encountered in laparoscopic surgery is navigating back to the target when changing instruments is necessary.

Navigational skills and intracorporeal suturing are cognitive skills, not visual skills. However, because of the paradoxical world in laparoscopy, the development of cognition in laparoscopic surgery is not intuitive and special training is required.

Specific repetitive tasks in laparoscopic surgery can be learnt until they become automatic or cognitive, and the rest will follow. Once skills such as navigation and suturing become cognitive, it will allow a surgeon to perform complex laparoscopic surgery with a minimum of effort.

COGNITIVE NAVIGATION

One can learn to navigate hand instruments with great precision by learning to 'triangulate' and by using 'gestalt' or mental spatial memory.

Triangulation

Triangulation is making use of two converging reference points to navigate your hands' instruments to the same point. Given that most laparoscopic operations require a telescope and at least two other hand instruments, the surgeon should be able to navigate any instrument to the convergent point by using the other two instruments, e.g. the telescope and one hand instrument as the external reference points. To do this, the surgeon needs to develop a mental spatial image of where the points converge and introduce the third instrument to this spatial point. This is best performed without visual guidance, such as looking at the video monitor, and is particularly useful when instrument bearing is lost.

Gestalt

This is also useful in allowing the surgeon to interchange instruments and to navigate instruments back to the exact spatial position without external or visual reference points by using their own mental spatial memory. To develop this skill, the surgeon needs to remember the spatial alignment of the instrument as it is removed from the port, and to follow this same path when reinserting a second instrument.

This spatial relationship will be altered if the surgeon's body moves relative to the patient, so it is extremely important that you do not move during the interchange of instruments.

LAPAROSCOPIC INTRACORPOREAL SUTURING

This is probably one of the most challenging laparoscopic tasks to master, but is especially important in reconstructive surgery. Because of the lack of freedom of movement imposed by having to work around the fulcrum, the correct positioning of this port is critical for fine laparoscopic suturing and the optimum position for this suturing port is to place it so that the laparoscopic needle driver is approximately in line with the intended anastomosis line. Placing the suturing port in any other position will severely restrict your ability to suture.

The limitations of not working with stereoscopic vision can largely be replaced by the superior fidelity and resolution of high definition camera systems which show far greater detail than is possible with the naked eye.

Fitt's law applies to laparoscopic suturing. Paul Fitt, a psychologist at Ohio State University studied rapid, aimed, human movement and is the pioneer of aviation safety. He stated that the time required to point or move rapidly from one point to another is dependent on the distance from, and the size of the target. If we apply Fitt's law to intracorporeal suturing, the optimum position for the telescope and hand instruments is to be as close to the suture line as is practicable. Likewise, laparoscopic suturing is greatly facilitated if the target is bigger. Translated, this means that for the surgeon to optimize their ability to suture, the biggest video monitor available should be used.

COGNITION IN LAPAROSCOPIC SUTURING

Laparoscopic intracorporeal suturing can be broken down into cognitive steps. Each of these steps requires the surgeon to learn to pronate or supinate both hand instruments synchronously and these movements can be practiced, just like tying a surgical knot, until it is automatic or cognitive. Once these actions are mastered and have become cognitive, then the ability to perform an intracorporeal knot becomes automatic.

The following points about laparoscopic suturing should be noted:

- Suturing is impossible if the needle holder is at right angles to the intended line of anastomosis.
- It is easier to suture towards a port.
- It is best to mount the needle at the halfway point.
- It is best to place the telescope as close as possible to the suturing point.
- It is best to form loops over the loose end rather than bringing the loop to the end.
- Use very short sutures (5–7 cm).

HEURISTICS

Heuristics are 'rules of thumb' that experts learn through trial and error. Heuristics are used in everyday surgical dissection and form a very important basic tool of surgery. Examples of rules of thumb which are equally applicable to both open and laparoscopic surgery include 'work from the known to the unknown'.

However, many rules of thumb used in open surgery may be completely inappropriate when applied to laparoscopic surgery. One such example is 'breaking the table' when performing open renal surgery. While it is logical to bring the kidney closer to an open incision, it will not assist laparoscopic exposure, as pushing the kidney closer to the abdominal wall only reduces the internal volume available for manipulating instruments.

In developing new 'rules of thumb' or heuristics for laparoscopic surgery, it is important to take into consideration the special and sometimes unique conditions created in a completely paradoxical world, where positional requirements may be counterintuitive and where conventional logic may only restrict your ability to perform advanced laparoscopy.

The thoracoscopic repair of esophageal atresia is a good example. Whereas in open surgery, the patient is positioned for right thoracotomy lying on the side, this positioning will severely restrict the surgeon's ability to visualize the esophagus thoracosopically. Thus, counterintuitively, the optimum position is to lie the patient prone. This will allow the lung to collapse away from the operating field and any potential bleeding or fluid to drain away from the operating field.

It is often said that the laparoscopic procedure must be identical to the open procedure. This is no longer true. Given that laparoscopy surgery allows the surgeon to operate on any organ *in situ*, it is no longer necessary to mobilize the organ, as you can gain direct surgical access to the operation with the telescope and hand instruments. An example is laparoscopic Heller's cardiomyotomy which can be performed without mobilization of the esophagus. By preserving the attachments of the esophagus, the cardio–esophageal junction is not disrupted and it is therefore not necessary to perform a fundoplication to repair the cardio–esophageal junction attachments which are left intact.

In summary, most surgeons perform everyday tasks using cognition. However, in a paradoxical environment, together with the restriction on freedom of movement, surgeons need to develop and adopt new rules of thumb or heuristic rules relevant to this paradoxical environment. An understanding of ergonomics, heuristics, and cognition is essential to master advanced laparoscopic surgery.

Suggested reading:

Leeder PC, Patkin M, Stoddard J, and Watson DI. Dissection efficiency during laparoscopic oesophageal dissection. *Minimally Invasive Therapy & Allied Technologies* 2005; **14**(1): 8–12.

Patkin M, Isabel L. Egonomics, engineering and surgery of endosurgical dissection. *Journal of the Royal College of Surgeons of Edinburgh* 1995; **40**(2): 120–32.

41

Abdominal surgery

NICHOLAS SY CHAO, DAVID A LLOYD, and HOCK LIM TAN

GENERAL PRINCIPLES OF ACCESS

David A Lloyd

PRINCIPLES AND JUSTIFICATION

Anatomic considerations

1a,b There are important anatomic differences between the abdomen of the newborn infant and that of the older child or adult. The following are characteristics of the infant.

- The shape of the abdomen is a square compared with the rectangular shape of the older child. A transverse mid-abdominal incision in an infant will therefore provide access to the whole peritoneal cavity, with the possible exception of the pelvis.
- The compliant ribcage and wide subcostal angle facilitate access to the upper abdominal organs and diaphragm.
- The rectus muscle is wider and extends further laterally.
- The liver is relatively large and extends from below the costal margin on the left down to the right lower quadrant.
- The umbilicus is relatively low and nearer the pubic symphysis, and the bladder extends up to the umbilicus. There is limited space for an incision below the umbilicus in the neonate.

Site and size of incision

The incision must be planned to provide optimal exposure for the surgeon whilst minimizing abdominal muscle damage. In a modern environment it is unusual to operate on a patient who is not stable, and the surgeon is able to place greater emphasis on the cosmetic aspects of the incision than was possible in the past. An incision that has been correctly sited does not need to be unduly long. Nonetheless, common reasons for a surgeon to experience difficulty are inadequate exposure due to an incision that is too small, poor retraction by the assistant, poor lighting, and inadequate muscle relaxation.

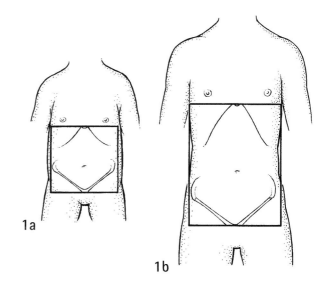

PREOPERATIVE

Anesthesia

General anesthesia with muscle relaxation and endotracheal intubation are required for abdominal operations on children.

Skin cleansing

A variety of topical preparations are in use for removing potential pathogens from the skin in the operative field. Alcohol-based solutions evaporate rapidly, promoting heat loss, and iodine-based preparations may irritate the skin. Aqueous chlorhexidine (Hibitane) has none of these potential disadvantages and has effective antibacterial activity. In newborn infants, the solution should be warmed. Excess fluid must not be used, as this may run under the patient, resulting in chemical or electrical burns, as well as promoting heat loss.

Draping

Sterile towels or drapes are used to provide a sterile environment around the incision. These are covered with a large, sterile, adhesive plastic sheet, which stabilizes the towels and also helps to keep the infant warm by reducing heat loss from the skin and by keeping the infant dry.

OPERATIONS

Transverse abdominal incision

The muscle-cutting transverse upper abdominal incision is suitable for most operations in infants, except when access is required to the distal colon and rectum. The incision may be limited to one side of the abdomen or can be extended across the midline, dividing both rectus muscles. For some procedures, such as reduction of an intussusception, a transverse incision lateral to the right rectus muscle will suffice.

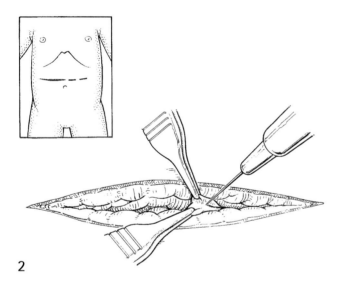

2

POSITION OF PATIENT AND INCISION

2 The patient lies supine. The skin incision starts in the midline, 1–2 cm above the umbilicus, and extends laterally across the rectus muscle. The subcutaneous fat is lifted with two pairs of fine-toothed forceps (one held by the surgeon and one by the assistant) and cut with diathermy to minimize blood loss, particularly in the small infant. Bleeding from small vessels in the skin edge will stop spontaneously with compression; larger vessels are touch-coagulated with needle-point diathermy or picked up accurately with fine-toothed forceps and coagulated, taking care not to damage the skin.

3 This exposes the anterior rectus sheath, which is incised transversely. A pair of artery forceps inserted deep to the rectus muscle is used to lift the muscle off the underlying fascia while cutting it with the diathermy. The vessels are identified and cauterized before being cut.

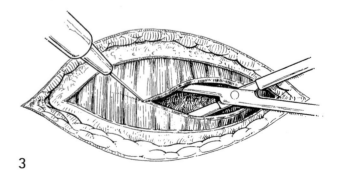

3

4 The posterior rectus sheath is picked up with two pairs of artery forceps placed about 1 cm apart, and a small incision is made between them, taking care not to damage the underlying bowel. Once air has entered the peritoneal cavity, the bowel falls away, unless it is distended or there are adhesions, and the incision can be completed safely using scissors. In the neonate, the transversalis muscle is well developed and vascular and may be divided using diathermy.

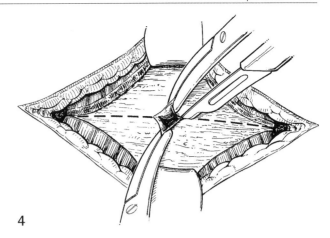

4

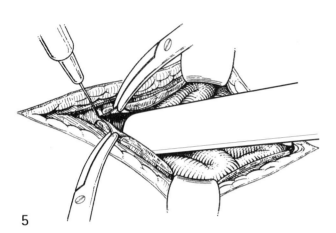

5

5 The incision is extended laterally by lifting the abdominal wall muscles with artery forceps applied to the upper and lower edges of the posterior rectus sheath, and cutting the external oblique, internal oblique, and transversalis muscle layers with the diathermy, while protecting the underlying bowel.

If the bowel is distended, it should be protected with a flat retractor or a swab. Adhesions must be carefully dissected off the peritoneum; when a pre-existing incision is being re-opened, it is advisable to begin the incision beyond the end of the scar so that the peritoneum is opened where it is 'normal' and underlying adhesions are unlikely to be present.

6 The incision may also be extended medially across the midline. The falciform ligament is cut with scissors and the ligamentum teres is ligated with absorbable ligatures and divided.

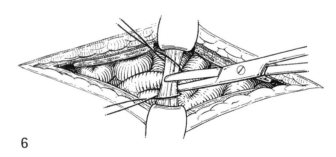

6

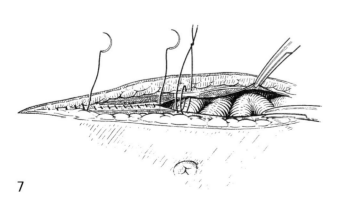

7

WOUND CLOSURE

7 The abdomen is closed in layers using absorbable sutures (4/0 or 3/0 sutures on a round-bodied needle for infants and 2/0 for children).

The margins of the peritoneum and transversalis muscle or fascia are grasped with artery forceps, elevated, and approximated with a continuous absorbable suture. In the older child, if the incision divides both rectus sheaths, closure of the midline (linea alba) is reinforced with a single figure-of-eight suture. No sutures are placed in the rectus muscle, which is adherent to the rectus sheath and does not retract.

The anterior rectus sheath is also repaired using a continuous suture. Lateral to the rectus sheath, the internal and extenal oblique muscles are repaired in separate layers.

When there is doubt about the ability of the abdominal wall muscles to retain sutures, as in very premature or malnourished infants, the abdomen may be closed in a single layer with sutures incorporating all the muscles and the peritoneum. The skin is closed as a separate layer. The same technique may be used when a pre-existing incision is closed.

8 Before closing the skin, local anesthetic is infiltrated into the layers of the abdominal wall surrounding the incision. In most infants, the subcutaneous fat falls together without the need for sutures, and the skin is approximated with adhesive strips. In older children, the deep fascia is repaired with 4/0 or 3/0 absorbable sutures. This takes the tension off the skin, which is approximated with adhesive strips or a subcuticular 5/0 absorbable suture. The incision is covered with a dressing, mainly to allay the anxiety of the child.

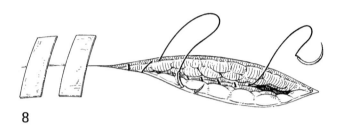

8

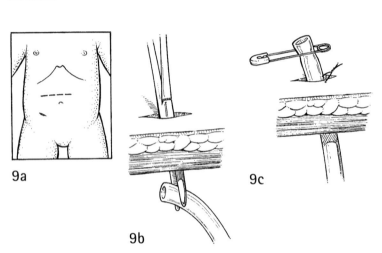

9a

9b

9c

9a–c If an abdominal drain is required, it must be placed through the abdominal wall before closing the incision. At a suitable site, depending on the area to be drained, a short transverse incision is made through the skin and external oblique muscle.

With a hand in the peritoneal cavity to protect the bowel, an artery forceps is pushed through the abdominal wall into the peritoneal cavity to grasp the drain. The type of drain will depend on the specific situation; a Penrose drain suffices for most situations.

The drain is pulled out through the abdominal wall and sutured to the skin. A safety pin is placed through the drain to prevent it from slipping into the peritoneal cavity.

Subcostal incision

The left subcostal incision is useful for access to the diaphragm (congenital diaphragmatic hernia), esophagus (fundoplication), or spleen. On the right, the incision is used for operations on the gallbladder and bile ducts; if the liver is to be exposed, the incision is extended to the left subcostal region.

10 Depending on the age of the patient, the skin incision is made 1.5–3 cm below and parallel to the costal margin. It should not overlie the costal margin when sutured. In the midline, the incision may be extended cranially to the xiphisternum for better access to the esophagus or diaphragm.

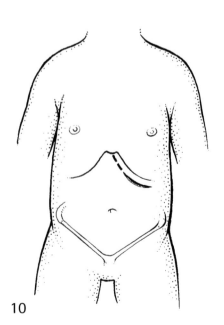

10

The layers to be divided are the same as for a transverse incision, but in an oblique direction.

WOUND CLOSURE

Closure is as for a transverse incision. If a gastrostomy tube has been inserted, ideally it should be brought out through a separate incision. On occasion, the most direct route is through the main incision; in this case the incision is closed in two halves, beginning on either side of the

tube. On each side of the gastrostomy the stomach must be securely anchored to the abdominal wall with a non-absorbable suture.

Bilateral subcostal (rooftop) incision

This is the preferred exposure for surgery of the liver and portal structures.

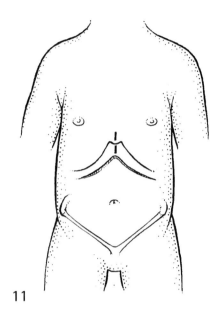

11 For initial exploration of the liver, a right subcostal incision is made; this is then extended to the left with a curve across the midline. If necessary, a further extension may be made cranially in the midline to enter the mediastinum.

WOUND CLOSURE

Closure is as for subcostal and midline incisions. A single 3-point suture is placed in the midline at the junction of the two incisions before closing the peritoneum.

Midline abdominal incision

The access offered by the upper abdominal midline incision in the infant is restricted by the relatively large liver, but this disadvantage is offset by the wide costal angle and the cosmetic scar. The incision is useful for pyloromyotomy, gastrostomy, and fundoplication. In the older child, this is the incision of choice for blunt abdominal trauma.

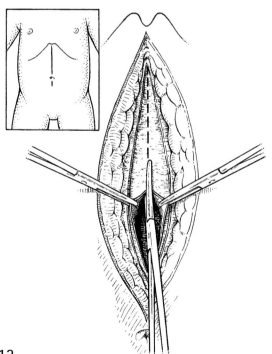

12 The skin is incised from xiphisternum to umbilicus. (For pyloromyotomy, a shorter incision is adequate.) If it is necessary to extend the incision caudally, it should be taken straight through the umbilicus and not around it. This gives a superior cosmetic result, and the risk of infection is not increased if the umbilicus has been properly cleaned. The subcutaneous tissues are cut with the diathermy down to the fascia.

A short incision is made in the linea alba using a scalpel, and the falciform ligament is entered. The edges of the incision are grasped with artery forceps and elevated. A plane is developed deep to the linea alba, which is incised with scissors. Near the umbilicus, the peritoneum fuses with the linea alba, and the peritoneal cavity will be entered as the incision is extended caudally. The left or right fold of the faciform ligament is incised, depending on the exposure required; if necessary, the ligamentum teres is ligated and divided.

11

12

WOUND CLOSURE

The falciform ligament/peritoneum may be repaired, but this is not essential. The linea alba is approximated with a continuous strong suture of slowly absorbable material such as polydioxanone (PDS), or with a nylon suture (3/0 for infants, 2/0 or 0 gauge for children). The knot at each end should be buried to avoid an unsightly nodule. A subcutaneous suture may be required. The skin is closed with adhesive strips or a 5/0 continuous subcuticular absorbable suture.

Grid-iron incision

The modified McBurney incision is the ideal incision for acute appendectomy in childhood.

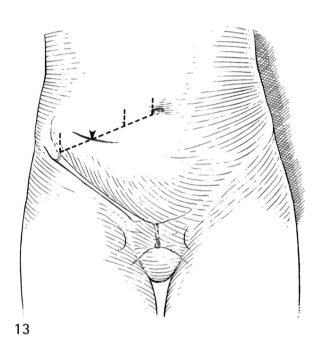

13 The traditional incision is centered over McBurney's point, which is two-thirds of the distance from the umbilicus to the right anterior superior iliac spine, and is aligned with the skin creases, which lie in a slightly oblique direction. It should be lateral to the rectus muscle, which is relatively broad in a child. A lower incision may be preferred for cosmetic reasons, but exposure of the appendix may be difficult if the incision is too low or too medial. If a mass can be palpated when the child is under anesthesia, this may influence the siting of the incision.

13

14 The subcutaneous tissues are divided with diathermy and swept aside with a swab to expose clearly the external oblique aponeurosis; this facilitates subsequent closure. The external oblique muscle is incised and then divided along the line of its fibers and separated from the underlying muscle.

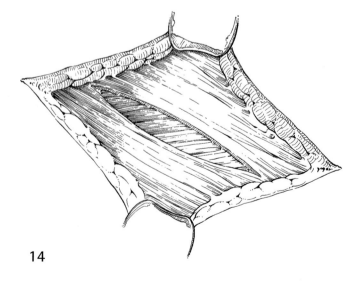

14

15 The internal oblique muscle is opened by passing blunt scissors or artery forceps into the muscle and spreading it at right-angles to the direction of the fibers. Two Langenbeck retractors are inserted into the space and used to separate the fibers widely. The underlying transversus abdominis muscle and the fatty layer covering the peritoneum are opened in a similar fashion.

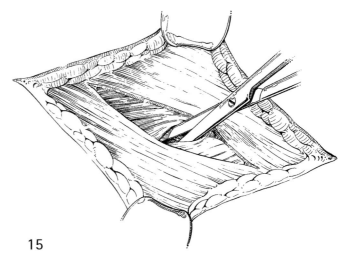

15

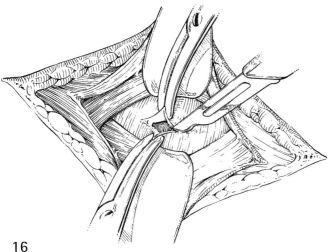

16

16 The peritoneum is grasped with two pairs of artery forceps, taking care to avoid the underlying bowel. The forceps are lifted and the peritoneum is incised transversely with a scalpel; the opening is enlarged using scissors.

WOUND CLOSURE

17 The edges of the peritoneum are grasped with artery forceps and closed with a continuous absorbable suture.

The fibers of the transversus and internal oblique muscles are closed as a single layer, using two or three interrupted sutures, which are tied loosely to avoid muscle ischemia. The external oblique muscle is closed with a continuous absorbable suture. The subcutaneous fat seldom requires sutures.

For skin closure, if adhesive strips alone are not adequate, a subcuticular suture of 5/0 absorbable material is used. In children, the skin is always closed after appendectomy, regardless of the degree of contamination; appropriate prophylactic antibiotic cover must be given.

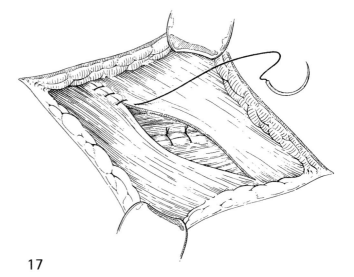

17

EXTENDING THE INCISION

Circumstances may require the incision to be extended laterally; this is done by dividing the abdominal muscles in layers using the diathermy, as shown in Figure 18.

18 To extend the incision medially, the incision in the external oblique muscle is continued onto the anterior rectus sheath. The rectus muscle is retracted medially. The internal oblique and transversalis muscles are divided medially and this incision is extended to open the posterior rectus sheath and peritoneum. If necessary, the rectus muscle is also divided. The incision is closed in layers, as for a transverse abdominal incision.

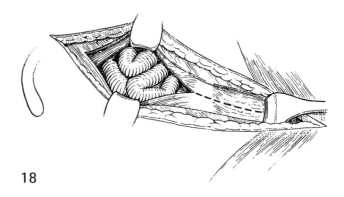

18

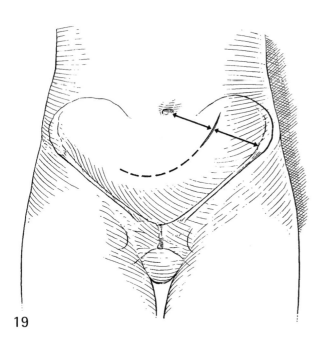

19

Pfannenstiel incision

This lower abdominal incision provides access to the pelvic organs, in particular the bladder, uterus, and ovaries, without dividing the rectus muscles.

20 The skin and subcutaneous tissues are incised transversely between the lateral borders of the two rectus muscles. The incision is slightly curved to follow the skin creases, and is centered about 2 cm above the pubic symphysis. The anterior rectus sheaths are divided transversely and dissected off the rectus muscles by blunt and sharp dissection, extending cranially well up to the umbilicus and caudally to the pubic symphysis. The rectus muscles are separated vertically in the midline and retracted laterally. The transversalis fascia and peritoneum are then opened vertically, taking care to avoid the bladder.

WOUND CLOSURE

The incision is closed in layers, as for a transverse upper abdominal incision. The rectus muscles are approximated in the midline with interrupted sutures.

Oblique muscle-cutting (Lanz) incision

In the left iliac fossa, this incision is used for colostomy formation. It may be extended medially as the 'hockey-stick' incision to provide access to the pelvis.

19 The skin is incised in an oblique direction at the midpoint of a line from the umbilicus to the anterior superior iliac spine. The external oblique muscle is incised along the line of its fibers, as for a grid-iron incision. The internal oblique and transverse muscles are cut obliquely in the same direction as the external oblique muscle, using the diathermy. For the 'hockey-stick' extension, the incision is continued medially, parallel to the skin creases. The rectus muscles and peritoneum are cut transversely.

WOUND CLOSURE

The incision is closed in layers, as for a transverse abdominal incision.

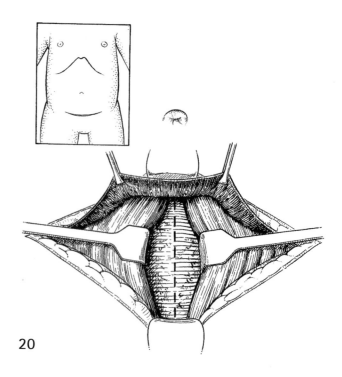

20

COMPLICATIONS

The intestine is at risk of injury while the incision is being made, by being cauterized by the diathermy while incising the muscle layers, particularly in the newborn infant, or by being crushed by artery forceps or incised with the scalpel when the peritoneum is opened. During wound closure, the intestine is also at risk of injury from artery forceps applied to the edges of the incision or the peritoneal suture.

The risk of wound infection is reduced by minimising trauma such as from retractors, meticulous hemostasis and prophylactic antibiotics where indicated. Wound dehiscence has become uncommon with the use of slowly degrading, absorbable sutures.

GENERAL PRINCIPLES OF LAPAROSCOPIC ACCESS

Nicholas SY Chao and Hock Lim Tan

INTRODUCTION

Because of its ability to visualize and access virtually the entire peritoneal cavity, laparoscopy has become an essential part of modern pediatric surgery for both diagnostic and therapeutic procedures. Its clinical application is as relevant in infants and young children, in whom the only other option to laparoscopy is a relatively large incision to access a small abdominal cavity. The usual advantages of small incisions: better cosmesis, reduced pain and surgical stress, less wound complications, and faster recuperation are equally applicable in small infants as they are to adults. As a result, a large number of laparoscopic procedures have evolved from being feasible alternatives to becoming the standard surgical care.

While the general principle of surgical exposure in open surgery is to site the incision as close to the surgical field as possible for optimal exposure, the principles in laparoscopic surgery are somewhat counter-intuitive and require an understanding of anatomy and ergonomics (see **Chapter 40**).

LAPAROSCOPY

The Veress needle versus the Hasson technique

Conventional transumbilical port insertion and creation of pneumoperitoneum with a blind Veress needle have been popularized by many adult surgeons and gynecologists, as well as many pediatric surgeons. However, especially in a small infant, there is an ever present risk of inadvertent visceral injury from blind techniques, and the authors' preference is to access the abdominal cavity via an open laparoscopy (Hasson) which guarantees a consistently safe and easy access, particularly in small infants and children.

The supra- and infraumbilical Hasson

1 The authors prefer the supraumbilical open laparoscopy approach. In neonates and infants particularly, the bladder is an intra-abdominal organ and the prominent umbilical arteries and urachus make for a very busy approach if the infraumbilical route is selected. The convergence of the trilaminar anterior and posterior rectus sheaths above the umbilicus provides sturdy tissue for sutures anchoring the Hasson, and the only anatomical structure of importance is the falciform ligament, or the umbilical vein which remains patent for a few weeks after birth.

It is important not to make a side rent or to open the umbilical vein (falciform ligament in the neonate) when placing the umbilical trocar. There have been reports of gas embolism in neonates when gas is inadvertently insufflated into a side hole in the umbilical vein at commencement of insufflation. This is at risk mostly from transumbilical Veress needle puncture.

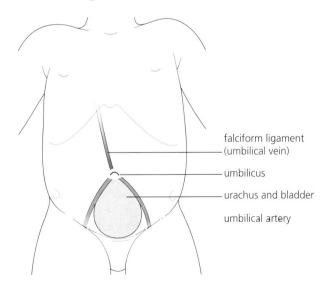

falciform ligament
(umbilical vein)

umbilicus

urachus and bladder

umbilical artery

1

Open laparoscopy or Hasson cannula insertion

2 There are many trocars and cannulae available for laparoscopy and our preference is for the Hasson trocar which has a moveable conical attachment to the shaft of the cannula to which a transfixion suture can be wrapped around to prevent accidental dislodgement.

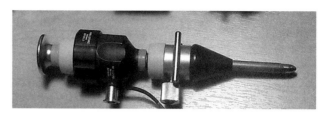

Figure 41.2 Neonatal Hasson Trocar

METHOD OF INSERTION

3 A supraumbilical full-thickness stab incision is made only in skin within the skin crease, and sharp-pointed iris scissors inserted into the stab incision and spread in the sagittal plane. This will split the circumumbilical skin along Langer's line and expose the underlying subcutaneous fat. This should be completely bloodless. The underlying linea alba should be grasped through the subcutaneous fat between two hemostats and lifted out to the surface by everting the two hemostats.

A transverse incision is then made in the linea alba between the two hemostats to expose the underlying peritoneum which is then opened.

A purse string should now be placed around the linea alba defect and the Hasson cannula inserted. The purse string should be firmly secured with a tight single throw to prevent gas leak and the purse string secured to the Hasson cone by winding it around the suture holder. This will hold the Hasson firmly in place.

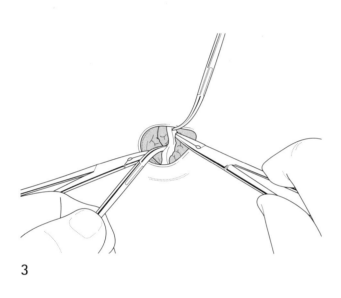

3

Pneumoperitoneum and anesthesia

Endotracheal intubation with sufficient muscle relaxation by the anesthetist is preferred, although the laryngeal mask may be used for short procedures. An experienced pediatric anesthetist should endeavour minimize prior 'bagging' which can lead to significant gaseous distention of the stomach and intestines. Likewise, nitrous oxide should be avoided.

Insufflation must be limited to 6–8 mmHg in low birthweight infants, to 10 mmHg in infants less than 10 kg, and 12 mmHg in older children to minimize diaphragmatic splinting. Excessive intra-abdominal pressure will result in splinting of the diaphragm impeding vital capacity, functional residual volume, as well as CO_2 elimination causing respiratory acidosis. Increasing the insufflation pressure in young children will not increase the internal working space and by the same token, reducing the pressure to much lower than 8 mm does not produce sufficient support for the abdominal wall when introducing the instrument trocars, and leads to tenting and the risk of inadvertent injury to the underlying viscera.

The laparoscope and the conventional working trocars

A 5-mm 30° angled scope is the laparoscope of choice in most instances, although a straight lens may be used in procedures which only require straight viewing. Smaller 4-mm telescopes are preferred for neonates and low birthweight infants, but are unsuitable for older children as they do not provide sufficient illumination in large celomic cavities.

Working instrument ports

A large variety of working instrument ports are available for pediatric laparoscopy, and it is best to choose the smallest diameter port suitable for the available instruments, to reduce gas leak during laparoscopic surgery particularly when using 3-mm instruments. However, it is often necessary to use at least one 5-mm port in order to accommodate 5-mm instruments, such as clip applicators or electrosurgical devices, in which case it is important to select a cannula which does not leak when 3-mm instruments are inserted through the same cannula. This may require using a washer with a smaller hole.

Working ports are ideally inserted under direct vision. It is best to make a full-thickness skin incision at the port site and to introduce the trocar under endoscopic control. This will reduce the risk of inadvertent visceral injury. It is of particular importance to avoid the inferior gastric vessels when inserting ports in either iliac fossa. The inferior epigastric artery will not stop bleeding spontaneously, because of the absence of the posterior rectus sheath to act as a tamponade.

It is possible in small infants usually less than 5 kg to insert the hand instruments directly into the celomic cavity without a port. A small full thickness stab incision is made with a size 11 blade and a straight hemostat introduced into this incisision to dilate it wide enough to just accommodate a 3- or 2-mm hand instrument. The small caliber of the stab incision minimizes gas leak and the advantage of not using a port is that there is no internal protrusion of a cannula sleeve to clash with the hand instruments, particularly when operating in a very confined space.

SECURING THE INSTRUMENT PORTS

4 A common problem during infant laparoscopy is for the instrument cannula to be dislodged during the operation because of the thinness of the abdominal wall. A popular method of securing the cannula is to attach a rubber sleeve and then transfix the sleeve to the abdominal wall with a transfixion suture.

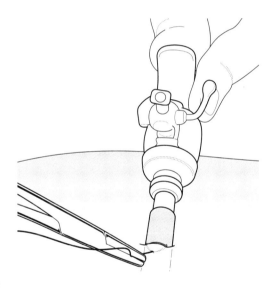

4

ACCESSING THE UPPER ABDOMEN

Preoperative preparation

A nasogastric tube is useful in reducing gastric distention especially if any degree of anesthetic bagging is required. Similarly, the colon may be very loaded especially in bed-ridden patients and a colonic washout will be useful as access to the upper abdomen may be impeded for example, by a very dilated transverse colon during fundoplication.

Patient position

For hiatal, gastric, and hepatobiliary operations, the child is positioned near the foot of the table with the video monitor 'cephalad' or near the head of the table, so that the surgeon at the table end is in line (see **Chapter 3**). The table should be tilted head up about 20°.

For splenic and transperitoneal renal access, the child should be positioned with ipsilateral elevation about 45°, without any hip flexion, as a flexed hip may otherwise hinder your ability to manipulate hand instruments in the lower quadrant.

Visceral exposure

5 It is often useful particularly when operating in a small child, to create more space by 'lifting' a large overhanging liver with a transabdominal 'hitch-stitch' wound around the falciform ligament. The liver can be lifted by the falciform ligament onto the undersurface of the abdominal wall, and securing the externalized suture with a hemostat placed precisely at their exit points..

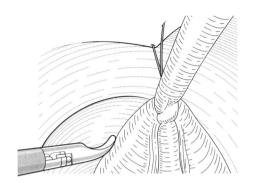

5

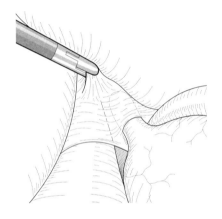

6

6 The left lobe of the liver may be retracted in the small child by inserting a grasper (blunt or tooth-ratcheted) through a right subxyphoid port (or 'portless stab') curling under the falciform to grasp the diaphragm above the hiatus for fundoplication and Hellers.

When extensile exposure is required, a 'Nathanson' retractor will provide more exposure.

ACCESS TO THE POSTERIOR ABDOMINAL CAVITY

Emerging procedures, such as laparoscopic pancreatic surgery and laparoscopic repair of duodenal atresia, will require access to the posterior abdomen.

This is best facilitated by positioning the patient at least 20–30° head up which will allow the transverse colon to fall away from the operative site by gravity, after the transverse colon is detached from the greater curvature of the stomach.

The pancreas is best exposed by lifting the stomach off the lesser sac with a Nathanson retractor.

7 Access to the duodenum in the lesser sac for duodenal repair can be challenging, and requires mobilization of the hepatic flexure. The hepatic flexure should be detached up to mid-transverse colon level. The most consistent method of gaining adequate exposure of the atretic duodenum is to follow the first part of the duodenum to its blind end and to lift it out of the posterior peritoneum with a hitch-stitch inserted through the abdominal wall.

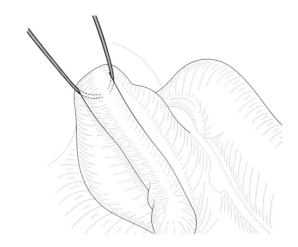

7

ACCESSING THE LOWER ABDOMEN AND PELVIS

Preoperative preparations

A distended bladder and sigmoid colon will impede surgical access. Except for brief and simple procedures such as inguinal hernia repair, bladder catheterization is essential to prevent accidental injury during insertion of working ports. Colonic enemas, where appropriate, may also help to maximize pelvic working space.

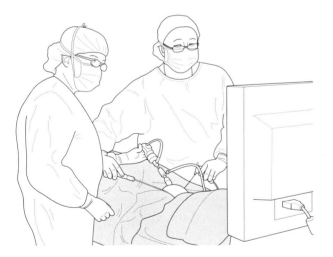

Positioning the patient

8 For most procedures in the low abdomen or pelvis, the surgeon and assistant may stand on each side of the table, with the video which is placed at the foot of the table.

Placing the patient in the Trendelenburg position will also allow abdominal viscera to be retracted from the pelvic cavity to provide an uninterrupted view.

8

RETROPERITONEAL (RENAL) ACCESS

Both the transperitoneal or posterior retroperitoneal approach are equally popular for access to the kidneys and adrenals, depending on the surgical indications and needs.

The transperitoneal exposure of the kidney has the advantage of better and more extensile exposure and can either be transmesocolic or retrocolic, by mobilizing the colon to expose the kidney. The authors' preference is to mobilize the colon because of the limited exposure offered by the transmesocolic approach.

Posterior retroperitoneal approach

9 The posterior retroperitoneal approach is similar to an open posterior lumbotomy approach. The patient is positioned prone or semi-prone and a 1-cm incision is made between the 12th rib and the iliac crest at the lateral margin of the quadratus lumborum. Additional ports for hand instruments can then be inserted under direct internal visualisation as per diagram.

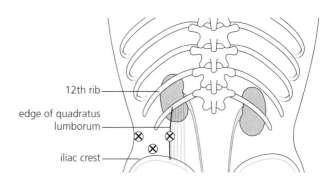

12th rib

edge of quadratus lumborum

iliac crest

9

Developing the space: the 'pneumoretroperitoneum'

A straight hemostat is introduced into this incision through the lateral edge of the quadratus lumborum, and this track is dilated sufficiently to introduce a balloon into the retroperitoneal space. A balloon, fashioned out of a digit of a large glove and feeding catheter, is inserted into the retroperitoneal space and this balloon is gently inflated with about 200 mL normal saline and kept inflated for about 8 minutes before it is deflated and removed. This will give sufficient time for the balloon to act as a tamponade to reduce bleeding from the wall of the space created. Some surgeons prefer to insufflate air, but this is compressible unlike saline and may not create the space necessary to manipulate instruments.

Two additional instrument ports are then inserted under direct vision to perform retroperitoneal surgery.

Delivering large viscera

Large cystic organs, such as benign ovarian cysts or non-functioning hydronephrotic kidneys can be punctured and the fluid aspirated before delivery through the port site.

The supraumbilical linea alba incision can be extended laterally on either side to remove reasonably large organs intact using the Tan–Bianchi approach originally described for open pyloromyotomy.

In older children, a laparoscopic bag retrieval can be introduced via a 12-mm port, and the organ placed in the bag, the neck of which is exteriorized, and the solid organ 'morcellated' inside the bag.

However, it is difficult, if not impossible, to place a giant spleen into a bag inside a small abdomen, and our preference is to perform a small Pfannenstiel incision to remove the solid organ in one piece.

Closure of port sites

Although laparoscopy wounds are seldom large enough for bowels to herniate through, omentum can herniate through a port site and cause internal herniation through a 'barber pole' adhesion. It is best to close the fascia of all 5-mm or larger ports to prevent omental herniation.

The Hasson port site can usually be closed by tightening the purse string previously placed to secure the port. However, before closing this port, it is necessary to lift the port away from the viscera to ensure that a slip of omentum is not caught in the port site.

The skin can be effectively closed with cyanoacrylate cement which also serves as a waterproof dressing.

Suggested reading:

Esposito C, Mattioli G, Monguzzi GL, *et al.* Complications and conversions of pediatric videosurgery: the Italian multicentric experience on 1689 procedures. *Surgical Endoscopy* 2002; **16**(5): 795–8.

Kalfa N, Allal H, Raux O, *et al.* Multicentric assessment of the safety of neonatal videosurgery. *Surgical Endoscopy* 2007; **21**(2): 303–8.

Dutta S, Langer JC. Minimal access surgical approaches in infants and children. *Advances in Surgery* 2004; **38**: 337–61.

McHoney M, Eaton S, Pierro A. Metabolic response to surgery in infants and children. *European Journal of Pediatric Surgery* 2009; **19**(5): 275–85.

McHoney M, Eaton S, Wade A, *et al.* Effect of laparoscopy and laparotomy on energy and protein metabolism in children: a randomized controlled trial. *Journal of Pediatrics* 2010; **157**(3): 439–44.

42

Nissen fundoplication

LEWIS SPITZ and AGOSTINO PIERRO

INTRODUCTION

Gastroesophageal reflux is more common in infancy and childhood than is generally recognized. Although in the majority of cases (>90 percent), the reflux resolves spontaneously within the first year of life as the lower esophageal sphincter matures, a small but significant proportion of cases develop complications requiring prolonged medical or surgical treatment.

HISTORY

In 1956, Rudolph Nissen of Basel, Switzerland, described the fundoplication procedure that he had been using for the previous 20 years to minimize postoperative reflux after resection of a peptic ulcer in the region of the cardia of the stomach. The technique did not involve division of the short gastric vessels, and the wrap extended for 4–6 cm on the esophagus. Subsequently, modifications have been made by Rossetti, Dor, Toupet, Donahue, and DeMeester.

PRINCIPLES AND JUSTIFICATION

Clinical presentation

EARLY INFANCY

The child presents with recurrent vomiting, which may be regurgitant or projectile. The vomitus may contain altered blood (the 'coffee-grounds' appearance) or traces of frank blood. The infant fails to thrive and may be constipated.

OLDER CHILD

Vomiting is a major feature. In addition, the child complains of heartburn and dysphagia and may occasionally present with iron-deficient anemia secondary to chronic blood loss.

MENTAL RETARDATION

Recurrent vomiting occurs in 10–15 percent of neurologically impaired children. It is often regarded as part of the neurologic problem, but around 75 percent of these children have significant gastroesophageal reflux. It is notable that there is a high failure rate of medical treatment in this group.

ANATOMIC ANOMALY

Gastroesophageal reflux is more common in infants with esophageal atresia, diaphragmatic hernia, anterior abdominal wall defects, and malrotation.

ASPIRATION SYNDROMES

There is a small but definite association of aspiration symptoms (asthma, pneumonitis, cyanosis, apneic episodes) and gastroesophageal reflux.

OTHER UNUSUAL PRESENTATIONS

Other presentations include rumination, Sandifer's syndrome (torsion spasms of the neck), protein-losing enteropathy, irritability, and hyperactivity.

Pathologic anatomy

Reflux may, or may not, be accompanied by an associated hiatus hernia. Two types of hiatus hernia are recognized.

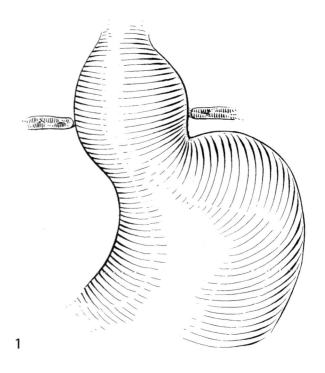

1 Sliding hiatus hernia, characterized by ascent of the cardia into the mediastinum.

1

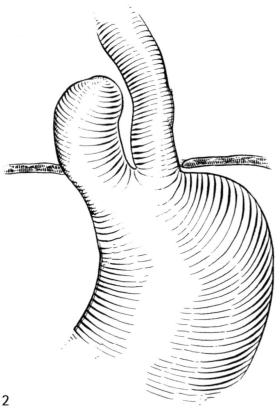

2

2 Paraesophageal or rolling hernia, in which the gastroesophageal junction remains in the abdomen while part of the gastric fundus prolapses through the esophageal hiatus into the mediastinum.

The sliding hernia is often associated with reflux, while gastric stasis in the paraesophageal hernia predisposes to peptic ulceration, perforation, or hemorrhage.

NORMAL MECHANISMS PREVENTING REFLUX

Physiologic control of reflux depends on the following factors:

- Anatomic:
  - length and pressure of the lower esophageal sphincter;
  - the intra-abdominal segment of the esophagus;
  - the gastroesophageal angle (angle of His);
  - the lower esophageal mucosal rosette;
  - the phrenoesophageal membrane;
  - the diaphragmatic hiatal pinchcock effect.
- Physiologic:
  - co-ordinated effective peristaltic clearance of the distal esophagus;
  - normal gastric emptying.

PATHOPHYSIOLOGY OF REFLUX

The squamous epithelium of the esophagus is unable to resist the irritant effect of gastric juices. The acid pepsin causes a chemical inflammation with erythema of the mucosa. With continued reflux, the mucosa becomes friable and bleeds easily on contact. Later, frank ulceration develops, which, with repeated attempts at repair and relapse, eventually leads to stricture formation. This process is summarized in **Figure 42.1**.

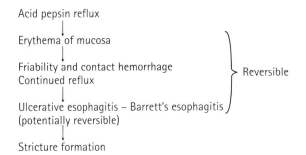

Figure 42.1 Pathophysiology of reflux.

INDICATIONS FOR ANTIREFLUX SURGERY

Antireflux surgery should be undertaken in the presence of an established esophageal stricture or when conservative measures of treatment have failed. Surgery may also be considered at an early stage (1) in the presence of an anatomic anomaly, e.g. esophageal atresia, malrotation, exomphalos and (2) in the presence of associated neurologic impairment, where the response to conservative measures is notoriously poor. Surgery may also be necessary if the patient is suffering from apneic episodes and repeated respiratory infections due to aspiration of refluxed material, or if the infant fails to thrive despite adequate therapy.

PREOPERATIVE

Investigations

A number of preoperative investigations should be performed.

- **Barium esophagogram**, with particular attention to the anatomy of the esophagus (presence of strictures, ulcerative esophagitis, abnormal narrowing or displacement); presence of a hiatus hernia; peristaltic activity of the esophagus and rate of clearance of contrast material; the degree of gastroesophageal reflux (grade I, distal esophagus; grade II, proximal/thoracic esophagus; grade III, cervical esophagus; grade IV, continuous reflux; grade V, aspiration into tracheobronchial tree); and evidence of gastric outlet obstruction.
- **Esophageal pH monitoring**. Continuous 24-hour monitoring of the pH in the distal esophagus is the most accurate method of documenting reflux. A pH of less than 4 is regarded as significant. During the 24-hour recording, the following parameters should be examined:
  - the number of episodes during which the pH falls below 4;
  - the duration of each reflux episode;
  - the number of episodes lasting more than 5 minutes;
  - the total duration of reflux, expressed as a percentage of recording time.
- **Esophageal manometry**. Pressure recordings are made with continuously perfused, open-tipped catheters or solid-state pressure transducers. A high-pressure zone is normally present in the distal esophagus. Individual pressure values are unreliable diagnostic indicators of reflux, but may be useful in predicting cases that will eventually require surgical treatment.
- **Endoscopy and biopsy**. Endoscopy will determine the degree of esophagitis; histology of the biopsy will provide pathologic grading of inflammatory cell infiltration. Four grades of esophagitis are recognized at endoscopy:
  - grade I, erythema of mucosa;
  - grade II, friability of mucosa;
  - grade III, ulcerative esophagitis;
  - grade IV, stricture.
- **Scintiscanning**. Technetium (^{99}Tc) sulfur colloid scans may be useful in documenting pulmonary aspiration.

MEDICAL MANAGEMENT

Small, frequent, thickened feeds should be given to infants with reflux. A 30° head-elevated, prone position is the most suitable posture for young infants. Antacids-alkalis with or without alginic acid (Gaviscon) should be administered. Histamine receptor antagonists (cimetidine, ranitidine) will suppress acid secretion and allow severe esophagitis to heal. Omeprasol (a proton pump inhibitor) is even more efficient. Metoclopramide and bethanechol increase lower esophageal pressure and stimulate gastric emptying.

ANESTHESIA

General endotracheal anesthesia is administered, with the patient supine. A single dose of prophylactic broad-spectrum antibiotics should be given after induction of anesthesia. The addition of epidural analgesia is extremely valuable in reducing postoperative pain and preventing respiratory complications.

OPERATION

Some surgeons insist on inserting a large-caliber bougie in the esophagus during the construction of the fundoplication to ensure that the wrap is not too tight. The author prefers a regular-size nasogastric tube and constructs a very loose wrap.

Incision

3 In the majority of cases, the ideal approach is via a mid-line upper abdominal incision extending from the xiphisternum to the umbilicus. Alternatively, a left subcostal muscle-cutting incision may be used.

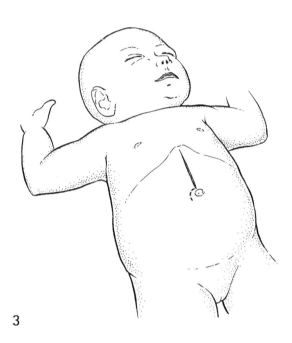

3

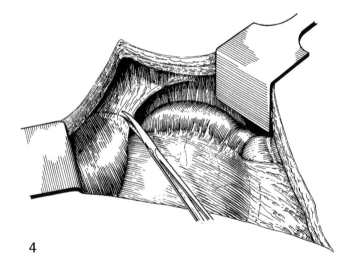

4

Exposure

4 Adequate exposure of the gastroesophageal junction will usually be obtained by retracting the left lobe of the liver anterosuperiorly. Additional exposure may be attained, if necessary, by dividing the left triangular ligament in the avascular plane and then retracting the left lobe of the liver to the right. In older children, especially children with kyphoscoliosis or obese children, the use of the self-retaining retractor is invaluable in obtaining adequate exposure of the operative field.

Mobilization of the fundus of the stomach

5a,b The proximal one-third to one-half of the greater curvature of the stomach is liberated from its attachment to the spleen by ligating and dividing the upper short gastric vessels in the gastrosplenic ligament. This is accomplished most safely by passing a right-angled clamp around each vessel in turn and ligating or coagulating with bipolar diathermy the vessel on the gastric and splenic side before dividing it.

When the vessels in the gastrosplenic ligament have been divided, the spleen should be allowed to fall back into the posterior peritoneum, thereby avoiding inadvertent trauma. Splenectomy should rarely be necessary in this procedure, even in revision fundoplication operations. The fundus is now sufficiently free to allow for a loose ('floppy') fundoplication.

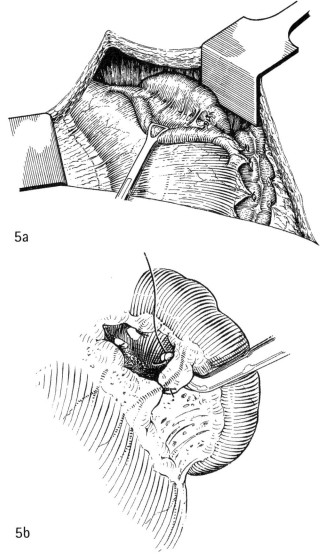

5a

5b

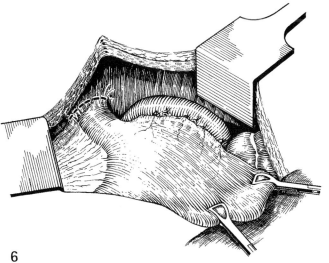

6

Exposure of the esophageal hiatus

6 The phrenoesophageal membrane is placed on stretch by downward traction on the stomach while the diaphragmatic muscle is retracted superiorly. The avascular membrane marked by a 'white line' is incised with scissors and the musculature of the esophagus displayed. The anterior vagus nerve will be seen coursing on the surface of the esophagus. It should be carefully protected and preserved.

Mobilization of the distal esophagus

7 Using a combination of sharp and blunt dissection, the lower end of the esophagus is encircled, avoiding injury to the posterior vagus nerve. A rubber sling is placed around the esophagus incorporating the posterior vagus nerve, which will be included in the fundoplication. The lower 2 or 3 cm of esophagus hiatus is completely exposed by dividing the upper part of the gastrohepatic omentum above the left gastric vessels.

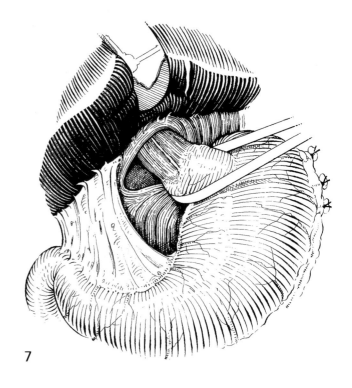

7

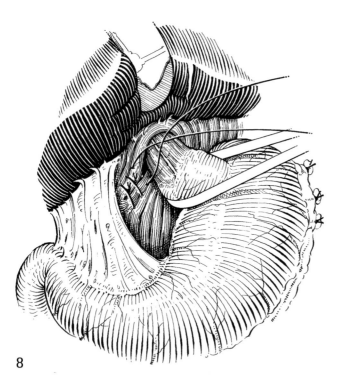

8

Narrowing of the hiatus

8 The esophageal hiatus is narrowed posterior to the esophagus by placing deep sutures through the crura of the diaphragm. The sutures are tied loosely to prevent them cutting through, but leaving sufficient space alongside the esophagus to allow the tip of a finger to pass. Two or three or more sutures may be required for this purpose.

Construction of the fundoplication

9a–c The mobilized fundus of the stomach is folded behind the esophagus so that the invaginated part of the stomach appears on the right side of the esophagus. It is important not to twist the stomach during this maneuver and to ensure that the stomach has been sufficiently mobilized to be able to fashion a loose wrap.

The length of the wrap varies from 1.0 cm in the infant to 2–2.5 cm in the older child. Commencing at the level of the gastroesophageal junction, three to four sutures of non-absorbable material (3/0 or 4/0) are placed through the stomach and esophageal muscle. Each suture passes from left to right through the anterior wall of the stomach, through the esophageal muscle (taking care not to enter the lumen of the esophagus), and through the wall of the mobilized portion of the fundus of the stomach, which has been folded behind the esophagus. Traction on the first (untied) suture brings the rest of the operating field clearly into view and facilitates the insertion of the remaining two or three proximal parallel sutures through the anterior wall of the stomach, esophageal muscle, and 'prolapsed' fundus. When all these sutures are in place, they are tied serially without tension on the wrap.

A second layer of non-absorbable sutures including the seromuscular surface of the stomach only may be placed superficial to the primary sutures to prevent disruption of the wrap.

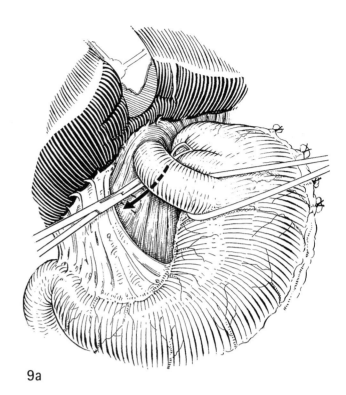

9a

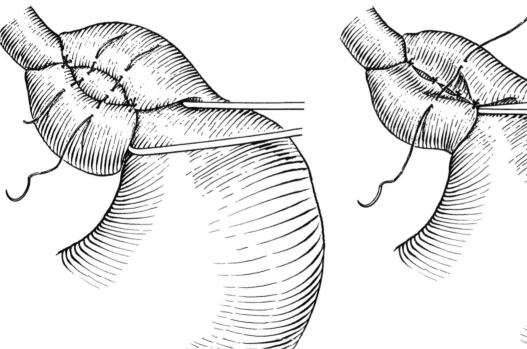

9b

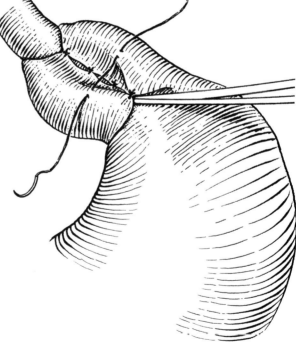

9c

10 The proximal suture of the second layer should be passed through the anterior wall of the esophageal hiatus in the diaphragm. An additional two or three sutures may be placed between the hiatus and the fundoplication to prevent the wrap migrating into the posterior mediastinum.

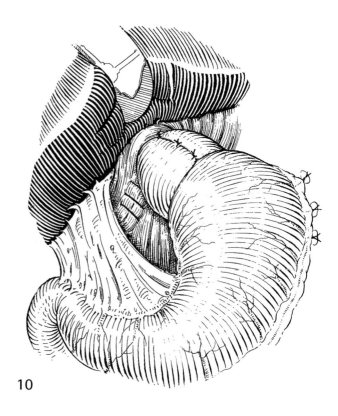

10

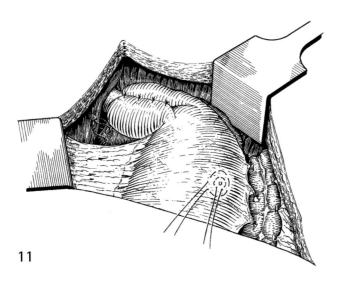

11

Closure

The wound is closed either in layers or with interrupted en-masse sutures. A subcuticular suture approximates the skin edges.

Gastrostomy

11 A feeding gastrostomy should be constructed in neurologically impaired children who are unable to eat normally. A suitable area on the anterior wall of the stomach is selected to permit the gastrostomy site to be anchored to the anterior abdominal wall without exerting traction on the fundoplication.

Two rows of circumferentially placed non-absorbable sutures are placed through the seromuscular layer of the stomach. A suitable-size Malecot catheter is inserted through a centrally placed gastrotomy into the stomach and the sutures are tied, invaginating the gastrotomy site. The tube is brought out through a separate stab incision in the left hypochondrium, and the stomach wall is sutured to the anterior abdominal wall at the exit site to prevent leakage.

POSTOPERATIVE CARE

Nasogastric decompression and intravenous fluids are continued until postoperative ileus has resolved (usually 48–72 hours).

Complications

- Death following this procedure is extremely uncommon. In severely retarded children, there is a small but not insignificant risk of mortality, related mainly to the underlying disease.
- Wound infection occasionally occurs.
- Respiratory complications, such as pneumonia or atelectasis, particularly affect severely retarded patients and patients undergoing fundoplication for chronic respiratory complications secondary to aspiration.
- Dysphagia may result from a wrap that is either too long or too tight.
- The gastroesophageal reflux may recur because of either disruption of the fundoplication or herniation of the fundoplication into the posterior mediastinum.
- Paraesophageal hernia occurs following inadequate approximation or disruption of the crural repair.
- Gas bloat, hiccup, retching, and dumping symptoms are usually transient.
- Adhesion intestinal obstruction is particularly common if an additional intra-abdominal procedure, such as gastrostomy, incidental appendectomy, or correction of malrotation is performed. It is important to alert the parents to the danger of intestinal obstruction, as the inability to vomit may result in inordinate delay in establishing the diagnosis.

LAPAROSCOPIC NISSEN FUNDOPLICATION

There are few contraindications to laparoscopic fundoplication and are mainly related to the cardiovascular or respiratory status of the child. Previous abdominal surgery is not necessarily a contraindication for laparoscopic surgery, as often the visceral adhesions are confined to the lower abdomen and, if present, in the upper abdomen can be divided by laparoscopy. The presence of previous gastrostomy makes the operation a little more difficult. In such cases, (1) the gastrostomy can be left in place and the operation is carried out above the gastrostomy or (2) the gastrostomy is taken down the opening on the stomach closed with intracorporeal sutures of 4/0 or 3/0 Prolene sutures. At the end of the procedure, a laparoscopic gastrostomy is fashioned again through a new opening in the anterior wall of the stomach.

Preoperative preparation

Particularly in neurologically impaired children, the transverse colon can be distended making the visualization of the stomach more difficult. It is recommended to perform a rectal washout a few hours before the operation to avoid over-distension of the colon and facilitate its retraction below the stomach.

Anesthesia

General anesthesia with full relaxation and endotracheal intubation is mandatory in children undergoing any form of laparoscopic surgery. The small attendant risk of breaching the left pleural cavity during esophageal mobilization and causing a tension pneumothorax is an additional reason for having complete airway control. A large nasogastric tube is inserted to ensure that the stomach is empty for the duration of the operation.

PATIENT POSITIONING

12a An infant is positioned at the foot of the table as per floor plan and the video monitor is placed at the head of the table. The table should be tilted head-up about 20–30°.

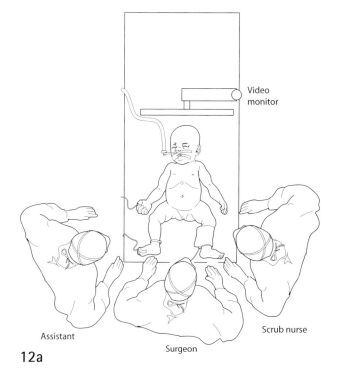

12a

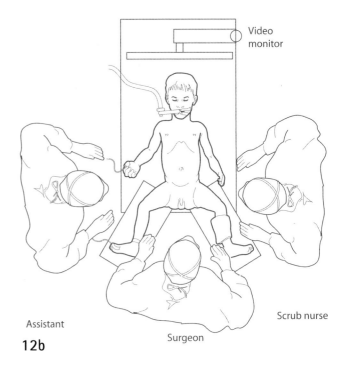

12b In older children, the legs are abducted using a special split table and the operator works between the legs at the lower end of the table; the position of the video monitor is as above.

Assistant

Surgeon

Scrub nurse

12b

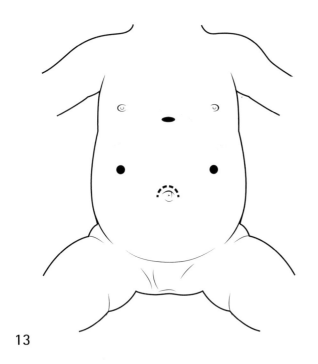

13

PORT PLACEMENTS

13 The operation is performed with three ports. A primary port for the telescope (5-mm Hasson) is usually placed above the umbilicus. Two ports for introduction of instruments are placed in the right and left upper quadrant of the abdomen; it is important to insert these ports quite laterally so that a wide angle is created that facilitates the intracorporeal suturing. The port on the right upper quadrant can be 3 or 5 mm depending on the size of the patient. The authors prefer a 5-mm disposable port in the left quadrant as it allows for the introduction of needles for suturing and can accommodate both 3- and 5-mm laparoscopic instruments. In the midline of the epigastrium, a small incision is made for the introduction of a Nathanson liver retractor without insertion of a port. The liver retractor size is decided on the basis of the size of child and that of the liver. The liver retractor is kept in position with the help of a fast clamp.

LAPAROSCOPIC INSTRUMENTATION

The following are the instruments required:

- 30° telescope
- 5-mm Hasson cannula
- Nathanson liver retractor

- Atraumatic intestinal grasper
- Kelly forcep
- 3-mm needle holder
- Scissors
- Hook diathermy or ultrasonic scalpel.

LIVER RETRACTION

14 Using the Nathanson liver retractor, the liver is retracted upwards, allowing dissection of the esophagogastric junction. Following a previous failed open or laparoscopic fundoplication, adhesions will be present between the stomach and the liver. These adhesions are carefully divided using hook diathermy as the liver retractor is moved into the desired position.

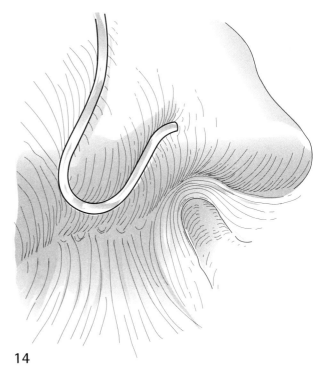

14

EXPOSURE OF THE CARDIOESOPHAGEAL JUNCTION

15 The key to this is to open the phrenoesophageal ligament and gastrohepatic omentum overlying the right crus. The right crus and esophagus are easily identified in this window created in the phrenoesophageal ligament. This dissection is made using hook diathermy (3 or 5 mm) inserted via the right upper quadrant port.

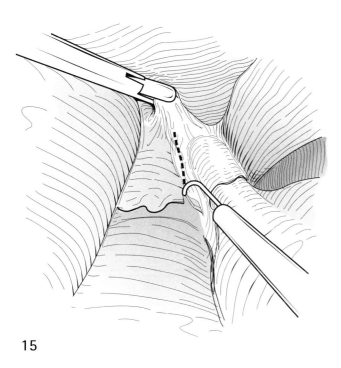

15

CRURAL EXPOSURE

16 The free edge of the right crus can then be separated from the esophagus by a combination of sharp and blunt dissection. The intra-abdominal esophagus should be exposed and separated from its surrounding adventitia and visceral peritoneum.

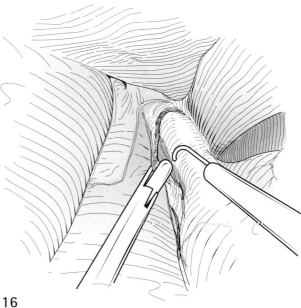

16

17 The left crus can be identified by following the edge of the right crus over the 'white line' where it merges with the left crus. The edge of the left crus should be exposed and separated from the esophagus. Some loose adventitial tissue attaching the fundus to the diaphragm and left crus can be identified by gentle downward traction on the fundus. The hook diathermy is the best instrument to avoid bleeding during dissection.

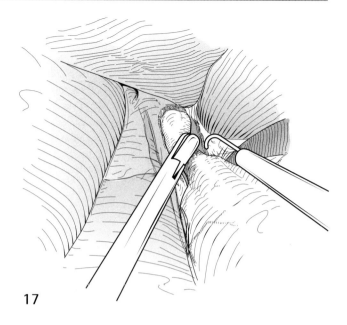

17

A too extensive dissection may result in an iatrogenic hiatus hernia and may predispose to failure of Nissen postoperatively due to disruption of the crura repair and herniation of the wrap. Recently, some surgeons have proposed minimal crural dissection to avoid disrupting the natural tissue planes and repairing of the crura only in the presence of hiatus hernia.

DIVISION OF THE SHORT GASTRIC VESSELS

Only the most cranial short gastric vessels are divided using the hook diathermy. Occasionally, the fundus is not completely mobile and does not allow a 360° wrap to be performed without tension; in these cases, it may be necessary to divide some additional short gastric vessels.

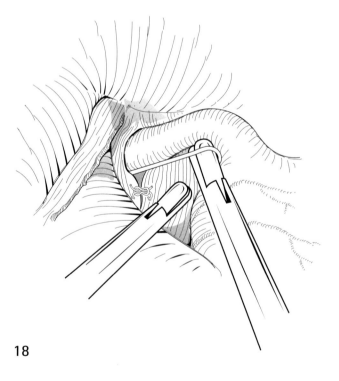

CREATION OF POSTERIOR ESOPHAGEAL WINDOW

18 The posterior esophageal window is created by opening the gastrohepatic omentum by blunt dissection. The esophagus is lifted anteriorly and the posterior vagus nerve identified. The left crus must be positively identified before creating the posterior window, otherwise there is a risk of breaching the left pleura, with resultant left tension pneumothorax. It is important to avoid damage to the crura during dissection and creation of the esophageal window.

18

APPROXIMATION OF THE CRURA POSTERIORLY TO THE ESOPHAGUS

19 The right and left crura are approximated posteriorly to the esophagus using interrupted sutures of non-absorbable monofilament (Prolene 4/0 or 3/0). To visualize the crura, the esophagus including the posterior vagal nerve, is lifted anteriorly. This maneuver is facilitated by insertion of a Nylon tape around the esophagogastric junction and elevation of the tape using a grasper inserted in the epigastrium without the need of inserting an extra port. In patients who need a gastrostomy, a 5-mm port can be inserted where the tube gastrostomy will be introduced (see below).

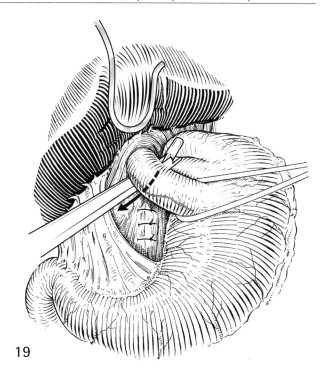

19

FUNDAL MOBILIZATION

The fundus can usually be identified through the posterior esophageal window created, and it should be grasped, and brought through the posterior window. This is considerably easier without a bougie in the esophagus.

CREATION OF THE WRAP

20a,b Non-absorbable monofilament sutures (Prolene 4/0 or 3/0) are then used to perform a 360° wrap of the fundus of the stomach around the distal esophagus. Do not be concerned if this first suture appears too tight or if it appears to be in an unsatisfactory position. The first suture can be replaced after placing a second suture in a more suitable position. The wrap can be completed with three interrupted, non-absorbable sutures, anchoring each of them to the anterior esophageal wall to prevent it from sliding.

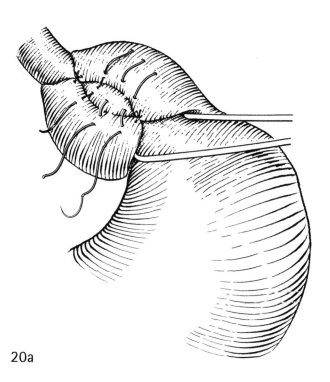

20a

21 The wrap should be floppy without any tension on the fundus or the sutures. This should avoid postoperative dysphagia.

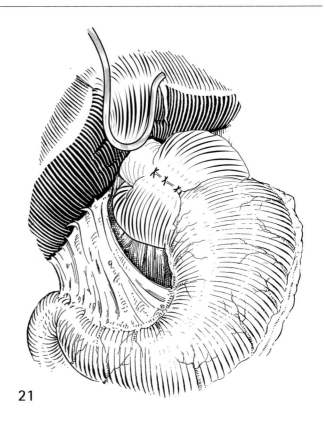

21

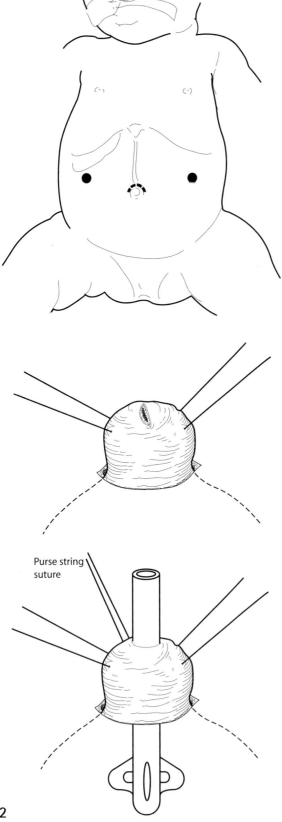

Purse string suture

22

INSERTION OF LAPAROSCOPIC-ASSISTED GASTROSTOMY

22 After performing the wrap, the anterior wall of the stomach midway between the wrap and the pylorus is grasped and brought out through an opening in the epigastrium. If a port was inserted in this position, it will be necessary to enlarge the opening to achieve at least a 1-cm opening in the fascia and the peritoneum. The selected area of the stomach is then retracted outside the epigastric incision/port site, and to facilitate this maneuver, insufflation is stopped. The anterior wall of the stomach is maintained outside the wound by insertion of two stay sutures of Vicryl 4/0 positioned approximately 3 cm apart. A small gastrotomy is made between these two stay sutures and a purse string of the same suture material is placed around the opening. A 12 Fr Malecot catheter is inserted and the purse string ligated around the catheter. The two stay sutures on the stomach are anchored to fascia. A bladder syringe is used to inject water in the stomach. Pneumoperitoneum is created again and by laparoscopy it is ascertained that (1) the stomach is anchored correctly to the anterior abdominal wall and (2) there is no leaking from the gastrostomy site. The gastrostomy tube is secured to the skin by using a non-absorbable suture.

Closure

The abdomen should then be desufflated and the fascia closed with absorbable sutures. The skin can be closed with Dermabond or skin glue.

Postoperative care

The nasogastric tube should be left on drainage overnight and removed the following day. If a gastrostomy tube is inserted, the nasogastric tube is removed at the end of the operation and the gastrostomy tube left on drainage. Oral or gastrostomy feeds are restarted on the first postoperative day. Patients should remain on a sloppy, semi-liquid diet for the first 2 weeks after fundoplication, gradually increasing the consistency of the food.

Outcome

Laparoscopic fundoplication generally has a good outcome, except in patients with neurological impairment in whom the incidence of wrap migration, disruption, and failure to correct reflux is higher. An immediate postoperative complication is dysphagia, which, if sufficiently symptomatic, can be relieved with an early flexible endoscopy or, if not responding, by performing single balloon dilatation. Retching postoperatively can occur, particularly in children with neurological impairment.

A randomized blinded controlled trial comparing open and laparoscopic Nissen fundoplication in infants and children indicated that there was no difference in the postoperative analgesia requirements and recovery after the two procedures. Early postoperative outcome confirmed equal efficacy, but fewer children had retching after laparoscopy.

FURTHER READING

Kubiak R, Spitz L, Drake D, Pierro A. Effectiveness of fundoplication in early infancy. *Journal of Paediatric Surgery* 1999; **34**: 295–9.

Leape LL, Ramenofsky ML. Surgical treatment of gastroesophageal reflux in children. Results of Nissen fundoplication in 100 children. *American Journal of Diseases of Children* 1980; **134**: 935–8.

McHoney M, Wade AM, Eaton S *et al.* Clinical outcome of a randomized controlled blinded trial of open versus laparoscopic Nissen fundoplication in infants and children. *Annals of Surgery* 2011; **254**: 209–16.

Pacilli M, Eaton S, Maritsi D *et al.* Factors predicting failure of redo Nissen fundoplication in children. *Pediatric Surgery International* 2007; **23**: 499–503.

Randolph J. Experience with the Nissen fundoplication for correction of gastroesophageal reflux in infants. *Annals of Surgery* 1983; **198**: 579–84.

Spitz L, Kirtane J. Results and complications of surgery for gastroesophageal reflux. *Archives of Disease in Childhood* 1985; **60**: 743–7.

Spitz L, Roth K, Kiely EM *et al.* Operation for gastrooesophageal reflux associated with severe mental retardation. *Archives of Disease in Childhood* 1993; **68**: 347–51.

St Peter SD, Barnhart DC, Ostlie DJ *et al.* Minimal vs extensive esophageal mobilization during laparoscopic fundoplication: a prospective randomized trial. *Journal of Pediatric Surgery* 2011; **46**: 163–8.

Tunnel WP, Smith EI, Carson JA. Gastroesophageal reflux in childhood: the dilemma of surgical success. *Annals of Surgery* 1983; **197**: 560–5.

43

Achalasia

LEWIS SPITZ and BENNO URE

OPEN ACHALASIA

LEWIS SPITZ

HISTORY

Achalasia was first described by Willis in 1672. He treated the patient by fashioning a rod out of a whale bone with a sponge on the end with which the patient was able to force food into his stomach. In 1877, Zenker and von Ziemssen, and in 1884 Mackenzie, suggested that achalasia was due to diminished contractile power of the esophageal musculature. In 1888, Meltzer and Mikulicz independently postulated that spasmodic contraction of the cardiac sphincter was the etiologic factor. In the same year, Einhorn proposed that the condition was due to failure of relaxation of the cardia on swallowing.

PRINCIPLES AND JUSTIFICATION

Achalasia is a motility disorder of the esophagus characterized by an absence of peristalsis and a failure of relaxation of the lower esophageal sphincter. The cardinal symptoms in childhood are vomiting, dysphagia, chest pains and recurrent respiratory infections, and weight loss. The child learns to eat very slowly and to drink large quantities of fluid to encourage food to enter the stomach. At first, there is only regurgitation of food, but later vomiting of undigested food eaten days earlier occurs. The child with achalasia is often first referred to a psychiatrist for treatment of food aversion or anorexia.

Histopathology

Strips of muscle from the distal esophagus reveal varying pathologies from complete absence of ganglion cells to chronic inflammatory changes through to normal ganglia. Histochemistry reveals a significant reduction in all neuropeptides, particularly vasoactive intestinal polypeptide, galanin, and neuropeptide Y.

Treatment

MEDICAL TREATMENT

Transient relief of symptoms can be achieved with nifedipine, a calcium antagonist that reduces the pressure at the lower esophageal sphincter.

FORCEFUL DILATATION

The aim of this treatment is to physically disrupt the muscle fibers of the lower esophageal sphincter by means of pneumatic or balloon dilatation. A fluid-filled (Plummer) or air-filled (Browne–McHardy, Rider–Moller, angioplasty catheter) bag of fixed diameter, or the balloon dilator, is radiologically positioned in the distal esophagus and gently inflated. Relief of symptoms in children is at best temporary, but may occasionally last for prolonged periods. Recently, it has been shown that botulinum toxin injected into the lower esophageal sphincter musculature results in symptomatic relief, but the effect is short lived.

SURGICAL TREATMENT

The basis of all surgical procedures is the cardiomyotomy described in 1914 by Heller. Controversies concern the length of the myotomy, the extent to which the myotomy extends onto the stomach, and the necessity for an antireflux procedure.

The principle of the procedure is to perform a myotomy over the distal 4–6 cm of esophagus, extending the incision for 1 cm onto the anterior wall of the stomach. The myotomy is covered by a short, floppy Nissen fundoplication to protect against subsequent gastroesophageal reflux.

PREOPERATIVE

Diagnosis

RADIOLOGIC FEATURES

1 A plain chest x-ray may show a dilated, food-filled esophagus with an air–fluid level. There may be radiologic signs of recurrent aspiration pneumonitis.

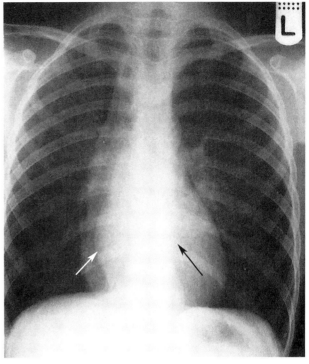

1

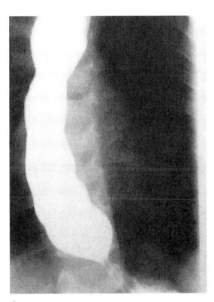

2

2 The diagnostic features of achalasia on barium swallow are a dilated esophagus, absence of stripping waves, incoordinated contraction, and obstruction at the gastroesophageal junction with prolonged retention of barium in the esophagus. Failure of relaxation of the lower esophageal sphincter gives rise to the classical 'rat-tail' deformity of funneling and narrowing of the distal esophagus.

ENDOSCOPY

The main value of esophagoscopy is to exclude an organic cause for the obstruction.

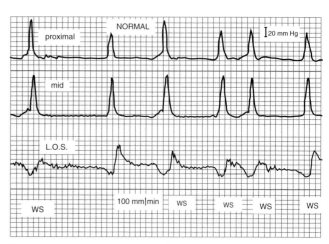

3a

ESOPHAGEAL MANOMETRY

3a,b The criteria for diagnosis include: (1) a high-pressure (>30 mmHg) lower esophageal sphincter zone; (2) failure of the lower esophagus to relax in response to swallowing; (3) absence of propulsive peristalsis; and (4) incoordinated tertiary contractions in the body of the esophagus.

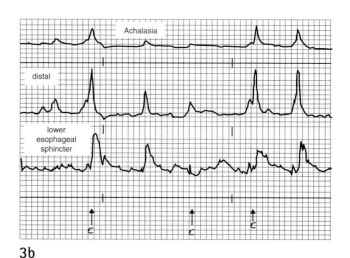

3b

Anesthesia

General endotracheal anesthesia is administered, with the patient supine on the operating table. Measures must be taken to avoid aspiration of esophageal contents during the induction of anesthesia. Preoperative esophagoscopy is recommended to ensure complete evacuation of retained food and secretions from the esophagus. A medium-caliber nasogastric tube is passed into the stomach.

OPERATION

Incision

4 The approach is via an upper abdominal midline incision extending from the xiphisternum to the umbilicus.

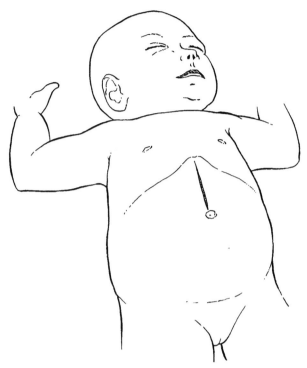

4

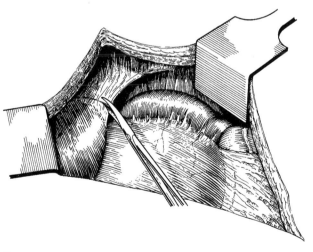

Exposure

5 In most cases, adequate exposure of the abdominal esophagus can be obtained by retracting the left lobe of the liver anterosuperiorly with a wide retractor. If necessary, additional exposure may be attained by dividing the left triangular ligament in the avascular plane and retracting the left lobe of the liver towards the midline.

5

Mobilization of fundus of stomach

6a,b As a Nissen fundoplication will be performed in addition to the extended gastroesophageal myotomy, the operative procedure for fundoplication should be followed at an early stage.

The proximal one-third of the greater curvature of the stomach is liberated from its attachment to the spleen by ligating or coagulating with bipolar diathermy and dividing the short gastric vessels in the gastrosplenic ligament. This is accomplished most safely using a right-angled forceps passed around each vessel in turn. When the vessels in the upper part of the gastrosplenic ligament have been divided, the spleen should be allowed to fall back into the posterior peritoneum, thereby avoiding inadvertent trauma. Splenectomy should never be necessary in this procedure. The fundus is now sufficiently free to allow for a loose (floppy) fundoplication. The esophageal hiatus is completely exposed by dividing the upper part of the gastrohepatic omentum above the left gastric vessels.

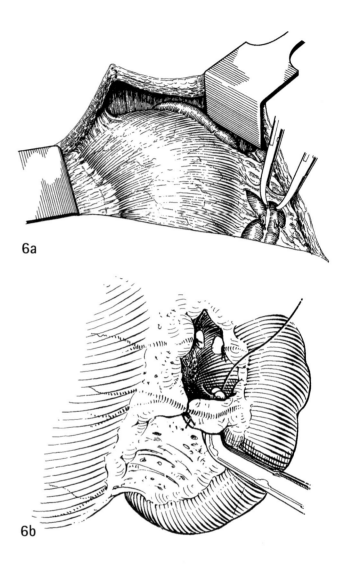

6a

6b

Exposure of esophageal hiatus

The phrenoesophageal membrane is placed on stretch by downward traction on the stomach while the diaphragmatic muscles are retracted superiorly. The avascular membrane is incised with scissors and the musculature of the esophagus displayed. The anterior vagal nerve will be seen coursing on the surface of the esophagus; it should be carefully protected and preserved.

Mobilization of the distal esophagus

7 Using a combination of sharp and blunt dissection, the lower end of the esophagus is encircled, taking care not to injure the posterior vagal nerve. A rubber sling is placed around the esophagus. The lower 5–8 cm of esophagus is now exposed through the esophageal hiatus into the posterior mediastinum using blunt dissection with either a moist pledget or right-angled forceps.

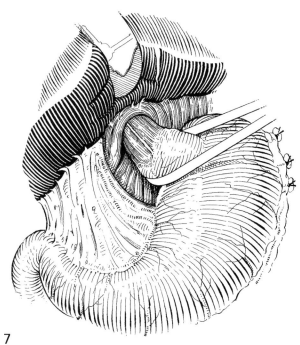

7

Gastroesophageal myotomy

8a–c The myotomy is performed on the anterior wall of the esophagus, extending for 1 cm onto the fundus of the stomach. A superficial incision (1–2 mm in depth) is made in the musculature of the distal 4–6 cm of the esophagus. The divided muscle is gently parted with a blunt hemostat until the underlying mucosa of the esophagus is encountered. The thickness of the muscle of the lower esophagus varies from a few millimeters to 0.5 cm or more. Great care must be taken to avoid opening into the lumen of the esophagus.

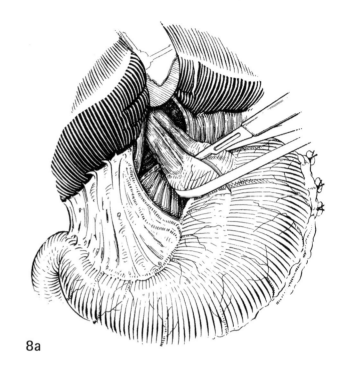

8a

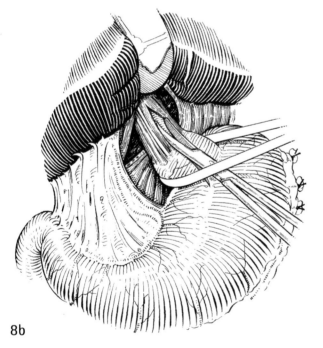

8b

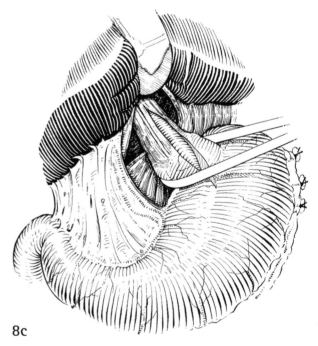

8c

9a,b The divided muscle is now separated from the underlying mucosa by blunt pledget dissection in the submucosal plane. The dissection is continued until at least 50 percent of the circumference of the esophagus is free of the overlying muscle.

The myotomy is extended through the gastroesophageal junction for 1 cm onto the fundus of the stomach and the musculature is similarly elevated from the underlying mucosa.

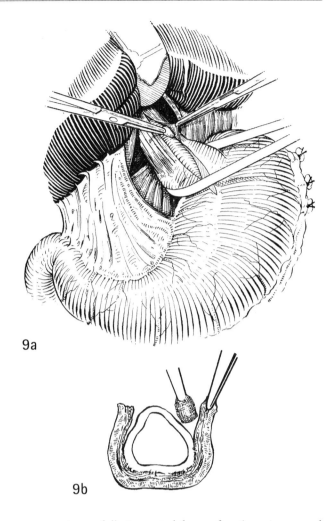

9a

9b

Testing for esophageal perforation

The stomach and esophagus are distended with air introduced through the nasogastric tube, and the exposed mucosa is carefully inspected for perforation. A mucosal defect should be carefully closed with fine polyglycolic acid sutures.

Narrowing of hiatus

10 The esophageal hiatus is narrowed posteriorly to the esophagus by placing deep sutures through the crura of the diaphragm. The sutures are tied loosely to prevent them from cutting through, leaving sufficient space alongside the esophagus to allow passage of the tip of a finger. Two or three sutures may be required for this purpose.

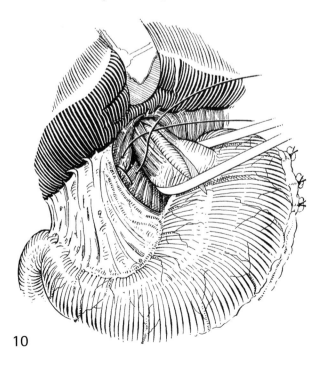

10

Fundoplication

11 A loose (floppy) Nissen fundoplication is now constructed over the distal 1–1.5 cm of the esophagus. The esophageal sutures are only placed through one side of the divided esophageal muscle in order to prevent reapproximation of the edges of the myotomy (see **Chapter 42**).

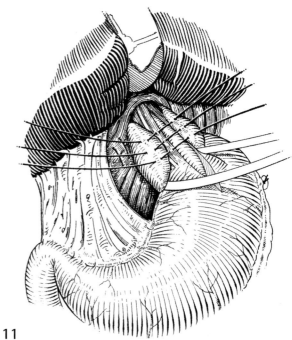

11

Wound closure

The wound is closed either in layers or with interrupted en masse sutures of 3/0 polyglycolic acid. A subcuticular suture approximates the skin edges.

POSTOPERATIVE CARE

Nasogastric decompression and intravenous fluids are continued until the postoperative ileus has resolved (mean of 3–4 days).

COMPLICATIONS

These can include mediastinitis due to failure to detect a mucosal perforation, and recurrence of symptoms if the muscle is not separated from the underlying mucosa for at least half the circumference of the esophagus. Gastroesophageal reflux is due to an inadequate fundoplication, and dysphagia for solids is due to too tight a fundoplication.

OUTCOME

After myotomy alone without an antireflux procedure, the long-term incidence of gastroesophageal reflux is around 15 percent. Relief of the dysphagia and respiratory problems is usually complete, but residual or recurrent pain may occur in 25 percent of patients and is due to diffuse esophageal spasm. The esophageal pain generally responds to pneumatic dilatation.

LAPAROSCOPIC ACHALASIA

BENNO URE

PREOPERATIVE PREPARATION OF THE PATIENT AND ANESTHESIA

Neither bowel preparation nor placement of a Foley catheter into the bladder is required. General anesthesia with full relaxation and endotracheal intubation is mandatory. It is recommended to perform esophageal endoscopy and clear the esophagus from retained food after induction of anesthesia. Thereafter, a medium size stiff nasogastric tube is inserted and left until the end of operation to fixate the esophagus and to ensure that the stomach is empty for the duration of the operation. Single shot intravenous perioperative antibiotic prophylaxis is given with induction of anesthesia.

Patient and team positioning

12 The patient is placed in a supine position at the lower end of the operation table. The operation is performed by the surgeon who stands between the legs of the patient and the camera assistant placed to his left. The scrub nurse is to the right hand of the surgeon. The laparoscopic tower including the video monitor is placed at the head or the left head of the table. The operation table is set in a reversed Trendelenburg position.

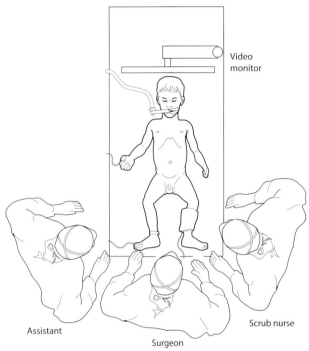

12

OPERATION

Laparoscopic instrumentation

Most patients with symptomatic achalasia are older than ten years of age. Therefore, 10-mm scopes and instruments with a diameter of 5-mm are used, however, the author prefers 3.5-mm ports in all children. The following instruments are required for laparoscopic Heller's cardiomyotomy:

- 30° telescope, 5- or 10-mm diameter
- One 5 or 10 mm infraumbilical trocar and cannula
- Two or three 3.5- or 5-mm trocars and cannulae
- One toothed, ratcheted grasper as liver retractor
- One curved scissors
- Two tissue forceps
- Two needle holders
- One monopolar hook
- One suction/irrigation device.

Port placements

13 A four-port technique is used. A 5- or 10-mm port for the telescope is inserted through or below the umbilicus with an open technique. Carbon dioxide is insufflated at a pressure of 8–10 mmHg. Two 3.5- or 5-mm instrument ports are inserted in the right and left mid-upper abdomen (one in each upper quadrant). A fourth trocar for the liver retractor may be introduced below the subcostal margin to the left of the falciform ligament. The grasper for liver retraction may also be introduced directly without using a trocar.

In case of difficulties with exposure, an additional 5-mm port may be introduced above the umbilicus right to the falciform ligament for the telescope. After changing the position of the telescope, an additional instrument may be used via the umbilical port for grasping the stomach and pulling it downward in these cases.

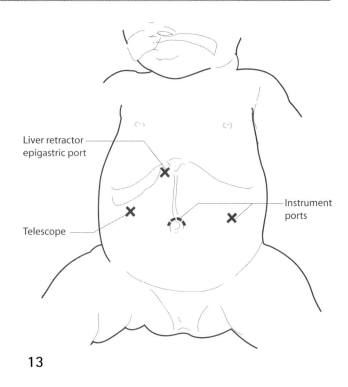

13

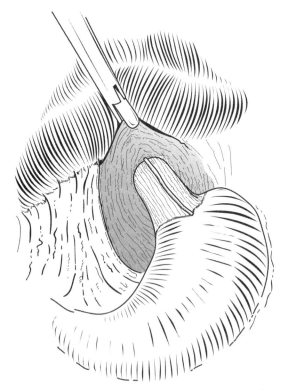

14

Liver retraction

14 The left lobe of the liver can be easily retracted upward with a single-toothed ratcheted grasper which is introduced through the subxyphoidal incision with or without use of a port. The grasper is fixed to the muscular diaphragm by grasping it just above the hiatus. It can then be left *in situ* during the duration of the operation.

Exposure of cardia and esophagus

15 The 'white line', which is the edge of the diaphragmatic crura, is easily identifiable by gentle downward traction of the stomach. The phrenoesophageal junction is divided using the monopolar hook and the anterior wall of the esophagus is freed. The dissection includes only the anterior and lateral esophagus and the posterior esophagus is not mobilized to prevent gastroesophageal reflux. The esophagus should be exposed from the crus down to the esophagogastric junction. The anterior vagal nerve should be identified, preserved, and pushed away from the myotomy incision.

Thereafter, the anterior crus is lifted away from the esophagus to gain entry into the mediastinal esophagus. An easy plane can be developed between the overarching crus and the esophagus, allowing the esophagus to be exposed in the mediastinum for up to 5 cm. Once an adequate length of intrathoracic esophagus has been exposed, attention should be redirected to the abdominal esophagus.

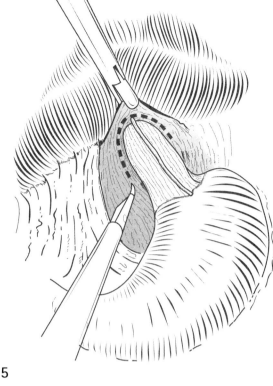

15

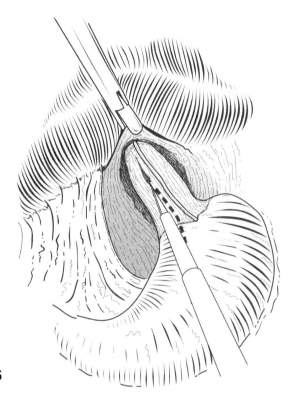

16

Esophageal myotomy

16 An esophageal myotomy is best started with a superficial incision on the anterior wall of the esophagus about 1 cm proximal to the esophagogastric junction. While it is possible to use monopolar diathermy or an ultrasonic scalpel to make this initial myotomy incision, both these instruments can produce deeper thermal damage, which may cause unrecognized damage of the underlying mucosa, resulting in delayed perforation.

17 Blunt curved scissor dissection is used and the longitudinal muscle layers are separated. The mucosa can be clearly seen as it herniates through the myotomy. The muscle layers should be spread further to the mediastinum for up to 5 cm using blunt dissection. Dissection is continued down to the gastric junction extending onto the fundus of the stomach, which can be identified when one sees the edge of circular gastric muscle fibers. The underlying mucosa should be allowed to pout outwards as much as possible. Bleeding from the esophageal muscle layers usually stops spontaneously and cauterization is unnecessary.

The mucosa is inspected for evidence of perforation and if there is concern, air may be instilled into the esophagus and stomach to check for mucosal leak. A mucosal leak can be repaired laparoscopically with an absorbable mucosal suture.

Intraoperative endoscopy may facilitate identification of the esophagogastric junction and dynamic manometry may identify the adequate length of myotomy, but the author considers these maneuvers unnecessary.

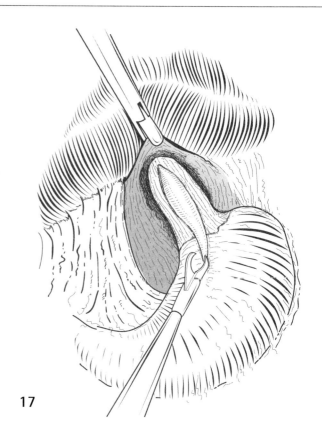

17

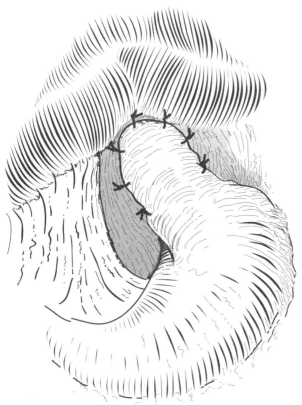

18

Fundoplication

18 A 180° anterior fundoplication is performed to prevent reflux and to protect the mucosa. The anterior gastric fundus is fixated to the anterior esophageal muscle layers with between four and six non-absorbable sutures. The upper sutures are attached to the anterior hiatus to prevent slipping of the wrap. There is no need to divide the short gastric vessels.

POSTOPERATIVE MANAGEMENT

The nasogastric tube is removed immediately after anesthesia. Patients can usually commence feeding with liquids immediately following the operation, with immediate relief of symptoms. A routine contrast study is not required before commencement of feeding. Oral feeding should be completed by day 3.

Long-term follow up is essential and clinical assessment is performed at 1, 6, and 12 months postoperatively. Contrast study, pH study, or manometry should only be used in case of persisting or new symptoms.

COMMON COMPLICATIONS AND THEIR MANAGEMENT

Bleeding from the myotomy site is common and usually stops spontaneously without further treatment.

Perforation of the mucosa during myotomy is rare and occurs mainly at the esophagogastric junction. The perforation site is closed by absorbable sutures. Patients with missed or delayed perforation present with sepsis and symptoms of peritonitis within 24–48 hours postoperatively. A contrast study is required to confirm perforation, and conventional surgical therapy via laparotomy is required. As with fundoplication, there is a small risk of breaching the left pleural cavity during dissection of the anterior wall of the mediastinal esophagus, and a tension pneumothorax may require immediate drainage.

Long-term dysphagia may occasionally require balloon dilatation to deal with incomplete myotomy or a too tight fundoplication.

FURTHER READING

Askegard-Giesmann JR, Grams JM, Hanna AM *et al.* Minimally invasive Heller's myotomy in children: safe and effective. *Journal of Pediatric Surgery* 2009; **44**: 909–11.

Berquist WE, Bryne WJ, Ament ME *et al.* Achalasia: diagnosis, management and clinical course in 16 children. *Pediatrics* 1983; **71**: 798–805.

Donahue PE, Schlesinger PK, Bombeck CT *et al.* Achalasia of the esophagus: treatment, controversies and the method of choice. *Annals of Surgery* 1986; **203**: 505–11.

Ellis FH, Gibb SP, Crozier RE. Esophagomyotomy for achalasia of the esophagus. *Annals of Surgery* 1980; **192**: 157–61.

Emblem R, Stringer MD, Hall CM, Spitz L. Current results of surgery for achalasia of the cardia. *Archives of Disease in Childhood* 1993; **68**: 749–51.

Mattioli G, Prato AP, Castagnetti M, Jasonni V. Esophageal achalasia. In: Bax NMA, Georgeson KE, Rothenberg S *et al.* (eds). *Endoscopic Surgery in Children*. Berlin: Springer, 2008: 245–52.

Vantrappen GD, Janssens J. To dilate or to operate? This is the question. *Gut* 1983; **24**: 1013–19.

Zaninoto GD, Annese V, Costantini M *et al.* Randomized controlled trial of botulinum toxin versus laparoscopic Heller myotomy for esophageal achalasia. *Annals of Surgery* 2004; **239**: 364–70.

44

Gastrostomy

MICHAEL WL GAUDERER

HISTORY

Gastrostomy is one of the oldest abdominal operations in continuous use and its history is closely associated with the evolution of modern surgery.

Gastrostomies are important in the management of a wide variety of surgical and non-surgical conditions of childhood. Although pediatric surgeons have become more selective in the use of gastrostomies for congenital malformations, there has been a marked increase in the use of feeding stomas in infants and children without associated surgical pathology, mainly those with an inability to swallow secondary to central nervous system disorders. This increase is reflected in the large volume of publications on the subject of the gastrostomy in the last couple of decades. Refinements in traditional procedures and the introduction of newer and simpler endoscopically, radiologically, ultrasonographically, and laparoscopically aided gastrostomies have enhanced the safety and expanded the applicability of this operation. It is perhaps fair to state that, over the years, few if any other commonly performed procedure has had as many different approaches as this seemingly simple access to the stomach. The use of softer, minimally irritating materials in the manufacture of gastrostomy catheters and the availability of several types of skin-level gastrostomy devices, commonly referred to as 'buttons', have greatly facilitated the long-term use of this type of enterostomy.

PRINCIPLES AND JUSTIFICATION

Gastrostomy is indicated in infants and children primarily for long-term feeding, decompression, or a combination of both. It is also commonly employed in conjunction with other interventions, notably antireflux procedures. Additional uses include gastric access for esophageal bougienage, placement of transpyloric jejunal feeding tubes, gastroscopy, and administration of medication.

TECHNIQUES

Three basic methods of constructing a gastrostomy are commonly used: (1) formation of a serosa-lined channel from the anterior gastric wall to the skin surface around a catheter; (2) formation of a tube from full-thickness gastric wall to the skin surface, a catheter being introduced intermittently for feeding; (3) percutaneous techniques, in which the introduced catheter holds the gastric and abdominal walls in apposition with or without the addition of fasteners. With certain modifications, each of these interventions can be performed by minimally invasive techniques or in conjunction with laparoscopy. Several of these approaches permit the primary insertion of a skin-level device or 'button'.

Channel formation around a catheter

In the first group of techniques, the catheter may be placed parallel to (Witzel technique) or perpendicular to (Stamm technique) the stomach with a laparotomy (see below under Operations). The stomach is usually anchored to the abdominal wall with sutures. The essence of the Stamm-type gastrostomy is the use of concentric purse-string sutures around the gastrostomy tube, producing an invagination lined with serosa.

Gastric tube brought to the surface

The gastric tube is constructed and then brought to the abdominal wall either as a direct conduit (Depage, Beck–Jianu, Hirsch, and Janeway methods) or interposing a valve or torsion of the tube to prevent reflux (Watsudjii, Spivack techniques). This conduit is secured to the layers of the abdominal wall and/ or the skin. The main appeal of the Janeway-type stoma is that the patient does not need a catheter between feedings. The use of automatic stapling devices, including those designed for laparoscopic use, has facilitated the construction of the tube from the anterior gastric wall.

Percutaneous catheter placement techniques

In this third group, the catheter is placed with endoscopic, radiologic, ultrasonographic, or laparoscopic assistance without a laparotomy. The percutaneous endoscopic gastrostomy (PEG) was the first of these methods and is still the most widely employed of these interventions. Depending on the method of introduction of the catheter, PEG may be performed using the original pull technique (Gauderer–Ponsky), a push technique (Sachs *et al.*) in which a semi-rigid catheter guide is advanced over a Seldinger-type wire instead of being pulled into place by a string-like guide from inside the stomach to the skin level, or the introducer technique (Russel *et al.*) in which a Foley catheter (or other balloon-type device such as one of the buttons) is advanced through a removable sheath from the skin level into the stomach. In some pediatric centers, non-endoscopic imaging-guided gastrostomies are also regularly employed.

Laparoscopic catheter placement techniques

Laparoscopically assisted gastrostomies are adaptations and/or modifications of the above basic types allowing surgeons numerous options either as single interventions or associated with other intracavitary procedures.

INDICATIONS

The type of gastrostomy, the preoperative work up, the technique, and the choice of gastrostomy device depend mainly on the indications for the procedure, the child's age and underlying disease, and the familiarity of the surgeon with the different operations.

Feeding and administration of medications

Placement of a gastrostomy for enteral feeding has two prerequisites: (1) the upper gastrointestinal tract must be functional and (2) the need for enteral feedings must be long term, at least several months. Children benefiting from gastrostomy fall into two broad categories: (1) those unable to swallow and (2) those unable to consume adequate nutrients orally. The first group is the largest and composed primarily of patients with neurologic disturbances. The second group includes patients with a variety of conditions in which the central nervous system is intact: failure to thrive, complex bowel disorders (e.g. short gut syndrome, Crohn's disease, malabsorption), malignancy and other debilitating illnesses, and various congenital or acquired diseases interfering with growth.

In selected patients, a gastrostomy is the most effective means of administering a non-palatable special diet (e.g. chronic renal failure) or ensuring compliance with medication (e.g. administering cholestyramine in Alagille's syndrome, anti-retroviral therapy in HIV infections).

All the gastrostomy types described above are suitable for this purpose (these are compared in **Table 44.1**). A comparison of devices used in all gastrostomy types (except gastric tube stomas) is given in **Table 44.2**.

Table 44.1 Comparison of the most commonly used gastrostomies.

	Serosa–lined channel	Gastric tube	Percutaneous techniques	Laparoscopic
Catheter/stoma device continuously *in situ*	Yes	No	Yes	Yes
Laparotomy	Yes	Yes	No	No
Laparoscopically feasible	Possible	Yes	Yes	Yes
Need for gastric endoscopy	No	No	PEG	No
Need for abdominal relaxation during operation	Yes	Yes	No	Yes and insufflation
Procedure time	Short	Moderate	Very short	Short
Postoperative ileus	Yes	Yes	Rare	Some
Potential for bleeding	Yes	Yes	No	Some
Potential for wound dehiscence/hernia	Yes	Yes	No	No
Potential for early dislodgment of catheter	Yes	No	Procedure dependent[a]	Some
Potential for gastric separation	Possible	Possible	Yes	Possible
Potential for infection	Yes	Yes	Yes	Yes
Potential for gastrocolic fistula	Possible	No	Yes	Possible
Incidence of external leakage	Moderate	Significant	Low	Low
'Permanent'	No	Yes	No	No
Suitable for passage of dilators for esophageal stricture	Yes	No	No	Possible[c]
Interferes with gastric reoperation (fundoplication)	No	Yes	No	No
Suitable for infants	Yes	No	Yes	Yes

PEG, percutaneous endoscopic gastrostomy.
[a]Low with PEG, high with imaging-guided procedures.

Table 44.2 Comparison of commonly used gastrostomy devices.

	de Pezzer, Malecot, T-tube	Foley (balloon type)	Skin-level (button type)
Suitable for initial insertion	Yes	Yes	Yes
Suitable for decompression	Yes	Yes	Yes[a]
Tendency for accidental dislodgment or external migration	Moderate[b]	Moderate	Very low
Tendency for internal (distal) migration	Moderate	High	Unlikely
Tendency for peristomal leakage (particularly large tubes)	Moderate	Moderate	Low
Balloon deflation	No	Yes	Depending on type
Reinsertion	Easy to moderately difficult	Easy	Easy to moderately difficult
Long-term (particularly ambulatory patients)	Adequate	Adequate	Best suited

[a]With special adaptor.
[b]High with Malecot.

Because of the high incidence of foregut dysmotility in the neurologically impaired patients, there has been an increase in the use of jejunal feeding through combined gastrostomy–jejunostomy long- or skin-level devices. However, because trans-gastrostomy jejunal feeding tubes are not ideal for long-term use, jejunostomies are, at times, added to gastrostomy procedures.

Decompression with or without enteral feeding

When a gastrostomy is placed in conjunction with another intra-abdominal procedure (such as fundoplication or repair of duodenal atresia), the tube is used initially for decompression and then for intragastric feedings. If prolonged gastric or duodenal dysmotility is anticipated, a smaller, more flexible catheter is advanced into the lumen of the jejunum, exiting either along the gastrostomy tube or through a counter-incision. Gastrostomies can be a temporary adjunct in the management of children with severe pathologic aerophagia and be of palliative value in the management of patients with intestinal obstruction secondary to unresectable malignancy.

All gastrostomy types, except gastric tubes, are suitable for these purposes.

CAVEATS AND CONTRAINDICATIONS

With all gastrostomy techniques, great care must be exercised in children with previous epigastric procedures, hepato- and/or splenomegaly, and patients with severe musculoskeletal abnormalities, notably scoliosis.

Contraindications to PEG are the inability to perform upper tract endoscopy safely or to identify transabdominal illumination and see an anterior gastric wall indentation clearly. Anatomic abnormalities, such as malrotation or marked scoliosis, ascites, coagulopathy, and intra-abdominal infection, if severe, may render the procedure inadvisable. In such cases, laparoscopic or radiologic control, a fully laparoscopic procedure, or gastrostomy with a conventional laparotomy may be indicated.

PREOPERATIVE

Gastrostomy for feeding

Gastroesophageal reflux, as a manifestation of foregut dysmotility, is a common problem in neurologically impaired children both before and after the placement of a gastrostomy. Evaluation for the degree of reflux in these patients is therefore necessary. Patients with severe reflux are best managed with an antireflux procedure and a gastrostomy. Children with mild or no reflux are candidates for gastrostomy only.

Gastrostomy as an adjunct in children with surgical lesions

The addition of a stoma to the surgical correction of a congenital or acquired lesion should be considered only if it will substantially facilitate perioperative or long-term care. Examples in neonatal surgery include complex esophageal atresia, certain duodenal obstructions, select abdominal wall defects in which long-term ileus is anticipated, and short gut syndrome. Indications in older children include severe esophageal stricture, complex foregut trauma, intestinal pseudo-obstruction, malignancy, and complex adhesive bowel obstruction.

OPERATIONS

Stamm gastrostomy

This operation is performed using general endotracheal anesthesia. The child is positioned with a small roll behind the back to elevate the epigastrium, then prepared and draped. The author prefers to use a silicone mushroom-type catheter ranging in size from 12 Fr (full-term neonates) to 20 Fr for adolescents, and a 10 Fr T-tube or Malecot catheter for preterm infants or neonates with very small stomachs, such as those found in children with esophageal atresia without distal fistula. The procedure may be modified slightly to accommodate the initial placement of a 'button'.

INCISION

1 The stomach is approached through a short, left, transverse, supraumbilical incision. Fascial layers are incised transversely and the muscle retracted or transected. The catheter exit site is approximately at the junction of the lower two-thirds and the upper one-third of a line from the umbilicus to the mid-portion of the left rib cage, over the mid-rectus muscle. A vertical incision may be useful in children with a high-lying stomach or a narrow costal angle.

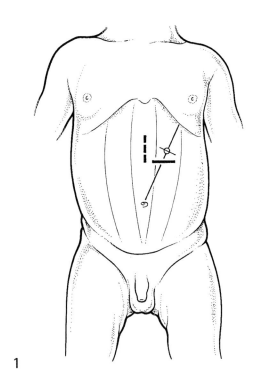

1

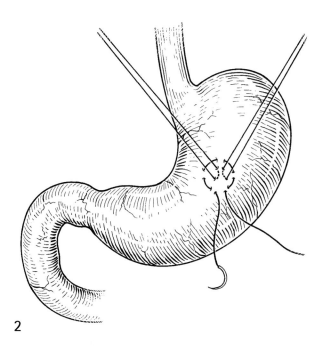

2

PRODUCTION OF A GASTROTOMY SITE ON THE ANTERIOR GASTRIC WALL

2 Traction guy sutures and a purse-string suture (synthetic, absorbable) are placed as shown. The opening should be away from the gastric pacemaker at the level of the splenic hilum; away from the greater curvature because that site may be needed for construction of a gastric tube for esophageal replacement; away from the fundus to allow for a possible fundoplication; and away from the antrum to prevent excessive leakage and pyloric obstruction by the catheter tip. If the catheter is to be placed cranially and close to the lesser curvature for a gastrostomy with antireflux properties, care must be taken to avoid the vagus nerve.

3 A lower guy suture pulls the stomach caudally, enhancing exposure and allowing better gastric access. The gastrotomy is performed with fine scissors or cautery, while the upper guy sutures are lifted to prevent injuring the back wall. The de Pezzer catheter is introduced using a simple stylet while these sutures are elevated. The insert shows a 'tulip' or 'dome' PEG-type catheter being stretched in the same manner for insertion.

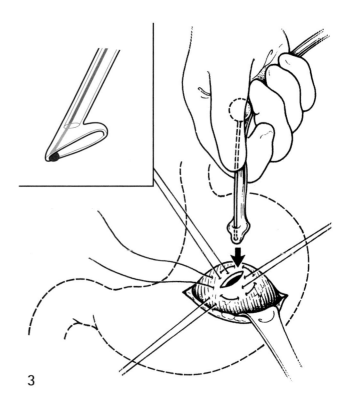

3

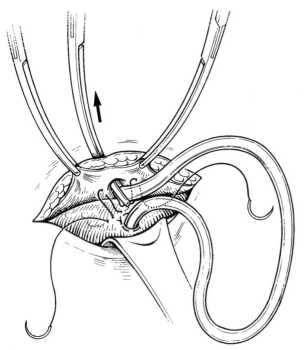

4

4 The purse-string suture is tied. A continuous, synthetic, absorbable, monofilament suture (polydioxanone) is used to anchor the stomach to the anterior abdominal wall. A Kelly clamp is placed through the counter-incision and the abdominal wall layers are pushed inwards. The posterior 180° of the anastomosis are completed, the peritoneum and fascia are incised, and the tip of the clamp is pushed through. The catheter end is grasped and the tube is brought out through the counter-incision.

5 Placement of the continuous monofilament suture is now completed. When tied, this suture provides a 360° fixation with a watertight seal. In most cases, this maneuver obviates the need for a second purse-string suture.

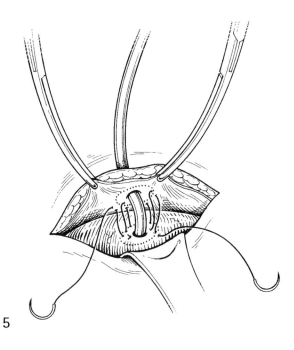

5

6 The abdominal wall layers are closed with synthetic absorbable sutures and the skin is approximated with subcuticular stitches and adhesive strips. The catheter is secured with synthetic monofilament sutures (polypropylene). These are removed 1–2 weeks after the operation, and a small crossbar is placed to prevent distal catheter migration.

6

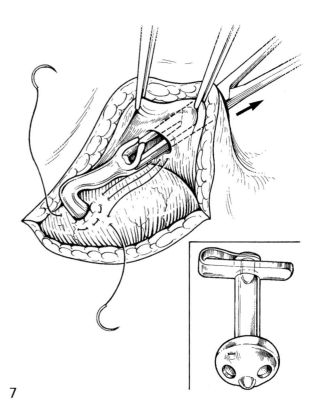

7

7 This standard procedure may be modified to allow the insertion of a skin-level gastrostomy device, the original 'button' (inset), a balloon-type skin-level device, or a changeable skin-level port-valve. These devices are available in different shaft lengths and diameters. The shaft length should encompass the invaginated gastric wall, the abdominal wall, and an additional few millimeters of 'play' to allow for postoperative edema, ease of care, and subsequent growth and weight gain.

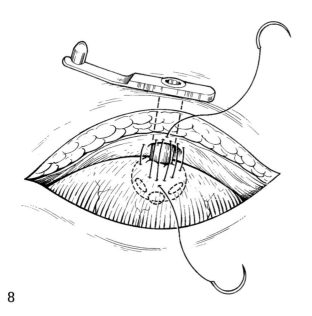

8

8 The stomach is vented with a nasogastric tube or a special decompression device, which, when inserted in the shaft, deactivates the one-way valve at the gastric end of the shaft.

Janeway gastrostomy

This procedure may be accomplished using either a conventional laparotomy or a gastrointestinal anastomosis stapler or employing an endoscopic stapler under laparoscopic control.

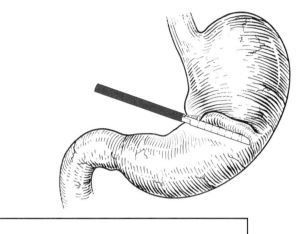

9 The stapler is employed to tubularize the gastric wall. The gastric tube is brought out away from the incision if the open technique is used or through one of the port sites if it is performed laparoscopically.

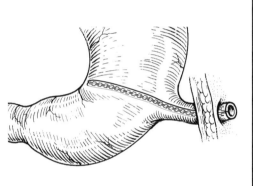

9

Percutaneous endoscopic gastrostomy ('pull' technique)

The procedure is best performed in the operating room. Older children and those able to tolerate endoscopy without compromising the upper airway receive local anesthesia with sedation as needed. Younger children require general endotracheal anesthesia, primarily because of anticipated difficulties with the airway management. A single dose of a broad-spectrum intravenous antibiotic is given shortly before the procedure. For the endoscopy, the smallest available pediatric gastroscope is used. The catheter and retaining crossbar or catheter head should be soft and collapsible enough to glide atraumatically through the oropharynx and esophagus. The 16 Fr silicone rubber catheter depicted in **Step figure 10** is suitable for most children. Hybrid catheters for primary implantation of skin-level devices are now also available.

A note of caution: In children with marked anatomical distortions, such as severe scoliosis, the stomach may be displaced cranially into the left chest. The transverse colon is then pulled upward and is more vulnerable to puncture. In these cases, laparoscopic control adds safety to the procedure.

The operative field is prepared in the usual sterile manner.

10 A pediatric catheter should be used, with a gastric retainer, markings on the shaft, and dilating tapered end with steel wire loop. Also shown in this illustration are a skin-level retainer (external crossbar) and a catheter adapter. The catheter is cut to an appropriate length after insertion.

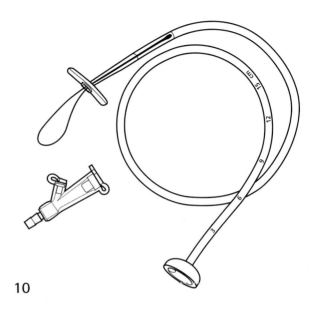

10

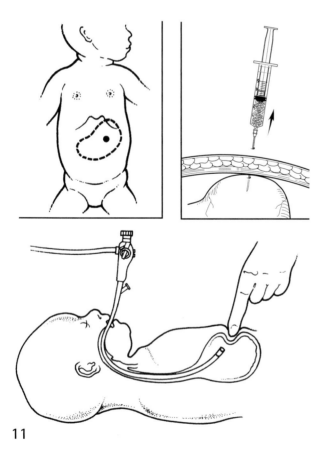

11

11a–c The gastroscope is inserted and the stomach insufflated. The stoma should be away from the ribcage. Under- or over-insufflation should be avoided to minimize the possibility of accidentally piercing the transverse colon. Insufflation of the small intestine tends to push the transverse colon in front of the stomach and should thus be avoided. Digital pressure is applied to the proposed gastrostomy site, which usually corresponds to the area where transillumination is brightest. Transillumination and clear visualization of an anterior gastric wall indentation are key points. Without these, an open or laparoscopic technique should be employed. Long-lasting local anesthetic is drawn into a syringe and the proposed PEG site injected. The needle is advanced further and continuous aspirating pressure is applied to the plunger. Air bubbles should be visible in the remaining fluid when the tip of the needle is seen by the endoscopist. If air bubbles are noticed before the needle tip is in the stomach, the colon or other intestinal loop may be interposed between the stomach and the abdominal wall (inset).

12 An incision of 8–10 mm is made in the skin and a Kelly-type hemostat applied to maintain the intragastric indentation. The endoscope is moved gently in small increments. The endoscopist then places the polypectomy snare around this 'mound'. The intravenous cannula is placed in the incision between the slightly spread prongs of the hemostat and then firmly thrust through the abdominal and gastric walls, exiting through the tip of the 'mound' into the loop of the polypectomy snare. The snare is partially closed, but not tightened around the cannula.

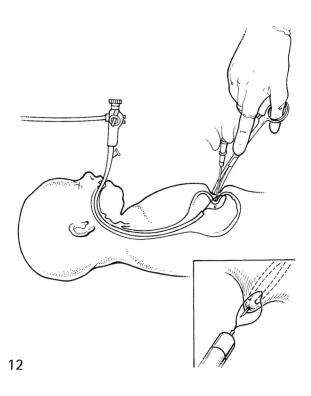

12

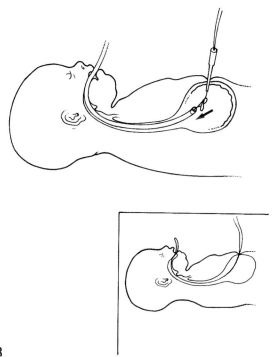

13

13 The needle is removed and the looped steel wire inserted through the cannula. The polypectomy snare is allowed to slide away from the cannula and is tightened around the wire. An alternative method is to retrieve the wire with alligator or biopsy forceps. The wire is then pulled back with the endoscope through the stomach and esophagus, exiting through the patient's mouth. A guiding tract is thus established.

14 The catheter is attached to the guidewire by interlocking the two steel wire loops. Traction is applied to the abdominal end of the wire, guiding the catheter through the esophagus and stomach and across the gastric and abdominal walls. The collapsed gastric retainer minimizes the risk of esophageal injury. (For diagrammatic purposes, a shortened catheter is shown.) The tapered end of the catheter exits through the abdominal wall before the gastric retainer enters the patient's mouth, allowing complete control of the catheter during placement. Traction is continued until the gastric and abdominal walls are in loose contact. The external crossbar is slipped over the catheter and guided to the skin level, avoiding pressure from the retaining crossbar on the mucosa or skin. The catheter is cut to the desired length and the feeding adapter attached. No sutures are used, and the catheter is connected to a small, clear plastic trap. A gauze pad and tape are applied.

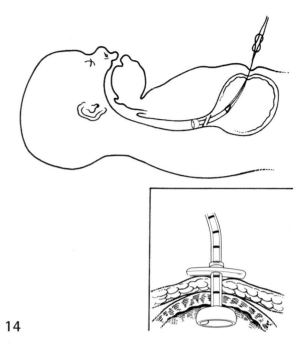

14

Hybrid gastrostomy

In children who have a markedly abnormal epigastric anatomy or dense adhesions because of previous abdominal operations or peritonitis, it may be impossible to perform a PEG or a laparoscopic gastrostomy safely.

At times, even a Stamm gastrostomy may be technically challenging. For these cases, a hybrid procedure was developed that combines the 'open' technique employing a mini-laparotomy with the 'pull' PEG insertion of a gastrostomy catheter.

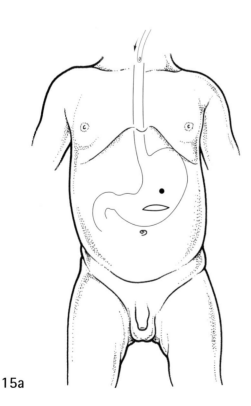

15a

15a–e A mini-laparotomy is made in the left upper quadrant (a). The anterior surface of the stomach is identified. A large (20–26 Fr) Nelaton-type catheter is inserted orally and advanced into the stomach, where it is clearly identified. A sturdy monofilament suture on a tapered needle is selected. The needle is pushed through the anterior gastric wall at the desired gastrostomy site, through the catheter, and then out of the stomach (b). The needle is then cut off. The catheter is pulled back with the suture embedded in it (c). The gastric end of the suture is brought out through a counter-incision (d). The oral end of the suture is attached to a PEG-type catheter, which is then pulled back in a manner similar to the 'pull' PEG illustrated above. Panel (e) demonstrates the completed procedure.

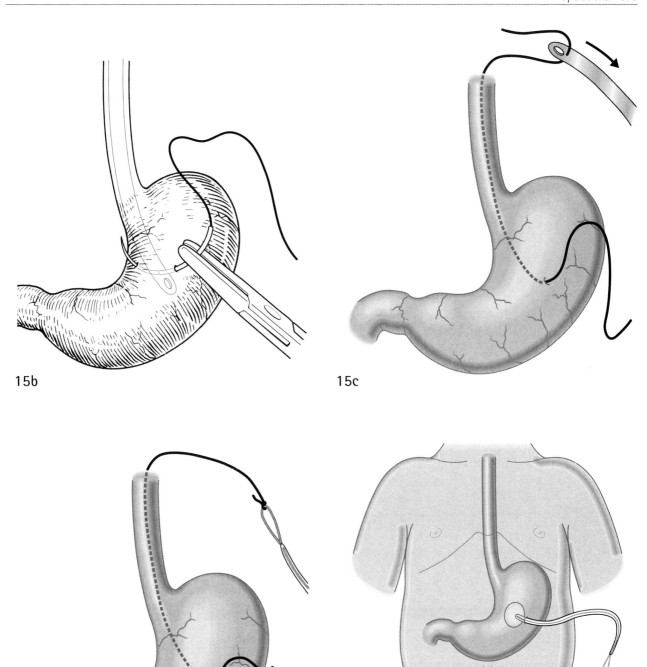

15b

15c

15d

15e

Laparoscopic gastrostomy

Several methods for establishing a laparoscopic gastrostomy, either alone or in conjunction with another laparoscopic procedure, such as a fundoplication, have been developed. In addition to the vidcoscopically controlled PEG, the two commonly employed methods are based on adaptations of the Stamm gastrostomy and modifications of the 'push' PEG using the Seldinger technique. Our preference is for the latter, because in order to place a purse-string suture through the exposed segment of the anterior gastric wall, the trocar site must be sufficiently enlarged. Bringing the gastrostomy catheter or skin-level device through this enlarged opening may predispose the site to leakage. In order to anchor the stomach to the abdominal wall temporarily, different approaches may be employed: T-fasteners, separate or continuous U-stitches. The double, separate U-stitch technique is illustrated here. This approach is, however, more difficult in older, overweight children. In these patients, additional trocars may be needed to suture the stomach to the abdominal wall. (An alternative is a laparoscopically controlled PEG.)

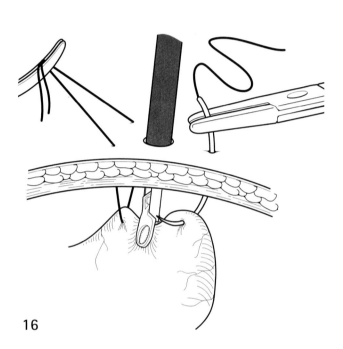

16

16 The most suitable site of a gastrostomy is selected in the left upper quadrant and marked. As in other types of gastrostomies, it should be away from the costal margin and the midline. A nasogastric tube is introduced. Pneumoperitoneum is established in the usual, age-appropriate manner and a 30° laparoscope introduced at the umbilicus. The left epigastric area is inspected. The previously marked site is infiltrated with a long-lasting local anesthetic. The needle is then pushed through the abdominal wall and the appropriate relation between the anterior gastric wall and the stoma site established. A small skin incision is made and a 5-mm trocar inserted. A bowel grasper is introduced and the stoma site on the anterior gastric wall is lifted toward the parietal peritoneum. (Alternatively, instead of placing a trocar through the gastrostomy site, as illustrated here, a small right lower quadrant incision is made under direct visualization and a 3-mm bowel grasper is inserted. The instrument grasps the gastric wall at the stoma site and lifts it against the parietal peritoneum.) A U-stitch of a 2/0 monofilament suture is passed through the abdominal wall, through the anterior gastric wall, and back out through the abdominal wall. A second U-stitch is passed parallel to the first one, 1–2 cm apart. The sutures are lifted, maintaining the stomach in contact with the abdominal wall. The grasper and the trocar are removed.

17 The stomach is insufflated with air through the nasogastric tube and a needle is inserted through the trocar site into the gastric lumen, between the two U-stitches. A Seldinger-type guidewire is passed through the needle into the stomach. The tract is sequentially dilated over the guidewire with tapered dilators (8, 10, 16, and 20) to the size required to insert either a Foley-type catheter or a balloon-type skin-level device. These are placed over the same guidewire. Stiffening of the catheter shaft with a thin dilator is helpful during this insertion.

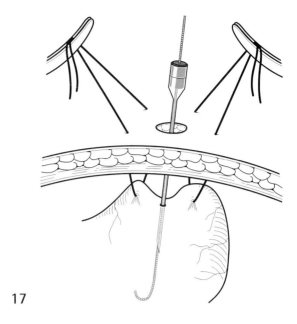

17

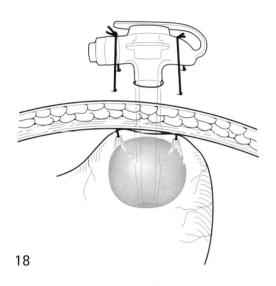

18

18 A balloon-type 'button' has been introduced and inflated under direct visualization to ensure adequate placement. The dilator and wire are removed. The previously placed U-stitches are tied over the wings of the 'button' securing the gastric wall to the parietal peritoneum and the device to the abdominal wall. Pneumoperitoneum is discontinued and the instruments are removed. The incisions are closed with absorbable sutures.

Percutaneous gastrostomy guided by fluoroscopy, computed tomography, or ultrasonography gastrostomy

These techniques are, in many ways, similar to the previously described methods of creating an approximation of the anterior gastric wall to the parietal peritoneum and inserting a self-retaining tube. For the fluoroscopic and computed tomography (CT)-guided procedures, the stomach is insufflated with air. In the ultrasonographic-guided gastrostomy, the stomach is filled with saline. In some techniques, the stomach is approximated and held in place by T-fasteners prior to the insertion of the catheter in an 'introducer' PEG variation, whereas in others a pig-tail catheter is used to gain access and retention. In both cases, a Seldinger-type technique is employed, followed by dilatation of the tract and catheter insertion. A fluoroscopically guided 'pull' PEG has also been described (see **Chapter 109**).

POSTOPERATIVE CARE

Enteral feedings begin following open gastrostomies once the ileus has resolved, and on the day after the operation for the minimally invasive procedures. The dressing is removed after 24 hours, the wound is examined, and the tension on the external immobilizers adjusted in order to avoid excessive pressure that could lead to tissue damage. The monofilament sutures used in the laparoscopic approach are removed after 5–7 days. Our preference is to leave the stoma uncovered. We avoid harsh antiseptic solutions and, after a few days, simply use soap and water for cleaning. Granulation tissue tends to form after a couple of weeks and is controlled with gentle applications of silver nitrate. If granulation tissue becomes excessive, it leads to leakage and needs to be excised. We have observed good results with the application of a triamcinolone and antifungal combination to prevent the recurrence of granulation tissue. Once the tract becomes epithelialized, no medication should be used.

If a 'button' has not been placed at the initial procedure, the long tube should be replaced with one of the skin-level devices as soon as a reliable adherence of the stomach to the abdominal wall has occurred.

Should a gastrostomy no longer be needed, the catheter is simply removed. The tract will usually close in a matter of days. If the gastrocutaneous fistula remains after several weeks, simple excision of the tract is performed.

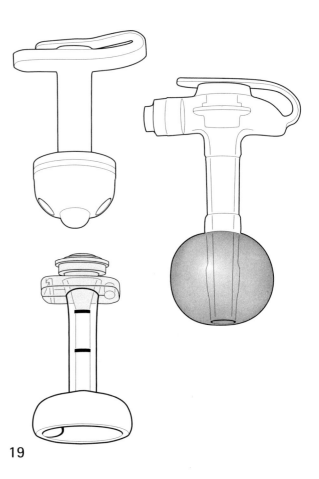

19 The three most commonly employed skin-level devices: the original 'button' (with a flapper-type one-way valve at the gastric end of the shaft), a balloon-type skin-level device (with a 'duck-bill' one-way valve in the upper shaft), and a changeable skin-level port valve (with an external valve mechanism).

19

COMPLICATIONS

Although generally considered a basic procedure, gastrostomy is associated with a long list of complications related to technique, care, and catheter use. Serious technique-related problems include separation of the stomach from the abdominal wall leading to peritonitis, wound separation, hemorrhage, infection, injury to the posterior gastric wall or other organs, and placement of the tube in an inappropriate gastric position. Separation of the stomach from the abdominal wall is usually due to inadvertent, premature dislodgement of the tube or a disruption during catheter change. It requires immediate attention. It is generally managed with a laparotomy, although in select cases a laparoscopic correction is possible. Most complications can be avoided by careful choice of the procedure and stoma device, considering it a major intervention, and using meticulous technique, approximating the stomach to the abdominal wall, exiting the catheter through a counter-incision, and avoiding tubes in the midline or too close to the rib cage.

Among the most serious long-term problems are the so-called 'buried-bumper syndrome' (or external catheter migration) and severe gastrostomy leakage. The first complication becomes apparent when there is difficulty with the administration of feeding that may also be associated with pain. This mishap can be avoided by always allowing sufficient 'play' between the skin-level device or external bumper and the skin. Severe leakage is initially managed using conservative measures. If these fail, the stoma should be relocated.

FOLLOW UP

All children with gastrostomies should be carefully followed up to prevent long-term catheter-related complications and monitored for manifestations of foregut dysmotility, particularly gastroesophageal reflux.

FURTHER READING

Aprahamian CJ, Morgan TL, Harmon CM *et al.* U-stitch laparoscopic gastrostomy technique has a low rate of complications and allows primary button placement: experience with 461 pediatric procedures. *Journal of Laparoendoscopic Advanced Surgical Techniques A* 2006; **16**: 643–9.

Chait PG, Weinbrg J, Connoly BL. Retrograde percutaneous gastrostomy and gastrojejunostomy in 505 children: a 4.5 year experience. *Radiology* 1996; **201**: 691–5.

Gauderer MWL. Percutaneous endoscopic gastrostomy (PEG) and the evolution of contemporary long-term enteral access. *Clinical Nutrition* 2002; **21**: 103–10.

Gauderer MWL. Experience with a hybrid, minimally invasive gastrostomy for children with abnormal epigastric anatomy. *Journal of Pediatric Surgery* 2008; **43**: 2178–81.

Gauderer MWL, Stellato TA. Gastrostomies: evolution, techniques, indications and complications. *Current Problems in Surgery* 1986; **23**: 661–719.

Sampson LK, Georgeson KE, Winters DC. Laparoscopic gastrostomy as an adjunctive procedure to laparoscopic fundoplication in children. *Surgical Endoscopy* 1996; **10**: 1106–10.

Yu SC, Petty JK, Bensard DD *et al.* Laparoscopic-assisted percutaneous endoscopic gastrostomy in children and adolescents. *Journal of the Society of Laparoendoscopic Surgeons* 2005; **9**: 302–4.

45

Pyloromyotomy

NIGEL J HALL and AGOSTINO PIERRO

HISTORY

Sabricius Hildanus first described pyloric stenosis in 1646. Harald Hirschsprung elaborated on the clinical presentation and pathology of the condition in 1888. At this stage, the preferred treatment was medical, using a combination of gastric lavage, antispasmodic drugs, dietary manipulation, and the application of local heat, because the surgical mortality was almost 100 percent. In 1908, Fredet advocated longitudinal submucosal division of the thickened pyloric muscle, but recommended suturing the defect transversely. In 1912, Ramstedt simplified the Fredet procedure by omitting the transverse suturing, leaving the mucosa exposed in the longitudinal subserosal defect. This operation was successful and its essential elements have remained virtually unmodified ever since. Surgery has now completely replaced medical measures for the treatment of pyloric stenosis.

The operative approach to the pyloromyotomy has also undergone a number of modifications in the last few decades. Up until the 1990s, the majority of surgeons approached the pylorus through either a transverse or midline incision in the upper abdomen. Frequently, the cosmetic result was unsatisfactory. In 1986, Tan and Bianchi reported the use of a paraumbilical incision to approach the pylorus with superior cosmesis and this has become the standard open approach in many centers. More recently, laparoscopic pyloromyotomy has been reported and has superseded an open procedure in many specialist pediatric surgical units.

PRINCIPLES AND JUSTIFICATION

Incidence

The incidence of pyloric stenosis among whites is 2–3 per 1000 live births. Blacks are less frequently affected. The male-to-female ratio is 4:1. The disorder often occurs in first-born boys, and there is a strong familial pattern of inheritance. Vomiting due to pyloric stenosis has been noted in twins, whose symptoms began within hours of each other.

Diagnosis

Symptoms usually commence at 2–4 weeks of age, but can sometimes be seen in neonates or infants close to two months of age. Symptoms consist of projectile vomiting of non-bilious material, constipation, dehydration, lethargy, or seizures, and failure to thrive. Hematemesis has been documented in a few cases.

Physical signs include variable degrees of dehydration, visible gastric peristalsis, and a palpable pyloric tumor.

If one takes the time to perform a proper clinical examination, the diagnosis can nearly always be made without further investigations, but more often patients will be referred to the surgeons with diagnostic images suggestive of pyloric stenosis.

Special investigations

While diagnostic images may be helpful in difficult cases, none is necessary if clinical examination demonstrates a palpable 'tumor' or 'olive'. When physical examination fails to identify a pyloric mass, ultrasonographic images should be obtained. If ultrasound is equivocal, barium swallow can be helpful, but is rarely required. Endoscopy should not be necessary to make the diagnosis of pyloric stenosis, but may be useful in symptomatic patients with other causes for gastric outlet obstruction.

Ultrasonography

1 This typically shows a thickened pyloric musculature with a central sonolucent area representing the lumen. The thickened muscle is easy to recognize as a donut or bull's eye. Ultrasonographers also use the following measurement criteria to make the diagnosis: pyloric channel >17 mm in length and pyloric thickness >4 mm.

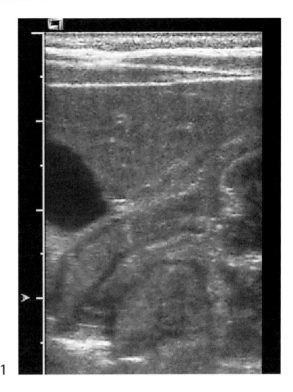

1

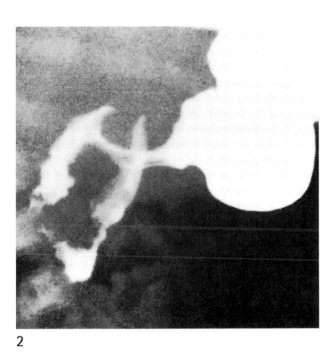

2

Barium swallow

2 The following features are diagnostic: 'string sign' of the narrow elongated pyloric canal; 'double track' in the pyloric canal owing to infolding mucosa; delayed gastric emptying; gastric hyperperistalsis; the mushroom effect in the duodenal cap due to indentation by pyloric 'tumor'.

PREOPERATIVE

Preparation of the patient

Pyloromyotomy is never an emergency; correction of dehydration and acid–base imbalance takes precedence. Parenteral correction of metabolic abnormalities is the safest way to prepare a patient for surgery. An intravenous infusion of isotonic saline (20 mL/kg) is administered over 60 minutes. Once urinary output has been established, potassium chloride (20–30 mmol/L) is added to the infusate of 5 percent glucose in 0.45 percent saline. The infusion is given at a rate of 120–150 mL/kg body weight per 24 hours.

It may take as long as 48–72 hours for rehydration to be complete and for the infant to be ready for surgery. The goal is to correct the serum electrolytes to nearly normal. Accordingly, the serum potassium should be at least 3–4.5 mEq/L, the serum CO_2 should be <27–30 mEq/L, and the serum sodium should be >130 mEq/L before surgery is considered. The serum chloride will usually correct itself to >100 mEq/L with the above measures.

Preoperatively, a nasogastric tube should be inserted, allowed to drain freely and aspirated every 4 hours. The volume of fluid drained should be replaced with an intravenous infusion of an equal volume of 0.9 percent saline containing 20 mmol/L potassium chloride.

Anesthesia

Although local anesthesia has been used successfully, general endotracheal anesthesia is now preferred, particularly if laparoscopy is performed. The stomach should be emptied immediately before induction to avoid vomiting and aspiration. An intravenous infusion is set up for the administration of perioperative fluids and other drugs.

OPERATION

Open pyloromyotomy

POSITION OF PATIENT

The patient is placed supine on the operating table, prepared and draped in the usual sterile fashion. A preoperative prophylactic antibiotic should be given at the time of the operation to minimize the risk of postoperative wound infection.

INCISION

3 A curvilinear incision approximately 2 cm long is made in the upper fold of the umbilicus, circumscribing the umbilicus itself. If the umbilicus is small, the incision may be extended laterally into an 'omega' shape to improve access. The incision is deepened through the subcutaneous tissues down to the linea alba which is stripped of overlying tissue longitudinally for approximately 2 cm above the umbilicus. The linea alba is then opened in a cephalad direction, the umbilical vein retracted to one side and the peritoneum opened longitudinally.

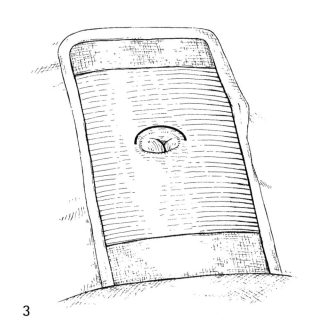

3

IDENTIFICATION OF THE STOMACH

With the peritoneum opened, the stomach may be visible but is often not. If it is, it is grasped with non-traumatic forceps and delivered gently into the wound where it is held with a moist gauze swab. No attempt should be made to grasp the pyloric tumor directly, as this leads to serosal tears and hemorrhage. If the stomach is not visible, gentle traction on the transverse colon or greater omentum will allow identification of the greater curve of the stomach.

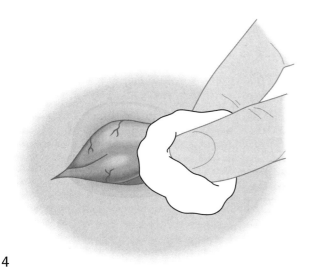

4

DELIVERY OF THE PYLORIC TUMOR

4 With the greater curvature of the stomach firmly drawn across to the left and exerting traction on the antrum, the pyloric tumor is delivered out of the incision by applying a gentle to-and-fro rocking traction on the pylorus. If this proves difficult, the likely cause is inadequate length of the skin incision. Extension of the incision will reduce the risk of serosal tearing and aid delivery of the pyloric tumor.

The pyloric vein of Mayo marks the distal extent of the tumor. Proximally, the tumor is less obvious where it merges with the hypertrophied stomach musculature. The tumor has a glistening, grayish appearance and is firm to palpation.

There is a relatively avascular plane in the middle of the anterior surface where the vessels entering the pylorus superiorly and inferiorly merge.

INCISION OF PYLORUS

5 A serosal incision is then made in the avascular area on the anterior surface of the tumor. It is carried distally as far as the pyloric vein of Mayo, which marks the pyloroduodenal junction, while proximally it extends well onto the anterior surface of the antrum of the stomach. The length of the incision is 2–3 cm.

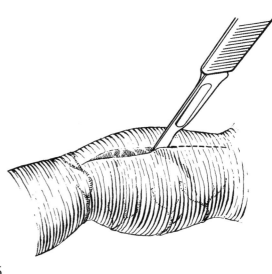

5

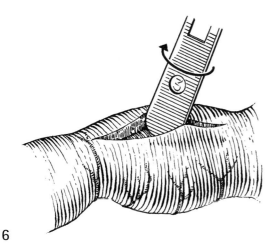

6

SPLITTING OF PYLORIC MUSCULATURE

6 Pressure with a blunt instrument, such as the back of the handle of a scalpel, into the incision with counter-pressure from a finger placed behind the tumor allows splitting of the hypertrophied muscle fibers down to the submucosa. This appears as a white, glistening membrane in the depth of the incision of the pylorus. A twisting movement on the blunt instrument produces an extension of the split proximally and distally and widens the incision. Alternatively, the blunt instrument is gently rubbed back and forth along the incision and over the muscle to split it.

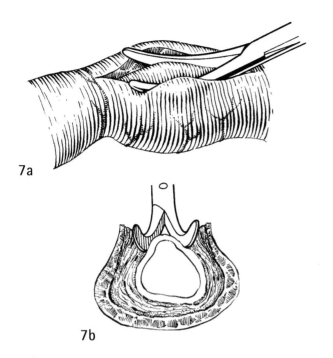

7a

7b

7a,b To ensure that all muscle fibers have been divided throughout the length of the incision, the edges of the split muscle are spread apart with either a pair of blunt forceps (ensuring that the points are held away from the mucosa) or a pyloric spreader (Dennis Browne or Benson and Lloyd) so that the submucosa bulges into the incision. Special care must be taken at the pyloroduodenal junction to avoid entering the lumen of the duodenum, which is particularly vulnerable because of the protrusion of the pyloric tumor into the duodenal lumen. The adequacy of the split is assured if the two halves of the muscle move independently of each other.

TESTING FOR PERFORATION

About 10–20 mL of air is introduced into the stomach via the nasogastric tube and then gently milked through the pylorus into the duodenum, and a gauze sponge is dabbed on the incision to detect any bile staining. Any perforation of the mucosa will become obvious at this juncture and should be closed by direct suture with 6/0 polydiaxonone or polyglycolic acid. Some surgeons advocate closing the pyloromyotomy completely and redoing the myotomy on the opposite side of the pylorus. In either case, the important point is to recognize the perforation and to repair any leak found.

Slight hemorrhage from the edges of the pyloromyotomy will cease once the tumor has been replaced into the peritoneal cavity and hence venous congestion relieved.

WOUND CLOSURE

The wound is closed with an interrupted suture of polyglycolic acid or polydiaxonone for peritoneum/muscle and fascia. The subcutaneous tissues are closed with continuous 4/0 polyglycolic acid suture and the skin is approximated with 5/0 polyglycolic acid subcuticular suture or surgical glue.

Laparoscopic pyloromyotomy

HISTORY

In 1991, Alain *et al.* described laparoscopic extramucosal pyloromyotomy for the first time. Since then, several other groups have reported their experience with the technique for laparoscopic extramucosal pyloromyotomy. However, the application of laparoscopy to the treatment of hypertrophic pyloric stenosis occurred late compared to other procedures in the pediatric population, as it was difficult to justify using it rather than the open technique. Tan and Najmaldin reported their initial experience in 1993 and 1995, with good results. Several high-quality prospective randomized controlled trials have now been performed comparing open and laparoscopic approaches.

OPERATIVE PROCEDURE

After the induction of anesthesia, the patient is placed in the supine position with the feet at the very bottom of the operating table and the table shortened if possible. The laparoscopic screen should be positioned over the patient's head facing the feet. The abdomen is prepared and draped in the usual sterile fashion, with special attention being paid to meticulous preparation of the umbilicus. A preoperative prophylactic antibiotic should be given at the time of the operation to minimize the risk of postoperative wound infection.

8 The surgeon and assistant should stand on either side of the patient initially. A stab incision is made in the supraumbilical skin crease using a No. 11 knife blade, and stretched along the contour lines to allow the passage of a 3-mm trocar. The subcutaneous tissues are divided to expose the linea alba which is opened followed by the peritoneum under direct vision. A purse-string-type absorbable suture is inserted around the defect, but not tied. A 3-mm trocar is inserted, the purse-string suture tightened to provide an airtight seal and a single throw of a knot placed on the suture to secure the port in position. A pneumoperitoneum is established keeping the pressure between 8 and 10 mmHg. A small-caliber 30° telescope is placed through the umbilical port. A general abdominal inspection is performed and the thickened pylorus is visualized. A small stab incision is made on the left side of the abdomen lateral to the mid-clavicular line, halfway between the umbilicus and the costal margin, and a small-caliber trocar is introduced for an atraumatic grasper passed directly through the abdominal wall. This is used to stabilize the pylorus either by supporting the duodenum distally or by grasping the stomach proximally. Another stab incision is made on the right side of the abdomen in a similar position but slightly higher on the abdomen. A 3-mm diathermy hook passed into the abdomen to initiate the pyloromyotomy. Some prefer to use a retractable, arthroscopic knife instead.

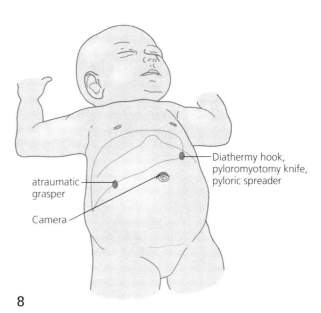

8

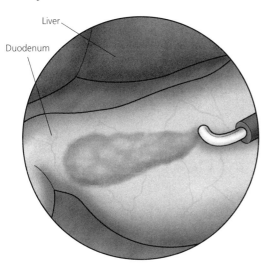

9 Pyloromyotomy made by diathermy hook

The pyloromyotomy site is then slowly widened under direct vision and an adequate myotomy is assessed by holding the edges of the myotomy using an atraumatic grasper and pyloric spreader and moving them independently to be certain that the two halves of the pylorus move independently.

The stomach should then be insufflated with air through a nasogastric/orogastric tube and milked through the pylorus into the duodenum to be certain that there are no leaks and that the air passes easily.

An incision is made using monopolar diathermy or the knife in an area of avascularity over the pylorus. The incision should extend from the anterior gastric wall to just proximal to the vein of Mayo.

The knife or diathermy hook is then withdrawn and a laparoscopic spreader introduced. The pyloric incision is deepened bluntly as in the open technique to expose the bulging mucosa.

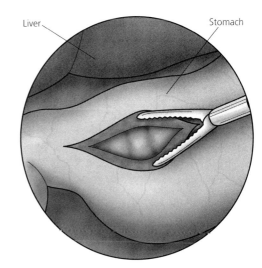

10 Pyloromyotomy showing split hypertrophied pyloric muscle with exposed intact mucosal layer in the depth of the split.

Following completion of the procedure, the stab incisions are closed with surgical glue. The supraumbilical port is removed, and the purse-string suture loosened and then retied to close the wound. The skin is closed with glue.

Postoperative analgesia can be achieved by infiltrating the closed wounds with 0.25 percent bupivicaine.

POSTOPERATIVE CARE

Patients are transferred from the recovery room to a regular hospital bed and intravenous fluids are continued. Feedings are begun and advanced as per surgeon preference. The authors find that, whereas in the past surgeons fed infants slowly, most of the time these infants can be advanced in their feedings quite rapidly once it is clear that they are tolerating oral intake, and start with an initial feeding of 15 mL (1 oz) of the infant's regular milk. If that is tolerated we commence *ad libitum* feeds 1 hour later. It is not unusual to see some occasional postoperative emesis. If this persists, it is usually due to curds of milk retained in the stomach, in which case, the authors lavage the stomach with a 10 percent solution of sodium bicarbonate and begin the feeding regimen again.

COMPLICATIONS

Other than the occasional postoperative emesis, the most frequently observed complication is wound infection. This is usually due to *Staphylococcus aureus* and is infrequently seen with the laparoscopic approach.

Mucosal perforation may occur as previously described. Following closure of the perforation, a nasogastric tube is left following the procedure and intravenous antibiotics given for 48 hours. The infant remains 'nil by mouth' for 24 hours postoperatively. If the infant remains well after this time, feeds are commenced. Incomplete pyloromyotomy is a rare complication (approximately 1 percent) and is due to an inadequate length of pyloromyotomy, usually at the gastric end. After initial improvement, the vomiting persists. This complication requires distinction from gastroesophageal reflux and the diagnosis is made by upper gastrointestinal contrast study. Repeat pyloromyotomy (open or laparoscopic) is curative.

FURTHER READING

Adibe OO, Nichol PF, Lim FY *et al*. Ad libitum feeds after laparoscopic pyloromyotomy: a retrospective comparison with a standardized feeding regimen in 227 infants. *Journal of Laparoendoscopic and Advanced Surgical Techniques* 2007; **17**: 235–7.

Alain JL, Grousseau D, Terrier G. Extramucosal pyloromyotomy by laparoscopy. *Surgical Endoscopy* 1991; **5**: 174–5.

Hall NJ, Pacilli M, Eaton S *et al*. Recovery after open versus laparoscopic pyloromyotomy for pyloric stenosis: a double-blind multicentre randomised controlled trial. *Lancet* 2009; **373**: 390–8.

Leclair MD, Plattner V, Mirallie E *et al*. Laparoscopic pyloromyotomy for hypertrophic pyloric stenosis: a prospective, randomized controlled trial. *Journal of Pediatric Surgery* 2007; **42**: 692–8.

Najmaldin A, Tan HL. Early experience with laparoscopic pyloromyotomy for infantile hypertrophic pyloric stenosis. *Journal of Pediatric Surgery* 1995; **30**: 37–8.

St Peter SD, Holcomb GW III, Calkins CM *et al*. Open versus laparoscopic pyloromyotomy for pyloric stenosis: a prospective, randomized trial. *Annals of Surgery* 2006; **244**: 363–70.

Tan KC, Bianchi A. Circumumbilical incision for pyloromyotomy. *British Journal of Surgery* 1986; **73**: 399.

46

Bariatric surgery: principles

SEAN J BARNETT and THOMAS H INGE

HISTORY

As the epidemic of pediatric obesity has been increasingly documented, and the efficacy and safety of bariatric surgery for adults has also become evident, more consideration has been given to bariatric procedures for clinically severely obese adolescents. Over the past 30 years, many bariatric procedures with various modifications have been introduced, including intestinal bypass (jejunocolic or jejunoileal), loop gastric bypass, horizontal and vertical gastroplasty, Roux-en-Y gastric bypass (RYGBP), biliopancreatic diversion (with or without duodenal switch), adjustable gastric banding, and most recently, sleeve gastrectomy. From the beginning of the subspecialty of bariatric surgery, the goal of the operation is to either restrict the intake of nutrients, interfere with the absorption of nutrients that are ingested, or both. The long-term goal is to maintain a degree of weight reduction which improves or eliminates obesity-related comorbidities and decreases the risk of future obesity-related medical complications and death.

PRINCIPLES AND JUSTIFICATION

Currently, minimally invasive techniques are being used for all of the modern weight loss procedures. These include RYGBP, the adjustable gastric band (AGB), the biliopancreatic diversion with duodenal switch, and the sleeve gastrectomy (SG). The procedure that has been used most commonly in this country and worldwide is the RYGBP, as this procedure has been associated with the safest side-effect profile, balanced with excellent long-term efficacy and maintenance of weight loss. Bariatric surgery effectively creates a 'tool' with which adolescents can lose one-third or more of their body mass and concomitantly reduce or eliminate most comorbidities of adolescent obesity.

This chapter focuses specifically on:

- the perioperative preparation of the patient and family once the decision for surgery has been made;

- technical aspects of the three most commonly performed bariatric surgeries in adolescents, namely the laparoscopic RYGBP, laparoscopic SG, and the laparoscopic AGB;
- postoperative management.

The NIH Bariatric Consensus Development Conference in 1991 concluded that two bariatric procedures, namely vertical banded gastroplasty and RYGBP, should be options for weight management for adults with morbid obesity given the recognized morbidity and mortality of uncorrected severe obesity. This conference concluded that there was insufficient data to make recommendations about bariatric surgery for patients <18 years of age. Significant, durable weight loss and long-term medical benefits have now been documented for adults who have undergone RYGBP. For this reason, current opinion holds that bariatric surgery should also be an option for highly selected adolescents with extreme obesity. Since relatively little is known about the long-term sequelae of bariatric surgery when performed in adolescence, conservative indications for operation have been recommended. Surgery should be reserved after at least six months of organized weight loss attempts have failed.

Recent best practice guidelines have been developed for pediatric/adolescent weight loss surgery. These new guidelines more closely mimic those for adult surgery than in previous years. Those considered for weight loss surgery include adolescents with a body mass index (BMI) ≥35 kg/m^2 and several specific obesity-related comorbidities for which there is clear evidence of short-term morbidity (type 2 diabetes, severe steatohepatitis, pseudotumor cerebri, and moderate to severe obstructive sleep apnea). Those adolescents with a BMI >40 kg/m^2 and other long-term medical co-morbidities should also be considered for weight loss surgery. Physical maturity should be documented by either history and physical examination or radiographic study, thus generally limiting surgery to those over the age of 12 years. The reader is referred to other sources for further discussion of the contraindications and preoperative decision-making for adolescent bariatric surgery.

Bariatric programs for adolescents should include expertise in adolescent obesity, nutrition, diet, and behavioral management. It is critical that thorough investigations be conducted to discover unrecognized coexisting obesity-related medical conditions. Minimally invasive surgery has significant advantages over open surgery, including a reduction in length of hospitalization and operative morbidity. Minimally invasive bariatric surgery is one of the most technically difficult operations to perform. Laparoscopic skills utilized in foregut surgery are not directly transferable to bariatric surgery. Expertise in minimally invasive surgery may not confer the same level of expertise in performing minimally invasive bariatric surgery. Surgeons performing bariatric procedures must be well trained as suggested by the American Society for Bariatric Surgery, American College of Surgeons, and the Society of American Gastrointestinal Endoscopic Surgeons. Prior to performing laparoscopic bariatric operations, surgeons must meet all local credentialing requirements for the performance of open bariatric procedures and advanced laparoscopic operations. Given the controversy centered on adolescent bariatric surgery, the aspiring adolescent bariatric surgeon, at a minimum, should take a course in bariatric surgery and perform his or her first five to ten procedures proctored by an experienced laparoscopic bariatric surgeon.

PREOPERATIVE ASSESSMENT AND PREPARATION

The preoperative education of the patient, family, and to some extent, the referring pediatrician, is of paramount importance. Information about the surgical procedure, alternative operations and the rationale for the operation to be performed, postoperative care, and the considerable lifestyle modifications required afterwards must be conveyed verbally and in writing to the patient and caregivers. The adolescent and parents must demonstrate understanding of the details of the procedure, its known and potential risks, and predictable consequences, and that understanding should be reflected in the archived responses to a written test. The referring pediatrician will need to become familiar with the anatomic and physiologic changes that occur after operation and develop an understanding of common postoperative complications to effectively partner with the surgeon in the care of the patient for years following the operation.

On the day prior to surgery, the patients are limited to clear liquids. No bowel preparation is required. Preoperative medications include low molecular weight heparin (40 mg s.c. and continued twice a day postoperatively while in hospital), and a second-generation cephalosporin (2 g i.v.); we prefer cefoxitin. Sequential compression boots are also used intra- and postoperatively and should be applied and functioning prior to induction of anesthesia. All patients should be considered candidates for the laparoscopic approach unless they have had extensive abdominal surgery in the past. There are no minimally invasive pediatric surgical procedures more technically challenging than bariatric surgical procedures.

Anesthesia

Patients undergo general anesthesia for all laparoscopic bariatric surgical procedures. There is generally no need for epidural analgesia. Routine preoperative consultation with the anesthesiologist and cardiologist is recommended to uncover potentially important information about the patient's airway, the patient or family's anesthetic history, and to determine whether occult cardiovascular disease is present. Preoperative anesthesia consultation also provides an opportunity for unhurried discussion of any concerns or questions the family or patient may have about the technique and risks of anesthesia.

Equipment

Although extra-long (45 cm) laparoscopic instrumentation is available for bariatric procedures, in general, laparoscopic bariatric procedures can be performed using standard 32-cm adult instrumentation. Various manufacturers supply the equipment required and the choice of one over another is largely a matter of surgeon preference. Specific instrumentation used at Cincinnati Children's Hospital for these procedures includes:

- All procedures:
  - 1 percent lidocaine, 10-cc syringe, and a long (spinal) needle
  - One 0°, 32-cm laparoscope (for initial abdominal access with ENDOPATH® XCEL™ Optiview trocar (Ethicon Endosurgery (EES))
  - One 30°, 32-cm laparoscope
  - One locking, atraumatic bowel grasper
  - Two non-locking atraumatic bowel graspers
  - One locking toothed grasper (used for liver retraction)
  - One hook scissor for cutting suture
  - One needle driver
  - One Wolfe bipolar electrocautery forceps
  - One Harmonic® scalpel (Ethicon Endosurgery)
  - Multiple 8 inch lengths of 2-0 silk and 3-0 dyed vicryl on SH needles
- Specific to RYGBP:
  - Three 10/12-mm ENDOPATH XCEL trocars (Ethicon Endosurgery)
  - Two to three 5-mm ENDOPATH XCEL trocars (Ethicon Endosurgery)

- One 15-mm ENDOPATH XCEL trocar (Ethicon Endosurgery)
- One Echelon Flex™ 60-mm Endocutter stapler (Ethicon Endosurgery, part No. LONG60A)
- Multiple blue (3.5-mm Ethicon part No. ECR60B) and white (2.5-mm Ethicon part No. ECR60W) staple loads
- One endoscopic curved circular stapler 25-mm (EEA) (Ethicon Endosurgery part No. ECS33)
- Gore SEAMGUARD® bioabsorbable staple line reinforcements, 25-mm EEA (WL Gore and Associates)
- One anvil grasper
- One articulating grasper (Richard Wolf)
- Carter-Thomason CloseSure System XL® (Cooper Surgical, part No. CTXL)
- One Jackson Pratt flat drain
- Specific to SG:
  - Two 10/12-mm ENDOPATH XCEL trocars (Ethicon Endosurgery)
  - Three 5-mm ENDOPATH XCEL trocars (Ethicon Endosurgery)
  - One 15-mm ENDOPATH XCEL trocar (Ethicon Endosurgery)

- One Echelon Flex 60-mm Endocutter stapler (Ethicon Endosurgery part No. LONG60A)
- One green (4.1-mm Ethicon part No. ECR60G) and multiple blue (3.5-mm Ethicon part No. ECR60B) staple loads
- Multiple Gore SEAMGUARD® bioabsorbable staple line reinforcements, 60-mm linear (WL Gore and Associates)
- One piece of umbilical tape measured to 6 cm in length
- One 34 Fr orogastric tube (Kimberly Clark, part No. 15034)
- Carter-Thomason CloseSure System XL (Cooper Surgical Inc, part No. CTXL)
- One Jackson Pratt flat drain
- Specific to AGB:
  - One 10/12-mm ENDOPATH XCEL trocar (Ethicon Endosurgery)
  - One 15-mm ENDOPATH XCEL trocar (Ethicon Endosurgery)
  - Two to three 5-mm ENDOPATH XCEL trocars (Ethicon Endosurgery)
  - One REALIZE® adjustable gastric band-C Pack with endodissector (Ethicon Endosurgery part No. RLZB32D1)

LAPAROSCOPIC ROUX–EN-Y GASTRIC BYPASS OPERATIVE PROCEDURE

1 This procedure is primarily a 'one surgeon' procedure, with the assistant's role largely that of tissue retraction. Thus, the experienced laparoscopic bariatric surgeon can perform this operation without another trained bariatric surgeon as an assistant. During laparoscopic RYGBP, the patient can be flat or in gentle reverse Trendelenburg position with legs together. The surgeon stands on the right, the scrub nurse to the surgeon's right side and the assistant on the left side of the patient. Given the patient's extreme girth, it is ergonomically advantageous to stand on a platform 20–40 cm above the floor. For initial abdominal access, the transparent, bladeless, direct viewing (XCEL Optiview®, Ethicon Endosurgery, Cincinnati, OH, USA) 12-mm trocar can be used safely and efficiently. This trocar is placed through the midline approximately 5–10 cm above the umbilicus. The exact site for this trocar is determined by lying a standard 10-mm adult laparoscopic telescope on the patient's abdomen, with the tip of the scope (the end which will be inside) at the nipple level, marking a skin site at the point beside the light cord insertion point on the scope. This skin site will provide optimal visualization of the upper and lower portions of the procedure. The two other 12-mm and up to two 5-mm trocar placement sites and the 5-mm subzyphoid site for liver retraction are shown.

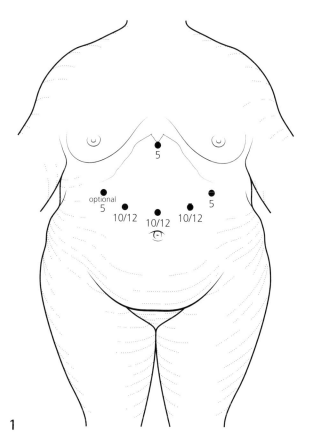

1

Roux limb construction

The omentum is first raised cephalad to expose the transverse mesocolon and origin of the jejunum (ligament of Treitz). Exposure of the small bowel is optimized if the table is placed into slight Trendelenburg position and the omentum is tucked carefully under the liver edge. The transverse mesocolon is grasped with a locking grasper just anterior to the duodenojejunal flexure and elevated anteriorly. The jejunum is divided generally 50 cm beyond the duodenojejunal flexure using the Echelon

60-mm linear stapler (EES, white load). The Roux limb is generally brought up to the pouch in the antecolic fashion, this requires at least 50 cm to comfortably reach the pouch in the epigastrium. The mesentery is minimally divided at this point using either half the length of a second stapler load or the Harmonic scalpel. Clamping the stapler jaws together for a 10-second count before firing mechanically thins the highly vascular tissue to reduce bleeding from the staple line. Bipolar electrocautery may be needed to achieve full hemostasis in this area.

2 There is no unanimity about the exact length of the Roux limb. Current practice employs a 150-cm Roux limb for most patients. With experience, the limb length can be visually estimated, by 'walking' hand over hand down the bowel with laparoscopic graspers. Precision in measurement can be increased by using a 0.25-inch Penrose drain of known length alongside the bowel if desired. Next, a single stay suture is placed to approximate the antemesenteric borders of the distal end of the biliopancreatic segment (the proximal jejunum) and the point 150 cm distal to the end of the roux limb. The Harmonic scalpel is used to make opposing enterotomies which are spread wide enough with a grasper to accept the stapler jaw. A side-to-side jejunojejunostomy is created using the 60-mm Echelon stapler with white load. The resulting enterotomy defect is closed either with a running 3-0 vicryl (SH needle) or by using another firing of the stapler (preferred method). There is an increased risk of narrowing the lumen if the stapled closure is not applied precisely. The mesenteric defect is next closed with a running 2-0 silk suture to avoid an internal hernial orifice.

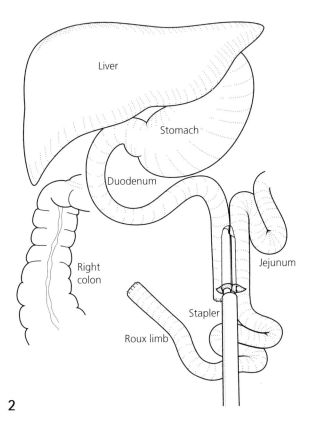

2

Since the antecolic technique is technically more straightforward and does not risk troublesome bleeding in the transverse mesocolon, it is a favored method by many high-volume bariatric surgeons. In the antecolic technique, the omentum must be draped back inferiorly, and often bivalved up to the transverse colon, to reduce the bulk of tissue that the roux limb will traverse. This omental division also reduces the tension (and thus risk of stricture) transmitted from the Roux limb to the anastomosis when the patient assumes an erect posture postoperatively. Finally, some surgeons have used the bivalved omentum to 'wrap' the gastrojejunal anastomosis at the conclusion of the operation. This technique has theoretical benefit in the event of leakage

of the gastrojejunal anastomosis, but is not commonly performed.

Gastric pouch construction

A locking, toothed grasper is next inserted below the xyphoid, applied to tissue just superior to the right crus of the diaphragm, and used to retract the left lobe of the liver anteriorly to expose the gastroesophageal junction. The lesser curve gastric pouch will be created beginning with the dissection at the angle of His. A sufficient plane is then created between the stomach and diaphragm at the angle of His, extending to the left crus, utilizing dissection both bluntly and with the Harmonic scalpel.

3 Next, a small gastrotomy is made along the greater curvature of the stomach with the Harmonic scalpel. The left upper quadrant (LUQ) 12-mm port site is then enlarged with a Kelly hemostat to allow passage of the 25-mm EEA stapler. The plastic tip of the anvil is dulled gently by the scrub assistant and a loop of vicryl suture is inserted through its end prior to its insertion. The anvil is then passed through the enlarged fascial defect in the LUQ and into the abdomen. Often a 15-mm XCEL trocar is needed to be placed within this newly created fascial defect to allow for adequate insufflations for the remainder of the procedure. The vicryl loop is then grasped with the articulating grasper and the entire anvil is placed through the previously made gastrotomy site. A site is chosen approximately 3–4 cm inferior to the esophageal hiatus along the lesser curvature of the stomach for the proposed gastrojejunostomy site. The point of the articulating grasper is then brought out through this proposed site with the aid of the Harmonic scalpel. Once this is accomplished, the suture is grasped and the connecting end (with the plastic insert) is brought out in its entirety through this site. The gastrotomy is then closed utilizing one or two loads from the blue stapler.

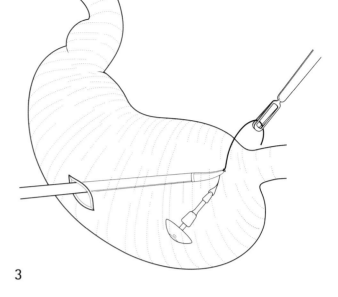

3

The creation of the gastric pouch begins with perigastric Harmonic scalpel dissection along the lesser curvature approximately 6–10 cm inferior to the gastroesophageal junction (usually just below the second major lesser curve vessel). The 'flat' side of the blade is used to ensure adequate hemostasis during this dissection. Bipolar electrocautery is also commonly needed. This dissection is continued posteriorly in close proximity to the gastric wall until the plane nearly reaches the lesser sac behind the stomach.

The greater curvature of the stomach is next elevated and a thin area of the gastrocolic ligament is chosen for entry into the lesser sac, using the Harmonic scalpel. Numerous posterior attachments between the lesser curve and retroperitoneum are divided to achieve continuity between the lesser curve dissection, which was performed anteriorly.

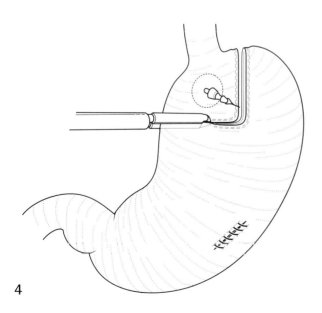

4

4 The dissection is continued gently such that the tip of the Harmonic scalpel traverses the posterior surgical plane to emerge anteriorly when the stomach is released. A tubular lesser curve pouch is next created using the Echelon 60-mm stapler with multiple blue loads. The first transverse cut across the lesser curvature, is achieved by abutting against the anvil of the EEA stapler, traversing the lesser curve dissection plane created above. Once in place across the lesser curve, the stapler is fired creating the inferior most margin of the pouch. Next, gentle dissection is performed at the apex of the staple line to completely break into the retrogastric lesser sac from above. This simple maneuver is critical since the procedure is far less difficult if the lesser sac is identified and entered from the anterior aspect at this point. The vertical staple line is advanced sequentially by multiple applications of the Echelon 60-mm stapler along the anvil of the EEA stapler. Once the angle of His is reached, the pouch is complete.

Gastrojejunal anastomosis

There are numerous techniques for laparoscopic gastrojejunostomy including handsewn, the end-to-end stapled technique with the anvil inserted orally (akin to the percutaneous endoscopic gastrostomy (PEG) method of gastrostomy), a linearly stapled technique, and the end-to-end stapled technique with anvil inserted into the pouch laparoscopically. When considering choices of technique, it is usually best to learn from someone who will be readily available for technical consultation, and adopt the technique that he or she employs. The remainder of this chapter will focus on details and pearls for performance of the EEA-stapled gastrojejunostomy technique.

5 With the gastric pouch created and the anvil of the EEA stapler in place and in full view, the previously fashioned Roux limb is brought up to the gastric pouch via an antecolic fashion. The end of the Roux limb is then opened along the antimesenteric border for approximately 4–6 cm with the Harmonic scalpel, enough space to accept the end of the 25-mm EEA stapler head. The EEA stapler is loaded with a Gore staple-line reinforcement insert and is introduced through the previously widened LUQ port. To protect the Gore staple-line reinforcement insert, a plastic sheath is placed over the stapler. This portion of the procedure can be tedious unless the port site has been widened appropriately. Once the stapler has been inserted, the plastic sheath is pulled away and the end of the EEA stapler is inserted into the open end of the Roux limb. Counter-traction is necessary to ensure that the entire stapler head is within the lumen. With continued traction, the stapler end is slowly opened until the internal mating device pierces through the small bowel (a). The pin is then removed from the end of the anvil. The anvil grasper is then used to mate the two ends of the stapler together. Gentle traction is applied below the proposed anastomosis to ensure that no stray tissue is within the final anastomosis. The stapler is then closed, fired, then removed from the port site with the anvil intact. One should check to ensure that two separate donuts of tissue are contained within the stapler complex at its inspection. The 15-mm trocar is then replaced to allow for adequate insufflation. The Harmonic scalpel is then used to take down the mesentery along the mesenteric border of the remaining section of the Roux limb lateral to the anastomosis. (b,c). An Echelon 60-mm stapler white load is then used to close the enterotomy, thus completing the anastomosis. The integrity and patency of the anastomosis is assessed laparoscopically with intraluminal air insufflation under saline. This pneumatic test is accomplished by temporarily obstructing the Roux limb just beyond the anastomosis and having the anesthesiologist rapidly bolus 60 cc of air into an orogastric tube.

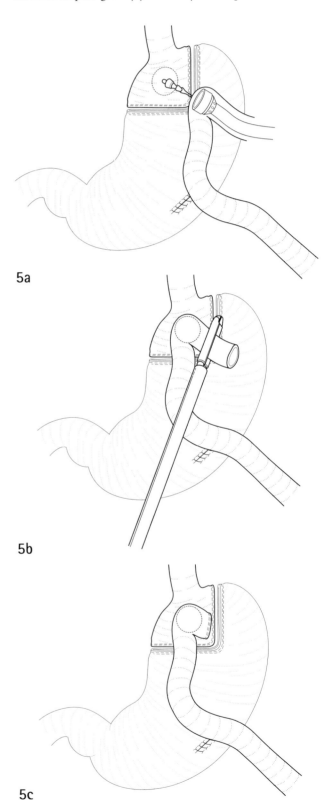

5a

5b

5c

A drain to prevent fluid collection within the abdomen and to provide for early identification of a leak is left near the anastomosis and exits via the patient's upper right trocar site. A temporary gastrostomy tube can be placed in the remnant stomach body if any intraoperative technical challenges are deemed significant enough to warrant deliberate decompression of the bypassed gastric remnant.

With the use of the bladeless trocars, the 5- and 12-mm port sites do not require fascial closure. The 15-mm port site is closed utilizing the Carter-Thomason CloseSure System in a figure-of-eight type fashion with 0 vicryl suture. The remaining skin incisions are closed in the standard surgical fashion.

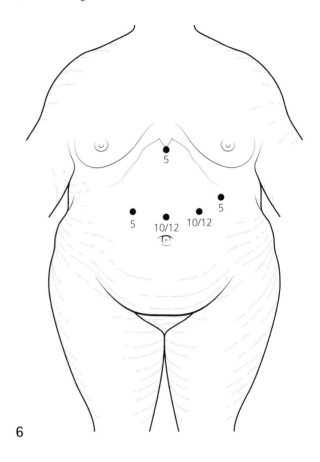

6

Laparoscopic sleeve gastrectomy operative procedure

6 The patient is positioned in a similar manner as previously described for the RYGBP procedure. Two 12-mm and three 5-mm trocars are utilized for the procedure and placed via a similar manner as previously described. A 34 Fr orogastric tube is placed by anesthesia at the beginning of the case and placed on suction to aid in the dissection. The liver retractor is placed in a similar manner as previously described.

Greater curvature dissection

7 An umbilical tape, cut to 6 cm in length, is placed within the abdomen and used to measure the distance from the distal extent of the pylorus along the greater curvature. This is the point where the dissection and initial resection will begin. The greater omentum is then carefully dissected away from the greater curvature of the stomach at this point until the lesser sac is entered. This dissection is carried to the level of the left crus of the diaphragm. The 34 Fr orogastric tube aids in the identification of the esophagus and the left crus during this portion of the procedure. The assistant is invaluable during this dissection, providing traction and counter-traction, given the often large size of the stomach in these cases. All attachments of the fundic portion of the stomach are taken down as this can sometimes be folded under the body of the stomach at its superior extent.

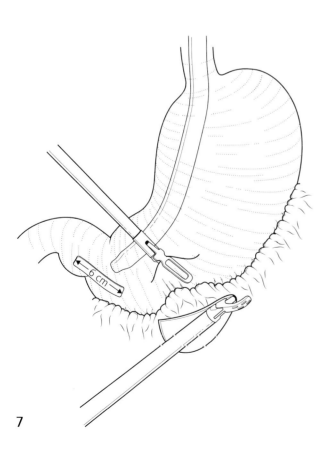

7

Gastric resection

8, 9 The resectional portion of the procedure is begun by once again measuring from the pylorus to the greater curvature/antrum of the stomach with the 6 cm of umbilical tape. The 34 Fr orogastric tube is then positioned into the antrum and along the lesser curvature of the stomach to act as a guide for the remainder of the procedure. Given its relative thickness, the Echelon 60-mm stapler with a green load, without Gore Seamguard® Bioabsorbable Staple Line Reinforcement, is used for the first fire across the antrum of the stomach abutting against the 34 Fr orogastric tube. The remainder of the stapler fires are carried out sequentially along the 34 Fr orogastric tube (adjacent to the lesser curvature of the stomach) with the Echelon 60-mm stapler, blue loads with Gore Seamguard Bioabsorbable Staple Line Reinforcement. As the esophagus is approached during the final stages of the resection, it is prudent to veer off slightly lateral to avoid its injury. This does leave a small triangular portion of stomach at the superior aspect of the resection margin, but ensures that the esophagus remains free from the staple line. This maneuver could potentially decrease the incidence of leaks at this site given the relative proximity of the thin esophageal tissue. The body and fundic portion of the stomach is now free and is removed from the abdomen by gently widening the LUQ 12-mm port site with a Kelly hemostat. The remnant can be placed in a laparoscopic retrieval bag prior to its removal, but in the authors' experience, we find that the remnant can be removed by simple traction with multiple Kelly hemostats through the widened port site alone.

The staple line can be tested and the enlarged LUQ 12-mm port is closed in a similar manner as described previously with a drain placed along its length. The skin incisions are once again closed in the standard surgical fashion.

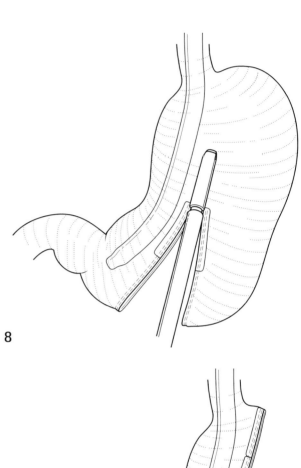

8

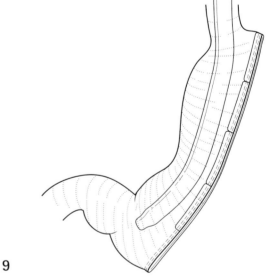

9

LAPAROSCOPIC ADJUSTABLE GASTRIC BAND OPERATIVE PROCEDURE

10 Although the adjustable gastric band is not currently approved by the Food and Drug Administration (FDA) for use in patients under the age of 18 years of age, there are certainly patients older than 17 who present to our institution for bariatric surgery. Because the weight loss seen in patients with the gastric band is less overall when compared to both the RYGBP and SG procedures, it is likely more suitable in those patients with a BMI of 45 kg/m^2 or less. One 15-mm, one 12-mm, and two 5-mm trocars are used to perform this procedure and are placed as previously described in the arrangement illustrated.

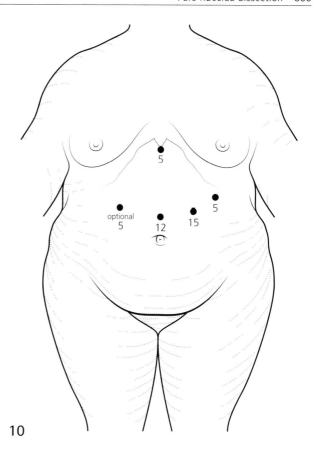

10

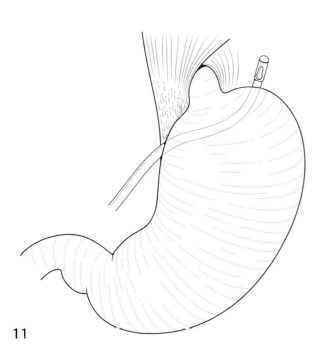

11

PARS FLACCIDA DISSECTION

11 The liver retractor is placed in a similar manner as described. The adjustable gastric band is first checked under saline for any evidence of leak at the balloon site prior to its insertion. All of the air is then removed from the balloon. The band is then gasped by its end, away from the balloon, stretched along the length of the laparoscopic grasper and placed through the LUQ 15-mm port site completely into the abdomen (this step can be performed before or after the pars flaccia dissection). The hook cautery or Harmonic scapel may then be used to dissect the angle of His carefully to expose the left crus of the diaphragm. A 5-mm blunt endoscopic dissector (supplied in the Realize® pack) is used, via the pars flaccida approach through the lesser omentum, to create a tunnel behind the superior portion of the stomach near the esophagogastric junction. Care must be taken to clearly identify the right crus of the diaphragm during this blind dissection under the stomach to avoid damage to the inferior vena cava (IVC) or aorta. Blunt dissection continues gently along the right crus to allow passage completely underneath the stomach. The hiatus is inspected at this time and a hiatal hernia should be repaired primarily before placement of the band. The dissector can then be articulated to be easily visualized on the patient's left of the esophagus/stomach. There is no need for any further dissection or to take down any of the short gastric vessels as this can lead to an increase in band slippage over time.

12 The suture end of the lock-end flap is then placed into the groove of the blunt dissector, the dissector straightened and pulled from left to right, through the created retrogastric tunnel, and into position around the stomach (a). A grasper is then placed through the buckle and the lock-end flap is pulled through the buckle and locked into place (b). The band is then rotated so that the buckle will eventually lie along the lesser curvature of the stomach. Rarely, a portion of the anterior paraesophageal fat pad (generally by the Harmonic scalpel) needs to be taken down to allow for correct placement. Three silk sutures are then placed to plicate the body of the stomach to the newly formed pouch, over the band to prevent band slippage (c).

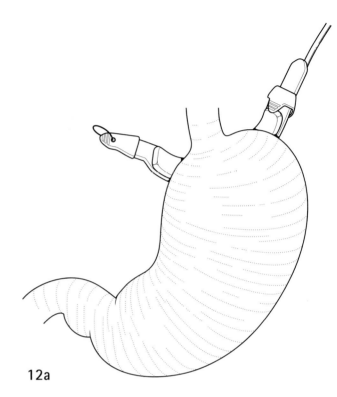

12a

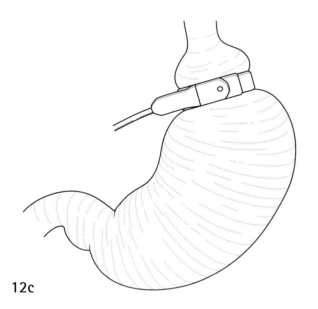

12c

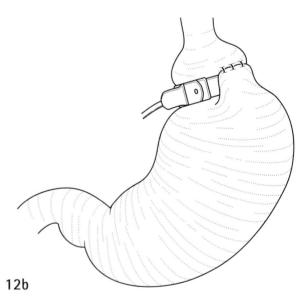

12b

13 The band tubing is then brought out through a separate site after a subcutaneous pocket is fashioned more towards the epigastrium. This not only allows for adequate visualization of the fascia for port placement, but also places the port in the same position each time to allow for easier identification for access in the clinic. The injector port is then attached to the tubing and transfixed to the fascia by an intrinsic staple device or by non-absorbable suture. Often the band is primed with up to 5 mL of sterile water at the conclusion of the procedure. There is no need for fascial closure of the 5- and 12-mm ports, but the 15-mm port site should be closed at the fascial level. The overlying skin of the port sites are closed in the standard fashion. In contrast to the two previously described procedures, there is no need for drain placement following the procedure and patients are generally discharged within 1 day postoperatively. Most adult programs will perform this procedure as an outpatient.

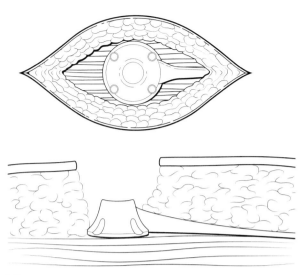

13

POSTOPERATIVE CARE

Postoperatively, the patients are typically extubated in the operating room after transfer to the hospital bed. They are cared for in a monitored, non-intensive care unit setting, and maintenance fluids are administered based upon lean body weight (typically 40–50 percent of actual weight). Early warning signs of complication include fever, tachycardia, tachypnea, increasing oxygen requirement, oliguria, hiccoughs, regurgitation, left shoulder pain, worsening abdominal pain, a feeling of anxiety, or acute alteration in mental status. These signs warrant aggressive attention and appropriate investigation since they may signal gastrointestinal leak (anastomosis or staple lines), pulmonary embolus, bowel obstruction, or acute dilation and impending rupture of the bypassed gastric remnant. Routinely, a water-soluble upper gastrointestinal (UGI) contrast study is obtained on postoperative day 1 following the RYGBP but only as needed for SG. After satisfactory passage of contrast is documented, patients are begun on clear liquids and subsequently advanced to a high protein liquid diet for the first month after operation. AGB patients are started on clear liquids immediately following the procedure and generally discharged home on post-operative day 1 without the need for a UGI study.

Postoperative monitoring

Bariatric surgery essentially results in surgically enforced very low-calorie, low-carbohydrate dietary intake, thus requiring attention to an adequate intake of important macro- and micronutrients postoperatively. Postoperative follow up after RYGBP and SG in adolescence is intensive – 2 week postoperative visit, then at 6 weeks, 3 months, 6 months, 9 months, 12 months, 18 months, 24 months,

then yearly. Serum chemistries, complete blood count, urine specific gravity, prothrombin time (evidence of vitamin K adequacy) and representative B complex vitamin levels (e.g. B1, B12, folate) are obtained at 3, 6, 9, and 12 months post-operatively then yearly. Body composition can be assessed with either bioelectrical impedance or dual energy x-ray absorptiometry analysis (DEXA; for patients weighing less than 300 lb (136 kg)). DEXA not only allows for the measurement of rate and relative amounts of fat and lean body mass loss, but also provides a quantitative assessment of bone mineral density changes. This body composition analysis can be used to modify dietary plans intended to preserve lean body mass during the period of dramatic weight loss.

The follow up for gastric banding is more frequent and labor-intensive given the need for frequent adjustments. Prior to the operation, patients are told to expect up to ten visits for adjustments of their band within the first postoperative year. Some adult programs will utilize fluoroscopy for adjustments to decrease this number of visits. Routine screening at six months and then yearly with esophograms is performed to evaluate for esophageal dilation.

Postoperative diet

For the first postoperative month, the diet is essentially a protein-rich liquid diet. Dietary advancement after the first month is a methodical process of introducing new items of gradually increasing complexity, toward the goal of a well-balanced, small portion (approximately one cup per meal) diet which ensures a daily intake of 1 g of protein per kg of ideal weight. Non-steroidal anti-inflammatory medications should be avoided to reduce the risk of intestinal ulceration and bleeding most commonly seen in RYGBP. Ranitidine is prescribed for six months postoperatively with some sleeve gastrectomy patients requiring the transition to a proton-pump inhibitor due to the increased incidence of reflux-type symptoms. Our program commonly prescribed urosodial in the past, but this practice has been abandoned due to conflicting literature of its use and efficacy and a lack of clinical evidence. Postoperative vitamin and mineral supplementation typically consists of two pediatric chewable multivitamins, a calcium supplement, and an iron supplement for menstruating females. B-complex vitamins are supplemented beyond that which is contained in multivitamin preparations, primarily to augment thiamine and folate supplementation, due to severe complications if deficiency develops. Adjustable gastric banding patients will start a more solid diet by postoperative weeks 2–4. They are instructed to eat small portions, slowly, and to wait at least 30 minutes to drink after eating. This allows for the expansion of the pouch and satiety.

Five basic 'rules' are routinely emphasized with patients and family at each visit: (1) eat protein first; (2) drink 64–96 oz of water or sugar-free liquids daily; (3) no snacking between meals; (4) exercise at least 30 minutes per day; and (5) always remember vitamins and minerals.

OUTCOME

Patient satisfaction has generally been very good with this surgical and postoperative approach. Weight loss at a rate of 2.5 kg per week for the first six months is not uncommon in both RYGBP and SG. Weight loss with the AGB will be slower. The RYGBP and SG operation results in a loss of 60–80 percent of excess weight over the first year postoperatively. When careful attention is given to adequate protein intake, significant improvements in body composition can be expected after operation. In a recent study from Australia, adolescents with the AGB can still lose from 50 to 70 percent of their excess weight over the span of two years, but did require a significant number of reoperations. At Cincinnati Children's Hospital, adolescents undergoing RYGBP and SG have an average BMI between 50 and 60. Using detailed body composition analysis, we find that these patients lose nearly 20 percent of both fat mass and lean mass in the first three months following RYGBP. Interestingly, absolute

fat mass decreases further by 40 percent from three to 12 months postoperatively, while absolute lean mass does not decrease further after three months. Consequently, body composition significantly improved over time, with mean percentage fat mass decreasing from 47 percent preoperatively, to 45 percent at three months to 35 percent at 12 months. Fat loss appeared to plateau by 12 months. This suggests that adolescents undergoing laparoscopic RYGBP dramatically and preferentially reduced body fat mass compared to more modest loss of lean body mass. Additionally, we have found no detrimental effects of RYGBP on bone mineral density after short-term follow up of one year. Further data have also demonstrated a resolution of diabetes and hypertension – well-known risk factors for cardiovascular disease, following RYGBP. Data at this time for the short- and long-term effects of the sleeve gastrectomy are limited in the adolescent, but the excess weight loss appears to mimic that of patients undergoing RYGBP in this cohort of patients at our institution. The current National Institutes of Health (NIH)-sponsored TEEN-LABS study hopes to answer many of the questions with regards to both short- and long-term effects of bariatric surgery on the adolescent.

FURTHER READING

Colquitt JL, Picot J, Loveman E, Clegg AJ. Surgery for obesity. *Cochrane Database of Systematic Reviews* 2009; **15**: CD003641.

DeLaet D, Schauer D. Obesity in adults. *Clinical Evidence* 2011; **3**: 604.

Inge TH, Jenkins TM, Zeller M *et al.* Baseline BMI is a strong predictor of nadir BMI after adolescent gastric bypass. *Journal of Pediatrics* 2010; **156**: 103–8.

Inge TH, Miyano G, Bean J *et al.* Reversal of type 2 diabetes mellitus and improvements in cardiovascular risk factors after surgical weight loss in adolescents. *Pediatrics* 2009; **123**: 214–22.

O'Brien PE, Sawyer SM, Laurie C *et al.* Laparoscopic adjustable gastric banding in severely obese adolescents: a randomized trial. *Journal of the American Medical Association* 2010; **303**: 519–26.

Pratt JS, Lenders CM, Dionne EA *et al.* Best practice updates for pediatric/adolescent weight loss surgery. *Obesity* 2009; **17**: 901–10.

47

Duodenoduodenostomy

ROBERT E CILLEY, SIMON CLARKE, and ARNOLD G CORAN

OPEN DUODENODUODENOSTOMY

Robert E Cilley and Arnold G Coran

HISTORY

The surgical correction of congenital duodenal obstruction was made difficult by a lack of appropriate suture material and the lack of understanding of the perioperative care needs of neonates. By the middle of the twentieth century, enteroenterostomy, typically using a retrocolic, side-to-side duodenojejunostomy, became the standard operation for this problem. Improved perioperative care of the sick neonate resulted in many survivors. More recently, duodenoduodenostomy has been used to bypass congenital duodenal obstruction in an effort to hasten the return of intestinal function after surgery and to promote duodenal emptying. Duodenoduodenostomy may be performed in either a standard side-to-side fashion or in an eccentric fashion commonly known as the 'diamond duodenoduodenostomy'. Video-endoscopic techniques for treating congenital duodenal obstruction are gaining popularity.

PRINCIPLES AND JUSTIFICATION

The choice of surgical procedure for the treatment of duodenal obstruction is largely based on the preference of the surgeon. There may be unusual anatomic variants that make one procedure obviously preferred at the time of surgery. Each surgeon should be familiar with options. The diamond duodenoduodenostomy may result in earlier postoperative feeding and shorter duration of hospitalization. The procedure may be performed using open surgical techniques or video-endoscopically. The duodenoduodenostomy is applicable to almost all cases of duodenal obstruction, whether caused by stenosis or atresia, with or without annular pancreas. It may also be used as a safe choice for the treatment of a duodenal web, since it does not risk damage to the pancreaticobiliary system, which may occur with web excision. In the hands of those experienced with the technique, almost any atresia is readily handled using the mobility afforded by the dilated proximal duodenum in combination with mobilization of the distal duodenum beneath the superior mesenteric vessels. A one-layer anastomotic technique is used most often. Although a decompressing gastrostomy was placed at the time of surgery in the past, this is no longer done routinely. In a child with multiple anomalies, in whom poor feeding is predictable, a gastrostomy may be added to the duodenoduodenostomy. The only contraindication to surgery is the presence of multiple severe anomalies incompatible with life.

PREOPERATIVE

Duodenal obstruction may be diagnosed prenatally by fetal ultrasound or fetal magnetic resonance imaging. A dilated stomach and duodenum are seen on imaging studies. Neonates with congenital duodenal obstruction most often present with obvious symptoms on the first day of life. Feeding intolerance and vomiting, which is usually bilious, are noted from the outset. Vomiting may be non-bilious when preampullary obstruction is present. Dehydration and electrolyte depletion rapidly ensue if the condition is not recognized and intravenous therapy begun. Secondary complications, such as aspiration and respiratory failure, may also be present. The presence of a 'double bubble' on a plain abdominal radiograph is essentially pathognomonic of duodenal atresia. Air may be seen distally in the gastrointestinal tract with an unusual double ampulla that opens both above and below the stenosis. Contrast radiography is confirmatory and may be especially helpful in confirming the pathology when duodenal stenosis (incomplete obstruction) is present or unusual pancreaticobiliary anatomy allows air into the distal intestinal tract. Differentiating intrinsic duodenal obstruction from malrotation with volvulus may be difficult, and contrast radiography may also be helpful. Duodenal obstruction is treated less urgently than malrotation by some surgeons and therefore differentiating between the two entities is critical.

Trisomy 21, occurring in one-third of affected infants, and congenital heart disease must be suspected in all children with duodenal atresia. Duodenal atresia also occurs as part of the Feingold syndrome and Joubert syndrome and has been reported in Goldenhar syndrome and 47XXX.

Concurrent malrotation and second intestinal atresias are gastrointestinal abnormalities that occur with increased frequency in patients with duodenal atresia. The utility of demonstrating distal bowel continuity is debated.

Rarely, duodenal atresia has occurred in association with esophageal atresia, hereditary multiple atresias, and developmental abnormalities of the bile ducts (including choledochal cysts and biliary atresia).

Diagnosis and treatment (timing and sequence) of simultaneous duodenal atresia and esophageal atresia may be difficult. Typically, duodenal repair is performed first, although simultaneous repair may be appropriate.

ANESTHESIA

General anesthesia with rapid sequence endotracheal intubation is required. Many pediatric anesthetists use epidural anesthetic supplementation for the operation, as well as for postoperative analgesia. Prevention of hypothermia is accomplished by heating the operating room, warming the anesthetic gases, external warming lights, operating table warmers, warming of the intravenous fluids, and the use of adhesive plastic drapes for surgical draping.

OPERATION

Incision and initial evaluation

1 A small, transverse, right upper quadrant incision provides adequate exposure. Alternatively, a transumbilical laparotomy may be performed. The type and location of the atresia, as well as any pancreatic abnormality or the presence of a rare preduodenal portal vein are noted. The patient is assessed for any abnormality of intestinal rotation; if present, a Ladd's procedure and appendectomy are performed. The presence of a normal gall bladder is noted.

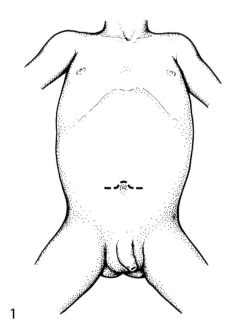

1

Mobilization and retraction

2a,b The hepatic flexure of the colon is mobilized sufficiently to expose the duodenum, and the proximal obstructed duodenum is freed from its retroperitoneal attachments. The requirements for distal mobilization vary according to the location of the atresia. If necessary, the entire distal duodenum may be mobilized from beneath the superior mesenteric artery. Rightward traction on the exposed distal duodenum allows these retroperitoneal attachments to be divided. A transpyloric tube may be passed to determine if a 'windsock' abnormality is present. Either hand-held or fixed, table-mounted retractors may be used.

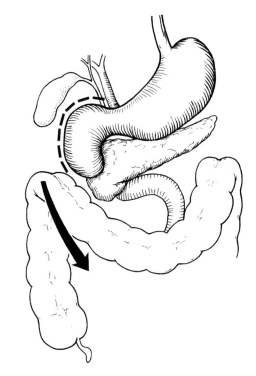

2a

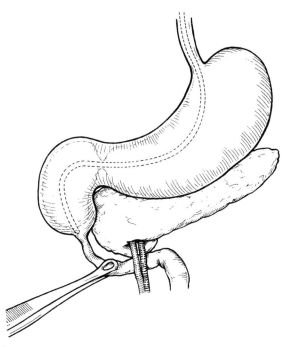

2b

Duodenoduodenostomy

3a–c A transverse duodenotomy is performed in the proximal segment. It is important that this incision be made 1 cm above the atresia to avoid any possibility of injury to the pancreaticobiliary system, which may enter anywhere in the vicinity of the duodenal web, stenosis, or atresia. Retrograde passage of a probe into the stomach confirms the absence of a duodenal web and eliminates the rare possibility of a concurrent gastric antral web. A longitudinal duodenotomy of the same length is created in the distal segment. Passage of a small tube distally confirms patency of the distal duodenum. Injection of air or saline into the distal segment is conveniently performed at this stage to rule out a second atresia if deemed necessary. A single layer of interrupted sutures with posterior knots tied inside and anterior knots tied outside ensures symmetry. The orientation of the sutures in the 'diamond' anastomosis is shown in (b) and the completed anastomosis is shown in (c).

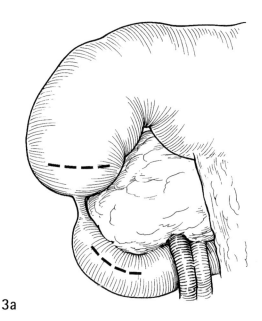

3a

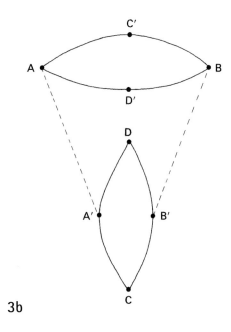

3b

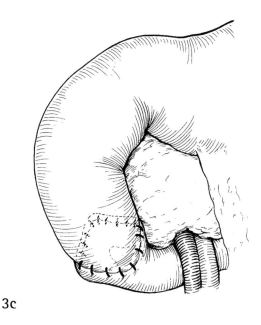

3c

If a long atretic segment is encountered or if it is difficult to mobilize the distal duodenum, a duodenojejunostomy may be performed. The first portion of the jejunum beyond the ligament of Treitz is passed through a small fenestration in the transverse colon mesentery for the duodenal–jejunal anastomosis. A gastrostomy may be performed if the need is anticipated.

Video-endoscopic approaches

Repair of duodenal atresia may be performed as a traditional open procedure, as a hybrid procedure using laparoscopy and a minimal incision, video-endoscopically, or robotically.

Laparoscopic duodenoduodenostomy has been shown to be both safe and effective. Three-millimeter instrumentation and three or four ports are typically used. Potential advantages include earlier postoperative feeding, less pain, and shorter hospitalization.

It is uncertain whether the video-endoscopic technique will be free of technical problems when adopted as a standard surgical practice. Higher leak rates have been reported. Technical changes in anastomotic techniques may minimize such problems. Advances in small articulating instruments will enhance the ability of pediatric surgeons to perform this procedure. It is difficult to confirm patency of the distal gastrointestinal tract during laparoscopy. However, the incidence of second atresias is very low and the need to inspect the remaining intestines has been questioned.

Robotic repair is unlikely to have greater benefit or applicability than standard video-endoscopic techniques.

POSTOPERATIVE CARE

Postoperative care consists primarily of supportive measures to provide nutrition while awaiting the return of intestinal function. Immediate enteral feeding can be started if a transanastomotic tube is placed at the time of the initial operation. Transanastomotic feeding may reduce parenteral nutrition use and improve the time to oral feeding. The disadvantages of transanastomotic feeding include tube dislodgment and intestinal injury. Parenteral nutrition may be used to provide nutritional support postoperatively. To minimize the risks of parenteral nutrition (especially hepatotoxicity), total calories, protein and fat intake should be kept at the lowest levels possible to allow growth. Placement of a central venous catheter at the time of surgery is often convenient. Peripherally inserted central venous catheters are used as well. Unless the child was septic before surgery, only a prophylactic course of antibiotics is indicated. Ventilatory support is provided as needed. Nasogastric or gastrostomy drainage is maintained until gastric emptying begins, as heralded by a change in the quality of the gastric drainage from bilious green to clear or yellow and a decrease in gastric residuals. Feeding is instituted slowly and may require a period of several weeks before full enteral nutrition is tolerated. Standard infant formulas or breast-milk are satisfactory, and expensive, partially digested formulas are usually unnecessary. The need and timing for postoperative contrast studies is debated. There is a trend toward earlier attempts at feedings.

OUTCOME

The outcome depends almost entirely on the presence of other anomalies. Anastomotic leak, intra-abdominal sepsis, and wound complications occur rarely. Missed second atresias are rare. Duodenal atony or paresis with a functional duodenal obstruction in the face of an anatomically patent anastomosis is a rare but frustrating problem. Plication of the duodenum or an alternative method of duodenal bypass is a surgical option if conservative observation is unsuccessful. Long-term complications are uncommon. Symptoms such as pain, vomiting, and feelings of fullness may be present in up to one-third of patients when studied as adults. The symptoms correlate poorly with objective findings on upper gastrointestinal radiographic studies and endoscopy. Late non-function may respond to duodenal plication. Long-term follow up of these patients is recommended.

LAPAROSCOPIC DUODENODUODENOSTOMY

Simon Clarke

As minimal access surgery in neonates became increasingly reported over a decade ago, preliminary reports of the laparoscopic approach being used to treat congenital duodenal obstruction began to emerge.

PRINCIPLES OF LAPAROSCOPIC DUODENODUODENOSTOMY

As in the open approach, adequate exposure with identification of the proximally dilated duodenum and the collapsed distal segment is essential, followed by the creation of a diamond-shaped anastomosis. Potential advantages of the laparoscopic approach are reduced bowel handling, earlier resumption of feeds, fewer adhesions, and improved cosmesis. The magnification of the anastomosis also allows for a significantly improved operative view. Completion of the procedure, however, requires advanced laparoscopic skills.

DIAGNOSIS

The diagnosis of duodenal atresia is usually made prenatally with a double bubble-type appearance on prenatal ultrasound and confirmed with a postnatal abdominal radiograph.

CONTRAINDICATIONS TO LAPAROSCOPIC REPAIR

Low birth weight may be considered a relative contraindication, though successful published reports are described in infants weighing 1.3 kg.

PREOPERATIVE PREPARATION

The diagnosis is confirmed usually with a postnatal radiograph. A double bubble appearance confirms the diagnosis. If sparse distal gas is seen then an incomplete stenosis is a possibility. Echocardiogram is often performed to exclude congenital heart disease.

ANESTHESIA

The procedure requires endotracheal intubation with general anesthesia in a suitably warmed operating theater environment.

PATIENT POSITIONING

The supine infant is either placed at the end of the operating table or across and at the end of the table. The operating surgeon stands at the infant's feet with the cameraman to the surgeon's left and scrub team on the right. A warming blanket surrounding the infant is advisable. The bladder is emptied by the Crede method of gentle suprapubic pressure.

LAPAROSCOPIC INSTRUMENTATION AND SUTURES

- 5-mm optical endoscope 30°
- 3-mm needle holder
- 3-mm Kelly forceps
- 3-mm scissors
- 3-mm soft bowel grasper
- 2-0; 4-0; 5-0 or 6-0 polydioxanone suture

OPERATION

4 Port placements are as follows:

- 1 × 5-mm supraumbilical port is placed under direct vision. A securing purse-string suture is advisable to avoid peritoneal leak of carbon dioxide and for port stability.
- 1 × 3-mm port in the left lateral quadrant just above the umbilicus with a latex catheter cuff to allow a securing suture.
- 1 × 3-mm port in the right lateral quadrant just below the umbilicus with a latex catheter cuff to allow a securing suture.

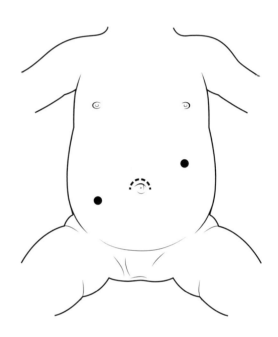

Insufflation

Insufflation is 5–8 mmHg CO_2 at a flow of 1L/min.

Procedure

The liver may obscure the initial view of the duodenum. To visualize the duodenum a 2-0 monofilament suture can be taken into the abdomen and out again through the upper abdominal wall gently hitching up the falciform ligament in its path. This is then tied onto the abdominal wall surface over a pledget to avoid marks on the abdominal wall skin. Alternatively, a 3-mm grasping instrument can be inserted into the left epigastric area to directly elevate the liver.

Once the liver is lifted the dilated duodenal pouch is usually visible. The hepatic flexure of the colon is mobilized to fully expose the duodenum. The dilated duodenum is then released from the surrounding anterior peritoneal attachments (kocherization) and the distal collapsed segment identified. The dissection is best carried out using the Kelly forceps and soft bowel grasper. Care must be taken to avoid injury to the pancreas and common bile duct.

5 Once identified, stabilization of the proximal pouch is essential by inserting one or two 4-0 stay sutures to the proximal pouch. Once inserted through the abdominal wall, the needle can be placed in the dilated duodenum and then taken back out and again tied onto a pledget on the abdominal wall. This now stabilizes the upper pouch ready for the anastomosis.

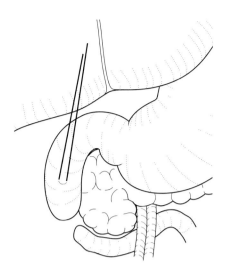

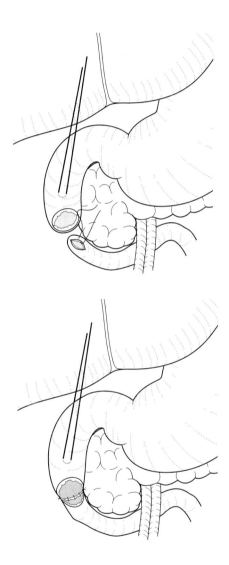

6a A transverse incision is initially made on the upper pouch using a 3-mm hook diathermy and then extended with scissors. Care must be taken not to generate too much heat with the hook as the ampulla may be nearby. A 3-mm sucker can be introduced if bile is seen. A 10–15-mm incision is usually sufficient and is followed by a similar sized longitudinal incision along the distal collapsed segment. Care must be taken when handling the delicate tissue of the distal bowel.

The bowel graspers can be used to gently prise open the two incisions. A separate 5-0 or 6-0 polydioxanone suture can be introduced at this point.

6b The distal collapsed duodenum can then be fixed to the upper pouch incision at the superior and inferior apical points of the intended anastomosis. If the initial superior apical suture is also brought out of the abdominal wall as a stay suture then further stability is afforded for the remainder of the anastomosis.

The posterior wall is then sutured using interrupted or a continuous suture layer with knots tied intracorporeally. Knots lie within the lumen of the bowel for the posterior layer. The anterior layer is then completed with extraluminal knots. If the operator's usual practice is to flush the distal bowel with saline then this can be attempted before final anastomotic closure although this can be cumbersome. An inspection by walking the bowel can also be carried out and obvious atresias identified. The association of distal atresia with duodenal atresia is less than 2 per cent.

Once the anastomosis is complete the abdomen should be desufflated and the ports removed under direction vision to avoid extraction of omentum. All wounds, including the 3 mm, are then closed with 4-0 Vicryl. Skin can be closed with either tissue glue or suture.

If at first the dilated duodenum and distal bowel appear in continuity, then an intrinsic web may be the obstructive cause. In this situation, duodenoduodenostomy is still preferred with partial web excision to allow for continuity and avoid injury to the ampulla.

POTENTIAL PITFALLS

Potential pitfalls include:

- injury to pancreas or common bile duct during kocherization;
- injury to ampulla during anastomosis;
- incomplete examination of distal bowel to exclude atresia or web;
- anastomotic leak.

POSTOPERATIVE CARE

Nasogastric tube decompression and intravenous feeding is continued until the volume of aspirates has reduced. Feeds are then usually introduced slowly. Medication for gastroesophageal reflux may be required.

FURTHER READING

Ein SH, Kim PC, Miller HA. The late nonfunctioning duodenal atresia repair – a second look. *Journal of Pediatric Surgery* 2000; **35**: 690–1.

Kay S, Yoder S, Rothenberg SS. Laparoscopic duodenoduodenostomy in the neonate. *Journal of Pediatric Surgery* 2009; **44**: 906–8.

Kimura K, Mukohara N, Nishijima E *et al.* Diamond-shaped anastomosis for duodenal atresia: an experience with 44 patients over 15 years. *Journal of Pediatric Surgery* 1990; **25**: 977–9.

Rothenberg SR. Laparoscopic duodenoduodenostomy for duodenal obstruction in infants and children. *Journal of Pediatric Surgery* 2002; **37**: 1088–9.

Spilde TL, St Peter SD, Keckler SJ *et al.* Open vs laparoscopic repair of congenital duodenal obstructions: a concurrent series. *Journal of Pediatric Surgery* 2008; **43**: 1002–5.

van der Zee DC. Laparoscopic repair of duodenal atresia: revisited. *World Journal of Surgery* 2011; **35**: 1781–4.

48

Malrotation

JOE CURRY and BHANUMATHI LAKSHMINARAYANAN

INTRODUCTION

The term 'malrotation' refers to a condition in which the midgut – that part of the intestine supplied by the superior mesenteric vessels extending from the duodenojejunal flexure to the mid-transverse colon – remains unfixed and suspended on a narrow-based mesentery.

HISTORY

The first description of intestinal development was written by Mall in 1898. Frazer and Robins in 1915 expanded on the observations of Mall, and in 1923 Dott extended the embryological observations to the problems encountered clinically. In 1936, William Ladd emphasized the importance of releasing the duodenum and placing the cecum in the left upper quadrant and, indeed, the principles of the modern procedure are almost unchanged from those of Ladd.

PRINCIPLES AND JUSTIFICATION

Embryology

The alimentary canal initially develops as a straight tube extending down the midline of the embryo. As it lengthens, the intestine extends into the extra-embryonic celom of the umbilical cord, but later returns to the abdominal cavity. The foregut (stomach and duodenum) is supplied by the celiac artery, the midgut (small intestine and proximal colon) by the superior mesenteric artery, and the hindgut (mid-transverse colon to the rectum) by the inferior mesenteric artery. Three stages of development of the midgut are recognized.

STAGE I

The first stage occurs during weeks 4–10 of gestation. Owing to rapid growth, the celomic cavity is unable to contain the midgut within its confines. The midgut is forced out into the physiologic hernia within the umbilical cord.

STAGE II

Stage II occurs at weeks 10–12 of gestation, during which the midgut migrates back into the abdomen. The small intestine returns first and lies mainly on the left side of the abdomen. The cecocolic loop returns last, entering the abdomen in the left lower quadrant, but rapidly rotating 270° counterclockwise to attain its final position in the right iliac fossa. The duodenojejunal loop simultaneously undergoes a 270° counterclockwise rotation, coming to rest behind and to the left of the superior mesenteric vessels. The cecocolic loop lies in front of and to the right of these vessels.

STAGE III

During week 12 of gestation, various parts of the mesentery and the posterior parietal peritoneum fuse, notably the cecum and the ascending colon, which become fixed in the right paracolic gutter.

CONSEQUENCES OF ERRORS OF NORMAL ROTATION

Errors may occur at any of the three stages, with varying consequences.

Stage I

Failure of the intestine to return into the abdomen results in the formation of an exomphalos/omphalocele.

Stage II

During this stage, a number of errors could occur:

- **Non-rotation**: rotation may fail to occur following re-entry of the midgut into the abdomen.
- **Incomplete rotation**: counterclockwise rotation is arrested at 180°. The cecum lies in a subhepatic position in the right hypochondrium. The duodenojejunal rotation is similarly arrested and the duodenojejunal flexure lies to the right of the midline and superior mesenteric vessels. The base of the midgut mesentery is compressed and narrow, and the entire midgut hangs suspended on the superior mesenteric vessels by a narrow stalk, which is prone to volvulus.
- **Reversed rotation**: the final 180° rotation occurs in a clockwise direction, with the colon coming to lie posterior to the duodenum and superior mesenteric vessels.
- **Hyper-rotation**: rotation continues 360° or more so that the cecum comes to rest in the region of the splenic flexure in the left hypochondrium.
- **Encapsulated small intestine**: the avascular sac that forms the lining of the extra-embryonic celom returns en masse into the abdomen with the intestine.

The most common error is incomplete rotation. Treatment of this condition forms the basis of the rest of the discussion.

Stage III

Rotation occurs normally but fixation is defective, resulting in a 'mobile cecum'. It is estimated that this situation is present in 10 percent of asymptomatic individuals, but it may predispose to cecal volvulus or to intussusception.

INCIDENCE

Approximately 60 percent of clinical cases present in the first month of life, and more than two-thirds of these within the first week. Sporadic cases occur throughout life. It is generally accepted that once the diagnosis of malrotation has been established, surgical correction is mandatory to prevent the development of volvulus, which occurs in 40–50 percent of cases not treated surgically. Malrotation forms an integral part of exomphalos/omphalocele, gastroschisis, congenital diaphragmatic hernia, and prune-belly syndrome. It has also been found in conjunction with intrinsic duodenal obstructions, esophageal atresia, Hirschsprung's disease, biliary atresia, congenital heart anomalies, and urinary tract anomalies. Associated anomalies are present in 30–45 percent of patients.

CLINICAL PRESENTATION

Neonatal period

Malrotation in early infancy may present either with acute strangulating obstruction or with recurrent episodes of incomplete intestinal obstruction.

Acute, life-threatening, strangulating intestinal obstruction occurs as a result of midgut volvulus. The infant presents in a shocked and collapsed state with bilious vomiting (which often contains altered blood), abdominal tenderness with or (more commonly) without distension, and the passage of dark blood rectally. Edema and erythema of the abdominal wall develop as the volvulus becomes complicated by intestinal gangrene, perforation, and peritonitis.

Infants and children

A wide spectrum of clinical symptoms has been ascribed to malrotation. The most common symptom is intermittent vomiting, which is often bile stained. Failure to thrive and malrotation may be a result of intestinal malabsorption secondary to lymphatic compression in the narrow-based mesentery of the small intestine. Older children may present with features of anorexia nervosa. Early satiety or pain associated with intake of food results in a reluctance to eat or food aversion.

PREOPERATIVE

Radiologic investigations

PLAIN ABDOMINAL RADIOGRAPHY

1 The features suggestive of a volvulus on the plain abdominal radiograph are an air-filled stomach and a paucity of gas in the rest of the intestine. In the infant presenting in shock with features of acute strangulating obstruction, further radiologic investigations only delay definitive treatment.

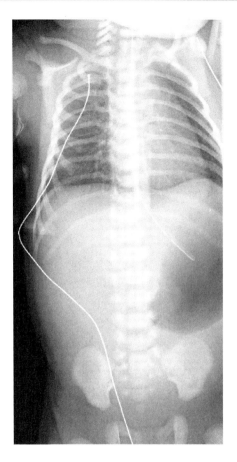

1

CONTRAST RADIOLOGY

2 The investigation of choice is an upper gastrointestinal contrast study. The features that should be elicited are an abnormal configuration of the duodenal C-loop, the identification of the duodenojejunal flexure to the right of the midline, and small bowel loops on the right side of the abdomen. A 'twisted ribbon' and 'corkscrew' appearance of the duodenum and upper jejunum indicates a midgut volvulus.

Contrast enema gives information only about the position of the cecum, which may occasionally be normally placed even in the presence of a volvulus.

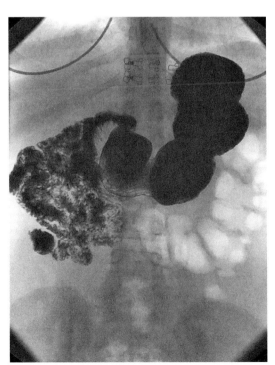

2a

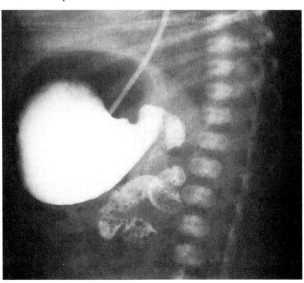

2b

ULTRASONOGRAPHY

Doppler ultrasound of the orientation of the mesenteric vessels can be a useful non-invasive radiological investigation. If the superior mesenteric vein is to the left of the artery this is diagnostic of malrotation. Other orientations are also known, such as the vein lying anterior to the artery. In some cases of malrotation, however, the orientation between the vessels is normal and this does not exclude malrotation.

The diagnosis of midgut volvulus on ultrasound can be made if a whirlpool sign is seen. This is frequently seen in cases that present beyond the neonatal period.

Preoperative resuscitation

Patients presenting with acute strangulating obstruction require rapid resuscitation before proceeding to surgery. This comprises rapid intravenous volume replacement (plasma 20 mL/kg body weight), nasogastric decompression, correction of electrolyte and acid–base imbalance, and administration of broad-spectrum antibiotics. Attempts should be made to correct hypothermia. The period of intensive resuscitation should not extend for more than 1–2 hours before proceeding to surgery, as prolonging the time will expose the intestine to increased ischemia and may result in more extensive bowel necrosis.

OPERATIONS

Surgical correction of the anomaly should always be regarded as an emergency, even in patients presenting non-acutely. Volvulus may supervene at any stage and the operation should be scheduled as early as possible.

Laparotomy

INCISION

3 A laparotomy is performed via an upper abdominal, transverse, muscle-cutting incision, extending mainly to the right side. The obliterated umbilical vein in the free edge of the falciform ligament is ligated and divided. The entire bowel is delivered into the wound for careful examination. A small volume of white to yellowish, free peritoneal fluid is usually present in any early intestinal obstruction, but blood-stained fluid is indicative of intestinal necrosis.

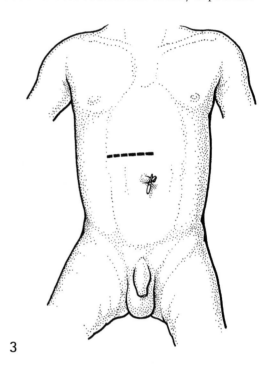

3

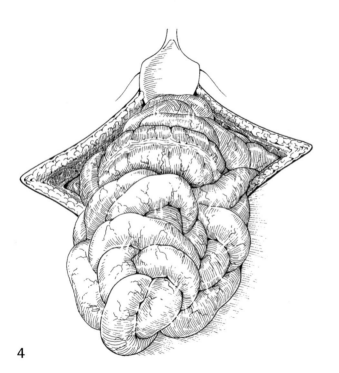

4

MIDGUT VOLVULUS

4 The volvulus occurs around the base of the narrow midgut mesentery. The twist usually occurs in a clockwise direction and is untwisted by as many counterclockwise rotations as required.

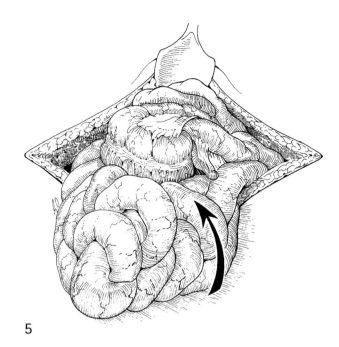

5

5 Moderately ischemic bowel, which appears congested and dusky, rapidly resumes a normal pinkish color on reduction of the volvulus. Frankly necrotic bowel is extremely friable and may disintegrate on handling. Bowel of questionable viability should be covered, after untwisting, with warm, moist swabs and left undisturbed for approximately 10 minutes before assessing the extent of ischemic damage. A Ladd's procedure for the malrotation is carried out (see below).

In patients with extreme gangrene, frankly necrotic bowel should be resected and the bowel ends either tied off or stomas fashioned with a view to performing a second-look laparotomy in 24–48 hours, when lines of demarcation will be clearly evident. At this stage, an end-to-end anastomosis may be feasible. In the intervening period, the patient is electively ventilated and resuscitative measures continued.

UNCOMPLICATED MALROTATION (LADD'S OPERATION)

The aim of this procedure is to restore intestinal anatomy to the non-rotated position with the duodenum and upper jejunum on the right of the abdomen and the cecocolic loop in the left upper quadrant.

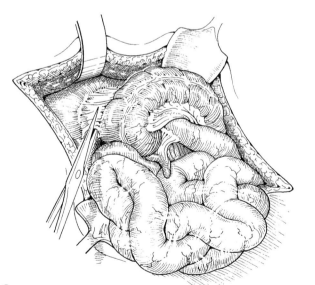

6

6 Folds of peritoneum extending from the cecum and ascending colon across the duodenum to the right paracolic gutter and to the liver and gallbladder are carefully divided. This maneuver leaves the cecocolic loop free laterally, but dense adhesions in the base of the mesentery must be divided before the cecum and ascending colon can be fully separated from the duodenojejunal loop. Separation is achieved by opening the serosa of the mesentery between the duodenum and cecum and exposing the anterior surface of the superior mesenteric vessels coursing in the narrow-based mesentery to the midgut.

The mesentery in this part is often thickened and edematous, especially if an associated midgut volvulus needs to be untwisted. Care should be taken to avoid trauma to the main vessels, and small branches may need to be ligated before being divided. Large, fleshy lymph and lymphatic channels that have been divided should be sealed by ligation or electrocoagulation to avoid postoperative chylous leakage.

7 The mesentery is widened peripherally to allow the right colon to be mobilized. Centrally, the dissection is continued into the base of the mesentery until the superior mesenteric artery and vein are freed of any fibrous compression.

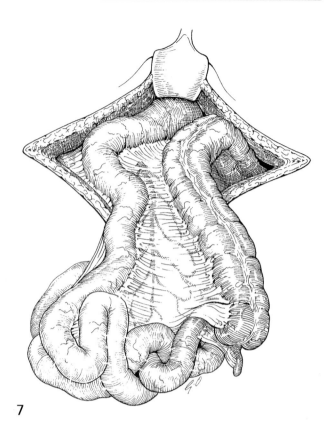

7

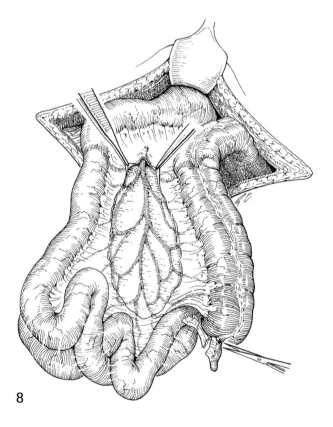

8

8 The duodenum is straightened by dividing the ligament of Treitz, following which the duodenum should be carefully inspected for the presence of any intrinsic obstruction. If there is any doubt, a balloon catheter should be passed per-orally through the duodenum into the proximal jejunum, inflated, and carefully withdrawn into the stomach. Inability to pass the catheter through the duodenum or hold up of the inflated balloon on withdrawal indicates an intrinsic obstruction.

An appendicectomy may also be performed at this stage as the cecum will be placed in the left upper quadrant of the abdomen and the diagnosis of subsequent appendicitis in later life could be difficult to establish. Appendicectomy can be performed either as a standard ligation of the appendix base and resection or as an inversion appendicectomy thus avoiding potential contamination. There are, however, reports of postoperative intussusception arising from inversion appendicectomy.

9 The intestine is replaced in the peritoneal cavity, commencing with the duodenum and proximal jejunum that lie on the right side and ending with the terminal ileum and cecum that are placed in the left hypochondrium. No attempt is made to fix the intestine in this position.

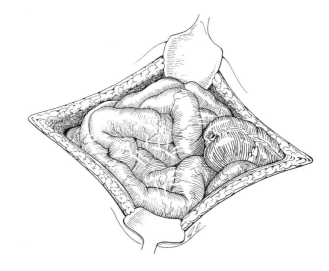

CLOSURE

The abdomen is closed in layers with continuous sutures. The skin is closed with a continuous subcuticular suture.

Laparoscopy

Laparoscopy has two potential roles in the management of malrotation:

1. The treatment of symptomatic malrotation in the newborn period
2. To determine in cases of doubtful malrotation whether or not surgical therapy is required.

TREATMENT OF SYMPTOMATIC MALROTATION IN THE NEWBORN PERIOD

It has been stated that volvulus is a contraindication for a laparoscopic approach. Volvulus is always present in the newborn with symptomatic malrotation and is amenable to laparoscopic correction. Strangulation with necrosis and/or perforation is a contraindication to laparoscopy.

The child is placed in a supine reversed Trendelenburg position on a short operating table (**Figure 48.1**). The child's right side is 15° elevated. The sheet covering the operating table is enveloped over the legs to prevent slipping of the child when the table is in reversed Trendelenburg position.

The surgeon is positioned at the bottom end of the table with the camera assistant to the left and the scrub nurse to the right. The laparoscopy column stands to the left of the child's head, the second screen to the right of the child's head (**Figure 48.2**).

The first cannula is inserted in an open fashion through the inferior umbilical fold. A purse-string suture is placed

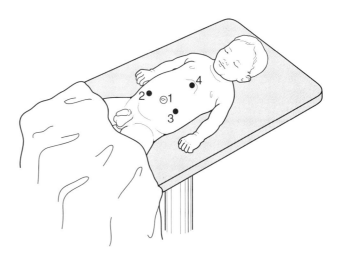

Figure 48.1 Positioning of the patient for laparoscopic exploration and treatment.

in the underlying fascia to narrow the aperture and prevent gas leak and is then attached to the cannula to prevent inadvertent removal (**Figure 48.1**).

Before starting CO_2 insufflation, the intraperitoneal position of the tip of the catheter is checked with the telescope. Pneumoperitoneum is established at a pressure of 8–10 mmHg using a flow of 1–2 L/minute. Optimal muscle relaxation helps to increase the working space.

Two working cannulae are inserted, one pararectally on the right at umbilical level and one in the left hypochondrium. An extra cannula is inserted subcostally on the left and is used for retraction (**Figure 48.1**).

The table is tilted to the left so that the bowel tends to move to the left by gravity. When the bowel is not critically ischemic, the volvulus should be left in place, as this keeps the bowel out of the way during the initial dissection of the proximal duodenum (**Figures 48.3, 48.4, 48.5, and 48.6**). Next, the volvulus, which is always in clockwise direction, is untwisted in counterclockwise direction.

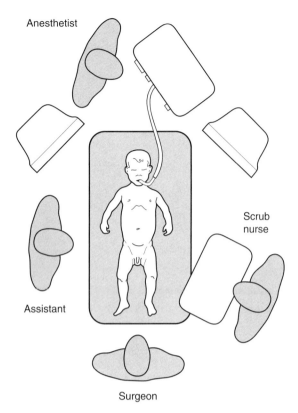

Figure 48.2 Positioning of the team and equipment for laparoscopic exploration and treatment.

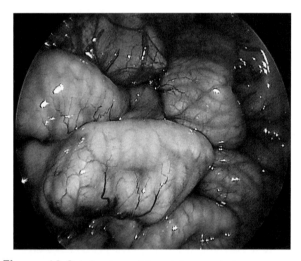

Figure 48.3 Ischemic small bowel due to volvulus.

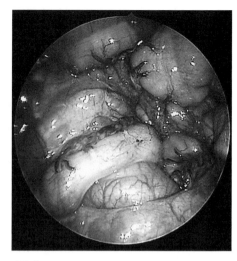

Figure 48.4 Volvulus of small bowel around the mesenteric stalk.

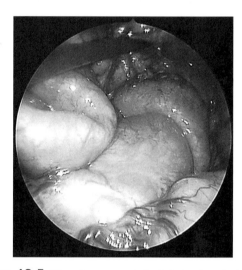

Figure 48.5 Edematous mesenteric stalk due to volvulus.

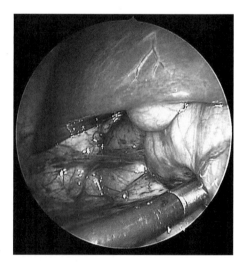

Figure 48.6 The colon is displaced to the left. Next, the duodenum is mobilized.

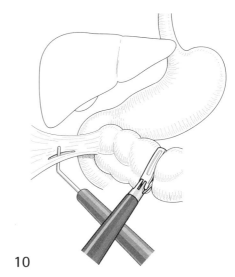

10 The cecum and ascending colon are dissected free and displaced to the left.

10

The kissing area between the ileocecal region and the duodenum should be undone by incising the anterior leaf of the mesentery (**Figures 48.7** and **48.8**).

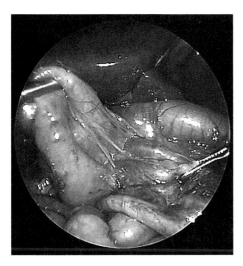

Figure 48.7 Separation of the duodenum and ileocecal region. Note the engorged veins.

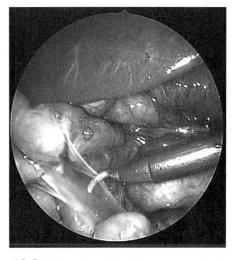

Figure 48.8 Transection of bands between the duodenum and ileocecal region.

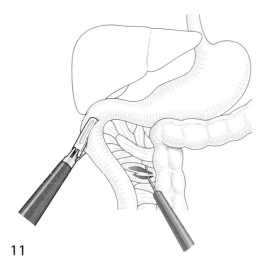

11

11 In doing so, the mesenteric stalk is enlarged. The duodenum is now followed downwards and freed. The last band to be divided is the remnant of the duodenojejunal flexure, which is to the right of the vertebral column.

At the end of the procedure, the anesthetist is asked to inject air into the stomach so that its passage in the proximal small bowel can be checked, thus excluding a membranous occlusion.

12 Removal of the appendix is optional. This can be done outside the body by exteriorizing the appendix through the porthole on the left (**Figure 48.9**).

The cannulae are removed under endoscopic control. The fascia at the umbilicus is closed with one absorbable suture. Skin is approximated with adhesive strips or tissue glue.

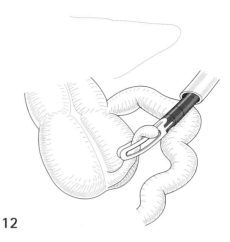

12

DOUBTFUL MALROTATION

The diagnosis of malrotation may be difficult to make. The position of the duodenojejunal flexure on upper gastrointestinal contrast study may be just on the left pedicle and not clearly to right or left. An inverted relationship between the superior mesenteric artery and vein may be present on ultrasound. The critical question is not whether there is malrotation, but whether the mesenteric stalk is narrow and not fixed to the posterior abdominal wall. In other words, is there a high likelihood of volvulus? Laparoscopy is an ideal tool to look at the broadness and the fixation of the mesenteric stalk.

The child is placed in a supine reversed Trendelenburg position on the operating table. The child's right side is elevated 15°. Small children are placed in a frog-like position with the legs enveloped in the sheet, which covers the operating table (**Figure 48.1**). The legs of larger children may be placed on abducted leg supports so that the surgeon stands in between them (**Figure 48.2**).

A three-cannulae technique is used as described above.

- The laparoscopic exploration should be systematic.
- Position and fixation of the cecal region to the lateral peritoneal wall (**Figures 48.10** and **48.11**).
- Position of the transverse colon and greater omentum (**Figure 48.12**).
- Position of the ligament of Treitz.
- Fixation of the mesenteric stalk.

More often than not, the diagnosis of 'dangerous malrotation' is excluded.

The cannulae are removed under endoscopic control, and the fascia defect at the umbilical level is closed with absorbable suture. Skin is approximated with adhesive strips or tissue glue.

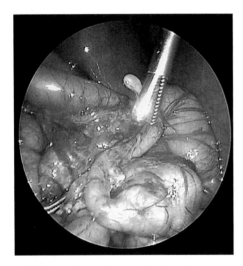

Figure 48.9 Grasping and exteriorization of the appendix through the port in the left hypochondrium.

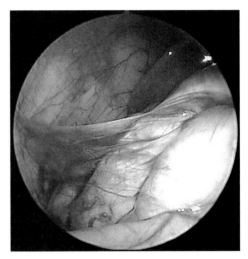

Figure 48.10 The ascending colon is securely attached to the lateral peritoneum.

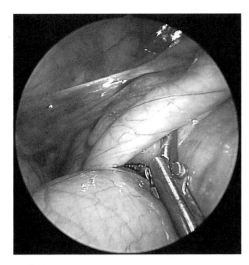

Figure 48.11 The appendix is securely attached to the lateral peritoneum.

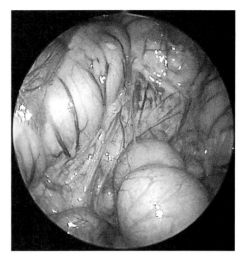

Figure 48.12 Normal position of the transverse colon and greater omentum. The duodenojejunal flexure lies to the left of the vertebral column and is securely attached, as is the mesenteric stalk (not shown).

POSTOPERATIVE CARE

Nasogastric aspiration and intravenous fluid and electrolyte support continue until bowel function returns. The period of ileus generally last less than 48 hours, during which time intestinal fluid losses should be replaced with an equivalent volume of 0.9 percent sodium chloride containing 10 mmol/L potassium chloride. Prophylactic antibiotics need not be carried on postoperatively if there is no contamination.

OUTCOME

Recovery is generally prompt and uncomplicated. Infants who have suffered extensive bowel loss following midgut volvulus may experience problems of short bowel syndrome with a prolonged requirement for parenteral nutrition. It is felt that performing an open Ladd's procedure may help to promote adhesions that effectively prevent recurrent volvulus, but adhesive intestinal obstruction is relatively common (3–5 percent). Conflicting evidence on the rate of recurrent volvulus following laparoscopic Ladd's procedure exists in the literature with some series showing higher rates and others lower when compared to the open counterpart. There are no trials comparing open and laparoscopic approach so far and long-term results from the laparoscopic approach are still awaited. Fixation of the cecum is usually not performed in the open procedure for the above-mentioned reasons and controversy exists over performing cecopexy in the laparoscopic approach.

As more and more minimal invasive surgical techniques are introduced into pediatric and neonatal surgery, there is ongoing debate about management for intestinal rotational abnormalities associated with other defects, such as congenital diaphragmatic hernia, abdominal wall defects, and heterotaxia syndromes. In the context of such abnormalities, it is recommended that an upper gastrointestinal contrast study be undertaken, and if malrotation is diagnosed then a laparoscopic examination of the intestine be performed and Ladd's procedure undertaken if required.

ACKNOWLEDGMENTS

The illustrations in the chapter have been reproduced from *Operative Newborn Surgery* (P Puri (ed.)), with permission from Butterworth-Heinemann.

FURTHER READING

El-Gohary Y, Alagtal M, Gillick J. Long-term complications following operative intervention for intestinal malrotation: a 10-year review. *Pediatric Surgery International* 2010; **26**: 203–6.

Fraser JD, Aguayo P, Sharp SW. The role of laparoscopy in the management of malrotation. *Journal of Surgical Research* 2009; **156**: 80–2.

Ladd WE. Surgical diseases of the alimentary tract in infants. *New England Journal of Medicine* 1936; **215**: 705–8.

Lampl B, Levin TL, Berdon WE, Cowles RA. Malrotation and midgut volvulus: a historical review and current controversies in diagnosis and management. *Pediatric Radiology* 2009; **39**: 359–66.

Skandalakis JE, Gray SW. *Embryology for Surgeons*, 2nd edn. Baltimore, MD: Williams & Wilkins, 1994: 184–200.

Stanfill AB, Pearl RH, Kalvakuri K *et al.* Laparoscopic Ladd's procedure: treatment of choice for midgut malrotation in infants and children. *Journal of Laparoendoscopic and Advanced Surgical Techniques* 2010; **20**: 369–72.

49

Congenital atresia and stenosis of the intestine

ALASTAIR JW MILLAR and ALP NUMANOGLU

HISTORY

In 1911, Fockens of Rotterdam reported the first successfully treated case of small intestinal atresia. Late presentation, dysmotility of the proximal dilated atretic bowel, the blind loop syndrome, malnutrition, infections, prematurity, and associated congenital abnormalities contributed to a high mortality. In a comprehensive review of the world literature up to 1950, Evans could find reports of only 39 successfully treated cases of jejunoileal atresia.

In 1952, Louw suggested that most jejunoileal atresias were probably due to a vascular accident rather than being the result of inadequate recanalization, as had previously been commonly accepted. At his instigation, Barnard perfected an experimental model in pregnant mongrel bitches and reproduced all types of atresia found in humans. This not only confirmed Louw's hypothesis, but also provided the opportunity to improve the technical aspects of corrective surgery, which involved resection of the dilated proximal blind-ending bowel and primary end-to-end anastomosis.

These factors, along with advances in neonatal care, have achieved survival rates greater than 90 percent.

PRINCIPLES AND JUSTIFICATION

Pathogenesis

1 Although several mechanisms have been postulated, the most feasible theory is that of a localized intrauterine vascular incident resulting in ischemic necrosis, liquefaction, and absorption of the affected devascularized segment(s). The ischemic hypothesis is further supported by additional evidence of incarceration or snaring of bowel in an exomphalos or gastroschisis, fetal intussusception, midgut volvulus, transmesenteric hernia, and thromboembolic occlusions. The anomaly is usually not genetically determined. The ischemic insult causes morphologic and functional abnormalities of the remaining proximal and distal bowel. The blind-ending proximal bowel becomes dilated and hypertrophied, resulting in functional abnormalities that include ineffective peristalsis. The distal bowel is unused and collapsed, with potential normal length and function. Multiple atresia may occur on a genetic basis and have been described occurring in families and associated with immune deficiency syndromes.

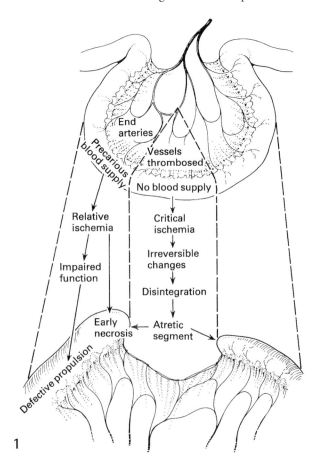

1

Classification

The most proximal atresia or stenosis determines whether it is classified as jejunal or ileal.

STENOSIS

2 The proximal dilated and distal collapsed segments of intestine are in continuity with an intact mesentery, but at the junction there is a short, narrow, somewhat rigid segment with a minute lumen which may mimic atresia type I. The small intestine is of normal length.

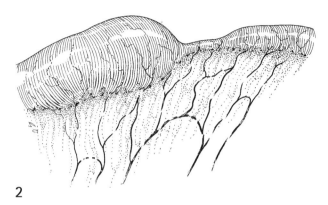

2

ATRESIA TYPE I (MEMBRANE)

3 The dilated proximal and collapsed distal segments of intestine are in continuity and the mesentery is intact. The pressure in the proximal intestine tends to expand the membrane into the distal intestinal lumen, so that the transition from distended to collapsed intestine is conical in appearance: the 'windsock' effect. The distal intestine is completely collapsed, but the bowel immediately distal to a 'windsock' may be dilated by the windsock. The small intestine is of normal length.

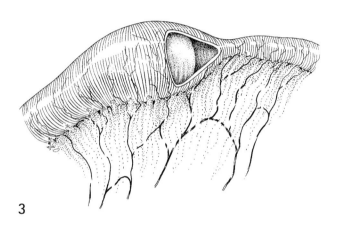

3

ATRESIA TYPE II (BLIND ENDS JOINED BY A FIBROUS CORD)

4 The proximal intestine terminates in a bulbous blind end that is grossly distended and hypertrophied for several centimeters, but more proximally assumes a normal appearance. This blind end is often hypoperistaltic. The distal completely collapsed intestine commences as a blind end that is occasionally bulbous, owing to the remains of a fetal intussusception. The two blind ends are joined by a thin, fibrous band, with the corresponding intestinal mesentery intact. The small intestinal length is usually normal.

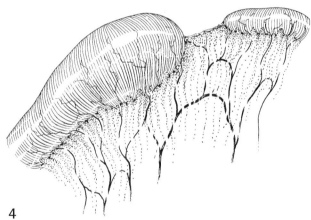

4

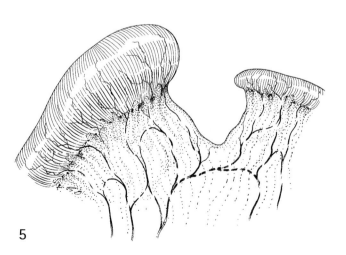

5

ATRESIA TYPE IIIA (DISCONNECTED BLIND ENDS)

5 The appearance is similar to that in type II, but the blind ends are completely separate. There is always a mesenteric defect of varying size, and the proximal intestine may, as a secondary event, undergo torsion or become over-distended with necrosis and perforation. The total length of intestine is reduced to a varying extent.

ATRESIA TYPE IIIB ('APPLE PEEL', 'CHRISTMAS TREE' ATRESIA)

6 As in type IIIa, the blind ends are unconnected and the mesenteric defect is large. The atresia is usually localized in the proximal jejunum near the ligament of Treitz, with absence of the superior mesenteric artery beyond the origin of the middle colic branch and absence of the dorsal mesentery. The distal intestine assumes a helical configuration around an attenuated, single artery of blood supply arising from the ileocolic or right colic arcade. Occasionally, further atresias of type I or II are found in the distal intestine, usually close to the blind end. Vascularity of the distal intestine may be impaired. There is always a significant reduction in intestinal length.

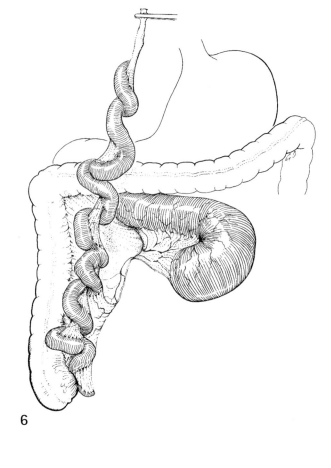

6

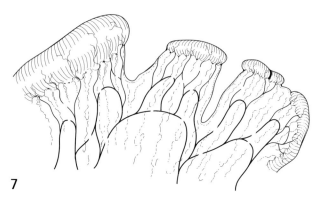

7

ATRESIA TYPE IV (MULTIPLE ATRESIA)

7 Multiple atresias can be combinations of types I–III and often present morphologically as a string of sausages.

Prognostic factors

- Prematurity and congenital anomalies are associated with increased mortality.
- Delayed diagnosis may precipitate ischemia and necrosis of the proximal atretic segment.
- Type III atresia has the highest mortality.
- Short bowel syndrome, which may be due to extensive intrauterine bowel loss, over-zealous bowel resection, ischemic injury to the bowel, or postoperative complications.

PREOPERATIVE PREPARATION

Clinical presentation

Many cases of intestinal atresia are now being diagnosed prenatally by ultrasonographic and magnetic resonance imaging investigation of the fetus, showing dilated fetal intestine, suggesting obstruction, particularly in pregnancies complicated by third trimester polyhydramnios. Postnatally, atresia or severe stenosis of the small intestine presents as neonatal intestinal obstruction with persistent bilious (green) vomiting dating from the first or second day of life, and varying degrees of abdominal distension. Erythema of the abdominal wall, tenderness, distension, and rigidity may signify bowel ischemia or peritonitis.

Radiology

The diagnosis of atresia is confirmed by radiologic examination. Erect and supine abdominal radiographs done after 6–8 hours of birth will reveal distended, air-filled small intestinal loops proximal to the obstruction and a gasless distal abdomen. In some cases, the first abdominal radiograph reveals a completely opaque abdomen due to a fluid-filled obstructed bowel. Emptying of the stomach by means of a nasogastric tube and the injection of a bolus of air will demonstrate the level of the obstruction. When intestinal stenosis is present, an abnormal differentiation in caliber of the proximal obstructed intestine and the distal collapsed intestine will be evident. When an incomplete small intestinal obstruction is diagnosed, an upper gastrointestinal contrast study is indicated to demonstrate the site and nature of the obstruction as the diagnosis may be difficult and is often delayed. When the radiograph suggests a complete low obstruction, a contrast enema is given to rule out associated colonic atresia or functional obstruction, e.g. total colonic aganglionosis or meconium ileus, which may be confused with atresia of the distal ileum.

Factors that can mimic jejunoileal atresia include midgut volvulus, meconium ileus, incarcerated hernia, Hirschsprung's disease, colonic atresia, birth trauma, prematurity, drugs, and hypothyroidism.

Preoperative preparation

- Proximal gastric and intestinal decompression to prevent aspiration.
- Fluid management:
  - maintenance;
  - replacement of deficiency/ongoing losses.
- Plain abdominal radiograph (air contrast).
- Contrast enema.
- Correction of hematological and biochemical abnormalities.
- Prophylactic antibiotics.

Anesthesia

The major anesthetic considerations are related to prematurity, fluid and electrolyte disturbance, abdominal distension, the risk of aspiration, and additional congenital anomalies. Rapid sequence induction and cricoid pressure may further reduce the risk. Invasive monitoring is indicated in sick or unstable infants, and a central line may be required for intravenous feeding postoperatively.

The anesthetic management is dictated by the condition of the infant and the available facilities. Light general and epidural anesthesia may avoid the need for postoperative ventilation.

OPERATION

Principles of surgery

- The operative procedure depends on the type of atresia.
- The whole length of the small intestine should be inspected carefully to determine the site and type of atresia and the most likely pathogenesis.
- Patency of the distal small and large bowel must be confirmed.
- Back resection of the proximal dilated bowel with primary, single-layer, end-to-end (end-to-back) anastomosis using interrupted sutures of 5/0 or 6/0 with or without tapering or plication is the preferred operative procedure.
- Residual bowel length must be documented.
- Ischemic or twisted bowel must be untwisted, and anastomosis may be delayed for 24 hours to assess viability.
- Every effort should be made to preserve bowel length in the presence of foreshortened bowel in type III or IV atresia.
- Proximal or distal stomas are rarely indicated.
- Bowel must be returned into the abdominal cavity, avoiding twisting or kinking of the anastomosis.
- Additional steps may include derotation of the proximal jejunum and duodenum in high intestinal atresia, with back resection of the dilated bowel followed by tapering or inversion plication of the megaduodenum.
- Gastric decompression is best achieved with a nasogastric tube and aspiration.
- Bowel-lengthening procedures should preferably not be performed at the initial operation.

Incision

Adequate exposure is obtained through a supraumbilical, transverse incision transecting the rectus muscles 2 cm above the umbilicus. Increasingly minimally invasive techniques are used with small circumumbilical incisions and extracorporeal anastomosis.

Exploration

8 In uncomplicated cases, the intestine can be delivered through the wound by gentle exertion of pressure on the abdominal wall. If free gas escapes on opening the peritoneum, or if there is contamination of the peritoneal cavity, the perforation should be identified immediately and closed before further exploration. The intestine proximal to the obstruction is distended, whereas the intestine distal to the obstruction is collapsed, tiny, and worm-like, and may contain intraluminal contents. The intestine is exteriorized to determine the site and type of obstruction and to exclude other areas of atresia or stenosis, as well as associated lesions, e.g. incomplete intestinal rotation or meconium ileus.

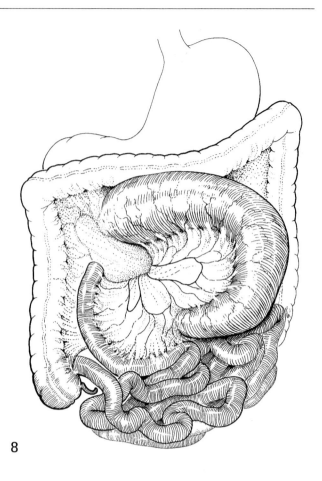

8

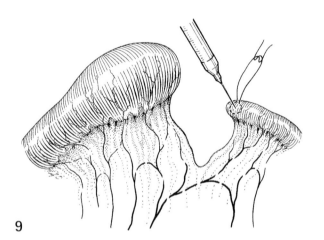

9

Detection of other atretic areas

9 After the type and location of atresia have been determined, the distal intestine is carefully examined. If a volvulus is present, the bowel should be untwisted. Other atretic segments should be excluded, which can occur in 6–21 percent of cases. Intraluminal membranes are best detected and localized by injecting normal saline into the lumen of the collapsed intestine and following the advancing fluid column down to the cecum. Colonic atresia is excluded by a similar procedure through the cecum or by a previously performed contrast enema. The total length of small intestine is measured accurately along the antimesenteric border. The normal length at birth is approximately 250 cm and in the preterm infant 115–170 cm.

Resection

10a,b The atretic area and adjacent distended and collapsed loops of intestine are isolated. After milking the intestinal contents into the proximal bulbous end, or in high jejunal atresia into the stomach, from where it is aspirated, an atraumatic bowel clamp is applied across the bowel a few centimeters proximal to the site selected for transection. To ensure adequate postoperative function, the proximal distended and hypertrophied intestine should be liberally resected. We usually resect 10–15 cm even if it appears viable. The mesentery adjoining the portion to be resected is clamped, ligated, and divided using bipolar diathermy. The proximal intestine is transected at right angles. The blood supply at this level should be excellent. Some 2–3 cm of the distal intestine is then resected using a slightly oblique line of transection to create a 'fish mouth' that renders the opening about equal in size to that of the proximal intestine. Alternatively, an extramucosal end-to-end anastomosis is possible with diameter discrepancy of up to 8:1. A culture swab is taken from the proximal gastrointestinal tract, which may have become colonized with bacteria.

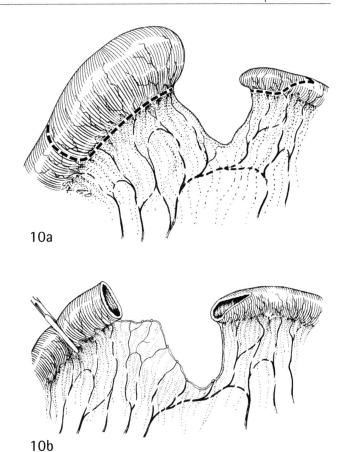

10a

10b

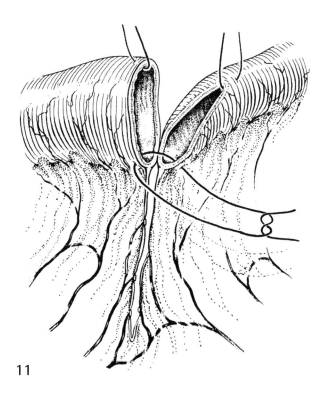

11

Uniting the mesenteric borders of bowel

11 A 5/0 or 6/0 monofilament, synthetic, absorbable, full-thickness suture unites the mesenteric borders of the divided ends, and temporary stay sutures are placed at the antimesenteric angles to facilitate accurate approximation.

Anastomosis

12a–c The 'anterior' bowel edges are joined by interrupted full thickness sutures, starting from the mesenteric side, and tied on the serosal surface. Once the anterior layer has been completed, the bowel is rotated 180° to expose the back wall. If there is size discrepancy between the transected proximal and distal ends, a short cut back along the antimesenteric border can be performed on the distal bowel.

A similar technique is used for stenoses and intraluminal membranes. Procedures such as simple enteroplasties, excision of membranes, and bypassing techniques are not recommended because they fail to remove the abnormal segment of intestine. Side-to-side anastomosis is avoided because of the increased risk of creating blind loops.

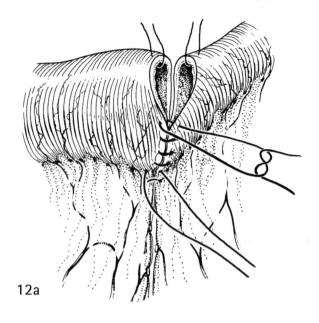

12a

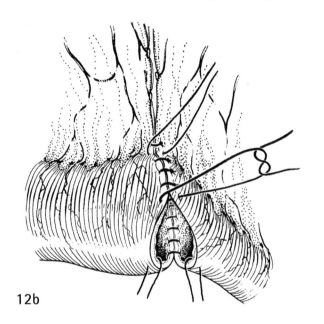

12b

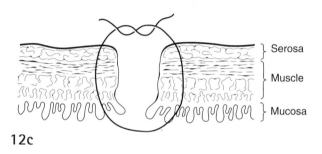

12c

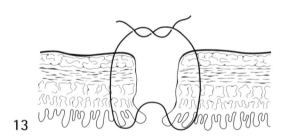

13

Completion of anastomosis and closure of mesenteric gap

13 Gambee interrupted inverting or extramucosal stitches may also be used instead of through-and-through stitches. This facilitates a more end-to-end anastomosis with size discrepancies of up to 8:1 accommodated. Alternatively, the posterior bowel edges are united with interrupted through-and-through or inverting Gambee sutures, with the knots tied on the mucosal surface. The anterior bowel edges are then joined in a similar fashion, with the knots being tied on the serosal surface.

14 The suture lines are inspected and additional stitches are placed if required to ensure a 'watertight' anastomosis. The defect in the mesentery is repaired by approximating (and overlapping if necessary) the divided edges with interrupted sutures, taking great care not to kink the anastomosis or to compromise the blood supply. Thereafter the intestines, well moistened with warm saline, are returned to the peritoneal cavity.

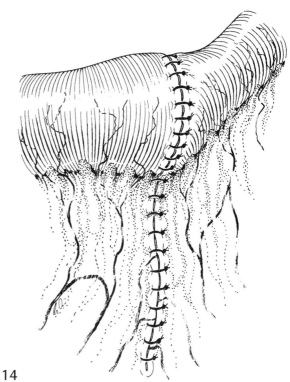

14

Closure of abdominal wound

Before closure, the whole peritoneal cavity is irrigated with warm saline and all blood clots and particulate matter removed. The anterior abdominal wound is then closed with a single-layer mass closure of sheath and muscle layers utilizing a continuous absorbable stitch, excluding Scarpa's fascia and skin. Scarpa's fascia and subcutaneous layers are approximated with absorbable sutures. The skin is closed with a continuous, synthetic, absorbable subcuticular suture or approximated with adhesive strips and then covered with a thin, sterile skin dressing. No drains are used.

BOWEL-SAVING PROCEDURES

Tapering duodenojejunoplasty or enteroplasty

15 This surgical procedure is indicated for bowel-length preservation, especially in type IIIb atresia and for high jejunal atresias. The bulbous, hypertrophied proximal bowel is derotated and resected back along the antimesenteric border into the third or second part of the duodenum. The tapering is performed over a 22–24 Fr catheter to ensure adequate luminal size. An intestinal autostapling instrument may greatly facilitate this procedure. The linear anastomosis is reinforced with interrupted absorbable 5/0 or 6/0 sutures. Tapering can safely be done over an extended 10–20 cm length.

The tapered bowel is then anastomosed to the distal bowel and replaced in a non-rotated position. Tapering is also indicated for equalizing diameter size for more distal atresias and for correction of a failed inversion plication procedure.

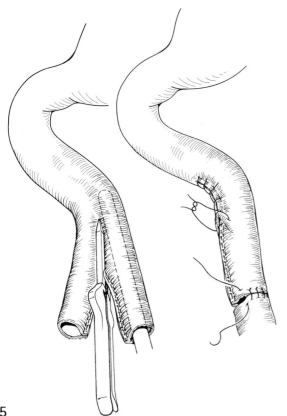

15

Plication or infolding enteroplasty

16 The same technique used for tapering enteroplasty is used, except that antimesenteric intestinal plication involves infolding of up to half or more of the intestinal circumference into the lumen over an extended length. The plication is performed by a running stitch up to 1 cm from the planned anastomotic site. The distal end is then completed by interrupted stitches to allow for additional surgical trimming if required. The keel created by the infolding should be sutured closed. Excessive infolding must be avoided and the patency of the lumen not compromised. The infolding is accomplished with non-absorbable sutures and the bowel is left in a position of non-rotation.

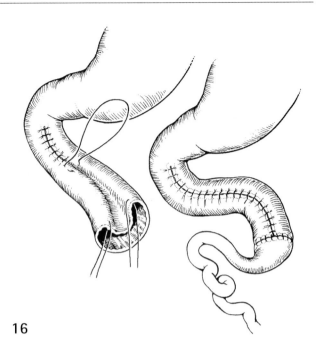

16

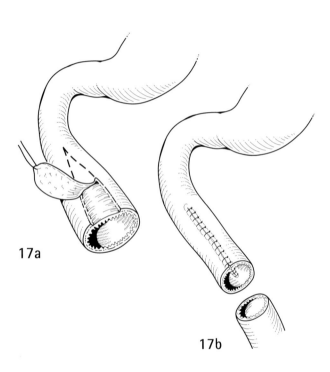

17a

17b

Antimesenteric seromuscular stripping and inversion plication

17a,b This technique tapers the dilated proximal bowel segment and prevents unraveling of a plication enteroplasty. An antimesenteric, seromuscular segment of the dilated proximal bowel is resected by blunt and sharp dissection from the underlying submucosa.

The muscular margins so created are approximated with interrupted sutures, with the underlying mucosa imbricated or inverted into the lumen of the bowel. The distal end of the created keel should be tapered and sutured closed. This technique prevents anastomotic leakage and enhances the establishment of prograde peristaltic activity.

SPECIAL SURGICAL CONSIDERATIONS

Multiple atresias

Multiple atresias are often localized to a short segment of intestine, and resection with one anastomosis is preferred if sufficient intestinal length remains. If the bowel length is critical, multiple anastomoses should be performed. Placing an intraluminal silastic or polyvinyl chloride tube facilitates ease of anastomosis.

Bowel lengthening

Bowel-lengthening procedures, such as the serial transverse enteroplasty procedure (STEP), and longitudinal intestinal lengthening and tailoring (LILT) procedures (described by Bianchi) have no place at the initial operation.

Exteriorization

Exteriorization of proximal and distal intestine may be required with established peritonitis or questionable vascularity of the remaining intestine. The authors do not favor the fashioning of stomas in situations other than these.

Intestinal atresia and gastroschisis

Primary anastomosis may be difficult and hazardous, and the favored option is reduction of the eviscerated intestine with the atresia left intact, closure of the abdominal wall defect, and delayed resection and primary anastomosis of the atresia at 14–21 days.

Colonic atresia

The incidence of colonic atresia is less than small bowel atresia (one in 66 000) and it is usually 5–8 percent of all atresias. Prematurity is common and they may be associated with other congenital abnormalities.

Colonic atresias may be seen distal to small bowel atresias and also may be associated with conditions such as gastroschisis and Hirschsprung's disease. Typically, they present with signs and symptoms of distal bowel obstruction. Plain abdominal radiographs show dilated intestines with air-fluid levels and as in distal ileal atresia there may be one very large loop. Contrast enema confirms the presence of a microcolon and is very helpful in assessing the level of atresia.

Colonic atresias may be located anywhere in the large bowel, both above and below the peritoneal reflection. The dilated proximal segment may undergo secondary volvulus. Malrotation may also be present.

Surgical options include resection and primary anastomosis or initial stoma formation and later closure of the stomas. It is important to establish presence or absence of the distal pathology, such as Hirschsprung's disease, if primary anastomosis is contemplated. The majority of studies recommend initial placement of colostomy followed by the bowel anastomosis in due course. Primary anastomosis may be feasible in cases where the caliber change proximal and distal to the atresia is not significant and pathology in bowel distal to the atresia has been excluded.

When colonic atresias are associated with gastroschisis extreme loss of small bowel may result in short bowel syndrome. These children may require intestine lengthening procedures. Outcome of colonic atresia is generally good.

POSTOPERATIVE CARE

Nasogastric decompression is usually required for 4–6 days after the operation (longer for high jejunal atresias). Therapeutic antibiotics are continued for 5–7 days or longer, and an oral antifungal agent is given prophylactically. Oral intake is commenced when the neonate is alert, sucks well, and there is evidence of prograde gastrointestinal function, i.e. clear gastric effluent of low volume, a soft abdomen, or when flatus or feces have been passed. Surveillance should continue until the infant has established normal gastrointestinal function.

If at any time there is suspicion of a leak at the anastomosis (suggested by ileus, abdominal distension, vomiting, and peritonitis), a plain erect or decubitus radiograph of the abdomen should be taken. If this reveals free air in the abdomen more than 24 hours after operation, laparotomy should be performed immediately and the leaking site sutured, or the anastomosis redone.

Complications

Although a survival rate of more than 90 percent can be expected, complications are not infrequent. These include anastomotic leaks and stricture formation, ischemia of the bowel due to the delicate blood supply, especially in type IIIb, adhesive bowel obstruction, the short bowel syndrome, and infections related to pneumonia and septicemia.

OUTCOME

Before 1952, the mortality rate for congenital atresias of the small intestine in Cape Town was 90 percent. Between 1952 and 1955, 28 percent of the neonates survived. At that stage, most were treated by primary anastomosis without resection. With liberal back resection of the blind ends and end-to-end anastomosis, the survival rate increased to 78 percent during the period 1955–58. During the 52-year period (1959–2011), 336 patients with jejunoileal atresia and stenosis were admitted to the Paediatric Surgical Service at the Red Cross Children's Hospital, of whom 35 have died, giving an overall mortality rate of 10 percent (Tables 49.1, 49.2, and 49.3). However, in line with the improved preoperative and postoperative care of newborns, our last 21-year mortality rate dropped to 4.5 percent (six deaths in 133 patients). Causes of death in these six patients were short bowel syndrome in two patients, moribund at presentation due to volvulus and necrotic bowel (IIIb), congenital syphilis, sepsis, and cot death at two months of age (each one patient).

Table 49.1 Jejunal atresia and stenosis: Red Cross Children's Hospital experience 1959–2011 (March 2011).

Type	Jejunum	Ileum	Total	(%)
Stenosis	21	13	34	10.12
Type I	63	18	81	24.11
Type II	19	13	32	9.52
Type IIIa	27	24	51	15.18
Type IIIb	61	0	61	18.15
Type IV	63	14	77	22.92
Total	254	82	336	100

Table 49.2 Mortality related to type of atresia.

Type	Patients	Mortality	%
Stenosis	34	0	0.00
Type I	81	4	4.94
Type II	32	4	12.50
Type IIIa	51	8	15.69
Type IIIb	61	10	16.39
Type IV	77	9	11.69
Total	336	35	10.42

Table 49.3 Jejunoileal atresia and stenosis: improvement in survival.

Authors	Years of study	n	Survival (%)
Fvans	1950	1498	9.3
Gross	1940–1952	71	51
Benson *et al.*	1945–1959	38	55
De Lorimer	1957–1966	587	65
Nixon and Tawes	1956–1967	62	62
Louw	1959–1967	33	94
Martin and Zerella	1957–1975	59	64
Cywes *et al.*	1959–1978	84	88
Danismead *et al.*	1967–1981	101	77
Smith and Glasson	1961–1986	84	61
Vecchia *et al.*	1972–1997	128	84
Millar *et al.*	1990–2011	133	95.5

FURTHER READING

Benson CD, Lloyd JR, Smith JD. Resection and primary anastomosis in the management of stenosis and atresia of the jejunum and ileum. *Pediatrics* 1960; **26**: 265–72.

Evans CH. Atresias of the gastrointestinal tract. *International Abstracts of Surgery* 1951; **92**: 1–8.

Kimura K, Perdzynski W, Soper RT. Elliptical resection of tapering the proximal dilated bowel in duodenal or jejunal atresia. *Journal of Pediatric Surgery* 1996; **31**: 1405–6.

Kling K, Applebaum H, Dunn J *et al.* A novel technique for correction of intestinal atresia at the ligament of Treitz. *Journal of Pediatric Surgery* 2000; **35**: 353–6.

Louw JH, Barnard CN. Congenital intestinal atresia. *Lancet* 1955; **269**: 1065–7.

Smith GHH, Glasson M. Intestinal atresia: factors affecting survival. *Australian and New Zealand Journal of Surgery* 1989; **59**: 151–6.

50

Meconium ileus

FREDERICK J RESCORLA and JAY L GROSFELD

ETIOLOGY AND CLASSIFICATION

Cystic fibrosis (CF) is the most common serious inherited defect affecting the Caucasian population. Cystic fibrosis is transmitted as an autosomal recessive condition with a 5 percent carrier rate and an incidence of approximately 1:2500 live births. The cystic fibrosis transmembrane conductance regulator (*CFTR*) gene is located on the long arm of chromosome 7. According to the Cystic Fibrosis Genetic Analysis Consortium, 13 mutations occur at a frequency of greater than 1 percent and account for 87 percent of CF alleles. The delta F508 mutation is the most common and is present in 70 percent of CF alleles in the United States. There are great differences among populations, and among African Americans delta F508 only accounts for 43 percent of the alleles. The CFTR protein controls sodium and chloride transport and in cystic fibrosis this results in abnormal luminal secretions. Neonatal intestinal obstruction due to inspissated meconium has been identified since the early reports concerning cystic fibrosis and is referred to as meconium ileus. This presentation is observed in 10–15 percent of infants born with cystic fibrosis. The etiology of this abnormal meconium (mucoviscidosis) is due to deficient pancreatic and intestinal secretions, as well as an abnormal concentration of the meconium within the duodenum and proximal jejunum. Instances of meconium ileus can be classified into uncomplicated and complicated cases.

Uncomplicated meconium ileus

CLINICAL PRESENTATION

1 In this condition, the abnormal thickened meconium causes a simple obturator obstruction of the terminal ileum. The distal 15–30 cm of terminal ileum is filled with inspissated meconium pellets, which are adherent to the bowel wall. The ileum just proximal to the obstruction fills with thick, putty-like meconium and dilates to 3–4 cm in diameter. The colon is unused and small (microcolon), because meconium has not yet entered this segment of bowel.

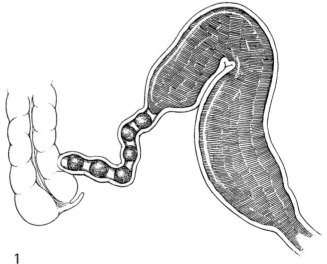

1

The typical neonate with meconium ileus may appear relatively normal for the first 12–18 hours of life and some tolerate several feeds. As the proximal bowel fills with swallowed air, however, abdominal distension and emesis (initially clear, later bilious) and failure to pass meconium are noted, heralding the presence of intestinal obstruction at 24–36 hours of age.

RADIOGRAPHIC EVALUATION

2 Plain abdominal x-rays and decubitus views usually demonstrate similar-sized dilated loops of intestine without air–fluid levels. A 'soap bubble' appearance is often noted in the right lower quadrant, a result of air mixing with the thick meconium.

INITIAL MANAGEMENT

The neonate with suspected bowel obstruction should be treated with oral gastric tube decompression of the stomach and intravenous fluids to replace pre-existing fluid deficits and ongoing losses. Antibiotics are administered, as the differential diagnosis of a newborn with this presentation includes sepsis.

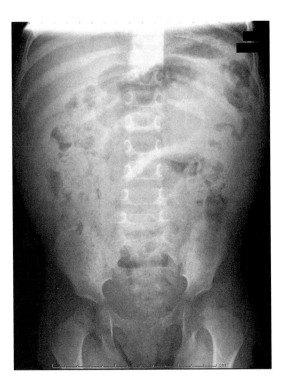

2

DIAGNOSTIC ENEMA

3 The initial diagnostic test is a contrast enema. If the diagnosis of meconium ileus is not apparent from the plain x-rays, a barium enema is the diagnostic procedure of choice. This will demonstrate a microcolon and may also document the presence of meconium pellets in the proximal ascending colon and terminal ileum.

This study will also exclude cases of colon atresia, small left colon syndrome, and meconium plug syndrome, and document the location of the cecum to rule out anomalies of rotation and fixation. Neonates with distal ileal atresia and total colonic aganglionosis may have similar appearance on a contrast enema examination, but these neonates usually have air–fluid levels in the dilated proximal small bowel and absence of pellets in the distal ileum and proximal colon. If the neonate is stable and there is no evidence of complicated meconium ileus (peritoneal calcifications, giant cystic structure, etc.), non-operative treatment with a hypertonic contrast material enema is recommended.

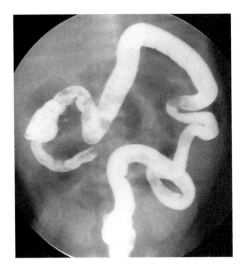

3

THERAPEUTIC ENEMA

The management of neonates with uncomplicated meconium ileus was significantly altered with the introduction of the diatrizoate meglumine (Gastrografin) enema by Noblett in 1969. The efficacy of this procedure is related to the hyperosmolar nature of Gastrografin (1100–1900 mOsm/L), which contains a wetting agent (Tween 80) and draws large volumes of fluid into the bowel lumen, thus washing out the obstructing meconium. Although initial reports used full-strength Gastrografin, most pediatric radiologists dilute the contrast material to approximately 3:1, and the Gastrografin currently used does not contain a wetting agent. Complications reported following Gastrografin enema include perforation, necrotizing enterocolitis, shock, and the occasional death. Most of these events are probably related to the hyperosmolar nature of the contrast material causing fluid depletion, which results in decreased intestinal blood flow and perfusion. Some radiologists prefer using other agents, such as diatrizoate sodium (Hypaque) or iothalamate meglumine (Conray), alone or in combination with *N*-acetylcysteine, but the authors prefer to use dilute Gastrografin. It is essential that the radiologists and clinicians are aware of the osmolality of the solution.

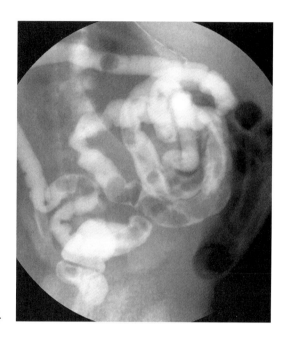

4 The enema is gently administered under fluoroscopic control and the contrast material flushed around the obstructing meconium pellets in the terminal ileum.

4

Before the enema, an intravenous route is established and the infant is appropriately resuscitated, and fluids are infused at a rate of 1.5 times maintenance during and after the procedure. The infant's pulse rate and urine output are carefully monitored in anticipation of fluid shifts into the bowel lumen. Meconium pellets, followed by loose meconium, generally pass through the rectum over the next 4–8 hours. If evidence of bowel obstruction persists and the infant remains clinically and hemodynamically stable, a second or third enema may be administered.

N-acetylcysteine (2.5–5 percent, 5 mL every 6 hours) may be administered by oral gastric tube to aid in clearing the thickened meconium from above. As the clinical evidence of obstruction resolves, the oral gastric tube is removed and feeding advanced. The Gastrografin enema is successful in resolving the obstruction in approximately 55 percent of cases. Survival for these infants at one year is nearly 100 percent. If these non-operative efforts fail, surgical exploration is required.

Complicated meconium ileus

CLINICAL PRESENTATION AND INITIAL MANAGEMENT

5a–c Complicated cases include instances of volvulus, bowel perforation, intestinal atresia, and giant cystic meconium peritonitis. Volvulus usually occurs when the distended segment of ileum twists at the level of the narrow, pellet-filled, distal small intestine (a). In some cases, volvulus can result in bowel perforation, leading to meconium peritonitis (b), and in others, the bowel may become necrotic and liquefy, resulting in a pseudocyst. This latter condition is referred to as a giant cystic meconium peritonitis. Bowel atresias are thought to arise when the base of the volvulus becomes ischemic (c).

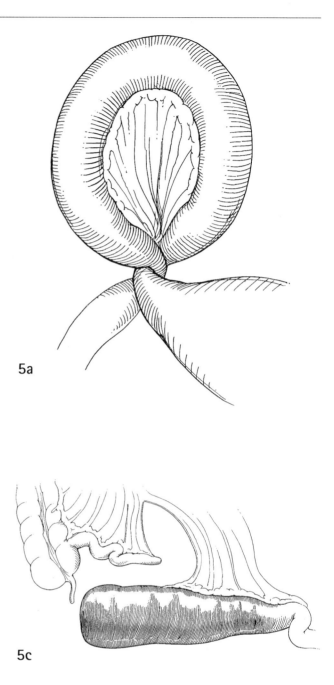

5a

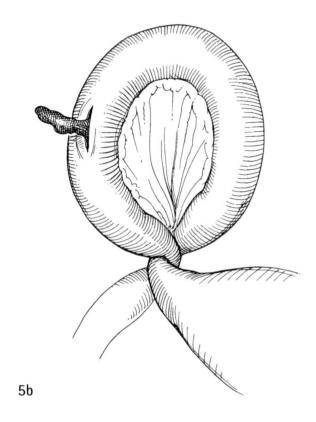

5b

5c

Neonates with complicated meconium ileus usually present with abdominal distension at the time of, or shortly after, delivery. In addition, bile-stained fluid is usually noted in the stomach. On physical examination, an abdominal mass may be noted. Neonates with meconium peritonitis occasionally have meconium in the scrotal sac or vagina as a result of passage of this material through a patent processus vaginalis or the fimbriated ends of the Fallopian tubes, respectively. In addition, in one unusual report, a meconium pseudocyst appeared as a buttock mass. The early management of these neonates includes intravenous hydration, antibiotics, and oral gastric tube decompression of the stomach.

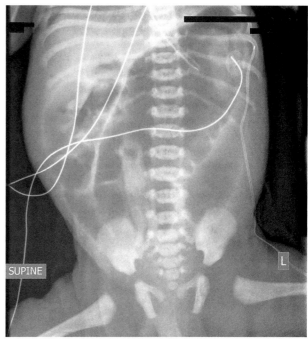

6a

DIAGNOSIS

6 In contrast to neonates with uncomplicated meconium ileus, flat and erect or decubitus x-rays of the abdomen in complicated cases may demonstrate distended loops of small bowel of different size with air–fluid levels. Intraperitoneal calcifications from the extravasated meconium, characteristic of meconium peritonitis, may be noted. A mass effect or ascites may also be observed.

Neonates who can be identified as complicated cases by plain abdominal radiographs are taken to the operating room for prompt exploration. In uncertain cases, a barium enema may be useful to exclude other causes of distal obstruction.

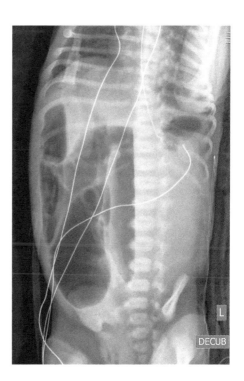

6b

OPERATIONS

Uncomplicated meconium ileus

MIKULICZ PROCEDURE

Meconium ileus was often considered a fatal condition until 1948 when Hiatt and Wilson reported a number of survivors after enterotomy and irrigation. This technique was not widely utilized and, in 1953, Gross reported successful outcomes in infants with meconium ileus following bowel resection and use of Mikulicz enterostomy.

7 The dilated bowel loop filled with thickened meconium is brought out of the abdomen and the small bowel proximal and distal to this segment is sutured together in a side-to-side fashion by interrupted seromuscular sutures. Following closure of the abdomen, the exteriorized dilated bowel is resected, thus avoiding the risk of peritoneal contamination. This results in an enterostomy through which the distal bowel can be irrigated in the postoperative period to wash out the obstructing meconium pellets. A Mikulicz spur-crushing clamp is applied, resulting in a common lumen, and the ostomy is then closed at a later date.

The disadvantages of this procedure are the loss of fluids from the mid-small bowel ostomy, the need for a subsequent procedure to close the stoma, and some reduction of bowel length due to initial resection.

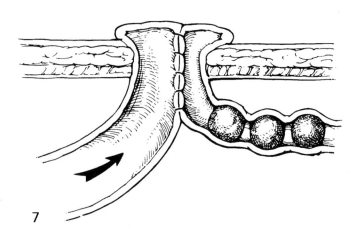

7

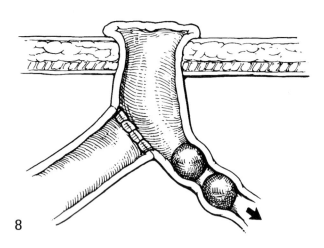

8

BISHOP–KOOP PROCEDURE

8 In 1957, Bishop and Koop reported resection of the large dilated loop followed by an anastomosis between the end of the proximal segment and the side of the distal segment. The end of the distal bowel is then brought out as an end ileostomy. A catheter is passed into the distal segment to allow postoperative irrigation. As the distal obstruction is relieved, the intestinal contents preferentially pass into the distal ileum and colon, thus decreasing loss of fluid and electrolytes from the stoma. The ostomy can be closed at a later date and, in some cases where it is trimmed beneath the skin, may close spontaneously.

The disadvantages of this technique include loss of bowel length at the time of the initial procedure, the need for an intraperitoneal anastomosis, and the need for a second operative procedure.

SANTULLI–BLANC ENTEROSTOMY

9 This modification of the Bishop–Koop procedure concept was reported in 1961. The operation involves resection of the distal dilated bowel segment followed by a side-to-end anastomosis with proximal enterostomy.

The disadvantages are similar to those noted for the Bishop–Koop procedure.

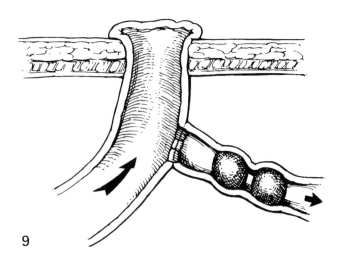

9

PRIMARY RESECTION AND ANASTOMOSIS

The use of resection with primary anastomosis in the management of meconium ileus was first reported by Swenson in 1962.

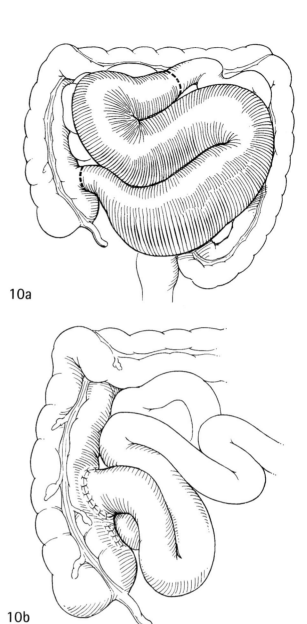

10a

10a,b After resection of the obstructed bowel segment, the remaining pellets in the distal bowel are irrigated clear and an ileocolonic anastomosis is performed.

The disadvantage associated with this procedure is resection of additional bowel, as the terminal ileum containing meconium pellets was usually resected along with the dilated segment of ileum. This, as well as concerns about an unvented intraperitoneal anastomosis, prevented wide acceptance of this procedure.

10b

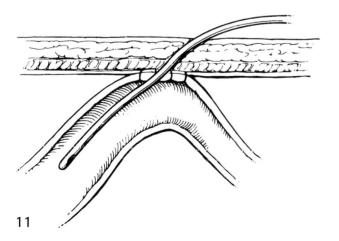

11

TUBE ENTEROSTOMY

11 In 1970, O'Neill and colleagues reported success with a simple procedure involving tube enterostomy with postoperative irrigation. Their initial report of five neonates was followed by a report by Harberg *et al.* concerning nine of 11 neonates who had successful meconium washout using this technique. Harberg and colleagues modified the technique slightly by utilizing a T-tube. A follow-up study of this technique noted success in 20 out of 23 patients with T-tube irrigation utilizing pancreatic enzymes or 1 percent *N*-acetylcysteine, 5–12.5 mL per dose. Unfortunately, three patients required a second procedure in the neonatal period due to inadequate treatment with the T-tube.

ENTEROTOMY AND IRRIGATION

The technique of enterotomy with irrigation has been one of the two procedures of choice at our institution since 1981. As previously noted, this procedure was originally described by Hiatt and Wilson in 1948. Reports by several other authors appeared in the literature between 1970 and 1990.

The infant is taken to the operating room and an endotracheal tube is placed before anesthesia to avoid aspiration.

12 After induction of general anesthesia, the procedure is carried out through a right-sided supraumbilical transverse abdominal incision. The right rectus abdominis muscle, as well as a portion of the right external and internal oblique and transversus abdominis muscles, is divided using electrocautery. The peritoneal cavity is entered and explored. The distended meconium-filled loops and pellet-filled distal small bowel are identified and delivered into the wound.

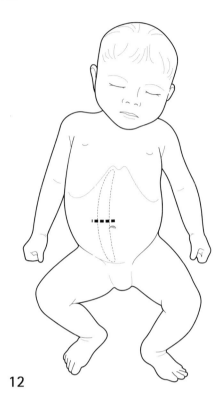

12

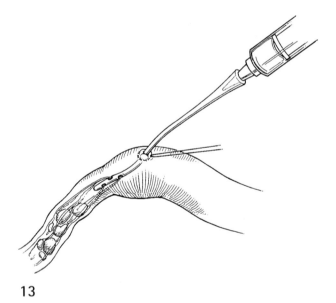

13

13 A purse-string suture of 4/0 silk is placed on the antimesenteric border of the dilated bowel 6–8 cm proximal to the narrow region containing the obstructing pellets. An 8–10 Fr red rubber catheter is placed through a small enterotomy, the purse-string suture is snugged, and the bowel lumen is irrigated by gently instilling saline through a syringe attached to an adapter and three-way stopcock. Fluid is irrigated into the proximal thick meconium and around the distal pellets.

With irrigation and gentle manual manipulation, the thick meconium from the distended loop and the distal pellets can be removed through the enterotomy or washed out distally through the colon. Occasionally, the enterotomy may need to be extended to a 1.5–2.0-cm opening to allow removal of the thick meconium and pellets. Numerous irrigations are usually required. Dilute Gastrografin or 2.5–5 percent *N*-acetylcysteine solution may also be used for irrigation. There have been occasional reports documenting hypernatremia with *N*-acetylcysteine. When the pellets are cleared, saline is irrigated through the distal ileum and into the colon to exclude the possibility of atresia and also to flush some of the distal pellet fragments into the colon. The enterotomy is then closed in two layers, using an inner full-thickness layer of absorbable 4/0 or 5/0 polyglactin (running or interrupted) and an outer seromuscular layer with interrupted 5/0 silk suture.

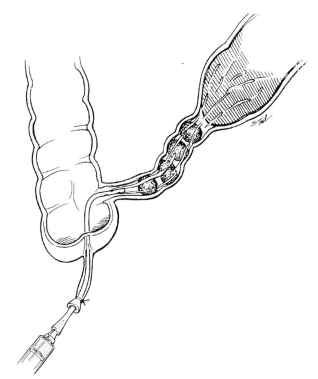

14a

APPENDICAL IRRIGATION

14a,b In 1989, Fitzgerald and Conlon reported the use of the appendix to instill dilute Gastrografin around the thickened meconium and pellets and flush the material into the colon. This has become the other preferred technique at our institution. The catheter can usually be advanced from the cecum retrogradely into the ileum, and saline is gently irrigated into the terminal ileum (a); the surgeon gently compresses the pellets and meconium to allow smaller particles to mix with the saline. The catheter is then withdrawn into the appendix and the surgeon 'milks' the material into the colon (b). This process must usually be repeated several times and as the material is advanced into the ascending colon, it is gently flushed into the distal colon and out of the rectum. After the ileal obstruction is completely relieved, the appendix is removed in the standard fashion.

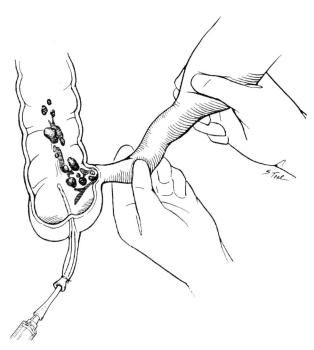

14b

Complicated meconium ileus

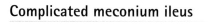

The anesthetic management is similar to that described for uncomplicated cases. The abdomen is entered through a transverse supraumbilical incision. The operative findings and ease of procedure may vary significantly, from volvulus and bowel atresia to meconium peritonitis or giant cystic meconium peritonitis. These conditions will, therefore, be discussed separately.

VOLVULUS AND ATRESIA

In instances of meconium ileus associated with bowel volvulus or atresia, the pathology is usually easily identified at laparotomy, and a primary anastomosis is nearly always possible.

15a–c In cases of volvulus, the involved loop is resected and an end-to-oblique anastomosis is constructed between the dilated proximal bowel and smaller distal bowel. The proximal bowel is divided at a 90° angle with respect to the mesentery and the distal bowel at a 45° angle. The distal meconium pellets should be removed through the open bowel, and the distal segment should also be irrigated to facilitate return of bowel function and to avoid a postoperative obturator obstruction distal to the anastomosis. The anastomosis is constructed with one or two layers of interrupted 5/0 silk sutures.

In cases of atresia, if adequate bowel length is present, the proximal dilated segment (usually 10–15 cm) is resected, as it is frequently atonic, and an end-to-oblique anastomosis is fashioned.

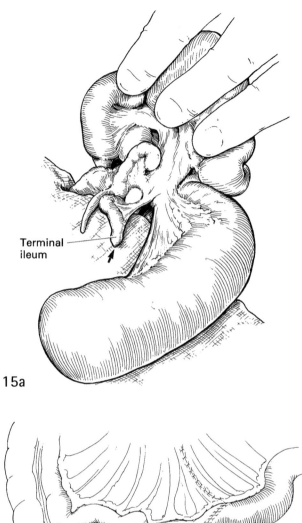

Terminal ileum

15a

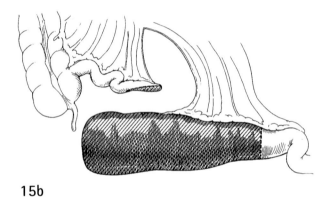

15b

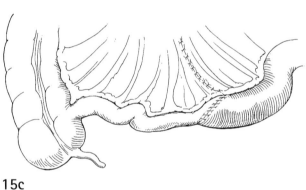

15c

MECONIUM PERITONITIS AND GIANT CYSTIC MECONIUM PERITONITIS

Neonates with these two disorders generally have numerous adhesions throughout the abdomen and may have significant blood and fluid losses during the operation. The abdomen is explored and the small bowel and colon carefully identified and dissected free from the numerous adhesions.

The necrotic dilated segment is resected and, if possible, an end-to-end or end-to-oblique anastomosis is constructed. In some cases, this is not possible and a temporary enterostomy is required. The bowel opening may be found within the pseudocyst. Most of the pseudocyst wall should be resected, if possible. This may result in some blood loss requiring transfusion. The

proximal end may be brought out as a temporary stoma through the corner of the wound or through a separate incision. The distal bowel can either be closed with sutures or staples and left in the abdomen, or brought out as a separate mucous fistula to allow irrigation, as well as refeeding of the effluent from the proximal ostomy into the distal bowel.

POSTOPERATIVE CARE

Uncomplicated meconium ileus

In the early postoperative period, an oral gastric tube is left in place until bowel function returns. Use of

N-acetylcysteine (2.5–5 percent, 5–10 mL in 6 hours) through an oral gastric tube may further aid passage of inspissated meconium. When bowel function returns, the tube is removed and enteral feedings are initiated along with pancreatic enzyme supplementation. The diagnosis of cystic fibrosis is confirmed by obtaining an elevated sweat chloride level on testing and the actual chromosomal defect is identified to assist in genetic counseling. The management of these patients requires a multidisciplinary team, including the pediatric respiratory physician, in order to optimize the pulmonary status, as pulmonary function deterioration is the major cause of morbidity and mortality.

LONG–TERM COMPLICATIONS

Gastrointestinal problems after the newborn period are relatively common in children with cystic fibrosis. These include intussusception, appendiceal distension with inspissated material and appendicitis, rectal prolapse, and gallbladder disease. In the early 1990s, colonic strictures were reported by several centers in association with high pancreatic enzyme replacement. One of the most common gastrointestinal disorders in children and adolescents with cystic fibrosis is the distal intestinal obstruction syndrome. The obturator obstruction often occurs after an intercurrent illness in which the child has a decreased oral intake and stops taking the pancreatic enzyme supplement.

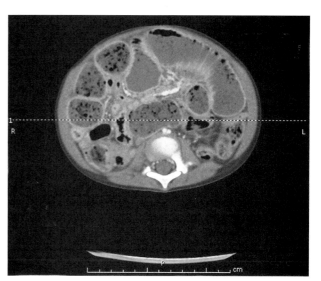

16a

16 The clinical presentation includes abdominal pain and decreased stool frequency. Plain x-rays frequently demonstrate large amounts of fecal material with the 'bubbly' granular appearance similar to meconium ileus (a). This may require treatment with Gastrografin enemas or administration of a balanced intestinal lavage solution orally or through a nasogastric tube. The obstruction usually responds to non-operative management with a balanced salt solution such as GoLytley (20 mL/kg per hour for 3–4 hours). If dehydration is present, intravenous hydration will be required. In some more advanced cases or if the diagnosis is not clear, a water-soluble contrast enema with Gastrografin or other solution may be both diagnostic and therapeutic (b). The use of oral or nasogastric Gastrografin has also been reported with a dose of 50 mL followed by at least 200 mL of water in children less than eight years of age, and 100 mL followed by at least 400 mL of water in children over eight years of age.

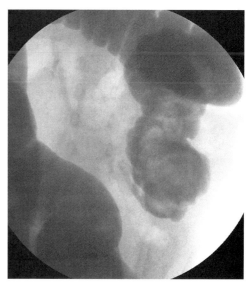

16b

Complicated meconium ileus

Neonates with complicated meconium ileus are managed in a similar manner to uncomplicated cases, although return of bowel function may be somewhat slower, particularly in cases of perforation. Some infants may require total parenteral nutrition if bowel function is slow to return, or if a proximal enterostomy does not provide an adequate absorptive surface to support the infant with enteral nutrition alone. Infants with both a proximal and distal stoma can often be managed with oral feeds combined with refeeding of the proximal ostomy effluent into the distal stoma. Enterostomy closure is generally performed 5–6 weeks after the initial procedure.

OUTCOME

The results of the medical and surgical management of 60 neonates with meconium ileus treated between 1972 and 1991 at the Riley Hospital for Children, Indianapolis, have been reviewed. The study included 20 girls and 40 boys. A family history of cystic fibrosis was present in six neonates.

Twenty-five neonates had uncomplicated meconium ileus due to intraluminal obstruction of the terminal ileum with concretions of abnormal meconium. The treatment of these patients can be divided into two time periods, 1972–1980 and 1981–1991. Ten infants presented during the first time period, and only two of them were successfully cleared with a diatrizoate meglumine (Gastrografin) enema. The eight remaining infants underwent resection, operative irrigation, and enterostomy formation. A Bishop–Koop stoma was constructed in two infants, and six had a double-barrel (side-by-side) enterostomy. Of the 15 neonates treated during the later time period, eight (53 percent) were successfully cleared with a Gastrografin enema. The remaining seven infants required laparotomy. Seven were treated with enterotomy and intraoperative irrigation with saline or dilute contrast agent (Hypaque or Gastrografin) and one with irrigation and double-barrel enterostomy.

Thirty-five neonates presented with 56 complications of meconium ileus, including volvulus (22), atresia (20), perforation (6), and giant cystic meconium peritonitis (8). Clinical presentation in these neonates included abdominal distension, bilious vomiting, and failure to pass meconium; these symptoms were usually noted earlier than in uncomplicated cases. Neonates with perforation and giant cystic meconium peritonitis often had abdominal distension at the time of delivery. Three were diagnosed by prenatal ultrasound.

Operative management of patients with atresia, volvulus, and perforation included resection and anastomosis in 15 and enterostomy in 12. The eight patients with giant cystic meconium peritonitis underwent excision of the pseudocyst and enterostomy.

The diagnosis of cystic fibrosis was confirmed in all cases by sweat chloride test. Pancreatic enzyme therapy was instituted, along with a routine formula feed. Enterostomy closure was usually accomplished between 4 weeks and three months of age. All patients have been followed by the Indiana University Cystic Fibrosis Clinic at Riley Hospital for Children. Survival at one year was 92 percent (23/25) in patients with uncomplicated meconium ileus, and 89 percent (31/35) in complicated cases. The mortality in the uncomplicated cases was due to pulmonary problems and both occurred during the early time period. Deaths in the complicated cases were the result of sepsis (2), renal failure (1), and severe cholestatic jaundice progressing to liver failure (1). Since this report, uncomplicated cases have been managed exclusively with either enterotomy and irrigation, or irrigation through the appendix.

FURTHER READING

Burke MS, Ragi JM, Karamanoukian HL *et al.* New strategies in nonoperative management of meconium ileus. *Journal of Pediatric Surgery* 2002; **37**: 760–4.

Fitzgerald R, Colon K. Use of the appendix stump in the treatment of meconium ileus. *Journal of Pediatric Surgery* 1989; **24**: 899–900.

Kerem BS, Rommens JM, Buchanan JA *et al.* Identification of the cystic fibrosis gene: genetic analysis. *Science* 1989; **245**: 1073–80.

Mak GZ, Harberg FJ, Hiatt P *et al.* T-tube ilestomy for meconium ileus: four decades of experience. *Journal of Pediatric Surgery* 2000; **135**: 349–52.

O'Halloran SM, Gilbert J, McKendrick OM *et al.* Gastrografin in acute meconium ileus equivalent. *Archives of Disease in Childhood* 1986; **61**: 1128–30.

Rescorla FJ, Grosfeld JL. Contemporary management of meconium ileus. *World Journal of Surgery* 1993; **17**: 318–25.

51

Vitellointestinal (omphalomesenteric) duct anomalies

SPENCER W BEASLEY

INTRODUCTION

The vitellointestinal (omphalomesenteric) duct is an embryonic communication between the yolk sac and the midgut. This communication normally disappears at about the sixth week of fetal life. Persistence of the duct between the intestinal tract and the umbilicus, or persistence of its embryonic blood supply, results in a variety of lesions that usually present in early infancy, but occasionally appear later in life.

TYPES OF ANOMALIES

A Meckel's diverticulum represents persistency and patency of the inner intestinal component of the vitellointestinal tract (see illustration 1). In a small proportion of patients there will be a fibrous band extending from the apex of the Meckel's diverticulum to the undersurface of the umbilicus (see illustration 2), but more often there is a band representing the remnants of the vitelline vessels joining the Meckel's diverticulum to the mesentery of the small bowel (see illustration 3). Meckel's diverticulum has diverse clinical presentations (**Table 51.1**), but frequently remains quiescent throughout life. The chances of an asymptomatic Meckel's diverticulum causing symptoms later in life are such that en passant removal of the structure when it is observed during operation for some other reason is arguably justified in children, but is probably not justified in adults in whom the chances of it becoming symptomatic are much less likely.

Table 51.1 Presentation of Meckel's diverticulum.

Melena and anemia	Ectopic gastric mucosa in the Meckel's diverticulum releases hydrochloric acid, which causes ulceration of adjacent ileum, producing major gastrointestinal bleeding
Abdominal pain (Meckel's diverticulitis)	Inflammation of a Meckel's diverticulum, particularly if long and with a narrow lumen, causes clinical features similar to those of acute suppurative appendicitis
	Perforation of an adjacent ileal ulcer may also cause an inflammatory mass, pneumoperitoneum and peritonitis
Intussusception	A Meckel's diverticulum may invert and act as a lead point for an intussusception
	This is responsible for about 2% of intussusceptions
Meckel's band obstruction	A band extending from a Meckel's diverticulum to the root of the small bowel mesentery or to the umbilicus may cause a loop of bowel to become entangled around it, producing a bowel obstruction
Incidental findings	A Meckel's diverticulum may be found during laparotomy for other conditions, e.g. appendicitis

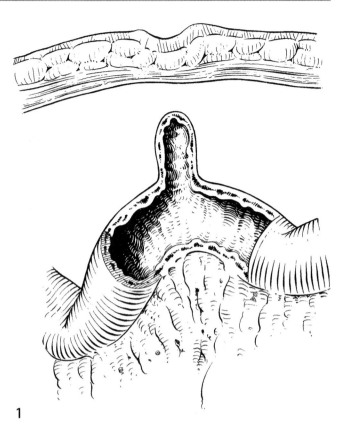

1 The typical appearance of a Meckel's diverticulum is shown in cross-section. Parts of the inner surface may contain ectopic pancreatic or gastric mucosa. Ectopic gastric mucosa produces hydrochloric acid, which can ulcerate adjacent non-gastric mucosa, either in the diverticulum itself or in adjacent ileum, and cause major bleeding. The child may present with 'brick-red' rectal bleeding (often without much abdominal pain), and anemia.

1

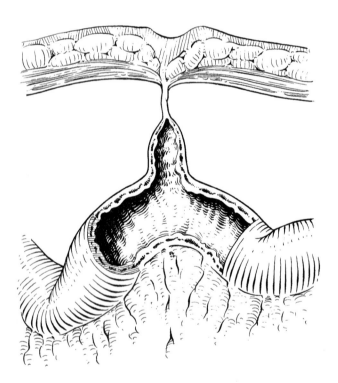

2 The vitellointestinal band (Meckel's band) is the remnant of the duct in which the lumen has been obliterated, but a fibrous cord or band persists. This runs from the deep surface of the umbilicus to the ileum or to a Meckel's diverticulum. There is always a risk that a loop of bowel may become entangled around it, producing intestinal obstruction.

2

3 The Meckel's diverticulum is often bound down by remnants of the vitelline vessels from its apex and is adherent to the mesentery of the ileum. (Division of the vessels at the apex of the peritoneal fold reveals its typical antimesenteric origin.) Loops of bowel can be trapped beneath this band, producing a closed loop obstruction.

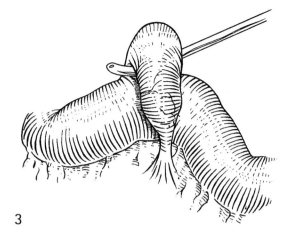

3

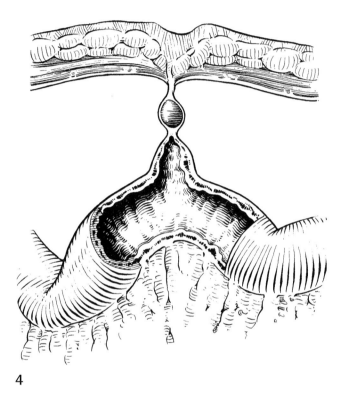

4

4 This form of Meckel's diverticulum has a cord containing a cystic remnant, which may slowly increase in size. The cyst is the result of partial obliteration of the duct. It may become infected and form an abscess; if it has a sinus, pus may discharge from the umbilicus.

BLEEDING MECKEL'S DIVERTICULUM

Principles and justification

This is the most common clinical presentation of a Meckel's diverticulum, and results from the presence of ectopic gastric mucosa in the lining of the diverticulum. Hydrochloric acid produced by the gastric mucosa causes ulceration of the adjacent small bowel mucosa and, less commonly, of the diverticulum itself. This may result in rapid hemorrhage, which usually presents as relatively painless but profuse 'brick-red' rectal bleeding. The resultant anemia may necessitate blood transfusion, but the bleeding usually stops spontaneously without the need

for emergency surgery. The definitive investigation is surgery, but a technetium scan may confirm the presence of ectopic gastric mucosa.

Indications

Surgery (open or laparoscopic) is indicated where the clinical presentation of major and painless intestinal hemorrhage is consistent with a bleeding Meckel's diverticulum, irrespective of the result of the technetium scan. One advantage of a laparoscopic approach is that the diagnosis can be confirmed using a minimally invasive technique.

Preoperative

ANESTHESIA

The procedure is performed under general anesthesia and muscle paralysis, using the same technique as for any acute abdominal procedure. Blood transfusion is required very occasionally in the perioperative period for major blood loss from the ileum, although the operative procedure itself is relatively bloodless. Electrolytes and fluid balance must be monitored. Perioperative antibiotics effective against bowel organisms are administered.

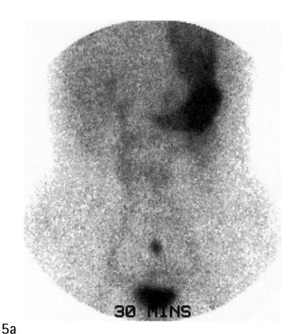

5a

Open operation

INCISION

5a,b The surgical approach is through a small, right transverse, infraumbilical, muscle-splitting or muscle-cutting incision. This can be extended medially by retracting the rectus toward the midline or even dividing the muscle if necessary. A Meckel's diverticulum can be excised easily through the standard incision used for an appendicectomy. Alternatively, laparoscopic-assisted Meckel's diverticulectomy through an umbilical incision can be employed (see below under Laparoscopic approach).

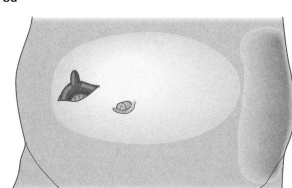

5b

IDENTIFICATION OF LESION

At laparotomy for bleeding, the Meckel's diverticulum will not usually be inflamed. A blue discoloration will be seen in the ileum and colon distal to the diverticulum if recent bleeding has occurred. The diverticulum causing bleeding is delivered through the wound.

CONTROL OF ILEUM AND ITS CONTENTS

6 Compression of the ileum with fingers or a non-crushing bowel clamp (fingers are preferred because they are less traumatic to the bowel) reduces the amount of bleeding and soiling that occurs when the ileum is opened and the diverticulum is excised. Packs are placed on either side of the loop of ileum containing the Meckel's diverticulum. Suction is kept nearby to reduce accidental spillage of liquid ileal contents when the ileum is opened. Stay sutures (3/0) are placed on the ileum on either side of the diverticulum.

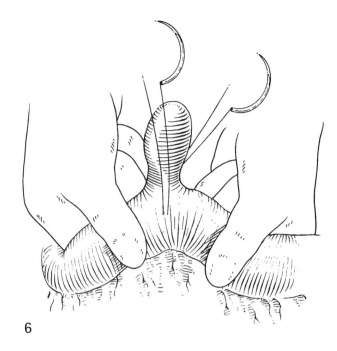

6

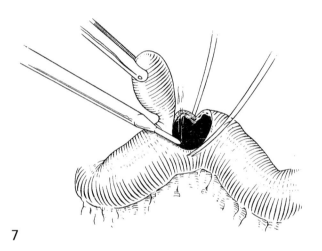

7

EXCISION OF DIVERTICULUM

7 A longitudinal or oblique elliptical incision is made in the ileum near the base of the diverticulum using scissors or diathermy. It is essential that the entire diverticulum is removed, because a remnant of acid-secreting mucosa left at the base of the diverticulum could continue to cause ulceration and bleeding of the adjacent ileum.

8 The stay sutures are then held apart to transform the longitudinal or oblique elliptical incision into a transverse one. This allows closure of the wound without narrowing the lumen of the ileum.

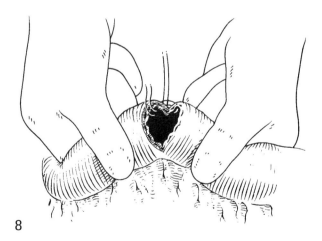

8

CLOSURE OF ILEUM

A 4/0 absorbable, continuous or interrupted, all-layers suture is used to close the bowel. A second seromuscular continuous layer is employed by some surgeons.

ALTERNATIVE METHOD FOR NARROW-NECKED DIVERTICULUM

9 A curved artery forceps or crushing clamp is placed across the base of the diverticulum at 45° or more to the long axis of the ileum. This avoids the narrowing that might be caused by an incision closed longitudinally. Mattress sutures of 3/0–4/0 absorbable material are inserted under the clamp and tied. The diverticulum is cut away at the distal border of the clamp.

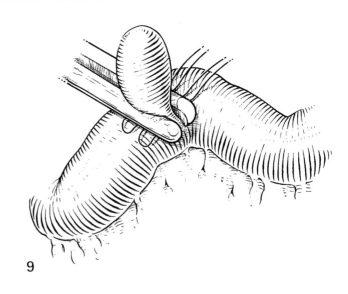

9

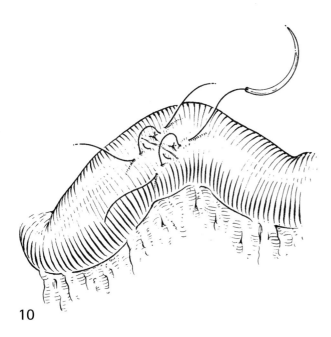

10

10 The clamp is removed and the line of section is buried by a second layer of sutures.

WOUND CLOSURE

The peritoneal cavity is irrigated with saline before closure. The wound is closed in layers with 2/0 or 3/0 absorbable sutures in the standard fashion.

Postoperative care

Oral fluids can be commenced on about the second day after operation when the abdomen is becoming soft to palpation and there is no nausea, i.e. no clinical evidence of ileus. Most children can be discharged on the second or third day after operation.

LAPAROSCOPIC APPROACH

This is now the preferred approach of many surgeons, and offers the advantage of being able to confirm the presence of a Meckel's diverticulum using a minimally invasive technique where there has been diagnostic uncertainty preoperatively.

11 Under general anesthesia and infiltration of local anesthetic with 0.25 percent plain bupivacaine, an infraumbilical incision is made. The linea alba is incised and the peritoneum opened under direct vision. A 5- or 10-mm 30° telescope is introduced through a 5- or 10-mm umbilical port and secured to the rectus fascia. An initial inspection of the peritoneal cavity is performed. One or two 3- or 5-mm working ports can be introduced on the left side of the abdomen, the size and location being determined by the age of the child.

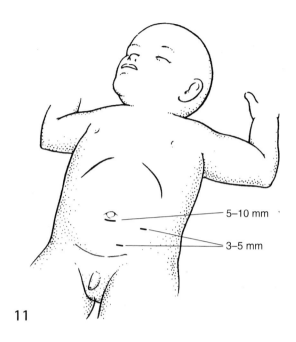

11

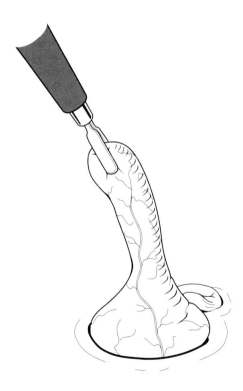

12 Once located, the Meckel's diverticulum can be delivered through the umbilical port opening (sometimes requiring enlargement) and the diverticulum is removed outside the abdomen using the same technique as described above.

13a,b Alternatively, particularly where the diverticulum is quite narrow at its base, it can be dissected from the ileum laparoscopically: the vitelline vessels are either divided by electrocautery or included in two endoloops placed around the base of the Meckel's diverticulum. Care is taken both to ensure the whole diverticulum is removed (to avoid leaving ectopic gastric mucosa behind) and to ensure that the caliber of the lumen of the ileum is not compromised. The Meckel's diverticulum is divided between the endoloops and removed through the umbilical port. An alternative and equally effective method involves resection using an endoGIA stapler.

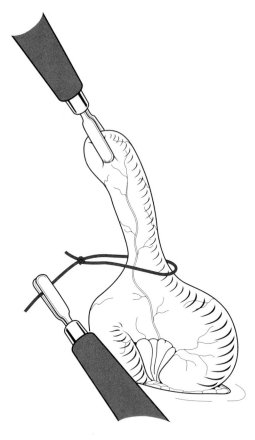

13a

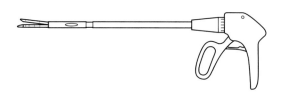

13b

MECKEL'S DIVERTICULITIS

Principles and justification

Meckel's diverticulitis is an unusual presentation in children. When it does occur, the child is assessed clinically as having acute appendicitis, but at laparotomy the appendix is found to be normal and there is an inflammatory process involving a Meckel's diverticulum. In all operations for suspected appendicitis in which the appendix is found to be normal at laparotomy or on laparoscopy, the distal 100 cm of ileum should be inspected to exclude inflammation of the Meckel's diverticulum as being responsible for the symptoms. The inflamed Meckel's diverticulum is often palpable in the abdomen on opening the peritoneum. An inflammatory mass around a Meckel's diverticulum may result from perforation of an ulcer in the ileum adjacent to the base of the diverticulum. Perforation may also cause pneumoperitoneum and peritonitis.

Indications

The indication for surgery for Meckel's diverticulum is when the appendix is found to be normal at the time of surgery for suspected appendicitis and an adjacent inflammatory mass (inflamed diverticulum) is identified.

Preoperative

ANESTHESIA

The procedure is performed under general anesthesia and muscle paralysis using the same technique as for acute appendicitis. Perioperative antibiotics are administered.

Operation

INDICATION AND EXPOSURE

When the diagnosis is known or suspected before the operation, a small, transverse, right infraumbilical incision can be used. If the diagnosis is made during operation at the time of exploration for suspected appendicitis, the inflamed Meckel's diverticulum and adjacent ileum can be delivered easily through the appendicectomy wound and the diverticulum excised outside the abdomen. If a laparoscopic approach to appendicectomy has been performed, the Meckel's diverticulum can be removed:

- laparoscopically;
- laparoscopically assisted, by delivering the diverticulum through the umbilical port; or
- by converting to an open approach, depending on the expertise and experience of the surgeon.

EXTENSIVE INFLAMMATORY MASS

14 If there is severe or long-standing inflammation of the diverticulum causing edema and involving the surrounding ileum, or if the base of the Meckel's diverticulum is very broad, it is appropriate to excise it with a small sleeve of ileum and perform an end-to-end small bowel anastomosis along conventional lines. Otherwise, the inflamed Meckel's diverticulum is excised in the same way as for a bleeding Meckel's diverticulum.

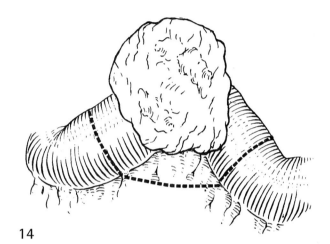

14

Indications

These children present with a distal small bowel obstruction, the exact cause of which usually cannot be determined clinically. Laparotomy is performed for obstruction. Closed loop obstruction is common. A laparoscopic approach can be used by the experienced laparoscopic surgeon, but the distended loops of small bowel may compromise visualization of the cause of the obstruction.

Operation

15 A right supraumbilical or subumbilical incision is standard where the pathology is not certain before operation. The band running from the Meckel's diverticulum is identified and divided, releasing the entrapped loops of bowel. Most commonly, the band runs to the root of the small bowel mesentery (see illustration 2), but may be attached to the undersurface of the umbilicus (see illustration 3).

Occasionally, the small bowel trapped by the band in a closed loop obstruction is found to be gangrenous and will need to be removed. The ends of viable bowel are reconnected with a standard end-to-end anastomosis.

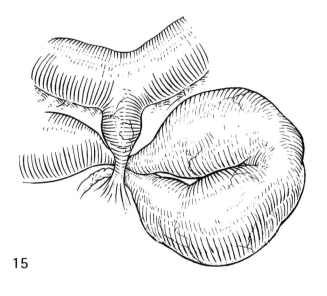

15

INTUSSUSCEPTION OF MECKEL'S DIVERTICULUM

Meckel's diverticulum is the most common cause of intussusception in which a pathologic lesion at the lead point is identified. It may occur at any age during childhood, but is most common in the first two years of life.

Indications

Peritonitis or other clinical evidence of the presence of ischemic bowel is an absolute indication for surgery in patients with intussusception. Otherwise, the child is treated initially by gas (or barium) enema. Where the intussusception is due to a Meckel's diverticulum, however, enema reduction is unlikely to be successful, and surgery is indicated because the enema has failed to reduce the intussusception.

OPERATION

INCISION

A right, transverse, supraumbilical incision is deepened as a muscle-cutting incision through the rectus abdominis muscle. Alternatively, a laparoscopic approach can be employed.

TECHNIQUE

16 The intussusception is located and an attempt is made to reduce it manually by gentle compression of the colon in a proximal direction at the level of the lead point. Much of the intussusception can be reduced, but when there is a Meckel's diverticulum at the lead point the final portion often cannot be reduced and must be resected in continuity with the diverticulum. On other occasions, the diverticulum will become evident once the intussusception has been fully reduced.

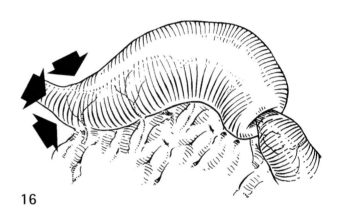

16

17

COMPLETE PERSISTENCE OF THE VITELLOINTESTINAL DUCT (FISTULA)

Principles and justification

17 When the entire vitellointestinal (omphalomesenteric) duct persists and remains patent, there is an open communication between the ileum and the umbilicus. This allows intermittent discharge of the contents of the ileum (gas and ileal fluid) and causes periumbilical excoriation. The tract may be of sufficient caliber to allow prolapse of the ileum as a 'pair of horns'.

Diagnosis

Escape of air and feces through an opening in the umbilicus is pathognomonic of a patent vitellointestinal tract. When there is doubt about the nature of the discharge from the umbilicus (often because it is intermittent), a sinogram will usually demonstrate direct communication with the ileum.

Indications

Surgery is indicated in all cases where a patent vitellointestinal tract has been demonstrated.

Operation

INCISION

18 A right transverse incision immediately lateral to the umbilicus through the rectus muscle allows adequate exposure of the vitellointestinal tract from within, avoiding the need to circumcise the umbilicus. After dissection of the tract, the defect in the umbilicus can be repaired from its deep surface.

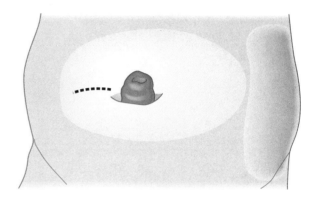

18

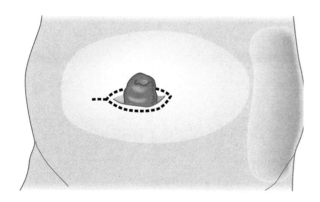

19

19 Alternatively, an incision in the umbilicus at the mucocutaneous junction, circumcising the external opening of the patent vitellointestinal tract, can be made. The tract is mobilized by separating it from the tough fascia of the linea alba surrounding it, and the peritoneum is opened. To improve exposure, the incision may need to be extended lateral to the umbilicus by dividing the medial 1–2 cm of rectus abdominis muscle, including the anterior rectus sheath, medial fibers of the rectus abdominis muscle, and the posterior rectus sheath.

DISSECTION OF TRACT

20 Dissection of the vitellointestinal tract is continued into the peritoneal cavity, where its communication with the ileum is identified.

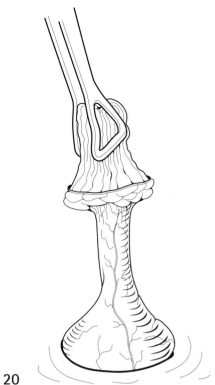

20

DIVISION AT JUNCTION WITH ILEUM

Two stay sutures are placed on the ileum and the vitellointestinal tract is divided at this point. The communication with the ileum may be narrow, resembling a fibrous cord, or broad, as in many patients with a Meckel's diverticulum. The ileum is closed in one or two layers with 3/0 or 4/0 absorbable sutures.

RECONSTRUCTION OF UMBILICUS

The defect in the umbilical ring is repaired in the same way as for an umbilical hernia. When the incision has been extended to the right, the posterior and anterior rectus sheath should be closed with 3/0 absorbable sutures.

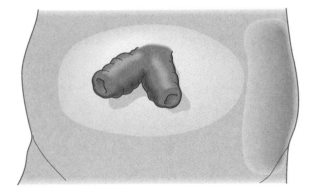

21

PROLAPSE OF PATENT VITELLOINTESTINAL TRACT

Principles and justification

21 When the channel is a short and broad vitellointestinal tract, the ileum may intussuscept through it onto the surface of the umbilicus, producing a double-horned 'Y-shaped' segment of bowel, inside out, with a lumen evident on each horn.

Operation

As long as the bowel is not necrotic (which is rare), it should be reduced manually, after which the vitellointestinal tract can be excised as a semi-elective procedure. In extremely rare situations, there is a single-horned prolapse of the vitellointestinal tract: this is seen in the neonatal period and suggests that there is an atresia of one horn, which will necessitate excision of the vitellointestinal tract and end-to-end ileoileostomy to reconstitute gastrointestinal continuity. This is usually an isolated lesion, not associated with other abnormalities.

ECTOPIC MUCOSA

Principles and justification

Discharge of mucus from the umbilicus may be caused by a small sequestrated nodule of ectopic alimentary mucosa (representing persistence of the external part of the vitellointestinal tract). It appears as a shiny, spherical, deep-red nodule in the depths of the umbilical cicatrix, but may be pedunculated. Crusts may form on the cicatrix and on the surrounding skin. It should be distinguished clinically from the more common umbilical granuloma, which presents as a small mass of heaped pink or grayish granulation tissue producing a chronic seropurulent discharge; the granuloma can be treated with topical application of silver nitrate.

Contraindications

If a sinus opening is evident, it is likely that all or part of the vitellointestinal tract is present and patent. Likewise, discharge of air or fecal fluid suggests complete patency of the vitellointestinal tract (vitellointestinal fistula). In this situation, surgical excision of the whole tract will be required.

Operation

22 Pedunculated ectopic mucosa can be ligated within the umbilical ring; alternatively, a wider based lesion may be excised by diathermy dissection across its base. Suture is required only occasionally.

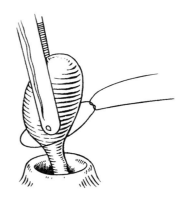

22

FURTHER READING

Campbell J, Beasley SW, McMullin N, Hutson JM. Clinical diagnosis of umbilical swellings and discharges in children. *Medical Journal of Australia* 1986; **145**: 450–3.

Loh DL, Munro FD. The role of laparoscopy in the management of lower gastrointestinal bleeding. *Pediatric Surgery International* 2003; **19**: 266–7.

Potts SR. Meckel's diverticulum. In: Najmaldin A, Rothenberg S, Crabbe D *et al.* (eds). *Operative Endoscopy and Endoscopic Surgery in Infants and Children.* London: Hodder Arnold, 2005: 273–7.

Saw RS. Appendix and Meckel diverticulum. In: Oldham KT, Colombani PM, Foglia RP (eds). *Surgery of Infants and Children: Scientific Principles and Practice.* Philadelphia, PA: Lippincott-Raven, 1997: 1224–8.

Valla JS, Steyaert H, Leculee R *et al.* Meckel's diverticulum and laparoscopy of children. What's new? *European Journal of Pediatric Surgery* 1998; **8**: 26–8.

52

Duplications of the alimentary tract

STIG SØMME and JACOB C LANGER

HISTORY

Duplications of the alimentary tract have also been termed giant diverticula, enterogenous cysts, ileum duplex, and inclusion cysts. Calder described the first case in 1733. Ladd introduced the term 'duplications of the alimentary tract' in 1937. He also listed a set of three criteria for the diagnosis: (1) the presence of a well-developed coat of smooth muscle; (2) epithelial lining that represents some part of the alimentary tract; and (3) an intimate attachment to some part of the alimentary tract.

PRINCIPLES AND JUSTIFICATIONS

Alimentary tract duplications are congenital malformations that may be found anywhere from mouth to anus. Duplications are found in about 1 in 4500 autopsies. The most common duplication is cystic and located on the mesenteric aspect of the small or large intestine. Multiple duplications are seen in about 10 percent of patients. As many as 30 percent of patients with thoracic or thoracoabdominal duplications have additional duplications below the diaphragm. Duplications are lined by alimentary tract mucosa and usually share a common smooth muscle wall and blood supply with the adjacent gut. Ectopic acid-producing gastric mucosa may be present in approximately 20 percent of duplications, and can cause peptic ulceration, bleeding, and perforation. Most duplications cause symptoms in infancy or early childhood and most are diagnosed by the age of two years, but some present as an incidental finding in patients with other conditions or may be identified on routine prenatal ultrasound; about 50 percent are diagnosed before five months of age. There is an overall equal sex distribution. In adults, duplications can rarely present with adenocarcinoma.

The pathogenesis for the development of duplications is unknown, but cystic duplications are thought to develop secondary to a split notochord mechanism and tubular duplications secondary to partial twinning. Cystic duplications may be associated with spinal cord and vertebral anomalies, and tubular duplications may be associated with urinary tract, spine, and central nervous system anomalies. Foregut duplications probably occur during the normal division of the foregut into respiratory and esophageal structures, and may therefore contain elements of respiratory tract, such as cartilage and bronchial epithelium (bronchogenic cyst), elements of esophagus such as smooth or striated muscle and squamous epithelium (esophageal duplication), or elements of both (foregut duplication).

DISTRIBUTION AND VARIETY

1 The distribution of 495 alimentary tract duplications in 455 patients shows that the most common location is in the midgut, and most of these duplications are located in the ileum.

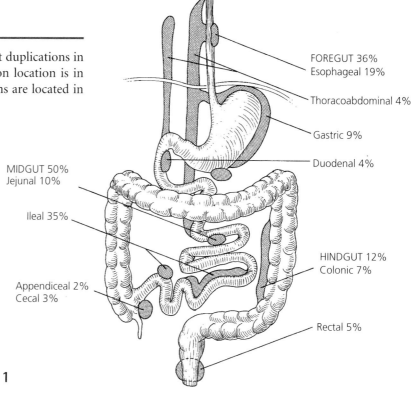

FOREGUT 36%
Esophageal 19%

Thoracoabdominal 4%

Gastric 9%

Duodenal 4%

MIDGUT 50%
Jejunal 10%

Ileal 35%

HINDGUT 12%
Colonic 7%

Appendiceal 2%
Cecal 3%

Rectal 5%

1

PRESENTATION

Patients may present with a mass or with symptoms related to the location and size of the cyst. Intestinal duplications can serve as a lead point for intussusception and can cause a localized volvulus of the small bowel. Ectopic acid-producing gastric mucosa can cause peptic ulceration of the normal intestinal mucosa, with resultant painless gastrointestinal bleeding or perforation. Duplication cysts may also cause intestinal obstruction due to mass effect, particularly those in the small bowel, which are located on the mesenteric surface between the leaves of the mesentery. Foregut duplication cysts may present with obstructive symptoms involving the esophagus, trachea, or both. Some duplication cysts are diagnosed on routine prenatal ultrasound. The differential diagnosis in these cases includes ovarian cyst, mesenteric or omental cyst, lymphatic malformation, choledochal cyst, and, less commonly, cysts of solid organs such as the kidney, spleen, liver, or pancreas. A pediatric surgeon should counsel the parents prenatally. Postnatally, the infant should be evaluated by a pediatric surgeon and should have a repeat ultrasound. If the child is asymptomatic and the cyst is still present and less than 4 cm in diameter, it is reasonable to manage it expectantly with repeated ultrasounds and a technetium scan to rule out ectopic gastric mucosa. Ovarian cysts will usually resolve over time, whereas duplication cysts will not. Symptomatic cysts should be resected expeditiously.

TREATMENT

Because alimentary tract duplications may be complicated by infection, bleeding, intestinal obstruction or volvulus, and may lead to the development of malignancy, many surgeons believe that they should be treated by early complete excision when possible. Sometimes complete excision is not achievable, e.g. in cases of long segmental tubular duplications or complex duodenal or retro-peritoneal duplications. Development of adenocarcinoma of the mucosal lining is rare, with only a few cases having been described in the literature. It is therefore acceptable to manage asymptomatic duplications that are not amenable to resection expectantly. Unresectable symptomatic duplications should be managed by partial resection in order to deal with the particular symptom. With close monitoring it is safe to wait until an infant is 3–6 months old before resecting asymptomatic duplication cysts. At 3–6 months infants are larger, tolerate the surgery well and are potentially less affected by anesthesia and risks of infection.

PREOPERATIVE ASSESSMENT AND PREPARATION

Associated anomalies

The associated anomalies can be predicted based on the location of the duplication. Foregut duplications may be associated with vertebral anomalies. Midgut duplications may have associated malrotation or atresia of the bowel. In patients with hindgut lesions, genitourinary duplications, anorectal malformations, and bladder exstrophy are sometimes seen. Associated anomalies are often identified clinically or with imaging. When multiple anomalies are found in the same patient, it is important that the management of the patient be planned carefully, since a multidisciplinary approach involving various specialists may be necessary.

Imaging diagnostics

ABDOMINAL RADIOGRAPHS

Radiographs of the abdomen may reveal a mass effect in the case of large abdominal cysts. Chest x-ray may show a mass, usually in the middle or posterior mediastinum, and associated vertebral anomalies.

ULTRASOUND

2 Ultrasound will determine whether a mass felt on physical examination is cystic or solid and its relationship to the intestine. Often a characteristic outer hypoechoic rim and an inner echogenic rim can be seen, a sign that is sometimes referred to as a 'bowel signature'.

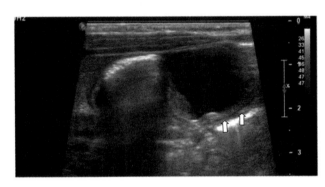

2

COMPUTED TOMOGRAPHY AND MAGNETIC RESONANCE IMAGING

Computed tomography (CT) or magnetic resonance imaging (MRI) may be helpful in cases where ultrasound is unclear or cannot be done for technical reasons. These modalities are particularly useful for the investigation and delineation of foregut duplications, duodenal duplications, and rectal lesions. Chest CT with contrast is useful for the visualization of foregut duplications, and provides important information for the preoperative planning of the procedure. MRI may be helpful in identifying and characterizing involvement of the spinal cord in cases of neurenteric cysts.

TECHNETIUM SCANNING

Technetium scanning is used to identify ectopic gastric mucosa in the cyst, which is present in about 20 percent of cases. This technique is most useful in the investigation of the child with painless rectal bleeding, for which the differential diagnosis includes both Meckel's diverticulum and intestinal duplication. It is also useful in the investigation of the child with an asymptomatic prenatally diagnosed duplication, in whom demonstration of ectopic gastric mucosa may push the surgeon to recommend excision rather than observation.

ESOPHAGOGASTRODUODENOSCOPY

Esophagogastroduodenoscopy may be helpful to identify ulcers or strictures, and better define the anatomy prior to operative excision of duplication cysts in the upper gastrointestinal tract.

CONTRAST RADIOGRAPHY

Upper and lower intestinal contrast radiography may be helpful for elucidating the anatomy. Barium swallow will demonstrate a typical anterior indentation of the esophagus in cases of foregut duplication cysts.

OPERATION

Esophageal duplications

3a–c Esophageal duplication cysts and foregut duplication cysts are usually intramural, non-communicating, cystic lesions. They are most commonly located to the right side of the esophagus (illustration a). Those in the proximal esophagus are often situated between the esophagus and the trachea. A posterolateral thoracotomy provides excellent exposure for most esophageal duplications, although many surgeons are now using a thoracoscopic approach (see below under Minimally invasive surgery for duplications). Proximal foregut duplications may be removed more easily through a supraclavicular cervical incision. The phrenic and vagus nerves and the thoracic duct should be carefully identified to avoid injury. Esophageal duplication cysts are excised by dissecting the duplication off the esophageal wall at the base; it is important to remove residual mucosa from the wall of the esophagus (illustrations b and c). If the esophagus is inadvertently entered, it can be repaired primarily and a pleural flap can be used to buttress the repair. If an esophageal stricture or ulcer was noted on preoperative esophagoscopy or swallow study, it may be necessary to perform a segmental resection of the esophagus.

Attempts should be taken to reapproximate the muscularis over the excised area, since weakness of the esophageal wall can occur if the submucosa is not contained.

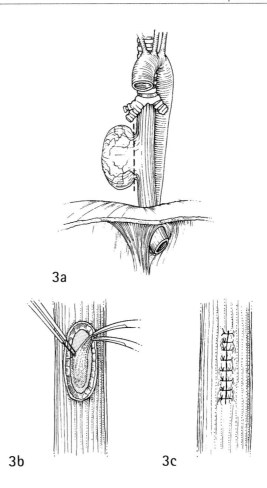

3a

3b   3c

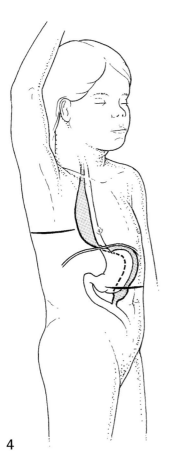

4

Thoracoabdominal duplications

4 Thoracoabdominal duplications are commonly located to the right of the esophagus in the posterior mediastinum. They may communicate with the stomach or small intestine through the diaphragm, and may also communicate with the spinal canal (neurenteric cysts). These lesions are best approached with a combination of thoracotomy/thoracoscopy and laparotomy/laparoscopy, or through a thoracoabdominal incision.

It is recommended to start with a posterolateral thoracotomy or thoracoscopy and to excise the intrathoracic component first. This involves dissecting the duplication off any attachments in the chest. Sometimes it is attached to the vertebrae and must be carefully dissected off the bone. If an intraspinal component is present and a laminectomy is necessary for complete removal, a neurosurgeon should be involved. After the duplication is free of any attachments in the chest, it is traced distally to the diaphragm, where it is divided between ligatures. Next, the resection is completed through a laparotomy or laparoscopy. The duplication is easier to identify below the diaphragm if the abdomen is opened prior to the completion of the dissection in the chest. That way pulling on the duplication will help identify its continuation in the abdomen. The diaphragmatic defect can usually be closed primarily. The abdominal part of the duplication is often a tubular lesion communicating with the small intestine, although it sometimes ends blindly along the greater curve of the stomach. Occasionally, thoracoabdominal duplications present with hemoptysis as peptic ulceration leads to erosion into the lung.

Gastric duplications

5 Duplications of the greater curvature can be treated by complete resection. As with esophageal duplications, most gastric duplications are contained within the stomach wall and can be resected without entering the gastric lumen. Laparoscopic or laparoscopic-assisted resection has been described.

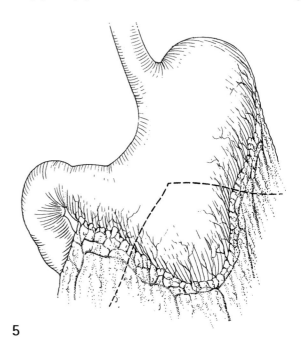

5

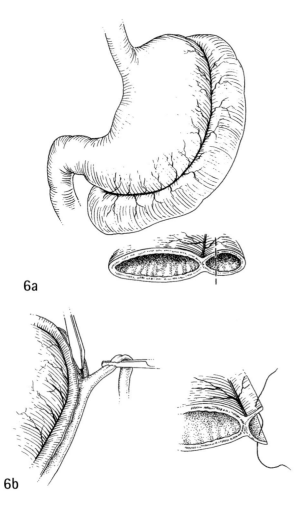

6a

6b

6a–c If the duplication cyst involves an extensive part of the stomach, partial resection and stripping of the residual mucosal lining is an alternative.

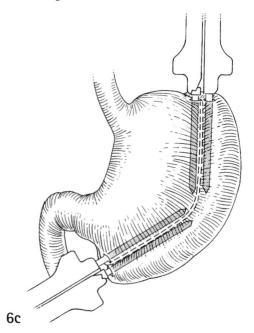

6c

Duodenal duplications

7 Duplications of the duodenum often present with vomiting and abdominal pain, but due to the close proximity to the biliary tree and pancreas, symptoms and findings related to these organs can be part of the initial presentation. Duodenal duplication cysts of the first, third, and fourth portion can usually be excised using a technique similar to that described for esophageal and gastric duplications. Duodenal duplications attached to the second portion of the duodenum should undergo preoperative and/or intraoperative radiographic visualization of the bile ducts and pancreatic ducts. If the biliary or pancreatic ducts are involved, complete excision will be difficult. Partial excision and mucosal stripping are an acceptable alternative in these cases. In some cases, a small bowel Roux-en-Y loop can be brought up and a cystenterostomy created, similar to what has been described for the treatment of pancreatic pseudocysts.

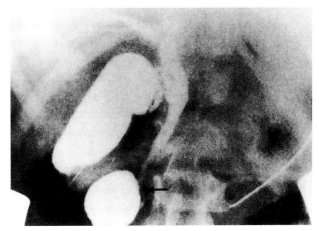

7

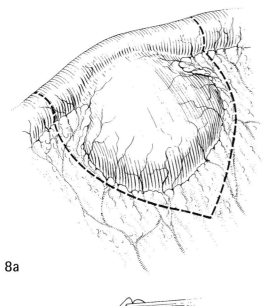

8a

Small intestinal duplications

8a–c Cystic lesions of the jejunum or ileum are the most common duplications and are usually excised without difficulty. Because cyst and normal bowel often share a common muscular wall and blood supply, they are usually resected as one specimen. This procedure can often be performed using laparoscopic techniques.

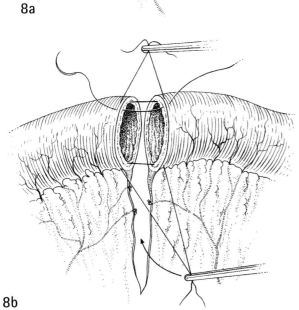

8b

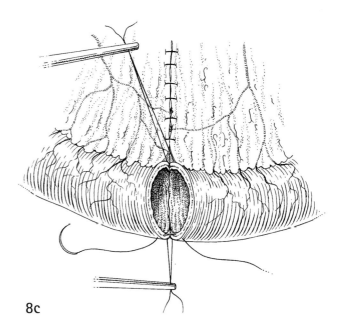

8c

9a–c Duplications that are separate from the intestine and located within the mesentery can be removed by careful separation of the two leaves of mesentery, division of the vessels on one side, and enucleation of the duplicated bowel.

Short tubular duplications can be excised in continuity with adjacent intestine, but care should be taken to obtain complete excision at the proximal and distal ends of the lesion, where the distinction between normal and duplicated bowel is difficult to detect. Very long tubular duplications, where the remaining intestinal length may be insufficient if completely excised, pose a greater surgical challenge. Treatment possibilities include the following:

- Submucosal resection, where the mucosal lining is stripped using multiple longitudinal seromuscular incisions.
- If a proximal communication exists, establish a distal communication by fenestration of the common wall to prevent a blind loop. In many cases, this will be the best option, as the shared blood supply makes resection very difficult.
- No surgical treatment and close follow up may be appropriate if the patient is asymptomatic and no communication exists between the cyst and the bowel.

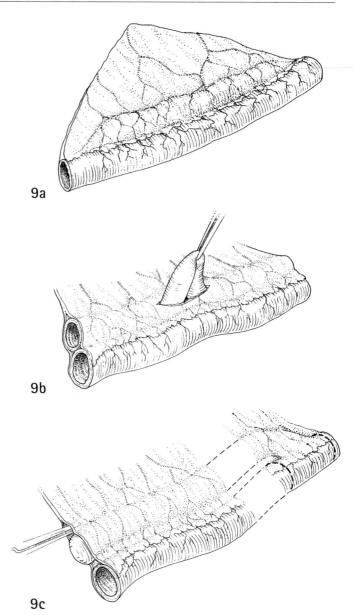

9a

9b

9c

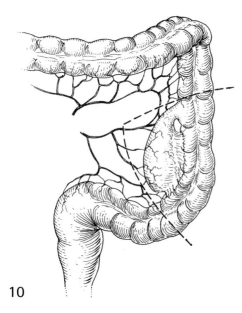

10

Colonic and appendiceal duplications

10 Cystic duplications and most short tubular duplications may be excised directly. The colon is then repaired with an end-to-end anastomosis.

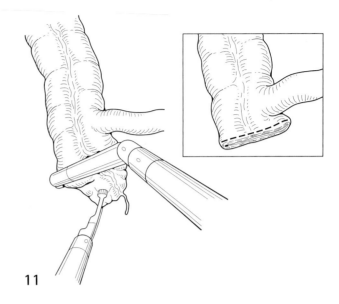

11 The operation can also be performed using a laparoscopic or laparoscopic-assisted technique (see below under Minimally invasive surgery for duplications).

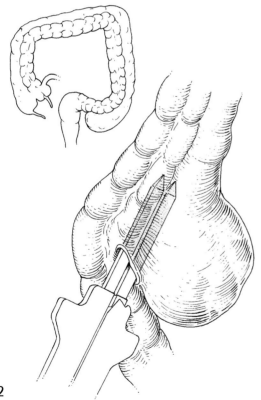

12 Total colonic duplications are long tubular duplications involving the entire colon. They are located on the antimesenteric border or medial to the normal colon and not in the mesentery. The duplication usually communicates proximally with the normal bowel. If the duplication also communicates distally and involves most of the colon and rectum, no treatment is necessary. If the tubular duplication does not communicate distally, a communication must be established, and if a small communication is present, this opening may need to be enlarged. Fenestration can be established by excising a piece of the common wall.

Rectal duplications

13 Rectal duplications are cystic and located in the retrorectal space. There is often a fistula to the anal canal or perineal region. The presentation may include constipation, rectal abscess, rectal bleeding, prolapse of the rectum, urinary tract infection, and hemorrhoids. If the cyst is infected, it should initially be drained and then later excised when the inflammation has resolved. Rectal duplication has been associated with a number of other anomalies, including spinal abnormalities, urethral duplication, and anorectal malformations. The abscess can be drained much like any pelvic abscess: transrectally, transgluteal, or transabdominal, depending on location.

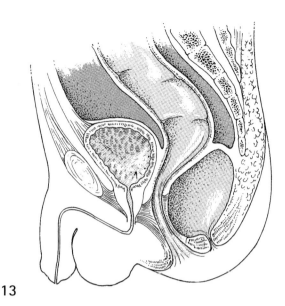

13

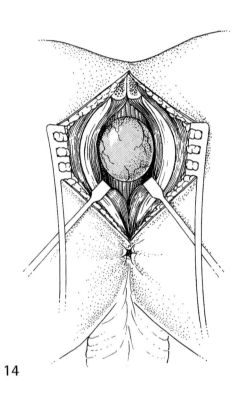

14

14 Treatment options include transanal or posterior sagittal exposure and excision, or transanal fenestration of the common wall if the cyst is large. Fenestration is a good alternative in cases where the cyst is infected or a fistula between the cyst and the rectum is already present. All patients should receive bowel preparation prior to the operation.

15 Small submucosal rectal lesions can be excised through a small incision in the mucosa over the cyst. To make the dissection easier, the cyst should preferably not be aspirated until the end. After excision, the mucosa is closed with absorbable sutures.

In most cases, rectal duplications can be safely excised without a defunctioning colostomy.

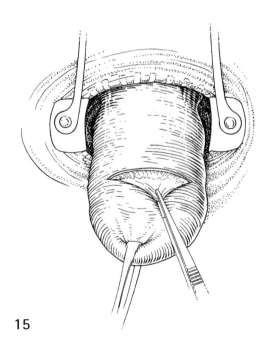

15

Minimally invasive surgery for duplications

THORACIC

Esophageal duplications are often amenable to thoracoscopic resection. Thoracoscopy minimizes postoperative pain, decreases hospital stay, and provides a better cosmetic result. Most commonly, the esophageal duplications are non-communicating, intramural, cystic lesions located on the right side of the esophagus. When deciding on an open versus thoracoscopic approach, it is important to rule out an extension to the spinal canal, which would necessitate an open approach.

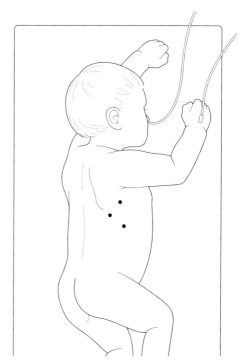

16 The child is positioned in a semi-prone position at approximately 30°; this gives the best access and exposure of the posterior mediastinum. The majority of esophageal duplications are approached through the right chest due to their location. It can be beneficial to use a bronchial blocker to minimize ventilation of the right lung.

16

The first port is placed in the mid-axillary line in the fourth or fifth intercostal space. The remaining two ports can be placed under direct visualization taking into consideration the location of the esophageal duplication. The middle port is placed in the posterior axillary line, while the lower port is placed in the anterior or mid-axillary line.

Esophagoscopy may be necessary to locate the lesion. A large oral-gastric tube or a Maloney dilator should be placed prior to starting the dissection to help with identifying the esophageal wall. Injury to the thoracic duct is a potential pitfall, especially if the duplication is located low in the chest.

The dissection of the lesion is performed with a combination of sharp dissection with hook cautery and gentle blunt dissection. The principles for the dissection are the same as for an open resection. If there is a weakness of the wall where the duplication was excised or if the esophagus was entered, this can be closed with several laparoscopic sutures. A chest tube is not necessary in most cases, but can be placed through the lower trocar site at the discretion of the surgeon.

ABDOMINAL

Most duplications in the abdomen can be approached using laparoscopic techniques or a laparoscopic-assisted approach. Initially, an umbilical port is placed. This is followed by the placement of two or three additional working ports, usually 3 or 5 mm. A 12-mm port is necessary if the endoscopic linear stapler is going to be used, and this port can also be used for removal of the specimen. If it is anticipated that a laparoscopic-assisted approach is necessary, one port site is placed over the location of the duplication so that it can be used as part of the open incision.

17 For resection of a small bowel duplication and primary anastomosis, it is often best to bring the duplication out through the umbilicus and perform an extracorporeal dissection and anastomosis. This often requires a short extension of the umbilical incision. Cystic small bowel duplications can be aspirated under direct visualization with a large gauge needle either transabdominally or at the umbilical incision prior to externalization. By aspirating the cyst the decrease in size will make it possible to use a smaller incision, often just confined to the umbilicus.

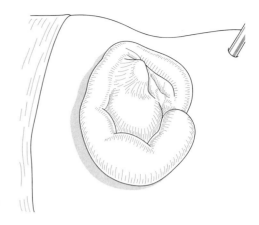

17

Retroperitoneal duplications and spinal involvement

Retroperitoneal duplications can be very large and difficult to remove. It is important to identify adjacent and involved structures to prevent inadvertent injury during the operation. The precise procedure and exposure are dictated by the location and symptoms of the duplication. Intradural and extradural spinal duplications should always be treated in collaboration with a neurosurgeon.

POSTOPERATIVE CARE

The patient should be monitored and followed up according to the extent of the procedure and the findings during the operation. Patients who are managed by incomplete excision or fenestration and have cyst tissue left behind should be followed closely, with repeat ultrasound examinations on a regular basis.

OUTCOME

Generally, patients with the most commonly found cystic duplications of the small and large intestine have an excellent outcome, with several series reporting no mortality or significant morbidity after surgical management. The same applies to short tubular gastric duplications and isolated rectal duplications. Patients who present with thoracoabdominal duplications, complete obstruction of the gastrointestinal tract, bleeding, perforation, and involvement of the mesenteric vessels often have a more difficult clinical course. Associated anomalies, when present, may have a significant impact on long-term outcome.

FURTHER READING

Azzie G, Beasley S. Diagnosis and treatment of foregut duplications. *Seminars in Pediatric Surgery* 2003; **12**: 46–54.

Diamond IR, Teckman J, Langer JC. Laparoscopy in the management of colonic duplications. *Pediatric Endosurgery and Innovative Techniques* 2003; **7**: 439–43.

Ladd WE, Gross RE. Surgical treatment of duplications of the alimentary tract: enterogenous cysts, enteric cysts, or ileum duplex. *Surgical Gynecology and Obstetrics* 1940; **70**: 295–307.

Norris RW, Brereton RJ, Wright VM, Cudmore RE. A new surgical approach to duplications of the intestine. *Journal of Pediatric Surgery* 1986; **21**: 167–70.

Stern LE, Warner BW. Gastrointestinal duplications. *Seminars in Pediatric Surgery* 2000; **9**: 135–40.

Stringer MD, Spitz L, Abel R *et al.* Management of alimentary tract duplications in children. *British Journal of Surgery* 1995; **82**: 74–8.

53

Intussusception

MELANIE HIORNS and JOE CURRY

INTRODUCTION

An intussusception is an invagination of one part of the intestine (the intussusceptum) into another part of the intestine (the intussuscipiens). It most commonly occurs in a proximal to distal direction. The most common area to be affected is the ileum intussuscepting into the cecum and ascending colon. The incidence is highest in infants between the ages of four and ten months, but it has also been reported in neonates and adults.

ETIOLOGY

The most common etiological factor in the so-called 'idiopathic group' is a preceding viral illness either of the upper respiratory tract or a gastroenteritis. The resulting viremia stimulates the gut-associated lymphoid tissue with enlargement and edema of Peyer's patches on the luminal surface of the distal small bowel. At the time of laparotomy, these enlarged Peyer's patches can be frequently found at the lead point of an intussusception along with marked lymphadenopathy in the mesentery. Between 2 and 12 percent of patients will have a pathological lead point. This most commonly is a Meckel's diverticulum but polyps, duplication cysts and solid tumors have also been described. A pathological lead point should always be suspected in a child who presents outside the normal range or who has multiple episodes. The condition is seen to occur more commonly in boys, unless there is a pathological lead point in which the incidence is equal.

CLINICAL PRESENTATION

Colicky abdominal pain with the infant characteristically 'drawing up the legs' is one of the first clinical signs of intussusception. The child will initially be well in between the spasms, but will later become pale and lethargic. As intestinal obstruction develops, the vomiting will become bilious. Bright red rectal bleeding mixed with mucus, the so-called 'red currant jelly stool' will be seen in a quarter of cases and more frequently if digital rectal examination is performed. A palpable mass is felt in the right upper quadrant or epigastrium along with a distinguishable feeling of emptiness in the right iliac fossa (Dance's sign). Tenderness with evidence of peritonism indicates ischemia or perforation of the intestine. Marked hemodynamic instability with depletion of the intravascular volume can be encountered in children with intussusception. Tachycardia and decreased capillary return should prompt vigorous resuscitation. The diagnosis of intussusception should always be borne in mind when dealing with a child with shock of unknown cause.

At the time of presentation, the findings on the plain abdominal x-ray are often variable and non-specific and may only be contributory in 50 percent of cases. The x-ray may have a normal appearance if the presentation is early, or may show a relative paucity of gas, possibly in the right iliac fossa. As time progresses, the features of small bowel obstruction with dilated gas-filled loops and the soft tissue mass of the intussusceptum may be seen (**Figure 53.1**). It is important to note that the possibility of intussusception is usually raised clinically, but the diagnosis is usually established radiologically, by ultrasound. Therefore if the diagnosis of intussusception is suspected, ultrasound is the first-line investigation.

ULTRASOUND IN THE DIAGNOSIS OF INTUSSUSCEPTION

Ultrasound is the technique of choice for establishing the presence of an intussusception and should be performed in all cases of suspected intussusception and especially those in which the clinical findings are equivocal. Ultrasound is highly accurate in the diagnosis of intussusception with a sensitivity of 98–100 percent and a specificity of 88–100 percent. The technique is universally available and does

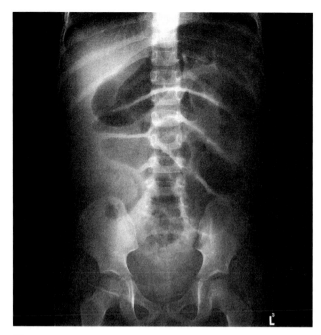

Figure 53.1 Plain abdominal x-ray of the abdomen of a child with intussusception showing small bowel obstruction with paucity of gas in the right iliac fossa.

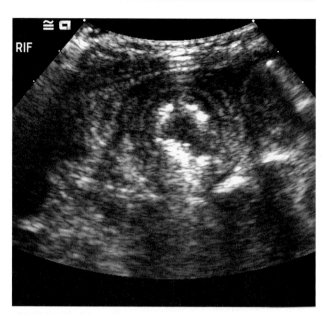

Figure 53.2 Ultrasound scan (transverse section) showing the typical 'target' sign of intussusception.

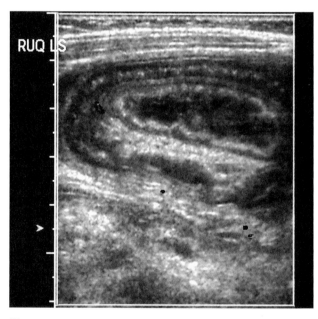

Figure 53.3 Ultrasound scan (longitudinal section) showing the oval-shaped intussusception ('pseudokidney') with echogenic mucosal walls.

not involve ionizing radiation. False-negative studies are rare, even for less experienced operators, and therefore the absence of intussusception on ultrasound should generally exclude the diagnosis. Ultrasound may also be able to give information on alternative diagnoses.

Ultrasound is performed with the child supine. The characteristic appearance of an intussusception is a series of concentric rings on the transverse view and of oval multilayered mass on the longitudinal view and (**Figures 53.2 and 53.3**) the layers representing the invaginated layers of the bowel wall and edematous mucosa. The most common site for an intussusception to be demonstrated is in the right hypochondrium, but the intussusception may extend as far down as the rectum. Ultrasound may not always be able to demonstrate the full extent of the intussusception as gas-filled loops of small bowel may exclude visualization in the mid-abdomen and the pelvis.

Color Doppler can be used to assess the vascularity of the intussusception. If no color flow is seen, the intussusception may be of longer duration and may be harder to reduce non-surgically, but the absence of color flow does not necessarily imply that the intussusception is avascular or necrotic and, all other factors being satisfactory, the patient should still have attempted radiological reduction. Fluid seen between the intussuscipiens and the intussusceptum, so-called 'interloop fluid' (**Figure 53.4**), is associated with increased failure of pneumatic reduction. Lymph nodes are a common finding on ultrasound and are usually a reflection of the underlying inflammatory process but may represent the lead point, especially if associated with mucosal thickening.

Ultrasound is also useful for assessing the presence and extent of free intraperitoneal fluid. Small amounts of fluid

are commonly seen on ultrasound, but larger amounts of fluid may indicate bowel perforation and if this is a clinical concern then a plain x-ray may be helpful.

NON-OPERATIVE MANAGEMENT

Once the diagnosis of intussusception has been confirmed, and after liaison between the surgeon and the radiologist, the patient would normally proceed to radiological reduction.

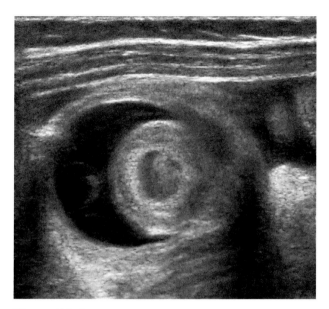

Figure 53.4 Fluid seen between the intussuscipiens and the intussusceptum.

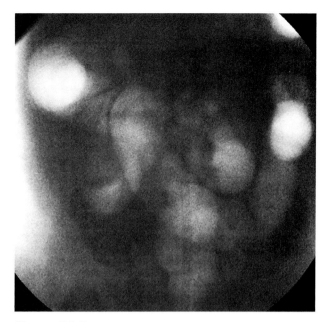

Figure 53.5 Appearance of colon during pneumatic reduction. The intussuscipiens can be seen as a filling defect on the left side of the image. Air fills the more distal colon.

Radiological reduction of intussusception

Once the diagnosis of intussusception has been confirmed on ultrasound, radiological reduction will be attempted, provided the patient is adequately resuscitated and there are no contraindications, such as free intraperitoneal air or signs of peritonism. A history longer than 24 hours or absent color flow on Doppler are not considered contraindications but may indicate that reduction may be more difficult and should be undertaken with caution, and there is no doubt that air enema reduction is more successful with a history of less than 24 hours. Radiological reduction should only be attempted in centers also offering pediatric surgery in case of complication or unsuccessful reduction.

Radiological reduction is performed using air under fluoroscopic guidance. It is also possible to use water or air under ultrasound guidance. Fluoroscopy allows visualization of the whole abdomen and therefore early detection of perforation, but uses ionizing radiation. Ultrasound uses no radiation, but can only follow the head of the intussusceptum. Hydrostatic reduction using barium or water-soluble contrast media is generally no longer used as air reduction has been shown to be safer, has a higher reduction rate and gives a lower patient radiation dose.

Before any radiological reduction, the patient must have good intravenous access and be fully resuscitated. A nasogastric tube should be passed and prophylactic antibiotics administered. Analgesia can be given at the surgeon's discretion.

When using air reduction a catheter or feeding tube is placed in the patient's rectum, the anus is occluded either by strapping the buttocks tightly together with tape or by the radiologist gripping the patient's buttocks together between the fingers. Some devices are becoming

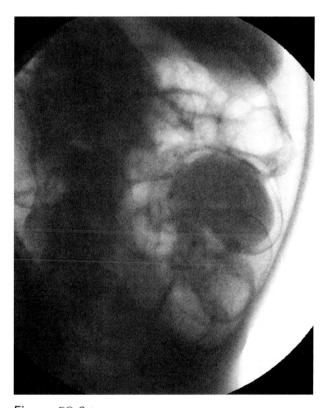

Figure 53.6 Pneumoperitoneum occurring during attempted reduction. Free air is seen over the right side of the image.

available to occlude the anus, but the value of these is not yet proven. The catheter is connected to a device or system which can deliver air at consistent pressure which can be set by the operator. The system must include a safety device to prevent the pressure unexpectedly exceeding that set by the operator. The child may be supine or prone, but it is easier to observe the child if he is supine. A control image is obtained and then air is slowly introduced into the large bowel until the first set pressure is reached, typically 80 mmHg equivalent (**Figure 53.5**). This slow start allows visualization of the head of the intussusceptum and prevents it being missed if reduction is very rapid. Multiple attempts will then be made to reduce the intussusception, usually for 3 minutes, each for three times at three increasing pressures: 80, 100, and 120 mmHg. This will be monitored very closely under fluoroscopic guidance so that if perforation does occur it is immediately detected (**Figure 53.6**) and the procedure can be stopped immediately before a pneumoperitoneum causes splinting of the diaphragm and respiratory arrest, or increased vasovagal stimulation causes a cardiac arrest. The procedure is also terminated if air is seen to track along the sides of the intussusceptum, the 'air dissection' sign, as this implies attempted reduction will be unsuccessful (**Figure 53.7**).

Reduction is achieved when air flows freely into the small bowel (**Figure 53.8**).

The procedure is often distressing for the child and its parents if they are present in the room. However, only a few centers in the UK give sedation as there is some evidence that when the child cries and performs a Valsalva maneuver the brief rise in intra-abdominal pressure assists the reduction while the Valsalva maneuver may provide a protective effect against perforation because external abdominal pressure decreases the transmural gradient. More importantly, if there is a sudden deterioration in the child's clinical condition, this is more likely to be detected in an unsedated child.

If the intussusception is reduced as far as the ileocecal valve but not through it (**Figure 53.9**), it is now considered worthwhile to allow the child to settle for a few hours as edema at the ileocecal valve may settle and a further radiological attempt at reduction can be made to avoid

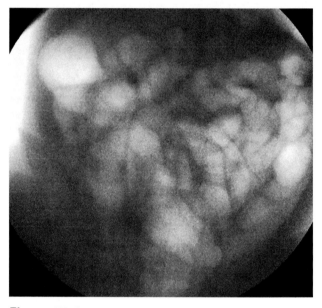

Figure 53.8 Filling of small bowel with air, indicating successful reduction.

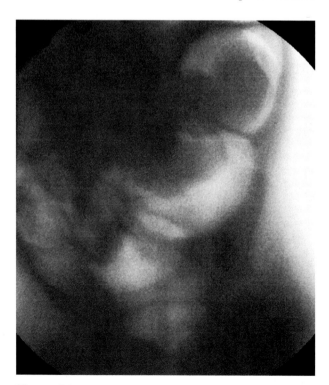

Figure 53.7 Air dissection along the side of the intussusception.

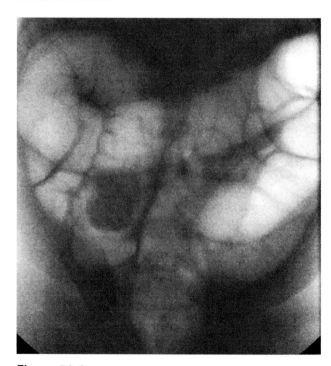

Figure 53.9 Persistence of intussusception at the ileocecal valve.

the need for surgery. A second attempt may be made at 4 to 6 hours if the patient is stable and the surgeon and radiologist agree, and if the intussusception has been partially reduced on the first attempt. Reported rates of 50–82 percent improved reduction suggest this may be an important technique in previously failed air enema reductions.

Success rates vary between institutions, but current guidelines suggest that a success rate of at least 70 percent should be achieved. Perforation rates are typically 1–2 percent and the consenting parents should be warned that this would necessitate immediate surgical intervention. A significant pneumoperitoneum requires immediate decompression by the radiologist, usually by the placing of an 18-G needle into the abdomen. Perforation with air reduction does not result in widespread contamination of the peritoneal cavity as the large bowel is usually empty of stool as a result of the preceding diarrhea and also because air escapes and rises to the top of the abdomen rather than washing contaminated contents around within the abdomen as fluids would do. Perforation is most likely secondary to bowel necrosis and not excessive pressures.

The principles outlined above also pertain to ultrasound-guided reduction. A tube is passed per rectum and a good seal is obtained at the anus. Water is introduced via the tube connected to a reservoir which is then raised above the patient. To generate a pressure equivalent to 120 mmHg, the reservoir must be 150 cm above the patient. The intussusceptum already identified is then followed on ultrasound as it passes back along the colon. Reduction is complete when fluid is seen to pass retrogradely into the small bowel. Ultrasound reduction can be technically difficult for the operator if there is marked small bowel obstruction, with distended gas-filled loops, as air does not allow the passage of ultrasound and the image may be difficult to obtain. Nevertheless, not needing to use ionizing radiation is a considerable advantage. Recent studies have demonstrated the possibility of using air reduction under ultrasound guidance with some success, but it is too early to know whether either of these ultrasound techniques will become the standard practice.

OPERATIVE REDUCTION

Indications for operative reduction include:

- initial evidence of peritonism or perforation;
- perforation during radiological reduction;
- failure of radiological reduction;
- third time presentation (presentation well beyond the usual age range).

PREOPERATIVE PREPARATION

Arrangements should be in place for emergency surgery in all infants undergoing attempted radiological reduction to minimize delay.

Fluid resuscitation should continue and the infant's hemodynamic status be regularly assessed. Broad-spectrum antibiotics should be administered if not previously given prior to attempts at radiological reduction and a nasogastric tube is passed.

Informed consent is obtained and should include the possibility of bowel resection especially the terminal ileum.

Anesthesia

General anesthesia with endotracheal intubation and muscle paralysis is used.

OPERATION

Incision

1 A right transverse skin incision is made either above or below the level of the umbilicus depending on the presence of a mass or radiological indication of the site of the intussusception. The lateral abdominal muscles, rectus sheath, and rectus muscle are divided to provide adequate and safe exposure. A sample of the peritoneal fluid is sent for microbiological analysis.

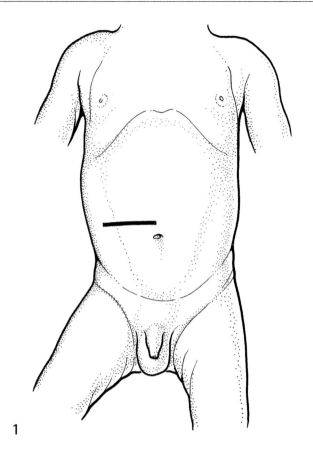

1

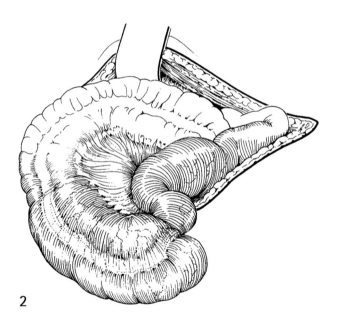

2

Reduction of intussusception

2 The affected bowel is delivered from the abdominal cavity to facilitate reduction. This often involves division of the peritoneal attachment of the right colon and cecum using sharp dissection.

3 Once the affected segment has been delivered, all other parts of the intestine are returned to the abdomen. Reduction is achieved by gently applying pressure on the apex of the distal part of the intussusception. Grip on the intestine can be facilitated by the use of a gauze swab. Traction on the proximal intestine should be avoided but a gentle pull may establish the direction in which to apply the reducing squeeze.

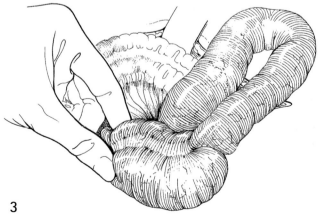

3

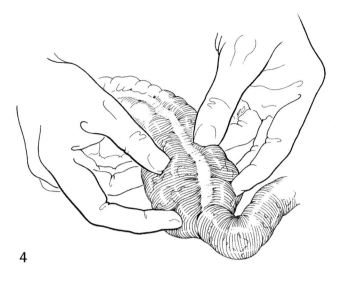

4

4 Reduction of ileum through the ileocecal valve requires patience. Forefingers and thumbs are used to apply gentle squeeze to the apex of the intussusception while pulling back the cecal wall. The gut should be palpated to rule out a pathological lead point bearing in mind that an edematous ileocecal valve or Peyer's patch can mimic an intraluminal mass. Careful palpation and knowledge of the likely etiology, particularly in the young infant, should prevent unnecessary resection.

Resection

5a–c Resection will be necessary if the intussusception cannot be reduced; there is necrotic or compromised bowel after reduction; there is a pathological lead point.

The intussusception should be reduced as far as possible to minimize the extent of any resection. Resection is usually segmental and rarely extends to formal right hemi-colectomy.

If the intussusception is extensive, i.e. beyond the splenic flexure, then consideration should be given to examining the duodenojejunal flexure for coexistent malrotation. If present, a formal Ladd's procedure should be performed.

In the presence of a transverse incision below the level of the umbilicus, it is acceptable to perform an incidental appendicectomy provided the adjacent cecal wall is normal.

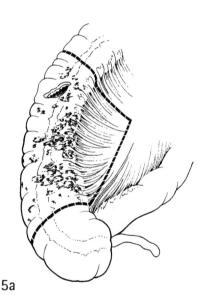

5a

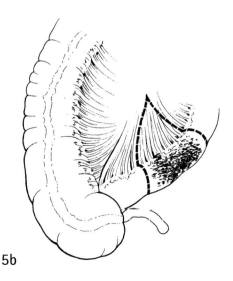

5b

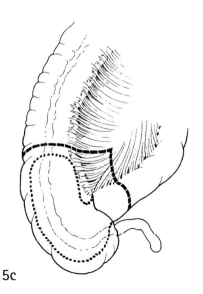

5c

Anastomosis

6 Suction of the proximal and distal bowel avoids the need for bowel clamps. Primary anastomosis is almost always possible and is performed with a single layer of interrupted extramucosal sutures. Knots are placed on the serosal surface. The choice of suture material will depend on the surgeon's preference. Any mesenteric defect is closed in a similar fashion. The need for expeditious surgery in a very sick infant, along with doubt about the viability of the resection margins, may require the formation of adjacent stomas. Closure is performed when the infant's condition has improved and the stomas are healthy.

It may be possible to oversew a perforation using interrupted extramucosal sutures provided the edges are clean and viable.

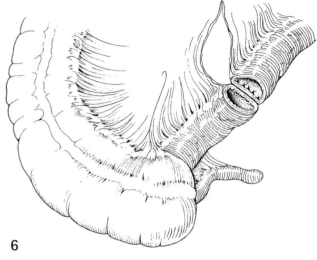

6

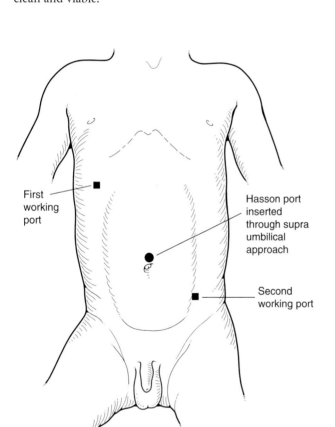

First working port

Hasson port inserted through supra umbilical approach

Second working port

7

Laparoscopic reduction

7 The techniques of minimally invasive surgery are currently being applied to infants with intussusception. Potential advantages are the ability to diagnose full reduction when this is unclear after pneumatic reduction thus avoiding full laparotomy or cases of recurrence. Reduction is more problematic, often due to the resulting small bowel dilatation, but if achievable, avoids the trauma of open access and significantly reduces the risk of intraperitoneal adhesions. Irreducible intussusceptions can be externalized through extension of the umbilical port or through a small and accurately placed incision.

Pneumoperitoneum is raised according to surgical preference (see **Chapter 41**). Access ports are inserted in the right upper quadrant and left lower quadrant, at right angles to the small bowel mesentery.

Attention is initially focused in the right iliac fossa. The small bowel and colon is examined to find the area of intussusception. Reduction is effected by a combination of taxis and traction using atraumatic graspers. Careful visualization of the bowel is necessary to avoid rupture and intraperitoneal contamination. In the case of successful reduction, the appendix should be left *in situ* as there is no scar in the right iliac fossa.

The lack of tactile clues to a pathological lead point should be remembered and consideration given to delivering the small bowel through the umbilical port after successful reduction in older children.

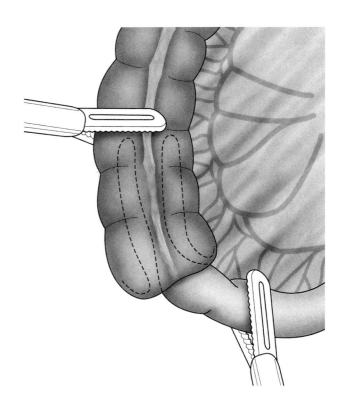

Figure 53.10 Laparoscopic atraumatic graspers applying taxis and traction to the bowel to reduce the intussusception

POSTOPERATIVE CARE

Appropriate intravenous fluids are continued postoperatively. Nasogastric decompression is continued until the volume decreases indicating the return of intestinal function. Oral fluids are commenced within 24 hours, but in the presence of resection may be delayed a further 24 hours. Continued antibiotic therapy is dictated by surgeon's preference and the presence of peritoneal contamination at the time of laparotomy.

A high temperature is common in the first 24–48 hours postoperatively and usually subsides without specific treatment.

OUTCOME

Recurrences following pneumatic reduction are reported in up to 8 percent of cases. Further radiological reduction should be attempted, but a third should raise the possibility of a pathological lead point.

Deaths from intussusception have been reported and relate to failure to make the diagnosis and inadequate resuscitation.

Excision of the ileocecal valve may rarely predispose to anemia secondary to depletion of vitamin B12 or the development of gallstones from loss of bile salts.

FURTHER READING

Applegate KE. Intussusception in children: evidence-based diagnosis and treatment. *Pediatric Radiology* 2009; **39** (Suppl. 2): S140–3.

del-Pozo G, Albillos JC, Tejedor D *et al*. Intussusception in children: current concepts in diagnosis and enema reduction. *Radiographics* 1999; **19**: 299–319.

Gartner RD, Levin TL, Borenstein SH *et al*. Interloop fluid in intussusception: what is its significance? *Pediatric Radiology* 2011; **41**: 727–31.

Kaiser AD, Applegate KE, Ladd AP. Current success in the treatment of intussusception in children. *Surgery* 2007; **142**: 469–75.

Ong NT, Beasley SW. The leadpoint in intussusception. *Journal of Pediatric Surgery* 1990; **25**: 640–3.

van der Laan M, Bax NM, van der Zee DC *et al*. The role of laparoscopy in the management of childhood intussusception. *Surgical Endoscopy* 2001; **15**: 373 6.

54

Appendectomy: open and laparoscopic procedures

RISTO J RINTALA and MIKKO P PAKARINEN

HISTORY

Medical descriptions of right lower quadrant peritonitis, perityphlitis, appeared more than 500 years ago. Inflammation of the appendix was conclusively demonstrated to cause this condition by Reginald Fitz in 1886. The first published report on appendectomy is attributed to Claudius Amyand from England who, in 1736, removed an inflamed perforated and fistulizing appendix from the scrotum of an 11-year-old boy. The first deliberate appendectomy for perforated appendix was performed by Morton in 1887.

In earlier centuries, appendicitis was frequently a fatal disease. The development of modern surgical care and antibiotic therapies has made this most common abdominal surgical emergency a much more benign condition. However, in the pediatric population, appendicitis continues to be associated with significant morbidity and occasional mortality. The overall lifetime risk of appendicitis is between 5 and 10 percent.

PRINCIPLES AND JUSTIFICATION

Indications

Prompt appendectomy is the generally recommended treatment of appendicitis. The indications are the same for open and laparoscopic procedure. Although operation without delay has been the gold standard, there is a trend away from immediate surgery, especially during the night. No increased incidence of complications or perforations has been reported between patients who have been operated within 6 hours or 6–18 hours after admission.

Early surgery has been advocated especially for young children because of higher risk of perforation before surgery.

Appendectomy is also the generally accepted treatment of perforated appendicitis. However, there is significant controversy regarding the treatment of a palpable appendix mass. Some surgeons advocate immediate appendectomy, others favor initial conservative therapy with intravenous antibiotics and interval appendectomy two to three months later. Interval appendectomy may be performed either by open or laparoscopic technique.

Appendectomy is also recommended for small (<2 cm) carcinoid tumors at the tip of the appendix, other benign conditions of the appendix, and as part of Ladd's procedure for midgut malrotation. Incidental removal of a normal appendix is a controversial issue, but may be beneficial in children taking into account the relatively high lifetime risk of appendicitis. Incidental appendectomy should not be performed in patients that may need the appendix for construction of continent stoma for the bladder or cecum.

Contraindications

Serious acute medical conditions causing appendicitis-like symptoms should be ruled out by clinical examination, laboratory tests, and imaging. These include right basal pneumonia, meningitis, urinary tract infections, Henoch–Schöenlein purpura, and acute diabetes. Every effort should be made to confirm the diagnosis of appendicitis before surgery. The formerly accepted rates of negative explorations (20–40 percent) are not supported by recent literature. Repeated clinical examinations and modern imaging techniques should reduce the negative appendectomy rates below 10 percent.

Appendix mass has been considered as a contraindication for laparoscopic surgery. Recent data, however, do not support this; laparoscopic early surgery for appendix mass is at least as safe as open surgery.

If ileocecal Crohn's disease is found to cause the symptoms of appendicitis, the appendix should not be excised because there is a significant risk of subsequent fistula formation.

A normal appendix should not be removed if prosthetic materials used or ventriculoperitoneal shunts are encountered during the operation.

PREOPERATIVE

The approach to the diagnosis of acute appendicitis in this era of sophisticated preoperative imaging still relies on a typical history that progresses to localized somatic findings in the right lower quadrant. In many instances, no further testing is required. Laboratory studies are unhelpful in arriving at a definitive diagnosis. Most patients have an elevated leukocyte count with left-shifted neutrophil count. Elevated C-reactive protein (CRP) values are helpful for the diagnosis but do not occur in the early phases of the disease.

When the diagnosis is questionable, ultrasonography is useful, not only to visualize an inflamed appendix, but also to exclude other abdominal and pelvic conditions, especially in teenage girls.

Plain abdominal radiography has a very low sensitivity and specificity in the diagnosis of appendicitis. Computed tomography has been shown to be better than ultrasonography. However, the radiation dose remains a significant concern, therefore, ionizing radiation studies should be used only if the diagnosis is unclear.

Children with appendicitis are evaluated for degree of sepsis and dehydration. Most will have vomited or not eaten for more than 24 hours. For this reason alone, intravenous isotonic fluid resuscitation before operation is mandatory for all patients with appendicitis. Superimposed sepsis will require closer attention to volume support before operation.

Infectious complications are best prevented and treated in all patients by using perioperative antibiotics. The regime is designed to control aerobes and anaerobes of the lower gastrointestinal tract and typically comprises second- or third-generation cephalosporins and metronidazol.

The most efficient way to control preoperative pain is immediate appendectomy, but if delayed, intravenous narcotics are acceptable. Nasogastric and bladder decompression prior to operation facilitate a laparoscopic procedure.

Psychological preparation of the child and family is essential for a successful procedure. For many patients, this is their first introduction to the hospital and surgery. The child and the family are informed of what to expect during the hospital stay, as well as of the resources available to them.

Informed consent includes the location of the incision, the expected postoperative course, the negative appendectomy rate, the possibility of drains, infectious, and hemorrhagic complications, and the remote chance of a stoma.

Anesthesia

Apart from pain control, premedication is generally unnecessary. A general anesthetic with muscle relaxation provides the best environment for surgical exposure.

OPERATION

Open appendectomy

1 The skin incision for appendicitis is a transverse or slightly oblique right lower quadrant skin crease approach that allows for extension medially or laterally. The incision is placed just above and slightly medial to the anterior superior iliac spine. The incision courses medially through or below McBurney's point. Lateral extension of the incision is possible to the flank, while medial enlargement crosses the rectus sheath. In a slender child, the appendix can be removed safely through a 3–4 cm skin incision. As a general rule, a higher and longer incision will provide more room for exploration and satisfactory and faster dissection, but a more prolonged and painful hospital stay.

The subcutaneous tissues above the external oblique aponeurosis are dissected sharply by using monopolar electrocautery.

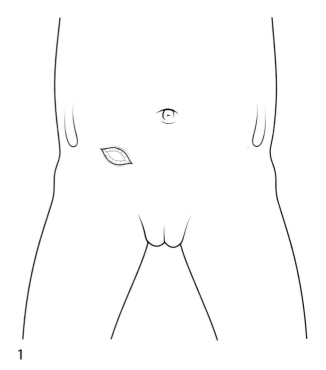

1

2 Following sharp dissection, the external oblique muscle is split along the direction of the fibers. A liberal split of the external oblique muscle will provide adequate operative exposure.

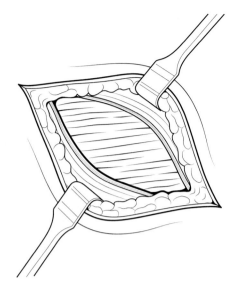

2

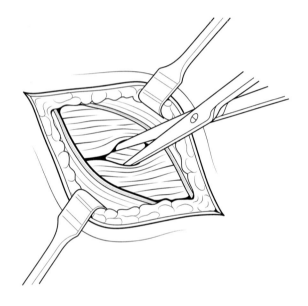

3

3 The internal oblique and transverse muscles are split in the direction of their fibers using blunt-tipped scissors or the fingers of the operating surgeon. Generally, both muscle layers are split in tandem, as the transverse muscle is nearly parallel with the internal oblique muscle. The aponeurosis of the transverse muscle occurs more laterally, and the fibers may run more obliquely from lower right to upper left than those of the internal oblique.

4 The peritoneum is grasped after blunt dissection of the transversalis fascia and preperitoneal fat. Edema from appendiceal inflammation may obscure the peritoneum laterally; it is best identified medially. On opening the peritoneum with a scalpel or monopolar cautery, free fluid is suctioned and may be sent for culture. The peritoneal opening is enlarged with cautery or scissors.

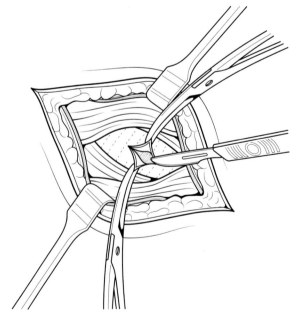

4

5 The key to successful exposure of the appendix is delivery of the cecum into the wound. The anterior tenia coli is grasped and the cecum delivered first pulling it down then up. If the cecum cannot be delivered easily, lateral peritoneal attachments may require dissection under direct vision using cautery.

An appendiceal mass is almost always bound down laterally and inferiorly. Medial attachments are usually to the terminal ileum and its mesentery. In most cases, a large appendix mass cannot be delivered through the wound. However, the appendix itself can usually be mobilized by blunt dissection to enable removal and safe ligation of the appendix base.

A difficult dissection becomes easier with wound extension. The muscle-splitting incision can be extended medially across the anterior and posterior rectus sheaths using cautery.

The rectus muscle is retracted and the inferior epigastric vessels are cauterized or ligated if required. Lateral incision enlargement may be helpful if further dissection is required in the flank.

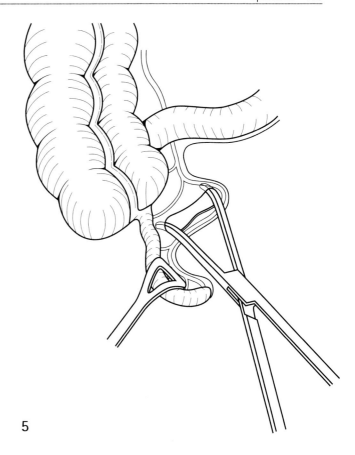

5

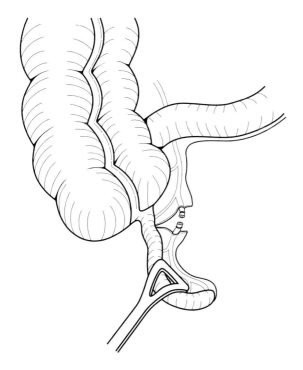

6

6 The inflamed appendix and any overlying omentum should not be allowed to touch the wound once delivered. Attached omentum is divided by cautery or between ties, and the mesoappendix is gently grasped with Babcock forceps. With traction on the Babcock forceps, the appendix is easily controlled and any further lateral attachments divided with cautery. The mesoappendix is then divided by cautery or between hemostats and ligatures. The mesenteric division should continue to the fold of Treves. Any residual small vessels may be controlled by cautery.

7a–c The base of the appendix is crushed 5 mm above its origin and the clamp is drawn distally a few more millimeters. The area crushed is then tied with an absorbable suture and the appendix removed by sharp division just proximal to the clamp. The mucosa of the remaining stump may be cauterized.

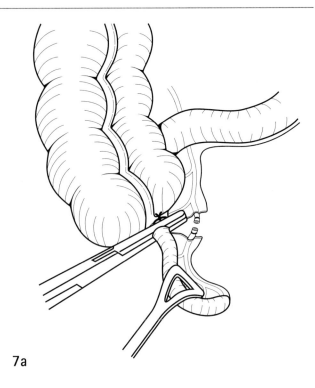

7a

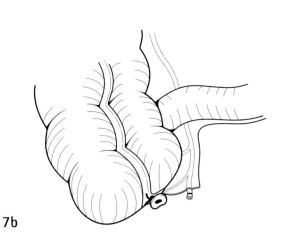

7b

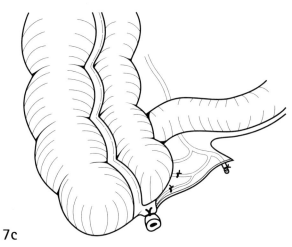

7c

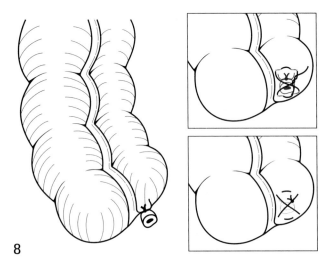

8

8 Stump inversion is not necessary but, if performed, an absorbable Z-stitch or purse-string suture is placed through the seromuscular base of the cecum. If the stump is inverted with the help of a hemostat or forceps, it is traditionally removed from the operating field. Rarely, the base of the appendix is so severely and widely inflamed that it cannot be safely ligated. In these cases, the whole inflamed base should be inverted by separate stitches that are taken through the healthy cecal wall.

Before replacing the cecum, the operative field and mesoappendix are inspected for hemostasis. The distended cecum may prove difficult to return to the abdomen. Gentle emptying of the cecum by milking with finger compression usually deflates the bowel to enable its safe repositioning within the abdomen.

The pelvis and right paracolic spaces are suctioned. In simple appendicitis, wound irrigation is not required. In perforated appendicitis, samples for bacterial culture are obtained and the operative field is irrigated to evacuate all visible pus, but separate wound drainage is not necessary.

The wound is closed in layers with absorbable sutures after irrigation of each consecutive layer. The perito-neum is run, and the internal oblique and transverse muscles are closed at the same time by apposition of the internal oblique epimysium using interrupted, absorbable sutures. The external oblique aponeurosis is closed with a running suture. Even when there has been perforation and gross contamination, the skin is usually closed with an absorbable, running, subcuticu-lar suture.

If a normal appendix is found, most surgeons would remove the appendix. Before this, the peritoneal cavity is formally explored for other conditions, such as Crohn's disease, Meckel's diverticulitis, mesenteric lymphadenitis, and gynecological conditions in adolescent females.

Laparoscopic appendectomy

9 The surgeon stands on the left side of the patient and a first assistant on the right with personal screens on the opposite sides. A short, 10–15 mm, semicircular incision is made to the upper edge of the umbilicus. The fascia is exposed and incised transversely. A 5- or 12-mm port for a laparoscopic camera is introduced under visual control. The abdomen is insufflated with carbon dioxide using up to 10–12 mmHg intra-abdominal pressure.

In addition to the umbilical camera port, two 5-mm working ports are introduced under laparoscopic visual control. One is placed to the right upper quadrant at or above the level of the umbilicus below the liver edge in order to provide enough working space and the other to the left lower quadrant to the level of the iliac spine.

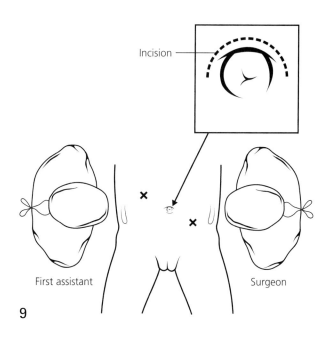

Incision

First assistant

Surgeon

9

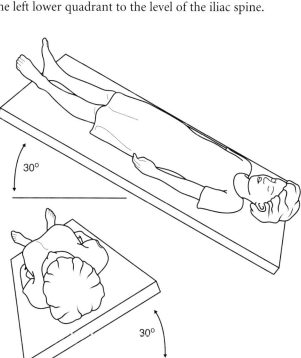

30°

30°

10

10 After the laparoscopic ports have been introduced, the patient is turned to a generous Trendelenburg position and rotated to the left for optimal laparoscopic exposure of the appendix.

11 The distal mesentery of the appendix is grasped by Maryland or Babcock forceps to expose the base of the appendix. In a case of an uninflamed appendix, the entire abdominal cavity is carefully assessed including the entire length of the small intestine from the ileocecal valve to the ligament of Treitz and ovaries in girls.

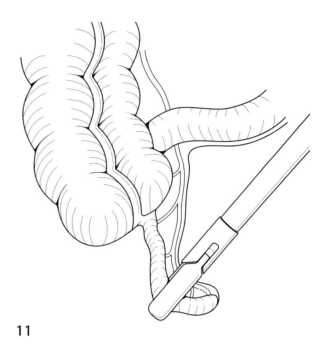

11

12a,b When needed, the appendix is mobilized by dividing inflammatory adhesions to the surrounding structures, such as the omentum or a loop of small bowel. Adhesions are divided with a diathermy hook or using blunt dissection by providing simultaneous counter-traction with forceps in another hand. In case of a retrocecal appendix, the cecum is mobilized first according to the same principles. The mesentery with its vessels are divided at the level of the base of the appendix using a diathermy hook.

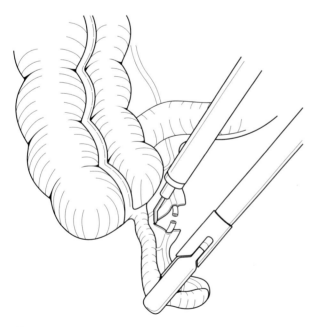

12a

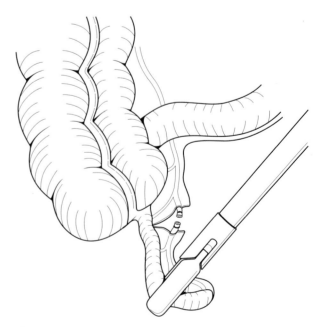

12b

13a,b Before division, the base of the appendix is ligated with a laparoscopic pre-tied loop suture. The appendix is grasped distal to a tightened loop suture and cut between them with scissors in order to avoid intra-abdominal spilling.

Rarely, when the entire appendix including the very base is necrotic, it is safer to use an endoscopic cutting stapler device by including the healthier tip of the cecum to the stapler line. Inversion of the appendiceal stump is not usually necessary.

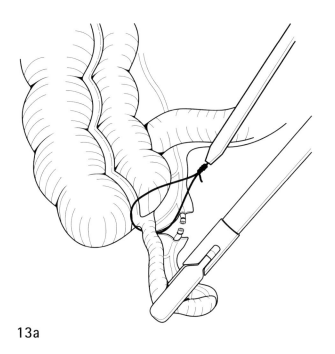

13a

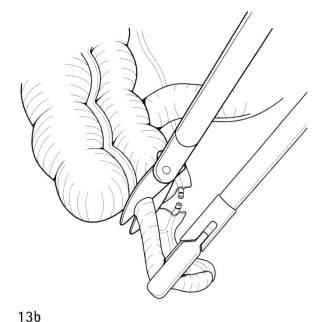

13b

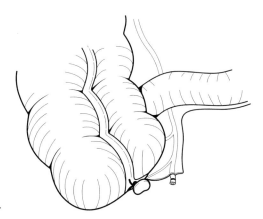

14

14 An inflamed appendix may be removed through a trocar or using a laparoscopic bag avoiding direct contact with port incisions. Visible pus is removed with a combination of irrigation and suction. The operative field is checked for hemostasis, the abdomen is desufflated and trocars are removed. Only the umbilical incision is closed with fascial sutures. The skin incisions are closed with intracutaneous sutures.

POSTOPERATIVE CARE

Nasogastric decompression is indicated only in cases with extensive intra-abdominal contamination or obvious associated small intestinal obstruction due to appendicitis. The need for abdominal drainage is exceptional. In non-perforated cases, the patients are allowed to resume oral intake once recovered from the anesthesia and the intravenous antibiotics are discontinued after three doses. Patients with uncomplicated appendicectomy are usually discharged within 2 days after both open and laparoscopic procedures. Following perforated appendicitis, intravenous antibiotics are switched to oral ones when the temperature has normalized and/or CRP concentration is clearly decreasing. Oral antibiotics are continued until CRP has normalized. Oral food intake is restarted along with resolution of intestinal paralysis and gradual reduction of intravenous fluid and energy replacement. Anti-inflammatory analgesics are usually sufficient for postoperative pain medication.

COMPLICATIONS

Generally, complications are more common after complicated appendicitis and include wound infection, intra-abdominal abscess formation, hemorrhage, intestinal obstruction, and prolonged paralytic ileus. Nowadays, stump leak is practically a non-existent problem. Wound infection is by far the most common complication with rates of less than 5 percent including complicated cases.

It heals almost invariably with local drainage and wound care. Frequency of postoperative intra-abdominal abscess formation is around 2 percent. Treatment includes systemic antimicrobial therapy with or without percutaneous computed tomography (CT)-guided drainage. Intestinal obstruction following appendicectomy occurs in less than 1 percent of patients with complicated appendicitis, which may necessitate early reoperation and adhesiolysis especially among preschool-aged children.

FURTHER READING

Berry J Jr, Malt RA. Appendicitis near its centenary. *Annals of Surgery* 1984; **200**: 567–75.

Bundy DG, Byerley JS, Liles EA *et al.* Does this child have appendicitis? *Journal of the American Medical Association* 2007; **298**: 438–51.

Morrow SE, Newman KD. Current management of appendicitis. *Seminars in Pediatric Surgery* 2007; **16**: 34–40.

Muehlstedt SG, Pham TQ, Schmeling DJ. The management of pediatric appendicitis: a survey of North American pediatric surgeons. *Journal of Pediatric Surgery* 2004; **39**: 875–9.

Puig S, Staudenherz A, Felder-Puig R, Paya K. Imaging of appendicitis in children and adolescents: useful or useless? A comparison of imaging techniques and a critical review of the current literature. *Seminars in Roentgenology* 2008; **43**: 22–8.

55

Necrotizing enterocolitis

NIGEL J HALL and AGOSTINO PIERRO

HISTORY

Necrotizing enterocolitis (NEC) is a devastating disease of infancy and the most common serious acquired gastrointestinal disease in the newborn infant. The term 'necrotizing enterocolitis' was first coined in the 1950s when used to describe infants who died with necrotic lesions of the gastrointestinal tract, but it did not become recognized as a distinct clinical entity until the 1960s, when a number of authors began reporting their experience with this disease. With improvements in neonatal intensive care over the past four decades, the incidence of NEC is increasing as more babies born at the extreme limits of prematurity now survive. Recent estimates place the incidence at approximately 0.5 percent of all live births and at between 3 and 5 percent of low birth weight infants born prematurely. Concurrent with this increase in incidence has been an extensive amount of time and energy devoted to exploring the etiology and pathogenesis of this disease by a number of individuals and groups worldwide. Despite these efforts, our understanding of the processes contributing to the development of NEC remains limited.

PRINCIPLES AND JUSTIFICATION

Necrotizing enterocolitis represents a disease state comprising a wide spectrum of intestinal pathology and resulting systemic manifestations. At one end of the spectrum lie infants with minimal systemic upset with a distended abdomen and in whom the diagnosis of NEC is made on the pathognomonic radiographic finding of pneumatosis intestinalis. In the absence of evidence of intestinal perforation or clinical deterioration, such infants are often managed conservatively by resting and decompressing the intestinal tract and administering broad-spectrum antibiotics. Following 7–10 days of such conservative management, feeds may be slowly reintroduced. While some of these infants may develop complications of NEC such as a post-inflammatory intestinal stricture requiring surgery, the majority recover without the need for operative intervention.

At the other end of the spectrum are infants with extensive intestinal involvement and gross systemic upset, often with failure of one or more organ systems. These infants almost invariably require surgical intervention and often require resection of one or more lengths of gangrenous intestine. Unfortunately, in these severely ill babies the intestinal involvement is only part of the overall disease process, and the development of multisystem organ failure requires prolonged periods of intensive care. Mortality in this severely affected group is as high as 20–40 percent.

There is a group of infants who present with similar, if not identical, abdominal and systemic symptoms and signs to those found in infants with NEC, but who are found to have a focal intestinal perforation, often in the terminal ileum, with preservation of the remainder of the gastrointestinal tract. This is often associated with indomethacin therapy used to encourage closure of a patent ductus arteriosus. Whether focal intestinal perforation is one end of the spectrum of NEC is frequently debated. The presentation and principles of management are identical to those of infants with NEC and they are often grouped together.

Symptoms and signs

The onset of symptoms of NEC appears to be inversely related to the gestational age at birth and birth weight, such that full-term infants who develop NEC (primarily but not exclusively those with congenital cardiac abnormalities) do so in the first few days of life, whereas preterm infants of low birth weight develop symptoms most commonly between 15 and 20 days of age. The etiological factors implicated in the development of NEC are an immature intestine, mesenteric hypoxia or ischemia, bacterial colonization of the intestine, and the presence of feed within the intestinal lumen. The precise pathogenesis remains poorly understood.

The physical condition of infants with NEC varies. Initial symptoms may be subtle, such as increased gastric aspirates, mild abdominal distension, and flecks of blood in the stool. However, some infants present with cardiovascular collapse, bilious vomiting, gross abdominal distension with tenderness, and the passage of frank blood per rectum. Additional presenting features include abdominal erythema or discoloration, the presence of an abdominal mass, and non-specific signs of sepsis, including fever and hypovolemia. In addition, abnormal laboratory tests are often present, including thrombocytopenia, raised C-reactive protein concentration, and high or low white blood cell count.

Radiographic findings

The radiographic findings in infants with NEC vary from one case to another, but the presence of pneumatosis intestinalis on abdominal radiograph is pathognomonic of NEC. Other radiographic findings include portal venous gas, dilated loops of intestine (one or more of which may appear to be 'fixed' on serial radiographs), ascites, and, in the presence of intestinal perforation, pneumoperitoneum (free gas within the peritoneal cavity). Radiographs of infants with focal perforation may have none of these findings other than pneumoperitoneum. The presence of pneumoperitoneum may be difficult to detect, and radiographs of infants with NEC or suspected NEC should be carefully examined for the presence of free gas.

Indications for surgery

The initial management of all infants with NEC consists of appropriate resuscitation and support of all failing organ systems. The majority of infants require mechanical ventilation and in many the cardiovascular, renal, and hematological systems also require support. Conservative management therefore comprises 7–10 days of intestinal rest and broad-spectrum antibiotic treatment, with frequent clinical review to identify those infants in need of surgical intervention.

Indications for surgery (**Box 55.1**) in the setting of acute NEC are contested among surgeons and remain based largely on clinical judgment and previous experience. Absolute indications for surgical intervention reported in the literature are the presence of free gas within the peritoneal cavity, the continued deterioration of an infant despite maximal medical therapy, and the presence of an abdominal mass with ongoing intestinal obstruction or sepsis. Among these, the most widely accepted indication for surgery is pneumoperitoneum. The other 'relative' indications for surgical intervention are controversial.

Box 55.1 Indications for surgery in infants with acute necrotizing enterocolitis

Absolute indications
Pneumoperitoneum
Clinical deterioration despite maximal medical treatment
Abdominal mass with persistent intestinal obstruction or sepsis

Relative indications
Increased abdominal tenderness, distension and/or discoloration
Fixed intestinal loop
Portal vein gas
Positive paracentesis
Thrombocytopenia

In addition to surgery during the acute stage of NEC, a number of infants require surgery at a later stage to treat complications of NEC regardless of whether they have had surgery during the acute stage of their illness. The most common indication is the presence of an intestinal stricture.

Surgical approach

There is little surgical consensus among surgeons concerning the ideal surgical management of NEC. Surgical options include primary peritoneal drainage (PPD) or laparotomy. Primary peritoneal drainage was first reported in 1975 by Marsh and Ein as a means of stabilizing and improving the systemic status of premature infants with intestinal perforation secondary to NEC. Since then, PPD has been reported as a definitive therapy rather than an intermediary for laparotomy. Two large multicenter randomized controlled trials have recently demonstrated no benefit of PPD over laparotomy even in very small infants (less than 1000 g). There may remain a role for PPD as a temporizing measure in infants with cardiorespiratory compromise as a result of a tense pneumoperitoneum. We believe this should always be followed by a 'salvage' laparotomy as definitive treatment.

Minimal access surgery has become commonplace in recent years within the field of pediatric surgery and is slowly being incorporated into the surgical treatment of infants with NEC. The principal limitation of minimal access surgery as definitive treatment for NEC is physical size of the child. Performing any of the operations outlined below in a neonate using a laparoscopic approach would be technically demanding and potentially unsafe. However, diagnostic laparoscopy may assist surgical decision making in infants with NEC. In infants who are critically unwell yet who lack a specific indication for surgery and for whom laparotomy may have disastrous consequences, laparoscopy allows visualization of the intestine and a more informed decision to be made concerning the need for laparotomy based on the condition of the intestine.

PREOPERATIVE ASSESSMENT AND PREPARATION

Infants with NEC are nursed on a neonatal intensive care unit with continuous monitoring. Prior to surgery, infants should be fully resuscitated and cardiovascularly stable with adequate blood pressure. Of particular importance in the setting of NEC is correction of coagulopathy and thrombocytopenia prior to surgery, ensuring that blood products are available for immediate use during and after the operative period if required. A proportion of infants with NEC develop T-antigen activation in which red cells become sensitive to hemolysis during blood transfusion. Hemolysis can be avoided by the administration of compatible blood products (low titer anti-T fresh-frozen plasma, washed platelets, and red blood cells). It is our practice routinely to test all infants with NEC for T-antigen activation prior to the administration of blood products.

OPERATIONS

Diagnostic laparoscopy

Laparoscopy may be performed on the neonatal intensive care unit under fentanyl anesthesia with muscle paralysis. High-frequency oscillatory ventilation and inhaled nitric oxide therapy do not preclude laparoscopy.

1 Following preparation of the abdomen, a 3-mm Hasson cannula is inserted in the right or left iliac fossa under direct vision and carbon dioxide pneumoperitoneum is established with a maximum pressure of 15 mmHg and maximal flow rate of 2 L/min. A 30° laparoscope is inserted and the intestine and intraperitoneal contents are inspected.

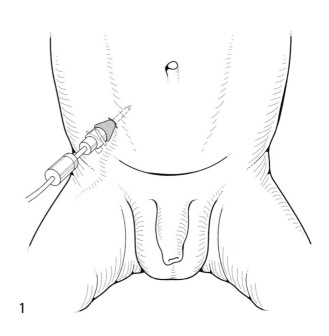

1

In cases in which there is perforation with peritoneal contamination, an additional incision may be made in the abdominal wall for the introduction of a peritoneal suction/irrigation device. Identification of frankly gangrenous intestine during laparoscopy may be considered an indication for laparotomy.

Primary peritoneal drainage

Primary peritoneal drainage can be performed at the cotside with the infant on the neonatal intensive care unit. The site of drain insertion is usually the left iliac fossa, although the right iliac fossa may also be considered if the lower border of the liver can clearly be palpated above the insertion site. The upper quadrants of the abdomen should be avoided to limit visceral damage.

2 With the infant sedated, local anesthetic is infiltrated into the skin and subcutaneous tissues. A small (0.5–1 cm) incision is made in the skin and blunt dissection used to expose first the fascia and then the peritoneum, which is carefully opened to avoid damage to the underlying bowel. Gas or meconium-stained fluid may be released from the peritoneal cavity and a microbiological swab should be taken to direct future antibiotic therapy. A soft drain, such as a Penrose drain, is inserted into the peritoneum and sutured in place to the skin to allow continued drainage of the peritoneal cavity. Stiff drains, including intravenous cannulas, are best avoided as they may perforate the intestine.

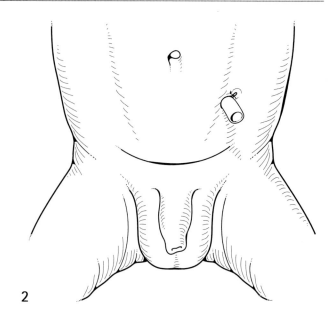

2

Laparotomy

The principal surgical objectives of laparotomy in acute NEC are to control sepsis, remove gangrenous bowel, and preserve as much bowel length as possible. Within these objectives, a number of options exist. The patient's weight and clinical status, as well as the extent of the disease, influence the choice of surgical procedure. At laparotomy, the extent of the disease can be classified as 'focal' when it is limited to a single intestinal segment, 'multifocal' if it includes two or more intestinal segments with more than 50 percent of the small intestine viable, and 'pan-intestinal' when the majority of small and large bowel is involved with less than 25 percent viable bowel remaining. Laparotomy is performed under general anesthesia and may be performed on the neonatal intensive care unit or in the operating room, depending on the stability of the infant and local practice and policy.

3 The authors' preferred approach to the operative management at laparotomy of infants with NEC is illustrated.

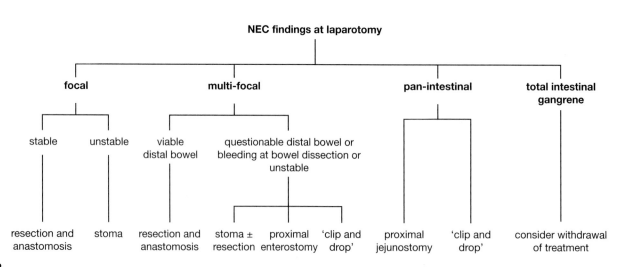

3

Incision

4 A standard transverse supraumbilical incision is used for laparotomy. This may be slightly to the right side initially, allowing for further extension of the incision to the left side if necessary.

Care should be taken to limit damage to the thin anterior abdominal wall in extremely premature infants. The skin is incised and the underlying subcutaneous tissues and muscle can be safely divided with point diathermy, which has the added advantage of providing a degree of hemostasis. When entering the peritoneal cavity, particular attention should be given to the liver, which is often very large and extremely fragile in infants with NEC. Capsular liver damage should be avoided at all costs, as hemorrhage from any injury to the liver may have disastrous consequences and result in death.

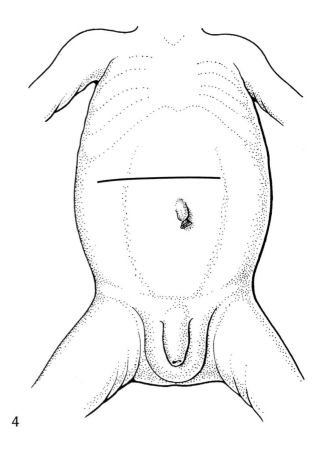

4

Operations for focal necrotizing enterocolitis

For infants with focal NEC, whether perforated or not, and for infants with a focal intestinal perforation with no evidence of NEC, there are two surgical options at laparotomy, namely resection followed by primary anastomosis and resection followed by stoma formation. Traditionally, the recommended surgical approach has been to perform resection followed by stoma formation. However, resection followed by primary anastomosis has been gaining popularity in recent years. It has the advantage of restoring intestinal continuity in one operation and avoids the potential complications associated with stoma formation. However, there is a risk of anastomotic leakage or stenosis with primary anastomosis. Infants selected for primary anastomosis should be stable during the perioperative period, and the resection margins and remaining intestine should be healthy with good perfusion. Neither the weight of the child nor the presence of peritoneal contamination secondary to intestinal perforation affects the decision of whether to perform primary anastomosis or to fashion a stoma. We eagerly anticipate the outcome of an ongoing randomised controlled trial comparing stoma formation with primary anastomosis in infants with NEC.

RESECTION WITH PRIMARY ANASTOMOSIS

The standard laparotomy incision is used. The affected segment of intestine is delivered through the wound and placed on povidone–iodine-soaked gauze to minimize the risk of further peritoneal contamination.

5a–d The affected segment along with its associated mesentery is resected, ensuring hemostasis of the mesenteric vessels, which can be satisfactorily achieved using bipolar diathermy. A single-layer extramucosal, seromuscular anastomosis is performed using an appropriately sized (6/0 in the premature neonate) interrupted monofilament suture. The first two stitches are placed on opposite sides of the intestine to give stability. The anastomosis is then completed, laying the knots on the outside of the lumen. Finally, the mesenteric defect is closed. In instances in which there is a discrepancy in the circumference of the two ends to be anastomosed, it may be necessary to cut one of the ends at an angle to increase the circumference for anastomosis.

Providing an adequate length of intestine remains, primary anastomosis may be used following resection of any part of the intestinal tract from the jejunum to the sigmoid colon, including cases of total colonic NEC requiring total colectomy and ileorectal anastomosis.

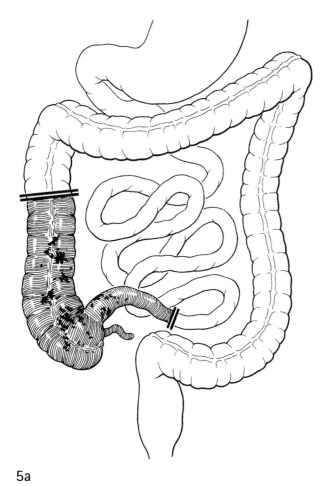

5a

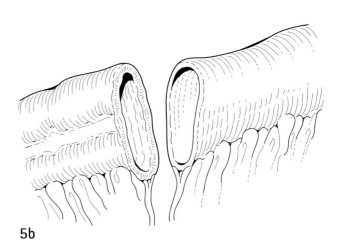

5b

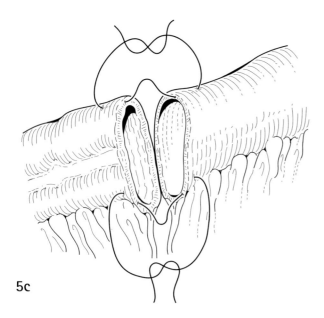

5c

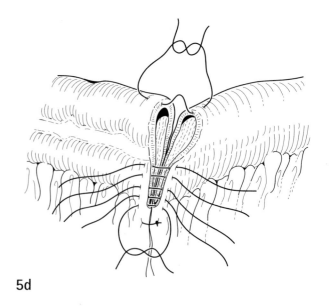

5d

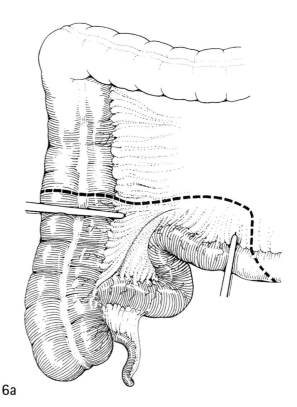

Resection and stoma formation

6a–e In infants with focal NEC who are too unstable to undergo the procedure of primary anastomosis, or when the resection margins or remaining intestine are of doubtful viability, or when it is not possible to ascertain the condition of the intestine distal to the resected region, a stoma is formed following resection. The stoma is fashioned into one end of the abdominal incision unless the mobility of the mesentery is inadequate, in which case the stoma may be positioned anywhere on the anterior abdominal wall. Whenever possible, a mucous fistula is also fashioned next to the proximal stoma. Wide separation of the proximal stoma and mucous fistula is to be avoided, as this would require a full laparotomy rather than a more limited procedure when restoring intestinal continuity. When it is not possible to bring the distal resection margin to the wound, it may be clipped or oversewn.

6a

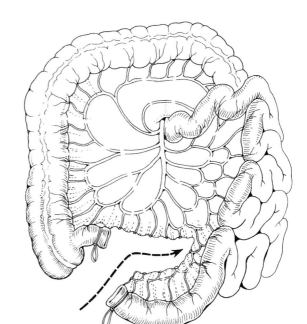

6b

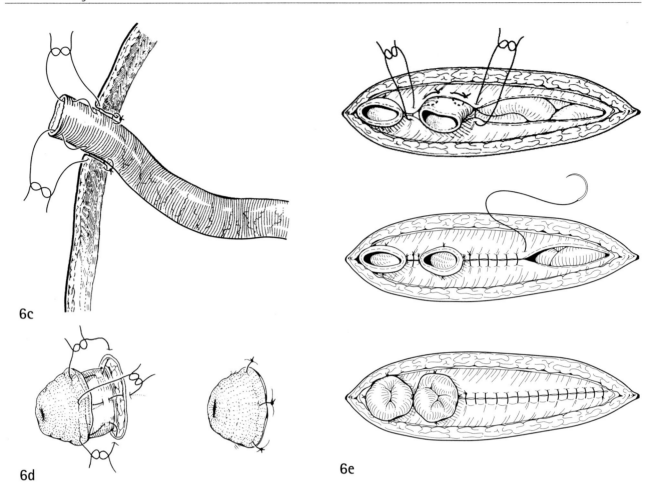

6c

6d

6e

When fashioning the stoma, a limited number of sutures is used to secure the intestine to the anterior abdominal wall to avoid compromising the blood supply. It is not mandatory to secure the serosa to the fascial layer of the abdominal wall, although some surgeons believe that this reduces the risk of stomal prolapse. Similarly, the choice of whether to evert the mucosa as a mature stoma is left to the individual. The mucous fistula is attached to the skin in a similar fashion, but may be left flush with the wound. When the stoma is fashioned away from the main incision and through a separate 'stab wound' type of opening, care must be taken when delivering the bowel through the anterior abdominal wall to ensure that the tract is neither too small (which may lead to stenosis) nor too large (which may predispose to prolapse) and that the bowel passes through en masse without stripping of the serosa.

Operations for multifocal necrotizing enterocolitis

When there are multiple separate segments of diseased intestine separated by lengths of healthy bowel, there are a number of surgical options at laparotomy, depending on the overall condition of the infant, the viability of any potential resection margins, and the mobility of the remaining intestine and mesentery. Of prime concern in such cases is the excision of all gangrenous intestine while preserving as much bowel length as possible. Measuring the remaining healthy intestine may be used as a guide to expected outcome. In a stable child with minimal peritoneal soiling and healthy resection margins, it is possible to perform multiple resections and multiple primary anastomoses. However, we advise against performing more than two anastomoses due to the increased risk of complications.

Stoma formation may also be used in such cases of multifocal disease. If this approach is selected, the most proximal resection margin should be brought out as a stoma. In some cases of multifocal disease, a combination of stoma formation and primary anastomosis may be most appropriate. Resection margins suitable for primary anastomosis may be joined and areas of more doubtful viability may be exteriorized as a stoma. Similarly, if an anastomosis has been performed following resection of one segment of diseased intestine, but it is not possible to determine the viability of the colon, a stoma may be formed below a primary anastomosis. This approach is preferable to the formation of multiple stomas and requires the closure of the stoma rather than a full laparotomy to restore intestinal continuity at a later stage.

In addition, the 'clip and drop' operation may be used in the presence of multifocal disease to preserve as much bowel length as possible.

'CLIP AND DROP' OPERATION

7a–c This technique allows for removal of gangrenous intestine and also avoids stoma formation. All segments of grossly non-viable or perforated bowel are resected and the peritoneal cavity irrigated. The ends of remaining bowel are clipped using Ligaclips and returned to the abdomen. This is followed by a second-look laparotomy, ideally with anastomosis, not longer than 72 hours later. This procedure may be combined with stoma formation as appropriate.

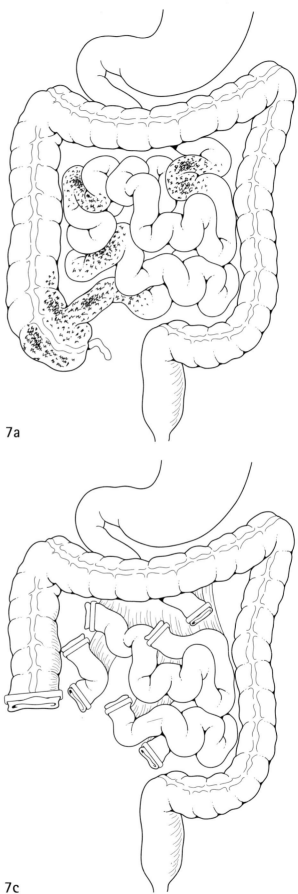

7a

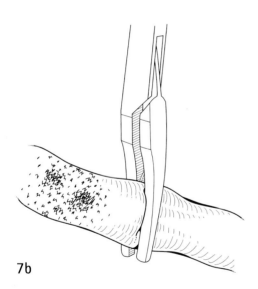

7b

7c

Operations for pan-intestinal necrotizing enterocolitis

The techniques described thus far are of particular use for the infant with one or more short segments of NEC. Infants with NEC affecting a large proportion of the gastrointestinal tract pose a particularly difficult problem, and treatment of this group remains controversial. The surgical principles in these children are difficult if not impossible to fulfill. Due to the length of bowel involved, it is often not possible fully to remove all gangrenous intestine, while salvaging adequate length for sustainable life. It is for these reasons that in the infant with pan-intestinal NEC who is unstable and critically ill, some surgeons would perform an 'open and close' laparotomy, ascertaining the futility of further treatment with subsequent withdrawal of therapy. However, when there is doubt, a number of techniques may be utilized with the aim of allowing time for stabilization of the infant's general condition and the chance of some healing of the gastrointestinal tract to occur. Due to the severity of the disease, the mortality in these cases remains high regardless of the surgical approach. The procedures available are the 'clip and drop' and 'patch, drain, and wait' approaches, as described above under Operations for multifocal necrotizing enterocolitis, and the formation of a proximal defunctioning jejunostomy.

PROXIMAL JEJUNOSTOMY

Surgical creation of a proximal jejunostomy in the presence of pan-intestinal disease allows decompression and defunctioning of the diseased intestine but does not remove gangrenous segments and may permit continued bacterial translocation. This procedure is useful in neonates with NEC affecting the majority of the intestine, but the high morbidity and mortality rates should be carefully considered.

8a,b The jejunum is divided proximally to the most diseased section of intestine and the distal resection margin oversewn. The proximal margin is exteriorized as a stoma as previously described, either through the end of the wound or at a separate site.

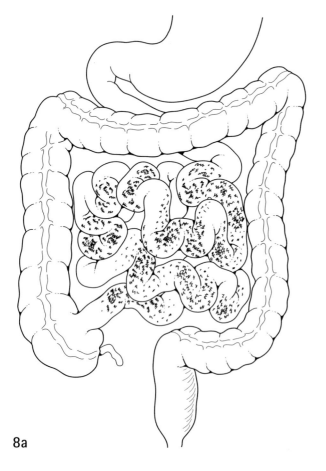

8a

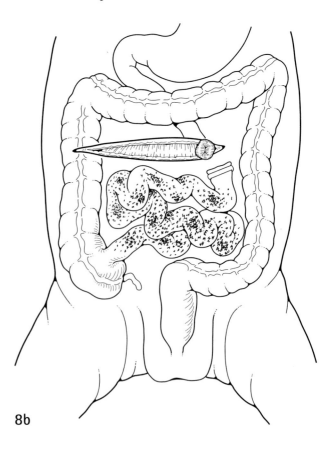

8b

Once the infant is more stable, the intestine has had a chance to recover from the initial insult, and the infant has had the opportunity to grow, a second laparotomy is performed. A definitive procedure is undertaken and the stoma closed. A specific complication of forming a high jejunostomy is the risk of massive stomal output resulting in fluid and electrolyte imbalance. This may expedite the need for second laparotomy and stomal closure.

POSTOPERATIVE CARE

The postoperative care of infants with NEC is invariably on the neonatal intensive care unit with continuous monitoring. Usually respiratory and sometimes cardiovascular support is necessary. A systemic inflammatory response often develops in response to either NEC or surgery (or a combination of both), and failure of one or more organ systems may ensue, requiring appropriate intervention. Sepsis is a common problem during the postoperative period, despite the routine use of broad-spectrum antibiotics for 10 days. Feeds are reintroduced 10 days following surgery, using a cautious regime and increasing as tolerated.

Intestinal stricture

Infants who do not tolerate feeds should be investigated for the presence of an intestinal stricture. Following anastomosis, a stricture at the anastomotic site should also be considered. In suspected cases, a gastrointestinal contrast study may prove the diagnosis. Treatment is by laparotomy, with resection of the strictured intestine and primary anastomosis.

Closure of stoma

Once the infant is thriving and has achieved satisfactory weight gain, any stoma may be closed and intestinal continuity restored. Typically, this is after a period of approximately two to four months but earlier stoma closure may be of benefit in preterm infants who may have difficulty in thriving with a stoma. Prior to closing any stoma, a contrast study should be undertaken of the distal intestine to ensure the absence of intestinal stricture requiring resection. The stoma is closed by performing an anastomosis between the two ends of bowel in an identical fashion to that described for primary anastomosis in the setting of acute NEC.

OUTCOME

Necrotizing enterocolitis appears to be associated with a significant long-term morbidity, although the long-term outcome for infants with NEC is poorly reported. The most serious gastrointestinal complication of NEC is short bowel syndrome, with an incidence of up to 23 percent in NEC survivors. Neurodevelopmental implications of NEC are being increasingly recognized as important although the mechanisms responsible remain to be elucidated. Only approximately 50 percent of the neonates with NEC are neurodevelopmentally normal. Further research is required to identify causative factors and improve neurodevelopmental outcome in this group of infants.

The mortality rate of neonates with NEC depends on the severity of the disease, associated anomalies, weight, and gestational age. Overall mortality in a study of 83 neonates from our institution requiring laparotomy for NEC was 30 percent. The acute mortality rate was higher (67 percent) in patients with pan-intestinal involvement of the disease compared to patients with multifocal NEC (30 percent) or focal disease (12 percent). Causes of death included multisystem organ failure ($n = 10$), sepsis ($n = 14$), and congenital cardiac abnormality ($n = 1$). In a recent study of 51 infants with NEC weighing less than 1000 g, including 44 who underwent surgery, outcome did not appear to be related to surgical procedure performed. However, the mortality in this group of extremely small infants was 27 percent during the acute illness and 49 percent at a median follow up of 24 months. While the surgical outcome of treatment for NEC may be successful in the majority of cases, the long-term morbidity and mortality associated with such premature infants should not be overlooked.

FURTHER READING

Kosloske AM. Indications for operation in necrotizing enterocolitis revisited. *Journal of Pediatric Surgery* 1994; **29**: 663–6.

Moss RL, Dimmitt RA, Barnhart DC et al. Laparotomy versus peritoneal drainage for necrotizing enterocolitis and perforation. *New England Journal of Medicine* 2006; **354**: 2225–34.

Pierro A, Hall N. Surgical treatment of infants with necrotizing enterocolitis. *Seminars in Neonatology* 2003; **8**: 223–32.

Rees CM, Eaton S, Kiely EM et al. Peritoneal drainage or laparotomy for neonatal bowel perforation? A randomized controlled trial. *Annals of Surgery* 2008; **248**: 44–51.

Vaughan WG, Grosfeld JL, West K et al. Avoidance of stomas and delayed anastomosis for bowel necrosis: the 'clip and drop-back' technique. *Journal of Pediatric Surgery* 1996; **31**: 542–5.

56

Anorectal malformations

MARC A LEVITT, ANDREA BISCHOFF, and ALBERTO PEÑA

HISTORY

Anorectal malformations have been described for centuries. Previously, most children with these malformations received an operation involving the creation of an orifice on the perineum. With this simple procedure, many children survived, probably because the rectum was located very close to the skin. However, many died, probably because the rectum was located high in the pelvis. In 1835, Amussat reported, for the first time, suturing of the rectal wall to the skin edges, essentially the first anoplasty.

For many years, surgeons performed a perineal operation, without a colostomy, for the so-called 'low malformations'. High imperforate anus, on the other hand, was usually treated with a colostomy performed during the neonatal period, followed by an abdominoperineal pull-through sometime later in life. The specific recommendation was to pull the intestine as close to the sacrum as possible to avoid trauma to the genitourinary tract. Stephens performed the first objective anatomic studies of human cadavers with these defects, and in 1953 proposed an initial sacral approach to separate the rectum from the urinary tract with preservation of the puborectalis sling (considered a key factor in maintaining fecal continence). He also suggested opening the abdomen, if necessary, after the sacral approach. Following Stephens' recommendations, several different surgical techniques were proposed. The common denominator in all these techniques was the protection and utilization of the puborectalis sling. In 1980, a new approach, the posterior sagittal anorectoplasty, allowed direct exposure of this important anatomic area by incising and then reconstructing the funnel-like sphincter mechanism. With this approach, it became possible to correlate the external appearance of the perineum with the operative findings, and subsequently the clinical results. The approach has implications for understanding the anatomy of these defects, terminology, classification, and most importantly, treatment.

PRINCIPLES AND JUSTIFICATION

Incidence

Anorectal malformations occur in 1 in 4000 neonates, slightly more commonly in boys than in girls. The most common defect in girls is a rectovestibular fistula followed by a rectoperineal fistula. Contrary to what is claimed in most of the published literature, girls with rectovaginal fistulas are rare. Most of the 'rectovaginal fistulas' reported in the literature are probably cases of misdiagnosed cloacas or rectovestibular fistulas. Therefore, the third most common defect in girls is persistent cloaca. The most common defect in boys is a rectourethral fistula, followed by a rectoperineal fistula. Rectobladderneck fistulas in boys represent 10 percent of the entire group of defects. Imperforate anus without fistula in both boys and girls is unusual and represents only 5 percent of the entire group of defects, although it is particularly common in patients who also have Down syndrome. The estimated risk of having a second child with an anorectal malformation is 1.4 percent, but when the first child is born with a perineal or vestibular fistula this incidence increases to 3 percent. There is less family transmission among patients with cloacas, rectobladderneck and rectourethral prostatic fistulas.

Classification

The classification shown in **Box 56.1** is proposed because it is therapeutically oriented.

Box 56.1 Classification of anorectal malformations

Boys
- Rectoperineal fistula
- Rectourethral fistula
  - Bulbar
  - Prostatic
- Rectobladderneck fistula
- Imperforate anus without fistula
- Rectal atresia

Girls
- Rectoperineal fistula
- Vestibular fistula
- Persistent cloaca
- Imperforate anus without fistula
- Rectal atresia

BOYS

Rectoperineal fistula

1 This type of defect is also known as a low imperforate anus. The rectum is located within most of the sphincter mechanism. Only the lowest part of the rectum is anteriorly displaced.

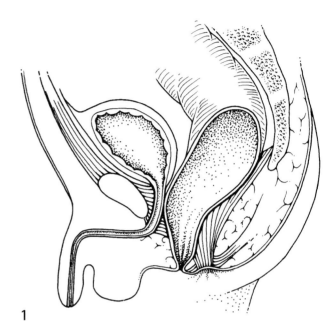

1

2, 3 Sometimes, the fistula follows a subepithelial midline tract opening along the midline perineal raphe, scrotum, or penis. The perineal findings in this kind of defect include a prominent skin tag, below which an instrument can be passed, known as a 'bucket-handle' malformation (Illustration 2),

a black or white, ribbon-like, midline structure that represents a subepithelial fistula filled with meconium, or a very well-formed anal dimple suggesting the presence of a very low defect (Illustration 3). The diagnosis is established by perineal inspection. No further investigations are required.

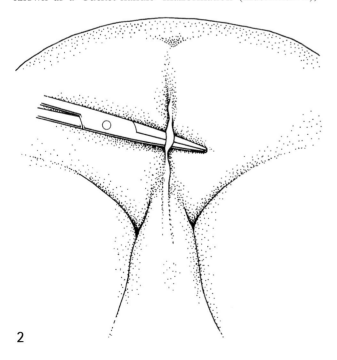

2

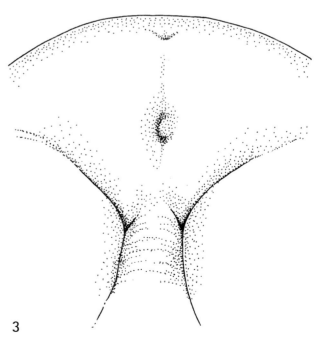

3

Rectourethral fistula

This is the most common defect in boys.

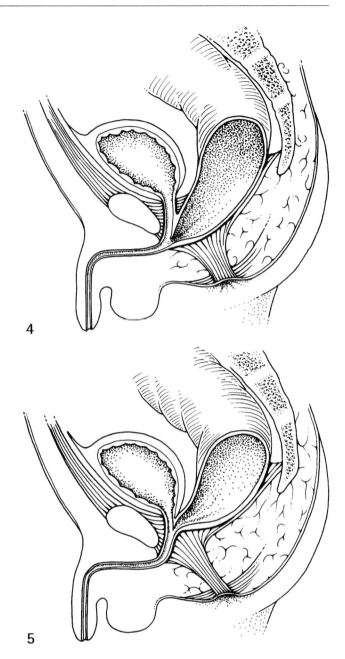

4, 5 The rectum may communicate with the lower part of the urethra (bulbar urethra) or with the upper urethra (prostatic urethra). Immediately above the fistula site, the rectum and urethra share a common wall with no plane of dissection. This anatomic fact has important technical implications. The rectum is surrounded laterally and posteriorly by the levator muscle mechanism. Between the end of the rectum and the perineal skin, there is a portion of striated voluntary muscle called the 'muscle complex'. The contraction of the levator muscle pushes the rectum forward. The contraction of the muscle complex elevates the skin of the anal dimple. At the level of the skin, and located on both sides of the midline, there is a group of voluntary muscle fibers called 'parasagittal fibers'.

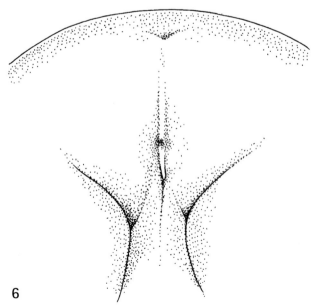

6 Patients with rectourethral bulbar fistulas usually have a normal sacrum and a 'good-looking perineum' consisting of a prominent midline groove.

7 Patients with rectourethral prostatic fistulas tend to have an abnormal sacrum, underdeveloped sphincter mechanism, and flat perineum. The anal dimple is often located very close to the scrotum. Exceptions exist, however. Neonates with rectourethral fistulas may pass meconium through the urethra, usually after 20 hours of life, which is an unequivocal sign of rectourethral fistula.

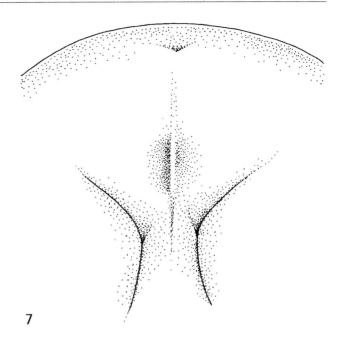

7

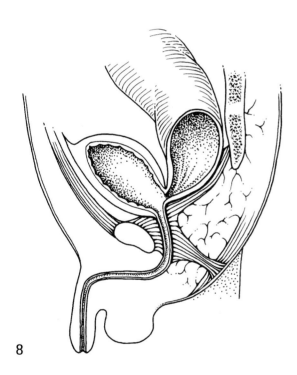

8

Rectobladderneck fistula

8 In these malformations, the rectum communicates with the urinary tract at the bladderneck. The levator muscle, muscle complex, and parasagittal fibers are often poorly developed. The sacrum is often deformed or absent. The entire pelvis seems to be underdeveloped, and its anteroposterior diameter seems to be foreshortened. The perineum is usually flat. For all these reasons, the prognosis for bowel function is poor.

Imperforate anus without fistula

In these cases, the rectum is completely blind and is almost always found at the same level as in cases with rectourethral bulbar fistula. The sacrum and sphincteric mechanism are usually normal and therefore these patients have a good prognosis. This is a common malformation in patients with Down syndrome.

Rectal atresia/stenosis

This is a very unusual defect, occurring in only 1 percent of cases. These are the only patients with imperforate anus who are born with a normal appearing anal canal. Externally, the anus looks normal, and the malformation is often discovered during an attempt to take a rectal temperature or after the onset of symptoms and signs of low intestinal obstruction. About 2 cm from the anal verge, there is an atretic or stenotic area. The upper blind rectum is usually located very close to the anal canal. The sacrum is normal, the sphincteric mechanism is excellent, and therefore the prognosis is good. This malformation is particularly associated with a presacral mass.

GIRLS

Rectoperineal fistula

9 This defect is equivalent to the rectoperineal fistula described for boys. The rectum and vagina are separated. The sphincteric mechanism is very good, and therefore the prognosis is also good.

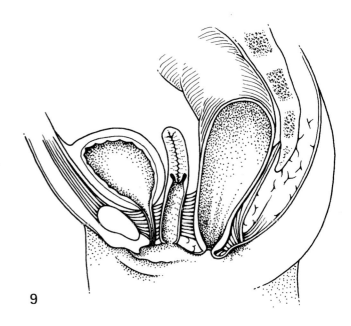

9

Rectovestibular fistula

This is the most common defect seen in girls. It has an excellent functional prognosis. Unfortunately, this is the most common type to suffer a failed repair.

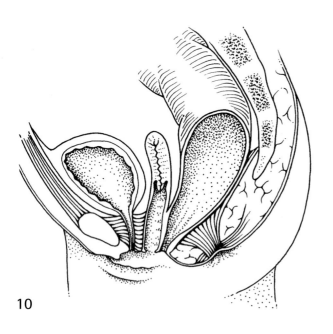

10

10 The intestine opens in the vestibule of the female genitalia immediately posterior to the hymen. The most pertinent anatomic characteristic of this defect is that immediately above the fistula site, the rectum and vagina share a very thin common wall. These patients usually have good muscles and a normal sacrum. The diagnosis is established by perineal inspection. These patients are commonly mislabeled as having a rectovaginal fistula, which only reflects an imprecise inspection of the newborn genitalia.

Imperforate anus without fistula and rectal atresia/stenosis

These defects in girls have the same anatomic characteristics as those described in boys, and therefore have similar prognostic implications.

ASSOCIATED DEFECTS

Sacrum and spine

The sacrum is often abnormal in anorectal malformations. There appears to be very good correlation between the degree of sacral development and the final functional prognosis.

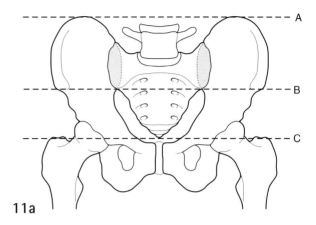

11a

11a,b In order to improve the prognostic accuracy based on sacral abnormalities, a sacral ratio was created that expresses the degree of sacral development. For this measurement, three lines are drawn: line A extends across the uppermost portion of the iliac crests; line B joins both inferior and posterior iliac spines and passes through the sacroiliac joint; and line C runs parallel to lines A and B and passes through the lowest radiologically visible sacral point. In 100 normal children, the ratio of the distances BC:AB was between 0.7 and 0.8 in both anteroposterior and lateral projections. Children with anorectal malformations suffer from different degrees of sacral hypodevelopment, with the ratio varying between 0 and 1.0. A ratio of less than 0.4 represents a poor functional prognosis, and all such patients have fecal incontinence.

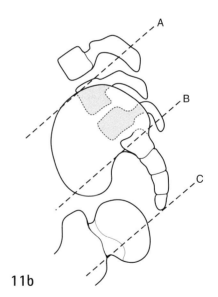

11b

12a,b Two different examples of sacral abnormalities and poor ratios.

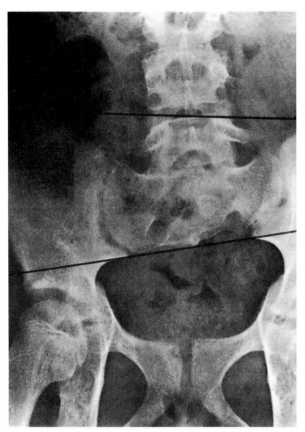

12a

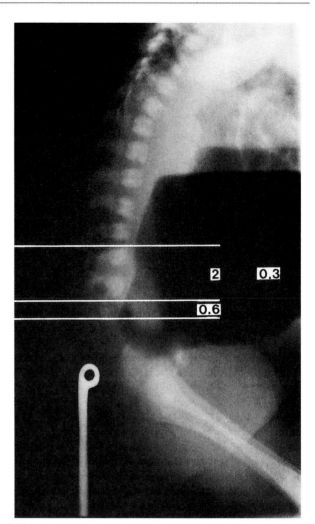

12b

Higher spinal abnormalities include hemivertebrae located in the lumbar or thoracic spine. The prognostic implications of these types of defects in terms of bowel and urinary control are not known. These patients often need treatment for scoliosis. Further, all neonates with anorectal anomalies require investigation of their spinal canal, generally with a spinal ultrasound.

Urogenital defects

The frequency of associated urogenital defects varies from 25 to 50 percent. The reported variation may reflect the accuracy and thoroughness of the urologic and gynecologic investigations in different institutions. Patients with persistent cloaca or rectobladderneck fistulas have a 90 percent chance of having significant associated urologic abnormality. Children with minor defects (rectoperineal fistula) have less than a 10 percent chance of suffering from an associated urologic defect. The most common urologic malformation associated with imperforate anus is absent kidney, followed by vesicoureteric reflux. Hydronephrosis, urosepsis, and metabolic acidosis from poor renal function represent the main sources of mortality in neonates with anorectal malformations. Patients with anorectal

malformations should have an ultrasonographic study of the abdomen during the first 24 hours after birth, and if this study shows some abnormalities, a thorough urologic evaluation is indicated. Gynecologic issues, such as a vaginal septum and absent vagina, are common (5–10 percent of rectovestibular fistulas), and inspection of the vaginal canal is important prior to proceeding with surgical intervention. In cloacas, duplicated Müllerian systems and hydrocolpos occur in 40 and 30 percent, respectively.

Other defects

Other congenital malformations are commonly associated with anorectal malformations including esophageal atresia, duodenal atresia, and cardiovascular defects.

Management of anorectal malformations during the neonatal period

Two important questions must be answered during the first 24 hours of life: what are the associated anomalies and what operation is required, a newborn pull-through or a colostomy?

BOYS

The decision-making algorithm for the management of newborn males with anorectal malformations is shown in **Figure 56.1**. Associated malformations must be investigated. In more than 80 percent of boys, perineal inspection and urinalysis provide enough clinical evidence to make a clinical diagnosis. If a rectoperineal fistula exists, the patient may be treated with a minimal posterior sagittal anorectoplasty in the newborn period. The presence of a flat bottom and the demonstration of meconium in the urine are an indication for a diverting colostomy. The colostomy decompresses the intestine in the neonatal period, provides access for a contrast study to define the anorectal anatomy, and will subsequently provide protection against infection during the healing process after the main repair.

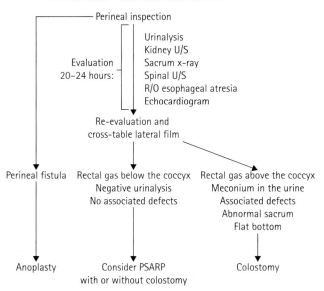

Figure 56.1 Decision-making algorithm for the management of newborn males with anorectal malformations.

It is important to wait 20–24 hours before making a decision, for these patients do not show abdominal distension during the first few hours of life. Even if a rectoperineal fistula is present, meconium is not usually seen on the perineum until 20–24 hours after birth, because a significant amount of intra-abdominal pressure is required for the meconium to force its way through a perineal or urinary fistula. A significant amount of intraluminal rectal pressure is required to reach a level high enough to overcome the voluntary muscle tone that keeps the most distal part of the rectum compressed. It must be remembered that, in most cases of anorectal malformation, the most distal part of the rectum is surrounded by a striated muscle mechanism that keeps the rectum collapsed (see illustrations 1, 4, and 5). To distend that most distal part of the rectum, it is necessary to exert significant intraluminal pressure. Radiologic evaluations

performed during the first hours of life are therefore unreliable, as they will show a falsely high rectum.

Shortly after birth, intravenous fluids should be administered and a nasogastric tube inserted to keep the stomach decompressed and thus avoid the risk of vomiting and aspiration. An ultrasonographic study of the abdomen is performed to rule out the presence of other anomalies (mainly urologic). A piece of gauze is placed on the tip of the penis, and the nurses are then instructed to check for particles of meconium filtered through this gauze.

If after 20–24 hours of observation there is no clinical evidence indicating the need for a colostomy or a primary perineal operation, the patient should have a cross-table lateral film performed in the prone position, to determine the position of the rectal pouch. The anal dimple is marked with radio-opaque material. If the rectum is visible below the coccyx, the patient can undergo a primary newborn repair, provided the surgeon is experienced with this technique. If the image is questionable, it is preferable to construct a diverting colostomy.

After recovering from the colostomy, the patient is discharged from the hospital. If the patient is growing well and has no other associated defects (cardiovascular or gastrointestinal) that require treatment, he is readmitted at one to three months of age for a posterior sagittal anorectoplasty.

Performing the definitive repair at that young age has important advantages for the patient, including less time with an abdominal stoma, less size discrepancy between proximal and distal stoma at the time of colostomy closure, simpler anal dilatation, and no recognizable psychologic sequelae from painful perineal maneuvers. In addition, at least theoretically, placing the rectum in the right location early in life may be an advantage in terms of acquired local sensation.

Some surgeons have proposed a primary repair of all anorectal malformations during the neonatal period without a protective colostomy. There is no question that this can be done and that it has the potential of avoiding the morbidity related to the formation and closure of a colostomy. However, diagnostic tests (other than a distal colostogram which obviously requires the presence of a colostomy), used to determine the level of the defect, are not accurate enough, and the surgeon is actually subjecting the patient to a blind exploration of the perineum. If the rectum is located high in the abdomen, the surgeon may damage other structures during the search for the rectum. Such structures include the posterior urethra, seminal vesicles, vas deferens, and ectopic ureters. In addition, there is a risk of dehiscence and infection because the stool is not diverted.

GIRLS

A decision-making algorithm for the initial management of female newborns is shown in **Figure 56.2**. Perineal inspection usually provides more information in girls than in boys. The principle of waiting 20–24 hours before making a decision is again valuable.

Newborn Female – Anorectal Malformation

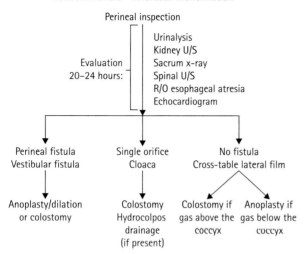

Figure 56.2 Decision-making algorithm for the management of newborn females with anorectal malformations.

13 The presence of a single perineal orifice is pathognomonic for a cloaca. Because of their complexity, these defects are dealt with separately in **Chapter 57**.

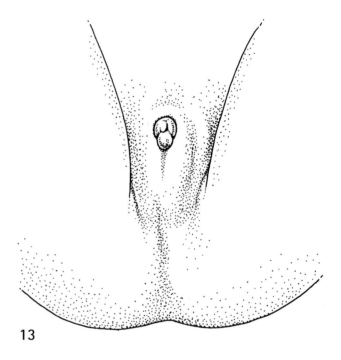

13

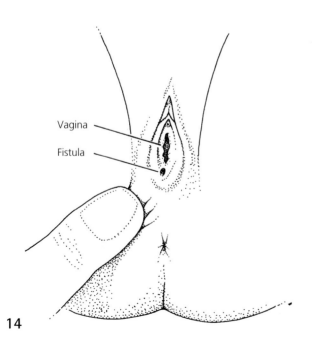

14

14 Perineal inspection may reveal the presence of a rectovestibular fistula, which is the most common condition in girls. In cases of imperforate anus with rectovestibular fistula, the rectal orifice is located within the vestibule and outside the hymen. A true rectovaginal fistula is an extremely rare anomaly.

These patients can undergo a primary repair via a posterior sagittal approach, either in the newborn period or following a period of dilatations provided the surgeon has adequate experience and a meticulous technique is utilized. The authors' preference is the newborn period. A colostomy followed by the definitive repair is also an acceptable and safe approach.

These fistulas are usually large enough to decompress the gastrointestinal tract. Occasionally, the fistula is too narrow and the patient will suffer from abdominal distension. In these patients, the fistula may first be dilated in order to facilitate emptying of the rectum. The defect is then repaired with a limited posterior sagittal operation.

Patients with rectovestibular fistula are the ones who most often suffer from a failed attempt at primary repair without a colostomy. In addition, patients with this defect are usually continent after a successful operation. Therefore, an infection and/or dehiscence is particularly problematic as it may damage the continence mechanism and change the final functional prognosis.

15 A rectoperineal fistula is the simplest defect in the spectrum of female malformations. These patients can be treated with a minimal posterior sagittal anoplasty, without a colostomy, during the neonatal period.

Most girls with imperforate anus have a fistula (95 percent). Sometimes, after 20–24 hours of observation, the neonate's abdomen may become distended and yet there is no evidence of meconium passing through the genitalia. In such a case, the baby likely has imperforate anus without fistula. The neonate should undergo a cross-table lateral radiograph using the same principles discussed for male neonates above (see **Figures 56.1** and **56.2**).

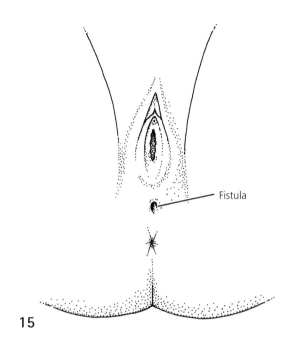

Fistula

15

OPERATIONS

Colostomy

A descending colostomy with separated stomas is preferable for the management of anorectal malformations. Transverse colostomies have several disadvantages: the mechanical preparation of the distal colon before the definitive repair is much more difficult and, in the case of a large rectourethral fistula or rectobladder fistula, the patient often passes urine into the colon, where it remains and is absorbed, leading to metabolic acidosis. Also, during the distal colostography, it is more difficult to distend the distal rectum and define the anatomy. Patients with transverse colostomies are more likely to develop a megarectosigmoid. A more distal colostomy does not allow significant absorption of urine. Loop colostomies often permit the passage of stool from the proximal stoma into the distal intestine, which can cause urinary tract infections and impaction of stool in the distal rectal pouch. Prolonged dilatation of the rectal pouch may translate into severe constipation later in life. Colostomy prolapse is more common with loop colostomies and those created in a mobile portion of the colon. A colostomy created too distally in the area of the rectosigmoid colon may interfere with mobilization of the rectum during the pull-through procedure. The incidence of prolapse in the proximal limb of descending colostomies is almost zero, due to the fact that the proximal stoma is opened immediately distal to where the descending colon is fixed to the left retroperitoneum.

During the opening of the colostomy, the distal intestine must be irrigated to remove all the meconium, preventing the formation of a megasigmoid.

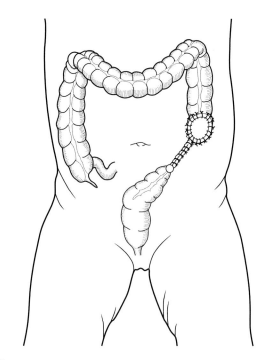

16   The colostomy is constructed through a left lower quadrant oblique or transverse incision. The proximal stoma is exteriorized through the upper and lateral part of the wound and the mucous fistula is placed in the medial or lower part of the wound. The colostomy should be made in the mobile portion of the colon, immediately distal to the descending colon taking advantage of its retroperitoneal attachments, and the mucous fistula is made very small to avoid prolapse. The stomas should be separated enough to allow the use of a stoma bag, which covers only the functional stoma.

16

High-pressure distal colostography

Before the definitive repair, distal colostography is performed. It is the most valuable and accurate diagnostic study to define the anatomy of the anorectal malformation. Water-soluble contrast medium is instilled into the distal stoma, which fills the distal intestine and enables demonstration of the location of the blind rectum and the precise site of a rectourinary fistula. The rectum is surrounded by striated muscle, which keeps it collapsed and prevents filling of the most distal part. This may give the erroneous impression of a very high defect and may prevent demonstration of a rectourinary fistula, which is always located at the most distal part of the rectum. To avoid this problem, the contrast medium must be injected with considerable hydrostatic pressure under fluoroscopic control. The use of a Foley catheter is recommended; it is passed through the distal stoma, the balloon is inflated (2–5 mL), and it is pulled back as far as possible to occlude the stoma during the injection of the contrast medium. This maneuver permits exertion of enough hydrostatic pressure (syringe manual injection) to overcome the muscle tone of the striated muscle mechanism, fill the rectum, and demonstrate the urinary fistula when present.

In cases of rectourethral fistula (prostatic and bulbar), the surgeon knows precisely where to find the rectum. In cases of rectobladderneck fistulas, the surgeon does not expect to find the rectum through the posterior sagittal approach and thus avoids a blind perineal dissection. In this latter case, the surgeon can prepare the patient for an additional laparoscopy or laparotomy to mobilize a very high rectum.

Definitive repair

INCISION

All anorectal malformations benefit from the use of the posterior sagittal approach. The length of the incision depends on the specific defect. The patient is placed in the prone position with the pelvis elevated. An electric stimulator is used to elicit muscle contraction during the operation as a guide to remain exactly in the midline. An incision that starts in the lower portion of the sacrum and extends anteriorly to the anal sphincter is necessary for rectoprostatic fistulas. Smaller incisions (limited posterior sagittal anorectoplasty) are adequate for defects, such as rectovestibular fistula. Rectoperineal fistulas require a very small posterior sagittal incision (minimal posterior sagittal anoplasty).

The anatomic relationship of the rectum to genitourinary structures is complex. The separation of the rectum from these structures represents the most risky part of the procedure.

About 90 percent of male defects can be repaired via the posterior sagittal approach without entering the abdomen.

Repair in boys

RECTOPERINEAL FISTULA

The repair of these defects consists of a small anoplasty with minimal mobilization of the rectum, sufficient for it to be transposed and placed within the limits of the sphincter. This is a meticulous operation and can be done during the neonatal period without a colostomy. The most common complication during the repair of this defect is a urethral injury, which can be avoided by placing a urethral catheter and taking particular care during the dissection of the anterior rectal wall. These patients, both boys and girls, have an excellent prognosis. These patients have problems with bowel control if they are subjected to an inadequate surgical technique, if they are not treated adequately to prevent constipation, fecal impaction, and overflow pseudo-incontinence, and if they have significant associated spinal or sacral problems. Others have described an alternative approach, a Pott's transplant anoplasty, whereby the majority of the perineal body is preserved, the mobilized fistula is brought through a separate incision which is confined to the size of the future neoanal canal.

RECTOURETHRAL FISTULA

A Foley catheter is inserted through the urethra. In about 5 percent of cases, this catheter goes into the rectum rather than into the bladder. To avoid this, the catheter must be intentionally directed anteriorly by the use of a Coude catheter or with a lacrimal probe inserted in the distal tip of the catheter to find its correct path. Occasionally, the catheter must be positioned intraoperatively under direct vision once the fistula is visualized. Cystoscopic insertion of a catheter over a glidewire is another option.

17 The skin is opened through a mid-sagittal incision, and the parasagittal fibers and muscle complex are divided exactly in the midline by use of fine-needle cautery. The fibers of the muscle complex run perpendicular and medial to the parasagittal fibers. The crossing of the muscle complex fibers with the parasagittal fibers represents the anterior and posterior limits of the new anus. These limits can be seen most clearly with the use of an electrical stimulator. The levator muscle, which lies deep in the incision, is then divided in the midline. The higher the malformation, the deeper the levator muscle is found. The levator muscle fibers run parallel to the skin incision. Levator muscle and muscle complex are in continuum.

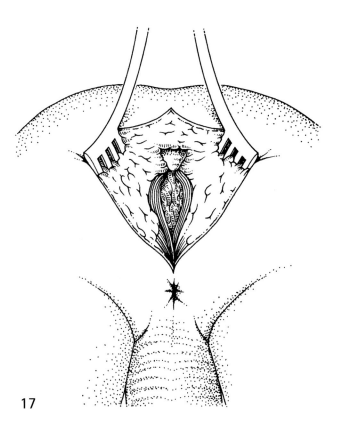

17

18 When all muscle structures have been divided, the rectum can be seen. In cases of rectourethral bulbar fistulas, the distal rectum is prominent and it almost bulges into the wound. In cases of rectoprostatic fistulas, the rectum is located much higher, just under the coccyx, and is not as prominent. In cases of rectobladderneck fistulas, the rectum is not visible through this approach, and searching for it risks injuring other structures.

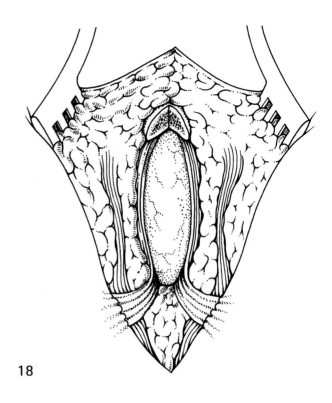

18

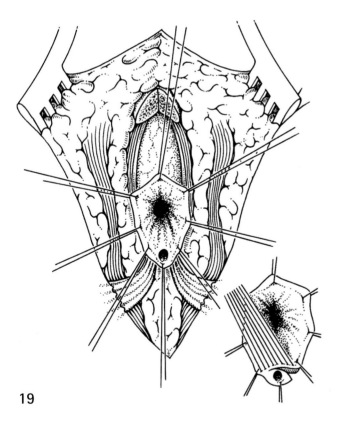

19

19 Two silk sutures are placed in the posterior rectal wall on both sides of the midline. The rectum is opened between the sutures and the incision is continued distally, exactly in the midline, down to the fistula site. Temporary silk sutures are placed on the lateral and anterior edges of the open posterior rectal wall for traction. One silk stitch is placed at the location of the fistula and it will serve as a guide to locate the fistula site after the rectum is completely separated from the urinary tract.

The anterior rectal wall immediately above the fistula is a thin structure. There is no plane of separation between the rectum and urethra in that area. A plane of separation must be created in the common wall. Multiple 6/0 silk sutures are placed through the rectal mucosa immediately above the fistula in a semi-circle. The rectum is then separated from the urethra, creating a submucosal plane for approximately 5–10 mm above the fistula site until the rectum is free from its adherence to the periurethral tissue. A typical areolar plane is then seen. During this delicate dissection, it is very helpful to dissect the rectum laterally first, very close to the rectal wall and then anteriorly, until both dissections (lateral and medial) meet, separating the rectum completely from the urinary tract. Once the rectum is fully separated, a circumferential perirectal dissection is performed to gain enough rectal length to reach the perineum. The rectum is surrounded by a conspicuous whitish fascia. The dissection must be performed between this fascia and the rectal wall to avoid damage to the innervation of the bladder and genitalia.

In cases of a fistula opening into the bulbar urethra, the dissection necessary to pull the rectum down to the perineum is minimal, whereas in cases of prostatic fistula the perirectal dissection is considerable. In both cases, enough rectal length must be gained in order to perform a comfortable, tension-free anastomosis between the rectum and the skin. As traction is exerted on the mobilized rectum, some grooves can be seen in the rectal wall, which demonstrate the tension lines that hold the rectum. These indentations are vessels that must be divided. For a high prostatic fistula, a laparoscopic approach may be helpful, similar to that described for rectobladderneck fistula.

20 Once the rectum has been fully mobilized, a decision must be made concerning the need for tailoring of the rectum. The size of the rectum can be evaluated and compared with the available space so that its size matches the limits of the sphincter. If necessary, the rectum can be tapered by removing part of the posterior wall, and reconstructing it with two layers of interrupted, long-lasting, absorbable sutures. We prefer a braided suture of 5/0 and 6/0. The tapering of the rectum must always be done on the posterior rectal wall. The part of the intestine that will be adjacent to the closed rectourethral fistula must be normal rectal wall to avoid a recurrent fistula. The anterior rectal wall is often damaged to some degree as a consequence of the separation between rectum and urethra. To reinforce this wall, both smooth muscle layers can be sutured together with interrupted 5/0 absorbable suture. The rectourethral fistula is then sutured longitudinally with a single layer of long-term, absorbable sutures.

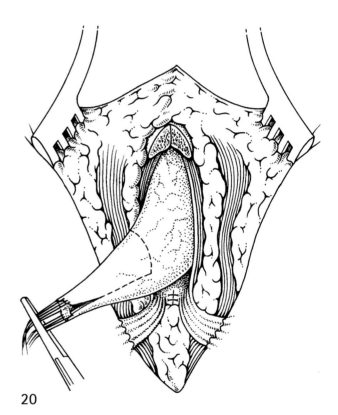

20

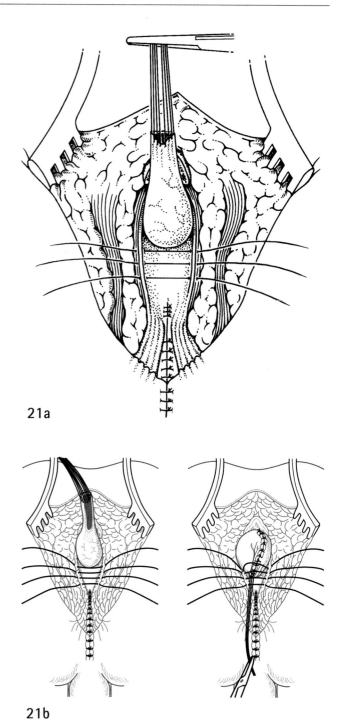

21a,b The rectum is placed in front of the levator muscle and within the limits of the muscle complex and external sphincter (illustration a). The electrical stimulator is helpful in identifying the limits of these muscle structures. Anterior and posterior limits of the external sphincter are temporarily marked with silk sutures. In cases in which the incision is extended anteriorly beyond the limits of the sphincter, it is necessary to repair the anterior perineum with interrupted, long-term, absorbable sutures to bring together both anterior limits of the external sphincter. Long-term absorbable sutures are placed on the posterior edge of the levator muscle. The posterior limit of the muscle complex must also be reapproximated behind the rectum (illustration b). These sutures should include part of the rectal wall in order to anchor it and help to avoid rectal prolapse.

21a

21b

22a–d The anoplasty is performed with 16 interrupted, long-lasting, absorbable sutures. Anoplasty sutures are placed under slight tension, so that once cut, the anus retracts slightly. The wound is then closed, bringing together corresponding sphincteric structures in the midline. Sutures used are absorbable and braided, 5/0, and 6/0, depending on the size of the child and rectum. The incision is then covered with antibiotic ointment.

The Foley catheter is left in place for 7 days. The patient receives broad-spectrum antibiotics for 1 day and prophylactic antibiotics while the Foley is in place.

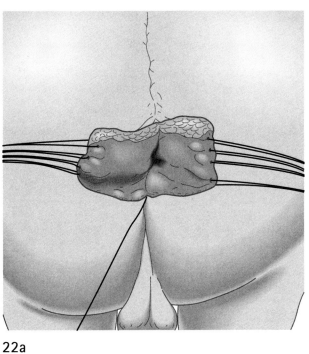

22a

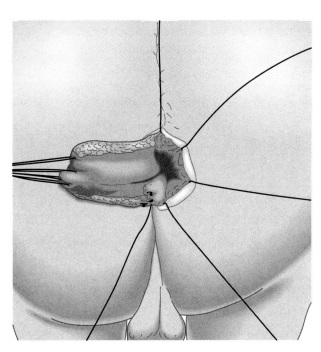

22b

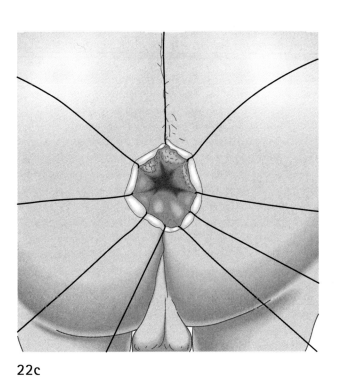

22c

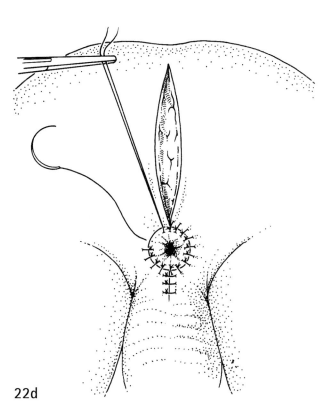

22d

RECTOBLADDERNECK FISTULA

23 For the repair of rectobladderneck fistulas, the entire lower part of the patient's body from chest down is included in the sterile field, so that the surgeon can work simultaneously in the abdomen and the perineum.

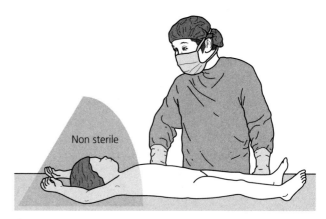

Non sterile

23

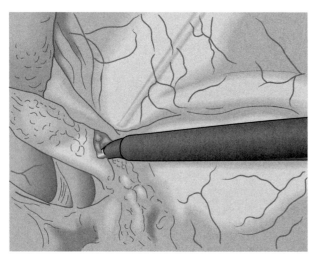

24a

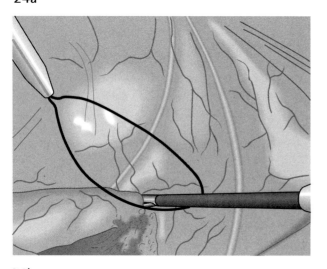

24b

24a–e The abdomen is entered either via laparotomy or laparoscopically, and the rectosigmoid colon is mobilized. The peritoneum should be divided around the distal rectum to create a plane of dissection to be followed distally. The dissection should stay right on the rectal wall. At the point where the rectum becomes narrow, where it communicates with the bladderneck, it should be divided. The bladder side of the fistula should be sutured or ligated with an endoloop (illustrations a–d). In this very high defect, the rectobladderneck fistula is located approximately 2 cm below the peritoneal reflection, and the rectum communicates with the urinary tract in a T fashion, which means that there is a minimal common wall between the distal part of the rectum and the urinary tract. The surgeon must be careful to avoid damage to the vas deferens, which run very close to the bowel (illustration d). With a laparoscopic technique, separation of the rectum from the bladderneck is straightforward. Gaining adequate length, particularly with a high rectum, is challenging, and must be meticulous so as to avoid devascularizing the distal rectum. The rectum is separated from the bladderneck and the bladder end of the fistula is closed with absorbable suture.

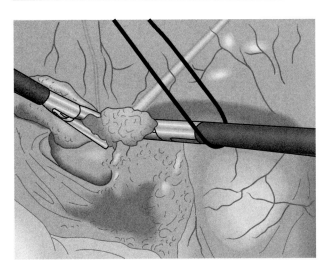

24c

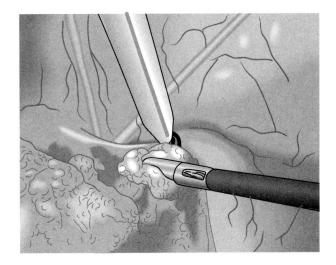

24d

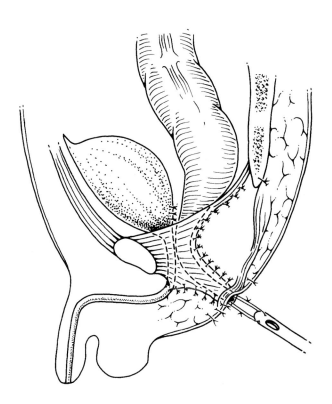

24e

25 As this is a very high defect, mobilization of the rectum to reach the perineum requires special maneuvers. Ligation of the inferior mesenteric vessels as high as possible, very close to their origin near the aorta, would mobilize the rectum, but would probably compromise the blood supply of the rectum because the arcades that connect the middle colic vessels with the inferior mesenteric ones may have been interrupted at the time of the colostomy creation. Instead, the surgeon must ligate the most distal branches of the inferior mesenteric vessels close to the rectum. If this is done, the more proximal branches of the inferior mesenteric vessels must be left intact to guarantee a good blood supply which runs intramurally to the rectum.

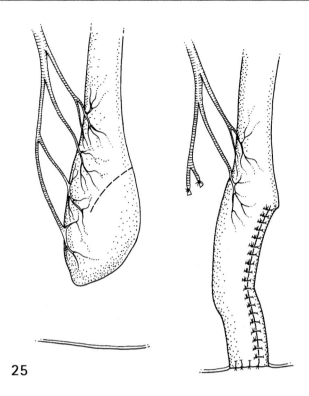

25

If it is necessary to gain extra length, a plasty of the distal dilated portion of the rectum can also be performed. A combination of these maneuvers usually allows the intestine to reach the perineum, provided the colostomy does not interfere with the pull-through of the rectum. This can be anticipated by the use of colostography, which demonstrates the precise length of intestine available from the colostomy to the end of the rectum. If the colostomy was placed too distal in the sigmoid, the surgeon may have to take down the mucous fistula and leave it as a Hartman's pouch or anastomose to proximal colostomy with or without a new diversion, to allow for the pull-through. The rectum should be preserved and never discarded as it performs a vital reservoir function. At this point with the legs lifted, a small perineal mid-sagittal incision is performed. The presacral space is dissected (a mosquito clamp dissects gently along the curve of the sacrum) and is visualized through the abdomen. The rectum is pulled through. Great care is taken to avoid urethral injury, as the course of the urethra is directly in front of the course of the future pull-through. Further laparoscopic dissection can be performed while pulling gently on the rectum. The rectum is tacked to the muscle complex and an anoplasty is performed as described previously.

Laparoscopy for this dissection can replace a laparotomy. It provides an excellent view of the peritoneal reflection, the ureters and the vas deferens; therefore it can be of use in cases of rectobladderneck fistula where a laparotomy is always needed. For high prostatic fistulas, it is also an option since the rectal dissection in a posterior sagittal approach may be very challenging.

IMPERFORATE ANUS WITHOUT FISTULA

About 5 percent of patients have imperforate anus without a fistula. This is the likely defect in patients with Down syndrome. In both boys and girls, the rectum lies about 2 cm from the perineal skin. Most of these patients have a very good sacrum and good muscles. The fact that these patients have no fistula does not necessarily mean that the repair is simpler. The rectum must be carefully separated from the urethra because the two structures have a common wall. The rest of the repair must be performed as described for the rectourethral fistula type of defect.

RECTAL ATRESIA AND STENOSIS

These defects are repaired through a posterior sagittal approach. The entire sphincteric mechanism is divided in the midline. The narrowed area of the distal rectum is opened posteriorly. The dentate line thus converts from a circle to a hemicircle. The posterior rectum is mobilized to reach the anal skin. No anterior dissection is needed. The sphincter mechanism posterior to the rectum is reconstructed. A presacral mass must be screened for and is removed during the same operation. The wound is closed following the principles already described.

Repair in girls

RECTOPERINEAL FISTULA

The treatment of rectoperineal fistula in girls is the same as that discussed for boys, except of course that the anterior rectal wall is mobilized off the area behind the vagina.

RECTOVESTIBULAR FISTULA

26 Most surgeons underestimate the complexity of this defect. Multiple 6/0 silk sutures are placed at the edge of the fistula in order to exert uniform traction on the rectum to facilitate its dissection. The incision used to repair this defect is shorter than that used to repair rectourethral fistulas in boys. The incision continues around the fistula into the vestibule. The sphincteric mechanism is divided in the midline until the rectal wall is located. A characteristic whitish fascia covers the rectum posteriorly and must be divided. This helps to locate the plane of dissection during mobilization of the rectum. Once the rectal wall has been identified, a lateral dissection is performed from the posterior midline, while placing traction on the fistula to make the plane of dissection more obvious. It is vital to be adjacent to the rectal wall, and clean away the thin white fascia that envelops it. The surgeon must be in this key plane in order to be able to mobilize the rectum.

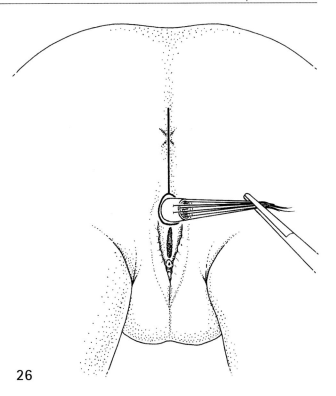

26

The most delicate part of this dissection is the anterior rectal wall. The rectum and the vagina share a common wall, which is often very thin. This thin wall has no plane of separation and the surgeon has to make two walls out of one. This dissection is performed using a fine needle cautery. It is continued up to the point where rectum and vagina separate and have full-thickness walls. A characteristic areolar tissue between the two full-thickness walls identifies this point in the dissection. The most common error in performing this operation is incomplete separation of the vagina and rectum. This may create a tense anastomosis between the rectum and the skin, which may provoke dehiscence and recurrence of the fistula.

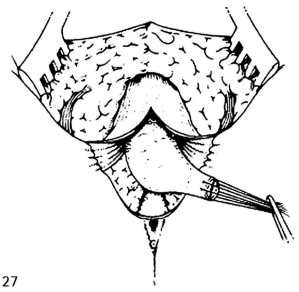

27 Once the dissection has been completed, the electrical stimulator is used to determine the limits of the sphincteric mechanism. The anterior limit of the external sphincter and the anterior edge of the muscle complex are reapproximated as previously described, creating the perineal body. The levator muscle is usually not exposed and therefore does not have to be reconstructed. The muscle complex is reconstructed posterior to the rectum. The anoplasty is performed as previously described.

27

RECTOVAGINAL FISTULA

Imperforate anus with a true rectovaginal fistula is extremely rare. The term is often misused, and patients with a rectovestibular fistula or cloaca are commonly incorrectly described as having a rectovaginal fistula. For a patient with cloaca that is misdiagnosed in this way, the surgeon might repair the rectum but leave the urogenital sinus intact, which would thereafter require a complete reoperation.

A true rectovaginal fistula requires a full posterior sagittal incision. The operation is essentially the same as that described for a rectovestibular fistula, except that it is necessary to dissect much more of the rectum to gain enough length to pull it down to the perineum.

POSTOPERATIVE CARE

Patients generally have a smooth postoperative course. Pain is not a prominent symptom, except in those patients who have undergone a laparotomy.

In cases of rectourethral fistula in boys, the urethral catheter is left in place for 7 days. If the urethral catheter is accidentally dislodged, the patient can be observed for spontaneous voiding, which usually occurs. Attempts to reintroduce a urethral catheter can be dangerous and must be avoided. A suprapubic tube is a better intervention if needed.

Intravenous antibiotics are administered for 24 hours. An antibiotic ointment is applied to the anoplasty for 5 days. The patient is discharged after 2 days in cases of a posterior approach without a laparotomy or laparoscopy, and after 3–5 days in cases of an abdominal approach. The parents are instructed to keep the incision clean, not to wipe, and to apply antibiotic ointment for 1 week.

Two weeks after the operations, anal dilatations are started. On the first occasion, a dilator that fits loosely into the anus is used to instruct the parents, who must carry out dilatation twice daily. Every week, the size of the dilator is increased until the rectum reaches the desired size, which depends on the patient's age (**Table 56.1**). Once the desired size is reached, the colostomy can be closed. The frequency of dilatations may be reduced once the dilator of desired size passes easily. This reduction should occur according to the following schedule: at least once a day for one month; every third day for one month; twice a week for one month; once a week for one month; and every 2 weeks for three months.

Table 56.1 Size of dilator required in different age groups.

Age group	Hegar dilator size
1–4 months	12
4–8 months	13
8–12 months	14
1–3 years	15
3–12 years	16
Over 12 years	17

After the colostomy is closed, patients often suffer from diaper rash as a consequence of multiple bowel movements. The number of bowel movements eventually decreases, and patients develop their own bowel movement pattern. This pattern has a very significant prognostic value by six months after the closure of the colostomy. A baby who has one to three bowel movements each day, remains clean between bowel movements, and pushes during each bowel movement (indicating that there is some feeling during the defecation process) has, in general, a good functional prognosis, and therefore is likely to respond to toilet training. On the other hand, an infant who passes stools constantly, without any evidence of feeling or pushing, usually has a poor functional prognosis and will need bowel management. In addition, on the basis of the results obtained in the authors' series, it may be possible to predict the final functional result from the precise anatomic diagnosis and the status of the sacrum and spine. In patients with good prognosis for bowel control (rectoperineal, vestibular, bulbar fistula, imperforate anus without fistula, cloaca with common channel <3 cm), constipation must be avoided and treated early in life.

FUNCTIONAL DISORDERS AFTER REPAIR OF ANORECTAL MALFORMATIONS

Most patients who have undergone repair of anorectal malformations suffer from some degree of functional disorder due to congenital deficiencies that are not correctable.

Deficiencies in sensation

Except for patients with rectal atresia, most patients are born without an anal canal. This means that they do not have the exquisite sensation that normally resides in this anatomic area. Most patients, however, still preserve a vague sensation called proprioception, generated from distension of the rectum, and therefore stretching of the voluntary muscles around it. Liquid stools, which do not distend the rectum, are not felt by most of these patients.

Sphincteric mechanism

Anorectal malformations are represented by a spectrum of defects. Most of these patients have a sphincteric mechanism comprising parasagittal fibers of the external sphincter, muscle complex, and levator muscle, with different degrees of development, which varies from almost non-existent muscles to an almost normal sphincteric mechanism. Therefore, most of these patients have a certain capacity to hold stool inside the rectum.

Coordinated rectosigmoid motility

Most patients with anorectal malformations suffer from abnormal rectosigmoid motility. Patients who have undergone a surgical procedure in which the rectosigmoid colon was removed, as in older endorectal procedures, do not have a normal fecal reservoir, but have a segment of sigmoid or descending colon pulled down to the perineum. They have a tendency to pass stool constantly, similar to patients with a perineal colostomy.

On the other hand, patients who have undergone repair in which the rectosigmoid colon was preserved (e.g. posterior sagittal anorectoplasty, sacroperineal pull-through, or simple anoplasty) behave as if their fecal reservoir is too large and floppy. Clinically, this translates into varying degrees of constipation. Mild cases of constipation can be treated very efficiently with laxatives, and the children usually live a normal life. Severe cases of constipation, particularly if they are not treated properly, may lead to fecal impaction, constant soiling, and therefore, overflow pseudo-incontinence. This constipation seems to be more severe in patients with lower defects. An ectatic distended colon (sometimes associated with a loop or transverse colostomy) leads to megarectosigmoid and eventually provokes severe constipation.

COMPLICATIONS

Wound infection

Wound infections and mild dehiscences of the posterior sagittal incision can occur. The infection usually affects only the skin and subcutaneous tissue, sometimes can be resutured, and will heal with local care.

Anal strictures

An anal stricture usually requires a secondary operation. A clear correlation exists with intraoperative devascularization of the distal rectum or excessive tension on the anoplasty.

Furthermore, if the protocol of dilatations is not followed, an anal stricture can occur. Such a stricture is only a ring-like fibrous band at the mucocutaneous junction, which is easily treated, and is different from a long, narrow stricture secondary to ischemia.

Before the advent of the posterior sagittal approach, most surgeons would try to create a very large neoanus to avoid strictures and cumbersome anal dilatations. With new concepts based on objective knowledge of the sphincteric mechanism obtained by direct visualization, the surgeon should create an anus no bigger than the size of the external sphincter. The new anus is surrounded by voluntary muscle that keeps it closed. If it is not dilated, the rectum will heal narrow or closed. Therefore, anal dilatations are necessary.

Constipation

This is the most common functional disorder observed in patients with anorectal malformations, particularly prevalent in lower malformations; rectoperineal, bulbar, and vestibular fistulas.

Transient femoral nerve pressure

Excessive pressure on the groin during a posterior sagittal operation can lead to this problem, which can be avoided by adequate cushioning of the patient's pelvis while in the prone position.

Neurogenic bladder

Difficulty voiding after a posterior sagittal approach should occur only in patients with a very abnormal or absent sacrum or with a tethered cord or myelomeningocele, in whom the presence of a preoperative neurogenic bladder can be predicted.

Neurogenic bladder following a posterior sagittal approach in patients with favorable anatomy can occur due to nerve damage during the rectal dissection, where the surgeon does not follow the principles of the posterior sagittal approach and veers off the midline. In addition, placing Weitlander's retractors deeper than is necessary may compress the nerves that come from the sacral area, causing a neurogenic bladder.

Medical management for fecal incontinence

As shown in **Table 56.2**, there remain a significant number of patients (approximately 25 percent) who suffer from fecal incontinence, despite optimal anatomic surgical reconstruction used for the repair of their malformations. For these patients, a program of bowel management is useful. This consists of training the parents and children to clean out the colon once a day with the use of enemas and to avoid bowel movements between irrigations by adherence to a specific diet and sometimes medication.

In addition to the over 2000 patients followed by the authors, more than 500 patients have been referred for management of fecal incontinence after they have undergone an operation for imperforate anus performed in another institution. All these patients are evaluated clinically and undergo a contrast enema, voiding cystourethrography, radiologic evaluation of their sacrum, and magnetic resonance imaging of the spine and pelvis. These evaluations allow the patients to be classified into the following groups.

Table 56.2 Clinical results in the most common defects.

Type of fistula	Perineal	Vestibular	Bulbar	Prostatic	Bladderneck
Total cases evaluated	39	97	83	71	29
Voluntary bowel movement (%)	100	92	82	73	28
Soiling (%)	21	36	54	77	90
Totally continent (%)[a]	90	71	50	31	13
Urinary incontinence (%)	None	4[b]	2[b]	8[b]	18[b]

[a]Voluntary bowel movement and no soiling.
[b]Patients with absent sacrum, tethered cord, meningocele, or severe associated urologic abnormalities.

MINIMAL TO NO POTENTIAL FOR BOWEL CONTROL

These are patients who have a poor sacrum, associated spinal problem, poor sphincters, a very high defect, and a poor bowel movement pattern. The best treatment for these patients is a bowel management program. Because of the nature of their original defect, these patients will nearly always suffer from fecal incontinence. Therefore, time should not be wasted on biofeedback programs, behavior modifications, or reoperations, and perhaps more importantly, false expectations should not be created for the family. The bowel management program allows the patient to remain clean all day in order to be socially accepted, and is successful in 95 percent of patients.

This group is usually divided into two categories:

1. **Constipated**. These patients have undergone a procedure in which the rectum was preserved, as in anoplasties, a sacroperineal approach or posterior sagittal approach. This group of patients tends to suffer from constipation in addition to their fecal incontinence, contrast study shows a megarectosigmoid. Management consists of the use of enemas with volumes of fluids large enough to clean a large rectosigmoid colon (400–750 cc of saline usually with added glycerin, castile soap, and/or phosphate). It is not usually necessary to use any kind of diet or medication, because the constipation contributes to the patients remaining completely clean between enemas.
2. **Patients with a tendency to have loose stool**. This group of patients has undergone a type of procedure in which their original rectosigmoid colon was resected, as in the Kiesewetter, Soave, or Rehbein types of operations. They have a natural tendency to suffer from the constant passing of liquid stools. A contrast enema shows that the colon runs straight from the splenic flexure down to the anus, and colonic haustrations are apparent all the way down to the perineum. They never suffer from constipation. This is the group that is most difficult to keep clean. Management consists of a small enema, a very strict constipating diet and agents that slow colonic motility, such as loperamide and water-soluble fiber. Patients in whom colonic motility fails to slow down are the rare candidates for a permanent colostomy.

POTENTIAL FOR BOWEL CONTROL

These patients were born with a favorable type of defect (rectovestibular fistula, rectoperineal fistula, rectourethral bulbar fistula), a good sacrum, a normal spine, and a good sphincteric mechanism, and underwent an operation that placed the rectum in the correct position. In addition, these patients have a good bowel movement pattern. They can undergo a behavior modification program to train them to have voluntary bowel movements, but they often need additional help with laxatives to treat their constipation.

CANDIDATES FOR A REOPERATION

These patients were born with a favorable type of defect, good sacrum, normal spine, and good sphincteric mechanism, and yet they underwent an operation that placed the rectum in the wrong place or left it strictured or prolapsed. Repositioning the rectum within the limits of the sphincteric mechanism may improve the functional result.

CANDIDATES FOR A SIGMOID RESECTION

There is a subgroup of patients who were born with a defect that has a good prognosis and who underwent a technically good operation but suffer from severe constipation and severe megasigmoid colon. Often such patients' constipation was not aggressively managed postoperatively as an infant. They are incapable of emptying the rectosigmoid colon and suffer from chronic soiling and overflow pseudo-incontinence. Prior to considering a sigmoid resection, a laxative test is performed. The test is carried out over a period of several days. First, the colon is disimpacted with enemas. This process is radiologically monitored. Then the laxative requirement is determined by trial and error. Once the right dose is reached, as demonstrated by an abdominal radiograph that shows a clean colon, the patient's ability to have bowel control can be determined. If the patient is continent, but in order to remain clean requires an enormous dose of stimulant laxatives, a sigmoid resection, preserving the rectum and creating an anastomosis between the descending colon and the rectum above the peritoneal reflection, can reduce that laxative requirement dramatically. If the patient is incontinent, a bowel management regimen is implemented and a sigmoid resection is contraindicated, because in an incontinent patient, looser stools are much more difficult to manage.

FURTHER READING

Bischoff A, Tovilla M. A practical approach to the management of pediatric fecal incontinence. *Seminars in Pediatric Surgery* 2010; **19**: 154–9.

Falcone RA, Levitt MA, Peña A, Bates MD. Increased heritability of certain types of anorectal malformations. *Journal of Pediatric Surgery* 2007; **42**: 124–8.

Hong AR, Rosen N, Acuña MF *et al.* Urological injuries associated with the repair of anorectal malformations in male patients. *Journal of Pediatric Surgery* 2002; **37**: 339–44.

Peña A, Grasshoff S, Levitt MA. Reoperations in anorectal malformations. *Journal of Pediatric Surgery* 2007; **42**: 318–25.

Peña A, Migotto-Krieger M, Levitt MA. Colostomy in anorectal malformations a procedure with serious but preventable complications. *Journal of Pediatric Surgery* 2006; **41**: 748–56.

Shaul DB, Harrison EA. Classification of anorectal malformations – initial approach, diagnostic tests, and colostomy. *Seminars in Pediatric Surgery* 1997; **6**: 187–95.

57

Cloaca

MARC A LEVITT, ANDREA BISCHOFF, and ALBERTO PEÑA

HISTORY

A persistent cloaca is a malformation in which the rectum, vagina, and urethra are fused into a single common channel. This defect is considered one of the most formidable challenges in pediatric surgery and represents the extreme in the spectrum of complexity of female anorectal and urogenital malformations. Treatments traditionally involved repair of the rectal component of the malformation, leaving the urogenital sinus alone, planning its repair in a second stage, or performing a combined abdominoperineal approach with vaginal and rectal pull-through. Some treatments were adequate for certain malformations, but not for others. The perineal approach to the urogenital sinus was useful for low defects but not for higher defects. Similarly, the abdominal approach was required for some anomalies but not for others. These approaches were often limited in their exposure and thus could not clearly define the complex anatomy of the defect, and as with surgery for anorectal malformations (**Chapter 56, Anorectal malformations**), the urinary and anorectal sphincters were matters of speculation because the precise anatomy was not visualized.

Hendren compiled the most comprehensive reports on the secondary reconstruction of these cases and emphasized a global approach to the simultaneous repair of the entire anomaly, with particular focus on the urologic reconstruction. The posterior sagittal approach for the repair of imperforate anus was used to repair a cloaca for the first time in 1982, and led to the operation known as the posterior sagittal anorectovaginourethroplasty (PSARVUP). This approach allowed for direct exposure of the complex anatomy and the voluntary muscles of urinary and fecal continence, and provided an approach to the entire spectrum of defects.

PRINCIPLES AND JUSTIFICATION

Incidence

Cloacal anomalies occur in approximately 1 in 20 000 live births. They occur exclusively in girls. Persistent cloaca was, in the past, considered an unusual defect, and a high incidence of rectovaginal fistulas was reported in the literature. In retrospect, it seems that cloaca is a much more common defect than reported, as imperforate anus with rectovaginal fistula is an almost non-existent defect, occurring in less than 1 percent of all cases. Most patients with persistent cloaca were probably erroneously thought to have a rectovaginal fistula. Many of those patients underwent surgery, had the rectal component of the malformation repaired, but were left with a persistent urogenital sinus.

The goals of treatment of cloaca include reconstruction of urethra, vagina, and rectum, and the achievement of bowel control, urinary control, and sexual function.

Classification

1 In cloacal malformations, the length of the common channel varies from 1 to 10 cm, which has important technical and prognostic implications. When the common channel is shorter than 3 cm, patients usually have a well-developed sacrum and good sphincters. When the common channel is longer than 3 cm, this usually suggests a more complex defect and the patient often has a poor sphincter mechanism and poor sacrum.

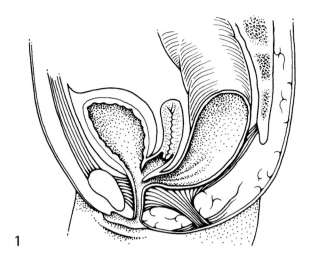

1

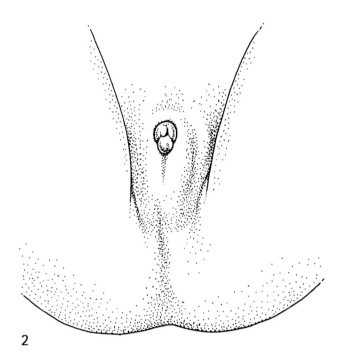

2

2 The diagnosis of persistent cloaca is a clinical one. Careful separation of the labia discloses a single perineal orifice, which is pathognomonic of a cloaca. These patients often have small external genitalia. Sometimes patients with cloacas have a palpable lower abdominal mass that represents a distended vagina (hydrocolpos). Failure to recognize the presence of a cloaca in a neonate may be dangerous, as more than 90 percent of these patients have important associated urologic problems.

Management of cloacal malformations during the neonatal period

Once the clinical diagnosis of a cloaca has been established, the next step is to perform a rapid urologic evaluation. Abdominal and pelvic ultrasonography is the most important screening test to rule out the presence of hydronephrosis, hydroureter, and/or hydrocolpos.

3 In 30 percent of these cases, the vagina is abnormally distended and full of urine and mucous (hydrocolpos). The distended vagina may compress the trigone, interfere with the drainage of the ureters, and produce megaureters. The most common error at this stage is to perform only a colostomy in a patient with severe obstructive uropathy, as this can lead to acidosis and urinary sepsis. The dilated vagina can also become infected, which is called 'pyocolpos' and may lead to vaginal perforation and peritonitis. Such a large vagina may ultimately represent a technical advantage at the time of the main repair, because having more vaginal tissue will facilitate its reconstruction.

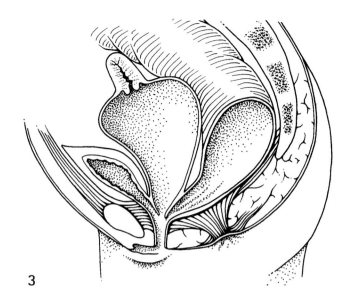

3

If a hydrocolpos is correctly identified and drained, obstruction of the urinary tract is usually relieved, making urinary diversions such as a vesicostomy, ureterostomy, or nephrostomy unnecessary. Rarely, a near-atresia of the urethra exists and a vesicostomy may be required.

Attempts to drain the urinary tract through the single perineal orifice (common channel) by way of intermittent catheterization or dilatations is not recommended, as it is unpredictable whether the catheter will enter the bladder or the vagina. This particularly applies in cases of long common channels. Blind dilatations of the single external orifice may also provoke damage that can interfere with the future repair.

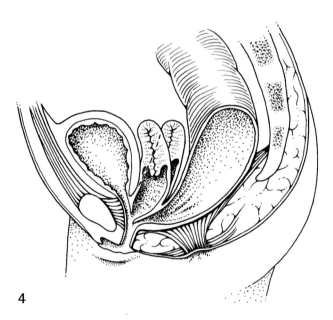

4 The vagina and uterus commonly show varying degrees of septation. The rectum usually opens in between the two hemivaginas.

4

ASSOCIATED DEFECTS

Genitourinary defects

Patients with persistent cloaca have a 90 percent chance of having an associated genitourinary abnormality. Hydronephrosis, urosepsis, and metabolic acidosis represent the main source of morbidity and mortality in newborns with anorectal malformations. Thus, a thorough urologic investigation is mandatory.

Müllerian anomalies

5 Some of these patients may also suffer from cervical or vaginal atresias or stenoses. When undetected, these may interfere with the drainage of menstrual blood during puberty. These patients can develop hematometra, hematocolpos, or intra-abdominal pseudocysts from retrograde menstruation. The gynecologic anatomy can be ascertained during the main repair (if the abdomen is entered) or at the time of the colostomy closure.

Associated spinal, sacral, cardiac, and gastrointestinal anomalies occur, as described for patients with anorectal malformations (see **Chapter 56, Anorectal malformations**).

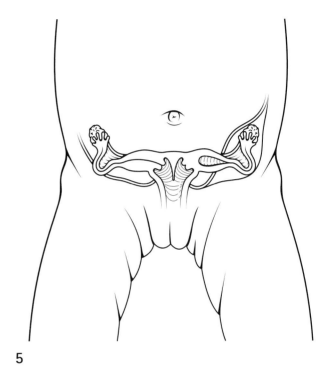

5

OPERATIONS

Endoscopy

An endoscopy is recommended for babies with cloaca to try to determine the anatomy. This is ideally done outside the newborn period during a separate anesthetic after the patient has recovered from the initial colostomy and/or drainage of a hydrocolpos. The specific purpose of this procedure is to determine the length of the common channel, the status of the bladderneck, and the presence or absence of one or two vaginas and cervices.

Two well-characterized groups of patients with cloaca exist. These two groups represent different technical challenges and must be preoperatively recognized (**Table 57.1**). The first comprises patients who are born with a common channel shorter than 3 cm. Fortunately, these patients represent about 55 percent of the entire group of cloacas. The cloacas in the majority of these patients can be repaired with a posterior sagittal approach only, without a laparotomy. The second group comprises patients with longer common channels. This group of patients usually needs a laparotomy, followed by a decision-making process that requires considerable experience to determine vaginal pull-through or replacement and technique of urologic reconstruction. Therefore, these patients should be referred to centers dedicated to the repair of these defects.

Table 57.1 Short versus long cloaca.

	Group A	Group B
Common channel	Short, <3 cm	Long, >3 cm
Type of operation	Only posterior sagittal	Posterior sagittal and laparotomy
Length of procedure	3 hours	6–12 hours
Hospitalization	48 hours	Several days
Associated urological defects (%)	59	91
Incidence in our series (%)	62	38
Voluntary bowel movements (%)	68	44
Urinary continence (%)	72	28
Average number of operations[a]	9	18
Intraoperative decision making	Relatively easy, reproducible operation	Complex, delicate and technically demanding[b]

[a]Including orthopedic, urologic, cardiac, and general.
[b]Bladder/vagina separation with or without the following procedures: ureteral catheter, ureteral reimplantation, vesicostomy, cystostomy, bladder neck reconstruction or closure, vaginal switch, vaginal replacement (rectum, colon, small bowel).

Colostomy

All babies with a cloaca need a colostomy. It is important to perform the colostomy proximally enough to avoid it interfering with the repair of the malformation. In other words, the surgeon must leave enough redundant distal rectosigmoid to allow a pull-through, and for potential use of colon for vaginal replacement (see the colostomy section in **Chapter 56, Anorectal malformations**).

DRAINAGE OF THE HYDROCOLPOS

During the opening of the colostomy, it is mandatory to drain the hydrocolpos when present. If the hydrocolpos is not large enough to reach the abdominal wall above the bladder, it can be drained with a transabdominal indwelling catheter that should be left in place until the time of the main repair. A pigtail tube is recommended to avoid displacement of the catheter after the vagina is decompressed, becomes less inflamed, and recedes away from the abdominal wall. Because a significant number of these patients have two hemivaginas, the surgeon must be certain that the tube inserted into the hydrocolpos is really draining both of them. Occasionally, a window in the vaginal septum needs to be created in order to drain both with a single tube. Sometimes, the hydrocolpos is so large that it may even produce respiratory distress; such giant vaginas may be drained directly, connecting the vaginal wall to the abdominal wall as a tubeless vaginostomy.

On rare occasions, patients with cloaca are unable to empty their bladders because they suffer from a near-atresia of the common channel. In such circumstances, the baby may require a vesicostomy or a suprapubic cystostomy.

DISTAL COLOSTOGRAPHY AND CLOACAGRAM

After the patient has recovered from the colostomy, a high-pressure distal colostogram and injection of contrast through the single perineal orifice will help define the cloacal anatomy. This is ideally performed with contrast injected into urinary, gynecologic, and colorectal tracts, and can be viewed in three dimensions with a rotating fluoroscopy machine. This study can demonstrate the location of the rectum, and demonstrate the vaginas or hemivaginas, and often assess for vesicoureteral reflux. It is a vital study to help plan the definitive repair.

Definitive repair

The goal of the operation is to separate the rectum from the vagina and place it within the sphincteric mechanism. The urethra and vagina need to be mobilized so that each is a separate orifice at the perineum.

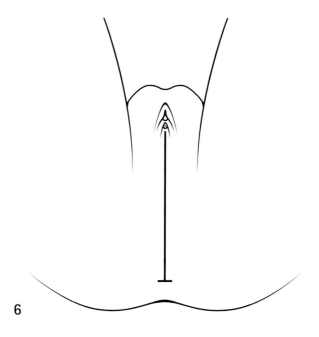

6

CLOACAS WITH COMMON CHANNEL SHORTER THAN 3 CM

6 With the patient in the prone position, a long midsagittal incision is performed that extends from the middle portion of the sacrum through the sphincter mechanism and down into the single perineal opening. All of the muscle structures are divided in the midline.

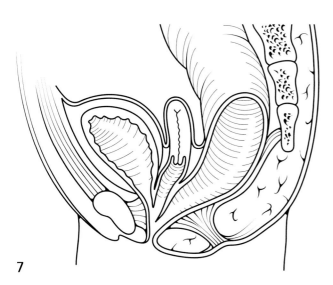

7

7 Low cloacal malformations (less than 3 cm common channel) are usually associated with a well-developed sacrum, a normal appearing perineum, and adequate muscles and nerves. Therefore, a good functional prognosis is expected.

8 The incision is continued all the way down to the single perineal orifice, exposing the entire malformation. The entire sphincter mechanism is divided in the midline.

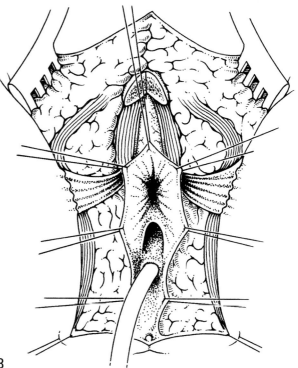

8

9 The first visceral structure to be found is usually the rectum. The surgeon must be prepared to find bizarre anatomic arrangements of rectum, vagina, and urethra.

At this stage, the surgeon has an objective idea of the complexity of the defect and can directly measure the length of the common channel. If the common channel is shorter than 3 cm, it will usually be possible to mobilize the entire urogenital sinus (vagina and urethra together, i.e. urogenital mobilization), as well as the rectum, without opening the abdomen.

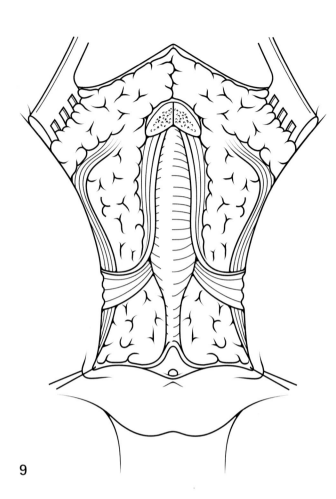

9

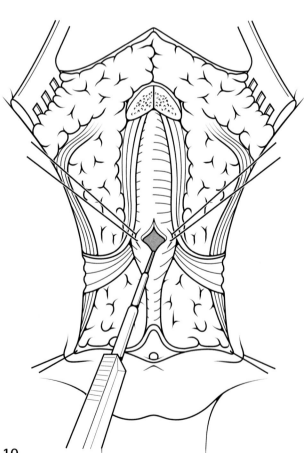

10

10 The rectum is opened in the midline and silk stitches are placed along the edges of the posterior rectal wall. The incision is extended distally through the posterior wall of the common channel.

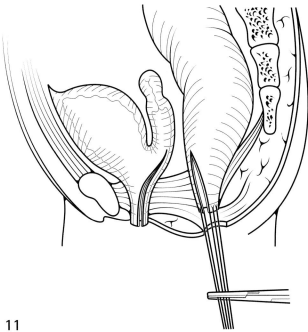

11 The next step consists of separating the rectum from the vagina. This is performed in the same way as described for the repair of rectovestibular fistula (see **Chapter 56, Anorectal malformations**). Rectum and vagina share a common wall.

11

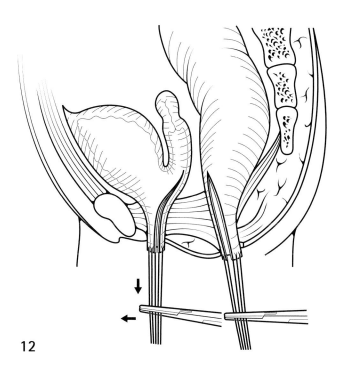

12

12 Once the rectum has been completely separated from the vagina, the total urogenital mobilization can be performed. This maneuver consists of the mobilization of both the vagina and urethra as a unit without separating one from the other. After the rectum has been separated, multiple silk stitches are placed, incorporating the edges of the vagina and the common channel, in order to apply uniform traction on the urogenital sinus.

13 Another series of fine stitches is placed across the urogenital sinus approximately 5 mm proximal to the clitoris. The urogenital sinus is transected full thickness between the last row of silk stitches and the clitoris, taking advantage of the fact that there is a natural plane between it and the pubis. Working in a bloodless field, one can very rapidly reach the upper edge of the pubis, where an avascular structure (the suspensory ligaments of the urethra and bladder) can be identified. While applying traction to the multiple stitches, these ligaments are divided, which immediately provides significant mobilization of the urogenital sinus. With this maneuver, one can gain between 2 and 3 cm of length.

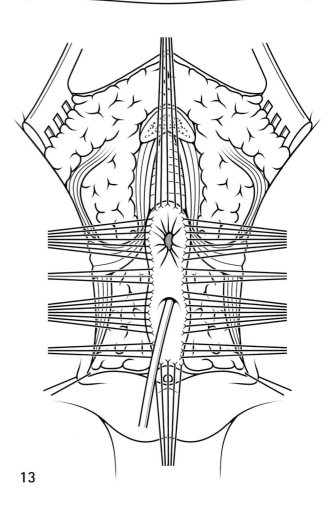

13

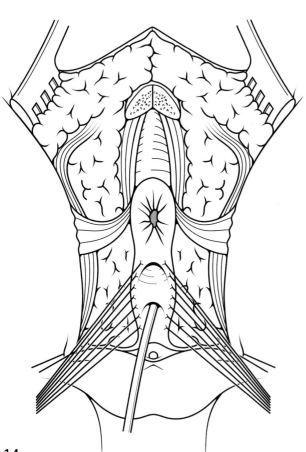

14

14 Additionally, one can then dissect the lateral and dorsal walls of the vagina. This dissection is enough to repair about 60 percent of all cloacas.

15 The urogenital mobilization has the additional advantages of preserving an excellent blood supply to both the urethra and vagina and of placing the urethral opening in a visible location and provides a smooth urethra which facilitates intermittent catheterization, necessary about 20 percent of the time in these lower cloacas. What used to be the common channel is divided in the midline, creating two lateral flaps that are sutured to the skin of the patient's new labia. The vaginal edges are mobilized to reach the skin to create the introitus. The limits of the sphincter are electrically determined. The perineal body is reconstructed, bringing together the anterior limit of the sphincter. The rectum is then placed within the limits of the sphincter.

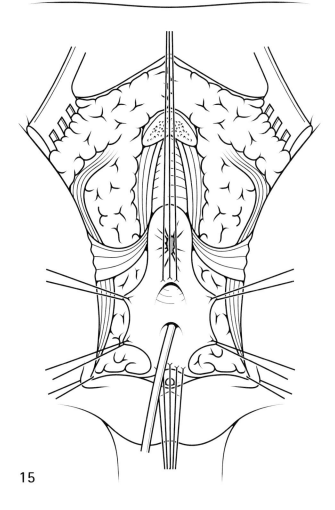

15

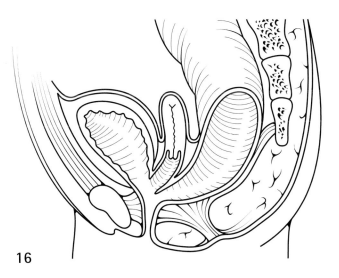

16

CLOACAS WITH A COMMON CHANNEL LONGER THAN 3 CM

16 When the endoscopy shows that the patient has a long common channel, the surgeon must be prepared to face a significant technical challenge.

The patient is prepared with a total body preparation so that the surgeon can switch between the prone position and an abdominal approach, as described for rectobladderneck fistula.

The rectum is separated from the vagina and urethra. A very long common channel (more than 5 cm) cannot be repaired by total urogenital mobilization alone, and therefore the channel should be left in place so that it can be used later for intermittent catheterization. In this situation, an attempt should be made to separate the vagina from the urinary tract first from below and then from the abdomen by placing multiple 6/0 silk stitches that take the vaginal wall to try to create a plane of dissection between the vagina and the urinary tract. This is a very delicate, meticulous, and tedious maneuver. With this dissection from the perineum one can gain a separation of the vagina from the urinary tract for approximately 2 cm. The rest of the separation must be completed through the abdomen.

A midline laparotomy is recommended; the bladder is opened in the midline and feeding tubes are placed into the ureters to protect them. A long common wall between the vagina and the bladder exists, and both the ureters run through this common wall. The ureters sometimes have to be skeletonized during this separation and therefore require protection.

The surgeon must be familiar with the different techniques of ureteral reimplantation because these patients may require this operation during the procedure. Once in the abdomen, the patency of the Müllerian structures can be confirmed by passing a No. 3 feeding tube through the fimbriae of the Fallopian tubes and injecting saline solution. If one of the systems is not patent, we recommend its excision, with very careful attention being paid to avoiding damage to the blood supply of the ovary. When both Müllerian structures are atretic, we recommend leaving them in place, and following the patient closely so that a decision can be made about them when she reaches puberty.

The procedure continues with the placement of traction sutures in the single uterus or in both hemiuteri. Traction sutures are also placed in the dome of the bladder. With the use of traction on both structures, dissection is initiated between the urinary tract and the vagina. This dissection is continued all the way down to meet the previous dissection initiated from below. The vagina is thus separated from the urinary tract, with care being taken to preserve its blood supply from the uterine vessels. Once the vagina(s) has been separated from the bladder and urethra, the surgeon has to make decisions based on the specific anatomic findings. The vagina at this point may reach the perineum. If it is found to be too short, some form of vaginal replacement or vaginoplasty is required.

Vaginal replacement

The vagina can be augmented or totally replaced with bowel when it is very small and is located very high, or in cases of absent vagina. The choices are rectum, colon, or small bowel.

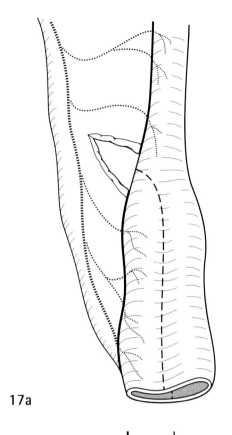

17a

RECTUM

17a,b Replacing the vagina with rectum is only feasible in patients who have a megarectum that is large enough or long enough to be divided into a portion with its own blood supply, which will form the new vagina, and a portion with enough circumference to reconstruct an adequate-sized rectum. The blood supply of the rectum will be provided transmurally from branches of the inferior mesenteric vessels.

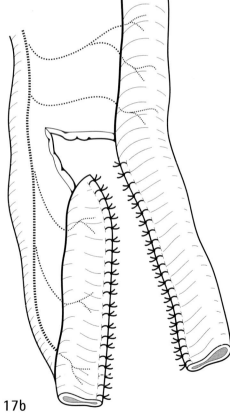

17b

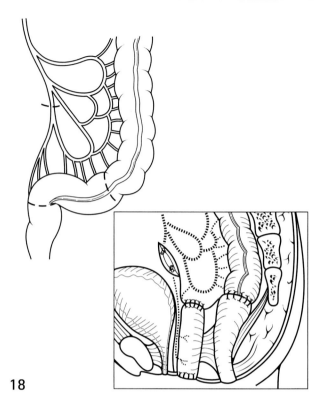

COLON

18 Although the colon appears to be an ideal substitute to replace the vagina, this type of reconstruction is sometimes inhibited by the location of the colostomy. The most mobile portion of the colon must be used in order to have a piece that has a long mesentery. Sometimes, the site of the colostomy can be pulled down to become a neovagina, with the more proximal colonic segment opened as a new colostomy. When the patient has internal genitalia or a little cuff of vagina or cervix, the upper part of the bowel used for replacement should be sutured to the upper vagina. When the patient has no internal genitalia (no vagina and no uterus), the vagina is created and left with its upper portion blind for use for intercourse only.

18

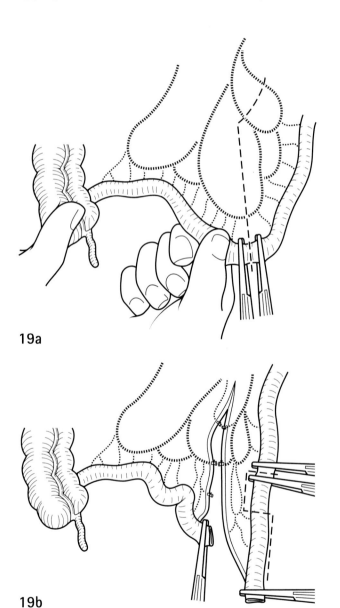

19a

19b

SMALL BOWEL

19a,b When small bowel is chosen for reconstruction, the most mobile portion is utilized. The mesentery of the small bowel is longer in an area approximately 15 cm proximal to the ileocecal valve. A segment of this portion of the small intestine is selected, preserving its mesentery.

20 The continuity of the small intestine is re-established with an end-to-end anastomosis. Two more anastomoses are necessary: the upper one between the segment of small intestine and the upper vagina, and the lower one between the lower part of the intestine and the perineal skin (new labia).

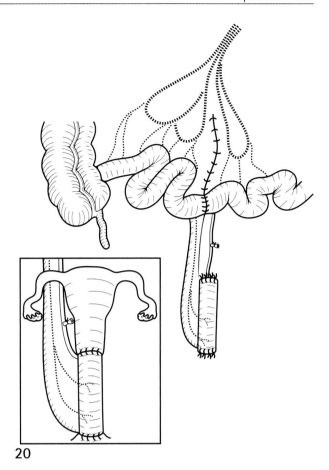

20

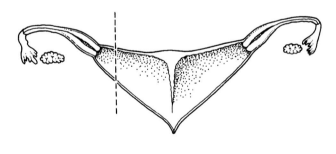

21

21 During separation of the vagina from the urinary tract, the blood supply to both hemiuteri and hemivaginas reaches the hemiuterus laterally and must be preserved until a decision is reached concerning the type of vaginal mobilization to be performed. The vaginal switch maneuver is applicable in cases with a specific anatomic variant consisting of a long common channel and two hemivaginas with bilateral hydrocolpos. After separation of the vagina from the urinary tract has been completed, the vagina may be too short to fill the gap between vagina and perineum, and it is therefore impossible to move the vagina down. The transverse diameter of both hemivaginas together may be long enough to reach the perineum, provided one of the hemiuteri is sacrificed. One of the hemiuteri and the ipsilateral Fallopian tube are resected, with particular care given to preserving the blood supply of the ovary. The blood supply of the hemivagina of that side is sacrificed, that of the contralateral hemivagina is preserved and is sufficient for both hemivaginas. The vaginal septum is resected, and both hemivaginas are tubularized into a single vagina, taking advantage of their combined long lateral dimension.

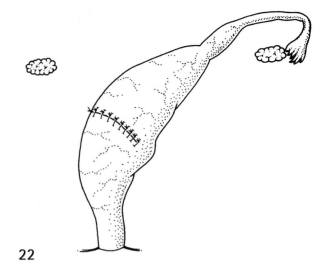

22 Then, what used to be the dome of the hemivagina where the hemiuterus was resected is turned down to the perineum. This is an excellent maneuver, but it can only be performed when the anatomic characteristics fulfill the requirements described.

22

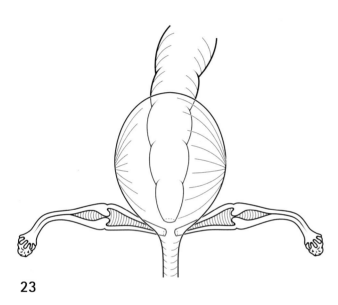

23

23 In the highest type of cloaca, one may find two little hemivaginas attached to the bladderneck or even to the trigone of the bladder. In these cases, the rectum also opens in the trigone. The separation of these structures is done abdominally. Unfortunately, when that separation is completed, patients are often left with no bladderneck or with a very severely damaged bladderneck. At that point, the surgeon must have enough experience to make a decision about whether to reconstruct the bladderneck or to close it permanently. In the first situation, most patients will need intermittent catheterization to empty the bladder, and there is no guarantee that the bladderneck reconstruction will work. In the second situation (permanent closure of the bladderneck), a vesicostomy is created, and the patient will require a continent diversion-type of procedure at the age of urinary continence (between three and four years of age). In this particular type of malformation, the patient also needs a vaginal replacement, which should be done in the way previously described.

COMPLICATIONS

Urethrovaginal fistula

Urethrovaginal fistula used to be the most common and feared complication in cases of persistent cloaca, but with the advent of the total urogenital mobilization maneuver, this complication has essentially been eliminated.

Acquired vaginal atresia

Ischemic vaginal fibrosis can occur secondary to an excessive dissection in an unsuccessful attempt to mobilize a very high vagina. To avoid this complication, adequate mobilization without tension or one of the described vaginal replacement maneuvers should be selected.

POSTOPERATIVE MANAGEMENT AND COLOSTOMY CLOSURE

Postoperatively, patients generally have a smooth course. Pain is not a problem, except for those who have undergone a laparotomy.

The Foley catheter is usually retained for 2–3 weeks. In our series, about 20 percent of the cloaca patients with a common channel shorter than 3 cm require intermittent catheterization to empty the bladder. Patients with common channels longer than 3 cm will require intermittent catheterization 70–80 percent of the time. Therefore, we leave the Foley catheter in place as long as the patient shows signs of edema in the genitalia, and if the urethral meatus is not perfectly visible, we prefer to keep the Foley catheter in place. Once we are able to see the urethral orifice, we remove the Foley catheter in the clinic and then observe the baby to see if she is capable of emptying the bladder. If the baby cannot pass urine, we teach the caregiver to pass the catheter intermittently. In cases of very long common channels, we prefer to leave a vesicostomy or suprapubic tube in place at the time of the cloaca repair.

Intravenous antibiotics are administered for 24 hours. Prophylactic antibiotics are administered orally to avoid urinary tract infections while the catheter is in. Antibiotic ointment is applied locally for 8–10 days. Most patients go home after 2 days, or after 3–4 days for those who required a laparotomy.

Two weeks after the repair, anal dilatations are started, following the protocol described for all patients with anorectal malformations.

For patients who had a suprapubic tube, a cystostogram is performed one month following surgery to verify the patency of the urethra and rule out the possibility of urethrovaginal fistulas or a urethral stricture. Intermittent clamping of the tube is commenced, and the residual urine is measured as an indicator of the efficiency of bladder function. The suprapubic tube remains in place until we have evidence of a good bladder function or the caregiver learns to catheterize the bladder when required. A vesicostomy can be similarly used.

At the time of colostomy closure, an endoscopy should be performed to ensure that the repair is intact. If the cloacal repair did not require an abdominal approach, inspection of the Müllerian structures (as already described) should be performed at the time of colostomy closure.

OUTCOME

A patient who has one to three bowel movements per day, remains clean between bowel movements, and shows evidence of feeling or pushing during bowel movements, has a good bowel movement pattern and usually a good prognosis. This type of patient is trainable. A patient with multiple bowel movements or one who passes stools constantly without showing any signs of sensation or pushing usually has a poor functional prognosis.

Cloacas represent a spectrum of defects that can be subclassified on the basis of potential for bowel and urinary control, for which the length of the common channel seems to be an important prognostic factor, along with the status of the patient's sacrum and spine.

Many patients suffer from a deficient emptying mechanism of the bladder. However, they do not have the typical 'Christmas tree' type of neurogenic bladder of spina bifida patients, but rather have a flaccid, smooth, large bladder that does not empty completely. Fortunately, most patients with cloacas have a very good bladderneck. The combination of a good bladderneck and a floppy, flaccid bladder makes these patients ideal candidates for intermittent catheterization, which keeps them completely dry. There are two exceptions. One is patients who have a very long common channel, in which the

hemivaginas are attached to the bladderneck, and, after these structures have been separated, the patients are left with no bladderneck or a very damaged bladderneck. The second exception is a small number of patients who are born with separated pubic bones. These patients have no bladderneck congenitally and they eventually require a continent diversion type of operation. These patients could be described as having a covered exstrophy.

Table 57.2 shows the clinical results obtained in our series of cases with cloacal malformations.

Table 57.2 Clinical results in cloacas.

Common channel	Short, <3 cm (%)	Long, >3 cm (%)
Bowel function		
Total cases evaluated	127	101
Voluntary bowel movement	65/99 (66)	26/73 (36)
Totally continent[a]	34/65 (52)	7/26 (27)
Soiling	61/95 (64)	47/56 (84)
Constipated	38/98 (39)	17/61 (28)
Urinary function		
Normal	76/103 (74)	28/87 (32)
Dry with intermittent catheterization	23/103 (22)	56/87 (64)
Through the urethra	18/23 (78)	28/56 (50)
Through Mitrofanoff conduit	5/23 (22)	28/56 (50)

[a]Voluntary bowel movement and no soiling.

Table based on our series of 539 cloacas, 228 of whom were available for follow up and above the age of potty training.

CLOACAL EXSTROPHY

Cloacal exstrophy represents the most complex of all anorectal and genitourinary malformations. The initial approach consists of the repair of the omphalocele, closure of the bladder (primarily or staged) with or without osteotomies, and the creation of an end colostomy utilizing all available colon. Then, we observe the patient for between three and five years since the ultimate goal for these patients should be to achieve dryness for urine, cleanliness for stool, and sexual function. With respect to fecal continence, most of these patients have a poor prognosis due to the presence of a dysplastic sacrum, significant vertebral defects, suboptimal anal sphincter and perineal muscle function, and different degrees of colon length, usually short, which leads to loose stool. Despite this poor prognosis, it is the capacity to form solid stool that allows for a successful bowel management program, where the child is kept clean for 24 hours with the use of one enema a day. To achieve this, it is vital that every piece of hindgut, no matter how small, is incorporated into the fecal stream, because it has been noted that these apparently useless small segments of colon will grow considerably with usage and time. Only after determining the potential for bowel control should a urological reconstruction be planned. With that unified approach, the majority of patients born with cloacal exstrophy can have a pull-through and are kept clean with bowel management, allowing for a better quality of life (**Figure 57.1**).

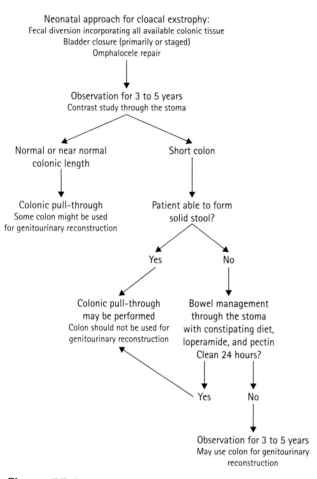

Figure 57.1 Decision-making algorithm for the management of newborns with cloacal extrophy.

FURTHER READING

Bischoff A, Levitt MA, Breech L *et al.* Hydrocolpos in cloacal malformations. *Journal of Pediatric Surgery* 2010; **45**: 1241–5.

Bischoff A, Levitt MA, Foong YL *et al.* Prenatal diagnosis of cloacal malformations. *Pediatric Surgery International* 2010; **26**: 1071–5.

Breech L. Gynecological concerns in patients with anorectal malformations. *Seminars in Pediatric Surgery* 2010; **19**: 139–45.

Hendren WH. Further experience in reconstructive surgery for cloacal anomalies. *Journal of Pediatric Surgery* 1982; **17**: 695.

Hendren WH. Repair of cloacal anomalies: current techniques. *Journal of Pediatric Surgery* 1986; **21**: 1159–76.

Levitt MA, Mak GA, Falcone RA, Peña A. Cloacalexstrophy – pull through or permanent stoma? A review of 53 patients. *Journal of Pediatric Surgery* 2008; **43**: 164–70.

Levitt MA, Peña A. Cloacal malformations: lessons learned from 490 cases. *Seminars in Pediatric Surgery* 2010; **19**: 128–38.

Levitt MA, Peña A. Pitfalls in the management of newborn cloacas. *Pediatric Surgery International* 2005; **21**: 264–9.

Peña A. Total urogenital mobilization – an easier way to repair cloacas. *Journal of Pediatric Surgery* 1997; **32**: 263–8.

Soffer SZ, Rosen NG, Hong AR *et al.* Cloacal exstrophy: a unified management plan. *Journal of Pediatric Surgery* 2000; **35**: 932–7.

58

Laparoscopic repair of anorectal malformations

JOHN BOUTROS and JACOB C LANGER

PRINCIPLES

The incidence, classification, and decision-making algorithms for the spectrum of anorectal malformations are detailed in **Chapter 56**. The authors will focus this chapter on the application of minimal access techniques to the repair of anorectal malformations.

Indications

The laparoscopic approach is not indicated for children with low anorectal malformations characterized by a perineal or vestibular fistula. In general, laparoscopic-assisted anorectal pull-through (LAARP) is most appropriate for high anorectal malformations in boys, including those with rectourethral fistula, recto-bladderneck fistula, and high imperforate anus without a fistula. Laparoscopy has also been used by several authors for selected forms of cloacal malformations, in order to evaluate the intra-abdominal anatomy and to perform mobilization of pelvic structures. The role of laparoscopy in this setting will not be addressed in this chapter.

The choice of posterior sagittal anorectoplasty (PSARP) versus laparoscopic pull-through remains controversial. Some authors advocate the laparoscopic approach for all high anorectal malformations, and believe that outcomes are better with this approach. We reserve the laparoscopic approach for children with proximal fistulas in the bladder neck or prostatic urethra, in which the PSARP is more difficult. In contrast, the PSARP is relatively easy in children with lower rectourethral fistulas, and the laparoscopic approach is correspondingly more difficult, making PSARP a better option for those patients. In children with high anorectal malformation without a fistula, the decision should be made based on the level of the rectal atresia.

Preoperative

Preoperative preparation is similar to that of patients being prepared for posterior sagittal anorectoplasty. This is detailed in **Chapter 56**.

OPERATIONS

The laparoscopic repair of high anorectal malformations can be completed in one, two, or three stages. The one-stage procedure is outlined first, followed by a description of the two- and three-stage procedure.

Primary pull-through procedure (one-stage procedure)

1 Following the institution of general anesthesia and administration of preoperative antibiotics (usually cefoxitin), cystoscopy is performed to identify the location of the fistula and a urinary catheter is inserted. The patient is positioned transversely at the foot of the operating table, and the child's entire torso, groin, perineum, and lower extremities are prepped. The authors use a split drape with the apex of the drape at the top of the patient's back and the two wings of the drape wrapped around the child's upper thorax at the level of the nipples, so that the patient's mid and lower thorax, abdomen and lower extremities are prepped and free-draped into the operative field. This allows easy access to the perineum and abdomen simultaneously.

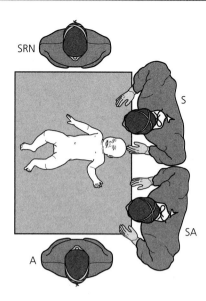

1

Following this, pneumoperitoneum is achieved. The authors' preferred technique is a semi-open approach using a radially dilating sheath and trocar system through the umbilicus. The umbilicus is everted and a 5-mm longitudinal incision is performed through the skin. At the center of the umbilical ring, a natural defect is identified,

the peritoneum is incised and passage of a mosquito clamp, without spreading, confirms entry into the abdominal cavity. The Veress needle and sheath are used to insufflate the abdomen to an intra-abdominal pressure of 8 cmH$_2$O with a flow of 0.1–0.5 cc/min. The pressure can be temporarily raised to 12 cmH$_2$O to facilitate exposure.

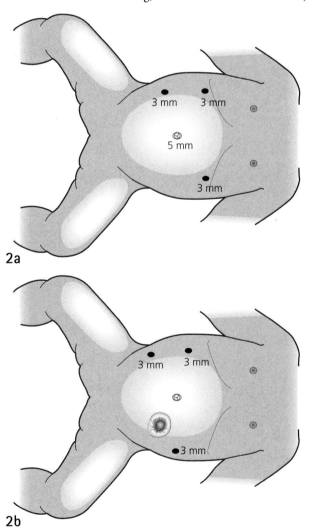

2a

2b

2a,b Then, 3-mm ports are placed in the left upper quadrant, right flank, and right upper quadrant along the anterior axillary lines. Care is taken that the right upper quadrant port is below the liver edge. An alternative approach is to pass the 3-mm instruments directly through the abdominal wall without trocars. The table is inclined left-side up to position the patient in the Trendelenburg position so that the small bowel is distracted cephalad exposing the rectum and pelvis.

3 Once position, access, and exposure have been achieved, rectal dissection follows, incising the peritoneum at the peritoneal reflection with hook cautery. Electrocautery is then used circumferentially to dissect the mesorectum off the rectum and the dissection is carried distally, making sure to stay right on the rectal wall. If the bladder obscures the surgeon's field of vision, a stitch can be passed through the abdominal wall, through the posterior wall of the bladder and back out of the abdominal wall to temporarily suspend the bladder anteriorly. It is important to identify the ureters and the vas deferens bilaterally to avoid injury to these structures during the rectal dissection. As the rectum tapers into the fistula, it is clipped and transected distal to the clip. The fistula to the genitourinary tract is then closed with a 2/0 PDS endoscopic loop, or sutured with an absorbable laparoscopic suture. The rectogenitourinary fistula is divided at the most distal point without injuring or encroaching upon the genitourinary tract. Opening the rectal fistula to identify the position of the urethra can sometimes be helpful.

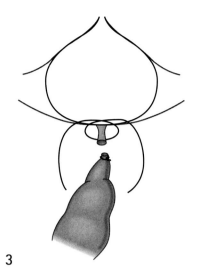

3

The rectum is then reflected cephalad and the pelvic floor is examined. The space from the apex of the pubococcygeus muscle extending posteriorly is identified and developed. This will be the space through which the rectum will be passed. The vas deferens medially points to the prostate, which aids the surgeon in locating the urethra so as to avoid inadvertently injuring it. The lateral attachments of the colon may need to be mobilized in order to allow the rectum to reach the perineum.

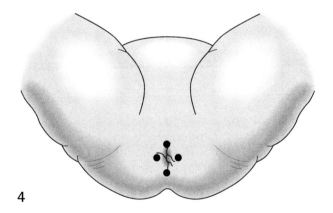

4

4 Attention is then turned to the perineum, where the center of the superficial anal sphincter is mapped with a muscle stimulator. The area of maximal contraction is marked at its anterior and posterior limits.

5 The patient's hips are flexed in such fashion that the knees are directed up to the patient's shoulders. This position straightens the path for the pull-through and neo-anus.

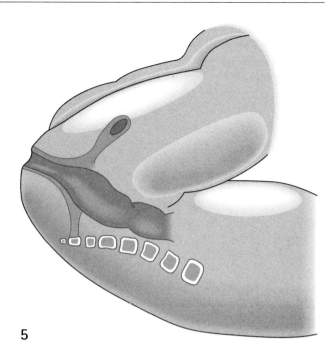

5

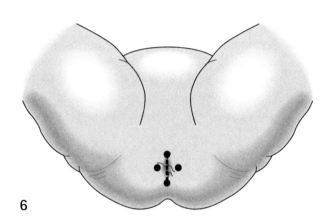

6

6 An 8-mm sagittal incision is made sharply in the center of the sphincter and the subcutaneous tissues are dissected bluntly, making every effort to stay in the midline. The laparoscopic transillumination is then seen at the site of perineal dissection and a 25-gauge, long needle is used to identify the correct tract for the pull-through, visualizing the needle laparoscopically from above.

7 Next, a radially dilating trocar is employed, to create the passage for the pull-through. The Veress needle and sheath are inserted under laparoscopic visualization, in the exact same axis that the finder needle had taken, pointing towards the apex of the 'V' of the pubococcygeus muscle, staying posterior to the urethra. The sheath is then dilated to a 12-mm port using the blunt trocars. A laparoscopic Babcock instrument is inserted through the perineal 12-mm port and the distal end of the rectum is grasped. The 12-mm perineal port, grasper, and rectum are gently pulled caudally, delivering the rectum through the sphincter complex to the perineal skin. The anastomosis is then fashioned with 4/0 Vicryl interrupted sutures. The neo-anus is calibrated with Hegar dilators and the size is recorded.

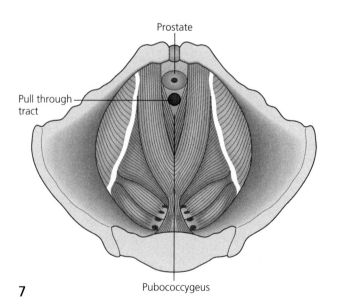

7

The abdominal cavity and pelvis are inspected laparoscopically for hemostasis, the pneumoperitoneum is released, and all the ports are removed. The linea alba at the level of the umbilical port is reapproximated with 2/0 Vicryl figure-of-eight suture and all the abdominal skin incisions are closed with a single horizontal mattress 5/0 chromic dermal suture. Steristrips are applied as a dressing to the abdominal incisions and polysporin to perineal incision.

Two- and three-stage procedure

TWO-STAGE REPAIR

The two-stage procedure involves neonatal repair and creation of neo-anus as described above, followed by the creation of a protecting descending colostomy. The second stage in this instance is closure of the colostomy.

THREE-STAGE REPAIR

A three-stage repair involves a preliminary colostomy performed in the neonatal period, followed by a pull-through several months later, and then closure of the colostomy as a third stage. There are several reasons for advocating a preliminary colostomy. First, the colon is often very dilated and full of meconium, which makes it difficult to dissect. Second, the creation of a stoma permits a contrast study to be done which can identify the location of the fistula to the urinary tract. Third, some surgeons prefer to do the pull-through when the child is larger and the anatomy may be clearer and the dissection easier.

The colostomy is fashioned once the diagnosis of a high anorectal malformation is confirmed, usually approximately 24 hours after birth. The colostomy may be done in the sigmoid, descending, or transverse colon, and can be a loop or a divided stoma. We prefer to do a divided stoma in the proximal sigmoid colon. Division of the stoma prevents spillover of stool with resultant dilatation of the distal rectum. The stoma must be done proximal enough that there will be adequate length to do the pull-through in the case of a proximal fistula to the urinary tract. The colostomy can be done in the left lower quadrant, left upper quadrant, or through the umbilicus, and can be done using a small incision or with a laparoscopic technique.

A thorough treatise on colostomy creation is available as a separate chapter in this volume (**Chapter 66**).

The second stage consists of the laparoscopic-assisted anorectal pull-through as described above, without closure of the colostomy. This is performed 4–6 weeks later. A distal contrast study through the colostomy or mucous fistula, and a simultaneous uretherogram should be performed preoperatively to define the anatomy of the fistula.

The third stage consists of closure of the colostomy, also detailed in **Chapter 66**. The colostomy closure is usually performed once the anus has been calibrated to the appropriate size, which usually requires an additional 4–6 weeks following the pull-through. A distal contrast study is often done prior to colostomy closure to ensure that there is no leak or recurrent fistula.

POSTOPERATIVE CARE

Following definitive repair and creation of the neo-anus, the urinary catheter is kept *in situ* for 5 days. The authors do not routinely obtain a vesicourethrogram before removing the catheter. If the catheter is inadvertently removed early, the patient is monitored for spontaneous passage of urine. The catheter should not be replaced blindly. If it becomes necessary to replace the catheter, this should be done under radiological guidance. The patient is maintained with intravenous fluids and bowel rest and is initiated on an oral diet once bowel function resumes. Postoperative antibiotics are not routinely administered. Postoperatively, the patient's perineum is monitored closely for perineal sepsis and the patient remains strictly nil per rectum for approximately 2 weeks. Furthermore, when the patient's perineum is exposed to feces for the first time, it is at high risk for contact dermatitis, which can be prevented with routine liberal application of a zinc-based protective barrier cream to the neo-anus and buttocks. Once the patient has resumed a full oral diet and is having bowel movements, or ostomy output, without difficulty, the patient is discharged to the community and is seen again in 2 weeks where the neo-anus is calibrated. The authors' preference is to continue with weekly dilatations in the surgeon's office, rather than have the parents perform dilatations at home, although many surgeons instruct the parents to dilate the neo-anus on a daily basis. Neo-anus size is directly dependent on age (**Table 58.1**). Once the desired neo-anus size and compliance is achieved, the dilatations are weaned.

Table 58.1 Age and Hegar size of neo-anus.

Age	Hegar size (mm diameter)
0–4 months	12
5–8 months	13
9–12 months	14
13–36 months	15
3–12 years	16
>12 years	17

59

Rectal biopsies

AUGUSTO ZANI and MARK DAVENPORT

INTRODUCTION

Hirschsprung's disease should be considered in neonates presenting with abdominal distension, delay in passage of meconium, and bile vomiting, and in older children with intractable constipation. Although the diagnosis may be suggested by a contrast enema showing the 'transitional zone' or by anorectal manometry, it can only be established with certainty by histologic examination of the affected, aganglionic bowel wall. This can be achieved most easily by obtaining a biopsy of the mucosa and, most importantly, the submucosa of the rectum.

RECTAL SUCTION BIOPSY

Principles and justification

Biopsy of the rectum using a suction biopsy tube is a common procedure in pediatric surgery and, especially in infants, has superseded the former techniques of open rectal biopsy and punch biopsy with a sigmoidoscope or speculum. The technique needs to be carried out with meticulous attention to detail in order to obtain a suitable diagnostic specimen of rectal mucosa with sufficient submucosa attached on each occasion. For this reason, the rectal suction biopsy (RSB) is not advised in children after three years of age, as it is less likely to provide adequate submucosa for identification of ganglion cells.

The procedure may be performed in the ward or clinic without anesthesia, and is painless provided it is taken at least 2.5 cm above the anal verge in the neonate and 3.5 cm in the older child (i.e. above the sensitive zone of the anal canal). It is general practice to give a prophylactic antibiotic, although there is no actual evidence base.

Preoperative care

It is advisable to perform a gentle bowel washout with 10 mL/kg of warm saline in order to increase the chance of success and decompress the bowel. No rectal manipulation should occur for the first 24 hours after RSB. In neonates, it is essential to confirm that vitamin K has been given.

Instrumentation

The original suction biopsy instrument was devised by Helen Noblett in 1969. Since then, some variants have been designed, including the Solo-RBT (SAMO Biomedica, Bologna, Italy) and the rbi2 (Aus Systems, Allenby Gardens, South Australia). Both instruments have a blunt-ended tube with a 3-mm side hole 2 cm from the tip (**Figs 59.1a** and **b**).

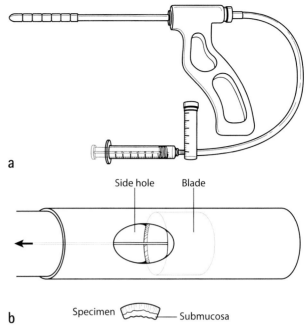

a

Side hole   Blade

b   Specimen   Submucosa

Figure 59.1

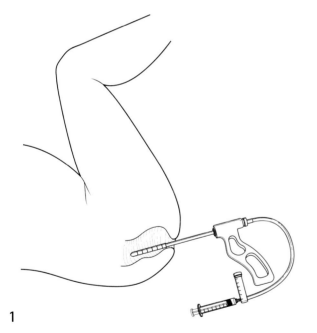

1

Operative technique

1 Infants are usually held in the lithotomy position, whereas the left lateral knees-bent position is more comfortable for older children. The lubricated instrument is inserted into the anus and the side hole positioned at 3 cm from the anal verge. This is the minimum distance and avoids the normal hypoganglionic zone and diagnostic confusion. The biopsy specimen should always be taken with the side hole facing the posterior or lateral walls of the rectum, because of the increased risk of perforation into the rectovesical or rectovaginal pouch of the peritoneal cavity if the biopsy is full thickness and anterior. It is advised to apply a gentle pressure on to the rectal wall in order to obtain an adequate sample.

Suction is then applied by withdrawing the syringe attached to the suction biopsy instrument to 3–5 mL (~150 cmH$_2$O). After 2–3 seconds, the knife is triggered. The syringe suction is released to neutral pressure before removing from the patient. The instrument is then withdrawn and the specimen removed. This is usually about 3 × 1 mm, and the critical submucosa can be recognized as a definite whitish layer. The procedure should then be repeated at 3.5 and 4 cm above the anal verge with between two and four specimens obtained.

The method of processing suction biopsies must be ascertained before the procedure, as dictated by specific laboratory requirements. Usually, fresh specimens are requested to carry out frozen sections. The biopsy material should be placed on a moistened filter paper or on wet gauze, as it is essential to avoid drying out during transport. The specimens must be marked with the level of collection. Although a presumptive diagnosis based on frozen sections is possible, definitive diagnosis usually requires a combination of paraffin section histology (conventional hematoxylin and eosin) and histochemistry (acetylcholinesterase). The diagnosis of Hirschsprung's disease is defined as an absence of ganglion cells in the submucosa, the presence of thick nerve trunks and marked acetylcholinesterase activity in the lamina propria. In previous times, acetylcholinesterase histochemistry has been one of the main methods used. However, a number of other techniques have been extensively reported in the literature and may well replace its use. These include neuron-specific enolase, nicotinamide adenine dinucleotide phosphate diaphorase (NADPH-d), α-naphtylesterase, succinic dehydrogenase (SDH), calretinin, peripherin, and S-100.

Postoperative care

A rectal examination should be carried out after completing the biopsy to exclude active bleeding. Observations should be continued for at least 2 hours, to ensure complete hemostasis.

Complications

The possible complications are as follows:

- **Inadequate specimen retrieval**. This has an occurrence rate of between 10 and 20 percent and is largely operator dependent, although newer single-use devices have improved this.
- **Perforation**. In one study, full thickness biopsies were identified histologically in 1 percent of 406 patients undergoing 1340 consecutive biopsies. Although these perforations can generally be treated conservatively with antibiotics, nasogastric suction, and intravenous fluid, a laparotomy may be needed.
- **Bleeding**. Some bleeding is to be expected usually immediately after the procedure post-biopsy, but this rarely requires blood transfusion or diathermy/stitching. Massive bleeding has been reported in the literature.
- **Pelvic sepsis**. This occurs as a result of perforation into the perirectal tissues.

OPEN RECTAL BIOPSY

Open rectal biopsy under general anesthesia is required when the specimen obtained with the RSB instrument is inadequate or the child is older.

Position

The infant is held in the lithotomy position while an older child will need to be placed in stirrups in the lithotomy position. Prophylactic antibiotics are given.

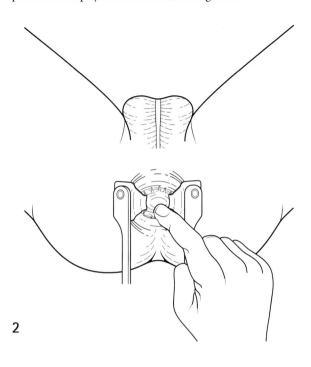

2

Procedure

2 The anal orifice is digitally dilated. It is held open either with a Parks' retractor (or similar self-retaining retractor) or by an assistant holding two small Langenbeck's retractors.

3 A stay suture is placed on the midline in the posterior rectal wall at least 2 cm above the dentate line. Applying traction on this stay suture, the operator places a further stay suture 2 cm higher, which is tied and the needle left intact. This is used to repair the defect once the specimen has been taken.

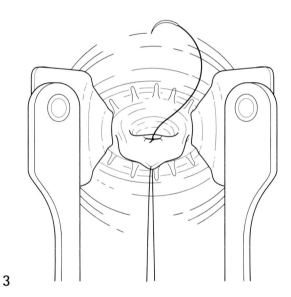

3

4 Using sharp-pointed scissors, a specimen comprising mucosa/submucosa or full thickness of the rectal wall is taken between the stay sutures.

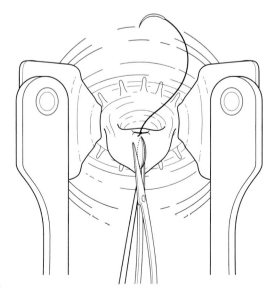

4

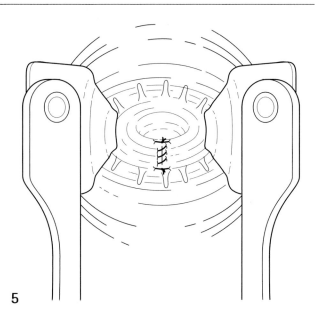

5 Hemostasis may be achieved with bipolar diathermy or, more usually, by suturing the defect with a running locking suture from above.

5

Complications

- Hemorrhage
- Infection

FURTHER READING

Alizai NK, Batcup G, Dixon MF *et al*. Rectal biopsy for Hirschsprung's disease: what is the optimum method? *Pediatric Surgery International* 1998; **13**: 121–4.

Croffie JM, Davis MM, Faught PR *et al*. At what age is a suction rectal biopsy less likely to provide adequate tissue for identification of ganglion cells? *Journal of Pediatric Gastroenterology and Nutrition* 2007; **44**: 198–202.

Hall NJ, Kufeji D, Keshtgar A. Out with the old and in with the new: a comparison of rectal suction biopsies with traditional and modern biopsy forceps. *Journal of Pediatric Surgery* 2009; **44**: 395–8.

Noblett HR. A rectal suction biopsy tube for use in the diagnosis of Hirschsprung's disease. *Journal of Pediatric Surgery* 1969; **4**: 406–9.

Pini Prato A, Martucciello G, Jasonni V. Solo-RBT: a new instrument for rectal suction biopsies in the diagnosis of Hirschsprung's disease. *Journal of Pediatric Surgery* 2001; **36**: 1364–6.

Rees BI, Azmy A, Nigam M *et al*. Complications of rectal suction biopsy. *Journal of Pediatric Surgery* 1983; **18**: 273–5.

60

Malone procedure (antegrade continence enemas) – open and laparoscopic

PADRAIG SJ MALONE and MUNTHER HADDAD

HISTORY

The ACE (antegrade continence enema) procedure is an established treatment for intractable fecal incontinence secondary to conditions such as spinal dysraphism and anorectal malformation. The successful use of the ACE has been described in numerous reports involving thousands of patients with follow up extending out to 20 years, and it has also been demonstrated that a successful ACE dramatically improves quality of life. Technical modifications which are illustrated in this chapter have been introduced over the years. It is no longer recommended to disconnect the appendix from the cecum as previously described, and the *in-situ* appendix is now the norm for the open ACE procedure. If no other procedure is required, a laparoscopic approach is recommended.

Where the appendix is absent or required for a simultaneous Mitrofanoff procedure, the Yang–Monti conduit is now the procedure of choice. The major ongoing complication associated with the ACE is stomal stenosis, which occurs in approximately 30 percent of patients, and this has led to a number of different techniques to construct the stoma.

PRINCIPLES AND JUSTIFICATION

The main indication for the procedure is fecal incontinence secondary to neuropathy and anorectal malformations which have not responded to conventional therapy. If an ACE is to be used for the treatment of chronic constipation, it may be best to site it in the left colon colonoscopically, as a clinical trial in the first instance. No child should have a colostomy without having the opportunity to consider the ACE as an alternative.

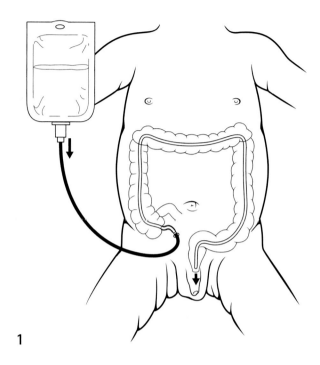

1 The ACE combines the principles of the Mitrofanoff continent, catheterizable conduit and antegrade colonic washout to produce a continent, catheterizable colonic stoma through which washouts are delivered to produce complete colonic emptying and thus prevent soiling.

1

PREOPERATIVE

Assessment and preparation

Motivation of children and their carers is essential for a successful outcome. Intensive counselling is required and it must be stressed that the ACE is not a 'magic' cure. A rigid, time-consuming regimen is required postoperatively and this is a lifelong commitment. A successful ACE takes approximately 45 minutes every day or on alternate days. Many children being considered for an ACE will also have a neuropathic bladder, and it is vital that management of the bladder is assessed simultaneously. In many cases, a combined lower urinary tract reconstruction and ACE is appropriate, and double continence rates have been reported in 79 percent of children with this approach. It is vital, therefore, to have a pediatric urologist involved in the assessment of these children and in the planning of the operative procedure. Investigations may include ultrasonography, renography, and videourodynamics. In the case of an isolated ACE, usually no special investigations

are required, but some authors recommend bowel transit studies to guide them as to where the conduit should be sited, in the cecum for isolated incontinence or in the left colon when performed for chronic constipation.

A preoperative full blood count is recommended, but cross-match is only required when a simultaneous bladder reconstruction is to be performed. For children with a neuropathic bladder or renal scarring, metabolic renal function should be assessed preoperatively. The author favors a 48-hour bowel preparation program using sodium picosulfate and rectal washouts, together with a 5-day course of antibiotics, such as co-amoxiclav. As the child loses a great deal of fluid with the bowel preparation, an intravenous infusion is administered on the night prior to surgery.

ANESTHESIA

The operation is performed under general anesthesia, but there are no special requirements.

OPERATION

Incisions

2 When an isolated ACE is performed, a laparoscopic approach is now recommended, but if an antireflux valve is to be created, a right or left lower quadrant muscle-cutting incision is used. A midline incision is better if a simultaneous bladder reconstruction is being carried out. For a cecal ACE, it is usually possible to site the stoma in the umbilicus, but for a left-sided conduit, the stoma is usually sited in the left lower quadrant. For patients who are wheelchair-bound, it may be necessary to site the stoma on the upper abdomen for ease of access.

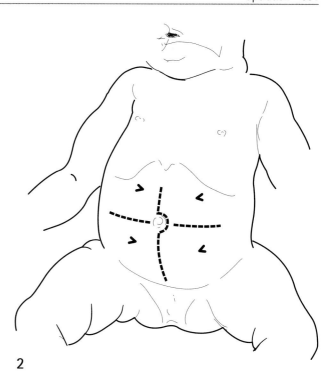

2

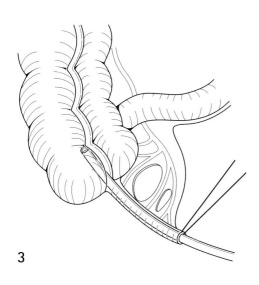

3

CREATION OF CECAL SUBMUCOSAL TUNNEL

4 A trough down to the submucosa is created along a tenia by a combination of sharp and blunt dissection. As the trough approaches the base of the appendix, a V-shaped incision is created around approximately 60 percent of its circumference; this allows the base of the appendix to be folded into the cecum without kinking. There is no need for a wide trough, as it is not planned to bury the appendix in it, it is simply there to fix the appendix when the cecum is wrapped around it.

The in situ appendix ACE

PREPARATION OF THE APPENDIX

3 The cecum is mobilized, the tip of the appendix is amputated, and a stay suture is inserted and the appendix stretched to reveal the mesentery. The mesentery is fenestrated between the vessels, as this allows the cecum to be wrapped around the appendix without compromising the blood supply. A 12 Fr catheter is passed through the appendix into the cecum.

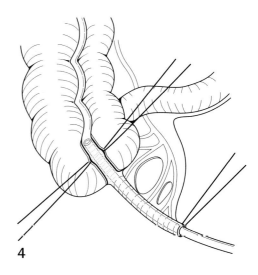

4

WRAPPING THE CECUM AROUND THE APPENDIX

5a–c The appendix is folded over on to the exposed submucosa and the cecum is loosely wrapped around the appendix through the fenestrations in the mesentery using a 4/0 polyglycolic acid suture. The suture picks up the seromuscular layer on the cecum on each side and the appendix to anchor it in the tunnel. The wrap is continued until only a short length of appendix sticks out from the tunnel. The stoma is then ready to be created. It is important to anchor the cecum to the back of the anterior abdominal wall where the appendix emerges to prevent twisting and kinking of the conduit.

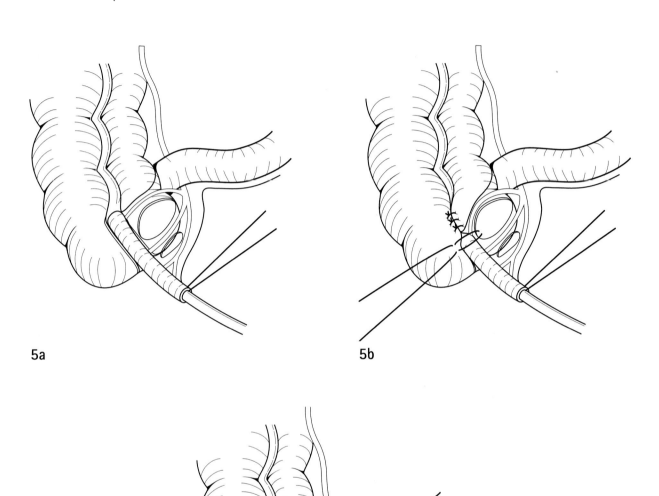

5a

5b

5c

Simultaneous Mitrofanoff procedure/absent appendix

SPLIT APPENDIX

6 When both a Mitrofanoff and ACE are required and the appendix is of sufficient length, it can be divided into two, provided the vascular anatomy is favorable. The ACE uses the *in-situ* technique as described above, and the distal end of the appendix is available for the Mitrofanoff.

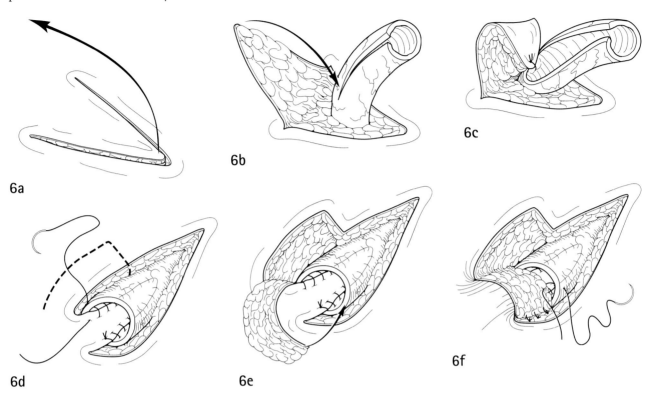

6a

6b

6c

6d

6e

6f

THE YANG–MONTI PROCEDURE

7 This technique can be used to create a conduit that can then be implanted into the colon at any site to create the ACE. It can be used when the appendix is absent and it is also used for a left-sided ACE. A 2-cm segment of ileum is isolated on its vascular pedicle. Bowel continuity is restored by a standard end-to-end anastomosis. The ileum is opened along the anti-mesenteric border. It can then be seen that the valvulae coniventes are now running in a longitudinal direction along the length of the bowel. The bowel is then tubularized over a 12 Fr catheter by a single-layer, interrupted, extramucosal anastomosis using 6/0 PDS suture. One end is then implanted into a submucosal tenial tunnel in the colon and the other is brought to the skin as the stoma.

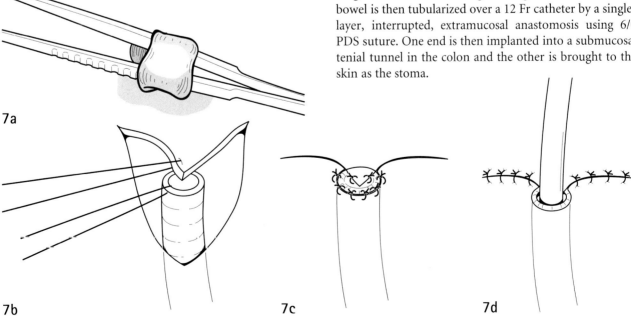

7a

7b

7c

7d

CREATION OF COLONIC SUBMUCOSAL TUNNEL

8 A tenia is stretched using proximal, distal, and two lateral stay sutures. The seromuscular layer of the tenia is incised with a scalpel down to the submucosa over a 5 cm length. The mucosa/submucosa is then freed from the overlying muscle using a combination of sharp and blunt dissection to leave an exposed strip of mucosa approximately 1 cm in width.

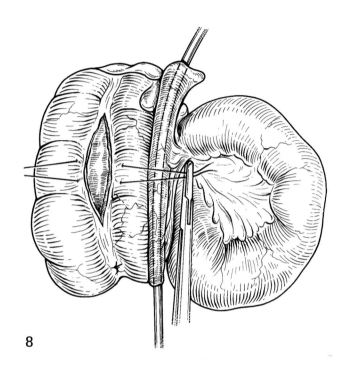

8

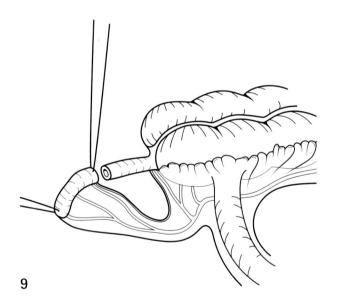

9

MONTI–MUCOSAL ANASTOMOSIS

9 A small hole is punched in the mucosa of the colon using artery forceps. This is usually placed at the distal end of the mucosal tunnel. The mucosa is anastomosed to the full thickness of the Monti tube using a 5/0 polyglycolic acid suture over the catheter in the conduit.

CLOSURE OF THE SEROMUSCULAR TUNNEL

10 The seromuscular wall of the colon is closed over the Monti tube using interrupted 4/0 polyglycolic acid sutures picking up partial thickness of the conduit wall to prevent it slipping out of the tunnel. (See also Figure 7a in Chapter 86.)

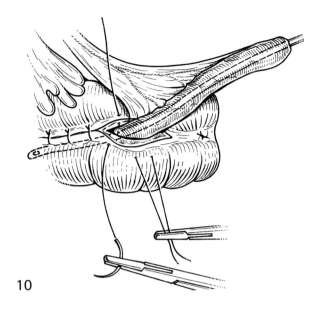

10

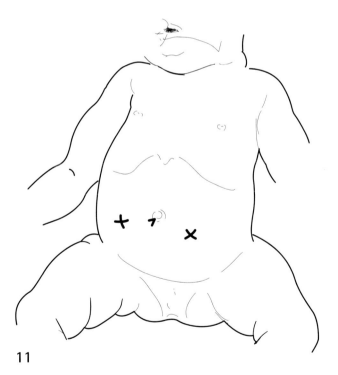

11

LAPAROSCOPIC ACE

11 In laparoscopic ACE (LACE), a 5-mm port is inserted at the umbilicus under direct vision. Two further 5-mm ports are inserted in both iliac fossae. The cecum is mobilized so the appendix can reach the umbilicus. The camera port is changed and the appendix is grasped with forceps and simply delivered through the umbilical port site, where a stoma is then created. The author does not usually create an antireflux valve during this procedure, and although leakage from the conduit is more common than when a valve is created, it is still not a common problem.

Percutaneous endoscopic colonic tube placement

12a–e Suction is then applied to the maximum of –300 cm H_2O by drawing on a 10 ml syringe attached to the suction tubing. A needle and thread is passed into the colon, grasped, and delivered through the anus. This is attached to a gastrostomy tube, which is pulled up into the colon until the flange on the tube pulls the colon to the abdominal wall. The tube is fixed externally to the abdominal wall and washouts can be commenced the following day. After a trial, if the ACE works, the patient has a choice of keeping the tube, changing to a button, or having a conduit constructed.

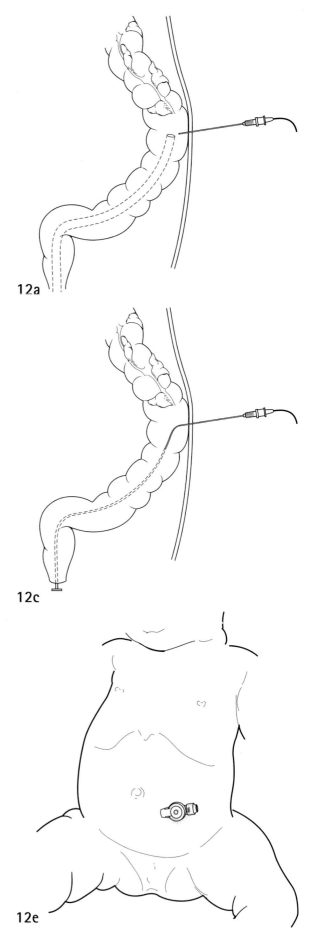

12a

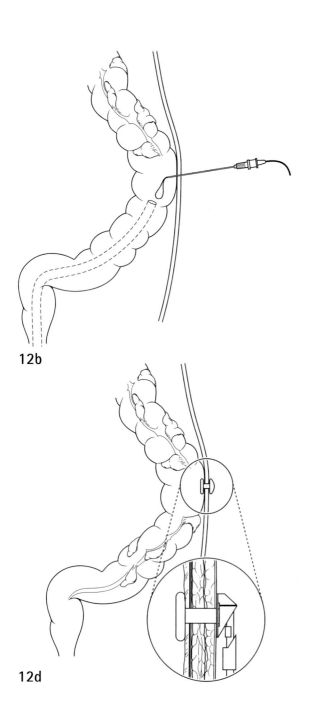

12b

12c

12d

12e

Fashioning the stoma

ABDOMINAL VQC STOMA

13a–g Two skin flaps (V and rectangular) are created at the site of the stoma. A hole is created in the abdominal wall that is sufficiently wide to allow the conduit to pass through freely. The cecum or colon is sutured to the anterior abdominal wall to prevent tension on the stoma or volvulus of the bowel on the conduit. The conduit is fish-mouthed and the apex of the V-flap is sutured into the defect using 5/0 Maxon™ sutures with the knots outside the catheterizing channel. The V-flap is gradually sutured into the defect until approximately 50 percent of the circumference of the conduit is complete. The rectangular flap is then sutured over the anterior circumference of the conduit until the anastomosis is complete. The resulting skin defect is closed in layers using 4/0 Maxon and 5/0 subcuticular polyglycolic acid sutures, resulting in a C-shaped wound (VQC stoma). A 12 Fr Silastic Foley catheter is left *in situ* for 4 weeks after the surgery prior to commencing catheterization.

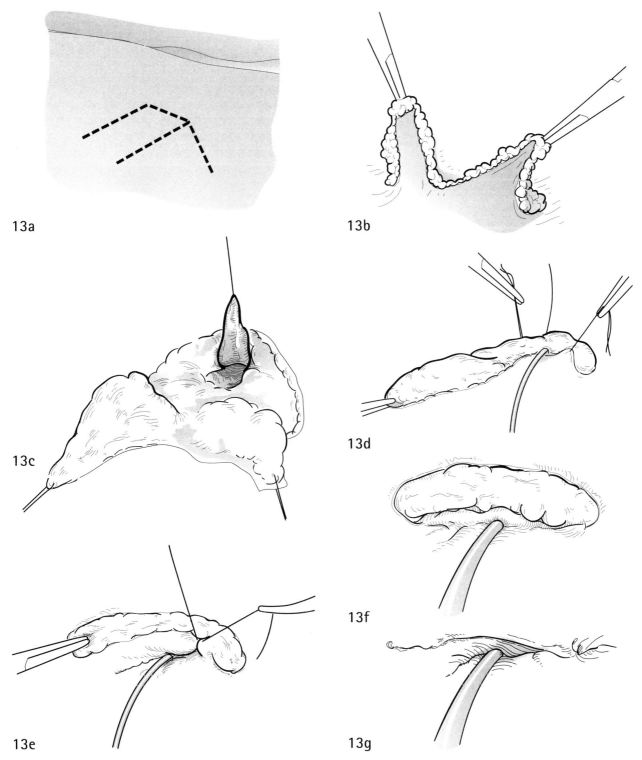

13a

13b

13c

13d

13e

13f

13g

UMBILICAL STOMA

14a–c The umbilicus is everted and a V-flap is created from the everted skin. This is sutured into the conduit as described above, and the remainder of the anastomosis is completed by suturing the conduit to the umbilical rim.

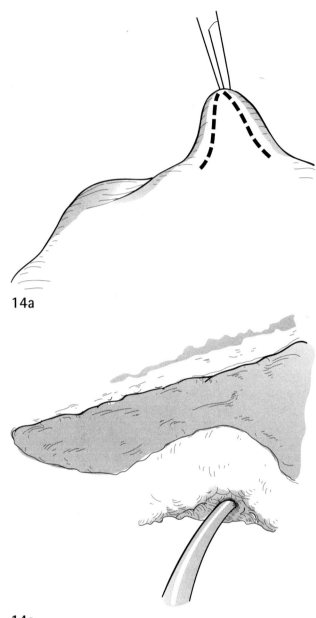

14a

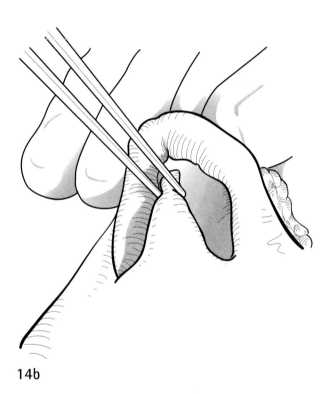

14b

14c

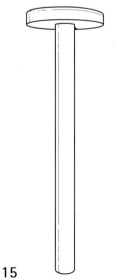

15

THE ACE STOPPER

15 Despite the improvement in stoma stenosis rates with the operative modifications described above, stenosis remains the most common complication. This led to the development of the ACE stopper. ACE stoppers are now commercially available in varying sizes, 10–14 FG diameters and 15–100 mm lengths (Medicina, Bolton, UK), and these are very helpful for patients who experience ongoing catheterization problems. The authors now leave this *in situ* for three months following the creation of the ACE and it has produced a further significant reduction in stenosis rates.

POSTOPERATIVE CARE

Following an isolated ACE, enteral feeding can commence the following day, and the first washout can be administered when the patient has recovered from the adynamic ileus. Once the child and carers are happy with the enema procedure, the child can be discharged with the indwelling catheter, to return 4 weeks later to learn intermittent catheterization, which seldom takes longer than 48 hours. An ACE stopper should be left *in situ* for a further three months.

A standard 12 Fr Nelaton catheter is used for washouts. The patient should be given some 8 Fr and 10 Fr catheters, because if catheterization becomes difficult, the smaller catheters can be used initially to help dilate the stoma. If severe stomal stenosis develops, dilatation under general anesthesia is recommended, following which a stopper can be left *in situ* for a period to reduce the risk of a further stenosis. Occasionally, stoma revision is required, and this usually takes the form of a Y–V plasty.

ENEMA REGIMENS

There is no single correct enema regimen, and each patient develops an individual practice by trial and error. The author starts with 1 mL/kg of phosphate enema (Fletchers' phosphate; Fleet Pharmaceuticals, Zaragoza, Spain) diluted to half-strength with an equal volume of tap water or normal saline. This is followed by a washout of tap water of between 10 and 20 mL/kg. A daily enema is given for the first few months, but after that about half the patients use the washouts on alternate days or, rarely, even less frequently than that.

Initially, many patients experience colicky abdominal pain, and this may be helped by reducing the concentration of the phosphate and the rate of enema infusion. If colic is persistent, the administration of mebeverine hydrochloride 30 minutes before the enema can help. Persistent pain may also be caused by constipation, and this can be managed by the administration of mineral oil via the ACE 4–6 hours prior to the washout.

If the enema does not produce a rapid result, the concentration of the phosphate can be increased in steps up to a full-strength enema, and in some patients this is used without a following washout. Most patients continue to use a washout, but if fecal leakage occurs between enemas, the volume can be reduced or increased and this usually resolves the problem.

Phosphate toxicity has been encountered, particularly in younger patients, and it is of vital importance that if there is no response from the enema after 6 hours, no further phosphate is administered until a result is obtained. Further washouts with tap water often help, but occasionally retrograde washouts are required.

ADMINISTERING ANTEGRADE COLONIC ENEMAS

Most patients use an infusion system such as a Kangaroo bag and pump set (Kendall, Tullamore, Ireland). The bag is filled with the required phosphate and infused over a 10-minute period. The bag is then refilled with water and infused over the next 15 minutes. Evacuation usually starts within 15 minutes and is complete 30 minutes later. As patients will spend a considerable time sitting on the toilet, the use of padded seat covers is recommended to reduce the risk of pressure sores.

COMPLICATIONS

The common complications and their management are discussed in the text. Uncommon complications include leakage of fecal fluid through the stoma, and if this occurs, the valve mechanism will need to be revised or a valve created, if this had not been done in the first instance.

OUTCOME

For patients with neuropathic conditions and anorectal malformations, the success rate of ACE procedures is 80–90 percent.

FURTHER READING

Chait PG, Shandling B, Richards HM. The cecostomy button. *Journal of Paediatric Surgery* 1997; **32**: 849–51.

Churchill BM, De Ugarte DA, Atkinson JB. Left-colon antegrade continence enema (LACE) procedure for fecal incontinence. *Journal of Paediatric Surgery* 2003; **38**: 1778–80.

Curry JL, Osborne A, Malone PS. How to achieve a successful Malone antegrade continence enema. *Journal of Paediatric Surgery* 1998; **33**: 138–41.

Gerharz EW, Vik V, Webb G, Woodhouse CRJ. The *in situ* appendix in the Malone antegrade continence enema procedure for faecal incontinence. *British Journal of Urology* 1997; **79**: 985–6.

Griffin SJ, Parkinsin EJ, Malone PSJ. Bowel management for paediatric patients with faecal incontinence. *Journal of Pediatric Urology* 2008; **4**: 387–92.

Monti PR, Lara RC, Dutra MA *et al.* New techniques for construction of efferent conduits based on the Mitrofanoff principle. *Urology* 1997; **49**: 112–15.

Wedderburn A, Lee RS, Denny A *et al.* Synchronous bladder reconstruction and antegrade continence enema. *Journal of Urology* 2001; **165**: 2392–3.

61

Hirschsprung disease

DANIEL H TEITELBAUM and ARNOLD G CORAN

PRINCIPLES AND JUSTIFICATION

Advances in our understanding of the embryogenesis and surgical care of Hirschsprung disease have advanced considerably over the past decade. Despite our increased knowledge of the disease, significant complications continue to be associated with this process. One must maintain a high degree of suspicion for the disease. Suction rectal biopsy and anal manometry studies have allowed for easier and less invasive methods of establishing the diagnosis; however, obtaining details of the infant's history is the most important first step. Failure to pass meconium within the first 48 hours of life, complaints of constipation and, finally, symptoms of enterocolitis should always be followed by a complete clinical examination for Hirschsprung disease.

The classic approach to the neonate diagnosed with Hirschsprung disease had been to perform a leveling colostomy and to wait until 6–12 months of age to perform the definitive pull-through. This approach has changed dramatically over the past three decades, and transition to primary pull-through is now predominant. Use of laparoscopy to facilitate both the diagnosis and the pull-through procedure has also become common. The transanal approach is now used by a large proportion of pediatric surgeons, and is discussed in this chapter.

FULL-THICKNESS RECTAL BIOPSY

Suction rectal biopsy, because of its relative ease and low morbidity, has become the most established diagnostic tool for Hirschsprung disease. Nevertheless, full-thickness rectal biopsies are occasionally required, and the technique of full-thickness biopsy is presented here to assist surgeons who are not familiar with the procedure. Perhaps the most common indication for a full-thickness biopsy is the child who has undergone more than one indeterminate suction rectal biopsy. Another indication is the older child whose mucosa is so thick that an adequate biopsy of the submucosa cannot be obtained using a suction method.

Preoperative

No formal bowel preparation is required. The child's rectum is irrigated with saline or very dilute povidone-iodine solution. A sponge is placed into the proximal rectal vault to prevent stool from entering the operative field. One dose of preoperative antibiotics is given. The child is placed in Trendelenburg to prevent spillage of stool into the operative field.

Operative technique

1 The patient is placed in the lithotomy position with the buttocks at the very end of the bed, supported with a folded towel. The feet are placed together (plantar surfaces adjoined) with a cotton roll, and both legs are suspended on an ether screen, or similar device. Flexion at the hips facilitates exposure.

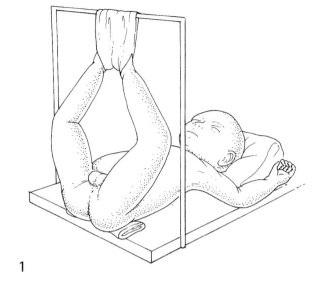

1

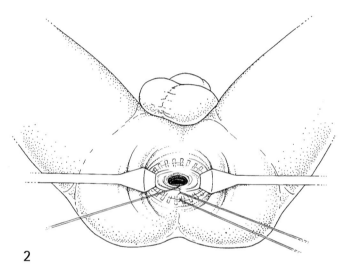

2

2 Digital dilatation is followed by placement of two narrow anal retractors. The superior aspect of the dentate line is identified and marked with a polyglactin suture (3/0), which is used for traction. Two additional polyglactin sutures are placed on the posterior wall of the rectum at 1 and 2 cm proximal to the dentate line. Retain the needle on the most cephalad of these sutures, as it can be used to begin the closure of the defect after the biopsy is obtained.

3 The surgeon's non-dominant hand holds the middle suture. Using sharp curved scissors, a full-thickness incision is made along the lower half of the rectal wall, between the dentate line and the middle suture. Once this is done, the scissors can be placed in the presacral space and gently spread. Bleeding can slightly obstruct the view at this point; however, by maintaining traction on the middle suture, the upper half of the rectum is incised with two smooth cuts of the scissors, each sweeping around one-half of the tissue suspended by the middle suture. The specimen is inspected and delivered off the table.

The rectal defect is closed in a single, full thickness running or interrupted layer with an absorbable suture (e.g. 4/0 polyglactin (Vicryl). Hemostasis is achieved fairly quickly once this suture has been placed.

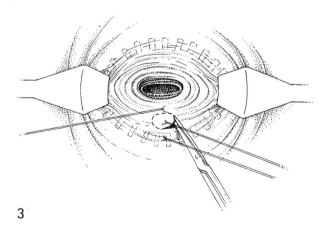

3

LEVELING COLOSTOMY

Although a primary pull-through is preferred in most infants, use of a leveling colostomy is required in infants presenting with a severe episode of enterocolitis at the time of diagnosis. A colostomy is also required in those patients with a delayed diagnosis of Hirschsprung disease, where the colon has become overly distended and not amenable to a primary pull-through. Although a right transverse colostomy has been advocated by some surgeons as the initial procedure, the authors prefer a leveling colostomy. This allows for the determination of the aganglionic level at the time of the colostomy, facilitating the subsequent pull-through. In addition, placement of a leveling colostomy allows the proximal bowel to grow, which will stretch the mesentery and simplify the subsequent pull-through procedure. Finally, this colostomy can be closed during the pull-through, thus avoiding a third operation. Placement of the ostomy is just proximal to the transition zone.

The incision is generally an oblique one in the left lower quadrant. If the level of aganglionosis is not readily apparent, this incision can be extended transversely across the midline. Use of laparoscopy, with serial seromuscular biopsies, has greatly facilitated the determination of the level of aganglionosis. This allows the surgeon to place the colostomy in the most optimal site.

Preoperative

Essentially, only the diagnosis of Hirschsprung disease is needed. Most diagnoses can be suspected based on the history alone, but confirmation is required by histopathologic examination of a suction rectal biopsy. The infant should receive rectal washouts and be placed on broad-spectrum, intravenous antibiotics just prior to the incision, but no formal bowel preparation is required or effective.

Operative technique

4 Once the peritoneum is entered, an attempt should be made to define a gross transition zone. The bowel proximal to the transition zone is normally dilated and has a diffuse hypertrophy of the muscular layer with no clearly distinguishable tenea. In neonates, such a transition often may not be seen. If this is the case, a good starting point is just above the peritoneal reflection.

A pair of fine, sharp scissors is used to make an incision only through the seromuscular layers. The muscular layer, which is fairly thick, even in the aganglionic section, makes this dissection fairly easy. Blunt dissection is used to strip off the muscle. In general, a 1×0.5-cm biopsy specimen is taken and interrupted silk or polyglactin sutures are placed to close the biopsy site.

Each biopsy specimen is sent for frozen section, progressively moving more proximally until both ganglion cells, as well as a loss of hypertrophied nerve bundles, are seen. Hypertrophied nerve bundles, despite the presence of ganglia, indicate that one is still in the transition zone. Another biopsy specimen should be taken several centimeters more proximally. Importantly, the transition zone varies from the anti-mesenteric and mesenteric sides of the bowel. Thus, the surgeon must confirm this correct level by sending a frozen section on the mesenteric side of the colon as well.

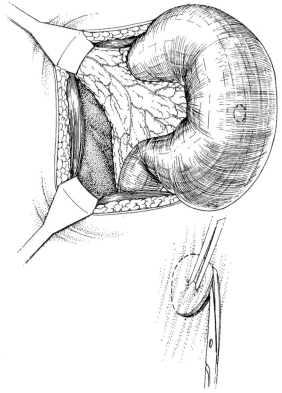

4

5 At this point, a loop colostomy can often be created at one of the normal biopsy sites. Because of the relatively large caliber of the bowel, stomal prolapse and peristomal hernias are common complications. It is extremely important to begin the colostomy by placing numerous fine polyglactin sutures both to the peritoneum as well as to the fascia. A stitch is placed between the proximal and distal loops of bowel, starting at the fascia, then to each limb of bowel, and finally back to the fascia. A portion of the fascia may be closed in the mid-portion of the defect between intestinal segments.

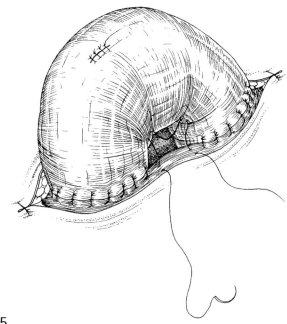

5

Postoperative care

The stoma usually begins to function within 24 hours, and feeding can begin shortly thereafter. It is occasionally helpful to perform intermittent dilatations of the proximal ostomy. These dilatations will prevent narrowing of the opening and allow the dilated proximal colon to return to normal size.

OPERATIONS

Duhamel

The Duhamel technique was advanced in 1956 to avoid the tedious pelvic dissection of the Swenson procedure, and to protect the nervi erigenti, which may be found lateral and anterior to the rectum. The procedure has undergone several modifications, the most important of which was by Martin and included the use of an automatic stapling device. It is fairly straightforward and continues to be popular today. Despite its relative simplicity, several key technical points must be followed.

As with other pull-through procedures, ganglionic bowel is brought down to less than 1 cm proximal to the dentate line. To preserve the autonomic nerve plexus to the genitourinary system, very little manipulation of the rectum is performed anteriorly.

The operation is generally performed when the child is 6–12 months of age with a weight of 10 kg. With the use of smaller endostapling devices, the procedure may also be performed primarily in the newborn period.

PREOPERATIVE

The child is admitted the day before the surgery for a mechanical bowel preparation as well as oral antibiotics. More recently, based on lack of evidence supporting its use, our group and others have deferred from the use of a bowel prep. Care must be taken to give adequate rectal and colonic washouts, as stool is often inspissated in the distal rectum. It is necessary to do a rectal examination on the child before the pull-through to ensure that no residual stool is present. Preoperative broad spectrum antibiotics should be given just prior to the skin incision.

OPERATIVE TECHNIQUE

6 A nasogastric tube is placed after induction of anesthesia. The child is placed in a supine position and prepared circumferentially from the abdomen to the feet. Stockinettes are placed around each foot and a Foley catheter is inserted in the bladder after the patient has been prepared and draped. Excellent exposure is obtained by assistants supporting and flexing the lower extremities at the hips during the anal anastomosis. Alternatively, the child can be placed in stirrups or on skis. A hockey-stick or oblique incision is made incorporating the colostomy (if present). The bowel is mobilized proximal to the former colostomy and the splenic flexure is brought down, if necessary, to ensure adequate length for the pull-through. In general, the ganglionated colon must reach just below the level of the perineum when drawn over the child's pubic symphysis with only modest tension. Occasionally, the mesentery is foreshortened and it is necessary to ligate the inferior mesenteric artery near the aortic root. By preserving the remainder of the arcades, the bowel should maintain its viability. The ureter is carefully identified and the peritoneal reflection between the rectum and bladder is incised. The distal rectum is mobilized for approximately 4 cm below the reflection. The colostomy site, if present, is removed with an automatic stapling device.

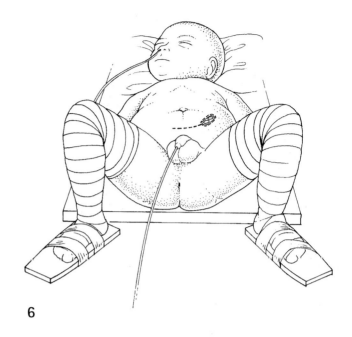

6

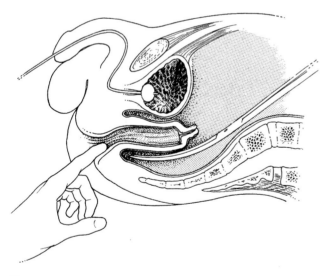

7

7 A retrorectal space is created, with dissection carried out directly in the midline. This dissection is carried down to the pelvic floor so that an assistant's finger can be felt when inserted no further than 1–1.5 cm into the anus. Dissection can be facilitated by a blunt clamp, but is also very easily performed with the index finger.

8 Once the retrorectal dissection has been completed, redundant aganglionic bowel is resected down to the peritoneal reflection with an automatic stapling device. Tacking sutures are placed on both left and right sides of the bowel so that it can be retracted anteriorly during the pull-through procedure.

The distal end of the ganglionic bowel is labeled mesenteric and antimesenteric with a separate polypropylene and polyglactin suture. This allows the surgeon working on the pulled-through segment to maintain correct orientation of the bowel as it is pulled into the anus.

At this point, the surgeon's attention is directed to the perineum. If not placed into skis, both the patient's legs are drawn upward, allowing a clear view of the anus. Narrow anal retractors are placed and held in position by the two assistants still working on the abdomen. No separate field is created, which allows improved communication and keeps surgeon and assistant on the same operative field. The authors have not found it necessary to have two completely different set-ups. However, all the instruments used in the perineal portion of the procedure are treated as dirty, and gloves are changed at the end of the anastomosis.

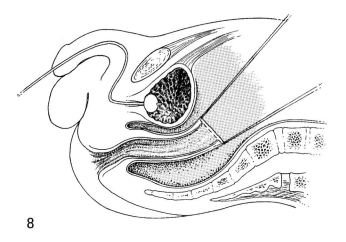

8

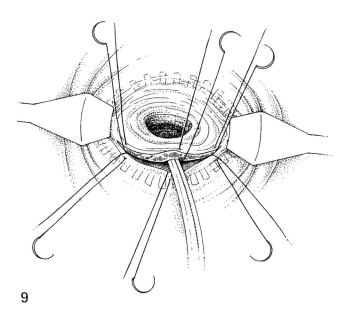

9

9 With the use of cautery, a full-thickness incision is made 0.5 cm proximal to the dentate line posteriorly. Care is taken to maintain this distance by curving the incision as one moves laterally in each direction. Three 4/0 undyed polyglactin sutures are placed on the inferior aspect of this incision, one in the midline and one each on the left and right sides. Three additional absorbable sutures (4/0 dyed polyglactin) are placed on the upper portion of this incision in similar positions. Needles are placed into the defect created by the incision and are retained for the initiation of the anastomosis. Each suture is held in position with hemostats. The different colored sutures prevent confusion of orientation once the ganglionic bowel is pulled through.

The surgeon operating on the anus inserts a long clamp into the retrorectal space towards the abdominal field.

10 The two tacking sutures on the distal ganglionic bowel are fed into this clamp and pulled down. The surgeon remaining in the abdominal field guides the bowel, and makes sure that it does not rotate as it is brought down.

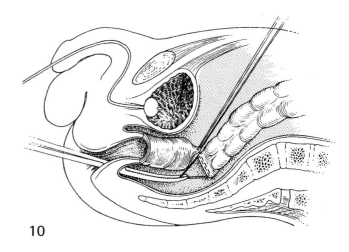

10

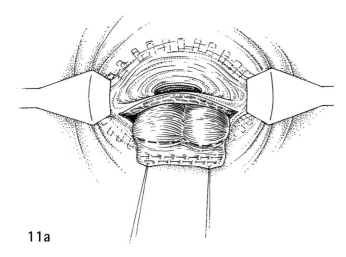

11a

11a,b Once the bowel is pulled through, the staple line is excised on the anterior half of the colon and a single-layered anastomosis is created, starting with the three previously placed polyglactin sutures. Care is taken with each stitch so that the anterior wall of the anus is not incorporated into any of the sutures.

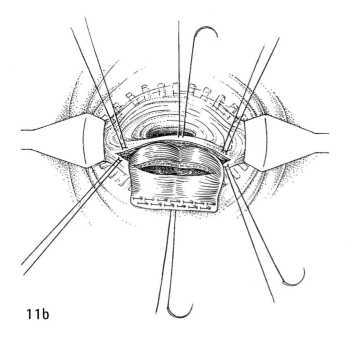

11b

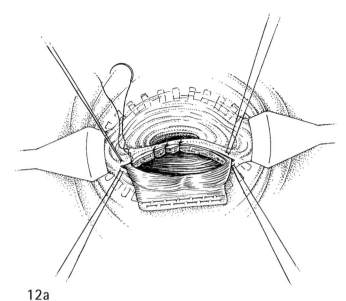

12a

12a,b Once the anterior half of the anastomosis is completed, the remainder of the staple line is excised, one quarter at a time, and the anastomosis is finished.

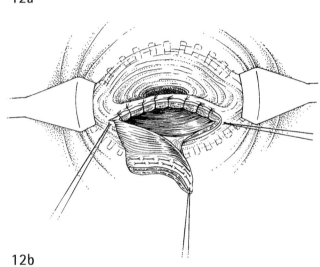

12b

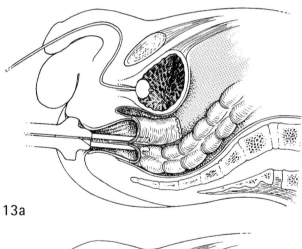

13a

13a,b An automatic stapling device is placed with one arm into the native anal canal and the other into the neorectum. The stapler is fired directly in the midline. Hemostasis along the suture line is checked. In general, a long (80 mm with 3.5 mm staples) device is preferred; a smaller endostapler is used in newborns.

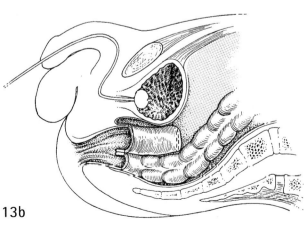

13b

14 Often a complete anastomosis between the ganglionic and aganglionic bowel cannot be achieved with a single staple application from below. A second firing from the abdomen will be necessary. The staple line of the remaining aganglionic rectum is opened and a small enterotomy is made in the ganglionic colon at a similar level. The abdominal surgeon places a reloaded automatic stapler between the two limbs of bowel to complete the anastomosis. This last step is critical. In the past, a proximal spur left between the bowel segments caused the eventual formation of huge fecalomas. It is critical for the surgeon to inspect the anastomosis digitally and make sure that the two limbs of bowel are completely anastomosed.

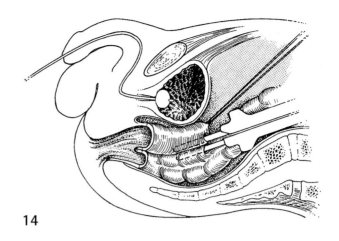

14

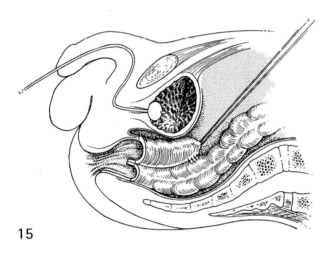

15

15 The anastomosis is completed by suturing the proximal end of the aganglionic rectum to the enterotomy in the ganglionic colon in two layers. The neorectum may or may not be reperitonealized, and the abdomen is closed.

Endorectal pull-through (Soave)

The Soave or endorectal pull-through was popularized by Franco Soave at the Institute G Gaslini in 1955. The procedure was modified by Boley by performing a primary anastomosis at the anus, and then further modified by Coran. This procedure is the most popular one used at the authors' institute, and has been further modified to facilitate the suturing of the anal anastomosis. The operation is now most commonly performed in the newborn period, with the complication rate being identical to that seen with the standard two-staged approach. Over the past decade, the operation has been performed with laparoscopic assistance and via a transanal route.

As with the Duhamel technique, this procedure avoids injury to the pelvic nerves and, by remaining within the muscular wall of the aganglionic segment, important sensory fibers and the integrity of the internal sphincter are preserved. Although one imagines that leaving aganglionic muscle surrounding normal bowel could lead to a high incidence of constipation, this is generally not the case.

PREOPERATIVE

Even in the neonatal period, serial rectal washouts and digital dilatations of the rectum are performed before beginning the pull-through, the last of the rectal irrigations containing 1 percent neomycin. Intravenous antibiotics are given before the beginning of surgery and are continued for two doses after surgery.

OPEN OPERATIVE TECHNIQUE

16 The child is placed in a supine position, with the buttocks brought to the end of the operating table, and propped slightly up with a folded towel. The legs are carefully padded and placed on wooden skis extending off the end of the table. A Foley catheter is placed after the entire field is prepared and draped. The operating table is placed in a slightly Trendelenberg position. A hockey-stick incision is made incorporating the leveling colostomy (if present). The same type of incision is made, however, for infants undergoing a primary pull-through operation. The level of aganglionosis is established by frozen section.

Ganglionic bowel is mobilized proximally and then transected above the transition level with a stapling device. The distal colon is mobilized and resected to about 4 cm above the peritoneal reflection. Traction sutures are placed on either end of the distal bowel. The endorectal dissection is then started about 2 cm below the peritoneal reflection.

The authors have progressively shortened the length of the endorectal dissection, because longer lengths of muscular cuff may lead to increased bouts of constipation and enterocolitis.

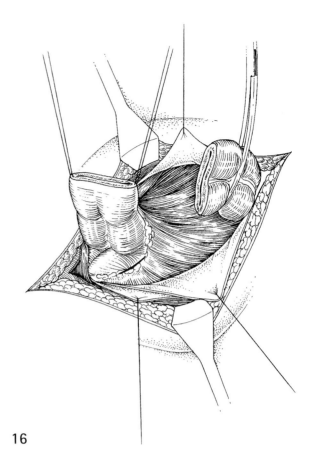

16

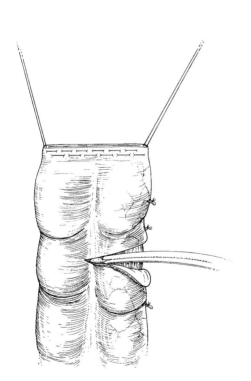

17

17 The endorectal dissection usually begins by completely clearing the serosa, mesentery, and fat over a 2 cm length of bowel. The seromuscular layer is incised with either sharp dissection or Bovie cautery. Once the submucosal layer is reached, the seromuscular layer is divided circumferentially using blunt dissection with hemostat or a Kitner dissector. In the neonatal period, a cotton-tip applicator is the most effective tool for this dissection.

18 After the plane is established, it is continued distally and facilitated by an assistant pulling upward on the already dissected mucosal/submucosal tube for countertraction. As the muscular cuff begins to develop, traction sutures are also placed in the muscle, one in each quadrant. Larger communicating vessels are coagulated; however, the majority of these are not cauterized during the dissection without resultant significant blood loss, particularly in the neonatal period. Dissection is carried down to within 1.5 cm of the anal opening in older children and approximately 1 cm in neonates.

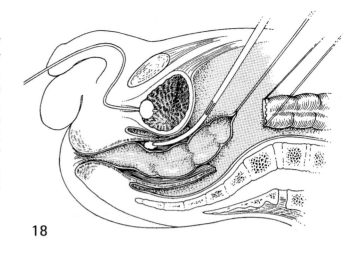

18

Some have advocated performing part of the endorectal dissection from the transanal approach, but the authors strongly advise against this if the dissection is started within the abdominal cavity. Once the endorectal dissection is started, it can proceed in a straightforward fashion. With appropriate traction and countertraction, the entire dissection can be performed in a child (and adult) of almost any size.

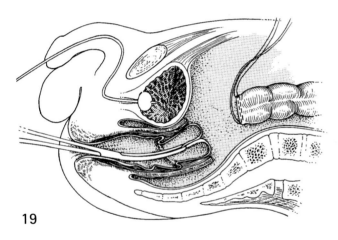

19

19 One of the surgeons then moves to the foot of the table. Narrow retractors (phrenic or army–navy) are placed at the anal mucocutaneous junction and a ring or Kelly clamp is inserted into the rectum. An assistant at the abdominal field places the end of the mucosal/submucosal tube into the clamp. The segment is then everted onto the perineum. The end of the everted tube is placed in a clamp and held on traction by an assistant to facilitate the anastomosis.

20 The mucosal/submucosal tube is incised on the anterior half, 0.5–1 cm above the dentate line.

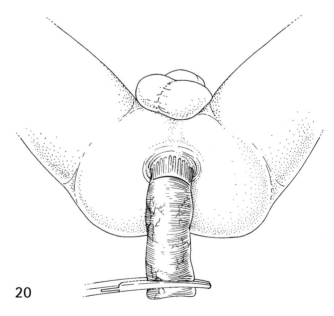

20

21 A Kelly clamp is inserted into this opening and the ganglionic bowel is brought down to this point by grasping the two previously placed traction sutures. Great care is taken not to twist the bowel as it is brought through the muscular cuff. As with the Duhamel procedure, different colored sutures on each side of the bowel are helpful in maintaining orientation.

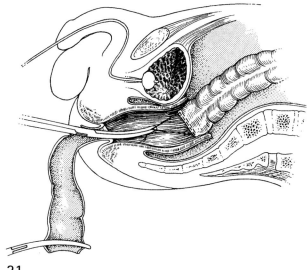

21

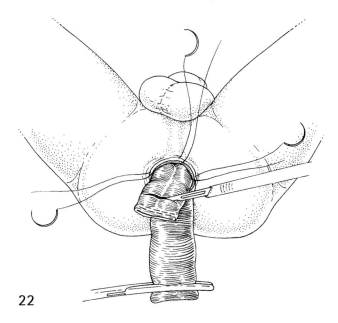

22

22 The anterior half of the ganglionic colon is incised and anastomosed to the anterior half of the anus with a 4/0 polyglactin suture. The first sutures are placed at each corner and in the midline, followed by interrupted sutures in between.

The assisting surgeon can facilitate visualization of the two edges of the bowel by putting outward traction on these initial quadrant sutures as the operating surgeon completes each quadrant.

23 One-quarter of the remaining ganglionic colon and one-quarter of the everted mucosal/submucosal tube are opened. A suture is placed in the posterior midline and this quarter of the anastomosis is completed. Throughout the anastomosis, countertraction applied by an assistant on the everted tube will help with the exposure.

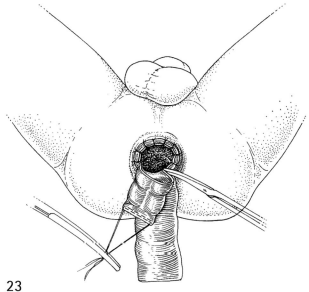

23

24 The final quadrant of the colon and submucosal/ mucosal tube are removed, and the anastomosis is completed and inspected.

The colon is pulled slightly upwards to invert the neorectum back into its correct position. Rectal examination at this point should reveal a well-formed anastomosis 1.5–2 cm above the anodermal junction. Gloves are then changed and attention directed to the abdominal field.

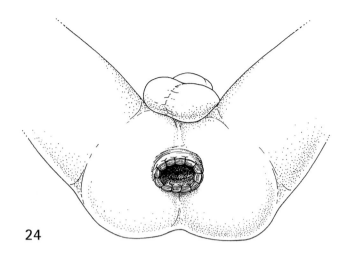

24

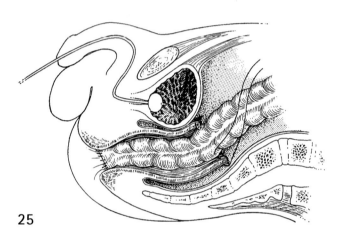

25

25 The pulled-through colon is attached with seromuscular bites to the muscular cuff to prevent the colon from prolapsing in the early postoperative period. No drain is placed, either through the anastomosis or from above in the muscular cuff, because there is rarely any significant oozing in the cuff (unlike the situation with ulcerative colitis in older patients). Posteriorly, the muscular cuff is split as distally as possible, and generally within 1 or 2 cm of the internal anal sphincter.

LAPAROSCOPIC APPROACH

26 The basic operative principles are virtually the same with the laparoscopic approach. Trocar placement consists of an initial umbilical trocar, followed by trocars in the right upper quadrant, and the remaining one in the suprapubic area.

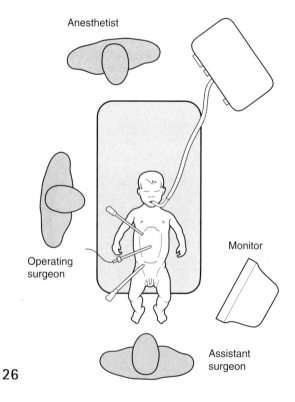

Anesthetist

Operating surgeon

Monitor

Assistant surgeon

26

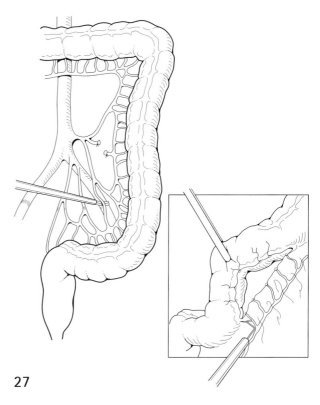

27 Dissection and leveling of the aganglionic segment are identical to the open technique. Blood vessels may be ligated with surgical clip appliers, or cautery for smaller vessels. Once mobilization is completed, the surgeon moves to the perineum, where a transanal dissection and anastomosis are performed (see below).

27

TRANSANAL APPROACH

28 The key element to beginning the case is placement of either a self-retaining retractor (e.g. Lone Star Medical Products, Houston, TX, USA) or a series of sutures that retract the anal verge.

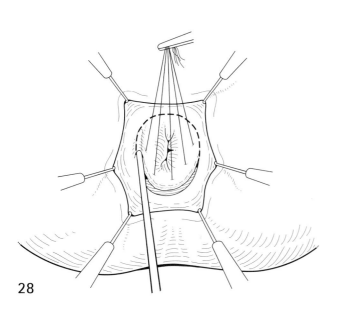

28

29 An incision 1 cm above the dentate line is begun with cautery in a circumferential fashion. A series of traction sutures are placed on the mucosa/submucosal tube, and dissection is carried proximally, primarily with blunt technique.

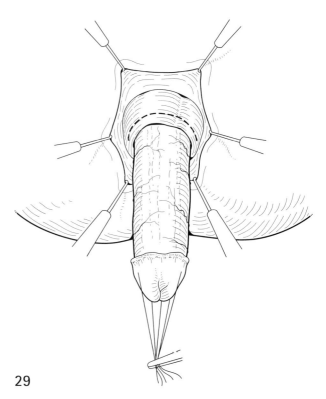

29

30 Once dissection is carried proximal to the peritoneal reflection, the muscular layer is entered, and the dissection becomes full thickness. This can be facilitated by placement of traction sutures on the muscular layer prior to dividing it.

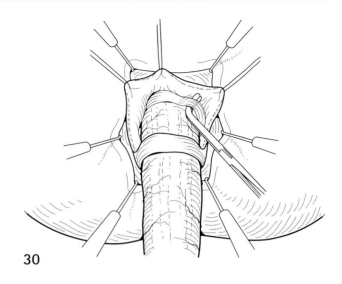

30

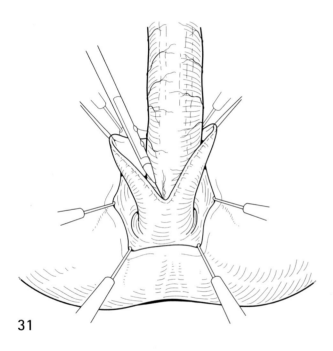

31

31 A key point is to split the muscular tube down to the top of the internal sphincter in the posterior midline. This splitting prevents the muscular cuff from creating a relative obstruction to the passage of stool. Although dissection of mesenteric vessels is easier with the laparoscopic approach, for rectosigmoid Hirschsprung disease, dissection of many of these vessels can be carried out via the transanal route. Biopsies are sent to determine the level of ganglionic bowel.

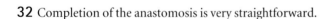

32 Completion of the anastomosis is very straightforward.

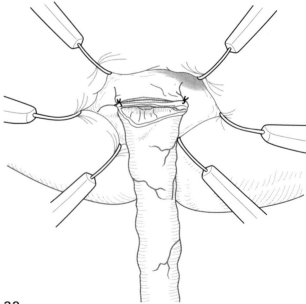

32

Swenson procedure

This technique was originally described by Swenson and Bill in 1948 and was the first successful method of treatment for children with Hirschsprung disease. They based their technique on the principle that the diseased portion of the bowel was the aganglionic distal rectum, and that removal of this segment was necessary to allow for normal stooling. The initial incidence of postoperative enterocolitis was fairly high (early 16 percent and late 27 percent), and this was attributed to leaving too much aganglionic rectum. The procedure has since been modified by Swenson by creating an oblique anastomosis, in which one resects virtually all of the posterior rectal wall (and some internal sphincter) while leaving 1.5–2 cm of anterior rectal wall.

The technique demands meticulous dissection of the rectum down to within 2 cm of the dentate line. If the dissection moves off the rectal wall, a significant incidence of injury to the genitourinary innervation may occur. Properly performed, the results with this procedure are quite good; however, because of the technical difficulties of the dissection, it has fallen into relative disfavor.

PREOPERATIVE

The child is admitted the day before surgery for a routine bowel preparation. Assessment and preparation are similar to those used in other pull-through operations.

OPERATIVE TECHNIQUE

33 The child is positioned in a fashion similar to that for an endorectal pull-through procedure. The incision was classically described as a left paramedian incision with take down of the colostomy; however, the modified hockey-stick incision will work equally as well.

The redundant aganglionic rectum is excised and proximal ganglionated colon mobilized past the splenic flexure, if necessary, as in the other two techniques. At this point, the peritoneal reflection over the rectum is incised.

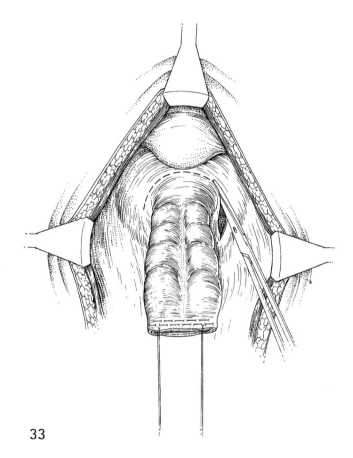

33

34 The operating surgeon then dissects the rectum caudally. This is a critical dissection, which demands the surgeon to stay directly on the bowel wall. Dissection is facilitated by the first assistant applying upward traction on the end of the aganglionic rectum. Multiple blood vessels enter directly into the bowel wall; each must be dissected out and can usually be coagulated. Dissection is carried down toward the anal verge, but is not carried as far anteriorly in order to avoid autonomic nerve injury. This dissection may be carried out with equal ease via a laparoscopic approach. Deeper pelvic exposure will often require an extra retractor lifting up the bladder, or an externally placed suture which grasps the bladder.

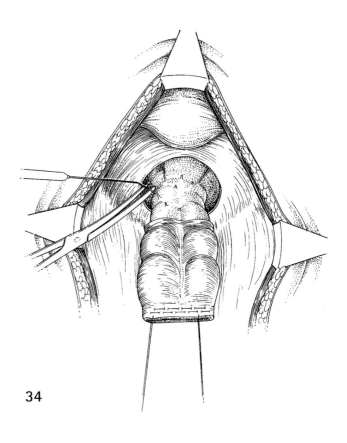

34

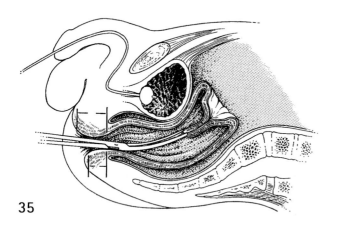

35

35 The perineal part of the operation is then started. The rectum is everted with the use of a long clamp. The anterior half of the everted rectal wall is cut 1.5–2 cm proximal to the anodermal junction. The posterior wall will be no longer than 1 cm in length. A gently curved incision, which is shorter posteriorly, is thus created along the anterior half of the bowel.

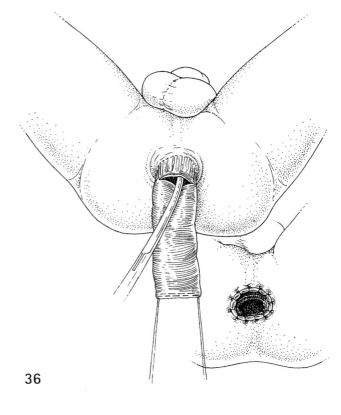

36 The ganglionic colon is pulled through and the anastomosis is virtually identical to that for the endorectal pull-through operation. Classically, silk sutures have been used, but the authors, however, have utilized polyglactin sutures with good results.

The anastomosis is allowed to recede and is gently pulled upward from the perineum. Closure is essentially the same as for the previous procedures.

36

Second pull-through

37 A child with an initial unsuccessful pull-through operation may present with severe constipation or significant incontinence. These children should undergo a thorough investigation of the details of the initial operation, as well as a review of the pathologic specimens. In most cases, an appropriate pull-through has been performed and an aggressive bowel program needs to be instituted. It is essential to rule out a retained segment of aganglionic bowel. Should this be the case, a second pull-through operation will usually be necessary. Because of its relative ease, a Duhamel is generally the procedure of choice. The authors quite commonly perform an endorectal pull-through in patients who have previously undergone this procedure. For those patients who underwent an initial Duhamel procedure, a Swenson pull-through should be used. For children who underwent an initial Swenson procedure, one could also successfully perform an endorectal dissection. If the patient has a stricture in part of the pull-through, one will generally be better off using a Duhamel approach for the 'redo' pull-through.

For the child with debilitating incontinence, a detailed history should be taken and an examination to rule out encopresis and to assess the degree of anorectal tone. Anal manometry is particularly helpful in this group, as a lack of normal muscular control is generally felt to be a poor indicator of a successful outcome for a repeat pull-through operation. An occasional child in this latter group may best be served by a diverting colostomy or placement of an appendicostomy tube.

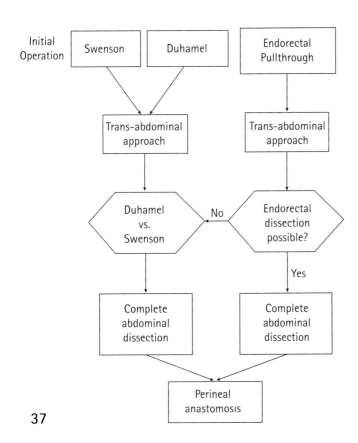

37

Ano/rectal myectomy

A child with short-segment Hirschsprung disease may be a candidate for an anal/rectal myectomy. The advantage of this procedure is that it avoids an abdominal operation. The procedure must be confined to very short-segment (4 cm or less including the transition zone) Hirschsprung disease. One must be certain that the myectomy is extended beyond the level of the transition zone. Because performing an inadequate myectomy may adversely affect the outcome of a subsequent pull-through operation, a myectomy should be avoided if there is any uncertainty as to the level of disease. More commonly, an ano/rectal myotomy or myectomy is performed for a child who, following a pull-through procedure, has persistent enterocolitis symptoms, or who has difficulty stooling after a pull-through procedure. The most satisfying results with a myectomy are for those children with long-standing enterocolitis after a pull-through procedure.

OPERATIVE TECHNIQUE

Transanal approach

38 The child is placed in an identical position to that for the full-thickness rectal biopsy.

Digital dilatation is performed, and two narrow anal retractors are inserted and held by assistants. The posterior aspect of the dentate line is identified. A 2 cm transverse incision through the mucosa and submucosa starting 0.5–1 cm above the dentate line is made. Following this, a submucosal dissection is carried upward for several centimeters. The mucosal/submucosal flap is held up with silk sutures and can be extended proximally with vertical incisions on either side.

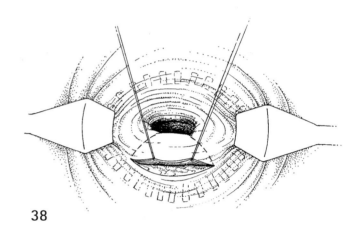

38

39 The myectomy is then performed by sharply incising the full thickness of the muscle layer and a 0.5–1 cm wide muscle strip is created in the midline. One should try to avoid the use of Bovie cautery until the specimen is obtained – preventing cautery artifact which may make pathologic interpretation difficult. The initial strip removed should be at least 5 cm in length.

Before transecting this strip, two silk sutures are placed proximal to the point of transection so that, should further dissection be necessary, the proximal muscle will not retract beyond the view of the surgeon. The strip should be mounted on a tongue depressor with mounting pins or suture; proximal and distal orientation must be clearly depicted.

A frozen section confirming ganglion cells at the proximal margin must be obtained before the procedure can be terminated. The dissection can be carried out in this manner for approximately 4–6 cm. If the surgeon suspects that the level of aganglionosis is longer than 4 cm, it may be advisable to forego this approach.

Once a sufficient length of muscle has been removed, hemostasis is achieved with cautery. The wound is irrigated and closed with fine, interrupted, absorbable sutures approximating the mucosa/submucosal dissection.

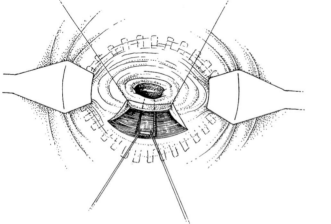

39

40 For patients who have had several procedures, obtaining a submucosal plane may be quite difficult and it is simpler to perform a vertically oriented, elliptical, full-thickness excision.

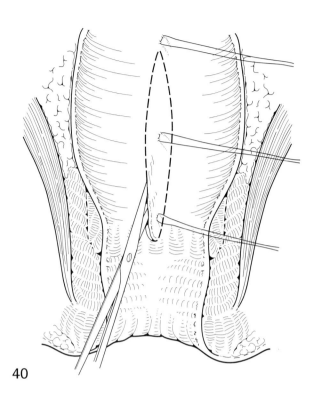

40

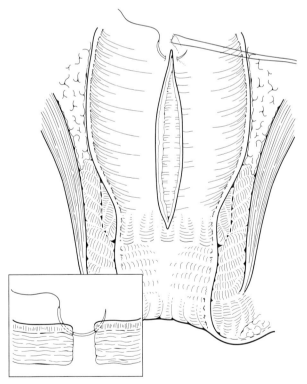

41

41 Closure is performed with a running absorbable suture that approximates only the mucosa and submucosa, leaving a defect in the muscular layer.

RIGHT-SIDED AGANGLIONOSIS

Pull-throughs in patients with extended colonic disease (to the right of the middle colic vessels) often create problems in maintaining the colon in the correct orientation, and are at greater risk for torsion of the pulled-through intestine. This problem was recognized by Duhamel early on.

42a,b This problem may be best approached by rotating the right colon in a counterclockwise fashion, as shown below. Because the small bowel then exits the colon from the patient's left side, it is sometimes necessary to follow this with a complete release of the ligament of Treitz (i.e. create a malrotation).

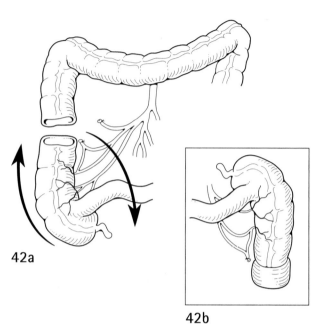

42a

42b

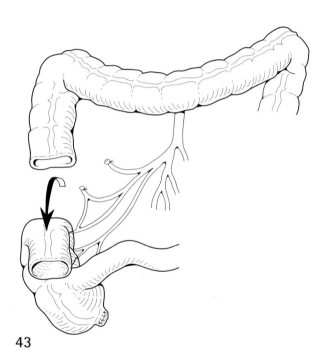

43

43 Alternatively, the colon may be flipped anteriorly, with reasonably good results.

POSTOPERATIVE CARE

Following all of the pull-through procedures, the nasogastric tube is removed on the first postoperative day, and feedings are begun once gastrointestinal activity returns. The Foley catheter can be removed on the second postoperative day following the endorectal and Duhamel procedures because bladder innervation has not been affected by the pelvic dissection. However, after the Swenson pull-through or redo pull-throughs, the Foley catheter should be left in for 4–5 days because of the possibility that there may be some bladder atony from the dissection. Antibiotics are continued for 24 hours after surgery. Most patients are commonly discharged by the third postoperative day.

Great emphasis is placed on examining the perineal region for the development of erythema or cellulitis, as this is an early sign of an anastomotic leak. Investigation of a leak consists of an enema contrast study or a computed tomographic scan with contrast medium. Although fairly uncommon, should a leak be found, the urgent placement of a diverting colostomy is needed.

For the endorectal pull-through, a gentle rectal examination with cotton-tip applicator is performed to ensure patency of the rectal anastomosis before discharge. Parents are given thorough instructions on perineal care and the potential development of enterocolitis. To avoid perineal excoriation, the parents are instructed to apply a thick coat of a zinc oxide-based ointment with each diaper change. If a significant rash develops, more intensified applications are used.

Digital or small Hegar calibrations are performed, starting on the third week after surgery. These are occasionally needed after the endorectal pull-through procedure, particularly in neonates. These dilatations are usually sufficient to prevent anastomotic stricturing.

Stool frequency is generally quite high (7–12 bowel movements per day) immediately after the pull-through operation, but this slowly decreases and is generally normal by 6–9 months.

Children should be followed up for several years. Occasionally, some develop intermittent bouts of constipation, occasional soiling, and enterocolitis. Most problems with constipation or soiling can be managed with changes in diet or enema regimens. Episodes of enterocolitis are managed with oral metronidazole; however, severe cases will necessitate admission, intravenous antibiotics, and rectal washouts. Increasingly, a large number of patients are started on rectal washouts, beginning at 3 weeks following the pull-through. This acts as a prophylactic method of avoiding enterocolitis, and may be continued for the first few months following the surgery.

With regard to children with total colonic Hirschsprung disease, large volumes of stool and electrolyte losses can occur after either a modified Duhamel or an ileoanal endorectal pull-through. These losses must be replaced and are usually controlled with dietary changes and the addition of an opioid agent (e.g. loperamide). Perineal excoriation is very common in these infants and demands constant attention. Normalization of stooling will take much longer than in children with classic Hirschsprung disease, and these children may sometimes require parenteral nutritional support for several months before full enteral feeding can be initiated.

OUTCOME

There is controversy concerning which procedure yields the best results. Long-term outcomes with the Duhamel, Soave, and Swenson techniques are basically similar, provided they are performed with meticulous technique. Depending on the anatomy and history of the patient, the surgeon should be familiar with all of these techniques, but should use one as the primary procedure. This is the only way that consistently good results can be achieved.

Of equal importance is the need to follow such patients over long periods of time, as many of the complications (e.g. enterocolitis, constipation, and urgency) may not become manifest until much later in the patient's life.

ACKNOWLEDGMENTS

Illustrations were drawn by Paul Richardson and Shayne Davidson. Illustrations 19, 21, and 24 are reproduced from Coran AG, Weintraub WH. *Surgery, Gynecology and Obstetrics* 1976; **143**: 277–82, with permission of the publishers.

FURTHER READING

Boley SJ. New modification of the surgical treatment of Hirschsprung's disease. *Surgery* 1964; **56**: 1015–17.

Coran AG, Weintraub WH. Modification of the endorectal procedure for Hirschsprung's disease. *Surgery, Gynecology and Obstetrics* 1976; **143**: 277–82.

El-Sawaf MI, Drongowski RA, Chamberlain JN et al. Are the long-term results of the transanal pull-through equal to those of the transabdominal pull-through? A comparison of the two approaches for Hirschsprung disease. *Journal of Pediatric Surgery* 2007; **42**: 41–7.

Georgeson KE, Cohen RD, Hebra A et al. Primary laparoscopic-assisted endorectal colon pull-through for Hirschsprung's disease: a new gold standard. *Annals of Surgery* 1999; **229**: 678–82; discussion 682–3.

Kim AC, Langer JC, Pastor AC et al. Endorectal pull-through for Hirschsprung's disease – a multicenter, long-term comparison of results: transanal vs transabdominal approach. *Journal of Pediatric Surgery* 2010; **45**: 1213–20.

Langer JC, Durrant AC, de la Torre ML et al. One-stage transanal Soave pull-through for Hirschsprung disease: a multicenter experience with 141 children. *Annals of Surgery* 2003; **238**: 569–76.

Martin LW, Caudill DR. A method for elimination of the blind rectal pouch in the Duhamel operation for Hirschsprung's disease. *Surgery* 1967; **62**: 951–3.

Swenson O, Bill AH. Resection of the rectum and rectosigmoid with preservation of the sphincter for benign spastic lesions producing megacolon. An experimental study. *Surgery* 1948; **24**: 212–20.

Wildhaber BE, Pakarinen M, Rintala RJ et al. Posterior myotomy/myectomy for persistent stooling problems in Hirschsprung's disease. *Journal of Pediatric Surgery* 2004; **39**: 920–6.

Inflammatory bowel disease

DANIEL H TEITELBAUM and ARNOLD G CORAN

HISTORY

The evolution of surgical procedures for inflammatory bowel disease has been one of trial and error. Based on previous successful and unsuccessful outcomes, a variety of procedures have been developed that allow for maximal preservation of bowel length, as well as function. These include proctocolectomy with end-ileostomy, endorectal pull-through, and stricturoplasty. The pediatric patient with inflammatory bowel disease presents with additional growth, nutritional, and psychologic problems that may not affect the adult patient. All of these factors must be considered when determining the timing and type of procedure.

Over the past 30 years, the use of the endorectal pull-through for ulcerative colitis has become increasingly popular. The operation was initially a modification of the endorectal pull-through technique for Hirschsprung disease. The procedure has taken time to become accepted by the general surgical community, principally because of unfamiliarity with the endorectal dissection and the significant incidence of complications associated with many of the original cases.

PRINCIPLES AND JUSTIFICATION

Protocolectomy with end ileostomy

This had been the standard procedure for children with ulcerative colitis and multiple polyposis, but can also be utilized in severe Crohn colitis. The abdominal colectomy portion of the procedure may also be performed in conjunction with an endorectal pull-through. For patients with ulcerative colitis, initial medical management is generally advised. In children with an acute exacerbation of ulcerative colitis, surgery is indicated in cases of severe hemorrhage or in those who fail to respond to intensive medical treatment after several weeks. The timing of an elective procedure is more difficult to establish. Some surgeons feel that resection is only indicated in those

children who show mucosal atypia on colonoscopic biopsy. Detecting these changes is difficult because one cannot routinely biopsy the entire colon, and the incidence of carcinomatous changes increases as the duration of the disease increases. In fact, carcinoma can be found in many surgical specimens when only atypia was found on colonoscopic biopsy. Many surgeons therefore recommend a colectomy once the disease process has been present for ten years. However, today many gastroenterologists recommend surveillance colonoscopy every year or every other year even if the disease has been present for more than ten years. Surgery should be performed sooner if atypia is identified or in those children with significant growth failure or lack of sexual maturation, and in those on chronic high doses of steroids in whom significant changes and complications due to medication use have occurred. In children with multiple polyposis, the timing can also be controversial. If all the polyps can be removed from the colon and the child is followed up every six months, surgery can be delayed at least until the child is past adolescence. If the polyps are too numerous to be removed, surgery should be performed earlier.

Endorectal pull-through

The endorectal pull-through is a curative procedure for patients with ulcerative colitis as well as colonic polyposis, while eliminating the need for a permanent ileostomy. An additional advantage of this procedure is the elimination of the extensive pelvic dissection outside the rectal wall, which can be associated with a significant incidence of injury to the nerves supplying the genitourinary system.

Stricturoplasty

Strictures secondary to Crohn disease of the small bowel do occur in children. Conventional approaches to their treatment have consisted of complete resections or side-to-side bypasses of the involved area. Multiple resections of these strictured areas have not uncommonly led to the development of the short bowel syndrome. Bypass of significant areas of the bowel usually results in bacterial overgrowth. Over the past 20 years, the use of stricturoplasty has therefore evolved. The technique has enabled patients to retain significantly greater lengths of bowel with adequate relief of the obstruction and is a modification of the Heineke–Mikulicz procedure for a pyloroplasty. Although the bowel length may appear shorter after the performance of multiple stricturoplasties, the functional length is the same. A few contraindications to this procedure exist, for example the occurrence of several small strictures very close together, which could be more simply managed with a resection, although it is not uncommon for a patient to have multiple stricturoplasties during one operation. If the stricture is associated with fistula or abscess formation, the bowel segment should be excised.

Ileocolectomy

Although ileocolectomy is commonly performed in the pediatric patient for Crohn's disease, the procedure is reasonably straightforward and an operative description is not included in this chapter. However, at the end of this chapter, a laparoscopic-assisted ileocolectomy is described.

PREOPERATIVE

Proctocolectomy with end ileostomy

The child is admitted the day before surgery and depending on surgeon preference may undergo a complete bowel preparation. Caution should be observed in those patients with severe colitis or Crohn disease. Overly aggressive laxatives may cause a perforation of the colon or an exacerbation of the disease process. In general, a balanced electrolyte solution should be slowly administered orally. Oral antibiotics and gentle enemas are given the day before surgery. An enterostomal therapist should mark the skin site of the ileostomy with indelible ink the day before surgery.

Endorectal pull-through

Before performing the procedure, the diagnosis of ulcerative colitis must be as firm as possible. If Crohn's colitis is present instead of ulcerative colitis, recurrent disease in the pulled-through ileum and fistula formation from this same segment of bowel are common. Repeat colonoscopy with biopsies along with a series of small intestinal contrast studies should be performed to rule out Crohn disease, and fully stage the disease process. If biopsies have been performed elsewhere, they should be re-read by pathologists at the center where the operation is to be carried out. Many of these children will have been on steroids during the previous year and will need stress doses of steroids in the perioperative period.

Stricturoplasty

Suspicion of a stricture is usually initiated by the patient complaining of symptoms consistent with a partial bowel obstruction. Most patients complain of cramping abdominal pain, with obstipation and nausea. The diagnosis is made with a small intestinal contrast series or magnetic resonance imaging (MRI) enterography. A thorough look for multiple strictures is necessary. No formal bowel preparation is needed, but intravenous antibiotics should be given.

OPERATIONS

Proctocolectomy with end ileostomy

POSITION OF PATIENT AND INCISION

1 The child is placed in the lithotomy position, with leg supports (without weight on the posterior portion of the leg) for older children and skis for smaller children. Careful padding of the lower extremities is critical to avoid neurovascular injury. The procedure is best carried out through a large midline or left paramedian abdominal incision, which extends from the pubis to a few centimeters above the umbilicus. Alternatively, the majority of the procedure can be done with the child in the supine position, and the legs can be placed in previously aligned stirrups at the time of the pull-through and transanal anastomosis. This may be of particular

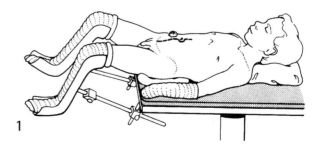

1

benefit with a laparoscopic-assisted approach, or for more prolonged dissections.

An alternative approach to an incision in a pre-adolescent or smaller teenage child is to perform a Pfannenstiel incision, with transection of the rectus muscles. Often one can perform the entire colectomy through this incision by carefully mobilizing the splenic and hepatic flexures.

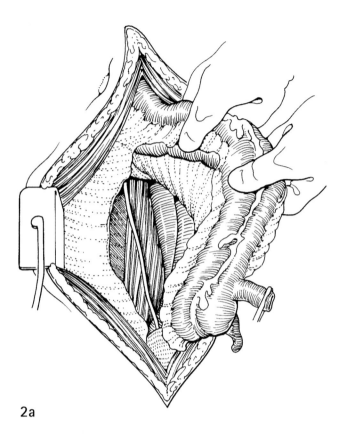

2a

MOBILIZATION OF COLON

2a,b The abdomen is explored and the right colon is mobilized by incising the line of Toldt and by dividing the terminal ileum approximately 1 cm from the ileocecal valve. Identification of the ureters is performed on both sides of the abdomen. The hepatic flexure and splenic flexure are then divided without putting traction on the spleen. The omentum is included in the transverse colectomy specimen.

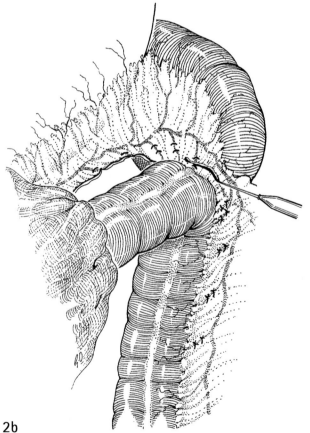

2b

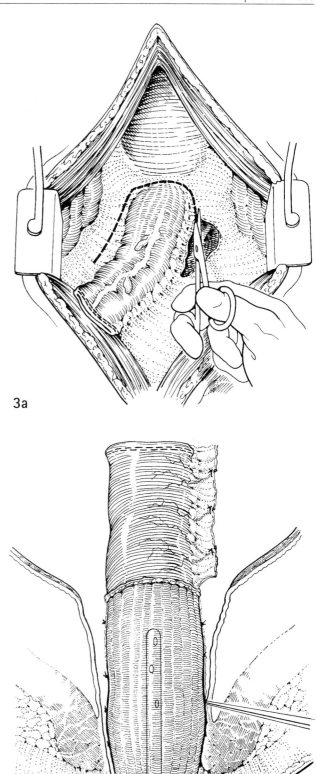

3a,b The descending colon is mobilized in a similar fashion by dividing its retroperitoneal attachment. The mesentery of the colon is then divided and the vessels are suture ligated with 2/0 or 3/0 silk suture, and smaller vessels with a Harmonic (Ethicon Endo-Surgery) or a Ligasure (Covidien) device. The colon is then divided at the rectosigmoid junction with an automatic stapling device. The peritoneal reflection of the rectum is incised and the dissection is continued directly on the muscular rectal wall. Deviation from the rectal wall will increase the chances of injuring the pelvic autonomic nerves, with subsequent impotence or bladder dysfunction. This portion of the operation is facilitated by superior countertraction on the remaining proximal rectum by the assisting surgeon (illustration b). Each individual vessel is grasped with forceps and either cauterized or ligated. Dissection should continue down as far distally as possible from the abdominal approach.

3a

3b

EXCISION OF RECTUM

4 The surgeon then moves to the foot of the table and an elliptical incision is made around the anus.

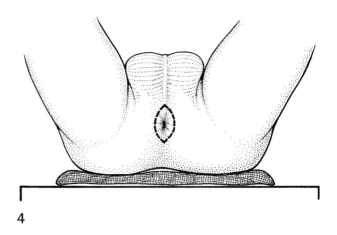

4

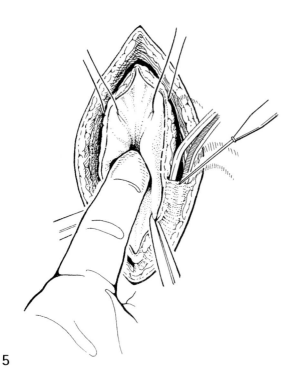

5

5 Dissection is carried upwards, remaining directly on the rectal wall. Skeletal muscles and the prostate should be avoided or considerable bleeding may arise.

6 Dissection continues until the presacral space is entered posteriorly. The remainder of the excision is carried out with the proximal rectum everted onto the perineum. Sometimes, in a thin patient, the entire proctectomy can be performed transabdominally, with the actual excision of the anus from the abdominal approach. The peritoneum is approximated from the abdominal side.

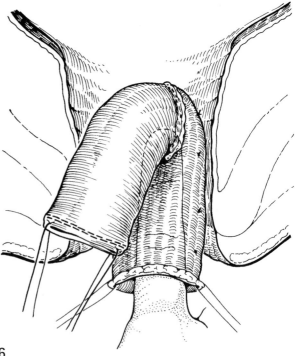

6

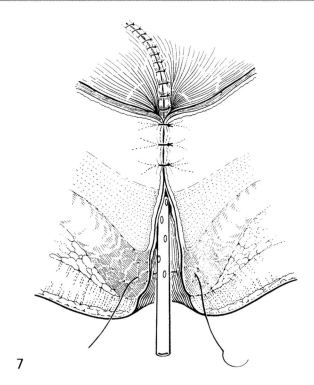

TISSUE APPROXIMATION

7 The levator complex and subcutaneous tissues are approximated through the perineal wound. A small, flat, closed suction drain is placed into the perineal wound.

7

FORMATION OF STOMA

8a,b The stoma is exteriorized at a previously marked site. The circle of skin about 2 cm in diameter is removed with cautery and the fascia is cruciated to allow the ileum to exit comfortably through it. The terminal ileum is prepared for creation of the ileostomy by ligating a few vessels along the most distal 3 cm of small bowel. The ileum is tacked to the peritoneum with interrupted sutures (polyglycolic acid). Once the abdomen and skin are closed, a classic Brooke stoma is formed.

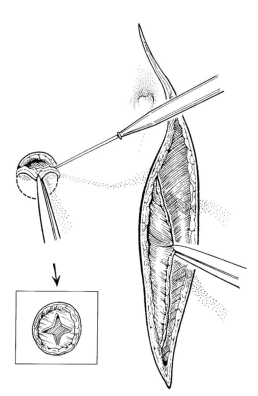

8a

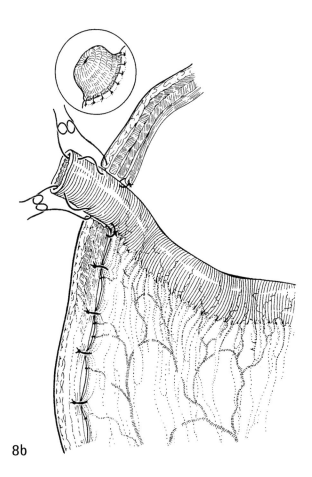

8b

Endorectal pull-through

POSITION OF PATIENT AND INCISION

Positioning for this procedure is essentially identical to that for proctocolectomy; however, because of the longer procedure, very careful attention must be paid to padding of the lower extremities to avoid neurovascular injury. A long midline or paramedian incision is made from the pubis to several centimeters above the umbilicus. The abdominal colectomy proceeds as already described. Alternatively, the legs can be prepped and draped and positioned so that the lower extremities fit properly in the stirrups; however, the legs are laid on the operative table until it is time to perform the pull-through portion of the case. This alternative approach can be very helpful with a laparoscopic pull-through where a longer period of time may occur for the colectomy.

MOBILIZATION OF ILEUM

The ileum is mobilized proximally to allow for an adequate length for the pull-through. In general, length is rarely a problem with a straight pull-through. With the J-pouch, more time must be spent in gaining bowel length. Adequate bowel length can also be difficult when the patient has had a previous ileostomy, as the mesentery may be scarred and foreshortened. In general, the main branch of the ileocecal artery can often be spared and the more proximal arcades ligated in the distal ileum. It is important to preserve the distal vascular arcade to the end of the ileum. If the ileocecal artery must be ligated, a bulldog clamp should initially be placed on this vessel to determine if a significant length of bowel will be lost. In such a case, one might opt for a straight pull-through which will not require as much mobilization and length.

ENDORECTAL DISSECTION

The authors prefer to do the entire endorectal dissection from the abdominal approach. It may be technically more difficult to develop the correct plane from the perineum and, although the initial portion of the dissection can be quite difficult in children with ulcerative colitis, once this correct plane is found the dissection proceeds fairly smoothly.

9 Countertraction of the dissected mucosal/submucosal tube, as well as traction in an upward and outward fashion on the muscular cuff (often with sutures retracted on all four quadrants), helps with the dissection.

The dissection involves greater blood loss than in cases of Hirschsprung disease. Any large penetrating vessels should be cauterized, but once the dissection is completed, bleeding usually stops spontaneously. If the correct plane is lost, the surgeon should turn to the opposite side of the bowel and work circumferentially until the dissection is distal to the area where the plane was lost. The level of the end of the dissection should be checked intermittently by feeling for an assistant's finger placed in the anus, just above the dentate line.

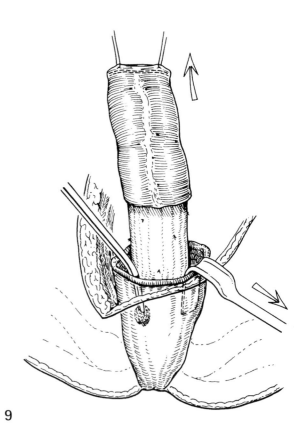

9

FORMATION OF RESERVOIR

The following description of the pull-through is applicable to all different types of ileal reconstructions (straight and reservoir procedures). Construction of the J-pouch, the lateral side-to-side ileal reservoir, and the S-pouch is subsequently described.

10 Once the endorectal dissection is completed, one of the surgeons moves to the foot of the table. Narrow retractors are placed at the anal mucocutaneous junction and a clamp is inserted into the rectum. An assistant working in the abdominal field places the end of the mucosal/submucosal tube into this clamp. The segment is then everted outside the perineum. The end of the everted tube is placed in a clamp and held on traction by an assistant to facilitate the anastomosis.

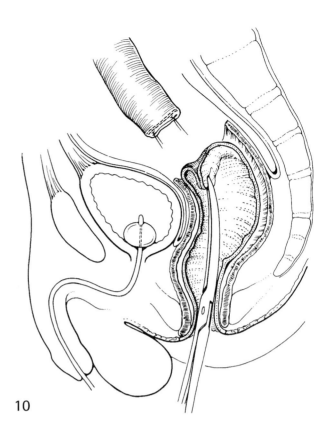

10

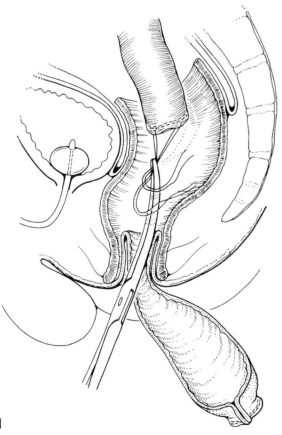

11

11 The submucosal/mucosal tube is incised on the anterior half, 1 cm proximal to the dentate line. A Kelly clamp is inserted into this opening and the ileum is brought down to this point by grasping two previously placed traction sutures. Great care must be taken not to twist the bowel as it is brought through the muscular cuff. Different colored sutures on the mesenteric and antimesenteric sides of the bowel are helpful in maintaining this orientation. Prior to bringing the bowel down, one should carefully examine the base of the ileal mesentery to ensure there is no torsion.

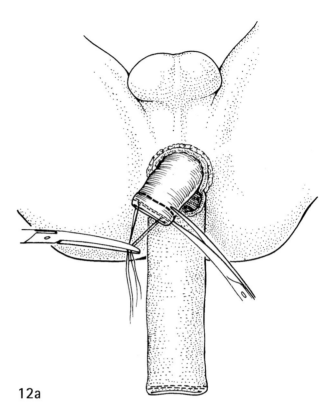

12a

12a,b The anterior half of the ileum is incised and is anastomosed to the anterior half of the anus with interrupted 3/0 or 4/0 absorbable sutures. The first sutures are placed at each corner and in the midline, and are followed by interrupted sutures placed in between.

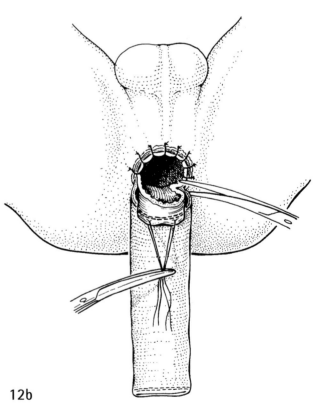

12b

13 One-quarter of the remaining ileum and the everted mucosal/submucosal tube are opened. A suture is placed in the posterior midline and this quarter of the anastomosis is completed. Countertraction, applied by an assistant on the everted tube and on the traction sutures on the ileum, will help with the exposure. The final quarter of the ileum and tube are removed and the anastomosis is completed and inspected. In many cases, bleeding is modest and no drainage is required. In those cases where a drain is chosen, it should be inserted before the last one or two sutures are placed using a thin, 3.5-mm closed suction drain between the rectal muscular cuff and the pulled-through ileum. The drain exits between the anastomotic sutures. It is placed most safely by advancing a small uterine sound retrograde through the anastomosis into the endorectal dissection. The drain can be secured onto this sound and then pulled through the anastomosis.

The ileum is pulled slightly upward, and this will invert the neorectum back into its correct position. Rectal examination at this point should show a well-formed anastomosis 1.5–2 cm above the anodermal junction. Gloves are then changed and attention is directed to the abdominal field. The pulled-through ileum is attached with seromuscular sutures to the muscular cuff to prevent it from prolapsing in the early postoperative period.

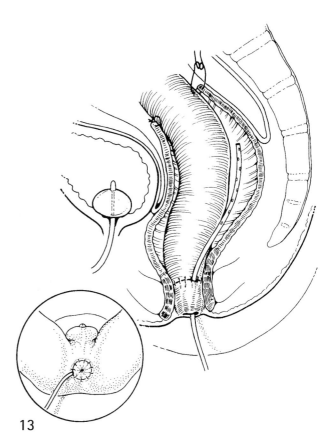

13

14a–c For the J-pouch, the ileum is folded back on itself (illustration a) for a length of 8–10 cm. The bowel is opened at the stapled end and at an adjacent position in the proximal ileum. An automatic stapling device is fired to create the anastomosis. A small section of ileum will remain separated at the apex of the J. The apex is opened and the stapler is fired (illustration b) in the opposite direction to complete the anastomosis. This open end is brought down for the anal anastomosis. It is critical that a septum is not left between the ileal limbs, as this will cause stasis, bacterial overgrowth, and a fecaloma.

Although the J-pouch is the most popular of all the reservoirs, some surgeons use other pouches, such as the lateral ileal reservoir, the S-pouch, and the W-pouch. The W-pouch is rarely used in adults or children and is not discussed here.

Increasingly, we have made the length of the J-pouch shorter (8–10 cm), in the hope of decreasing the incidence of pouchitis. In those patients where an 8 cm long pouch is created, a single firing (or at times two firings) of the stapler from the bottom of the pouch may be all that is required. This step eliminates the need to open the staple line; however, care must be taken to ensure that almost the entire length of the J-pouch is opened between the two lumens of bowel (illustration c).

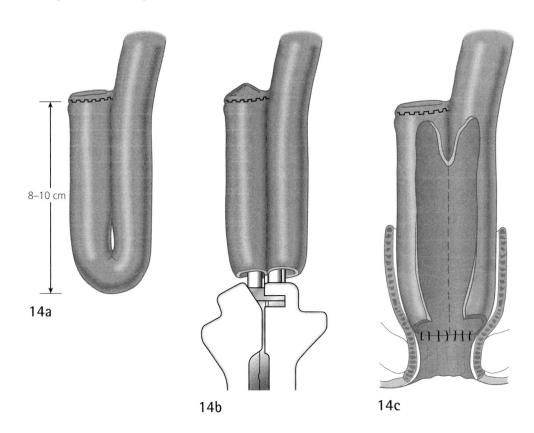

8–10 cm

14a

14b

14c

LAPAROSCOPIC ASSISTANCE

The use of laparoscopy has been increasingly popularized in recent years. Two approaches have been advocated: complete laparoscopic proctocolectomy and endorectal pull-through, or a laparoscopic-assisted approach. The authors advocate the latter approach, as the total use of laparoscopy has been associated with a significant increase in operative time and blood loss.

15 The approach to the laparoscopic proctocolectomy consists of the placement of an initial umbilical port, followed by four 5-mm Innerdyne ports (Salt Lake City, UT, USA), placed as shown here. The umbilical port initially contains the camera with a 30° telescope.

This is followed by an epigastric port and then left and right lateral ports. The colon, from the terminal ileum to the distal rectum, is mobilized and released from the peritoneal attachments and the splenic and hepatic flexures. Initial mobilization of the lateral attachments is facilitated by 'airplaning' the patient to the contralateral side, with traction on the colon, with a blunt bowel grasper through either the epigastric or the contralateral trocar sites, and using cautery scissors via the remaining trocar site. The ureters are identified early during this dissection. Depending on the site of mobilization, the camera and operating ports will vary.

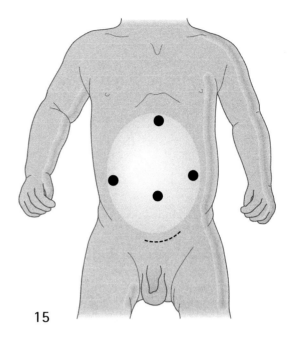

15

The more time-consuming aspect of the dissection is the mobilization of the omentum off the transverse colon. A pair of 5-mm ultrasonic scissors or the use of an endogastrointestinal anastomosis (endo-GIA) stapling device will help at this point in the dissection. Care is taken to identify and staple or ligate the middle colic vessel. Alternatively, the omentum may be spared by retracting it superiorly and using electrocautery dissection between the stomach and colon.

Once the colon is fully mobilized, a low transverse suprapubic incision is made, using a Pfannenstiel-type incision. The operating surgeon pulls the entire colon out through this incision and sequentially ligates the mesenteric

vessels. The ileum is divided, and an optional ileal pouch may be created. The endorectal dissection is then performed.

ALTERNATIVE STAPLED ANASTOMOSIS

One of the major restrictions in performing a J-pouch pull-through is the difficulty in bringing down the end of the pouch sufficiently out of the anal canal to perform a hand-sewn anastomosis. Strategies of placing the patient in reverse Trendelenburg and extensive dissection of the mesenteric vessels may help; however, in some cases this may not be sufficient. A conventional stapled anastomosis has the limitation of leaving an excessive amount of rectum. The great advantage of the modification shown here is that the anastomosis of the pouch is performed within the anal canal, taking a tremendous amount of tension off the anastomosis.

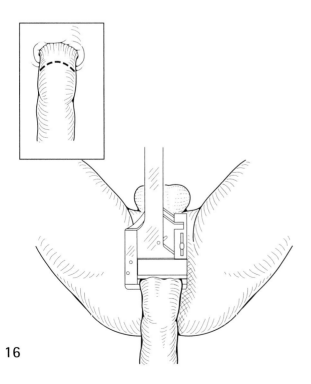

16 The endorectal dissection is carried out in an identical fashion to the open technique and the mucosal/submucosal cuff is prolapsed out onto the perineum. At this point, a stapling device is used to staple and transect the bowel approximately 1 cm above the dentate line. In obese patients with a very deep gluteal cleft, an endo-GIA-type stapling device allows better positioning of the stapler.

16

17,18 The residual anorectum is placed back into the anal canal and the largest possible circular stapler is inserted. The assisting surgeon from the abdominal field places the anvil into an opening in the end of the J-pouch. Care is taken to ensure that this opening is away from mesenteric vessels, which may be injured during the subsequent anastomosis. A suture is placed in purse-string fashion and tied to secure the anvil. The abdominal surgeon then helps guide the J-pouch down toward the pelvis. At the same time, the surgeon on the perineal side turns the stapling device to fully advance the trocar through the mucosal/submucosal tube into the peritoneal cavity. Great care must be taken to ensure correct alignment of the two sides, and to make sure both ends are cleared of adjacent tissues. Once this is done, the stapling device is fired and removed. Both tissue donuts are inspected and, in some patients, a sigmoidoscopy with air insufflation is done to assess the integrity of the completed anastomosis. A transanastomotic Penrose drain should be left in place to allow drainage of mucous for 2–3 postoperative days.

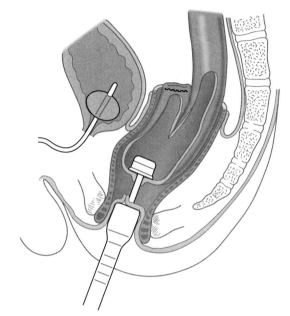

17

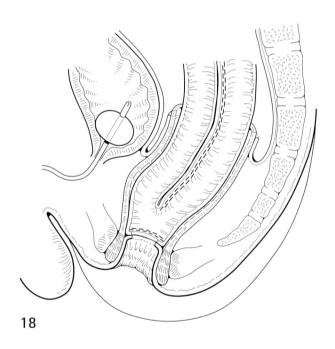

18

ADDITIONAL CONSIDERATIONS

The addition of a laparoscopic dissection will add time to the procedure. Thus the procedure may not always be desirable. Because of this increased time, care in patient positioning, as with all patients, is critical. In some cases, the authors elect to prepare the abdomen, buttocks, and entire lower extremities, with the legs placed in well-padded stockinettes. The legs are left supine and not placed in the stirrups until the ileoanal anastomosis is performed. The decision to perform a protective ileostomy is highly debatable. The advantage of eliminating the ileostomy is the ability to forego a subsequent surgery and the potential complications associated with an ostomy. In most cases an ileostomy should be given if the patient has been on anti-TNF-alpha therapy, or those with poor nutritional status. Ideally, the right-sided port can be used as the site of ileostomy.

Using the stapled technique will save tremendous time in the operating room, but will almost inevitably result in a narrowing of the anastomosis, which will require two to three dilatations to alleviate.

S-pouch reservoir

19a–c The S-pouch is created in a manner very similar to the J-pouch, except that there are two overlapping limbs of ileum. Each limb is 10 cm long with a 2 cm spout, which is used for the ileoanal anastomosis.

For all types of pull-through operations, a loop ileostomy is placed proximally. Care is taken to place this in an appropriate location marked before the operation. The ileum is carefully sutured to the peritoneum to prevent prolapse and twisting of it at the site of the ileostomy.

An advantage of an S-pouch is that the end of the spout can easily reach the outside of the perineum.

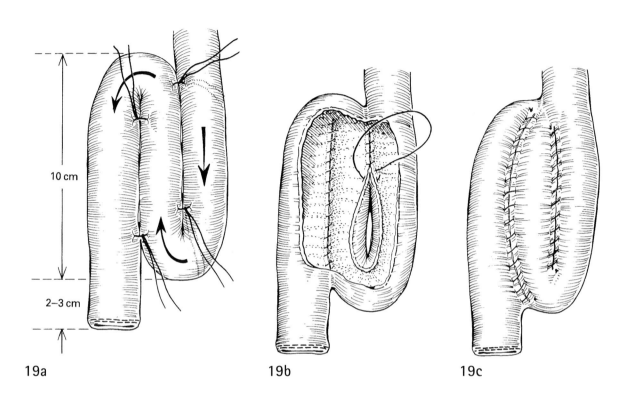

10 cm

2–3 cm

19a   19b   19c

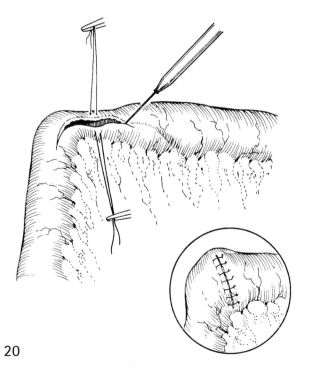

20

Stricturoplasty

20 The entire small and large bowel is inspected. Each stricture is identified and marked with a silk suture. A typical short-segment stricture is managed by placing traction sutures above and below the stricture on the antimesenteric surface of the bowel.

Using cautery, the bowel is opened longitudinally along the antimesenteric surface. It is then approximated transversely using interrupted 4/0 absorbable or non-absorbable sutures, and a second layer of Lembert sutures is placed.

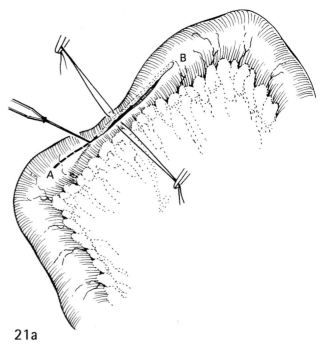

21a For strictures that are longer, the bowel is folded upon itself so that the stricture is at the apex and opened along a portion of both proximal and distal limbs.

21a

21b,c The limbs are anastomosed using an inner layer of running 4/0 absorbable sutures and interrupted Lembert sutures on the outside.

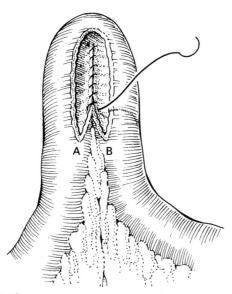

21b

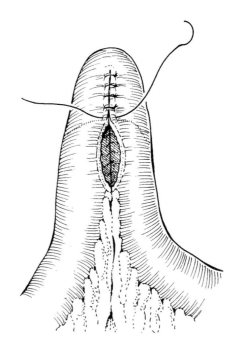

21c

Laparoscopic ileocolectomy

INDICATIONS AND WORK UP

Resection of the terminal ileum for Crohn's disease is quite commonly indicated for persistently strictured and fibrosed segments which are resistant to medical management. Not uncommonly, a partial obstruction of the small bowel is present in these children with associated significant malnutrition. Work up for these lesions was conventionally performed with contrast upper gastrointestinal series with small bowel follow-through. However, magnetic resonance enterography is increasingly used as it eliminates radiation and often can give greater information regarding associated fistulas and extent of the disease process. An open approach should be considered if the patient has a significant associated fistula, as scar formation may complicate the dissection. Should the fistula go to the retroperitoneum, great care must be taken to identify and protect the ureters and vasculature.

A bowel prep is typically not indicated, and the patient may well be obstructed and not tolerate this preparation. Preoperative second-generation cephalosporin is given prior to the incision, and no Foley catheter is used, unless the bladder may be involved with the dissection. Children of 14 years of age and older need sequential stockings to prevent deep vein thrombosis, and strong consideration should be given for perioperative low molecular weight heparin at prophylactic doses.

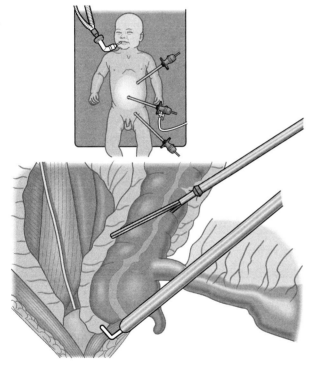

22

TECHNIQUE

22 Three to four 5-mm laparoscopic ports are placed as shown in the right upper and left lower quadrants, as well as an umbilical port. These should allow adequate triangulation of the working ports to facilitate dissection. A fourth port may be needed for additional traction. Prior to beginning the dissection, one should intraoperatively stage the extent of the disease. Running of the small bowel with two atraumatic graspers should be performed looking for other areas of stricture or inflammation.

The procedure is similar to the open approach, with one working port grasping the bowel with an atraumatic instrument and a hook cautery instrument or scissors used to initially mobilize the right colon and ileum.

Once full mobility has been done, two approaches may be taken. First, the bowel can be removed via one of the laparoscopic ports, or a right mid-abdomen transverse incision. The incision should be just big enough to allow the inflamed bowel and colon to be eviscerated. The mesentery can be ligated and bowel resected extraluminally, anastomosis performed and bowel returned to the peritoneum. An alternative approach is the complete laparoscopic excision and anastomosis performed intraluminally. While the latter approach is advocated by surgeons, because the abdominal incision used to remove the specimens is often the same size as the incision for the laparoscopic-assisted approach, the authors do not advocate this technique.

After closure of peritoneum and fascia, ports are removed and incisions are injected with 0.25 percent bupivicaine. In general, the 5-mm incisions do not require fascial closure.

POSTOPERATIVE MANAGEMENT

Antibiotics are given for two doses postoperatively. Nasogastric tube is optional, but should typically be removed by the first postoperative day. Other management is routine, and bowel function should return within 4 to 5 days postoperatively.

POSTOPERATIVE CARE

Following proctocolectomy or pull-through, a nasogastric tube is maintained overnight and the child is not fed until gastrointestinal activity returns. The Foley catheter can usually be removed in 2–3 days, but occasionally is left longer if the pelvic dissection was difficult. An additional dose of steroids is given on the day of surgery, and then slowly tapered down over the next few weeks. Routine stoma care must be thoroughly learned by the family before discharge. The ileostomy is generally closed after two months.

Postoperative care after stricturoplasty is routine. Nasogastric decompression is used overnight, and feedings are started once gastrointestinal activity returns. The child is given supplemental steroid therapy in the perioperative period. If the child has been malnourished for a prolonged period of time, consideration should be given to perioperative parenteral nutrition.

COMPLICATIONS

Complications associated with the endorectal pull-through are not uncommon. Diarrhea, with 7–15 bowel movements a day initially after closure of the ileostomy, is expected and this should be explained to the child and family before the operation. Most patients slowly normalize their stooling pattern over the first few months after the pull-through. Major losses of fluids and electrolytes may occur at first, as well as excoriation of the perineum. Diarrhea is best controlled with loperamide hydrochloride as needed. Occasionally, Metamucil may be added. Cholestyramine is occasionally added to this regimen.

Pouchitis is a well-described complication of an ileoanal pull-through. The presumed etiology is stasis of stool in the ileal segment, with subsequent bacterial overgrowth. The incidence is around 25–50 percent if reservoirs are employed, but with a straight pull-through the incidence is lower (<5 percent). Treatment of this condition consists of serial washouts of the pouch, sitz baths, and oral metronidazole.

The incidence of adhesive obstruction after any type of surgery for ulcerative colitis is 20–25 percent, irrespective of the type of procedure done. In the authors' series, however, adhesive obstruction occurred in 10 percent of cases, with only half of these requiring an enterolysis.

ACKNOWLEDGMENTS

Illustrations 16, 17, and 18 are reproduced from *Surgery* 2003; **134**: 492–5, with permission of the publishers, Elsevier, New York, NY, USA.

FURTHER READING

Coran AG. A personal experience with 100 consecutive total colectomies and straight ileoanal endorectal pull-throughs for benign disease of the colon and rectum in children and adults. *Annals of Surgery* 1990; **212**: 242–8.

Fonkalsrud EW. Update on clinical experience with different surgical techniques of the endorectal pull-through operation for colitis and polyposis. *Surgery, Gynecology and Obstetrics* 1987; **165**: 309–16.

Geiger JD, Teitelbaum DH, Hirschl RB, Coran AG. A new operative technique for restorative proctocolectomy: the endorectal pull-through combined with a double-stapled ileo-anal anastomosis. *Surgery* 2003; **134**: 492–5.

Martin LW, Sayers HJ, Alexander F *et al.* Anal continence following Soave procedure: analysis of results of 100 patients. *Annals of Surgery* 1986; **203**: 515–30.

Seetharamaiah R, West BT, Ignash SJ *et al.* Outcomes in pediatric patients undergoing straight versus J-pouch ileoanal anastomosis: a multi-center analysis. *Journal of Pediatric Surgery* 2009; **44**: 1410–17.

Teitelbaum DH, Lelli JL, Hirschl RB *et al.* Laparoscopy-assisted proctocolectomy for ulcerative colitis: a more rational approach. *Pediatric Endosurgical Innovative Techniques* 2001; **5**: 229–33.

63

Rectal polyps

JOSEPH L LELLI JR

PRINCIPLES AND JUSTIFICATION

Although the incidence of juvenile polyps is unknown, they are believed to occur in approximately 1 percent of all preschool children. Most appear in the first decade of life, with the peak incidence between three and five years. Polyps are solitary in 50 percent of cases, with the remainder having between two and ten polyps. Forty percent of juvenile polyps are found in the rectum or sigmoid colon. The remaining 60 percent are found evenly distributed throughout the colon.

Juvenile polyps are also known as retention, inflammatory, or cystic polyps. Such polyps are generally considered hamartomas or a malformation in which normal colonic tissue has become arranged in a haphazard manner. Grossly typical polyps have a glistening, smooth, spherical, reddish head and range from 2 mm to several centimeters in diameter. Polyps often have an ulcerated surface, which accounts for the rectal bleeding. A cross-section shows cystic spaces filled with mucus. Juvenile polyps are typically attached by a long, narrow stalk covered by colonic mucosa. This stalk predisposes the polyp to torsion, which results in venous congestion, surface ulceration, bleeding, and autoamputation.

Clinical features

Recent data suggest that juvenile polyps result from a structural rearrangement of the mucosa secondary to an inflammatory process. The initial event is probably ulceration and subsequent inflammation of the mucosa, leading to obstruction of regional, small colonic glands of the mucosa. The obstructed glands enlarge with mucous secretion and push up into the lumen. The fecal stream and peristalsis push the mass down the lumen, causing the stalk to elongate, resulting in the typical pedunculated appearance of the juvenile polyp. Ulceration of the surface or autoamputation leads to the bright red blood noted on presentation. Occasionally, polyps prolapse through the anal canal and present as dark, cherry red protrusions at the anus. Although many of the polyps are within reach of a digital rectal examination, they may not be easy to feel due to their mobility. Clinical symptoms of intermittent bright red blood warrant an investigation.

The diagnosis and treatment of juvenile polyps require a combination of history, digital rectal examination, and colonoscopy. The historical shift of juvenile polyps to the more proximal colon and the concern for the presence of juvenile polyposis (more than five juvenile polyps), with its increased risk of malignancy, mandates that the entire colon be surveyed. Polyps in the rectum can be removed easily during anoscopy. More proximal surveillance needs to be done by pancolonoscopy.

Differential diagnosis

The differential diagnosis of juvenile polyps encompasses all of the causes of rectal bleeding in toddlers and children up to the age of six years. Anal fissures and rectal prolapse cause rectal bleeding, but are easily distinguished from polyps on physical examination. Bleeding from a Meckel's diverticulum or duplication of the intestine usually causes more substantial blood loss than that from a polyp, and the blood usually mingles with the stool rather than coating it. Bleeding from an intussusception is accompanied by abdominal pain that is substantially worse than that seen with polyps. Inflammatory bowel disease is usually accompanied by diarrhea, which is not seen with polyps. Blood dyscrasias, such as Henoch–Schönlein purpura, should also be considered in the differential diagnosis. Rectal polyps occur in up to 15 percent of children with Peutz–Jeghers syndrome, and this condition should be considered.

OPERATION

Anoscopy with polyp removal and pancolonoscopy can be performed as an outpatient procedure. Standard bowel preparation for a colonoscopy is performed by the patient's parents at home prior to surgery. Suitable premedication is given and general anesthesia is induced. The child is turned into the left lateral position with the sacrum at the edge of the operating table. The anus and perineum are inspected and digital rectal examination is performed. Polyps in the anorectal area can usually be removed at this point if they are found at the anal verge (see illustration 1).

If a polyp is not identified on digital examination, an appropriately sized anoscope is lubricated and inserted.

Since complete bowel preparation and cleansing have been performed, the presence of formed stool is unlikely. If stool is present, removal can be accomplished with a moistened cotton swab. When a polyp is identified deeper in the rectum, a chromic or Vicryl endoloop is placed around the base of the stalk and cinched down. A second endoloop is placed at a distance distally on the stalk, tightened down, and the stalk cut. This allows for accurate placement of sutures and easy removal of the polyp once cut (see illustration 2).

After all polyps have been removed within the area of the anoscope or if no polyps are found in the most distant rectum, pancolonoscopy is performed. All polyps are removed endoscopically by the standard snare technique. The location of each polyp is recorded.

1 A polyp in the lower rectum or at the anal canal verge can often be brought out through the anus by digital examination. The stalk is then ligated by an absorbable suture and then cut. Often the stalk is torsed and the blood supply thrombosed. These polyps are occasionally avulsed during the maneuver to bring them out of the anal canal. Avulsion may cause minor bleeding, which will usually stop spontaneously or by applying pressure with a cotton-tipped applicator. Persistent bleeding can usually be controlled by the application of electrocautery.

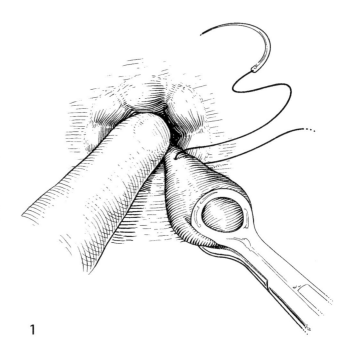

1

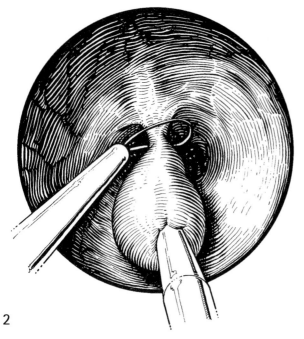

2

2 Polyps further up in the rectum can be visualized using an anoscope or nasal speculum placed in the anal canal. An absorbable endoloop snare is looped over the polyp and tightened down at the mucosal base. A second endoloop is placed distally on the stalk and the stalk is then transected with scissors, electrocautery, or a scalpel. The polyp should be recovered for histologic examination, and this is easily accomplished by holding on to the distal endoloop when the stalk is transected.

POSTOPERATIVE CARE

Most children can return home as soon as they have recovered from anesthesia. Parents should be warned that there may be some blood in the stool for a few days. The surgeon should follow up with the parents, verifying the type of polyp found on histologic examination. The parents should also be counseled to return should new bleeding occur.

Complications

Perforation and hemorrhage can occur, but they are extremely rare complications that are usually self-limiting.

OUTCOME

Most children with juvenile polyps will not have a recurrence of the problem. Pancolonoscopy should be performed, however, for any child with recurrent bleeding. In children with between two and four polyps, juvenile polyposis syndrome, with its increased risk of malignancy, should be considered. These children should undergo pancolonoscopy again a year after their initial polyp removal.

FURTHER READING

Franzin G, Zamboni G, Dina R *et al.* Juvenile and inflammatory polyps of the colon: a histological and histochemical study. *Histopathology* 1983; **7**: 719–28.

Jass JR. Juvenile polyposis. In: Phillips RKS, Spigelman AD, Thomson JPS (eds). *Familial Adenomatous Polyposis and Other Polyposis Syndromes.* Boston, MA: Little Brown, 1994.

Mestre JR. The changing pattern of juvenile polyps. *American Journal of Gastroenterology* 1986; **5**: 312–14.

Morson BC. Some peculiarities in the histology of intestinal polyps. *Diseases of the Colon and Rectum* 1962; **5**: 337–44.

Nelson EW, Rogers BM, Zawatsky L. Endoscopic appearance of auto-amputated polyps in juvenile polyposis coli. *Journal of Pediatric Surgery* 1977; **12**: 773–6.

64

Anal fissure and anal fistula

PAOLO DE COPPI

ANAL FISSURE

History

The first description of the treatment of anal fissure was by Boyer in his 1825 *Traité des Maladies Chirurgicales* and included the use of dorsal sphincterotomy without distinguishing the internal sphincter. Récamier described the use of anal dilatation in 1829. Since then, various methods have drifted in and out of vogue, including longitudinal incision of the base of the fissure (Lane, 1865), application of a sclerosant, anal dilatation, and radical excision of the fissure (Gabriel, 1930), and dorsal sphincterotomy (Morgan and Thompson, 1956). Dorsal internal sphincterotomy was occasionally observed to cause fecal leakage, and the lateral internal sphincterotomy was developed by Parks (1967).

Principles and justification

Anal fissure presents commonly to both general practitioners and surgical outpatient clinics, with peak incidence between 6 and 24 months. It is a tear to the squamous epithelial mucosa of the anal canal between the anocutaneous junction and the dentate line, and is thought to result from trauma by the passage of hard stool. Anal fissure is the most common cause of rectal bleeding in infants. More significantly, it can cause pain on defecation, initiating a vicious cycle of pain, reluctance to defecate, development of a large and hard stool with further tears to the anal mucosa accompanied by more pain. Counseling after treatment is required to break the cycle of pain and apprehension.

Other contributing factors implicated in the formation of anal fissures are hypertonicity of the internal anal sphincter, anodermal ischemia, infection, and chronic constipation. Chronic anal fissures may indicate Crohn's disease.

The majority of children can be managed medically with dietary advice (increasing dietary fluids and fiber) and stool softeners. Unresponsive anal fissures can be treated with topical glyceryl trinitrate (GTN) paste applied to the lower anal canal. The GTN paste has been shown to reduce the resting anal pressure while increasing the anodermal blood flow. Doses of between 0.05 and 0.2 percent have been used in children. Headaches secondary to systemic absorption and vasodilatation have been reported in over half of patients. Future therapies whose efficacy is yet to be established include topical diltiazem (2 percent gel) and botulinum toxin injection.

Alternatively, transcutaneous needle-free injection of botulinum toxin into the external anal sphincter has been successfully used for the treatment of chronic idiopathic constipation and anal fissure in children.

Preoperative assessment and preparation

Diagnosis of an anal fissure can be made by careful history and examination of the anus with gentle traction on the perianal skin to expose the lesion, most commonly found midline posteriorly. If the fissure is chronic, a sentinel tag may be visible at its base, representing epithelialized granulomatous tissue from chronic inflammation. No specialized investigations are required.

ANESTHESIA

General anesthesia is given. A caudal block is very useful for postoperative pain.

Operation

ANAL DILATATION

1 The patient is placed in the lithotomy position if an infant, or in the left lateral position if a larger child.

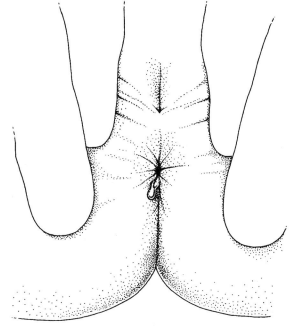

1

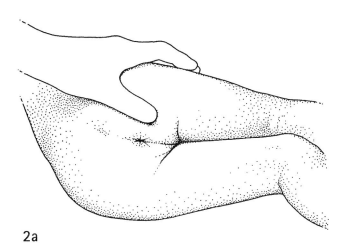

2a

2a The anal region is inspected and a digital examination performed. If the fissure appears suspicious, a biopsy should be taken.

2b Dilatation is performed using the index fingers, with gentle traction with one digit posteriorly followed by the second digit in countertraction anteriorly.

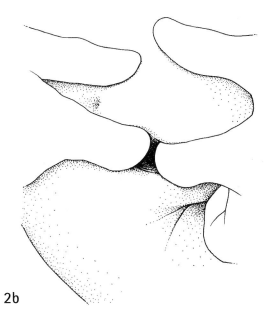

2b

3 The hands are rotated; gentle traction is now applied laterally. If any hard feces are found, these can be manually evacuated. Following gentle dilatation, the mucosa may appear more engorged, but there should be no further mucosal tears or bruising.

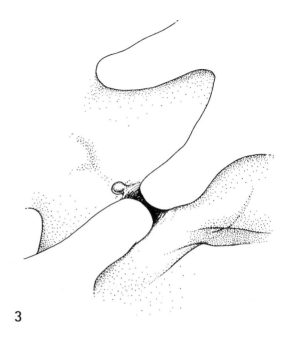

3

LATERAL ANAL SPHINCTEROTOMY

The patient is placed in the lithotomy position. An inspection of the anal region and digital examination are performed.

A rigid sigmoidoscopy is performed to confirm the diagnosis. A lubricated Park's retractor is then inserted and opened to expose the anal canal. The intersphincteric groove at the 3 o'clock position is palpated at the inferior border of the internal and external anal sphincters. This region is infiltrated with 1:250 000 epinephrine (adrenaline) with lidocaine (lignocaine) up to the dentate line and outside the internal sphincter.

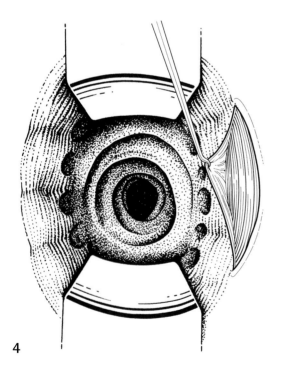

4 A 2-cm curvilinear incision is made outside the anal verge, raising a flap of skin off the internal sphincter as far as the dentate line.

4

5 A similar flap is raised on the other side to expose the internal sphincter. The lower third of the internal sphincter is incised to the dentate line. The skin is closed. If the fissure appears suspicious, a biopsy should be taken. The sentinel tag may be removed, taking care that no damage to the external sphincter occurs.

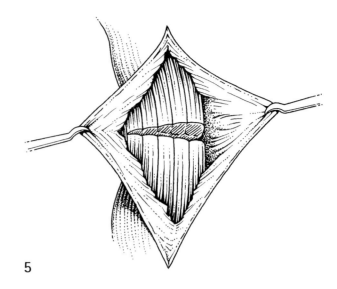

5

Postoperative care

Patients should continue dietary modification and stool softeners. The child can be weaned off stool softeners once defecation is comfortable. Mild analgesia should be given as required.

Outcome

Complications may include some postoperative rectal bleeding and perianal pain. Local infection is rare. Incontinence has been reported in adults but not in children undergoing these procedures.

Data describing the long-term outcomes of the two surgical procedures are lacking. Anal dilatation usually provides prompt pain relief. Recurrence of symptoms has been reported in 5–30 percent of patients. More than one attempt may be required for permanent relief of symptoms. Lateral anal sphincterotomy has a reported recurrence rate of 0–10 percent.

ANAL FISTULA

History

Documentation of anal fistula dates back as far as Hippocrates (460BC), who described treatment using a seton. Arderne (1307–1390), an English surgeon, described the application of a seton and provided the first report of laying open of the fistula in 1337. Further classification systems and theories of etiology were documented during the late nineteenth and early twentieth centuries. In 1976, Parks refined the classification system, which is still in use today.

Principles and justification

Anal fistulas commonly present in infants as recurrent perianal abscesses, which sometimes discharge spontaneously. They are hollow tracts lined with granulation tissue, probably originating as an infected anal canal gland. Unlike in adults, the tracts usually run radially and straight from their anal canal origin to the site of the abscess. Anal fistulas occur most commonly in males and in infants.

Perianal abscesses are common in infancy and occur with equal frequency in males and females. Fluctuant abscesses should be incised and drained. Superficial non-fluctuant infections may be treated conservatively with sitz baths. One-third of these will resolve without further treatment, but the majority will become fluctuant and require surgery. Almost 50 percent of all perianal abscesses develop a perianal fistula. A history of recurrent abscesses should alert the surgeon to possible underlying inflammatory bowel disease or chronic granulomatous disease and the child should be examined under general anesthetic.

Preoperative assessment and preparation

No special preoperative investigations are required.

ANESTHESIA
A general anesthetic is given with caudal block.

Operation

6 The child is placed in the lithotomy position. A careful inspection of the anal region is performed, looking for induration and signs of underlying pathology. Any suspicious lesions should be biopsied.

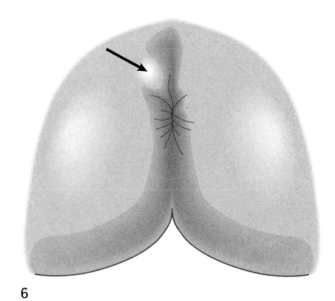

6

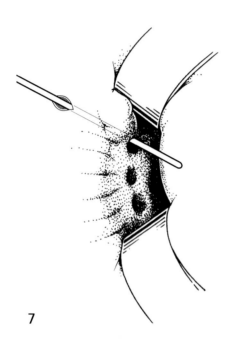

7

7 A lubricated Park's retractor is inserted to visualize the anal canal and the origin of the anal fistula. The abscess is incised and drained and a silver probe is gently inserted into the opening of the fistulous tract, taking care not to form a false tract. The opening in the anal canal is therefore visualized.

8 A knife or electrocautery is used to cut down onto the probe, laying the fistula open. If there is a great deal of granulation tissue in the floor of the fistula or the abscess cavity, this may be curetted. To ensure the tract can drain freely, excess overhanging skin should be excised.

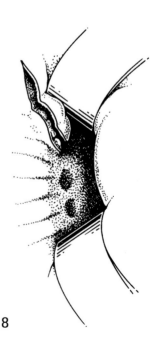

8

Postoperative care

Patients should be given stool softeners and dietary advice to reduce discomfort from trauma to the wound. They should also be advised to bathe carefully, using a shower jet to keep the wound clean.

Outcome

Wounds usually heal in 4–6 weeks. Recurrence should prompt further investigation into possible underlying disease.

FURTHER READING

Cohen A, Dehn TCB. Lateral subcutaneous sphincterotomy for treatment of anal fissure in children. *British Journal of Surgery* 1995; **82**: 1341–2.

Festen C, van Harten H. Perianal abscess and fistula-in-ano in infants. *Journal of Pediatric Surgery* 1998; **33**: 711–13.

Keshtgar AS, Ward HC, Clayden GS. Transcutaneous needle-free injection of botulinum toxin: a novel treatment of childhood constipation and anal fissure. *Journal of Pediatric Surgery* 2009; **44**: 1791–8.

Nelson R. A systematic review of medical therapy for anal fissure. *Diseases of the Colon and Rectum* 2004; **47**: 422–31.

Nelson R. Non surgical therapy for anal fissure. *Cochrane Database of Systematic Reviews* 2006; (**4**): CD003431.

Simpson J, Lund JN, Thompson RJ *et al.* The use of glyceryl trinitrate (GTN) in the treatment of chronic anal fissure in children. *Medical Science Monitor* 2003; **9**: 123–6.

65

Rectal prolapse

PAOLO DE COPPI

PRINCIPLES AND JUSTIFICATION

Rectal prolapse is a relatively common problem in young children, with a peak incidence of 1–3 years. In this age group, most cases are idiopathic and frequently self-limiting. A decision to operate is based on the frequency of recurrent prolapse (>2 episodes requiring manual reduction) along with symptoms of pain, rectal bleeding, and perianal excoriation because of recurrent prolapse. Prolapse is also associated with tenesmus and excessive straining at stool associated with diarrhea, constipation, parasitic worms, and rectal polyps. Children with neuromuscular problems, such as meningomyelocele or exstrophy of the bladder, often have rectal prolapse. There is an increased incidence of rectal prolapse in children with cystic fibrosis associated with tenacious stool, chronic cough, and loss of perirectal fat.

Appearance

1 Most commonly, the prolapse is incomplete, limited to 2–3 cm of mucosa protruding from the anus and classically displaying radial folds.

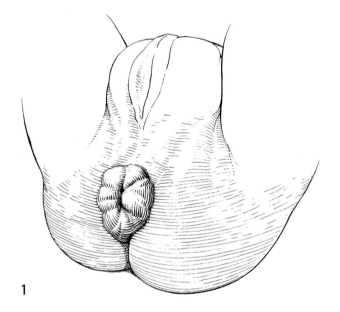

1

2 Complete, full-thickness rectal prolapse is more unusual. The mucosal folds in the acute complete case are circumferential. However, in both types, the mucosal definition is lost with time as the mucosa becomes edematous, smooth, and featureless. The size and palpable thickness of the wall will differentiate the two types.

Rectal prolapse may present initially as a pouting rosette of rectal mucosa typically occurring following straining at defecation. The prolapse may reduce spontaneously or require manual reduction. Prolapse may also present as mucosal bleeding.

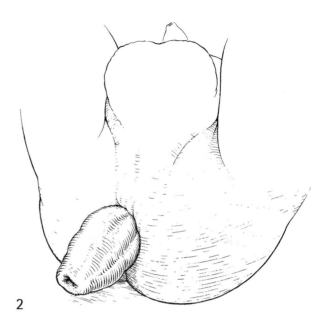

2

Assessment

The assessment of children presenting with rectal prolapse should include a general history and physical examination to exclude associated etiological factors. Initial investigations should include a sweat test or gene probe to exclude cystic fibrosis. Stool analysis should also be performed.

NON-OPERATIVE MANAGEMENT

The initial management of rectal prolapse is non-operative and aims to facilitate normal stooling without excessive straining by: (1) prescribing a laxative (e.g. lactulose); (2) encouraging a high-fiber diet; (3) encouraging regular, prompt defecation from a sitting, not squatting, position.

Additional support to the perianal region during defecation has been recommended in the past; however, there is no evidence that this prevents recurrence. The parent may provide support at defecation by placing their hands under the child's buttocks, fingers just inside the ischial tuberosities beside the anus. More prolonged support can be given by strapping the buttocks together. The authors do not recommend the use of external support as a definitive treatment.

Operative management is indicated when conservative measures have repeatedly failed to prevent recurrent prolapse.

PREOPERATIVE ASSESSMENT AND PREPARATION

Under general anesthesia, an initial rectal examination and proctoscopy are performed to exclude rectal polyps. If the rectum is loaded with hard stool, this should be evacuated. The specific goals of surgical management of full-thickness rectal prolapse are to eradicate the external prolapse of the rectum, improve continence, improve bowel function, and reduce incidence of recurrence.

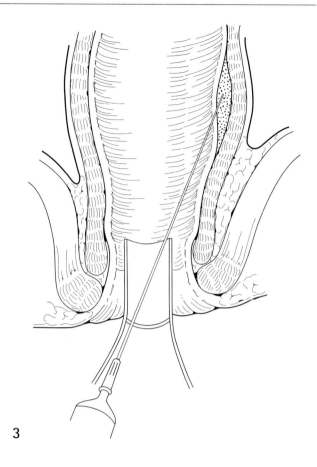

3

OPERATIONS

Injection of mucosal prolapse

3 A proctoscope of appropriate size is gently introduced into the lower anorectal region. A long, 23-gauge needle is placed under vision into the submucosal plane of the lower rectum approximately 4 cm from the anal verge. Then, 1–2 mL of 5 percent phenol, 30 percent saline solution, or 5 percent ethanolamine oleate is injected into the submucosal space into each of the four quadrants. A bulge at the injection site or blanching of the mucosa will indicate that sufficient sclerosant has been injected.

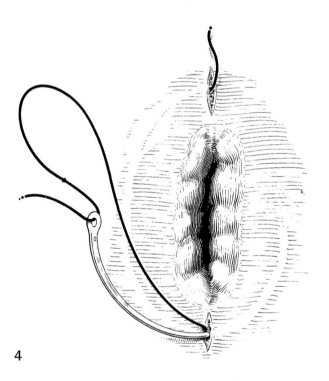

4

Thiersch operation (modified)

4 The child is placed in the lithotomy position and the perianal area is prepared and draped. Two small incisions are made 2 cm from the anal verge at 12 o'clock and 6 o'clock. A length of absorbable (e.g. 0 caliber polydioxanone (PDS)) suture material is threaded from the posterior incision to the anterior incision around the anus, just deep to the external sphincter muscle. The suture is continued from anterior to posterior so that eventually a ring is placed around the anus.

5 With an assistant's finger or a Hegar's dilator held inside the anal canal, the suture is pulled and tied inside the posterior incision. Absorbable sutures are used to close the two incisions. Thiersch's procedure acts by narrowing the anal orifice and thereby mechanically supporting the prolapse.

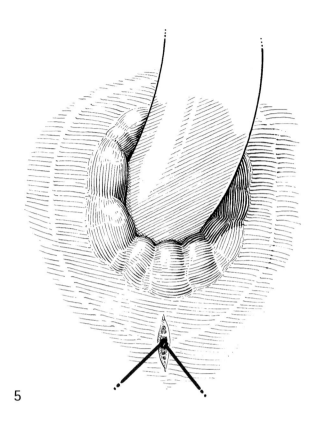

5

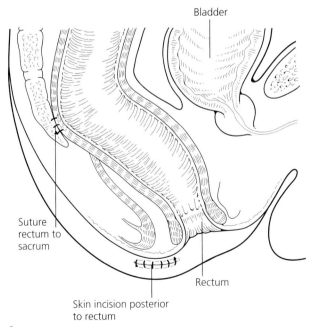

Bladder

Suture rectum to sacrum

Skin incision posterior to rectum

Rectum

6

Posterior plication

6 The patient is placed in the jack-knife position. A midline skin incision is made from the coccyx and extended halfway to the anus. This incision is deepened towards the coccyx, which, if the distance from the coccyx to the anus is short and the operating field limited, may be excised. The parasagittal fibers and levator muscle are divided exactly in the midline using cautery, taking care not to incise the muscle complex. The rectum is then dissected free for two-thirds of the circumference and up to 10–15 cm vertically. Three or four permanent seromuscular sutures (3/0 or 4/0 polypropylene (Prolene)) are then placed in a longitudinal, U-shaped, mattress pattern. When these sutures are pulled together, the redundant rectum is drawn together. A further set of sutures may then be passed through the last segment of the sacrum and tied on its surface. The muscle layers are then approximated and the wound closed.

Transanal mucosal sleeve resection

7a–d The patient is placed prone in the jack-knife position. The prolapse is gently drawn out and four quadrant traction sutures are placed through the submucosa at the apex. Epinephrine solution (1:200 000) may be injected to separate the mucosal and submucosal from the muscular layers, defining the plane of dissection (illustration a). A circumferential incision is made through the mucosal and submucosal layers approximately 1 cm proximal to the pectinate line, and blunt dissection is used to strip this layer from the underlying muscle (illustration b). The denuded muscle layer is gradually reduced into the pelvis while the traction sutures are used to pull the mucosal sleeve in the opposite direction. When the submucosal has been separated from the entire length of the prolapse, it is divided longitudinally into two halves (illustration c). As the sleeve is incised circumferentially, single absorbable sutures are placed to approximate the edges of the proximal and distal mucosal cuffs. Traction is maintained on the sleeve until the resection is complete; the sutures are then cut and the anastomosis retracts into the pelvis (illustration d).

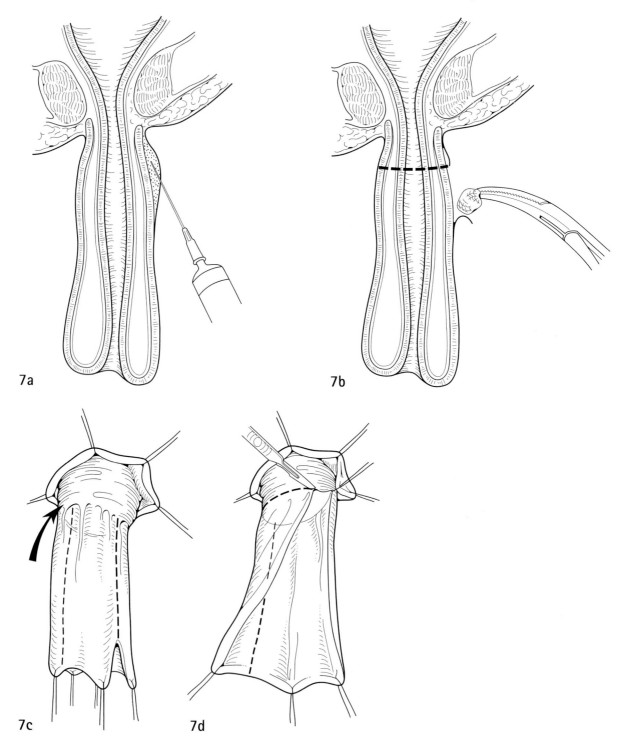

7a

7b

7c

7d

Laparoscopic abdominal rectopexy

Many open abdominal procedures previously advocated for severe recurrent rectal prolapse are now performed using laparoscopic techniques, such as the suture rectopexy and the modified sling rectopexy using a polypropylene mesh to secure the rectum.

8 The patient is placed in the lithotomy position. A nasogastric tube and urethral catheter are placed. A pneumoperitoneum is established under direct vision by placing a Hasson cannula. A 5-mm 0° laparoscope is passed to inspect the intra-abdominal contents. Three further 5-mm trocars are then inserted under direct vision, two in the right paraumbilical region and one in the left paraumbilical region. Laparoscopic technique includes a retrorectal dissection, starting from the peritoneal reflection on the right side of the rectum, extending from the sacral promontory to the pelvic muscular floor in the rectosacral bloodless plain. Great care is given to the identification of iliac vessels and ureter. In the absence of pelvic floor laxity, suture rectopexy to the sacral promontory and suture sigmoidopexy to the left lateral peritoneum are done without mesh. In cases with laxity and weakness of the pelvic floor and in patients with neuropathic conditions (spina bifida and meningomyelocele), additional retrorectal mesh is recommended. The mesh is tailored to fit the retrorectal space, where it is fixed to the rectum by between two and four non-absorbable stitches. Then, the mesh and the rectum are dragged up and fixed to the sacral promontory with closure of the peritoneal defect.

The growing body of literature supports the concept that laparoscopic surgical techniques can safely provide the benefits of low recurrence rates, improved functional outcome, less postoperative pain, short hospital stay, and early return of bowel function for patients with full-thickness rectal prolapse.

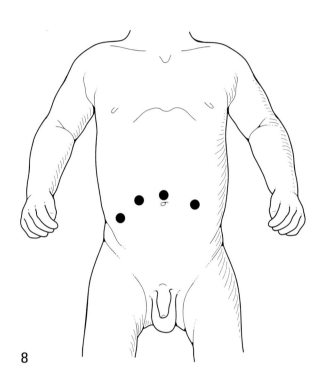

8

POSTOPERATIVE CARE

Mucosal injection and Thiersch suture can be performed as a day-case procedure. Regular bowel habit is encouraged, as in non-operative management. Stool softeners may be advocated for between three and six months, with advice to avoid sitting on the toilet for long periods.

Complications

All of the above procedures may be associated with infection and perianal abscess formation. Usually these complications resolve fully with conservative treatment, including antibiotic therapy; occasionally incision and drainage may be required. Rarely, serious scarring and stricture formation may result, causing deformity of the rectum and leakage of mucus or fistula formation. The Thiersch suture may cause stool retention and fecal impaction if tied too tightly, in which case suture removal

should be performed. Disruption of the skin wounds and exposure of knots may occur if they have not been buried sufficiently.

OUTCOME

Most patients presenting with a simple mucosal rectal prolapse respond to conservative, non-operative management. For recurrent rectal prolapse, the authors recommend the approach outlined in **Figure 65.1**.

Following injection of sclerosant, recurrence occurs in 10–20 percent of cases. In these cases, injection therapy may be repeated 4–6 weeks later. Many different treatments have been suggested for those persistent or severe cases that are resistant to injection therapy. Encircling procedures, abdominal rectopexies, and abdominal–perineal bowel resections have a recurrence risk of approximately 25 percent. Posterior sagittal and transanal procedures have a higher success rate of between 80 and 100 percent.

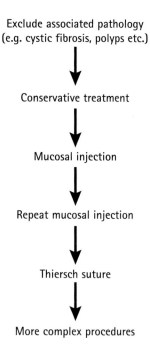

Exclude associated pathology
(e.g. cystic fibrosis, polyps etc.)

Conservative treatment

Mucosal injection

Repeat mucosal injection

Thiersch suture

More complex procedures

Figure 65.1 Management of recurrent rectal prolapse.

FURTHER READING

Ashcraft KW, Garred JL, Holder TM *et al*. Rectal prolapse: 17-year experience with the posterior repair and suspension. *Journal of Pediatric Surgery* 1990; **25**: 992–4.

Chan WK, Kay SM, Laberge JM *et al*. Injection sclerotherapy in the treatment of rectal prolapse in infants and children. *Journal of Pediatric Surgery* 1998; **33**: 255–8.

Chwals WJ, Brennan LP, Weitzman JJ, Woolley MM. Transanal mucosal sleeve resection for the treatment of rectal prolapse in children. *Journal of Pediatric Surgery* 1990; **25**: 715–18.

Ismail M, Gabr K, Shalaby R. Laparoscopic management of persistent complete rectal prolapse in children. *Journal of Pediatric Surgery* 2010; **45**: 533–9.

Laituri CA, Garey CL, Fraser JD *et al*. 15-Year experience in the treatment of rectal prolapse in children. *Journal of Pediatric Surgery* 2010; **45**: 1607–9.

Sander S, Vural O, Unal M. Management of rectal prolapse in children: Ekehorn's rectosacropexy. *Pediatric Surgery International* 1999; **15**: 111–14.

Solomon M, Young C, Eyers A, Roberts R. Randomized clinical trial of laparoscopic versus open abdominal rectopexy for rectal prolapse. *British Journal of Surgery* 2002; **89**: 35–9.

Tsugawa C, Matsumoto Y, Nishijima E *et al*. Posterior plication of the rectum for rectal prolapse in children. *Journal of Pediatric Surgery* 1995; **30**: 692–3.

66

Colostomy: formation and closure

JOE CURRY

HISTORY

Alexis Littre (1658–1726), the Parisian anatomist, is credited with being the first to propose a planned colostomy, or artificial anus. This occurred in 1710 during an autopsy on a child with anal atresia, when he explained how, after making an incision in the abdomen, it would be possible 'to bring the superior part of the bowel to the abdominal wound, which should never be closed and which would perform the function of the anus'. It was not until 1776 that this concept was applied, when a colostomy was performed by Pillore of Rouen on an adult with rectal carcinoma. In 1783, Dubois is said to have been the first to construct a colostomy in an infant, but the patient, who had anal atresia, died after 10 days. The first long-term survivor was an infant, also with imperforate anus, who had a colostomy made by Duret in 1793 and was still alive 45 years later. During the nineteenth century, the procedure was introduced at centers across Europe and various modifications were developed, including loop colostomy over a rod by Maydl (1888). Operation 'à deux temps' reported in 1885 by Davies-Colley of Guy's Hospital, London, consisted of suturing the bowel to the skin followed by delayed opening once the wound edges had sealed; this was an important development in an era when infection was the major cause of morbidity. The Hartmann procedure, described in 1923 for use following rectal excision for carcinoma at a time when anastomosis of the colon to the rectum was still dangerous, is still widely used in pediatric surgery.

Colostomy closure, too, was a dangerous procedure with a high risk of leakage and fecal peritonitis. This led to the introduction of techniques to minimize the risk of peritoneal contamination, such as extraperitoneal closure. With the Mikulicz technique, the common walls of a double-barrelled colostomy are crushed using an enterotome or forceps, and the resulting fecal fistula is closed later, leaving the suture line extraperitoneal if desired.

Today, colostomy formation and closure are safe operations provided basic surgical principles are adhered to, but the risk of potentially serious complications is ever present and must not be underestimated.

PRINCIPLES AND JUSTIFICATION

A colostomy is used to divert the fecal stream from the distal colon and rectum, and may be temporary or permanent. A temporary colostomy may be a primary procedure in the management of a congenital anorectal anomaly, distal obstruction as with Hirschsprung's disease, or an injury, severe inflammatory condition, or infective disease of the distal colon, rectum, or anus. It may also be a secondary procedure to protect a distal anastomosis. A permanent colostomy is required following radical excision of the anorectum for disease or debilitating fecal incontinence, for example due to anal sphincter dysfunction or colorectal dysmotility.

The following types of colostomy are in common use.

- **Divided colostomy**. This has the advantage of complete fecal diversion and a low risk of prolapse or retraction. The colon is transacted and the distal end exteriorized as a mucous fistula and either placed adjacent to the proximal stoma so that both stomas may be enclosed within the same colostomy bag, or the stomas are widely separated by placing them at opposite corners of the incision so that the proximal, but not the distal, stoma lies within the colostomy bag in order to prevent feces entering the distal colon. Alternatively, the distal stoma is closed and placed within the abdominal cavity (Hartmann procedure) (see illustration 10).
- **Loop colostomy**. A loop of colon is exteriorized and opened, but not divided. The procedure has the advantages of being simple and quick to perform and is of particular value in seriously ill patients, but it carries a higher risk of prolapse and retraction. The extent of fecal diversion is variable, which is a disadvantage in the presence of a complete anal occlusion, when the rectum cannot be washed out, or with an anorectal fistula, where there is a risk of recurrent urinary tract infection from rectal organisms.

Siting the colostomy

An elective colostomy is usually sited either in the proximal transverse or in the proximal sigmoid colon, where the colon is readily accessible and sufficiently mobile to be exteriorized without tension. The sigmoid colostomy has the advantage that there is a greater length of proximal colon available for fluid and electrolyte absorption, and the stools are thicker.

Optimal placement of the colostomy is important and will depend on the clinical situation. The colostomy bag must fit comfortably over the proximal stoma and, to avoid leakage, the surrounding skin surface must be flat, avoiding bony prominences, to ensure watertight adherence of the bag. Patients who manage their own colostomy, particularly those who are wheelchair bound, must be able to access the stoma easily; this requires preoperative planning with a stoma therapist.

PREOPERATIVE MANAGEMENT

Colostomy formation is a major operation and the patient's condition must be optimized before operation. Nasogastric drainage and intravenous fluid therapy are indicated in the presence of obstruction. Prophylactic antibiotics are given preoperatively.

Anesthesia

General anesthesia is employed with muscle relaxation.

OPERATIONS

Divided colostomy

1 For a transverse colostomy, a right upper transverse incision is planned so that a colostomy bag can be placed on a flat surface away from the costal margin. A transverse muscle-sparing incision is used for the sigmoid colostomy, centred about midway between the umbilicus and the left anterior superior iliac spine.

After incising the skin and rectus sheath, the rectus muscle is parted in the line of its fibres; laterally, the abdominal wall muscles are divided if extra space is needed (see **Chapter 41**). The peritoneal cavity is entered and the colon identified and exteriorized. This may be difficult when the colon is severely distended and a rectal washout is not possible, particularly as the sigmoid often falls to the right side of the abdomen. If locating the sigmoid colon is difficult, consideration should be given to performing a formal laparotomy.

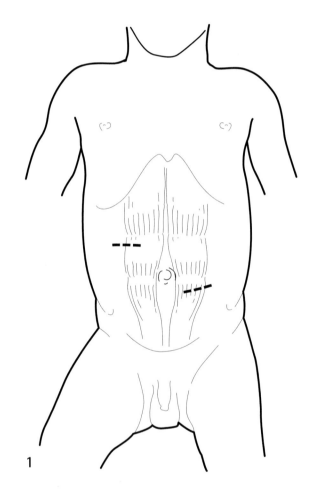

1

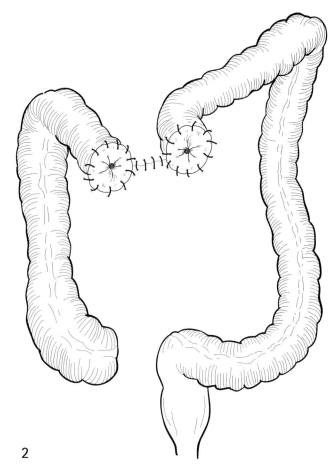

2 A transverse colostomy is placed towards the right side of the transverse colon. If the sigmoid colon is distended, it may lie in the upper abdomen and must be distinguished from the transverse colon by the presence of the fatty tenia coli, which are not found on the transverse colon.

2

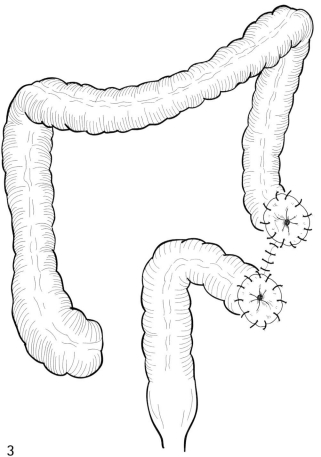

3

3 A sigmoid colostomy is usually placed nearer the proximal sigmoid colon, particularly for neonates with anorectal anomalies so as not to compromise the subsequent pull-through procedure, whereas for Hirschsprung disease the stoma is sited proximal to the transition zone as determined by intraoperative seromuscular biopsy. Note that for cloacal anomalies, a transverse colostomy is recommended to allow sufficient distal colon for vaginal reconstruction.

4 At the proposed point of transecting the colon, the marginal artery is divided between ligatures, and smaller branches to the colon are coagulated using bipolar diathermy.

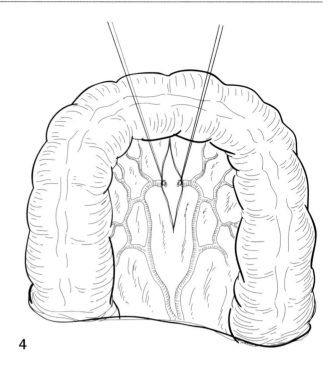

4

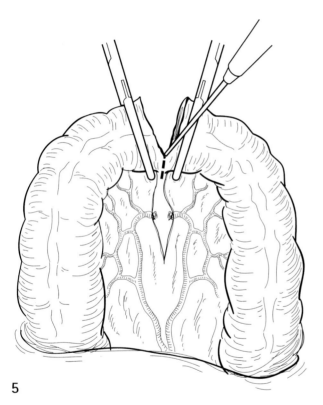

5

5 The colon is then divided using a scalpel or diathermy. Alternatively a GIA stapler may be used in older children.

6 The proximal and distal limbs of the colon are positioned at opposite corners of the incision, with sufficient distance between them to enable a colostomy bag to enclose the proximal stoma. Each limb is anchored to the abdominal wall with interrupted absorbable sutures in layers. The first layer is to the colon, peritoneum, and transversalis fascia; these sutures must be sufficiently close together to prevent loops of small intestine from prolapsing between them and should not penetrate the colonic mucosa as this may result in a fecal fistula.

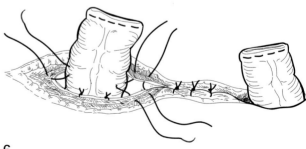

6

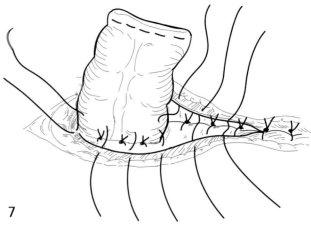

7   For the second layer, the colon is sutured to the surrounding external oblique aponeurosis taking care not to constrict the colon. The abdominal wall layers are approximated between the two limbs of the colostomy.

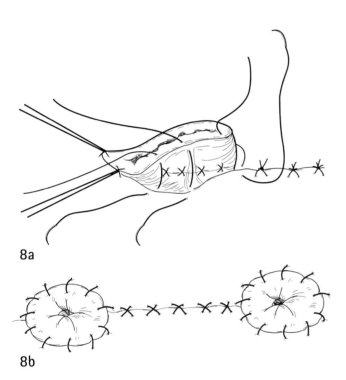

7

8a

8b

8a,b   Each limb of the colostomy is then opened. Full thickness, interrupted sutures approximate the cut edge of the colon to the adjacent edges of the skin incision.

9a,b   If required, the proximal stoma may be constructed with a spout that will protrude into the colostomy bag. Three-point interrupted sutures are placed through the abdominal wall muscle, the seromuscular wall of the colon and the cut edge of the colon to evert the end of the colostomy.

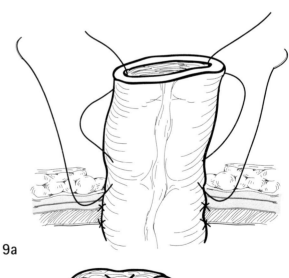

9a

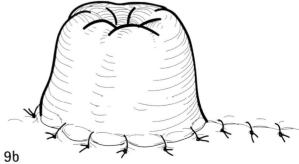

9b

10 Where there is no obstruction distal to the colostomy, the distal limb may be closed transversely in two layers and placed within the peritoneal cavity (Hartmann procedure). To enable the blind end to be located easily for subsequent reconstruction, it can be anchored to the undersurface of the peritoneum when the wound is closed.

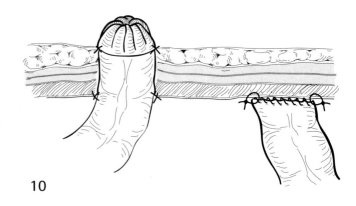

10

Loop colostomy

A muscle-splitting incision is used as for a divided colostomy, but the shape of the skin incision will depend on whether the exteriorized colon is to be supported by a catheter tube, in which case a standard straight skin incision is used (see illustration 1), or with a skin flap, for which an inverted V-incision is made (see illustration 13).

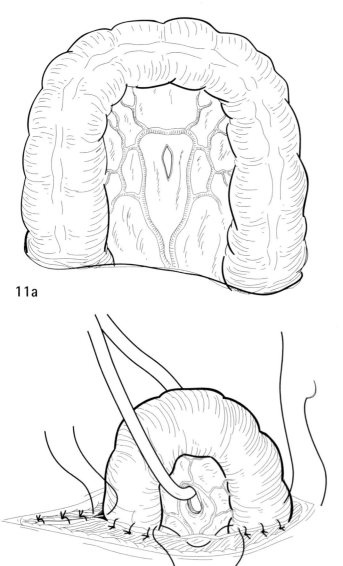

11a

11b

11a,b The colonic loop is exteriorized and elevated using a soft catheter passed through a window in the mesentery at the point of the proposed stoma. The mesenteric artery is not divided. The two limbs of the colon are secured to the abdominal wall in layers using absorbable sutures as described for a divided colostomy. The space between the two limbs is closed with interrupted sutures to prevent the small intestine prolapsing between them, taking care to avoid damaging the mesenteric blood vessels.

12 The catheter is shortened and anchored to the skin on either side of the loop of colon using non-absorbable sutures. The catheter must be short enough to be enclosed by the colostomy bag. The stoma is opened through a transverse incision at the apex of the colonic loop.

First, a short incision is made so that the edges of the colon can be lifted to avoid damaging its closely opposed opposite wall, particularly if diathermy is used to incise the colon.

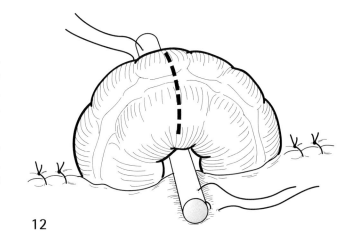

12

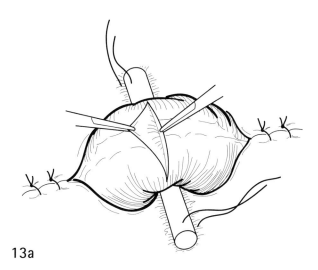

13a

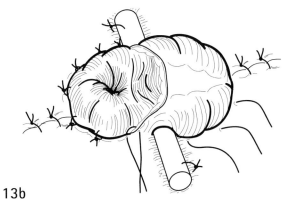

13b

13a,b The edges of the stoma are everted and sutured to the skin incision. A Hegar dilator is used to confirm that the stoma has not been constricted (transverse rather than longitudinal incision).

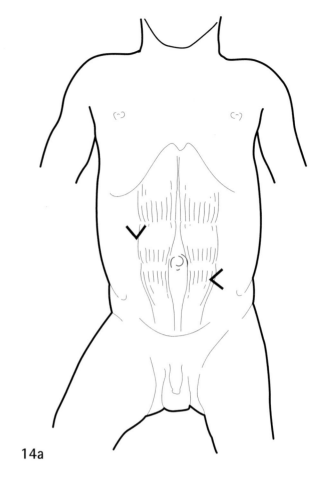

14a

14a–e If a skin flap is used to support the colostomy, the flap is drawn through the window in the mesentery and sutured as illustrated.

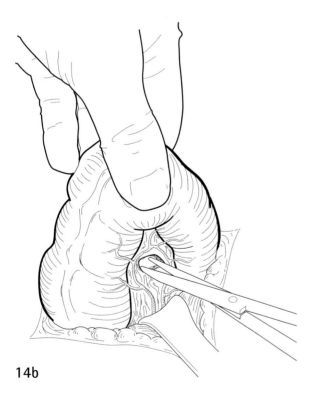

14b

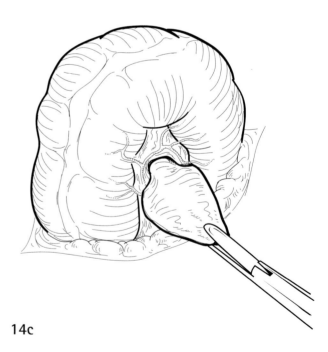

14c

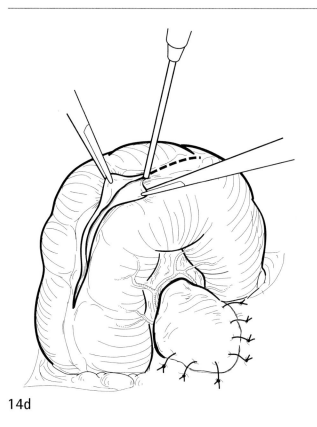

14d

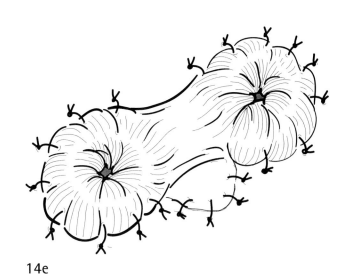

14e

Intraoperative colostomy

If a colostomy is required following intestinal resection, it should ideally be brought out through a separate incision. An exception is when the remaining intestine is fragile and compromised (as in neonatal necrotizing enterocolitis) and exteriorizing the colonic loops through separate incisions would be traumatic and risk further loss of valuable intestinal length. In this situation, the colonic loops may be brought out at either end of the main abdominal incision and carefully anchored to the abdominal wall. It is not necessary to evert and 'mature' the stoma as this will occur spontaneously.

COMPLICATIONS

Following colostomy formation, colostomy-related complications have been reported in up to 80 percent of patients. These include peristomal skin excoriation, prolapse, stomal obstruction/stenosis, parastomal herniation, and stomal bleeding.

Peristomal excoriation is very common and requires meticulous attention to skin care using specific protective preparations under the supervision of a stoma therapist. Prolapse from either loop may be troublesome, requiring repeated manual reduction and occasionally, stomal

revision. Stomal stenosis resulting in intestinal obstruction may require dilatation or revision. Parastomal hernia occurs as a result of small intestine herniating between the sutures anchoring the colostomy to the abdominal wall. Diversion proctitis, characterized by a mucopurulent rectal discharge, bleeding, and tenesmus, is a late effect of colonic diversion with characteristic endoscopic and histological features.

Colostomy closure

PREOPERATIVE PREPARATION AND ANESTHESIA

Prior to closing the colostomy, the integrity and patency of the bowel distal to the stoma must be confirmed by preoperative contrast radiology and, if appropriate, by digital rectal examination at the time of operation. Bowel preparation to empty the colon and rectal irrigation to evacuate residual stool may be necessary. Clear enteral fluids for 24 hours preoperatively can be used to reduce fecal residue.

General anesthesia is employed with muscle relaxation. A nasogastric tube is inserted, but removed at the end of the procedure. Prophylactic broad-spectrum antibiotics are administered at induction of anesthesia. Any colostomy bags are removed and residual adhesive paste is removed from the skin with solvent.

15 The incision encircles the two stomas and intervening skin scar. The skin should be incised in stages as there may be brisk arterial oozing from the margins of the incision. Monopolar diathermy can be employed for the skin incision to minimize blood loss if the skin is particularly inflamed.

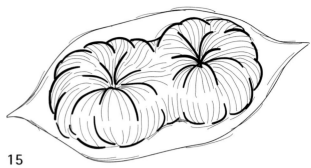

15

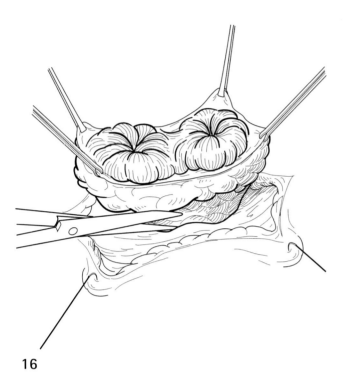

16

16 The incision is deepened to expose the external oblique aponeurosis and the margins of the opening in the abdominal wall are identified. With careful dissection using a combination of sharp dissection and monopolar diathermy, a plane is developed between the colonic loop and the abdominal wall to enter the peritoneal cavity, dividing the anchoring sutures and inevitable scarring without breaching the colonic wall or damaging the adjacent adherent loops of small intestine. This may be a difficult process and patience is essential. With a divided colostomy, the incision between the stomas is opened completely.

17 Once the two limbs of the colostomy have been mobilized sufficiently to allow them to be exteriorized, the stomas are resected back to healthy bowel and approximated by end-to-end anastomosis.

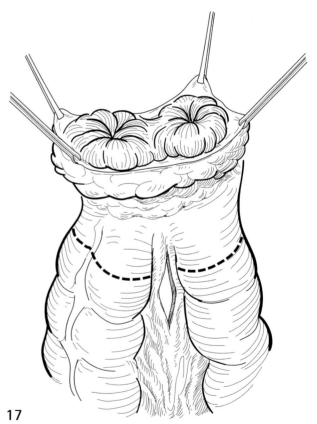

17

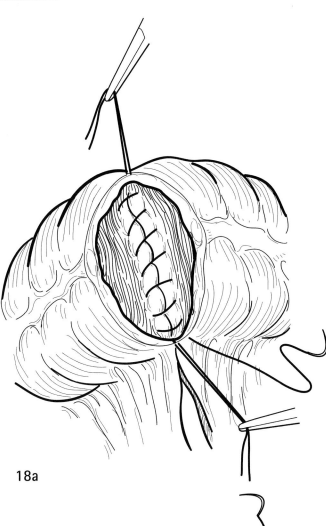

18a,b A single-layer of interrupted extramucosal sutures is suitable for all ages.

18a

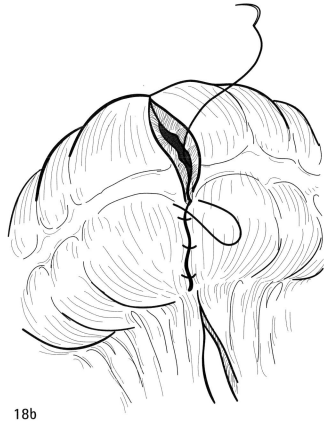

18b

19a,b In the older child, a loop colostomy may be closed without resecting the stoma. After mobilizing the colostomy, the edges are trimmed and the colon is closed transversely. In the infant, resection and end-to-end anastomosis are recommended.

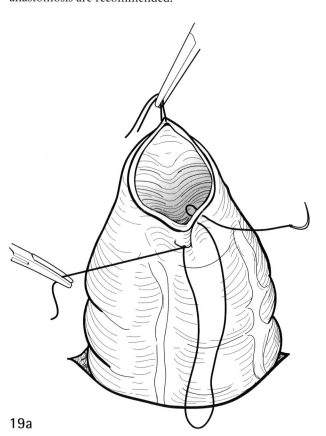

19a

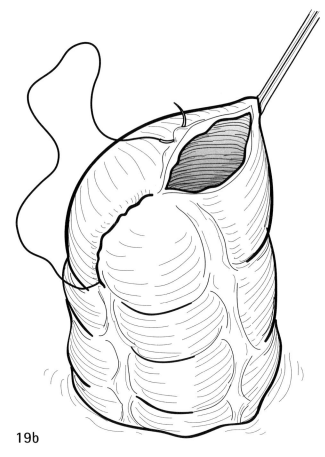

19b

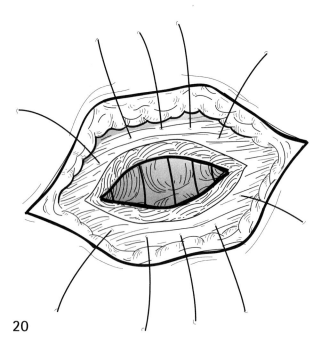

20

20 Interrupted, full-thickness sutures are used for the peritoneum and muscle layers if the tissue planes are not distinct, otherwise the abdominal incision can be closed in layers. If regional anesthesia has not been used, the muscle layer and wound are infiltrated with local anesthetic.

POSTOPERATIVE CARE

Intravenous fluids are continued until an adequate oral fluid intake is tolerated. Nasogastric tubes are not always required postoperatively, especially in infants. Enteral feeds are commenced usually within 24 hours and increased cautiously until flatus or stools are passed. Systemic analgesia is maintained as required.

COMPLICATIONS

Early complications following colostomy closure include wound infection, the risk of which is reduced by prophylactic antibiotics, and anastomotic leak. The latter is uncommon provided the bowel is healthy and well-vascularized; there is no tension on the anastomosis, and no distal bowel obstruction. Meticulous operative technique is required to ensure healthy bowel wall edges at the time of anastomosis. Late stenosis at the suture line is also uncommon if the colon is healthy. Adhesive small bowel obstruction has been reported in 6.5 percent of children following colostomy closure, and a mortality of less than 1 percent.

FURTHER READING

Bischoff A, Levitt M, Lawal TA, Pena A. Colostomy closure: how to avoid complications. *Pediatric Surgery International* 2010; **26**: 1087–92.

Chandramouli B, Srinivasan K, Jagdish S *et al.* Morbidity and mortality of colostomy and its closure in children. *Journal of Pediatric Surgery* 2004; **39**: 596–9.

Cigdem MK, Onen A, Duran H *et al.* The mechanical complications of colostomy in infants and children: an analysis of 473 cases in a single centre. *Pediatric Surgery International* 2006; **22**: 671–6.

Kiely EM, Ajayi NA, Wheeler RA, Malone M. Diversion procto-colitis: response to treatment with short chain fatty acids. *Journal of Paediatric Surgery* 2001; **36**: 1514–17.

Pena A, Migotto-Krieger M, Levitt MA. Colostomy in anorectal malformations: a procedure with serious but preventable complications. *Journal of Paediatric Surgery* 2006; **41**: 748–56.

Scharli WF. The history of colostomy in childhood. *Progress in Pediatric Surgery* 1986; **20**: 188–98.

67

Bowel-lengthening procedures

ADRIAN BIANCHI, TOM JAKSIC and KRISTINA M POTANOS

INTRODUCTION

The short bowel state is characterized by inadequate absorption from insufficient mucosal surface area. It follows extensive small bowel loss from antenatal or postnatal volvulus complicating malrotation or gastroschisis, and postnatal bowel loss or extensive resection for necrotizing enterocolitis. Other less common causes include long segment Hirschsprung disease extending high into the jejunum, and vascular accidents (embolism), tumors, or injury. The impact of extensive bowel loss reflects not only on the absorptive capacity of the small bowel, but also on gut-associated immunity, such that short-gut patients are at greater risk of gut-related infection and associated liver injury. Long-term survival will depend on the natural intestinal adaptation response within the residual 10–30 percent of absorptive small bowel, the presence of the ileocecal valve, and a greater length of colon.

Antenatal bowel loss presents as atresia with the typical obstructed, massively dilated proximal segment, and the defunctioned undeveloped distal bowel, usually the distal colon. End-to-end anastomosis between the two segments is followed by a failure of propulsion with stasis, sepsis, and portosystemic bacterial translocation from the proximal loop. Liver dysfunction follows gut-related sepsis, and is exacerbated by hyperalimentation, parenteral nutrition-related toxicity largely from plant phytosterols in lipid preparations, and possibly from a lack of small-bowel-related 'hepatoprotective factors'. In a high percentage of short-gut children, rapidly progressive liver injury leads to cholestasis and hepatocyte loss, with end-stage liver failure within a few months. However, liver dysfunction may be reversible if bowel adaptation is sufficient to shift the balance toward enteral nutrition and better gut-associated immunity. Bowel reconstructive procedures are designed to reduce the stasis and sepsis within the poorly propulsive dilated segment and to enhance the intestinal adaptation process toward enteral autonomy.

The child with short bowel: initial surgery

The child with short bowel presents a difficult, complex, multifaceted problem that requires close cooperation between the local team and a designated 'intestinal failure center' combining particularly pediatric gastroenterology and nutrition, autologous gastrointestinal reconstruction, and liver and bowel transplantation. Immediately at diagnosis, a 'management plan' is jointly developed, initially concentrating on survival and growth, liver protection, and preservation of venous access. Once stable, the child is best managed within his or her family and social environment, being hospitalized only for specific assessments or procedures.

1 At first surgery, all available bowel is preserved, and minimal, if any, bowel reconstruction is undertaken. A large-size Malecot catheter (16 Fr) is placed in the distalmost jejunum, and is brought out on the abdominal wall as a tube jejunostomy. This allows free drainage of the dilated bowel, thereby avoiding stasis, sepsis, and bacterial translocation. It is then also possible to commence oral (enteral) feeding, thus stimulating the child to become 'food-wise' and inducing small-bowel mucosal adaptation. Intermittent occlusion of the Malecot jejunostomy tube allows 'controlled bowel expansion', developing more autologous bowel for subsequent planned reconstruction. A smaller size Malecot catheter (10 Fr) is placed in the distal bowel (usually colon) to allow for recycling of jejunostomy losses, to maximize absorption, and to stimulate adaptation also in the distal colon.

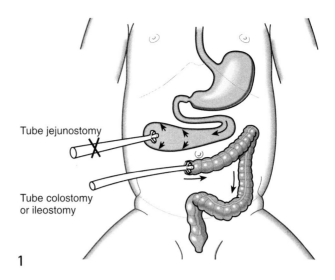

1

Autologous gastrointestinal reconstruction

Table 67.1 highlights the surgical techniques now available to enhance absorption and adaptation in the residual autologous bowel. These may be relevant alone or in various combinations.

Table 67.1 Procedures for bowel reconstruction.

Delay transit and increase contact time	Reversed antiperistaltic segments
	Prejejunal or pre-ileal colon transposition
	Intestinal valves
	Intermittent occlusion tube jejunostomy
Improve propulsion	Antemesenteric tailoring
	Plication (de Lorimer, Harrison)
Bowel expansion	Tube jejunostomy for 'controlled occlusion–recycle' (Bianchi)
	Nipple valve (Georgeson)
Bowel lengthening	Longitudinal intestinal lengthening and tailoring (LILT) (Bianchi)
	Serial transverse enteroplasty (STEP) (Kim et al.)
Antemesenteric blood supply	Isolated bowel segment Iowa model (Kimura)
	Composite bowel loops (Bianchi)
	Isolated segment + LILT (Georgeson)
Sequential and combined techniques	LILT + reversed segment (Bianchi)
	LILT + STEP (Kim et al.)

Such procedures are not an end in themselves, but should form part of a structured management plan specific to a particular child. Thus the bowel reconstructive plan may commence with a period of jejunostomy tube drainage of the dilated loop. The Malecot tube is then clamped for graded intervals to increase mucosal contact time for absorption and to induce bowel expansion, thereby creating more autologous tissue for eventual autologous gastrointestinal reconstruction (AGIR). This may take the form of longitudinal intestinal lengthening and tailoring (LILT), possibly combined with reversed antiperistaltic segments or colon transposition. In the event of bowel redilatation after LILT, a serial transverse enteroplasty (STEP) reduces bowel diameter to assist propulsion and further increases length to aid absorption.

Bowel-lengthening procedures

Bowel-lengthening procedures aim to reduce the diameter of dilated bowel without loss of absorptive mucosa, to establish effective propulsion, and to use the tailored bowel to create additional isoperistaltic length for increased mucosal contact and enhanced absorption. Since publication of the original technique in 1980, experience with LILT has been increasing. Results have been variable and largely dependent on the extent and quality of the residual bowel, and the condition of the child at the time of surgery. The procedure does not 'guarantee a cure', but has often been followed by enteral autonomy or by a significant reduction in parenteral nutrition requirements.

OPERATION

Longitudinal intestinal lengthening and tailoring (Bianchi 1980)

2 The abdomen is opened through an already existing scar or through a transverse supraumbilical incision, and the whole of the small and large bowel is dissected free of adhesions and exteriorized. During this phase, careful attention is given to avoiding damage to the mesenteric vessels supplying the dilated bowel. It is often easier to take down a previous anastomosis between the dilated proximal bowel (to be lengthened) and the distal bowel (often the colon). The bowel diameter and bowel length, measured along the antemesenteric border, are recorded. Bowel division may be undertaken using a manual technique or the endoscopic GIA stapler. The authors prefer, and recommend as safer, a manual division-and-suture technique.

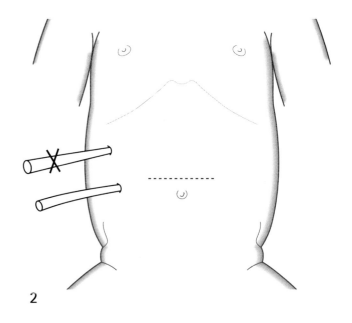

2

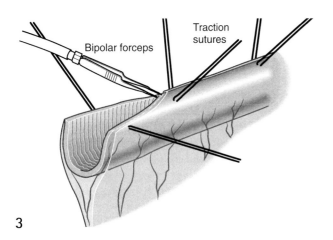

3

3 Traction sutures are placed along the antemesenteric border to the right and left of the midline at about 10-cm intervals, and the bowel is drawn upwards and outwards against the base of the mesentery.

4 With the 'cutting wave' of the bipolar diathermy, the bowel is divided longitudinally for a comfortable working length, passing between the traction sutures along the antemesenteric border to the right and left of the midline for about 10 cm.

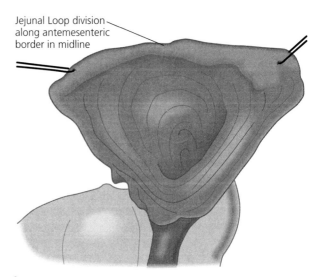

4

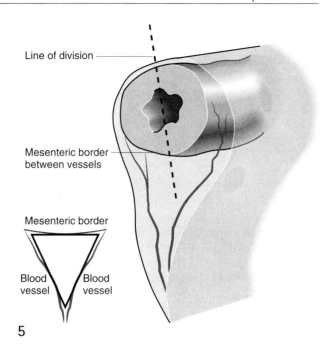

5   Outward and upward traction on the opened bowel loop against the base of the mesentery gives access to the blood vessels between the leaves of the mesentery. This natural plane is developed by blunt dissection, such that the mesenteric border of the bowel of approximately 1 cm width between the vessels forms the base of an inverted triangle. The mesenteric border is divided longitudinally in the midline with cutting bipolar diathermy, passing between the blood vessels, which can be safeguarded.

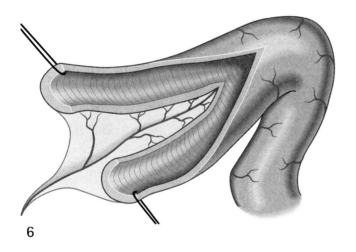

6   Stages 3, 4, and 5 are repeated moving proximally until the dilated bowel is divided into two fully vascularized hemi-segments.

7   One hemi-segment is completely detached by division along the lateral wall. The other hemi-segment is tubularized, in continuity with the duodenum, with a continuous horizontal inverting mattress suture of 5/0 absorbable material, tying a securing knot every fourth throw. The sutures are placed some 2 mm from the cut edge of the bowel, turning the edges into the lumen. It is important to avoid injury to consecutive blood vessels, which are more clearly seen when using a manual suture technique as compared to the stapler.

The second hemi-segment may be tubularized and then anastomosed isoperistaltically to the first. Alternatively, to ensure a safer hemiloop anastomosis, the second hemi-segment, while still open, is anastomosed to the end of the first, and is then tubularized in continuity.

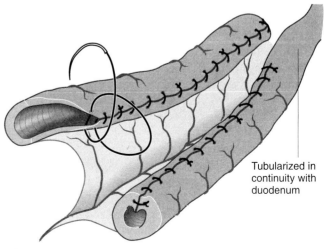

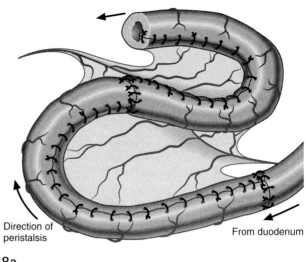

8a,b Isoperistaltic anastomosis requires apposition of opposite ends of the hemiloops. This can be performed in the shape of a Bianchi-S (a) with the bowel lying over the mesentery, or as an Aigrain Spiral (b) with one loop passing beneath the other. The distal end of the second hemiloop is anastomosed to the distal bowel (often the colon) to establish bowel continuity to the anus.

The abdomen is closed in layers, and abdominal drainage is optional. Blood loss is not usually significant; however, fluid and colloid losses may be appreciable and require appropriate replacement intraoperatively and postoperatively.

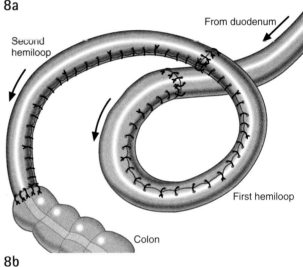

POSTOPERATIVE CARE

The child is managed with nasogastric aspiration, antibiotics, and intravenous alimentation until return of bowel function, often by the third to fifth day, when oral/enteral feeding is slowly reintroduced. Initial delay in passage through the lengthened bowel and intermittent vomiting are not uncommon and resolve rapidly. Parenteral nutrition is progressively reduced over several weeks in line with improving absorption.

Complications

There has been no operative mortality. Morbidity, which has been minimal, has been largely related to stenosis at the hemiloop anastomosis, occasional external fistula formation from suture line disruption, and the rare event of hemiloop loss from compromised blood supply during the surgery. Over the longer term, areas of significant stenosis and recurrence of bowel dilatation with stasis and sepsis may require further surgery. Despite the apparent lack of morbidity, bowel-lengthening procedures have the potential for serious complications and should not be undertaken lightly. Inappropriate and ill-timed application may compromise the child's only chance for enteral autonomy on autologous bowel and may precipitate the need for bowel or liver/bowel transplantation.

LONG-TERM OUTCOME

A period of at least 3–24 months is often necessary for steady progress to enteral autonomy. However, intestinal adaptation often continues for several years, and referral for bowel transplantation should not be hasty. Once enteral autonomy has been achieved, it is likely to be sustained, with relatively normal growth and development. Loss of the ileum with its specific binding sites will necessitate lifelong vitamin B12 supplements. Interruption of the enterohepatic circulation and loss of bile salts into the colon generate abnormal bile with an increased incidence of gallstones, and a greater absorption of free uric acid with the formation of renal calculi.

Failure to establish enteral autonomy will lead to consideration of 'life with parenteral support' or bowel transplantation, largely determined by quality of life and the ability to sustain parenteral feeding (venous access). Bowel transplantation still carries significant short-term and, particularly, long-term hazards and should not be regarded as the 'easier' primary option, but rather as a back up when all prospects for enteral autonomy on autologous bowel have been exhausted.

OTHER BOWEL–LENGTHENING PROCEDURES

The isolated bowel segment 'Iowa' models (Kimura 1993) and the composite bowel loop (Bianchi 1995)

These procedures import a new blood supply to the antemesenteric border of the dilated bowel by grafting the bowel to the liver and abdominal wall (Kimura – isolated bowel segment), or to a vascularized muscle flap from the greater curve of the stomach or a mucosally denuded colonic muscle patch (Bianchi – composite loop).

9 A longitudinal seromuscular myotomy incision is made in the midline along the antemesenteric border of the dilated bowel and the seromuscular layer is peeled back to expose the submucosa.

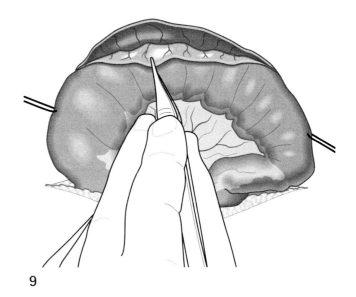

9

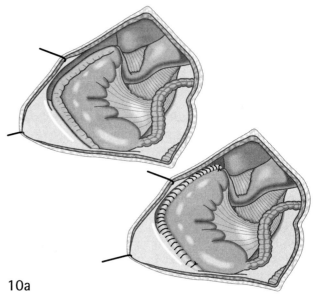

10a

10a,b For the Kimura procedure, the exposed submucosal surface is grafted to the undersurface of the liver and the abdominal wall (a). In constructing a composite loop, a 2–4-cm wide mucosally denuded, vascularized gastric muscle flap based on the right gastroepiploic artery is raised from the greater curve of the stomach and is grafted to the submucosal surface of the dilated jejunum (b). A similar vascularized, mucosally denuded colonic muscle patch can be prepared by removing the mucosa along the submucosal plane.

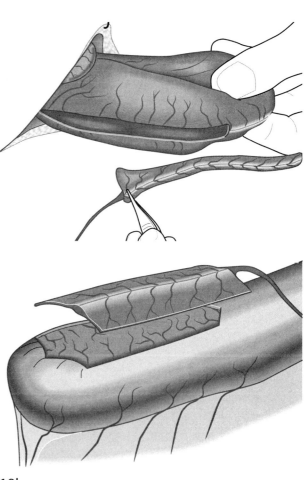

10b

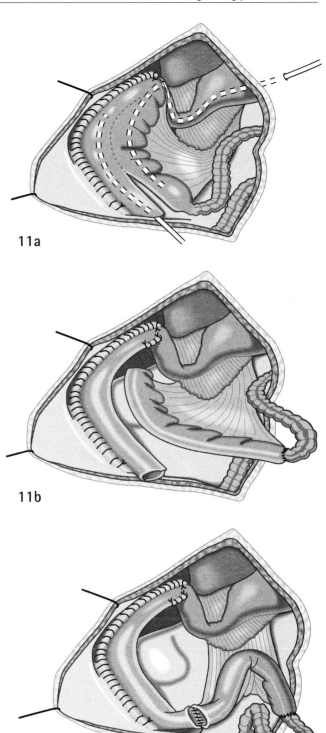

11a–c After 12 weeks to allow neovascularization, the bowel loop is divided horizontally, creating an isolated antemesenteric segment vascularized from adhesions to the liver and abdominal wall (Kimura isolated segment – illustration a) or from the gastric or colonic muscle flap (Bianchi composite loop – illustration b). Isolated segments are tubularized and anastomosed in continuity with the distal bowel (illustration c).

11a

11b

11c

12 A combination of the conventional Bianchi LILT and the Kimura isolated bowel segment (Georgeson sequential lengthening 1994) or the Bianchi composite loop allows the development of a third length of bowel. Clinical application has been limited, and these procedures should be applied with caution and only within specialized units experienced in the advanced management of the short bowel state.

12

SERIAL TRANSVERSE ENTEROPLASTY

A more recent development in autologous intestinal reconstruction surgery is the STEP. First described by Kim *et al.* in a porcine model in 2003, the STEP has since gained wide acceptance by pediatric surgeons as an option for the initial reconstruction of dilated bowel and as a repeat operation for redilation. In fact, the first human STEP was performed on a two-year-old with SBS (short bowel syndrome) from gastroschisis and midgut volvulus who had previously undergone LILT. In STEP, a stapler is placed perpendicularly to the mesentery and applied at intervals from opposite sides to create a zigzag channel. The surgeon determines bowel caliber by the position of the staple lines. In contrast to LILT, which decreases the bowel circumference by half regardless of the degree of dilation, STEP facilitates autologous reconstruction in patients with varying degrees of bowel dilation. Additional advantages of STEP include the absence of intestinal anastomoses, reduced potential for vascular compromise, and decreased technical complexity when compared with other bowel-lengthening procedures.

Indications for STEP

The indications for STEP are not absolute, but specific populations have been identified in whom the procedure may be most beneficial. SBS with intestinal failure and failure to progress toward enteral autonomy is the most common indication for STEP today. The STEP procedure is also well-suited for neonates with marginal bowel length due to atresia. Additionally, segmental dilation and bacterial overgrowth have been identified as indications for STEP.

STEP: operative technique

13 Laparotomy may be performed through an existing surgical incision, or transverse or midline exposure. The entire small bowel is freed of adhesions to define all areas of dilation. There is often need for extensive lysis of adhesions from previous operative interventions. The dilated bowel is measured and marked along the antemesenteric border to facilitate the perpendicular application of the stapler to the mesentery. The distal bowel is addressed first in the procedure, and then proximal progress is made.

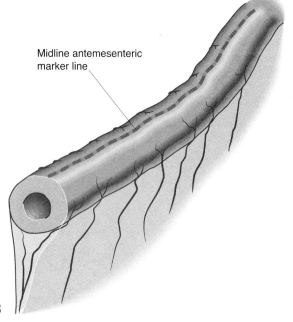

Midline antemesenteric marker line

13

14a,b A window is created in the mesentery to accommodate passage of a GIA stapler. In larger children and adults, a GIA stapler is utilized. In neonates and smaller children, the endo-GIA is preferred. The stapler is inserted through the window at a 90° angle to the mesentery and fired. A size 18 red rubber catheter can be placed on the lower anvil of the stapler to guide it through the defect and reduce the chance of vascular injury. The degree to which each staple line crosses the mesentery is determined by the surgeon, according to desired channel width and extent of bowel dilation. The non-dilated duodenum often provides a guide for the appropriate diameter. In neonates, the STEP channel is usually 1.5–2.0 cm.

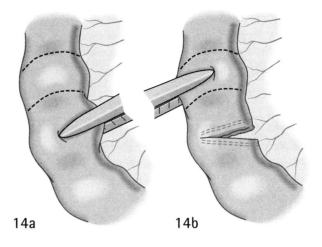

14a   14b

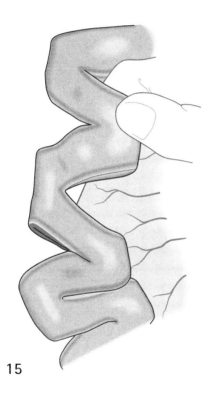

15

15 The process of creating a mesenteric defect, passing, and firing the stapler is repeated at intervals throughout the length of the dilated bowel. Each staple line approaches the bowel from the opposite direction of the previous staple firing, creating a zigzag channel. The distance between staple lines is again affected by the bowel dilation and desired channel width, and varies based on age and caliber of normal bowel. As the bowel becomes less dilated, there is decreased overlap of staple firings. A fine figure of eight PDS suture is placed at the staple line apex to decrease the risk of leak from the weakest area.

Outcomes of the STEP procedure

Although new bowel is not created from STEP, it is hypothesized that tapering and lengthening of the previously dilated bowel facilitates gut adaptation and allows enterocyte mass to increase. This is supported by the demonstration of increased levels of citrulline, a non-protein amino acid that correlates with enterocyte mass, in both animals and humans following STEP. Additionally, increased levels of the gut growth factor GLP-2 have been noted in rodents which have undergone a modified STEP operation. Small bowel motility in porcine models of SBS was preserved following STEP, when compared with control animals.

Similar complications to those that occur in LILT, including staple line leaks, have been reported in STEP. Although there are no anastomoses with the STEP, bowel obstruction and prolonged ileus have been reported. Sepsis, abscess formation, catheter-related bacteremia, and gastrointestinal bleeding as a result of portal hypertension have also been described. In the LILT or STEP procedures, recurrent dilation of the bowel can occur. In these instances, repeat STEP has been shown as a viable option for management, with progression to enteral autonomy after the repeat STEP reaching 43 percent in one series.

When outcomes from 43 LILT and 34 STEP procedures from a single institution were compared, survival and complication rates were not significantly different between the two procedures. There was a trend towards increased rate of total parenteral nutrition (TPN) weaning in STEP patients, but this was not statistically significant. Shorter duration of follow up for STEP patients had an unclear effect on study results.

INTERNATIONAL STEP REGISTRY

In order to better track STEP outcomes worldwide, a web-based International Data Registry for patients undergoing STEP was established in 2004 (www.stepoperation.org). Early reports of the voluntary registry, with a median follow-up 12.6 months, demonstrated an 8 percent mortality and an increase in mean enteral tolerance from 31 to 67 percent. The most recent report from this registry was published in 2013, summarizing the largest experience to date of the STEP procedure in 111 patients from 50 centers in 14 countries. The most common underlying disease process was gastroschisis, with or without concomitant volvulus (45 percent), followed by intestinal atresia (34 percent) and necrotizing enterocolitis (8 percent). Of the 97 registry patients with adequate follow-up following first STEP, 87 (89 percent) were transplant-free survivors. Over half of these patients achieved enteral autonomy and an additional 16 percent had improved enteral tolerance. A subgroup analysis of patients undergoing STEP for SBS with PN dependence identified longer small bowel length as the most significant preoperative factor associated with attainment of enteral autonomy following STEP. Median time to reach enteral autonomy in the entire cohort was 21 months (95 percent CI: 12–30). As with LILT, deaths following STEP were secondary to concomitant liver disease and sepsis. Multivariate analysis of the entire cohort identified significantly higher preoperative serum direct bilirubin and significantly shorter preoperative bowel length in patients who progressed to transplantation or death, when compared with transplant-free survivors. These identified factors, along with the median time needed to wean from PN, must be weighed when considering a candidate for STEP. Patients unlikely to survive long enough for sufficient bowel adaptation post-STEP should be strongly considered for small bowel transplantation in lieu of STEP or other bowel lengthening procedures.

STEP: CONCLUSION

Serial transverse enteroplasty has proven successful in increasing enteral tolerance in patients with intestinal failure through mechanisms thought to involve enhanced motility, reduced bacterial overgrowth, increased enterocyte mass, and improved nutrient absorption. It remains the preferred management at many centers for initial surgical reconstruction and repeat operation for bowel dilation. As in LILT, progression of intestinal failure-associated liver disease (IFALD) and sepsis remain the major sources of morbidity and mortality in patients undergoing STEP.

FURTHER READING

Bianchi A. Autologous gastro-intestinal reconstruction. *Seminars in Pediatric Surgery* 1995; **4**: 54–9.

Bianchi A. Longitudinal intestinal lengthening and tailoring: results in 20 children. *Journal of the Royal Society of Medicine* 1997; **90**: 429–32.

Chang RW, Javid PJ, Oh JT et al. Serial transverse enteroplasty enhances intestinal function in a model of short bowel syndrome. *Annals of Surgery* 2006; **243**: 223–8.

Georgeson K, Halpin D, Figueroa R et al. Sequential intestinal lengthening procedures for refractory short bowel syndrome. *Journal of Pediatric Surgery* 1994; **29**: 316–20.

Jones BA et al. Report of 111 consecutive patients enrolled in the international serial transverse enteroplasty (STEP) data registry: a retrospective observational study *Journal of the American College of Surgeons* 2013; **216(3)**: 438–46.

Kim HB, Fauza D, Garza J et al. Serial transverse enteroplasty (STEP): a novel bowel lengthening procedure. *Journal of Pediatric Surgery* 2003; **38**: 425–9.

Kim HB, Lee PW, Garza J et al. Serial transverse enteroplasty for short bowel syndrome: a case report. *Journal of Pediatric Surgery* 2003; **38**: 881–5.

Kimura K, Soper RT. A new bowel elongation technique for the short bowel syndrome using the isolated bowel segment Iowa models. *Journal of Pediatric Surgery* 1993; **28**: 792–4.

Modi BP, Javid PJ, Jaksic T et al. First report of the international serial transverse enteroplasty data registry: indications, efficacy, and complications. *Journal of the American College of Surgeons* 2007; **204**: 365–71.

Piper H, Modi BP, Kim HB et al. The second STEP: the feasibility of repeat serial transverse enteroplasty. *Journal of Pediatric Surgery* 2006; **41**: 1951–6.

Sudan D, Thompson J, Botha J et al. Comparison of intestinal lengthening procedures for patients with short bowel syndrome. *Annals of Surgery* 2007; **246**: 593–601.

68

Portal hypertension

JONATHAN P ROACH and FREDERICK M KARRER

INTRODUCTION

The treatment of portal hypertension in both children and adults remains the subject of considerable controversy. Therapeutic options now include a broad range of pharmacologic, endoscopic, interventional, and surgical procedures. The etiology of portal hypertension is different from that in adults, however. In adults, the vast majority of cases are caused by cirrhosis (usually due to alcohol abuse or viral infection), whereas in children portal hypertension is due to portal vein thrombosis (PVT) in up to 50 percent of cases. When cirrhosis is the cause in children, it is usually secondary to biliary atresia (BA). The differing etiologies of portal hypertension compel a distinct management approach.

1 The main clinical manifestation of portal hypertension is the same, namely esophageal variceal hemorrhage. Esophageal varices develop as a consequence of increased resistance to flow through the portal circuit. In an attempt to increase outflow from the splanchnic circulation, collateral vessels dilate. Many collateral pathways develop, including (1) left gastric (coronary) vein and short gastric veins to esophageal veins and thence to azygous/hemiazygous veins in the thorax; (2) superior hemorrhoidal veins to the middle and inferior hemorrhoidal veins and ultimately to the inferior vena cava; (3) umbilical vein to superficial veins of the abdominal wall and superior/inferior epigastric veins; (4) intestinal veins to the branches of the inferior vena cava (IVC) in the retroperitoneum (veins of Retzius); and (5) through the perihepatic veins of Sappey from the inferior side of the diaphragm to the superior side. The most clinically important collaterals are the submucosal esophageal varices. These have a propensity to rupture as a consequence of dilation of the lumen, leading to increased wall tension from vessel wall thinning and increased intraluminal pressure secondary to coughing or straining or from ulceration secondary to esophagitis.

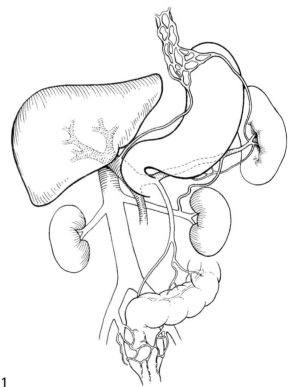

1

HISTORY

The management of esophageal bleeding has evolved dramatically over the last three decades. The use of surgical techniques employing a direct attack on the bleeding varices and portosystemic shunt procedures have been increasingly supplanted by the use of endoscopic means (sclerotherapy and banding) and transjugular intrahepatic portosystemic shunts (TIPS), as well as pharmacologic therapy. The success of liver transplantation has also dramatically altered the way in which we approach those patients with end-stage liver disease. Most patients with cirrhosis as a cause of portal hypertension are now listed for liver transplantation and bleeding from esophageal varices is managed by non-surgical means.

PRINCIPLES AND JUSTIFICATION

Bleeding from esophageal varices typically occurs suddenly, without warning, as massive hematemesis. This is often the disconcerting initial presentation of portal hypertension in children. Occasionally, the bleeding is more insidious, with melena, or more rarely hematochezia, as the first sign. When the cause of portal hypertension is portal vein thrombosis, the onset is typically in a previously healthy young child, by the age of six years in 80 percent of cases. Other stigmata of liver disease are usually absent, except for an enlarged spleen. The hemorrhage usually stops spontaneously, partly because coagulation is normal.

Conversely, in those children with portal hypertension caused by cirrhosis, the liver disease is usually known about and physical findings of chronic disease are obvious (e.g. caput medusa). Esophageal variceal bleeding in this setting should not be surprising or unexpected.

The choice of management technique is highly dependent on the etiology, as well as the experience and expertise available. In general, bleeding in patients with PVT is managed with medical therapy, endoscopic techniques, portosystemic shunts, or a combination of all three. Bleeding in patients with end-stage liver disease is managed by methods that do not interfere with subsequent liver transplantation, such as endosclerosis/banding or radiologic techniques. Shunts in these patients have a high morbidity rate and can make liver replacement very difficult or impossible. Non-shunting surgical procedures (ligation of varices, esophageal transection, Suigura's procedure) have largely been abandoned and are not recommended as primary surgical therapy. The only role for these procedures may be in cases where shunts and transplantation are not possible and endoscopic methods have failed.

2 The use of non-operative shunts for adults has gained widespread popularity. Transjugular intrahepatic portosystemic shunts have not been widely applied to children, but they avoid some of the surgical complications and should not interfere with future transplantation. Complications include those arising from the technical aspects of the procedure (bleeding and hepatic capsule perforation), those arising from the shunt itself (encephalopathy), and the development of shunt stenosis, occlusion, and infection. Continued shunt surveillance and periodic dilation are necessary to maintain patency. Therefore, TIPS is generally used as a bridge to liver transplantation and should be considered for short-term use only.

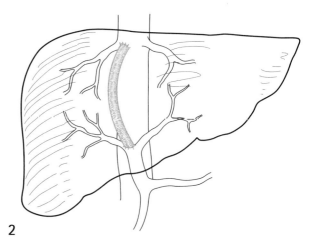

2

PREOPERATIVE ASSESSMENT AND PREPARATION

The first priority in the treatment of gastrointestinal bleeding is volume replacement and stabilization. Two large-bore intravenous catheters should be placed for volume repletion. Until blood is available, crystalloid and colloid solutions can be judiciously administered. The appropriate blood products should be used to replace shed blood and correct coagulopathy as needed. The goal of resuscitation is to restore tissue perfusion, which is best judged clinically by urine output monitored by Foley catheter placement. Invasive monitoring with central venous catheters and arterial catheters may also be helpful to judge volume status and maintain adequate perfusion pressure. Monitoring of these parameters is important as over-resuscitation can be detrimental by increasing portal venous pressure thereby exacerbating an active bleed, or cause rebleeding. Somatostatin and octreotide can be helpful in acute variceal hemorrhage to reduce portal pressure and promote the cessation of persistent bleeding.

Routine laboratory parameters (bilirubin, albumin, and prothrombin time) are used to assess the patient's liver function. Other liver enzymes (transaminases, alkaline phosphatase, gamma-glutyl transferase) are helpful in suggesting liver injury or hepatitis. Viral serologies are determined if indicated by history or preliminary evaluation.

Once the patient is stabilized, upper intestinal endoscopy should be performed to assess the source of bleeding and potentially provide therapeutic interventions. Even in patients with cirrhosis, up to 50 percent of upper gastrointestinal bleeding is from sources other than esophageal varices (gastritis, peptic ulcer disease, Mallory-Weiss tears).

As part of the work up, portal venous anatomy should be assessed in all patients by Doppler ultrasound. Ultrasonography should show the main portal vein (PV), superior mesenteric vein (SMV), splenic vein, and intrahepatic veins. Although suitable to demonstrate

patency and flow, patients being considered for shunting should also be evaluated by angiography. Both arterial and venous anatomy should be visualized. Injection of the superior mesenteric artery and splenic artery with venous phase images will identify the major splanchnic veins, and venography of the IVC and left renal vein is required, as these veins will be used for various shunting procedures. Computed tomography angiography (CTA) has sufficiently evolved to the point that it has replaced invasive angiography and venography in many institutions. Magnetic resonance angiography (MRA) is also a non-invasive alternative to traditional angiography. The surgeon should work closely with the radiologists to ensure that the necessary anatomy is clearly demonstrated prior to proceeding with operative therapy.

OPERATIONS

Endosclerosis

3 Originally described using a slotted, rigid esophagoscope, most sclerotherapy is currently performed with a flexible endoscope. The advantages of flexible endoscopy are the superior optics and the ability to visualize the stomach and duodenum in order to assess further the source of hemorrhage. Most of these procedures are performed under general anesthesia to protect the airway during the operation. A variety of sclerosing agents have been used in children, including 5 percent ethanolamine, 1 percent tetradecyl sulfate, and 5 percent sodium morrhuate.

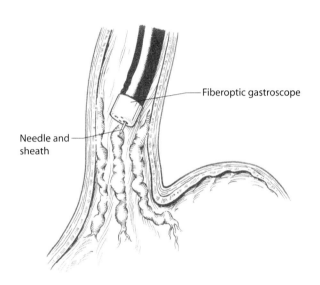

Fiberoptic gastroscope

Needle and sheath

3

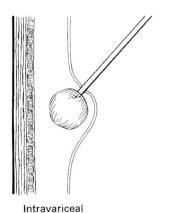

Intravariceal

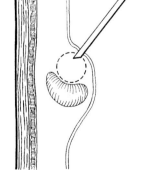

Paravariceal

4

4 Both intravariceal and paravariceal injection techniques have been reported. Intravariceal injection may be better than paravariceal because it is associated with better control of acute variceal hemorrhage. Usually no more than three varices are injected at each session, and sclerosis is repeated every few weeks until the varices are obliterated. The interval between endoscopic sessions can then be gradually lengthened up to annual surveillance examinations. When compared to endoscopic band ligation, sclerotherapy was found to be as efficacious in controlling hemorrhage. However, sclerotherapy posed greater risk of post-procedural fever, retrosternal pain, esophageal ulceration, or stricture. Therefore, band ligation has become the endoscopic procedure of choice to control variceal hemorrhage.

Variceal banding

5a–d Endoscopic variceal band ligation, first reported in 1989, utilizes mechanical ligation and strangulation of varices with elastic O-rings. The device consists of two fitted cylinders attached to the tip of a standard flexible endoscope. The inner cylinder has the small elastic O-ring stretched over the end, which is released as the inner cylinder is drawn into the hood by a tripwire running through the biopsy channel of the endoscope. When the varix to be ligated is identified, it is drawn into the cylinder by applying suction. The O-ring is released by pulling on the tripwire, resulting in strangulation of the varix and thrombotic obliteration of the submucosal venous channels. Usually, between one and three elastic band ligatures are placed at each session. The bands and varices slough off after 5–7 days. The procedure is repeated, similar to endosclerosis, until the varices are obliterated, and the frequency is gradually reduced to annual surveillance. Because the addition of the band ligation device to the endoscope limits the size of scope that may be utilized, smaller children may still require sclerotherapy for variceal control.

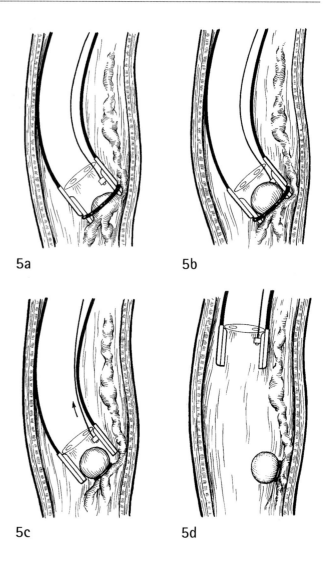

5a   5b

5c   5d

Mesocaval shunt

6 The classic mesocaval shunt, described by Clatworthy, was designed specifically for children in whom the portal vein is not usable because of PVT. It is easier to perform than some other shunts in children because the veins used are larger. A midline incision is preferred to avoid interruption of venous channels in the abdominal wall that serve as important collaterals after division of the IVC. The transverse colon is retracted cephalad and the small intestine is retracted inferiorly. A vertical incision in made in the mesentery of the small intestine over the SMV, which lies to the right of the arterial pulsation. Identification of the SMV can be aided by following the veins in the transverse mesocolon. Once located, the SMV is dissected free for about 5 cm below its passage behind the pancreas.

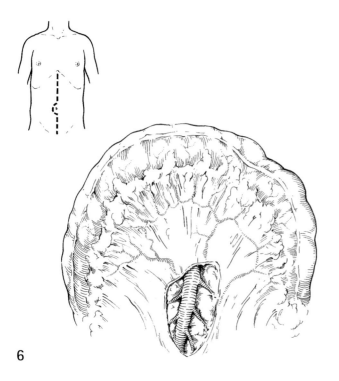

6

7 Next, the IVC is exposed by mobilizing the right colon. The duodenum is reflected medially by a Kocher maneuver to expose the junction of the renal veins and the IVC. The IVC is freed from the renal veins to the bifurcation. Individual lumbar veins are ligated. A tunnel is made in the posterior mesentery, which is often thick and edematous, to reach the SMV.

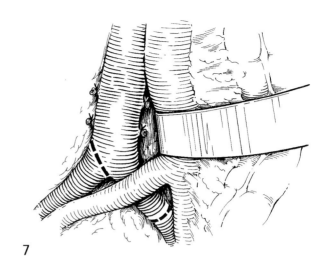

7

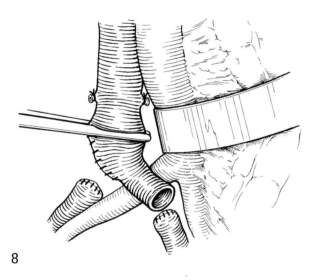

8

8 At this stage, a critical decision must be made about the length of the IVC needed to reach the SMV. Often, it is advisable to gain additional length by dividing the left iliac vein at some distance below the bifurcation of the IVC. The right iliac vein is oversewn flush with the bifurcation. The cava/iliac vein is then brought through the mesenteric tunnel and fashioned to appropriate length.

9 A small ellipse is cut in the SMV before the anastomosis with fine monofilament suture (6/0 polypropylene). Special attention to alignment of the venotomy and anastomosis is necessary to prevent kinking. The retroperitoneum and mesentery are reapproximated with a few absorbable sutures.

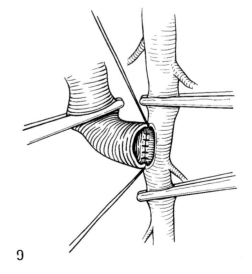

9

10 Because Clatworthy's classic mesocaval shunt requires division of the IVC, it can result in swelling of the lower extremities. Although usually temporary, an alternative procedure avoids this disadvantage by utilizing an interposition graft between the SMV and IVC. Synthetic vascular grafts have been used, but autologous graft (internal jugular or saphenous vein) offers the best chance of long-term patency. For wound closure, the abdomen is closed in a watertight fashion, without drains.

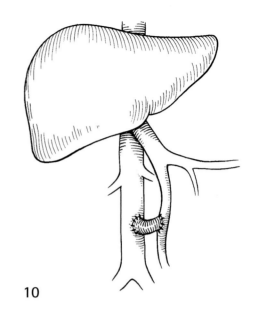

10

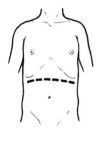

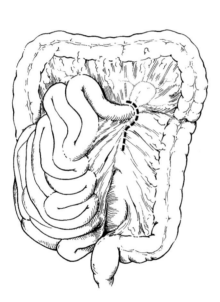

11

Side-to-side splenorenal shunt

11 A wide transverse upper abdominal incision is made. The transverse colon is retracted cephalad and the small intestine to the right to expose the base of the transverse mesocolon and duodenum. The ligament of Treitz is incised and the inferior mesenteric vein divided at its junction with the splenic vein. This allows the duodenojejunal junction to be swept cephalad and to the right. The operation is often modified to a splenectomy and central end-to-side splenorenal shunt in patients with very large spleens.

12 The left renal vein is exposed from the kidney hilum to the IVC. The left gonadal and left adrenal veins are ligated and divided. At the base of the transverse mesocolon, the inferior edge of the pancreas is dissected transversely. In long-standing portal hypertension, the retroperitoneum can be thick and edematous with numerous small collateral veins. With cephalad traction on the transverse mesocolon, the pancreas is rotated along its long axis to expose the splenic vein. The splenic vein is dissected out for a distance of 4–5 cm by ligation of small tributaries. Numerous small pancreatic veins must be meticulously ligated and divided to provide sufficient mobility of the splenic vein.

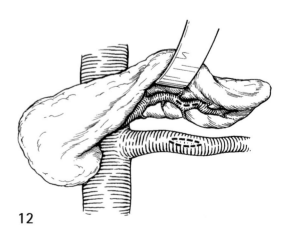

12

13 Vascular clamps are placed on both the splenic and left renal veins. The splenic vein is opened transversely in its most dependent portion, extending into the stump of the inferior mesenteric vein if necessary, to create a larger anastomosis. The left renal vein is opened in a similar way. The anastomosis is performed with loop magnification using fine monofilament suture (6/0 polypropylene). The posterior wall is completed first from the inside, then the anterior wall. The completed anastomosis should be 1.5–2.5 cm in length. The retroperitoneum is closed with absorbable sutures and the incision is closed in layers without drains.

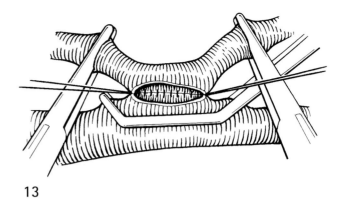

13

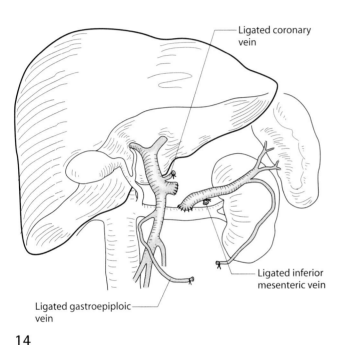

Ligated coronary vein

Ligated inferior mesenteric vein

Ligated gastroepiploic vein

14

Distal splenorenal shunt

14 The distal splenorenal shunt (Warren's shunt) is a selective shunt. The portal circulation is divided into two components: one maintains antegrade portal flow toward the liver via the SMV, and the other shunts flow away from the esophageal varices to the short gastrics then through the splenic vein into the renal vein.

Through a generous midline or bilateral subcostal incision, the body of the pancreas is mobilized in a fashion similar to that used for a central splenorenal shunt. Once mobilized, the splenic vein is divided just before its junction with the SMV. The distal splenic vein is then swung inferiorly and anastomosed with fine vascular suture to the left renal vein without angulation. Another essential step in the performance of Warren's shunt is division of the left gastric (coronary) vein, the umbilical vein, and the gastroepiploic arcade. This completes the division of the portal circulation. The wound is closed in layers in a watertight fashion.

Mesentericoportal shunt

15 The last type of shunt that deserves mention is an SMV to intrahepatic left portal vein shunt (the Rex shunt). The shunt was originally developed for the treatment of portal vein blockage following liver transplant, but has increasingly been used for PVT in the absence of a transplant, with good success. Uniquely, this shunt restores flow from the portal circuit back to the liver via the intrahepatic left portal vein. This vein remains patent in about two thirds of patients with cavernous transformation of the portal vein.

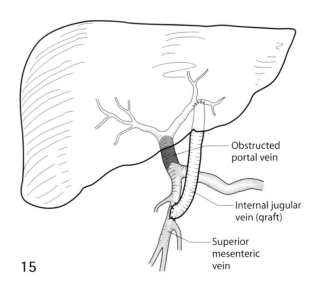

Obstructed portal vein

Internal jugular vein (graft)

Superior mesenteric vein

15

Both the neck and abdomen are prepped because a graft of internal jugular vein is often used to bridge the gap between the SMV and left portal vein. A wide transverse subcostal incision is preferred. The SMV is located where patent, as determined by preoperative angiography. Usually, the SMV can be located near the confluence with the splenic vein behind the head of the pancreas. The left portal vein is located by following the ligamentum teres (umbilical vein remnant) into the umbilical fissure, Rex's recess. Once the length of the gap is known, a segment of internal jugular vein is harvested, usually from the left neck. Anastomosis to the SMV or confluence is then completed before connecting to the left branch of the portal vein. Both are performed with fine monofilament suture (6/0 polypropylene). Once flow is restored and hemostasis is assured, the wound is closed in layers, with no drains.

POSTOPERATIVE CARE

Children treated by endoscopic techniques for acute hemorrhage must be monitored closely for ongoing or recurrent bleeding. Once initial control has been achieved, follow-up band ligation may be performed on an ambulatory outpatient basis. With more children receiving band ligation rather than endosclerosis, complications such as ulceration, perforation, hyperpyrexia, and bleeding have become rare. When significant pain or fever present in the postoperative setting, these signs must be taken seriously and prompt chest radiography and a contrast study. While the role of primary and secondary medical prophylaxis has gained widespread acceptance in the treatment of adults with esophageal varices, its role in the pediatric population is still controversial. The use of β-blockade allows for unopposed α-adrenergic stimulation decreasing flow through the portal system, thereby decreasing portal pressure and the subsequent risk of variceal hemorrhage. There are insufficient data in the pediatric literature to recommend primary and secondary prophylaxis with β-blockade and ambulatory band ligation.

For all portosystemic shunt procedures, nasogastric decompression should be maintained until normal bowel function has returned. Peptic ulcer prophylaxis is routine. Early ambulation and the use of elastic stockings may prevent lower extremity edema, which is occasionally seen after end-to-side mesocaval shunts. Vitamin K supplementation may be indicated based on prothrombin times. Dietary protein should initially be restricted and advanced only gradually to prevent hepatic encephalopathy. Ascites, which is common, may require salt restriction, diuretics, and the administration of exogenous albumin. Most surgeons use some type of anticoagulation postoperatively and then administer aspirin (81 mg) daily for antiplatelet effect.

OUTCOME

The authors' results and those of others have shown good control of variceal hemorrhage using endoscopic band ligation with regular surveillance and repeated banding as needed to eradicate varices. Especially in children with portal vein obstruction, the tendency towards variceal hemorrhage decreases with time, as spontaneous retroperitoneal shunts develop. Death is rare, except when related to cirrhosis and liver failure.

A properly performed portosystemic shunt is highly effective in controlling bleeding varices; however, because of the size of the vessels and the propensity to thrombosis, rebleeding rates of 15–25 percent have been reported. The Rex shunt restores normal portal flow to the liver, and therefore, with the distal splenorenal shunt, carries the theoretical advantage of decreased encephalopathy. The incidence of encephalopathy in children is difficult to estimate because different standards have been used to determine its presence and severity. In children with extrahepatic portal venous thrombosis, the risk of encephalopathy is directly related to liver synthetic function. The long-term prognosis for children undergoing portosystemic shunts also largely depends on the severity of hepatic dysfunction. Probably, those patients with advanced cirrhosis are best referred for liver transplantation and esophageal variceal bleeding managed by endoscopic means. For those patients with PVT, variceal bleeding can be successfully managed by endoscopic means, with low morbidity but with repeated visits and anesthetics. Shunts are associated with some surgical morbidity and mortality, but provide good control and usually improve growth retardation and hypersplenism. The most important factor in the choice of management is the expertise and experience available. Thoughtful application of the various options can decrease the complications and mortality associated with variceal hemorrhage from portal hypertension.

FURTHER READING

De Ville de Goyet J, Alberti D, Clapuyt P *et al*. Direct bypassing of extrahepatic portal venous obstruction in children: a new technique for combined hepatic portal revascularization and treatment of extrahepatic portal hypertension. *Journal of Pediatric Surgery* 1998; **33**: 597–601.

Huppert PE, Goffette P, Astfalk W *et al.* Transjugular intrahepatic portosystemic shunts in children with biliary atresia. *Cardiovascular Interventional Radiology* 2002; **25**: 484–93.

Karrer FM, Narkewicz M. Esophageal varices: current management in children. *Seminars in Pediatric Surgery* 1999; **8**: 193–201.

Ling SC, Walters T, McKiernan PJ *et al.* Primary prophylaxis of variceal hemorrhage in children with portal hypertension: a framework for future research. *Journal of Pediatric Gastroenterology and Nutrition* 2011; **52**: 254–61.

Ryckman FC, Alonso MH. Causes and management of portal hypertension in the pediatric population. *Clinics in Liver Disease* 2001; **5**: 789–818.

Zargar SA, Javid G, Khan BA *et al.* Endoscopic ligation compared with sclerotherapy for bleeding esophageal varices in children with extrahepatic portal venous obstruction. *Hepatology* 2002; **36**: 666–72.

69

Cholecystectomy

BAYANI B TECSON and HOCK LIM TAN

HISTORY

Open cholecystectomy has been performed for over a hundred years and was the gold standard until the early 1990s. However, a paradigm shift occurred when Dr Phillippe Mouret, a French gynecologist, reported the first laparoscopic cholecystectomy in 1987, quickly followed by reports from Drs Reddick and Olsen in North America and Drs Dubois and Perissat in France. Laparoscopic cholecystectomy has since become the operative procedure of choice.

PRINCIPLES AND JUSTIFICATION

Cholelithiasis is uncommon in children. While most pediatric gallstones are idiopathic, haemolytic disorders, such as spherocytosis and sickle cell disease are relatively common causes. Predisposing factors include congenital anomalies of the biliary tract, prolonged fasting, diuretic administration, phototherapy, antibiotics, umbilical catheterization and salmonella infections.

Cholelithiasis is increasingly being diagnosed in adolescents, but it may be as a result of earlier detection because of the widespread use of diagnostic ultrasound.

PREOPERATIVE ASSESSMENT AND PATIENT PREPARATION

A preoperative high-resolution diagnostic ultrasound should be performed to exclude common bile duct dilatation. A dilated common bile duct should raise suspicion of common bile duct stones particularly in the presence of jaundice, pancreatitis, elevated liver enzymes, amylase or lipase. However, it should be noted that jaundice alone without common bile duct dilatation in children with hemolytic disorders may just be a manifestation of significant ongoing hemolysis.

Magnetic resonance cholangiopancreatography (MRCP) is the investigation of choice to exclude common bile duct stones. If common bile duct stones are evident, our preference is to perform ERCP stone extraction, as laparoscopic common bile duct exploration in a child is challenging.

Preoperative preparation

It is important to ensure that the large intestine is empty immediately prior to the procedure, especially for the laparoscopic operation.

OPEN CHOLECYSTECTOMY

The 'traditional' open cholecystectomy procedure is still being offered in situations where the necessary experience, facilities, and appropriate instruments for a safe pediatric laparoscopic cholecystectomy procedure are lacking.

Anesthesia

General endotracheal anesthesia is the standard of care for most situations.

Patient position

The patient is placed in the supine position with abducted arms extended.

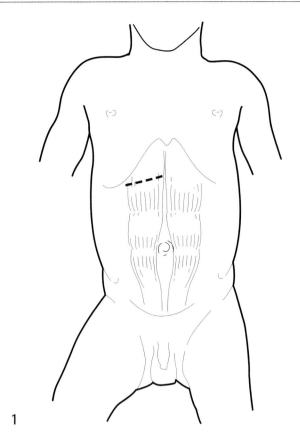

Incision

1 A right subcostal transverse muscle-cutting incision is usually adequate for open cholecystectomy. This incision can be extended if necessary.

1

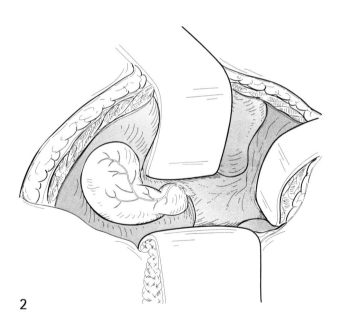

2

EXTENSILE EXPOSURE

2 A moistened rolled visceral pack is placed on the transverse colon which is retracted inferiorly, while the undersurface of the liver is retracted superiorly.

A 4 × 8 gauze pad with radio-opaque strip is placed into the Morisson's pouch to absorb any intraoperative ooze.

3 Hartmann's pouch is grasped with a Babcock forcep and retracted latero-inferiorly to expose Calot's triangle. Divide the peritoneum over Calot's triangle starting at the free edge of Hartmann's pouch and cystic duct junction. The cystic duct is identified and exposed, and the dissection is extended to expose the cystic artery. The cystic lymph node often overlies the cystic artery. It is not necessary to dissect and expose the cystic duct – common bile duct junction as this will avoid injury to the common bile duct.

The cystic artery should be ligated and divided at this stage.

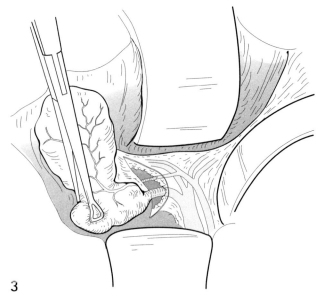

3

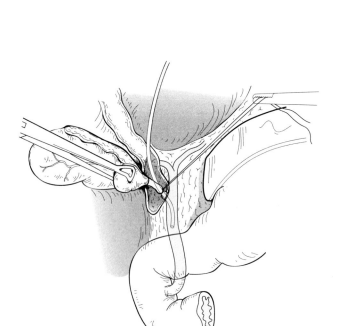

4

The gallbladder can now be removed from its fossa by grasping the fundus of the gallbladder and applying constant countertraction between it and the fossa to develop the tissue plane. Monopolar diathermy is best for this.

The fossa is then inspected for any oozing and the cystic duct for bile leak.

The abdominal wound is then closed without drainage.

Postoperative care

Most patients are able to tolerate a full meal 24 hours postoperatively. Postoperative pain is initially controlled with intravenous non-steroidal anti-inflammatory drugs (NSAIDs) followed by oral analgesia. Combination oral analgesia, NSAIDs plus mild opioid will be required in some patients for adequate pain control. Patients are usually discharged on the second or third postoperative day.

Intraoperative cholangiogram

4 If an intraoperative cholangiogram is indicated, a side hole is made in the cystic duct close to Hartmann's pouch and the cystic duct cannulated with a cholangiocatheter or a fine feeding tube. The catheter should be primed with normal saline to avoid creating a 'bubble' artifact during contrast injection. Diluted contrast will satisfactorily visualize the biliary tree and there should be free flow of contrast into the duodenum. On completion of cholangiography, the catheter is removed and the cystic duct ligated and divided.

LAPAROSCOPIC CHOLECYSTECTOMY

Contraindications

There are few contraindications to laparoscopic cholecystectomy. Even the presence of adhesions from previous abdominal operations is not a contraindication in the hands of the experienced pediatric laparoscopic surgeon who is adept at laparoscopic adhesiolysis.

Anesthesia

General anesthesia via endotracheal intubation with full muscle relaxation is the standard of care and a nasogastric tube must be inserted to decompress the stomach and duodenum.

Patient positioning

5a,b There are two common positions for laparoscopic cholecystectomy: (1) the French position has the surgeon standing between the legs, while (2) the American position has the surgeon standing on the left of the patient. While both are equally popular, the French position is more ergonomic, especially if you have to perform a splenectomy concurrently.

The video monitor is positioned at the head of the table allowing the surgeon, camera, and monitor to be in line to optimize the ergonomics. It is not necessary to use two video monitors when using the French position.

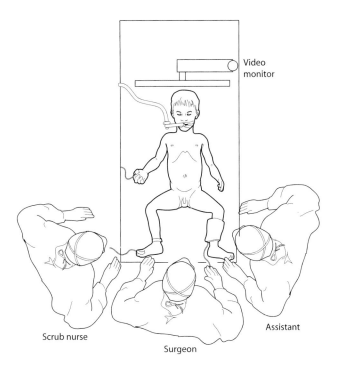

5a The French position

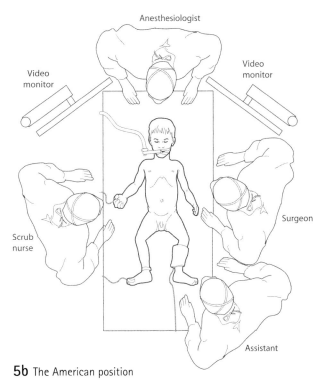

5b The American position

Laparoscopic instrumentation

Few instruments are required for laparoscopic cholecystectomy. In the modern era of 'needlescopic' surgery, 3-mm instruments are now sufficiently rigid to be used even in large adolescents.

- 0° or 30° 5-mm telescope
- 11-mm Hasson port (cannula and blunt tip trocar)
- 6-mm instrument ports (one) and 3-mm instrument ports (two)
- 3-mm hand instruments including blunt 'Reddick Olsen' graspers, toothed ratched grasper for Hartman's pouch, and Kelly's or small 3-mm (Maryland) dissectors
- 3- or 5-mm monopolar hook cautery
- 5-mm endoscopic clip applier: Hemolock clip is preferred (different sizes)
- 3-mm endoscopic scissor
- Suction–irrigation tube

Operative procedure

Ensure that the stomach and duodenum are completely empty to minimize the risk of damage to the duodenum, particularly when using the monopolar hook to dissect Calot's triangle. Open laparoscopy using the Hasson cannula is our preferred option, although many surgeons will use the Veress needle to develop the pneumoperitoneum.

It is seldom necessary to use more than 12 mm insufflation pressure when operating on children as this will lead to diaphragmatic splinting, and does not increase the intra-abdominal volume appreciably.

6 Three instrument ports are inserted under direct visualization. An instrument is required in the epigastrium for retraction, and two other ports for the hand instruments are inserted on either side of the umbilical trocar. The liver is relatively larger in young children and can overhang the subcostal margin making it necessary to position these ports lower than in an adult, to optimize the room to manipulate hand instruments inside the abdomen.

The patient is tilted head up about 30° to allow the transverse colon to fall by gravity away from the operative field.

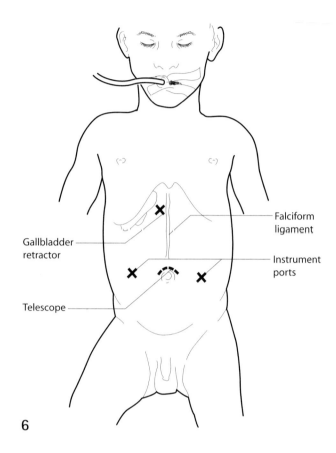

Gallbladder retractor

Falciform ligament

Instrument ports

Telescope

6

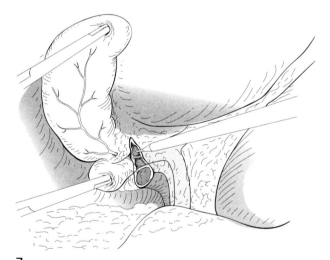

7

EXPOSURE OF THE GALLBLADDER AND CALOT'S TRIANGLE

7 The fundus of the gallbladder, easily visualized, is grasped with a toothed, ratcheted grasper in the epigastric port. The Hartmann's pouch is grasped with a toothed grasper and retracted laterally and inferiorly to display Calot's triangle.

EXPOSURE OF CALOT'S TRIANGLE

8 The peritoneum overlying the Calot's triangle is opened using monopolar hook diathermy, starting at the Hartmann's pouch end of the cystic duct. In developing this window, it is not necessary to extend the cystic duct dissection medially to avoid damaging the common bile duct.

The cystic artery should be similarly identified in Calot's triangle and displayed to develop two windows in Calot's triangle, one with the cystic duct and the other with the cystic artery forming one side of a smaller triangle. In the case of the cystic artery, it is only necessary to develop enough length to apply two clips on the medial side. Being an end artery it is unnecessary to clip the distal end. In the case of the cystic duct, sufficient length is freed to apply two clips on the common bile duct end and a single clip at the Hartmann's pouch end. We stress the importance of not chasing the cystic duct to the common bile duct junction to avoid common bile duct injury. Most reported cases of common bile duct injuries occur during this dissection.

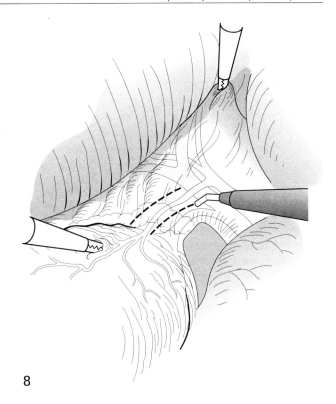

8

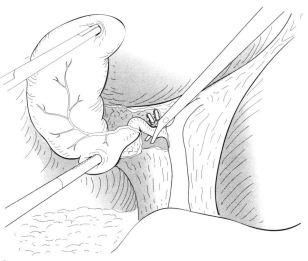

9

DIVISION OF THE CYSTIC ARTERY AND CYSTIC DUCT

9 The cystic artery is obliterated either with two vascular clips or vessel-sealing devices. While it is generally only necessary to apply a single clip for biliary tract, we prefer to apply two clips on the common bile duct side of the cystic duct for added safety. The single clip on the gallbladder side is to prevent bile spillage. The cystic artery must always be divided before the cystic duct, as there is risk of avulsing it if it is still in continuity during manipulation of the cystic duct.

The cystic duct is then divided and carefully checked for a bile leak.

GALLBLADDER DISSECTION

10 The gallbladder is best removed from its fossa using monopolar hook diathermy. It is important to maintain constant countertraction between the gallbladder and fossa at all times to identify the correct loose connective tissue plane attaching the gallbladder to its fossa. It is best to mobilize Hartmann's pouch first and work towards the fundus.

The operative site is then inspected for bleeding and bile leak. Bleeding from the fossa can generally be controlled with monopolar or bipolar coagulation.

If there is concern about ooze, a closed suction drain can be placed in Morrison's pouch and brought out through the right-sided port.

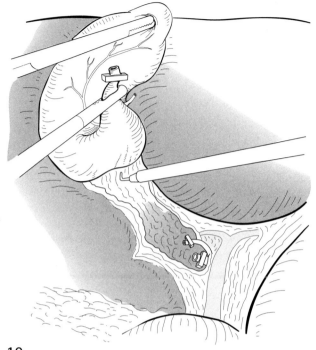

10

GALLBLADDER EXTRACTION

The gallbladder is extracted through the 10-mm umbilical by inserting the 5-mm telescope into the 6-mm port. It is best to grasp the gallbladder firmly with a 5-mm grasper and the gallbladder removed together with the port.

If the gallbladder was perforated during the dissection, it is best to place the gallbladder into an endobag for extraction through the umbilical port. Large gallstones inside the gallbladder may be entrapped in the umbilical incision and render extraction difficult. With intact gallbladders, Hartmann's pouch should be delivered through the incision, the bile aspirated, and sufficient stones extracted to disimpact the gallbladder so that it can be delivered through the umbilical incision.

With perforated gallbladders, the endobag is partially delivered to disimpact the contents before removing it through the 10-mm umbilical port.

WOUND CLOSURE

The abdomen should be desufflated before removing instrument trocars to avoid omental herniation through the puncture sites.

The umbilical incision is closed using the purse string suture previously used to secure the Hasson port. The fascia of the instrument port sites are closed with a single absorbable suture and cyanoacrylate is used to approximate the skin.

POINTS OF TECHNIQUE

If Hartmann's pouch is adherent to the duodenum because of previous episodes of cholecystitis, care should be taken when separating these two. It is best to use either the heel or hook in short bursts while maintaining gentle constant countertraction on the adhesions.

FURTHER READING

Chan S, Currie J, Malik I, Mohamed A. Paediatric cholecystectomy: shifting goal posts in the laparoscopic era. *Surgical Endoscopy* 2008; **22**: 1392–5.

St Peter SD, Keckler SJ, Nair A *et al*. Laparoscopic cholecystectomy in the pediatric population. *Journal of Laparoendoscopic and Advanced Surgical Techniques. Part A* 2008; **18**: 127–30.

Sicklick J, Camp M, Lillemoe K *et al*. Surgical management of bile duct injuries sustained during laparoscopic cholecystectomy perioperative results in 200 patients. *Annals of Surgery* 2005; **241**: 786–95.

Wesdorp I, Bosman D, de Graaff A *et al*. Clinical presentations and predisposing factors of cholelithiasis and sludge in children. *Journal of Pediatric Gastroenterology and Nutrition* 2000; **31**: 411–17.

70

Surgery for biliary atresia

MARK DAVENPORT and ATSUYUKI YAMATAKA

HISTORY

Thomson from Edinburgh described an infant dying from cirrhosis secondary to congenital biliary obstruction in 1891. Surgical exploration was advocated from the 1930s and the terms 'correctable' and 'non-correctable' became prevalent to describe what could be done with a conventional surgical operation (e.g. hepaticojejunostomy). However, as most cases of biliary atresia were anatomically 'non-correctable', their outlook was poor and true survivors were exceptional.

During the 1950s and 1960s, Kasai, a surgeon working in Sendai, Japan, developed a more radical approach to the dissection, exposing residual microscopic bile ductules within the apparently solid parts of the porta hepatis. This operation (portoenterostomy) resulted in a much larger proportion of children who lost their jaundice, following restoration of bile flow. Nevertheless, most still developed chronic liver disease. Liver transplantation became a practical option during the 1980s in the UK and North America, and in the 1990s in Japan. Initially, this was for older children with life-threatening complications of liver disease (e.g. portal hypertension), but then it became available for infants who had had no response to a Kasai operation or were deemed to have established cirrhosis.

PRINCIPLES AND JUSTIFICATION

Biliary atresia remains a rare disease with a frequency of between 1 in 10–18 000 live births. It is more common in Japan and China, than in Europe or the United States; although the reasons are not apparent. There is a slight female preponderance in most large series.

There appear to be a number of variants of biliary atresia; probably with differing etiology. For instance, there is a consistent association (approximately 10 percent of all cases) with other non-biliary anomalies, such as polysplenia, asplenia, cardiac malformation, situs inversus, absence of the IVC, preduodenal portal vein and malrotation, for which we have used the term 'biliary atresia splenic malformation'. Such cases may result from some 'insult' within the first trimester of pregnancy that causes abnormal development of susceptible organ systems. Although such insults are hard to define, maternal diabetes, maternal thyrotoxicosis, and drug abuse have been reported. In about 5 percent of cases, there is obvious cyst development within an otherwise obliterated biliary tree; these are also likely to be developmental in origin as up to half may be detected on an antenatal ultrasound scan, as far back as week 20 of gestation. In most cases, however, only the biliary tree is abnormal and no obvious prenatal cause is identified. This has led to speculation that a perinatal hepatotropic virus infection (e.g. rotavirus, reovirus, cytomegalovirus) has been able to damage an otherwise normally developed biliary tree. Certainly, the group of infants who demonstrate IgM antibodies to cytomegalovirus can be distinguished clinically by having a more 'hepatitic' histological appearance in the liver and a reduced expectation of bile flow postoperatively.

Biliary atresia is a cholangiopathy of the extra- and intrahepatic parts of the biliary tree which, if untreated, leads to hepatic fibrosis and ultimately cirrhosis. The histological appearance of the liver is characterized by portal tract edema, bile duct plugging and proliferation, a small cell infiltrate and variable amount of giant cell formation. Bridging fibrosis is a late feature, but in some cases may be present even at diagnosis.

1 The lumen of the extrahepatic duct is obliterated at a variable level and this forms the basis for the most common classification in use. There are three main types of biliary atresia: type 1 (5 percent) where the level of obstruction is within the common bile duct (the gallbladder therefore contains bile); type 2 (3 percent) where the level is within the common hepatic duct; and type 3, the most common (>90 percent), where there is no visible bile-containing proximal lumen and the obstruction is within the porta hepatis. Cystic change can be seen in all types; some contain mucus, while others contain bile and this invariably causes diagnostic confusion with a choledochal cyst. In such cases, the wall is thickened and communicates poorly with abnormal non-dilated intrahepatic ducts, demonstrable on cholangiography.

The porta hepatis of the most common variant, type 3, contains microscopic epithelial-lined bile ductules up to 300 µm in diameter. Partial destruction and desquamation of the epithelium occurs and the ductules are surrounded by a fibroinflammatory stroma. Large ductules are typically absent, but serial sectioning has shown that even small channels may communicate with intrahepatic ducts.

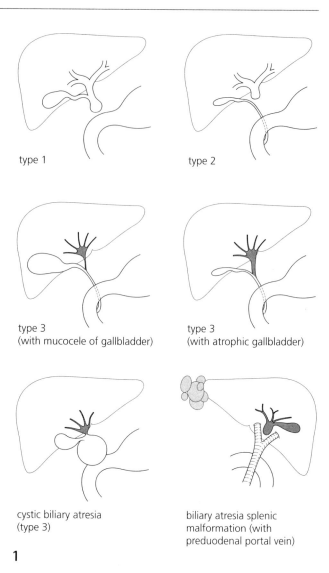

type 1

type 2

type 3
(with mucocele of gallbladder)

type 3
(with atrophic gallbladder)

cystic biliary atresia
(type 3)

biliary atresia splenic
malformation (with
preduodenal portal vein)

1

PREOPERATIVE ASSESSMENT AND PREPARATION

All infants with biliary atresia will be clinically jaundiced, and have pale stools and dark urine when looked for. This is due to the inability to excrete conjugated (i.e. water-soluble) bilirubin into the gastrointestinal tract, which is then excreted into the urine causing its color to darken. Such alternative pathways of bilirubin excretion are more developed (or perhaps better retained) in the neonate and very high levels of bilirubin (>300 µmol/L or >17 mg/dL) are not a feature (as might be seen in adults with complete biliary obstruction). Some infants with cystic biliary atresia will have had an abnormal antenatal maternal ultrasound scan.

The differential diagnosis of conjugated jaundice in infants is long and can be complicated to work out. Surgical causes, other than biliary atresia, are uncommon, but include obstructed choledochal malformation, spontaneous perforation of the bile duct and the inspissated bile syndrome (as seen particularly in preterm infants with other problems). The medical causes include biliary hypoplasia (as seen in Alagille syndrome), neonatal hepatitis, 1-antitrypsin deficiency, giant-cell hepatitis, and cystic fibrosis.

The diagnostic work up should always include ultrasonography, biochemical exclusion of α1-antitrypsin deficiency and cystic fibrosis, and (in the authors' institution) a percutaneous liver biopsy. Using this, about 80 percent will have a positive diagnosis prior to laparotomy. Other techniques which have been described include endoscopic retrograde cholangiopancreatography (ERCP), percutaneous cholangiography, duodenal intubation, and measurement of bile. MRCP (magnetic resonance cholangiopancreatography) is not detailed enough to confidently diagnose biliary atresia, although is valuable for the more obvious structural problems, such as a choledochal cyst. Radio-isotope hepatobiliary imaging (e.g. using IDA derivatives) was formerly a popular investigation in distinguishing biliary atresia from neonatal hepatitis, but lacks specificity.

Most infants presenting within 80 days will not show clinical features of cirrhosis or irretrievable liver damage (e.g. gross ascites, nodularity on ultrasonography, or histological cirrhosis on liver biopsy) and should undergo laparotomy with the intention of performing a Kasai portoenterostomy. Others, who do show these features, may be considered for liver transplantation as a primary procedure. Nevertheless, it should be realised that prognosis is difficult to predict with any certainty and even a poorly functioning Kasai operation may delay the need for a donor organ.

The blood investigations should include coagulation tests (e.g. international normalized ratio (INR)) to exclude a vitamin K-dependent coagulopathy and all infants coming to surgery should have parenteral vitamin K (phytomenadione, 1 mg/day) supplementation. The choice of parenteral antibiotics depends on local policies, but should be broad spectrum with reasonable bile penetration (e.g. second- and third-generation cephalosporins). In our institution, these are given intravenously for 5 days and then orally for a further 25 days.

OPEN KASAI PORTOENTEROSTOMY

The aim of the surgery is to excise all extrahepatic biliary remnants to allow a wide portoenterostomy reconstruction onto a portal plate, denuded of all tissue. This should be the object not only in type 3 biliary atresia, but also in those who do have a visible bile-containing proximal communication. It should be obvious therefore that frozen section, formerly used to confirm patent ductules, is not necessary because it should not be possible to resect any further biliary tissue.

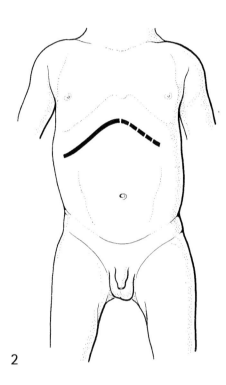

2

2 A short right (or left if situs inversus), upper quadrant muscle-cutting incision should be performed initially to confirm the suspected diagnosis or, if not immediately obvious, to perform an on-table cholangiogram. If there is no bile, or only clear mucus, in a collapsed, atrophic gallbladder, then it is invariably biliary atresia. In those circumstances where there is obvious bile in the gallbladder then an on-table cholangiogram is indicated.

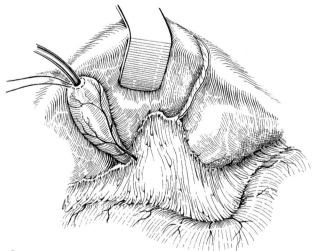

3

3 This is done by inserting a small feeding tube (4 Fr) into the gallbladder secured by a purse-string suture.

4 The demonstration of a patent common bile duct and intrahepatic ducts excludes a diagnosis of biliary atresia.

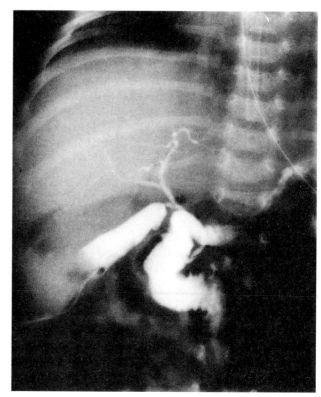

4

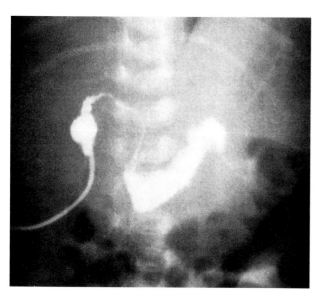

5

5 Sometimes, proximal passage of contrast into intrahepatic ducts can be difficult to show as typically it preferentially fills only the distal duct and duodenum. This can be prevented by a small vascular or 'bulldog' clamp on the common bile duct.

The incision can then be lengthened after confirmation of the diagnosis to cross the midline and ligate and divide the falciform ligament. The laparotomy should look carefully for other anomalies (e.g. polysplenia, preduodenal portal vein, absence of the inferior vena cava, and malrotation) which may alter the subsequent technique.

Mobilization of the liver

6 The liver should be fully mobilized by dividing the falciform ligament, coronary ligaments, and right and left triangular ligaments such that the organ can then be everted outside the abdominal cavity. This is a crucial step, which allows full exposure of the portal hepatis and facilitates the subsequent detailed dissection. It is necessary to warn the anesthetist at this stage as the maneuver impairs venous return to the heart by kinking the cava and will need an increase in intravenous volume support.

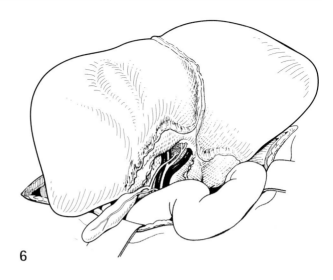

6

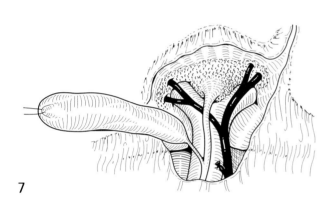

7

Mobilization of the gallbladder and bile ducts

7 A stay suture on the gallbladder allows its elevation and this is then separated with bipolar diathermy off its bed. The peritoneum overlying the portal triad (the hilar plate) is then divided and the various vascular (hepatic artery and portal vein) and biliary structures positively identified. Parts of the biliary tract may be missing, but usually there is an intact biliary structure conforming to the usual arrangement of gallbladder, cystic duct, common hepatic and common bile duct. The distal common bile duct is ligated and divided and the proximal part elevated from the underlying connective and lymphatic tissue. Following the divided end of the cystic artery should lead to identification of the right hepatic artery, which may be superficial or deep to the common duct and may need slinging.

Dissection and exposure of the porta hepatis

8 Gradual separation of the biliary remnant will lead proximally to the porta and its relationship to the bifurcation of the portal vein will become clearer.

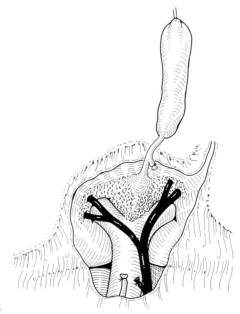

8

9 The bifurcation is gradually freed from the porta, typically by careful division of small veins crossing into the central portion. In the posterior part, the caudate lobe should become visible. The dissection is then extended to both right and left aspects. On the left, consideration should be given to exposing the so-called 'recessus of Rex' by dissecting the umbilical vein down to its origin from the left portal vein. An isthmus of liver parenchyma (from segment III to IV) may need division by coagulation diathermy to achieve this. This then becomes the proximal extent of the left-sided dissection. On the right side, remnant biliary tissue can be identified almost hemi-circumferentially around the right vascular pedicle and into the origin of the gallbladder fossa. Some authors advocate slinging the right and left portal veins, but the authors feel that this may compromise subsequent liver blood flow (risking portal vein thrombosis) and simple judicious retraction should give more than adequate exposure.

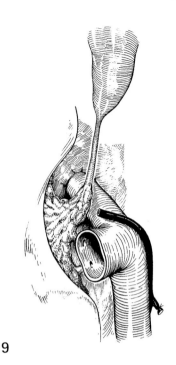

9

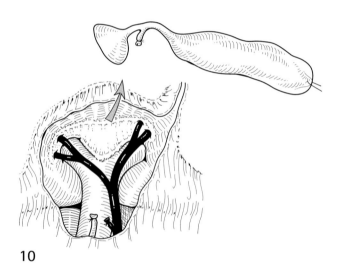

10

Formation of Roux loop

11 The duodenojejunal junction should be identified and a point about 10 cm from this should be freed to be the site of the jejunal anastomosis. The bowel is then divided using a stapled linear cutter, and a Roux loop, measured along the anti-mesenteric border at approximately 40 cm, constructed. This loop can then be brought through a right-sided window in the transverse mesocolon. An end-to-side jejunal anastomosis is constructed, using whatever technique the operator is comfortable with. The end of the Roux loop should have enough length to reach the porta without undue tension.

Excision of biliary remnants

10 The remnant can now be removed. Beginning at the right side and using a combination of scalpel and small curved sharp tenotomy scissors, a plane is developed between solid white biliary remnant and the underlying liver, flush with the capsule. The appearance at the transected portal plate should be almost translucent, denuded of tissue, but not actually transgressed. Actually excising liver parenchyma does not improve bile drainage, presumably because any divided ductules simply become obliterated by subsequent scar tissue. At this stage, untoward attempts at hemostasis of the porta by diathermy should be avoided. The area should be packed and the liver returned to the abdominal cavity, which will relieve venous congestion.

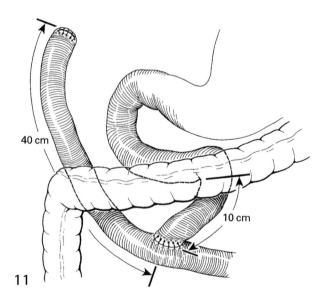

40 cm

10 cm

11

Portoenterostomy

12 The liver is again everted outside the abdominal cavity. A non-crushing bowel clamp placed along the jejunal loop keeps this part steady and an opening is made in the anti-mesenteric aspect about 1–2 cm from the stapled end.

It is easier if the posterior row of sutures (e.g. 6/0 polydioxanone (PDS: Ethicon, Somerville, NJ, USA) is placed sequentially and held with mosquito clips until the row is complete. The jejunal loop can then be 'parachuted' down to porta and the sutures then tied. The anterior row is then completed. The anastomosis should be wide, measuring about 2 cm, if there has been an adequate dissection of right and left sides.

The mesocolic window around the Roux loop is closed, avoiding any kinking. A drain can be left, particularly if there has been more than a small quantity of ascites, but is not essential. The wound closure though needs to be secure and watertight.

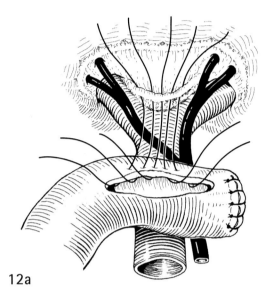

12a

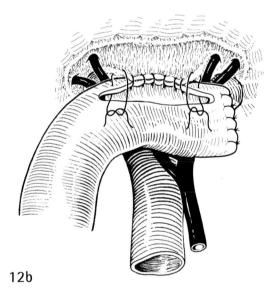

12b

LAPAROSCOPIC KASAI PORTOENTEROSTOMY

Positioning

13 The infant is positioned at the foot of the operating table, the surgeon at the patient's feet, an assistant with a camera beside the surgeon on his right, and an assistant either on the left or right side of the operating table. A 30° 5- or 10-mm laparoscope is used, inserted through a 10-mm trocar placed supraumbilically using the open Hasson technique. Three additional ports are used (two 5-mm ports are placed on either side of the upper quadrant port, for the surgeon's right and left hands, slightly above the umbilical level, just lateral to the rectus abdominis, and another 5-mm port is placed between the umbilical port and the left upper quadrant port, slightly below the umbilicus. The use of a Nathanson retractor (NR: Teleflex Medical, High Wycombe, UK), placed through the epigastrium, is crucial to expose the porta hepatis for anastomosis. Percutaneous stay-sutures (Ps) are also used to improve exposure and elevate the liver: one is introduced just below the xiphoid process to snare the falciform ligament and two are inserted into both right and left lobes.

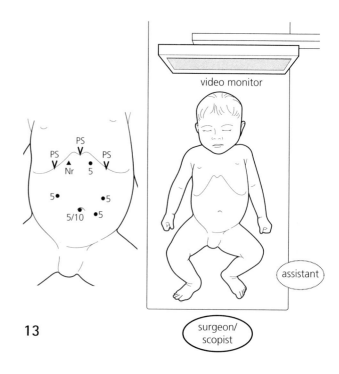

13

Gallbladder and porta hepatis dissection

Hook diathermy and tissue forceps are used to dissect the cystic duct and the distal biliary remnant. This is then transected at the level of the duodenum. The distal end of the biliary remnant is elevated to visualize key structures of the porta hepatis, that is, the fibrous biliary remnant cone.

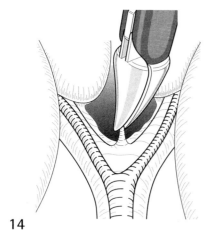

14

14 A further 5-mm trocar is placed in the epigastrium, specifically for a Ligasure device (Valley Laboratories, Boulder, CO, USA). This is used to dissect the proximal biliary remnant, especially when dividing portal vein branches at the porta hepatis draining into the caudate lobe.

15 This is used to minimize thermal injury to microscopic bile ductules in the biliary remnant cone during dissection. In this laparoscopic variant (illustration a), the level of transection is more akin to that of Kasai's original description (illustration b) and does not attempt to emulate the extended dissection described above in the open variant (illustration c).

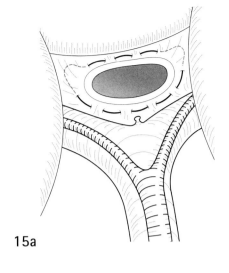

15a

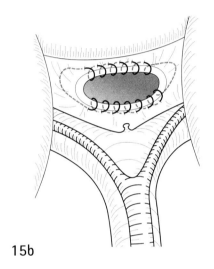

15b

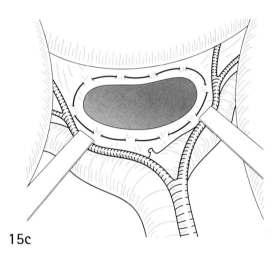

15c

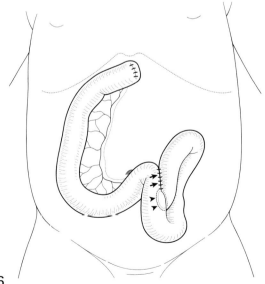

16

Extracorporeal transumbilical jejunal Roux-en-Y

16 The ligament of Treitz is identified and proximal jejunum about 15 cm from this is exteriorized through the umbilical port and divided. The length of the Roux limb is then determined by bringing it above the xiphoid process on the anterior abdominal wall. A jejuno-jejunostomy (arrowheads) is performed extracorporeally. The length of Roux limb is not predetermined to be, for example, 30, 40, or 50 cm.

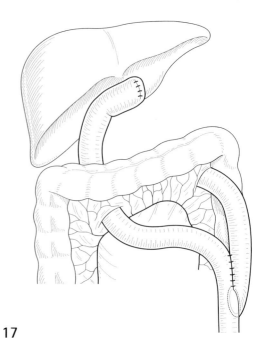

17

17 This 'short' Roux limb is approximated to the native jejunum for 8 cm cranially (arrows) to prevent intestinal contents of the native jejunum into the Roux limb (illustration 16) and the jejuno-jejunostomy will fit naturally into the splenic flexure. Finally, an antimesentric enterotomy 10 mm in length is made near the closed end of the Roux limb and the jejunum returned to the abdominal cavity. This is passed through a retrocolic window to lie without tension at the porta hepatis.

Portoenterostomy

Anastomotic sutures (5/0 or 6/0 PDS) are placed between the enterotomy and liver parenchyma around the margins of the transected portal plate. Except at the 2 and 10 o'clock positions, these should be deep enough to prevent leakage, but shallow enough to avoid residual ductules. At the 2 and 10 o'clock positions, no sutures are placed where the original left and right bile ducts were, but if needed to prevent leakage, sutures are placed to the connective tissues over the hepatic arteries or hepatoduodenal ligament (illustration 15a).

Surgical alternatives

There have been many alternatives proposed following the original description of the Kasai operation. The crucial part (i.e. the portal dissection) has certainly become more extensive and widened on both right and left sides, although the principle of complete excision has not been superseded. The laparoscopic approach above does not attempt to replicate this extended dissection. In the author's hands, good results can still be achieved, although published results from other laparoscopic specialists do not match their results with the open alternative and many have reverted.

Most other alternative techniques have involved variations of Roux loop construction; either involving creation of stomas or interposed 'anti-reflux' valves. The aim of these has been to reduce postoperative cholangitis. None has stood the test of time however, and a straightforward long (≥40 cm) Roux loop reconstruction is all that is required.

POSTOPERATIVE CARE

Intravenous fluids and nasogastric aspiration are continued until return of bowel function (3–4 days). Careful monitoring of blood glucose, electrolytes and INR is important in the early phase. Liver biochemistry (including bilirubin) may well worsen in the first week whatever the eventual outcome, but by about the fourth week there should be a definite fall in bilirubin and consistently pigmented stools in those who will do well.

The role of corticosteroids and ursodeoxycholic acid is unproven, although widely prescribed.

Strict attention to nutritional needs is important and all infants need regular vitamin supplementation. Medium-chain triglyceride formula milk (e.g. Caprilon®; SHS, Liverpool, UK) is advocated to maximize calorie input and facilitate lipid absorption.

OUTCOME

There are many factors, which will influence surgical outcome in biliary atresia. Some are unalterable (e.g. degree of cirrhosis at presentation; absence of, or paucity of bile ductules at the level of section) and some are subject to change (e.g. surgical experience, untreated cholangitis). In large centers with experienced surgeons, about 50–60 percent of all infants will clear their jaundice and achieve a normal (<20 μmol/L or <1.5 mg/dL) bilirubin. These should do well and have a good quality of long-term survival with their native liver. In those with no effect from the Kasai (usually apparent within two to three months), then active consideration should be given to early liver transplantation.

The relationship of surgical outcome to age at surgery is complex. While there is no doubt that with increasing age the liver becomes more fibrotic and ultimately cirrhotic, outcome might be more related to exposure of transected biliary ductules within reasonable age-limits.

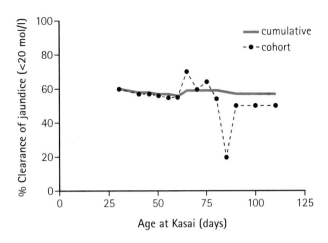

18a Effect of age at surgery in isolated biliary atresia (n = 177) (adapted from Davenport *et al.* 2008).

18a,b A large series of infants with isolated biliary atresia where the cumulative age plot against clearance of jaundice rate is relatively unchanged from 40–100 days and there is no obvious 'cut-off' and should be compared to illustration b in infants with cystic biliary atresia where there is a marked reduction in clearance of jaundice with increasing age. Other measures of outcome (e.g. native liver survival) show a similar effect.

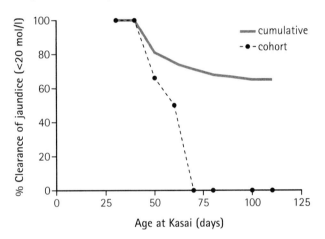

18b Effect of age at surgery in cystic biliary atresia (n = 23) (adapted from Davenport *et al.* 2008).

COMPLICATIONS

The two principle complications which can be life-threatening are cholangitis and the development of esophageal varices.

Cholangitis occurs most commonly in the year following primary surgery in about 40–50 percent of children. Paradoxically, it only occurs in children with some degree of bile flow, not in those with early failure. Clinically, it is characterized by worsening jaundice, fever, and acholic stools. The diagnosis may be confirmed by blood culture or by percutaneous liver biopsy, but it is important to treat suspected cases early with broad-spectrum antibiotics effective against Gram-negative organisms.

Increased portal venous pressure has been shown in virtually all infants at the time of the Kasai operation, however subsequent portal hypertension depends both on the degree of established fibrosis and, most importantly, the response to surgery. There is a relationship with biochemical liver function and variceal development and

in those who fail and need early transplantation about 30 percent will have had a significant variceal bleed. In those who respond well to initial Kasai, but who have established fibrosis, then variceal development can be delayed and presentation with bleeding perhaps only occurring at two to three years.

FURTHER READING

Caponcelli E, Knisley A, Davenport M. Cystic biliary atresia; an etiologic and prognostic sub-group. *Journal of Pediatric Surgery* 2008; **43**: 1619–24.

Davenport M, Caponcelli E, Livesey E *et al.* Surgical outcome in biliary atresia: etiology affects the age at surgery. *Annals of Surgery* 2008; **247**: 694–8.

Davenport M, Tizzard S, Underhill J *et al.* The Biliary Atresia Splenic Malformation syndrome: A twenty-eight year single-centre retrospective study. *Journal of Pediatrics* 2006; **149**: 393–400.

Davenport M, Ville de Goyet J, Stringer MD *et al*. Seamless management of biliary atresia. England and Wales 1999–2002. *Lancet* 2004; **363**: 1354–7.

Hartley J, Davenport M, Kelly D. Biliary atresia – review. *Lancet* 2009; **374**: 1704–13.

Howard ER, MacClean G, Nio G *et al*. Survival patterns in biliary atresia and comparison of quality of life of long-term survivors in Japan and England. *Journal of Pediatric Surgery* 2002; **36**: 892–8.

Kasai M, Suzuki H, Ohashi E *et al*. Technique and results of operative management of biliary atresia. *World Journal of Surgery* 1978; **2**: 571–9.

Koga H, Miyano G, Takahashi T *et al*. Laparoscopic portoenterostomy for uncorrectable biliary atresia using Kasai's original technique. *Journal of Laparoendoscopic Advanced Surgical Techniques* 2011; **21**: 291–4.

Nakamura H, Koga H, Wada M *et al*. Does the placement of sutures and extent of dissection during portoenterostomy affect outcome? Comparison of current portoenterostomy with Kasai's original procedure. *Journal of Pediatric Surgery* (in press).

71

Choledochal cysts

NGUYEN THANH LIEM, MARK D STRINGER AND HOCK LIM TAN

PRINCIPLES AND JUSTIFICATION

Congenital bile duct dilatation is a better description of this spectrum of congenital anomalies of the biliary tree, but 'choledochal cyst' is the traditional term.

1 The following classification is commonly used.

- Type I – cystic (Ic) or fusiform (If).
- Type II – diverticulum of the common bile duct.
- Type III – choledochocele (dilatation of the terminal common bile duct within the duodenal wall).
- Type IV – multiple cysts of extrahepatic and intrahepatic ducts (IVa) or multiple extrahepatic duct cysts (IVb).
- Type V – intrahepatic duct cyst (single or multiple [Caroli's disease]).

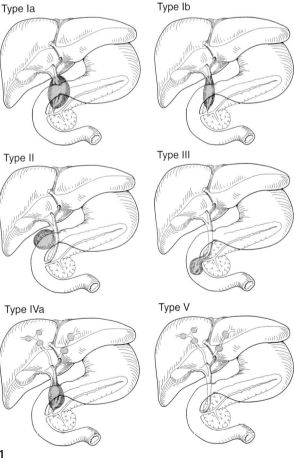

Type Ia Type Ib

Type II Type III

Type IVa Type V

1

Type I choledochal cysts predominate. Together with type IVa cysts, they account for more than 90 percent of cases. Intrahepatic duct dilatation that resolves after successful treatment of a type I cyst should be distinguished from the irregularly dilated intrahepatic ducts found with type IVa cysts. Caroli's disease is characterized by segmental saccular dilatation of the intrahepatic bile ducts; it may affect the liver diffusely or be localized to one lobe.

Pathology

There are three components to the pathology of a choledochal cyst: the cyst, which may be inflamed and thick-walled, and any abnormal bile ducts; the associated liver histology, which varies from normal to fibrotic or cirrhotic; and the existence of pancreatobiliary malunion, which is present in most but not all cases (Fig. 71.1). In the last, the terminal common bile duct and pancreatic duct unite to form a common channel well outside the duodenal wall. Since this common channel is not surrounded by the normal sphincter mechanism, pancreatic juice refluxes into the biliary tree and high concentrations of pancreatic amylase and/or lipase are typically present in the bile. Occasionally, bile refluxes into the pancreatic duct causing pancreatitis. In most cases, the common channel represents a simple union of the two ducts, but in some patients the anatomy is complex. Rarely, pancreatobiliary malunion occurs without biliary dilatation.

Whenever possible, the preoperative and intraoperative assessment of a choledochal cyst should include an evaluation of all three pathologic features. Additional biliary tract abnormalities can occur, such as distal duodenal displacement of the papilla of Vater and, in type IVa cysts, hilar duct strictures. Associated anomalies outside the biliary tract are uncommon.

Clinical features

Girls are affected more often than boys. Typical presenting symptoms are abdominal pain and/or obstructive jaundice. The classic triad of abdominal pain, jaundice, and a mass is rare. Abdominal pain is often associated with hyperamylasemia due to pancreatitis or diffusion of pancreatic amylase from the cyst. A choledochal cyst should always be considered in the differential diagnosis of obstructive jaundice or pancreatitis in children. The bile duct dilatation of a fusiform type I cyst may be relatively subtle.

An increasing proportion of cystic type I choledochal dilatations are detected by routine prenatal ultrasonography. If these infants are jaundiced and a cystic variant of biliary atresia has not been excluded, surgery should be performed promptly. If the infant is otherwise well, surgery can be safely deferred until about 3 months of age. Delaying treatment further exposes the infant to the risks of developing liver fibrosis, cholangitis, or cyst perforation.

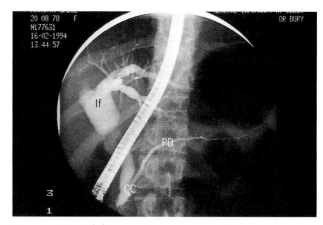

Figure 71.1 (a) Pancreatobiliary malunion with a fusiform type I choledochal cyst. CC, common pancreatobiliary channel; If, type I fusiform choledochal cyst; PD, pancreatic duct.

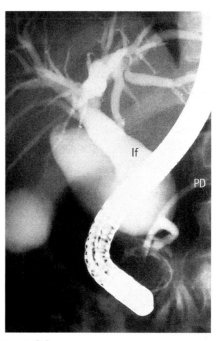

Figure 71.1 (b) Complex pancreatobiliary malunion. Reproduced with permission from Stringer MD. Choledochal cysts. In: Howard ER, Stringer MD, Colombani PM (eds). Surgery of the Liver, Bile-Ducts and Pancreas in Children, 2nd edn. London: Arnold, 2002: 149–68.

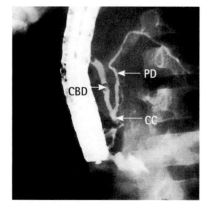

Figure 71.1 (c) Pancreatobiliary malunion without choledochal dilatation. Note filling defects in common bile duct. PD = pancreatic duct, CC = common pancreatobiliary channel, CBD = common bile duct.

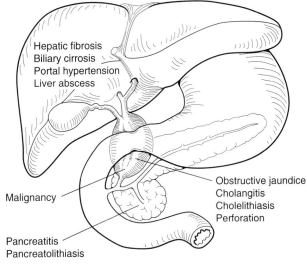

Complications

2   Choledochal cysts are prone to complications. Perforation is rare and presents with an acute abdomen. Malignant change is a late complication, mostly described in adults, but has been recorded in teenagers. It is much more likely to occur after cystenterostomy than if the cyst has been excised. Prompt surgery consisting of radical cyst excision and biliary reconstruction eliminates or reduces the risk of complications.

2

PREOPERATIVE ASSESSMENT AND PREPARATION

Biochemical liver function tests may be normal or show evidence of biliary obstruction. The plasma amylase level may be elevated during episodes of abdominal pain. A prolonged prothrombin time secondary to cholestasis should be corrected with intravenous vitamin K. Routine preoperative blood tests should also include a full blood count and blood group and save.

Modern imaging methods provide an accurate diagnosis. Ultrasonography is the initial investigation of choice – the size, contour, and position of the cyst, the proximal ducts, vascular anatomy, and hepatic echotexture can all be evaluated (Fig. 71.2). Percutaneous transhepatic cholangiography and endoscopic retrograde cholangiopancreatography (ERCP) give excellent definition of the cyst and duct anatomy, including the pancreatobiliary junction. However, both investigations are invasive and have a small risk of inducing complications such as pancreatitis and biliary sepsis, and both require general anesthesia and antibiotic prophylaxis. Endoscopic retrograde cholangiopancreatography should be avoided during an episode of acute pancreatitis.

Magnetic resonance cholangiopancreatography (MRCP) is non-invasive and can be performed under sedation in small children without the use of contrast agents or irradiation (Fig. 71.3). However, definition of the pancreatic duct and common channel may be suboptimal in infants and small children.

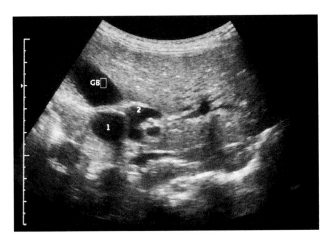

Figure 71.2 Ultrasound scan of a type I choledochal cyst in a three-year-old girl. GB, gallbladder. 1 and 2 are dilated extrahepatic bile ducts.

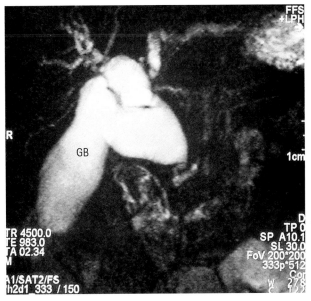

Figure 71.3 Magnetic resonance chalngiopancreatography of the type I choledochal cyst shown in Figure 71.2. Note the common pancreatobiliary channel (CC). GB, gallbladder.

Hepatobiliary scintigraphy with technetium-^{99}m iminodiacetic acid is useful in selected cases by confirming biliary excretion into the cyst or when assessing biliary drainage after surgery. Contrast enhanced computed tomography may be indicated in some patients with pancreatitis or if an associated tumor is suspected.

In most patients, a detailed ultrasound scan supplemented by MRCP or intraoperative cholangiography provides sufficient anatomical information.

Consent

Radical cyst excision and reconstruction by hilar hepaticoenterostomy is the optimum treatment for the common types of choledochal cyst. This disconnects the pancreatic and biliary ducts. In experienced units, this operation can be performed safely at any age with a very low morbidity. Complications are rare, but early problems may include an anastomotic bile leak, bleeding, intra-abdominal sepsis, injury to adjacent structures, and wound complications. Potential late complications are a bilioenteric anastomotic stricture, stone formation (more common within ectatic intrahepatic ducts in type IVa cysts), pancreatitis from residual abnormalities in the common channel, and adhesive small bowel obstruction. Even after adequate cyst excision, malignancy may very rarely affect residual extrahepatic ducts (e.g., the terminal common bile duct) or abnormal intrahepatic ducts (type IVa cysts).

3 Internal drainage of the cyst by cystenterostomy has a prohibitively high long-term morbidity from cholangitis, stone formation, malignant degeneration, etc., and should be avoided. Definitive surgical excision may be unsafe in a critically ill child with perforation, uncontrolled biliary sepsis, or serious concomitant ill-health. In such cases, temporary external drainage of the choledochal cyst and delayed surgery once the patient has improved and the anatomy has been defined is safer.

Anesthesia

Endotracheal intubation, muscle relaxation, and temporary nasogastric tube drainage are standard. Epidural analgesia can provide excellent perioperative pain relief. Broad-spectrum intravenous antibiotics are best given at induction of anesthesia and continued for 2–5 days postoperatively.

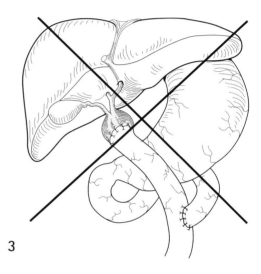

3

OPERATIVE TECHNIQUES

4 A high transverse or oblique right upper quadrant incision gives excellent exposure. The duodenum and head of pancreas may be displaced forward over the cyst. The appearance of the liver, spleen, and pancreas is noted. An intraoperative cholangiogram should be performed if the anatomy has not been clearly defined preoperatively. Bile is aspirated from the cyst and sent for culture and measurement of amylase/lipase. With large cysts, cholangiography is often best performed by the injection of contrast directly into the lower end of the common bile duct and into the common hepatic duct using a butterfly needle. Direct injection into a large cyst may fail to outline the intrahepatic ducts and obscure filling of the distal duct. It is important to try to identify the junction of the pancreatic and bile ducts.

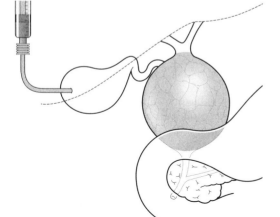

4

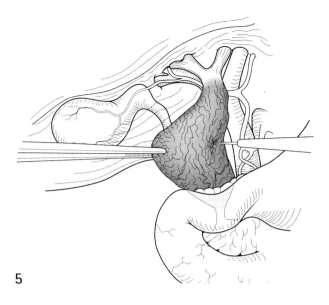

5 A plane is developed between the overlying peritoneum and the anterior wall of the cyst. The dissection extends inferiorly between the duodenum and the cyst and medially and laterally, keeping close to the cyst wall, using precise bipolar cautery to achieve safe and accurate hemostasis. Large cysts can be decompressed to facilitate dissection. The gallbladder and cystic duct are mobilized and the cystic artery ligated.

5

6 Where the bile duct begins to narrow down inferiorly, it is dissected circumferentially and encircled. In this region, small vessels arising from the pancreas need careful cautery. The distal common bile duct is dissected to just within the head of the pancreas and transected. The operative cholangiogram gives a useful guide to the distal level of bile duct transection. Protein plugs or calculi within a common channel should be removed using a combination of saline irrigation, balloon catheters and, when possible, intraoperative endoscopy using a pediatric cystoscope. The distal bile duct stump is then over-sewn with an absorbable monofilament suture (e.g., polydioxanone [PDS]).

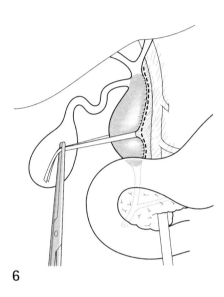

6

7 The cyst and gallbladder are lifted forward, exposing the portal vein behind. Sometimes the right hepatic artery crosses in front of the cyst and is adherent to its wall – it must be carefully freed and preserved. The common hepatic duct is divided at the level of the bifurcation, where it should appear healthy and well vascularized. Any dilated proximal intrahepatic ducts are cleared of debris by catheter irrigation with normal saline and, in larger ducts, with the aid of choledochoscopy.

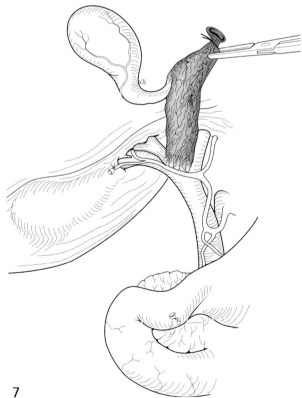

7

8 The left hepatic duct is incised for a variable distance (5–10 mm) to allow a wide hilar hepaticoenterostomy. Anastomosis to a narrow common hepatic duct should be avoided because of the long-term risk of stricture.

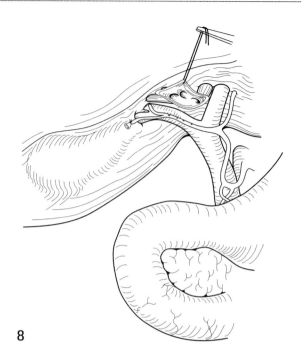

8

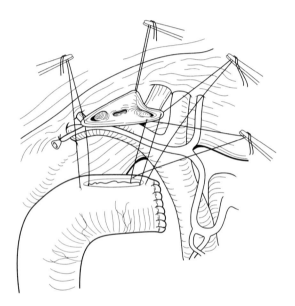

9

9 The duodenojejunal flexure is identified and the jejunum divided with a linear stapler approximately 15–20 cm downstream. At this point, there is a suitable vascular arcade to create a Roux loop that will reach the hilum of the liver without tension. The stapled end of the Roux loop is over-sewn with an absorbable suture and passed through a window in the transverse mesocolon to the right of the middle colic vessels. The Roux loop of jejunum is widely anastomosed to the hepatic duct bifurcation at the hilum of the liver using fine, interrupted, absorbable monofilament sutures (6/0 or 7/0 PDS). Magnifying loupes help to ensure a precise anastomosis. The anastomosis is constructed a few millimeters from the end of the Roux to avoid the development of a blind pouch with future growth of the bowel.

10 A 40 cm Roux loop is adequate in most cases, but a shorter (30 cm) loop is adequate in infants. The proximal stump of jejunum is anastomosed in an oblique end-to-side fashion to the distal jejunum using a single layer of interrupted extramucosal PDS sutures. Mesenteric defects in the transverse mesocolon and small bowel mesentery are closed with sutures. A liver biopsy is performed at the end of the operation to document hepatic histology. The operative field is washed with warm saline and, in straightforward cases, the abdomen is closed without drainage. If a drain is left in place, it should be placed in Morison's pouch and not in direct contact with the anastomosis.

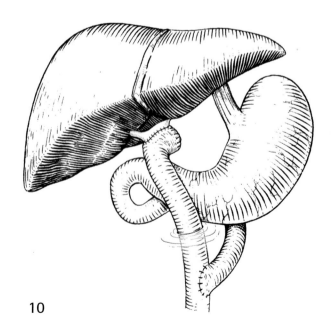

10

Alternative operative techniques

- Alternative biliary reconstructive techniques include an end-to-end hilar hepaticojejunostomy (in contrast to end-to-side) and hepaticoduodenostomy. Proponents of the latter argue that it is more physiological, associated with less risk of adhesion obstruction, and minimizes the loss of absorptive mucosa, but duodenogastric reflux of bile can be a problem and there are concerns about a long-term risk of anastomotic malignancy. Excellent results can be achieved with hepaticojejunostomy. The appendix should not be used as a conduit (hepatico-appendico-duodenostomy) because of a high incidence of subsequent biliary obstruction. An intussusception 'valve' offers no advantage in the Roux loop.
- Hilar ductal strictures may necessitate some form of ductoplasty or extended anastomosis.
- The addition of a transduodenal sphincteroplasty should be considered if the common channel is very dilated and contains debris.

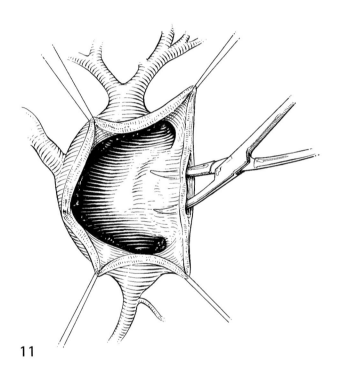

11

11● Occasionally, portal hypertension or dense inflammation from previous infection or surgery makes radical excision hazardous. Intramural resection of the posterior wall of the cyst (excising only the mucosa and inner wall) can help to avoid damage to the portal vein. The cyst lining is completely removed, but a portion of the outer wall remains posteriorly.

- Endoscopic sphincterotomy or transduodenal sphincteroplasty alone cannot be recommended for fusiform choledochal cysts because the majority of these patients have a common pancreatobiliary channel, which results in an ongoing risk of recurrent pancreatitis and later biliary tract malignancy.
- Type II cysts: excision of the diverticulum and repair of the common bile duct is a satisfactory procedure for this rare variety of choledochal cyst.
- Type III cysts: large choledochoceles can be removed transduodenally. Smaller choledochoceles can be treated by sphincteroplasty or endoscopic sphincterotomy if there is no pancreatobiliary malunion.
- Type V cysts: if the cysts are multiple and confined to one side of the liver, hepatic lobectomy may be curative. If multiple cysts are distributed throughout the liver, recurrent cholangitis and stone formation are common. Antibiotics and drainage procedures are helpful, but liver transplantation should be considered in progressive cases.

Laparoscopic operation

LAPAROSCOPIC COMPLETE CYST EXCISION AND HEPATICOJEJUNOSTOMY

12 A nasogastric tube, rectal tube, and Foley urinary catheter are used to decompress the stomach, the colon, and bladder, respectively. The patient is placed in a 30° head up supine position. The surgeon stands at the lower end of the operating table between the patient's legs.

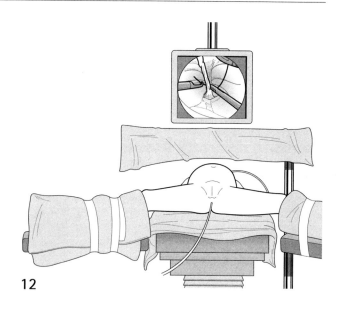

12

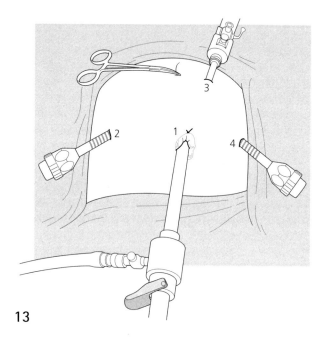

13

13 A 10-mm trocar is inserted through the umbilicus for the telescope. Three additional 5- or 3-mm trocars are placed for instruments: one at the right flank, one at the left flank, and the final one in the left hypochondrium.

14 A carbon dioxide pneumoperitoneum is maintained at a pressure of 8–12 mmHg. The ligament of Treitz is identified by laparoscopy. A 5/0 silk stay-suture is placed 30 cm distal to the ligament of Treitz. A second 5/0 PDS suture is placed 2.0 cm below the first sutures to mark the jejunal limb, which will be anastomosed to the hepatic duct. The jejunal segment with two sutures is grasped with an intestinal grasper. The transumbilical vertical incision is extended 1.0 cm above the umbilicus. The jejunum is exteriorized, and the jejunojejunostomy is carried out extracorporeally. The jejunum is then reintroduced into the abdominal cavity. The extended incision is closed. The laparoscopic instruments are repositioned.

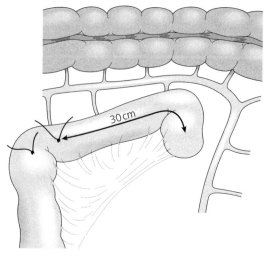

14

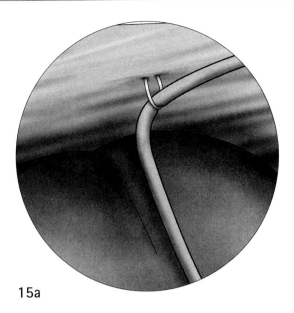

15a

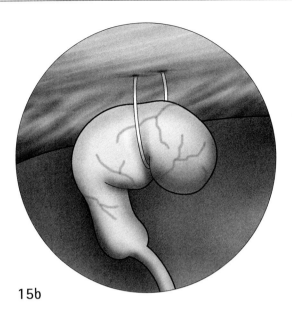

15b

15a,b The liver is secured to the abdominal wall by a stay suture placed at the round ligament. The cystic artery is identified, clipped, and divided. The cystic duct is also isolated, clipped, and divided. A second traction suture is placed at the distal cystic duct to elevate the liver and splay out the liver hilum.

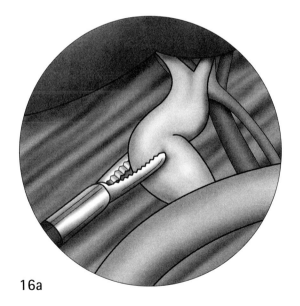

16a

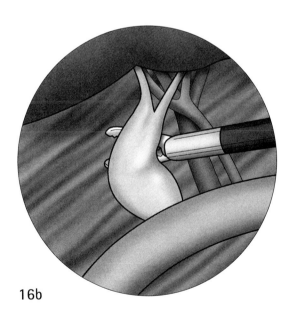

16b

16a,b The duodenum is retracted downward using a dissector through the fourth trocar site. The mid-portion of the cyst is dissected circumferentially. Separation of the cyst from the hepatic artery and portal vein is carried out meticulously (16a) until a dissector can be passed through the space between the posterior wall of the cyst and portal vein proceeding from left to right (16b).

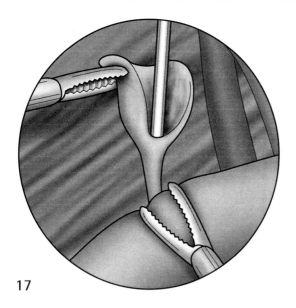

17

17 The cyst is then divided at this site. The lower part of the cyst is detached from the pancreatic tissue down to the common biliary–pancreatic duct using a 3-mm dissector for cautery and dissection. The distal part of the cyst is removed progressively. Protein plugs or calculi within the cyst and common channel are washed out and removed. The distal part of the cyst is opened longitudinally. The interior of the cyst is inspected to identify the orifice of the common biliary–pancreatic channel. A small catheter is inserted into the common channel. Irrigation with normal saline via this catheter is performed to eliminate any protein plug until the catheter can be passed down to the duodenum.

18 The inspection and irrigation may be performed through a pediatric cystoscope if the the common channel is wide enough. The distal choledochal cyst is clipped and divided at the level of the orifice of the common channel.

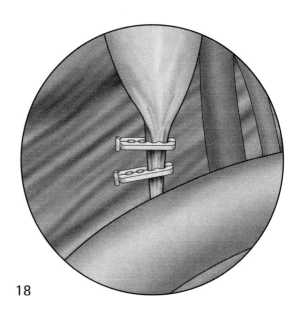

18

The upper part of the cyst is now dissected up to the common hepatic duct and divided. The choledochal cyst is initially divided at the level of the cystic duct, and after identifying the orifice of the right and left hepatic ducts, the definitive division is performed.

The common hepatic duct is irrigated with normal saline to wash out biliary debris and calculi. Irrigation with normal saline through a small catheter inserted into the right and then into the left hepatic duct is performed to wash out the protein plugs or calculi until the fluid from those ducts is clear.

With a large cyst, the dissection is started at the middle portion, proceeding distally. The distal portion of the choledochal cyst is separated from the portal vein. The distal common bile duct is divided above the biliary–pancreatic duct. The distal choledochal cyst is inspected from inside to identify the orifice of the common biliary–pancreatic duct. Irrigation with normal saline in the remnant is carried out to wash out debris and calculi. The distal common bile duct is then clipped and transected at the level of the common channel orifice.

When the cyst is intensely inflamed and extensive pericystic adhesion is present, the dissection of cystic wall from the portal vein is carried out carefully while viewing the cyst internally and externally. After dividing the mid-portion of the cyst, the upper and lower parts of the cyst are removed as described above.

The Roux limb is passed through a window in the transverse mesocolon to the porta hepatis. The jejunum is opened longitudinally on the antimesenteric border a few millimeters from the end of the Roux loop. Hepaticojejunostomy is fashioned using two running sutures of 5/0 PDS. (Interrupted sutures are used when the diameter of the common hepatic duct is less than 1.0 cm.) Sutures are inserted from the left to right with 3-mm instruments. Ductopasty is performed by opening the common hepatic duct and incising the left hepatic duct longitudinally for a variable distance if the common hepatic duct is too small.

Mesenteric defects in the transverse mesocolon and small bowel mesentery are closed with sutures.

The gallbladder is detached from its bed and surrounding tissues. Different parts of the cyst and gallbladder are removed through the umbilicus. The operative field is washed with warm saline. A subhepatic drain is inserted.

LAPAROSCOPIC CYST EXCISION AND HEPATICODUODENOSTOMY

The cyst excision is carried out as described above. The duodenum is mobilized, and a hepaticoduodenostomy is constructed 2.0 cm from the pylorus using two running sutures of 5/0 PDS. Interrupted sutures are used when the diameter of the common hepatic duct is less than 1.0 cm. The rest of the operation is performed as described above.

While the mainstay of surgical management is roux-en-Y jejunostomy, hepaticoduodenostomy is finding increasing favor as a surgical option.

POSTOPERATIVE CARE

Oral feeding is resumed after the fluid from the gastric tube becomes clear, usually on day 2 or 3 after the operation. The abdominal drain is removed on day 5 if there is no anastomotic leakage. Early postoperative complications include bleeding, intestinal obstruction, anastomotic leakage, and pancreatic fistula. The anastomotic leakage and pancreatic fistula can be resolved with abdominal drainage, intravenous antibiotics, nasogastric decompression, and parenteral nutrition.

Cholangitis, anastomotic stricture, and intrahepatic calculi are late complications. Cholangitis without anastomotic stricture or intrahepatic calculi is treated with antibiotics, whereas radiological intervention or surgery is considered for anastomotic stricture or intrahepatic calculi.

OUTCOMES

Between January 2007 and December 2010, laparoscopic surgery for 353 patients with choledochal cyst was performed at the National Hospital of Pediatrics, Hanoi, Vietnam, including 215 patients with cystectomy plus hepaticoduodenostomy and 138 with hepaticojejunostomy. Conversion to open surgery was required in two patients. Intraoperative complications included perforation of the right portal vein and perforation of the right hepatic duct in one patient each. Laparoscopic repair was successful in both patients. Early postoperative complications included biliary fistula in seven patients (2 percent) and pancreatic fistula in four patients (1.1 percent).

FURTHER READING

Farello GA, Cerofolini A, Rebonato M et al. Congenital choledochal cyst: video-guided laparoscopic treatment. Surgical Laparoscopy and Endoscopy 1995; 5: 354–8.

Iwai N, Yanagihara J, Tokiwa K, Shimotake T, Nakamura K. Congenital choledochal dilatation with emphasis on pathophysiology of the biliary tract. Annals of Surgery 1992; 215: 27–30.

Li L, Feng W, Jing-Bo F et al. Laparoscopic-assisted total cyst excision of choledochal cyst and Roux-en-Y hepatoenterostomy. Journal of Pediatric Surgery 2004; 39: 1663–6.

Liem NT, Hien PD, Dung LA, Son TN. Laparoscopic repair for choledochal cyst: lessons learned from 190 cases. Journal of Pediatric Surgery 2010; 45: 540–4.

Santore MT, Behar BJ, Blinman TA, et al. Hepaticoduodenostomy vs hepaticojejunostomy for reconstruction after resection of choledochal cyst. Journal of Pediatric Surgery 2011; 46(1): 209–213.

Stringer MD. Choledochal cysts. In: Howard ER, Stringer MD, Colombani PM (eds), Surgery of the Liver, Bile-Ducts and Pancreas in Children, 2nd edition. London: Arnold Publishers, 2002, 149–68.

Tan HL, Shankar KR, Ford WD. Laparoscopic resection of type I choledochal cyst. Surgical Endoscopy 2003; 17: 1495.

Todani T, Watanabe Y, Narusue M et al. Congenital bile duct cyst: classification, operative procedure, and review of 37 cases including cancer arising from choledochal cyst. American Journal of Surgery 1977; 134: 263–9.

72

Splenectomy

MARCUS JARBOE and JAMES GEIGER

PRINCIPLES AND JUSTIFICATION

There are several indications for splenectomy in children, including many hematologic diseases and uncontrolled hemorrhage from trauma. Removing the spleen has immunologic consequences and therefore benefits of the procedure should always be weighed against the risks of post-splenectomy sepsis. For this reason, partial splenectomy is being explored by some surgeons as an alternative in some of these disease states. Laparoscopic splenectomy has emerged as one of the most frequently performed laparoscopic solid organ procedures in children. Studies in children comparing laparoscopic splenectomy and open splenectomy have shown that the laparoscopic approach is safe and has several advantages, including reduced postoperative pain, a shorter stay in hospital, early return of normal activity, and improved cosmesis. Still, there are many instances where open splenectomy may be a more prudent choice for a variety of reasons, such as splenic trauma or severe splenomegaly among others.

Indications

Splenectomy or partial splenectomy is often required in children with hematologic disorders, such as sickle-cell disease, hereditary spherocytosis, thalassemia major, and idiopathic thrombocytopenic purpura. Rarely, splenectomy is indicated for trauma or other pathology.

OPERATIVE PROCEDURE

Preparation of the patient

If possible, vaccinations to *Streptococcus pneumoniae*, *Neisseria meningitidis*, and *Haemophilus influenzae* should be given before the operation, with adequate time to develop a full immunologic response. When removing the spleen electively for disease, a right upper quadrant ultrasound should be performed. If there is gallbladder disease, a cholecystectomy can be done at the same time. In the operating room, the stomach should be emptied with an orogastric or nasogastric tube, and the urinary bladder should be emptied either by a Credé maneuver or by placing a Foley catheter.

OPEN SPLENECTOMY

Positioning of the patient

The authors have found the right lateral decubitus position provides excellent exposure for an elective splenectomy, but if preferred, the supine position can also be utilized.

Operation

When in the right lateral decubitus position, a transverse incision starting off the 11th rib and extending medially is used. Midline or left subcostal incisions are also used especially in the setting of trauma. A Bookwalter, Thompson or other suitable retractor is placed to give exposure (in the trauma setting, a Richardson retractor may be preferred).

Splenic disease

1 The sequence of the operative steps for splenectomy can vary depending on the clinical condition and the surgeon's preference. In general, the authors complete the operation in this order. The spleen is mobilized by incising the splenocolic and splenophrenic ligaments. The short gastric vessels are divided and ligated, being careful to protect the stomach. The spleen and tail of the pancreas are delivered out of the peritoneum. The branches of the splenic artery and vein are divided with a suture or energy device with careful attention to protect the tail of the pancreas. The spleen is removed. The greater curve of the stomach and the pancreatic tail is inspected for any injury. Any areas of concern should be sutured or stapled. The area of the pancreatic tail, kidney, bowel mesentery, gastrosplenic ligament, and pelvis should be inspected for accessory spleens. Closed suction drainage is only used in cases of suspected pancreatic injury.

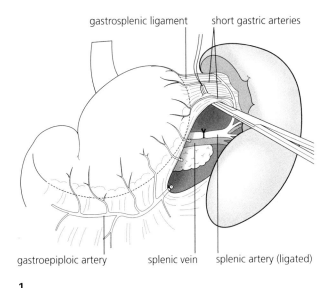

gastrosplenic ligament   short gastric arteries

gastroepiploic artery   splenic vein   splenic artery (ligated)

1

If operating in the presence of splenic vein thrombosis and varices, ligation of the main splenic artery before dissection of the hilum and ligamentus attachments is begun can help decrease the size of the spleen and reduce the size of the varices, thereby reducing the risk of massive blood loss.

Splenic trauma

TRAUMA SPLENECTOMY

2a–d While standing on the patient's right, the spleen should be retracted medially with the left hand and the splenorenal, splenophrenic, and splenocolic ligaments divided either sharply or bluntly. The hilus should be dissected bluntly by sliding the right hand posteriorly and underneath the pancreas and the spleen lifted into the wound. Rapid hemostasis should be provided by occluding the splenic artery and with the surgeon's fingers. The retroperitoneum should be packed with lap pads. The vessels in the hilus should be carefully exposed posteriorly and the vessels ligated with suture ligatures, with care being taken to avoid the tail of the pancreas. Then, the short gastric vessels should be ligated. The packing should be removed, whereupon complete hemostatis is obtained. Due to the expediency of splenectomy for trauma, careful inspection of the greater curve of the stomach and pancreatic tail for injury is mandatory.

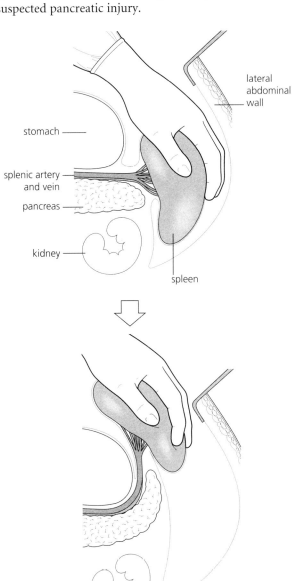

lateral abdominal wall

stomach

splenic artery and vein

pancreas

kidney

spleen

2a

lateral gutter

TRAUMA SPLENORRHOPHY

If the spleen is lacerated, but still viable, and hemodynamic and clinical variables allow, splenorrhaphy is an option that controls hemorrhage, but also preserves the immunologic benefits of having a spleen.

2b Using absorbable mesh such as Vicryl, a rectangular piece large enough to wrap around the spleen should be cut. Then the mesh should be cut at opposite ends in the middle of the mesh as shown. The mesh should be wrapped around the spleen with the tails of the mesh oriented towards the tail of the pancreas.

2c In this orientation, the cuts made in the mesh allow room for the vessels to enter the spleen.

2d Next, a stapling device should be used to staple the tails of the mesh together at the medial border of the spleen. The stapling should be done close enough to the splenic edge to make the mesh moderately tight around the spleen to provide hemostasis. Care should be taken not to make the mesh too tight and thereby cause venous and arterial insufficiency to the entire spleen.

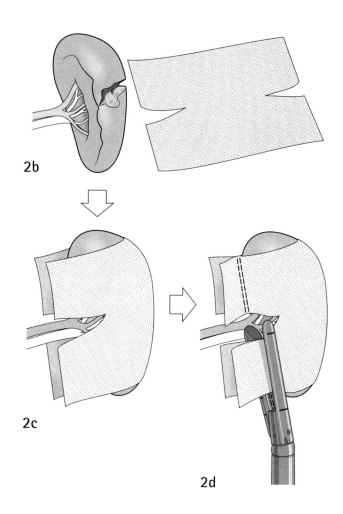

2b

2c

2d

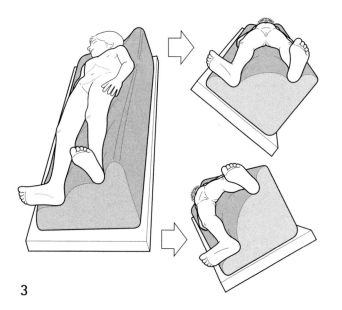

3

LAPAROSCOPIC TOTAL SPLENECTOMY

Positioning of the patient

3 The patient can be placed in a supine position on the table and then bumped up on the left with a bean bag or other means to about a 45° angle. Alternatively, the patient can be placed in the right lateral decubitus position with some rotation back towards the left. If the umbilicus is to be used for the camera port, the patient must be positioned as close as possible to the right side of the bed so that the camera can achieve the correct angle. The patient should be well secured to the table to allow for aggressive positioning during the operation.

Trocar insertion sites

4 A 5-mm 30° laparoscope should be placed through a 5-mm umbilical cannula. A 12-mm cannula is placed in the midclavicular line on the left side of the abdomen below the tip of the spleen. This is later enlarged to allow placement of a large laparoscopic retrieval bag. One to two additional 5-mm cannulae are placed. Their exact location may vary depending on the size of the spleen and the patient. In general, one 5-mm cannula on the patient's right side is usually placed near the midline in the epigastric area. An additional 5-mm port can be placed in the subxiphoid area just above the other port. The placement may need to be slightly modified if a cholecystectomy is to be performed at the same time. Airplaning the table to the left to place the ports is often helpful. The table then can be rotated to the right to obtain a lateral position and adding reverse Trendelenburg may be helpful to move the bowel away from the spleen (illustration 3).

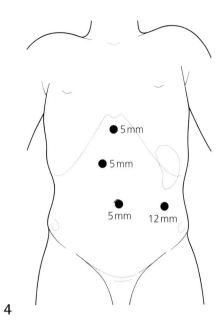

4

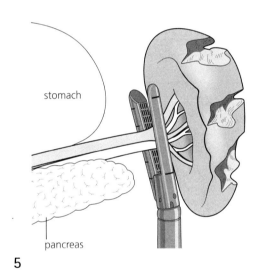

5

Dividing short gastric vessels

5a The greater curvature of the stomach should be grasped gently with an atraumatic grasper or Babcock clamp passed through the epigastric port on the right. In this way, the gastrosplenic ligament is retracted to expose the short gastric vessels. These vessels should then be divided with an energy device or between clips passed through the port on the left.

Freeing the spleen posteriorly

Once the short gastric vessels are divided, the spleen is retracted to the right and the splenocolic attachments are divided allowing retraction of the colon inferiorly. Following this, the posterolateral fascial attachments are divided to free the spleen so that its only remaining attachments are the splenic hilar vessels.

Dissection of the splenic vessels

Once mobilized, the spleen can be elevated and essentially suspended by a retracting instrument(s). The splenic artery and vein at the splenic hilum just beyond the tail of the pancreas should now be identified using gentle dissection with a curved dissector. These vessels should be separately and carefully divided between ligatures or with a bipolar electrosurgical device in small children. Alternatively, clips can be used to ligate each vessel, or the vascular load of an endoscopic stapler can be used to divide both vessels at once. The endoscopic stapler is hemostatic and diminishes the operative time significantly, but care should be taken to avoid the tail of the pancreas during stapling.

Dissection of ligamentous attachments

After the major splenic vessels have been divided, there are often some ligamentous attachments at the upper pole of the spleen that should be carefully divided using Metzenbaum-type scissors or cautery. At this point, the spleen should be completely mobilized and free in the peritoneal cavity.

Morcellating the spleen

6 The neck of the sac should be opened and the spleen should be broken up in the bag using a finger, sponge holder, or ovary forceps. We find use of the suction machine and attachments used for suction curettage facilitate morcellation. The organ can then be morcellated until it is sufficiently small to enable the entire pouch with any residual tissue to be withdrawn through the trocar site. Care should be taken not to tear the bag and thereby allowing splenic tissue to drop into the abdomen. This potentially can seed the abdomen with splenic tissue.

Accessory spleen

The port should be replaced and the abdomen insufflated again. Hemostasis should then be ensured. In addition, the area of the pancreatic tail, kidney, bowel mesentery, gastrosplenic ligament, and pelvis should be inspected for accessory spleens.

LAPAROSCOPIC PARTIAL SPLENECTOMY

The patient should be positioned supine with a bump to 45° or in the lateral decubitus position identical to the total splenectomy described above (illustration 3). A 5-mm 30°

Laparoscopic retrieval bag for the isolated spleen

A 15-mm laparoscopic retrieval bag should then be inserted through the 12-mm port site (with the port removed). When deployed in the abdomen, the freed spleen can be maneuvered into the sac and then the neck of the sac can be exteriorized through the trocar site.

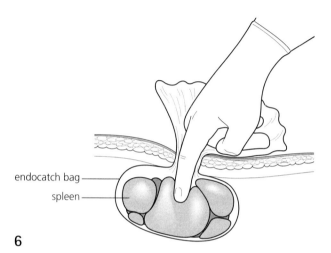

endocatch bag
spleen

6

laparoscope should be placed through a 5-mm umbilical cannula. A 12-mm cannula is placed in the midclavicular line on the left side of the abdomen below the tip of the spleen and one to two additional 5-mm cannulae are placed in the upper midline, as described above for the total splenectomy (see illustration 4).

Freeing the spleen

This step is similar to what was described above, except that many of the ligamentous attachments to the upper portion of the spleen are preserved in order to avoid postoperative volvulus of the remnant spleen.

Dissection of the splenic vessels and transecting the spleen

7 The identification of the main splenic vessels and their branches is crucial during a partial splenectomy. The majority of spleens (86 percent) have two lobar arteries branching off the splenic artery, while 12 percent have three.

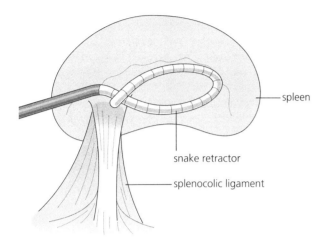

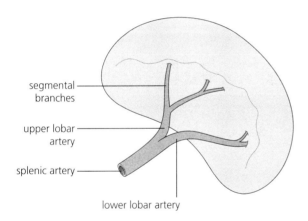

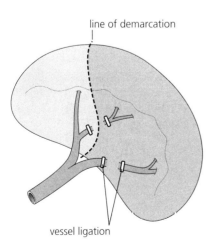

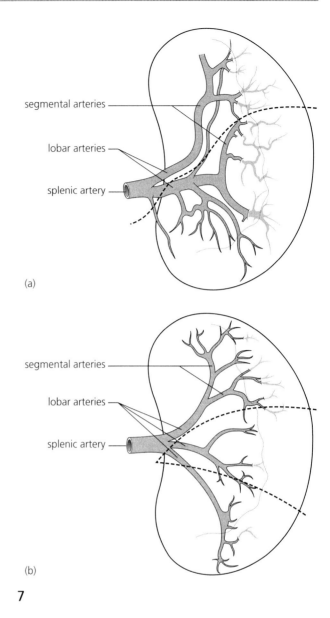

(a)

(b)

7

8 During a partial splenectomy, the splenic hilum is dissected and the splenic vessels and their branches are exposed. The spleen is partially devascularized by ligating one or more lobar arteries and segmental branches (depending on what the anatomy allows). In some cases, the lobar arteries branch before entering the splenic parenchyma allowing further ligation. The anatomy limits what percentage of the spleen can be left behind with good blood flow. After ligating the vessels, the devascularized portion of the spleen is allowed to demarcate. The splenic parenchyma is then divided approximately 1 cm from the line of demarcation using an electrosurgical energy device. Following parenchyma transection, if there is residual bleeding from the splenic bed it can be controlled with an argon beam coagulator, electrocautery, and topical hemostatic agents. The goal is to leave approximately 25 percent of the spleen intact and viable, although anatomy is often the limiting factor. The splenic tissue is then

8

removed via a laparoscopic retrieval bag. Ligamentous attachments are preserved to stabilize the splenic remnant and prevent volvulizing on its vascular supply. If vessels to the preserved pole are absent or if severe intraoperative bleeding is encountered, conversion to a total splenectomy is required. Conversion to total splenectomy is required in less than 5 percent of cases.

FURTHER READING

Buesing KL, Tracy ET, Kiernan C et al. Partial splenectomy for hereditary spherocytosis: a multi-institutional review. *Journal of Pediatric Surgery* 2011; **46**: 178–83.

Geiger JD, Dinh VV, Teitelbaum DH et al. The lateral approach for open splenectomy. *Journal of Pediatric Surgery* 1998; **33**: 1153–7.

Hirshberg A, Mattox KL. The 'take-outable' solid organs. In: *Top Knife: The Art and Craft of Trauma Surgery*. Harley: tfm Publishing Ltd, 2005: 100–14.

Kuhne T, Blanchette V, Buchanan GR et al. Splenectomy in children with idiopathic thrombocytopenia purpura: a prospective study of 134 children from the Intercontinental Childhood ITP Group. *Pediatric Blood Cancer* 2007; **49**: 829–34.

Lobe TE, Presbury GJ, Smith BM et al. Laparoscopic splenectomy. *Pediatric Annals* 1993; **22**: 671–4.

Minkes RK, Lagzdins M, Langer JC. Laparoscopic versus open splenectomy in children. *Journal of Pediatric Surgery* 2000; **35**: 699–701.

Murawski M, Patkowski D, Korlacki W et al. Laparoscopic splenectomy in children – a multicenter experience. *Journal of Pediatric Surgery* 2008; **43**: 951–4.

Reinberg O. Partial splenectomies by laparoscopy in children. In: Bax K, Georgeson KE, Rothenberg SS et al. (eds). *Endoscopic Surgery in Infants and Children*. Heidelberg: Springer, 2008: 455–61.

Rescorla FJ. Splenectomy. In: Bax K, Georgeson KE, Rothenberg SS et al. (eds). *Endoscopic Surgery in Infants and Children*. Heidelberg: Springer, 2008: 449–54.

Rescorla FJ, Breitfeld PP, West KW et al. A case controlled comparison of open and laparoscopic splenectomy in children. *Surgery* 1998; **1224**: 670–6.

Smith BM, Schropp KP, Lobe TE et al. Laparoscopic splenectomy in childhood. *Journal of Pediatric Surgery* 1994; **29**: 975–8.

Tulman S, Holocomb GW, Karamanoukian HL et al. Pediatric laparoscopic splenectomy. *Journal of Pediatric Surgery* 1993; **28**: 689–92.

SECTION VI

Tumors

73

Liver resections

JOHN A SANDOVAL and FREDERICK M KARRER

HISTORY

Liver resection has evolved to an established treatment for various hepatic tumors and other conditions. This evolution was opened by anatomists who paved the way for modern anatomically oriented liver resection which is based on the intrahepatic segmentation according to the portal structure branching and the course of major hepatic veins. The first successful, elective hepatic resection is credited to Langenbuch (1888). A year later, Konig performed the first partial hepatectomy in a child. In 1952, Lortat-Jacob and Roberts reported the technique of extrahepatic ligation of vessels to control hemorrhage to perform an anatomic hepatic lobectomy. In 1953, Quattlebaum described transecting the liver with the handle of a knife, and clamping the vessels within the plane of transection. Contemporary work by Ton That Tung, Couinaud, and Bismuth provide the basis for present techniques that allow for a controlled anatomic liver resection. Intraoperative high-resolution ultrasonography, introduced by Makuuchi, combined with the Glissonian pedicle ligation technique popularized by Launois, facilitated performance of segmental and sectoral hepatic resections. The advances in surgical technique together with surgical instrumentation, anesthesia, and diagnostic tests demonstrating the details of anatomy have revolutionized liver surgery. Successful liver surgery requires a fundamental understanding of liver anatomy, disease pathophysiology, and modern hepatic resection techniques. These foundations have allowed hepatic resections to be performed with an increased level of safety with decreased mortality and morbidity.

PRINCIPLES AND JUSTIFICATION

Indications

Primary tumors of the liver may be either malignant or benign. Hepatoblastoma (HB) and hepatocellular carcinoma (HCC) are the two most common malignant liver tumors which are rare and account for 0.5–1.5 percent of all childhood malignancies with a total annual incidence of 0.5–1.5 cases per million US children. Benign liver tumors comprise approximately one-third of hepatic pathology and include hemangiomas, hamartomas, hepatic adenomas, and focal nodular hyperplasia (FNH). Hepatic resection is a fundamental modality for many of these lesions in addition to selected cases requiring metastatectomy.

Preoperative considerations

1 Because of the rarity of primary liver pathology in children, affected patients should have liver surgery performed in centers with sufficient experience and modern equipment suitable for major surgery. Prior to any operation, two questions need to be addressed when contemplating hepatic resection surgery: (1) Can the lesion technically be resected, and (2) should the lesion be resected? To assess resectablity, staging of the liver tumors is important. There are two standard surgical staging systems for pediatric liver tumors. The Childhood Liver Tumor Strategy Group (SIOPEL) uses a presurgical-based staging system, while the Children's Oncology Group (COG) uses a postsurgical-based staging system. The staging systems support different treatment strategies. The presurgical staging system is used with neoadjuvant chemotherapy followed by definitive surgery (with the exception of Pretreatment Extent of Disease (PRETEXT) stage 1), while the postsurgical staging system has surgery as the initial strategy. It is worth emphasizing the desirability of avoiding very difficult liver resections that carry a high probability of leaving residual tumor. This recommendation applies mainly to tumors in close proximity to the major hepatic vessels which, in order to be preserved, would have to be peeled off the tumor or would require complex vascular resection and reconstruction. As anatomic features of the lesion may preclude safe liver resection, liver transplantation (LT) has been incorporated into the treatment armamentarium for pediatric liver tumors deemed unresectable by conventional surgical resection (see **Chapter 107**). The most frequent liver malignancies requiring LT include HB, HCC, hepatic epithelioid hemangioendothelioma (HEHE), and other rare tumors including undifferentiated, embryonal, and rhabdoid sarcomas, and angiosarcoma. Current recommendations for LT in advanced pediatric HCC include: (1) LT should be offered to children with any size or number of tumors, provided that they remain confined to the liver; (2) LT to children with vascular invasion should be offered as long as the features of diagnosis, treatment, and outcome are prospectively recorded and reported; (3) LT should not be offered for HCC that has metastasized outside the liver. The role of LT in unresectable HB includes: (1) Neoadjuvant chemotherapy should be provided before LT with early referral to a pediatric LT program, as LT is the treatment of choice. (2) LT is appropriate for children with metastatic HB when the distant disease appears to have been cured with chemotherapy alone. (3) LT as an option after surgical metastasectomy remains a controversial issue. Furthermore, in exceptional cases when LT is not a viable option, total vascular hepatic exclusion is of particular value for tumors located very close to the inferior vena cava (IVC), hepatic veins and/or portal vein because it allows dissection of the tumor from the vessel or resection of the tumor with a portion of the vascular wall and its subsequent reconstruction in a relatively bloodless field.

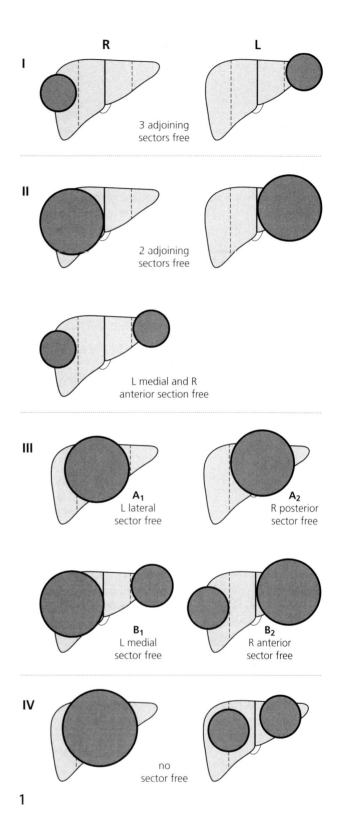

1

Whether the hepatic lesion should be resected is weighed against a variety of factors that may limit the feasibility of the procedure including preoperative factors that may affect the outcome of a planned procedure. Preoperative risk assessment involves evaluation of remnant liver volume, hepatic functional reserve, age, and the medical condition of the patient. Medical suitability to undergo liver resection is generally based on the underlying liver disease (cirrhosis and/or biliary pathology) or the effects and toxicity of chemotherapy (i.e. ototoxicity and nephrotoxicity related to cisplatin and cardiotoxicity due to doxorubicin). Another consideration in the case of large tumors is whether preoperative chemotherapy should precede the operation even when there is the possibility of resection. This strategy helps to preserve more mass of healthy hepatic tissue, decrease intraoperative/postoperative complications, and avoids sacrifice of normal hepatic tissue. In contrast, a rationale proposed for upfront surgical resection is that advanced gastric cancer (AGC) patients may achieve long-term survival with less intensive chemotherapy and less chemotherapy-related toxicity.

Children with HB generally respond to chemotherapy and have an overall survival of more than 90 percent in the setting of localized disease, and between 30 and 60 percent even in the presence of lung metastases. With the addition of cisplatin to the chemotherapy in the late 1980s, overall survival in hepatoblastoma increased from 30 to 70 percent. When compared to the outcome of pediatric patients with HB, the chemotherapy response rate of patients with HCC is less than 50 percent. In fact, the role of chemotherapy in pediatric HCC remains controversial. Current guidelines do not advocate chemotherapy for children with resectable localized HCC. Moreover, neoadjuvant chemotherapy has a very limited role in localized unresectable HCC, and should only be offered in the context of a clinical trial. Alternatives to cytotoxic therapy include radiofrequency ablation, cryotherapy, and transcatheter arterial chemoembolization. New therapies like sorafenib, a tyrosine kinase inhibitor, are being investigated in children with advanced HCC as an alternative to chemotherapy for palliation. Chemotherapy used for palliation of patients with metastatic HCC demands consideration of the goals of such therapy, and the understanding that such therapy is based on limited data.

Given the variable nature of benign liver tumors in children, the decision to proceed with surgery for benign hepatic lesions should take into consideration the presence of symptoms, diagnostic uncertainty, the known natural history, and the complication risks of the disease process (hemorrhage, rupture, or degeneration). Hemangioma is by far the most common benign tumor of the liver in infancy. Initial medical intervention for these lesions has been with corticosteroids and propranolol and may involve other treatment options like ε-aminocaproic acid, tranexamic acid, low-molecular-weight heparin, vincristine, cyclophosphamide, interferon 2-alpha, and AGM-1470. Surgical resection or enucleation of hemangioma should be the treatment of choice only when medical treatment or other less invasive measures, such as hepatic artery ligation or embolization, fail.

Preoperative laboratory investigation should be guided by the patient's clinical situation. Most children with liver tumors have normal liver function. A complete blood count and clot for crossmatch are useful for all children. Children who undergo neoadjuvant chemotherapy are more prone to anemia and thrombocytopenia as a result of bone marrow suppression. Anemia and thrombocytopenia should be identified and corrected prior to operation, and two units of crossmatched red blood cells should be available at the time of operation. These children should also have a complete chemistry panel preoperatively, as platinum-based regimens can be nephrotoxic. Impairment of hepatic synthetic function may lead to a potentially correctable coagulopathy. Children with underlying parenchymal liver disease should have liver function tests, as well as a prothrombin time and partial thromboplastin time, prior to operation. Alpha-fetoprotein is a tumor marker that is expressed by most hepatoblastomas and some HCCs. A baseline alpha-fetoprotein (AFP) level should be obtained for all children with these tumors, as it can be an indicator of tumor response to therapy, and it can be an early marker of tumor recurrence.

As the liver is a highly vascular organ, depending on the extent of resection, it is not unheard of to lose up to a blood volume of 80 mL/kg in a major liver resection. Therefore, a thorough and honest discussion should be held with the patient and family about the likelihood and risks of transfusion. Despite the accuracy of current imaging, the most accurate assessment of tumor resectability is operative exploration, and the possibility of being unable to resect the tumor should also be discussed preoperatively, particularly if imaging suggests possible hepatic vein or IVC involvement. Biliary injury, due either to direct mechanical injury or to indirect ischemic injury, should be mentioned. Postoperative risks include hemorrhage requiring transfusion or re-exploration, infectious complications (wound infection, subphrenic abscess) biloma or bile leak, pulmonary complications, wound complications, and long-term complications (e.g. hernia or adhesive small bowel obstruction). Postoperative hepatic insufficiency is rare, but it should be mentioned prior to liver resection in patients with cirrhosis. Overall mortality related to major liver resection should be less than 5 percent.

Imaging

2 The choice of a liver resection should be guided by the need to obtain a negative margin around the tumor and the need to preserve functional liver parenchyma. Accurate imaging can prove invaluable in the planning of a successful liver resection. Computed tomography (CT) scanning is the favored imaging study for the assessment of liver tumors in children. It is a high-resolution study that can be completed quickly, minimizing the need for sedation. The CT scans demonstrate the size and anatomic location of the liver tumor. The administration of intravenous contrast can give additional information, as scanner timing can be coordinated to image the liver during hepatic arterial and portal venous phases of the contrast. Contrast-enhanced scans reveal the relationships of the tumor to the hepatic veins, IVC, and portal structures. These relationships are pivotal, as an anatomic liver resection is defined by the preservation or sacrifice of hepatic veins and portal structures. In order to classify the tumor in the PRETEXT system, the patient must undergo imaging with spiral CT followed by contrast administration (including an angio-computed tomography reconstruction of hepatic vessels, when necessary). Computed tomography scans may not reveal with certainty whether a tumor merely abuts or truly invades a vascular structure, but it does reveal the proximity of this relationship. Contrast CT scanning may reveal aberrant hepatic arterial anatomy, although it is not as accurate as conventional arteriography or intraoperative exploration. The presence of aberrant arteries, if noted, is helpful for operative planning. In addition, preoperative CT scans inform the surgeon about possible involvement of the tumor with extrahepatic structures (e.g. vena cava, diaphragm, retroperitoneum, kidney, stomach, and regional lymph nodes). A chest CT scan should be performed in children with potentially malignant liver tumors in order to evaluate for pulmonary metastases. Magnetic resonance imaging (MRI) can be useful for the evaluation of large, complex, or multifocal liver tumors. It may more accurately delineate hemangiomas than CT, as some hemangiomas have a radiodensity similar to that of normal liver parenchyma. When combined with magnetic resonance angiography (MRA) using gadolinium, it reveals the relationship of the tumor to the major vascular structures of the liver and can reveal aberrant

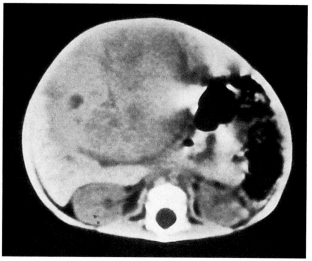

2

hepatic arterial anatomy. In addition, magnetic resonance cholangiopancreatography (MRCP) can be helpful in elaborating the patient's biliary anatomy in cases where a biliary reconstruction is anticipated, such as the patient with a previous Kasai procedure for biliary atresia.

Doppler ultrasound studies are of particular value in children, allowing real-time investigation of the tumor and its relationship to the main hepatic veins and portal branches, including an assessment of their patency or possible invasion by tumor. Duplex ultrasonography can be helpful if invasion or patency of the hepatic veins or vena cava is questioned. Conventional angiography is no longer routinely performed in patients with liver tumors. It is most useful in a patient with a vascular malformation for the performance of angioembolization as primary therapy. Conventional angiography may also be helpful to determine the hepatic arterial anatomy in cases where a hepatic artery infusion pump may be placed. Intraoperative ultrasonography (IOUS) is also a useful modality to determine the extent of disease, to assess margin control in the management of tumors involving the hepatic veins, and to guide hepatic resection, where the relationship between the dissection plane and the tumor edge can be followed and the direction of the dissection plane can be modified when needed.

Anatomy

3 The ligamentum teres is the fibrotic remnant of the fetal umbilical vein, and it runs from the umbilicus within the inferior edge of the falciform ligament, through the umbilical fissure, where it joins the left portal vein. Similarly, the ligamentum venosum is the remnant of the fetal ductus venosus and travels from the left portal vein to the left hepatic vein. The falciform ligament extends to the diaphragm, where it is continuous with the left and right triangular ligaments. These ligaments demarcate the bare area on the dome of the liver. The true anatomic left lobe and right lobe are separated by an imaginary line (Cantlie line) that runs from the gallbladder fossa to the suprahepatic vena cava. The middle hepatic vein lies in this plane. The anatomic left lobe is divided into a left lateral sector and a left medial sector by the umbilical fissure and falciform ligament externally and by the left hepatic vein internally. The right lobe is divided into a right anterior sector and a right posterior sector by the right hepatic vein.

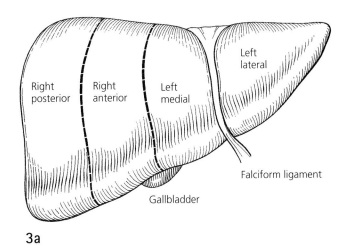

3a

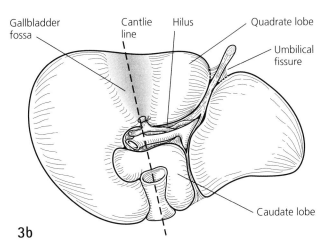

3b

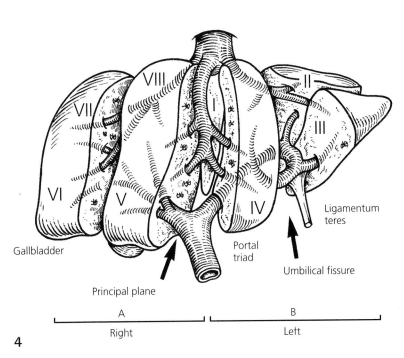

4

Gallbladder

Principal plane

A — Right

B — Left

Ligamentum teres

Umbilical fissure

Portal triad

4 The liver can be further divided into eight anatomic segments. Each segment is supplied by a portal pedicle, and each drains into a tributary of a hepatic vein. Segment I is synonymous with the caudate lobe. It is supplied by branches off the left and right portal triads, and its venous drainage is directly into the IVC. Segments II and III comprise the left lateral sector, and segment IV comprises the left medial sector. Segments V and VIII form the right anterior sector, and segments VI and VII form the right posterior sector. Appreciation of the segmental anatomy of the liver serves as the basis for liver resection, as it is preferable to obtain extrahepatic control of vascular structures prior to the division of liver parenchyma. Although lesser resections may be performed on the basis of this anatomy, the five most commonly performed liver resections are right hepatectomy (right lobectomy), left hepatectomy (left lobectomy), extended right hepatectomy (right trisegmentectomy), extended left hepatectomy (left trisegmentectomy), and left lateral lobectomy (left lateral segmentectomy).

Anesthesia

A general endotracheal anesthetic is administered. In appropriate patients, an epidural catheter is placed to facilitate analgesia in the intraoperative and postoperative periods. A Foley catheter is placed for intraoperative monitoring of urine output. A nasogastric tube is placed to decompress the patient's stomach. In light of the possibility of significant hemorrhage, vascular access is secured in the form of two large-bore intravenous lines in the upper extremities or neck. It is important to secure vascular access above the nipples in case the IVC needs to be cross-clamped for total hepatic vascular exclusion. A central venous catheter in the internal jugular or subclavian vein may be helpful for this purpose. In addition, central venous pressure (CVP) monitoring can help the anesthesiologist with intraoperative fluid management. Elevated CVP may increase blood loss from tributaries to the hepatic veins and the IVC; therefore, we favor judicious infusion of intravenous fluids as long as the patient is well perfused. A radial arterial line is placed for continuous blood pressure monitoring. This line is also useful in blood sampling for arterial blood gases, blood counts, and coagulation profiles during the operation. The patient's temperature requires close attention throughout the operation. Hypothermia can have deleterious effects on coagulation, particularly in the face of a large incision and significant blood loss. Normothermia is maintained through ambient room temperature, warming blankets, and infusions of warmed fluids and blood products.

OPERATION

5 The patient is placed supine on the operating table with a small rolled towel serving as a bump under the upper lumbar spine. The operating table should be placed in a slight Trendelenburg position, to minimize the risk of air embolism. The table can be rotated with the patient's right side up to facilitate exposure. A single dose of a first-generation cephalosporin is given prior to incision. The patient's abdomen and chest are both prepared and draped in the event that a median sternotomy or thoracoabdominal extension is needed to expose the tumor or obtain control of the IVC within the pericardium. A bilateral subcostal incision is made one finger's breadth below the costal margins. The incision extends from the lateral border of the left rectus sheath to the right anterior axillary line (dashed line). This incision allows for an extension superiorly in the midline or thoracoabdominal if additional exposure is needed (dotted line). A median sternotomy is advised if it is difficult to control the IVC within the abdomen.

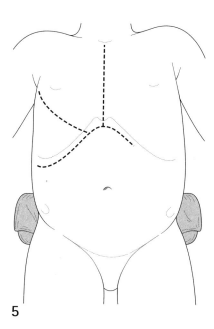

5

Dissection

6 Upon entry into the peritoneal space, the abdomen is explored by inspection and palpation. Particular attention is paid to the size and location of the primary tumor, adhesions to adjacent structures, enlarged lymph nodes, or additional tumor elsewhere in the liver. The ligamentum teres is ligated and divided. The liver is mobilized by sharply dividing the falciform ligament along its course up to the diaphragm. This dissection is continued along the left and right triangular ligaments in order to free the liver from the diaphragm. A self-retaining retractor is used to optimize exposure. The liver is manually retracted inferiorly to expose the suprahepatic IVC. The anterior and lateral surfaces are dissected free of loose connective tissue. The liver is then rotated to the patient's left side to expose the posterolateral aspect of the IVC. A blunt instrument is used to dissect the IVC circumferentially and encircle it with an umbilical tape above the hepatic veins. Some dissection of the hepatic veins outside of liver can be performed at this point, but, in general, dissection of the hepatic veins is postponed until the portal dissection is completed. Similar to the dissection above the liver, the IVC below the liver is circumferentially dissected and encircled with an umbilical tape above the level of the renal veins. This maneuver should be performed with care not to injure the lumbar veins as they enter the posterior aspect of the IVC, as bleeding from these veins can be difficult to control. A window is created into the lesser sac adjacent to the porta hepatis. The hepatogastric ligament is inspected and palpated for an aberrant left hepatic artery. The portal structures are encircled with a vascular tape. This allows for occlusion of the portal vein and hepatic artery (Pringle maneuver) if needed for the control of hemorrhage. Palpation along the posterior surface of the portal vein may reveal the pulse of an aberrant right hepatic artery.

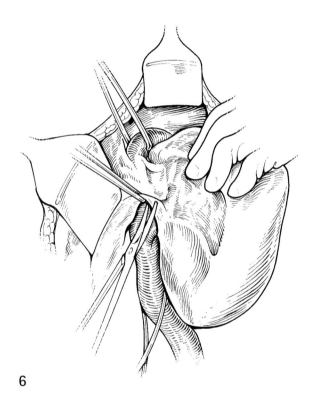

6

Right hepatectomy

7a–d Portal dissection is begun with a cholecystectomy. The cystic artery and cystic duct are divided between ligatures, and the cystic duct stump is followed to its confluence with the common hepatic duct. The common hepatic duct is followed into the hilum of the liver, where it bifurcates into right and left hepatic ducts. During this dissection, care is taken not to dissect the common hepatic duct extensively or circumferentially in order to minimize disruption of the blood supply of the duct, with the subsequent risk of ischemic stricture. The right hepatic duct is circumferentially dissected and divided between ligatures. The right hepatic artery typically runs

just deep to the right hepatic duct. It is circumferentially dissected, ligated, and divided. The right portal vein is the most posterior structure of the portal triad. It is circumferentially dissected and occluded proximally and distally with vascular clamps. The vein is divided between the clamps, leaving a longer cuff on the side adjacent to the confluence. This end is suture ligated with a running polypropylene suture. The hepatic side of the divided right portal vein is also suture ligated. Once the right portal structures are divided, the right lobe of the liver will become ischemic, with a line of demarcation extending up the liver towards the vena cava along the path of the middle hepatic vein.

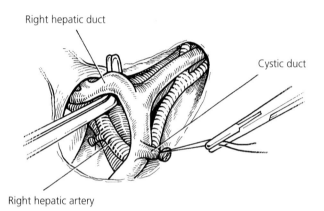

7a

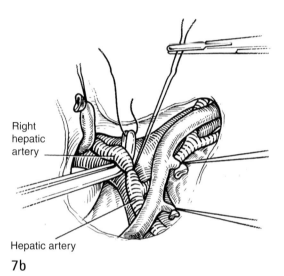

7b

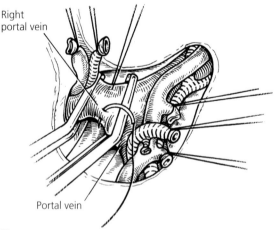

7c

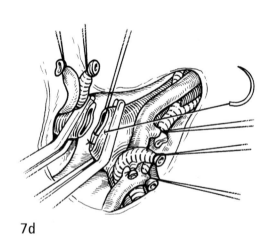

7d

8 Dissection and division of the right hepatic vein require great care, as an injury to the vein or adjacent vena cava can be accompanied by significant bleeding, which may be difficult to control. The course of the right hepatic vein may be very short as it exits the liver and enters the vena cava. If the tumor is not immediately adjacent to the hepatic vein, additional length can be obtained by cautiously dividing a small amount of liver parenchyma that overlies it. If the right hepatic vein can be circumferentially dissected, it is divided between vascular clamps and oversewn.

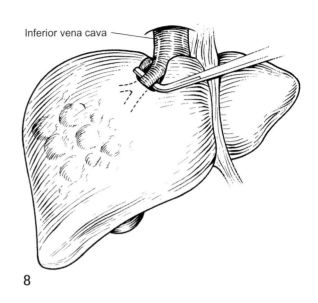

Inferior vena cava

8

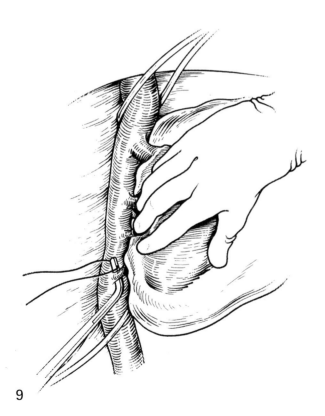

9

9 The right lobe of the liver is retracted to the patient's left side, to expose the length of the retrohepatic IVC. Numerous unnamed hepatic veins empty directly into the vena cava from the right and caudate lobe of the liver. These veins are divided between 4/0 silk ties, beginning with the most inferior veins and progressing superiorly toward the main hepatic veins. If the right hepatic vein cannot be safely controlled from an anterior approach, it can be approached from this posterolateral exposure. With the unnamed hepatic veins divided, the liver can be retracted anteriorly away from the IVC. A right-angle is used to dissect cautiously along the medial aspect of the right hepatic vein. The first clamp is removed, revealing additional venous cuff for suture ligation. If bleeding is encountered during these maneuvers, vascular clamps can be applied to the IVC directed by the previously placed umbilical tapes. A Pringle maneuver may be performed to occlude inflow to the left lobe of the liver, and thereby decrease blood flow through the left and middle hepatic veins.

10 At this point, the major vascular structures to the right lobe of the liver have been divided, and the parenchymal dissection is begun. Glisson's capsule is scored in the interlobar fissure using the electrocautery. The surgeon and first assistant compress the hepatic lobes adjacent to the line of transection during the division of the parenchyma. Although different methods may be used to divide the hepatic parenchyma, we favor the use of the ultrasonic scalpel, as it seals small vessels and ducts as it divides the parenchyma. Only modest amounts of liver parenchyma are divided with each application of the ultrasonic scalpel. This piecemeal transection exposes larger vessels and ducts. Vessels and ducts larger than 5 mm are ligated with 4/0 silk ties or sutures. Hepatic venous tributaries from segments V and VIII are encountered before they join the middle hepatic vein. These are divided between suture ligatures. Care is taken to avoid injury to the middle hepatic vein during the transection of the liver parenchyma. The parenchymal dissection tends to be accompanied by ongoing blood loss, and if this becomes excessive, a Pringle maneuver can be performed.

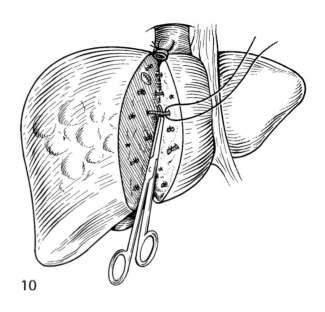

10

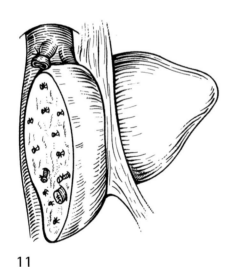

11

11 With the right lobe of the liver removed, attention is directed to the cut surface of the left lobe. Points of bleeding or bile leakage that were not controlled during the parenchymal dissection are closed with 4/0 suture ligatures. The argon beam coagulator is applied to the raw surface to coagulate small points of bleeding not amenable to ligation. Horizontal mattress sutures to compress the liver edges are not routinely used. Topical hemostatic agents are not routinely used either, but these may be useful to reduce the diffuse ooze of blood from the cut surface while the coagulopathy is being corrected. A clean surgical sponge is packed against the cut surface during the remainder of the operation until just prior to closure of the abdomen. This sponge acts as a monitor for a small bile leak that may not be apparent on initial inspection. When the sponge is removed, it is inspected for small bile staining, which would direct the surgeon to a point on the cut surface for suture ligation. The left lobe of the liver is allowed to lie in its 'resting' position. As long as the remaining hepatic venous and portal structures are without kinks or twists, no hepatopexy to the diaphragm or retroperitoneum is routinely performed.

Extended right hepatectomy

This operation is used for large right-sided tumors that extend across the interlobar fissure but do not involve segments II and III (the left lateral segment). The conduct of this operation is similar to the right hepatectomy, but segments I and IV are resected in addition to segments V to VIII.

12 As with the right hepatectomy, the portal dissection proceeds with division of the right hepatic duct, the right hepatic artery, and the right portal vein. Dissection proceeds along the anterior surface of the left hepatic duct towards the falciform ligament. This dissection is carried out within Glisson's sheath, which surrounds the portal structures as they enter the liver and bifurcate within it. The overlying hepatic parenchyma may need to be divided to facilitate this exposure. Branches of the portal structures come off the main trunks superiorly to enter segment IV. Branches to the caudate lobe come off posteriorly. These superior and posterior branches are ligated and divided from the main trunks up to the falciform ligament and the umbilical fissure. The left hepatic duct is particularly vulnerable, and it must be painstakingly preserved. No structures are divided to the left of the umbilical fissure and falciform ligament, in order to minimize the risk of damage to the left hepatic vein, which runs deep to these structures. The ligamentum teres serves as a posterior landmark that leads to the left portal vein. As these structures are divided, a zone of ischemia should develop, extending to, but not beyond, the umbilical fissure. The right hepatic vein is divided as previously described. Veins from the caudate lobe that empty directly into the IVC are divided as well. The middle hepatic vein may join the left hepatic vein within the liver before emptying into the IVC. Thus, extrahepatic ligation of the middle hepatic vein is sometimes not possible. It is secured during the parenchymal dissection. The liver parenchyma is divided to the right of the falciform ligament and umbilical fissure. This division proceeds superiorly towards the IVC. During the upper part of this dissection, the middle hepatic vein is exposed. At this point, it is divided and suture ligated. The parenchymal dissection is completed and the specimen is removed. Because of its small size, the remaining liver (segments II and III) may be more prone to torsion than would a larger section of liver. This may be especially true if this section of liver is supplied by an aberrant left hepatic artery off the left gastric artery. The falciform ligament and the ligamentum teres may be tacked to the diaphragm and retroperitoneum to maintain the liver in a neutral position.

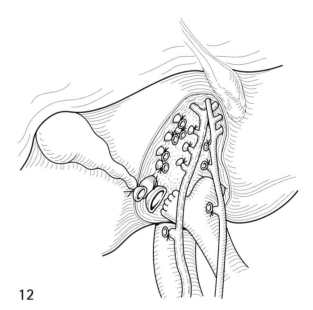

12

Left hepatectomy

13 Initial dissection proceeds in a similar fashion to the right hepatectomy. Again, we underscore the use of IOUS to aid in guidance of resection and using to create an accurate three-dimensional reconstruction of the relationships between the tumor, the hepatic veins, and the branches of the portal vein and hepatic arteries. Portal vein branches are used as landmarks in the definition of the resection line; localization of the portal vein branches is fundamental for planning the surgical strategy. Cholecystectomy does not necessarily need to be performed, but it is customarily done. The portal dissection proceeds, and the left hepatic duct, the left hepatic artery, and the left portal vein are divided near their bifurcations. If the caudate lobe is to be preserved, the left portal structures are divided distal to the posterior branches to the caudate lobe. Division of the vascular inflow to the left lobe should produce a zone of ischemia to the left of the interlobar fissure. The gastrohepatic omentum is explored, and aberrant left hepatic artery is ligated if present. The remainder of the gastrohepatic ligament is divided to permit full mobilization of the left lobe. With the liver rotated anteriorly and to the patient's right side, dissection along the ligamentum venosum will lead to the left hepatic vein. The left hepatic vein is explored. If the left hepatic vein passes outside the liver before it becomes confluent with the middle hepatic vein, it can be divided and suture ligated prior to the parenchymal dissection. If the two veins join within the liver, the extrahepatic confluence can be encircled with a vascular tape by passing a right-angle to the right of the termination of the ligamentum venosum, at the top of the caudate lobe. This can be used to occlude the hepatic veins if significant hepatic venous bleeding is encountered during parenchymal dissection.

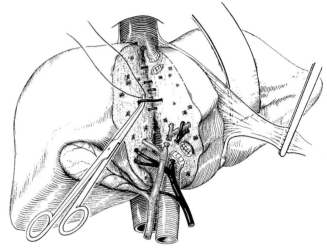

13

Division of the hepatic parenchyma proceeds just to the left of the interlobar fissure. The middle hepatic vein is preserved, and tributaries from segment IV are suture ligated as they are encountered. As the parenchyma is divided superiorly, the left hepatic vein is identified before its confluence with the middle hepatic vein. The left hepatic vein is suture ligated and the middle hepatic vein is preserved. The parenchymal dissection is then completed and the specimen is removed.

Non-anatomic liver resections

Wedge resections are generally performed for small, peripheral, or incidentally discovered liver tumors. They are usually done for diagnostic purposes. However, in certain circumstances, a wedge resection with an appropriate margin (generally 1 cm) may be used as a therapeutic operation. Large wedge resections and central wedge resections are discouraged, as bleeding may be excessive and difficult to control deep in the apex of the parenchymal defect. Inadvertent division of large intrahepatic vessels may unnecessarily jeopardize segments of the liver distant to the site of resection.

14 Because wedge resections are generally performed for smaller tumors, the liver is typically not mobilized extensively. The surgeon should not hesitate to enlarge an existing incision or divide ligaments of the liver if doing so would facilitate safe control of the liver during the resection. Dissections of the IVC and hilum of the liver are not performed in order to obtain segmental vascular control. In the case of a modest sized tumor (2–5 cm), the porta hepatis may be dissected in the hepatoduodenal ligament in order to perform a Pringle maneuver, if needed. The peripheral liver tumor is grasped and gently retracted. The liver capsule is divided in the path of intended resection using the scalpel or electocautery. The liver is manually compressed proximal to the margin of resection. Small lesions near the edge of the liver are sharply excised with a clamp or scalpel. The use of electocautery for excision of small lesions is discouraged, as thermal artifact may adversely affect subsequent histology. Vessels and ducts larger than 5 mm are still ligated in continuity and divided. The cut surface of the liver is coagulated with the electrocautery or argon beam coagulator. The current on the cautery can be increased to create an electrical arc to the liver surface. This facilitates coagulation of the surface without the cautery tip adhering to the coagulum from direct contact. Besides techniques applied during resection, several topical agents have been developed to improve hemostasis of the resection surface. Topical hemostatic agents can be divided into two groups. The first group consists of agents that only provide a matrix for endogenous coagulation; available matrices include those made of collagen (Tissufleece®, Novacol®, Lyostipt®, Antema®, Avitene®, Duracol®), cellulose (Gelfoam®, Spongostan®, Gelita®), or gelatin (Nu-knit®, Surgicell®). These agents do not contain active components. The second group consists of agents that do contain active components, the fibrin sealants (Tisseel® or Tissucol®, Quixil® or Crosseal®, Vivostat®, Beriplast®, Biocol®, Bolheal®, Hemaseel®) or carrier-bound fibrin sealants (FloSeal®, Tachosil®, Costasis®). These agents mimic endogenous coagulation.

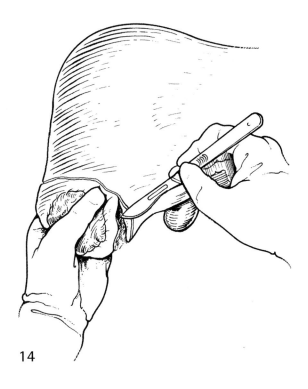

14

Wound closure

For most resections, a closed suction drain is brought through a stab incision below the subcostal incision. The drain is placed adjacent to the cut surface of the liver. The purpose of this drain is to identify and potentially control a delayed bile leak. The field is irrigated with warm saline. The abdominal wall is closed in two layers with running, absorbable, monofilament sutures. The skin is closed with a running, subcuticular, absorbable, monofilament suture.

POSTOPERATIVE CARE

Following major liver resection, patients are admitted to the pediatric intensive care unit (ICU) for continuous hemodynamic monitoring. Intraoperative resuscitation is continued in the ICU to target a temperature >36.5°C, urine output of 0.5–1 mL/kg per hour, hematocrit >22 percent, platelets >100 000/mL, and international normalization ratio (INR) <1.5. Over-resuscitation is avoided, and a CVP <8 mmHg is preferred, provided other indicators of perfusion are appropriate. The closed suction drain is monitored for volume and quality of output. The drain is kept in place to monitor for bile leak until the patient is tolerating a regular diet. The nasogastric tube is continued until abdominal distension resolves and appetite returns, at which time a clear liquid diet is started. Perioperative antibiotics are continued for 24 hours following the operation. In the absence of coagulopathy, an epidural catheter is the preferred means of postoperative analgesia. It is continued until the patient is able to tolerate oral analgesics. The patient's urinary catheter is removed once the epidural is turned off.

Complications

Hemorrhage is the most potentially catastrophic postoperative complication. It should be suspected in a patient with poor perfusion, labile hemodynamics, inappropriate response to transfusion, or failure to improve with resuscitation in the ICU. The closed suction drain is not a reliable indicator of intra-abdominal hemorrhage. Significant bleeding can occur even when small volumes of serosanguinous fluid are noted in the drain. The surgeon should maintain a low threshold for operative re-exploration and accept the possibility of a negative exploration rather than delay the operative control of significant bleeding. Metabolic derangements are unusual following liver resection in children with normal preoperative liver function. Hypoglycemia may occur for the first few days following a large liver resection, and this can be avoided or treated with 10 percent dextrose until hepatic glucose metabolism returns to normal. Patients with an elevated prothrombin time postoperatively may benefit from the administration of exogenous vitamin K. Hepatic function may be transiently impaired and patients may have delayed clearance of medications, such as analgesics and sedatives, which are metabolized by the liver. Hepatic function tests are abnormal in the early postoperative period and may not return to normal until several weeks following operation. Hepatic regeneration is remarkably fast and most patients will have a normal liver volume within three months of liver resection. Fever in the postoperative period can have a number of causes. Necrotic liver at the margin of the resection can cause fever. As long as the necrosis is not extensive or infected, the symptoms are self-limiting. An undrained bile leak can cause fever, whether or not it is infected. Once drained, most small bile leaks stop over time without any further intervention. Prolonged or recurrent fever approximately 1 week after resection should raise the suspicion of a subphrenic abscess. Once identified, most subphrenic abscesses can be drained percutaneously, with ultrasound or CT guidance.

OUTCOME

Hepatic resections are complex operations that require vigilant care both inside and outside the operating room. With advances in anesthesia, intraoperative/postoperative support, and surgical instruments, mortality from major liver resection is 5 percent or less in contemporary series. In patients with favorable risk factors, this mortality should be less than 3 percent. Overall outcome is related to the patient's underlying diagnosis. Successful liver resection is generally curative for benign disease, while resection remains the cornerstone of therapy for primary hepatic malignancies. Treatment results for affected children with HB have been markedly improved over the last decades due to evolution of therapy from surgery alone to a multimodal approach combining neoadjuvant chemotherapy regimens and surgery. The relapse-free survival rates for all HB increased from 25–40 percent 25 years ago to 75 percent currently. Low-stage tumors even achieve a long-term survival probability of over 90 percent. Liver transplantation is a useful adjunct in otherwise unresectable tumors. In contrast, HCC is relatively chemoresistant and therefore carries a poor prognosis with a dismal 15 percent cure rate. As HCC is more prone to metastasis and multifocality than HB and typically occurs on a background of underlying liver disease, complete surgical resection or transplantation of localized disease is often the only hope. Clearly, much work remains to be done to improve patient outcome with this disease.

FURTHER READING

Bismuth H, Castaing D. Peroperative echography in hepatobiliary surgery. *Annales of Gastroenterologie et Hepatologie (Paris)* 1984; **20**: 221–3.

Bismuth H, Houssin D, Castaing D. Major and minor segmentectomies 'réglées' in liver surgery. *World Journal of Surgery* 1982; **6**: 10–24.

Couinaud C. Lobes des segments hépatiques: notes sur architecture anatomique et chirurgicale du foie. *Presse Medicale* 1954; **62**: 709–12.

Gupta AA, Gerstle JT, Ng V *et al*. Critical review of controversial issues in the management of advanced pediatric liver tumors. *Pediatric Blood and Cancer* 2011; **56**: 1013–18.

Lehmann K, Clavien PA. History of hepatic surgery. *Surgical Clinics of North America* 2010; **90**: 655–64.

Malek MM, Shah SR, Atri P *et al*. Review of outcomes of primary liver cancers in children: our institutional experience with resection and transplantation. *Surgery* 2010; **148**: 778–82.

Meyers RL, Rowland JR, Krailo M *et al*. Predictive power of pretreatment prognostic factors in children with hepatoblastoma: a report from the Children's Oncology Group. *Pediatric Blood and Cancer* 2009; **53**: 1016–22.

Meyers RL. Tumors of the liver in children. *Surgical Oncology* 2007; **16**: 195–203.

Otte JB. Progress in the surgical treatment of malignant liver tumors in children. *Cancer Treatment Reviews* 2010; **36**: 360–71.

Tung TT, Quang NG. A new technique for operating on the liver. *Lancet* 1963; **1**: 192.

74

Wilms' tumor

PEDRO-JOSE LOPEZ and PETER CUCKOW

INTRODUCTION

In 1899, Max Wilms described a group of children with kidney tumors and since that time his name has been applied to nephroblastoma. The first nephrectomy for this malignancy was reported by Jessop in 1877 and the first radiation treatment given in 1915. In 1956, Farber introduced the chemotherapeutic agent actinomycin and the modern treatment protocols began.

Wilms' is the most common solid abdominal tumor of childhood and in 90 percent of cases presents as a painless mass in a well child. The annual incidence in children under 15 years of age is 7–10 cases per million, being 6–7 percent of all childhood cancers. Eighty percent of cases are diagnosed before five years of age and 6 percent present with bilateral disease. With modern treatment protocols, combining chemotherapy, surgery, and selective use of radiotherapy, 85 percent of children can expect long-term survival. Management is by a multidisciplinary team of surgeons, oncologists, radiologists, pathologists, pediatricians, and specialist nurses.

PRINCIPLES AND JUSTIFICATION

Indications for surgery

In continental Europe and the UK, all tumors are treated with vincristine and actinomycin before surgery. In the UK, all tumors are biopsied before chemotherapeutic treatment; this does not occur in the rest of Europe. In the United States, radical nephrectomy is still the primary treatment for unilateral operable Wilms' tumor. Secondary deposits, caval tumor, bilateral disease, or tumor in a solitary kidney are indications for Trucut biopsy, chemotherapy, and delayed partial or total nephrectomy.

PREOPERATIVE

Blood

- Full blood picture: to monitor the effects of chemotherapy.
- Coagulation studies: to detect the bleeding disorder von Willebrand's disease – a typical abnormality in Wilms' tumor.
- Liver function tests: performed to monitor the effects of chemotherapy.
- Overall kidney function: measured by serum creatinine.
- Tumor markers alpha-fetoprotein and beta-human chorionic gonadotropin (HCG), not raised in Wilms' but associated with hepatoblastoma and embryonal tumors that are part of the differential diagnosis.

Urine

A sample is monitored to measure vanylmandelic acid (VMA), which is raised in the presence of neuroblastoma – another important differential of Wilm's tumor.

Radiology

Ultrasound is usually the first imaging modality to be used and will demonstrate a solid tumor arising from the kidney and also involvement of the renal vein or vena cava with the help of Doppler studies. It can also identify liver or abdominal secondaries and survey the contralateral kidney, where smaller deposits may denote bilateral Wilms'. Chest radiography (anterior and lateral) is still used in European trials to identify pulmonary metastatic disease, but computed tomography (CT) scanning is more sensitive and provides more complete information about the lungs, both kidneys, the vasculature, and other abdominal involvement. Although in the past exploration of the contralateral kidney was a mandatory part of all Wilms' surgery, CT has eliminated the need for it. However, one limitation of imaging is the ability to determine resectability; it is a surgeon's role to determinate inoperability at surgical exploration.

OPERATION

Biopsy of the tumor

1 With the patient in the lateral oblique position, Trucut biopsy is usually performed with ultrasound guidance. Problems arise if the tumor is very cystic and bleeding occurs occasionally, although tumor seeding into the biopsy track is rare. Minimally invasive laparoscopy has the potential of a more active role, particularly is assessing and biopsying intra-abdominal tumor spread.

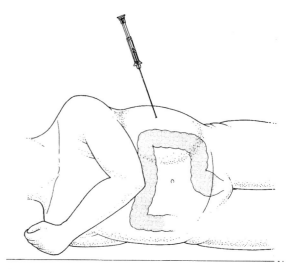

1

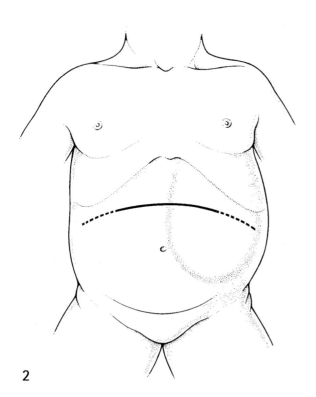

2

2 A generous transverse upper abdominal incision on the side of the tumor, extending across the contralateral rectus muscle, allows complete exposure of the kidney and access to its pedicle in particular. A longitudinal incision extending from the xiphoid to below the umbilicus may be more suitable in older patients.

The rectus sheath is incised with diathermy. Both rectus muscles are completely divided. The falciform ligament is divided between ligatures. The peritoneum is entered, with care to avoid breaching the anterior surface of the tumor or damaging the liver, and the incision extended laterally under direct vision.

3 The abdominal contents are carefully examined for liver and peritoneal secondaries.

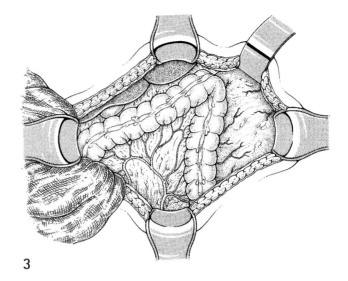

3

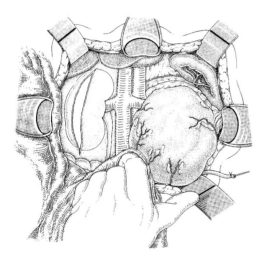

4

4 The contralateral kidney may be mobilized and examined in both anterior and posterior surfaces to detect possible bilateral disease. If a CT scan had been performed, the visual and manual inspection of the contralateral kidney is at the discretion of the surgeon. If unsuspected bilateral disease is detected, the main tumor and contralateral lesion are biopsied with no further excisional surgery. The patient is subjected to chemotherapy with subsequent nephron-sparing surgery.

5 The colon with its mesentery is dissected carefully from the anterior surface of the tumor after first dividing the lateral peritoneal attachment.

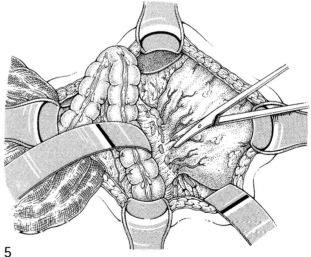

5

6 The ureter and gonadal vessels are ligated well below the kidney and may now be transected. The renal vessels cross in front of the ureter and renal pelvis, so this is used as a guide to find them as dissection continues cranially. If possible, the tumor is not mobilized at this stage, although large tumors which cross the midline can distort the anatomy. Lateral mobilization of the kidney can create more medial space in these cases and may require a further lateral extension of the incision.

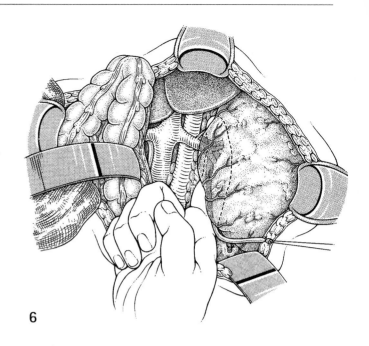

6

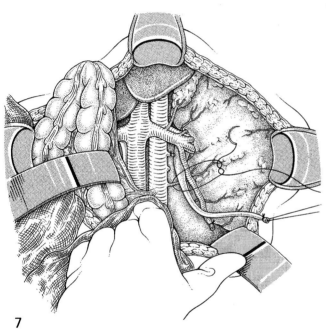

7

7 Dissection begins caudally, sweeping adventitial tissue and lymph nodes laterally off the great vessels, if necessary dividing it between ligatures. The renal vein and its branches are gently exposed. Careful palpation of the vein may detect venous extension of the tumor, although this should have been noted on preoperative investigations. Early mobilization of the inferior vena cava and renal vein may be required to prevent embolization of the tumor into the inferior vena cava, heart, and pulmonary artery. On the right side, the second part of the duodenum is encountered during this dissection and is reflected medially off the vessels.

8 The renal vein is gently mobilized and elevated with a vascular sling to expose the renal artery, which is typically situated behind the upper border of the renal vein. It is preferable to ligate and divide the renal artery first so as to prevent swelling of the kidney with arterial blood. Due to the size of the tumor, this sequence of ligation is not always possible.

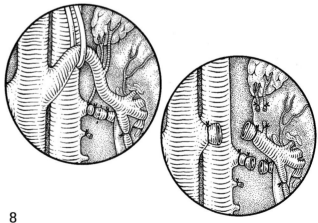

8

9 The posterior aspect of the kidney is partially mobilized by blunt dissection.

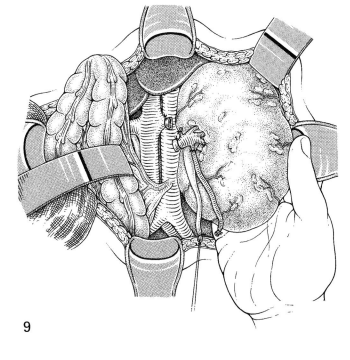

9

10 The superior dissection is hazardous on the left side, and damage to the spleen and tail of the pancreas must be avoided. On the right side, the tumor may be stuck to the undersurface of the liver, but rarely infiltrates it. Care is taken in separating them to avoid breaching the liver capsule. The adrenal gland is removed only if the tumor is in the upper pole of the kidney. In this circumstance, the adrenal vessels should be carefully controlled with ligatures.

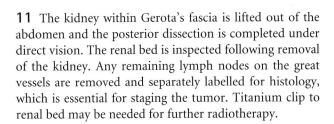

10

11 The kidney within Gerota's fascia is lifted out of the abdomen and the posterior dissection is completed under direct vision. The renal bed is inspected following removal of the kidney. Any remaining lymph nodes on the great vessels are removed and separately labelled for histology, which is essential for staging the tumor. Titanium clip to renal bed may be needed for further radiotherapy.

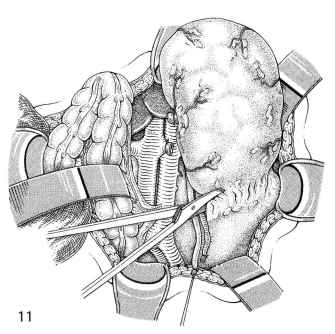

11

12 If the tumor is small and confined to the kidney, laparoscopy offers an alternative to open surgical removal. Three to four ports are used and the tumor is removed intact through a Pfannenstiel incision. Currently, less than 5 percent of patients with unilateral Wilms' tumor would be candidates for partial nephrectomy.

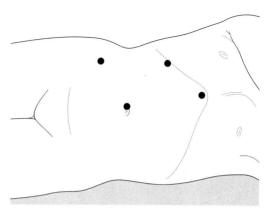

12

PRE- AND POSTOPERATIVE CHEMOTHERAPY

Unilateral disease

Vincristine and actinomycin are administered for 4 weeks and surgery is performed on week 5–6. The type and duration of postoperative chemotherapy is related to the surgical stage and histologic type of tumor. In a completely excised tumor that is confined to the kidney with a low-risk histology, no further treatment may be necessary. Combination treatment with actinomycin and vincristine is usual however, with the option to add doxorubicin with or without abdominal radiotherapy for higher grade tumors.

Metastatic disease

Pulmonary metastases documented on x-ray or CT of the chest preoperatively mandate pretreatment with vincristine, actinomycin, and doxorubicin. This will be followed by the same triple chemotherapy after surgery, with or without radiotherapy, if there has been a poor response.

Bilateral disease

Biopsy is performed and then combination chemotherapy is started. Subsequent surgical management may include a total or partial nephrectomy, bilateral partial nephrectomy, or bilateral nephrectomy with dialysis and delayed renal transplantation. Such decisions are complex and require a team approach.

Complication rates

The most common intraoperative complication is bleeding. Intraoperative tumor spill is an important complication with a markedly decreased incidence in the SIOP patients, 2.2 percent, compared to the NWSTG patients, 15.3 percent ($p < 0.001$). The most common complication after surgery is small bowel obstruction due to intussusception of the small bowel or adhesions (>5 percent). Chylous ascites is a less common but significant complication.

CONCLUSION

The management of Wilms' tumor consists of chemotherapy combined with surgery and, less frequently, radiotherapy. Radiotherapy is mainly administered in the presence of high-risk tumors, local spillage, or secondaries in the lung that do not respond adequately to chemotherapy. The management of Wilms' tumor includes a team consisting of a surgeon, oncologist, and histopathologist.

FURTHER READING

Duarte RJ, Dénes FT, Cristofani LM, Srougi M. Laparoscopic nephrectomy for Wilms' tumor. *Expert Reviews in Anticancer Therapy* 2009; 9: 753–61.

Duffy PG, Sebire N. Genitourinary malignancies. In: Thomas D, Duffy PG, Rickwood AMK (eds). *Essentials of Paediatric Urology*. London: Martin Dunitz, 2008: 295–305.

Ko EY, Ritchet ML. Current management of Wilms' tumor in children. *Journal of Pediatric Urology* 2009; **5**: 56–65.

Ritchey ML, Coppes MJ. The management of synchronous bilateral Wilms' tumor. *Hematology/Oncology Clinics of North America* 1995; **9**: 1303–15.

Wilms M. *Die Mischgeshwueiste der Niere*. Leipzig: Arthur Georgi, 1899: 1–90.

75

Neuroblastoma

EDWARD KIELY

HISTORY

Neuroblastoma is the most common abdominal malignancy of childhood, the annual incidence being about six cases per million children. These tumors arise in primitive precursors of the sympathetic nervous system and consequently are seen in the adrenal medulla and sites of sympathetic ganglia. Almost one-third are detected in the first 12 months of life and a further 50 percent between the ages of one and four years. Only 5 percent occur in children over the age of ten years.

The majority of tumors are locally extensive or metastatic at the time of diagnosis. The first successful excision of a neuroblastoma was reported over 90 years ago by Dr Willard Bartlett of St Louis, MO, USA but, until recently, surgery has been helpful only in the management of those with localized disease. With the advent of more effective chemotherapy, primary tumors have been rendered smaller, more fibrotic, and more amenable to resection. Consequently, macroscopic clearance of disease is now a realistic expectation.

PRINCIPLES AND JUSTIFICATION

Clinical presentation

Less than 3 percent of such tumors are detected on antenatal ultrasound. Post-natally, the majority present with non-specific symptoms, such as malaise, anorexia, weight loss, fever, and sweating. Bone and joint pain as a result of skeletal involvement may lead to an erroneous diagnosis of juvenile arthritis. Periorbital ecchymosis and proptosis may occur as a consequence of secondary disease in the skull. Less common presentations include massive hepatomegaly in stage 4S disease, or paraplegia as a consequence of spinal cord compression.

The diagnosis is usually suspected on clinical grounds alone. It is confirmed by the finding of elevated levels of catecholamine metabolites in the urine together with histologic examination of tumor biopsy specimens.

Cross-sectional imaging together with bone scanning and examination of bone marrow aspirates or trephines complete the initial work up.

Ultrasound examination is almost always performed and is of limited use. Computed tomography (CT) or magnetic resonance imaging (MRI) is essential.

The typical appearance of an abdominal neuroblastoma on CT scan is of an irregular mass arising in the suprarenal or para-aortic region which enhances after the administration of intravenous contrast medium. Cross-sectional imaging will also help to evaluate the extent of vascular encasement, and serial scanning after therapy will document the response to treatment.

1a,b A representative scan is shown in illustration 1a – a 4-year-old boy with Stage 4 neuroblastoma. The extent of vascular displacement and envelopement by the tumor is readily apparent, with the aorta lifted off the vertebral bodies. In addition, there is bilateral hydronephrosis.

A further scan of the same child after chemotherapy shows the extent of tumor regression and resolution of hydronephrosis (illustration 1b).

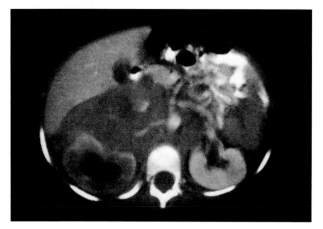

1a

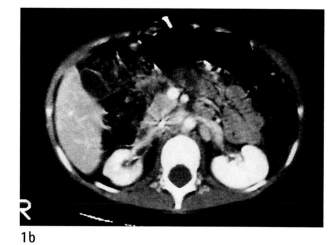

1b

2a,b Radionuclide scanning is also considered essential in the evaluation of distal disease. Skeletal imaging with 99mTc methylene diphosphonate is more accurate than conventional radiology in demonstrating skeletal metastases. More recently, MIBG scanning (131meta-iodobenzylguanidine) is used for the same purpose. Representative scans from the same child as shown on the CT images are demonstrated in illustrations a and b. Limb and skull involvement is clearly seen on both images.

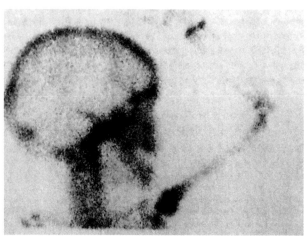

2a

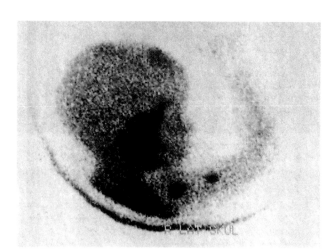

2b

Staging

Staging systems are used to document disease extent and to stratify treatment accordingly. The most common such system in use is the International Neuroblastoma Staging System (INSS) (**Table 75.1**). About 25 percent of patients have stage 1 or 2 disease, 60–70 percent have stage 3 or 4 disease, and about 10 percent present with stage 4S disease.

At the present time, the biological profile of the tumor is not included in the staging system.

Table 75.1 International Neuroblastoma Staging System criteria.

1	Localized tumor with complete gross excision, with or without microscopic residual disease; representative ipsilateral lymph nodes negative for tumor microscopically (nodes attached to and removed with the primary tumor may be positive)
2A	Localized tumor with incomplete gross excision; representative ipsilateral non-adherent lymph nodes negative for tumor microscopically
2B	Localized tumor with or without complete gross excision, with ipsilateral non-adherent lymph nodes positive for tumor; enlarged contralateral lymph nodes must be negative microscopically
3	Unresectable unilateral tumor infiltrating across the midline,[a] with or without regional lymph node involvement or Localized unilateral tumor with contralateral regional lymph node involvement or Midline tumor with bilateral extension by infiltration (unresectable) or by lymph node involvement
4	Any primary tumor with dissemination to distant lymph nodes, bone, bone marrow, liver, skin, or other organs (except as defined for stage 4S)
4S	Localized primary tumor (as defined for stage 1, 2A, or 2B), with dissemination limited to skin, liver, bone and marrow[b] (limited to infants younger than one year)

[a]The midline is defined as the vertebral column. Tumors originating on one side and crossing the midline must infiltrate to or beyond the opposite side of the vertebral column.

[b]Marrow involvement in stage 4S should be minimal (i.e. <10% of total nucleated cells identified as malignant on bone marrow biopsy or on marrow aspirate). More extensive marrow involvement would be considered to be stage 4. The meta-iodobenzylguanidine scan (if performed) should be negative in the marrow.

Pathology

The typical untreated tumor is rounded or lobulated and of varying consistency. More aggressive tumors are frequently friable and hemorrhagic.

After chemotherapy, tumors are substantially harder and less vascular. Calcification is generally present at the time of diagnosis and may be quite dense after chemotherapy.

Microscopic examination shows sheets of undifferentiated, small, blue nuclei. More differentiated tumors show varying numbers of ganglion cells.

TREATMENT

Surgery is the optimal treatment for those with stage 1 and 2 disease.

Patients with stage 3 and 4 disease are generally managed by initial chemotherapy followed by attempted surgical excision when metastases have been ablated.

Further therapy with bone marrow ablation and bone marrow transplant is used for those with high-risk disease, depending on local chemotherapy protocols.

Treatment protocols continue to evolve and are increasingly directed by adverse biological features.

Surgical management

Early surgery is appropriate for localized tumors where resection can be undertaken safely. For those with locally advanced or disseminated disease, the initial use of chemotherapy followed by surgery allows for a more complete resection.

The operation described here was developed to deal with the problem of vascular encasement. It also allows a planned and systematic approach to tumor excision and minimizes the risk of vascular accidents while achieving complete tumor clearance.

As neuroblastomas rarely invade the tunica media of major blood vessels, the dissection may be performed in the subadventitial plane with a scalpel. The success of the procedure depends entirely on the attitude and persistence of the surgeon.

The operation consists of three phases: vessel display, vessel clearance, and tumor removal. Vessel display is taken to mean the display of part of the circumference of each blood vessel that traverses the tumor, in continuity.

If this can be accomplished, these vessels can generally be cleared of tumor. Once the vessels are free, the tumor can be removed piecemeal.

The order in which the vessels are displayed and cleared depends on the site and size of the tumor together with the surgeon's preference.

Anesthesia

Full intubated general anesthesia is employed with intravascular pressure monitoring. Epidural anesthesia is often considered to reduce operative blood loss and provides very effective pain relief in the postoperative period.

Operation

3 The following refers to stage 1 tumors which are rare, but when encountered are amenable to simple complete excision. The abdomen is opened through a transverse supraumbilical incision. For right-sided tumors, the ascending colon and duodenum are reflected medially. The inferior vena cava below the limit of the tumor is exposed by incision of the tunica adventitia longitudinally along the middle of the vessel. The dissection advances proximally, exposing the anterior wall in the 12 o'clock position. If tumor is encountered anterior to the vena cava, it is incised down to the tunica media. This dissection is advanced proximally until the liver is reached.

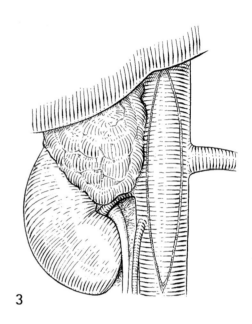

3

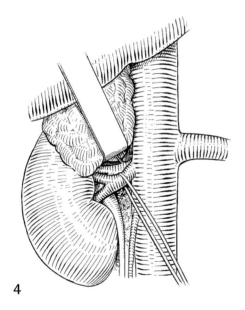

4

4 Subsequently, the right renal vein is displayed in similar fashion. The cava is then cleared of tumor and elevated to expose the right renal artery.

5 Once the right renal artery and vein are displayed, the cava above the renal vein may be cleared of tumor until the right adrenal vein is reached. It is as well to suture ligate this vein before the tumor is removed.

The more common situation is where an extensive residual tumor remains following intensive chemotherapy.

A key feature of the operation involves the systematic dissection of major vessels which abut or traverse the tumor. Dissection is commenced below the tumor where the vessel emerges – usually an iliac vein on the right or iliac artery on the left side. Optical magnification for surgeon and assistant is mandatory.

All tissue is divided under tension produced by the assistant and the surgeon picking up tunica adventitia and retracting laterally. The knife then divides the tissue down to the tunica media in a perpendicular direction. The dissection commences where the vessel is normal and not surrounded by tumor. The dissection then continues proximally dividing tumor and adventitia and keeping the vessel wall in view all the time. The technique remains the same – division of tissue under tension in lengths or 1–2 cm at a time. The dissection moves from what is visible to what is not visible.

Hemostasis is achieved using bipolar diathermy. In general, the tissue is divided first – initial coagulation may obliterate tissue planes and make the procedure more difficult.

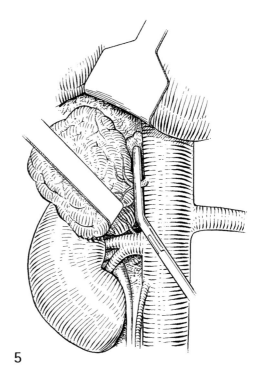

5

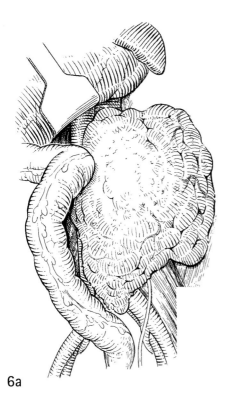

6a

6a For extensive retroperitoneal and left-sided tumors, the descending and sigmoid colon are mobilized, together with the spleen, pancreas, and stomach, and placed in an intestinal bag. The dissection commences just distal to the tumor edge along the middle of whichever artery is present.

6b The dissection commences at the left common iliac artery of the tumor exposing the subadventitial layer of the left common iliac artery in this case. The dissection then advances proximally, dividing the tumor and adventitia down to the tunica media of the vessel.

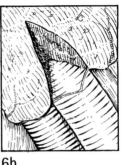

6b

7 The dissection continues proximally until the aorta is reached and then progresses upwards along this vessel. The inferior mesenteric artery is soon encountered and the division of the tumor and adventitia continued until the left renal vein is reached. Once the renal vein is encountered, a segment of 4–5 cms of the vein is cleared so that it can be retracted. Cautious dissection will bring the origin of the left renal vein into view. The plane of dissection then changes from the 12 o'clock position to the 2 o'clock position to avoid the superior mesenteric and celiac arteries. The operation proceeds until the superior limit of the tumor is reached and this may entail division of the median arcuate ligament to enter the posterior mediastinum.

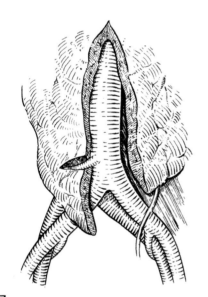

7

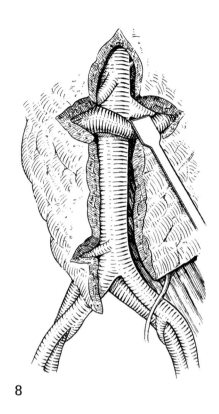

8 Each of the encased visceral arteries is dissected in turn – left renal, superior mesenteric, and celiac. The dissection advances distally on these vessels as far as is necessary. It is not unusual to have to dissect left gastric, hepatic, and splenic arteries for some distance.

8

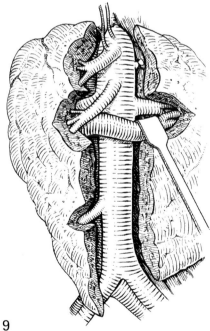

9

9 Once these vessels are safe and in view, they may be cleared circumferentially of tumor prior to removal of the residual tumor.

10 This illustration shows the final appearance of the operative field showing the inferior vena cava and aorta and associated branches completely cleared of tumor.

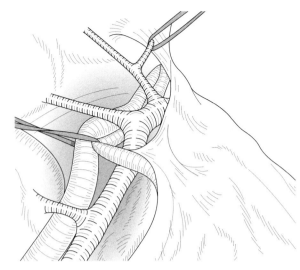

10

POSTOPERATIVE CARE

Postoperative care follows the same principles as for any other major laparotomies. Intravascular monitoring is continued for 24–48 hours. Urine output is carefully measured, and intravascular volume adjusted accordingly.

Blood sugar levels are checked 4-hourly initially and subsequently less frequently.

Effective pain relief is delivered in the form of either epidural infusion or intravenous opiate infusion. Enteral feeding usually resumes after about 3 days. Diarrhea is not uncommon when celiac and superior mesenteric arteries have been cleared of tumor.

OUTCOME

The surgical morbidity after this operation is similar to that encountered after other major procedures. Wound dehiscence or incisional hernia occurs in less than 1 percent of cases.

Chylous ascites is not unusual in the days following operation, but generally settles without the need for specific treatment. Five of the author's patients have required a peritoneovenous shunt for resistant ascites, having failed to respond to other measures.

The operative mortality is 1 percent. The effects of age, tumor stage, and changes in chemotherapy protocols confuse attempts to analyze the influence of surgery on the long-term prognosis.

Of 255 patients operated on by the author, six had stage 1 disease and 42 had stage 2 disease. All those with stage 1 disease survived, and for those with stage 2 disease, the survival was in excess of 95 percent.

For those with stage 3 disease, complete resection resulted in over 80 percent survival, as opposed to 40 percent with incomplete resection. Of those with stage 4 disease, roughly one-third survived regardless of the extent of resection.

For many years, it has not been clear whether or not surgical excision contributes to survival in those with metastatic disease, who constitute the majority of children with neuroblastoma. However, as there has been no prospective evaluation of the role of surgery, it cannot be assumed that those who undergo successful surgery necessarily have the same type of disease as those in whom resection was unsuccessful. More recent results suggest a trend toward improved survival where surgery has been complete.

FURTHER READING

Ambros PF, Ambros IM, Brodeur GM *et al.* International consensus for neuroblastoma molecular diagnostics: report from the International Neuroblastoma Risk Group (INRG) Biology Committee. *British Journal of Cancer* 2009; **100**: 1471–82.

Kiely EM. The surgical challenge of neuroblastoma. *Journal of Pediatric Surgery* 1994; **29**: 128–33.

Kiely EM. A technique for excision of abdominal and pelvic neuroblastomas. *Annals of the Royal College of Surgeons of England* 2007; **89**: 342–8.

La Quaglia MP, Kushner BH, Su W *et al.* The impact of gross total resection on local control and survival in high-risk neuroblastoma. *Journal of Pediatric Surgery* 2004; **39**: 412–17.

Tsuchida Y, Honna T, Kamii Y *et al.* Radical excision of primary tumor and lymph nodes in advanced neuroblastoma: combination with induction chemotherapy. *Pediatric Surgery International* 1991; **6**: 22–7.

76

Rhabdomyosarcoma

PHILLIP A LETOURNEAU and RICHARD J ANDRASSY

BACKGROUND

Rhabdomyosarcoma is a primary malignancy in children and adolescents that arises from embryonic mesenchyme with the potential to differentiate into skeletal muscle. Tumors may arise in any location, with prognosis affected by site, histology, local control, and metastatic speed.

Current management favors less radical surgical intervention together with the neoadjuvant chemotherapy with or without radiation. Since rhabdomyosarcoma is chemosensitive, some tumor locations (i.e. head and neck) require biopsy only, followed by chemotherapy. In other locations (i.e. extremities), the goal is complete tumor excision as primary therapy or following neoadjuvant chemotherapy. Pediatric surgeons play a role in diagnosis, staging, resection, and access to chemotherapy. Survival in patients with rhabdomyosarcoma continues to improve, with less radical or mutilating operations and a refinement of chemoradiation protocols.

PRINCIPLES AND JUSTIFICATION

Rhabdomyosarcoma is the most common soft-tissue sarcoma in pediatric patients and represents the third most common solid malignancy in this age group, following neuroblastoma and Wilms' tumor. Rhabdomyosarcoma accounts for 4–8 percent of all malignant disease and 5–15 percent of all solid malignancies in childhood. Approximately 70 percent of patients will be cured, but those who have metastatic or recurrent disease may suffer poor outcomes. Although rhabdomyosarcoma may occur in any anatomic site, only a few selected surgical sites are discussed in this chapter. Primary tumors in the head and neck are common and usually only require biopsy. Surgical resection of these tumors is generally reserved for persistent or recurrent cases. The clinical manifestations of rhabdomyosarcoma vary with the site of origin, the age of the patient, and the presence or absence of metastases.

Head and neck primary tumors are the most common, comprising 35–40 percent of all primary sites. The second most common primary site is genitourinary structures, which comprise 25 percent of primary tumors. These are subdivided into either bladder/prostate tumors (10 percent) or non-bladder/prostate tumors, which may include paratesticular sites, the perineum, vulva, vagina, and uterus. Other sites include the extremities, trunk, and buttocks. The goal of diagnostic evaluation for rhabdomyosarcoma is to determine the histologic variant of the tumor, its primary site, and the extent of disease (local and systemic). Evaluation may include computed tomography (CT) and/or magnetic resonance imaging (MRI) of the primary area and chest, bone marrow evaluation, and, in select sites, lymph node evaluation. Metastatic spread may occur to the lungs, bone marrow, lymph nodes, and skeleton. It is critical during diagnosis to obtain an adequate amount of tissue for histologic and cytologic diagnosis and classification. Percutaneous needle or core biopsies have been selectively utilized, but do not generally provide enough tissue for complete evaluation.

Preoperative staging

Staging for rhabdomyosarcoma is performed in order to determine the specific intensity of treatment and to compare outcomes. Staging evaluates the primary site, tumor invasiveness, tumor size, lymph node status and metastases. Pretreatment size is determined from measurement on MRI or CT, depending on the anatomic location. CT may evaluate nodal status, but this carries a high risk of false negativity.

Survival rates are significantly affected by primary tumor sites. Tumors located in the orbit, vagina, vulva, or near the testicles have a favorable prognosis. Primary sites in the extremities, bladder, prostate, uterus, and non-parameningeal head and neck locations have an intermediate prognosis. Relatively poor prognosis is associated with primary tumors located in the parameningeal region, head and neck sites, the retroperitoneum, the buttocks, the trunk, and the perineal and perianal locations, as well as in patients with metastatic disease. Primary tumor site is, therefore, considered in pretreatment staging (**Table 76.1**). Chemotherapeutic regimens have been directed at all risk classifications, including low, intermediate, and high-risk groups.

Biology and pathology

Rhabdomyosarcoma cells arise from undifferentiated mesodermal tissue and may appear anywhere in the body, including areas that do not usually contain striated muscle. Histologically, rhabdomyosarcoma is classified within the category of small, round, blue cell tumors of childhood. This category also includes neuroblastoma, Ewing's sarcoma, small-cell osteogenic sarcoma, and non-Hodgkin's lymphoma. Horn and Enterline classified rhabdomyosarcoma into four different pathologic types: embryonal, botryoid, alveolar, and pleomorphic. Today, the histologic variance of childhood rhabdomyosarcoma is grouped by a modification of the Horn and Enterline system which includes favorable-prognosis, intermediate-prognosis, and poor-prognosis groups. Favorable-prognosis tumors include botryoid and spindle-cell variants. Botryoid tumors are best described as appearing as 'clusters of grapes' in gross appearance. This variant appears primarily in young children and in visceral cavities, such as the nasopharynx, vagina, and biliary tree, and has the best prognosis of all types of rhabdomyosarcoma. Spindle-cell rhabdomyosarcoma is commonly found in paratesticular sites and also has a favorable outcome. Embryonal tumors have an intermediate prognosis and are composed of small, round, or spindle-shaped cells with variable cellularity and myogenous differentiation. Embryonal histology is the predominant type seen in infants and young children. Botryoid and spindle-cell variants are considered subvariants of embryonal rhabdomyosarcoma, but are now classified in the favorable-prognosis category.

Unfavorable-prognosis tumors include alveolar and undifferentiated rhabdomyosarcomas. Alveolar variants are characterized by prominent alveolar arrangement of stroma and dense, small, round tumor cells resembling lung tissue. Alveolar tumors frequently arise from the extremities, trunk, or perineum; they account for roughly 20 percent of rhabdomyosarcomas diagnosed in children. Undifferentiated sarcoma is a poorly defined category of sarcomatous tumors whose cells show no evidence of myogenesis or other differentiation. This sarcoma variant occurs most commonly in the extremities or head and neck, and has a very poor prognosis. Pleomorphic sarcoma is categorized by large pleomorphic cells with multinucleated giant cells, and is often seen in the extremities or trunk; it is rare in the pediatric population.

Table 76.1 Tumor node metastasis (TNM) pretreatment staging classification.

Stage	Sites	T	Size	N	M
1	Orbit	T_1 or T_2	a or b	N_0 or N_1 or Nx	M_0
	Head and neck (excluding parameningeal)				
	Genitourinary (non-bladder/non-prostate)				
2	Bladder/prostate	T_1 or T_2	a	N_0 or N_x	M_0
	Extremity				
	Cranial				
	Parameningeal				
	Other (includes trunk, retroperitoneum, etc.)				
3	Bladder/prostate	T_1 or T_2	a	N_1	M_0
	Extremity		b	N_0 or N_1 or N_x	
	Cranial				
	Parameningeal				
	Other (includes trunk, retroperitoneum, etc.)				
4	Any	T_1 or T_2	a or b	N_0 or N_1	M_1

Definitions

Tumor	T (site)$_1$, confined to anatomic site of origin; (a) ≤5 cm in diameter, (b) >5 cm in diameter
	T (site)$_2$, extends and/or fixed to surrounding tissue; (a) ≤5 cm in diameter, (b) >5 cm in diameter
Regional nodes	N0: nodes not clinically involved
	N1: nodes clinically involved
	Nx: clinical status of nodes unknown
Metastasis	M0: no distant metastases
	M1: metastases present

A number of genetic derangements have been identified in rhabdomyosarcomas. Embryonal rhabdomyosarcomas are known to demonstrate a loss of heterozygosity on the short arm of chromosome 11. Alveolar rhabdomyosarcomas are associated with a characteristic translocation between the long arm of chromosome 2 and the long arm of chromosome 13.

Tumor-specific markers have also been identified in rhabdomyosarcoma. Antibodies to desmin, muscle-specific actin, sarcomeric actin, and myoglobin are useful in the diagnosis of rhabdomyosarcoma. Non-myogenous proteins identified in rhabdomyosarcomas include cytokeratin, neuron-specific enolase, S-100 protein, and Leu-7.

Chemotherapy

The primary chemotherapeutic regimen is a combination of vincristine, dactinomycin, and cyclophosphamide (VAC). Published studies with this regimen have demonstrated five-year failure-free survival in low-risk groups of around 90 percent, and near 70 percent in the intermediate-risk category. High-dose chemotherapy with stem cell rescue has been used with some success in patients with high-risk tumors or recurrent disease.

Anesthesia

Biopsies, resections, and operative staging are generally done under general anesthesia. If indicated, bone marrow biopsies and placement of central venous catheters are carried out during the same procedure.

OPERATIONS

Biopsy and general principles of operative resection

Surgical treatment of rhabdomyosarcoma is site specific. General principles of resection include that: (1) complete total excision of the primary tumor and surrounding uninvolved tissues should be performed while preserving cosmesis and function, where possible, and (2) incomplete excision or tumor debulking as a general primary procedure is generally not helpful and suggests a need for neoadjuvant chemotherapy. Severely mutilating or debilitating excisions should not be performed as a primary procedure. Secondary excision after initial biopsy and neoadjuvant therapy has a better outcome than partial or incomplete initial resection and should be planned when primary excision is not possible. In these cases, incisional biopsy alone is employed, with biopsy of clinically suspicious lymph nodes as indicated. Certain sites, such as the extremities and trunk, may have a high incidence of regional node positivity (40–50 percent), and sentinel lymph node mapping is helpful in these patients. Positive sentinel lymph nodes will direct regional radiotherapy.

Clinical grouping is determined by the extent of biopsy and/or resection, as well as presence of metastatic disease. Biopsy may be best performed by needle, excisional or incisional, depending on the site. Incisional biopsies are typically made in the head and neck, while excisional biopsies are typically done in paratesticular tumors. Most rhabdomyosarcomas are treated with biopsy followed by chemotherapy and operative resection with or without radiation to the primary site or regions where positive nodes were found. Locations suspected as possible metastatic sites may warrant biopsy as well. Open or thorascopic techniques may be used if the lung is involved. Solitary pulmonary nodules are usually not metastatic disease in rhabdomyosarcoma and should be biopsied to rule out an infectious process.

Principles of surgical management of rhabdomyosarcoma include wide local excision of the tumor without destroying function. The likelihood of gross or microscopic residual neoplasm remaining after resection of an undiagnosed soft-tissue tumor is so high that reoperation is considered the initial approach to management. Re-excision of residual disease has demonstrated improved disease-free survival. Primary re-excision should be considered in cases where initial margins are negative, if the procedure was not a 'cancer operation' or when malignancy was not initially suspected. Clinical grouping is shown in **Table 76.2**.

Second-look procedures have been used to evaluate therapeutic response and these procedures performed along with re-excision have been shown to improve outcome. Furthermore, if a second-look procedure demonstrates a complete response to therapy, further toxicity of continuing chemotherapy or radiation may be avoided.

Site-specific surgery

HEAD AND NECK

The head and neck are the most common sites for primary rhabdomyosarcoma in children. Operative intervention is generally limited to biopsy alone. The incidence of cervical lymph node metastases is low and routine lymph node biopsy is not required unless there are clinically suspicious nodes.

GENITOURINARY TRACT

Rhabdomyosarcoma is the most common malignancy of the pelvis seen in the pediatric population. These tumors are classified into two different categories based on their different prognoses. Bladder and prostate tumors may be difficult to differentiate from each other, which may be related to the size and location of the tumor and difficulty of resection. Bladder and prostate rhabdomyosarcomas have a poorer prognosis compared to other pelvic rhabdomyosarcomas. Paratesticular, vulvovaginal, and uterine tumors have a better prognosis because of their high sensitivity to chemotherapy.

Table 76.2 Intergroup Rhabdomyosarcoma (IRS) clinical grouping classification.

Group I	Localized disease, completely resected
	Regional nodes not involved – lymph node biopsy or dissection is required except for head and neck lesions
	(a) Confined to muscle or organ of origin
	(b) Contiguous involvement – infiltration outside the muscle or organ of origin, as through fascial planes
	Notation: This includes gross inspection and microscopic confirmation of complete resection. Any nodes that may be inadvertently taken with the specimen must be negative. If nodes are positive, the patient is moved to group IIb or IIc (see below)
Group II	Total gross resection with evidence of regional spread
	(a) Grossly resected tumor with microscopic residual disease. (Surgeon believes that he/she has removed all of the tumor, but pathologist finds tumor at margins and additional resection is not feasible.) No evidence of gross residual tumor. No evidence of regional node involvement. Once radiotherapy and/or chemotherapy have been started, re-exploration and removal of area of residual tumor does not change the patient's group
	(b) Regional disease with involved node completely resected with no microscopic residual disease. Notation: Complete resection with microscopic confirmation of no residual disease makes this different from groups IIa and IIc. In contrast to group IIa, regional nodes (which are completely resected) are involved, but the most distal node is histologically negative
	(c) Regional disease with involved nodes, grossly resected, but with evidence of microscopic residual involvement of the most distal regional node (from primary site) in the dissection. Notation: The presence of microscopic residual disease makes this group different from group IIb, and nodal involvement separates this group from IIa
Group III	Incomplete resection with gross/residual disease
	(a) After biopsy only
	(b) After gross or major resection of primary tumor (>50%)
Group IV	Distant metastatic disease present at presentation
	(Lung, liver, bones, bone marrow, brain, and distant muscle and nodes.) Notation: This excludes regional nodes and adjacent organ infiltration, which places the patient in a more favorable grouping (as noted above in group II). The presence of positive cytology in cerebrospinal fluid, pleural or abdominal fluids, as well as pleural or peritoneal implants are indications of group IV status

Paratesticular

1 A paratesticular mass should be resected by inguinal orchiectomy, with complete resection of the spermatic cord to the level of the internal ring. Biopsy of rhabdomyosarcoma through the scrotum requires subsequent resection or radiation to the biopsy site. Biopsies or excision of masses through the inguinal approach do not require scrotal resection unless the mass is fixed. Proximal positive margins require higher resection than the internal ring. Patients over the age of ten years with the diagnosis of rhabdomyosarcoma should undergo ipsilateral retroperitoneal lymph node dissection. Those under the age of ten may be serially evaluated by thin-slice CT scans to monitor node status. Positive nodes warrant radiotherapy.

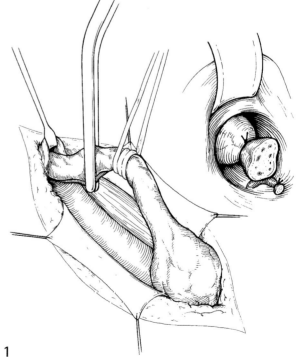

1

Vaginal

2 Vaginal rhabdomyosarcoma presents with vaginal discharge, bleeding, or prolapse of a polypoid mass. Diagnosis is made by vaginoscopy and biopsy of the lesion. Occasionally, tumors may present with a stalk, which facilitates primary resection or biopsy. Most patients require biopsy only with subsequent chemotherapy, with little or any surgical intervention. Partial vaginectomy or sleeve resection may be indicated on occasion. Persistent or recurrent disease in this region may require vaginectomy/ hysterectomy. Bladder salvage is almost always possible. Vaginal tumors most commonly arise on the anterior vaginal wall and may invade the vesicovaginal septum or bladder wall due to proximity. Follow-up vaginoscopy with repeat biopsy generally demonstrates an excellent response to chemotherapy, with no need for further resection. Lymphatic metastases are rare, and lymph node evaluation is not routinely performed.

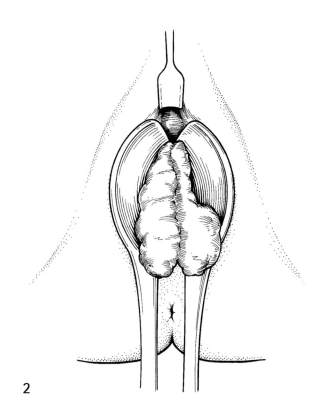

2

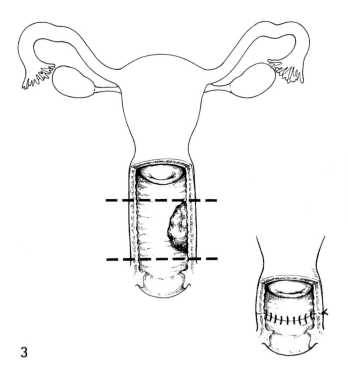

3

3 Tumors of the cervix and uterus are more common in older patients and may require hysterectomy. Persistent or recurrent tumors in the vagina can also be dealt with by local vaginal wall resection (as shown), or sleeve resection.

Extremities

4,5 Rhabdomyosarcomas arising in the extremities are seen in 20 percent of patients. Alveolar histology and poorer prognoses are common in these locations. Biopsy of extremity lesions should be undertaken with consideration of possible need for reoperation and wide local excision. Therefore, longitudinal incisions for biopsy are indicated. Patients with alveolar rhabdomyosarcoma are considered for post-chemotherapy radiation.

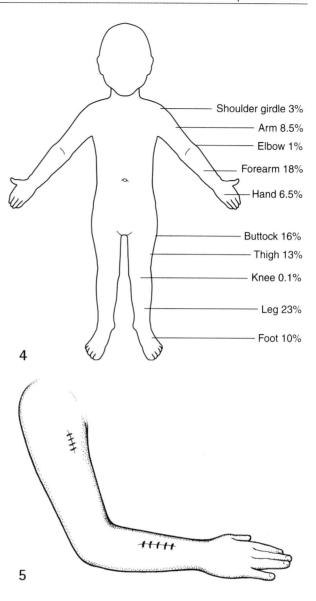

- Shoulder girdle 3%
- Arm 8.5%
- Elbow 1%
- Forearm 18%
- Hand 6.5%
- Buttock 16%
- Thigh 13%
- Knee 0.1%
- Leg 23%
- Foot 10%

4

5

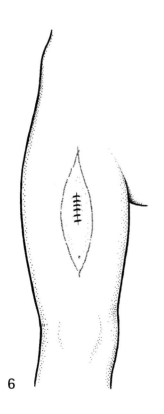

6

6 Small lesions may lend themselves to primary resection with sentinel lymph node evaluation. Wide local excision with negative margins is the operative goal in these rhabdomyosarcomas. Clear margins provide the best prognosis, although no minimum distance is required. Larger tumors are best treated with neoadjuvant chemotherapy with subsequent second-look operations to evaluate treatment success. Limb-sparing surgery is a paramount issue, with very few patients requiring amputation. Primary re-excision may also be of benefit, if indicated.

7 Regional lymph nodes of extremities and truncal lesions should be evaluated with sentinel lymph node mapping, as physical examination and CT are unreliable in extremity rhabdomyosarcomas. The sentinel lymph node is the first node in the regional basin that correlates with the nodal basin status. Positive sentinel lymph node mapping is followed by regional nodal radiation. Delayed second-look surgeries ensure a complete response, or indicate the need for further resection.

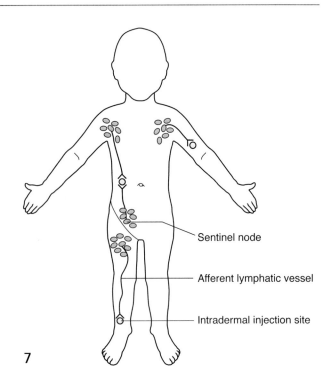

Sentinel node

Afferent lymphatic vessel

Intradermal injection site

7

FURTHER READING

Hayes-Jordan A, Doherty DK, West SD *et al.* Outcome after surgical resection of recurrent rhabdomyosarcoma. *Journal of Pediatric Surgery* 2006; **41**: 633–8; discussion 633–8.

Huh WW, Skapek SX. Childhood rhabdomyosarcoma: new insight on biology and treatment. *Current Oncology Reports* 2010; **12**: 402–10.

Meza JL, Anderson J, Pappo AS, Meyer WH. Analysis of prognostic factors in patients with nonmetastatic rhabdomyosarcoma treated on intergroup rhabdomyosarcoma studies III and IV: the Children's Oncology Group. *Journal of Clinical Oncology* 2006; **24**: 3844–51.

Neville HL, Andrassy RJ, Lally KP *et al.* Lymphatic mapping with sentinel node biopsy in pediatric patients. *Journal of Pediatric Surgery* 2000; **35**: 961–4.

Raney RB, Maurer HM, Anderson JR *et al.* The Intergroup Rhabdomyosarcoma Study Group (IRSG). Major lessons from the IRS-I through IRS-IV studies as background for the current IRS-V treatment protocols. *Sarcoma* 2001; **5**: 9–15.

Rodeberg DA, Paidas CN, Lobe TL *et al.* Surgical principles for children/adolescents with newly diagnosed rhabdomyosarcoma: a report from the Soft Tissue Sarcoma Committee of the Children's Oncology Group. *Sarcoma* 2002; **6**: 111–22.

77

Sacrococcygeal teratoma

AGOSTINO PIERRO and MIGUEL GUELFAND

INTRODUCTION

Sacrococcygeal teratomas (SCT) were first described by Virchow in 1869 and were called 'teratomas' from the Greek *teratos onkoma*, meaning 'monstrous tumor'. They represent the most common germ-cell tumors of childhood (40 percent), with an incidence of approximately 1 in 35 000–40 000 live births, and a female preponderance of 4:1.

Pathology

Embryologically, they arise from totipotent primordial endodermal germ cells, but may contain tissues originating from all three germ layers, including dermal elements (e.g. skin), muscle, glial tissue, intestinal mucosal, and pancreas. Ninety percent of lesions are benign at birth, but risk of malignancy increases with age at diagnosis (up to 50 percent malignancy at six months and up to 75 percent at one year of age), gender, the anatomical type of the lesion (American Academy of Pediatrics anatomical classification, see below; risk of malignancy is 8 percent in type I compared to 38 percent in type II), in recurrent lesions, and in those with incomplete resection. Histologically, teratomas are classified as mature (70 percent), immature with embryonic components (20 percent), or immature with malignant components (10 percent). Malignant sacrococcygeal teratomas almost exclusively arise from embryonal carcinomas or yolk-sac tumors.

Staging

Sacrococcygeal teratomas are currently staged using The Children's Cancer Study Group and Pediatric Oncology Group staging system for extragonadal germ-cell tumors (**Table 77.1**).

Table 77.1 Staging system used for sacrococcygeal teratomas.

Stage	Extent of disease
I	Complete excision with coccygectomy
	Negative tumor margins
	Tumor markers positive, but fall to normal if negative at diagnosis
	Lymphadenectomy must be negative for tumor
II	Microscopic residual tumor
	Lymph node negative
	Tumor markers positive or negative
III	Gross residual tumor
	Retroperitoneal nodes negative or positive
	Tumor markers positive or negative
IV	Distant metastases, including liver

Etiology

The precise etiology of the development of sacrococcygeal teratomas remains unclear. Several theories have been postulated, including the following:

- Presacral lesions occurring at sites of incomplete migration of endodermal cells along their normal pathway from near the origin of the allantois to the gonadal ridges.
- Postsacral lesions originating from remnants of Hensen's node (the midline primitive streak that comprises an aggregate of totipotential cells that are the primary organizers of embryonic development). These migrate caudally from the posterior embryo, finally resting anterior to the coccyx, and normally disappear by the end of the third week.
- Incomplete twinning theories. A familial link is found in 57 percent of cases, with an autosomal dominant mode of inheritance.

DIAGNOSIS

Prenatal diagnosis

The routine application of prenatal ultrasound has increased the prenatal diagnosis of sacrococcygeal teratomas and allowed for accurate identification of their site and details of any intrapelvic extension or urinary tract obstruction. Repeated ultrasound assessment of tumor size also helps determine the mode of delivery. Cesarean section delivery is advocated for tumors larger than 5 cm, as dystocia during vaginal delivery may cause tumor rupture, tumor avulsion, hemorrhage, and sometimes may result in the death of the infant. Finally, ultrasound may be used to prognosticate lesions. Polyhydramnios (27 percent), placentomegaly, and hydrops fetalis are poor prognostic indicators. Recent-onset polyhydramnios is associated with premature labor. Twenty percent of tumors diagnosed prenatally develop hydrops from high-output cardiac failure secondary to vascular steal of blood flow through arteriovenous channels within the tumor, which is associated with a near-100 percent mortality.

Diagnosis in the neonate and children

CLINICAL

1 Most sacrococcygeal teratomas are visible externally and are therefore diagnosed clinically at birth.

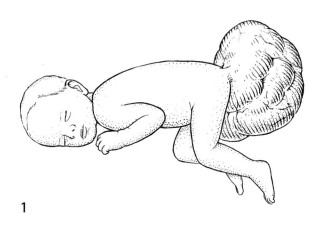

1

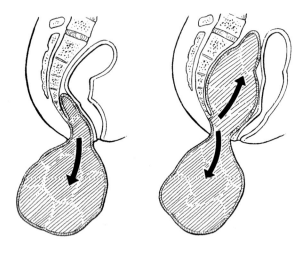

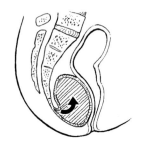

2

2 The tumor is classified anatomically according to the criteria of the Surgical Section of the American Academy of Pediatrics.

- Type I (47 percent of lesions): a pedunculated tumor predominantly external with minimal extension into the presacral region.
- Type II (34 percent of lesions): a type I tumor with significant intrapelvic extension.
- Type III (9 percent of lesions): a predominantly pelvic tumor with abdominal extension, but minimal external component.
- Type IV (10 percent of lesions): a completely internal presacral tumor without external evidence of disease.

The tumor is always attached to the coccyx (therefore the necessity of coccygectomy during tumor excision), and may project to a varying degree into the presacral space between the sacrum and the rectum. Although most neonates with sacrococcygeal teratomas are asymptomatic, this upward extension into the pelvic space may compress and elevate the rectum, vagina, bladder, and uterus. Displacement of these pelvic organs may cause presenting symptoms of constipation, large bowel obstruction, urinary retention, an abdominal mass, or symptoms of malignancy, such as failure to thrive.

Most lesions are isolated; associated anomalies are identified in up to 18 percent of patients. The most common anomalies are those of the central nervous system (26 percent) and musculoskeletal system (24 percent); the most common being Currarino syndrome: a triad of anorectal malformation (either anal stenosis or agenesis), sacrococcygeal bony defect (hemisacrum with preservation of the first sacral vertebra), and a presacral mass (usually a presacral teratoma or anterior meningocele, although duplication cysts and dermoid cysts have also been described). Other associated anomalies include urogenital anomalies (hypospadias, vesicoureteric reflux), duplications of the vagina or uterus, orthopedic anomalies (congenital dislocation of hips in 7 percent, vertebral anomalies), central nervous system lesions (e.g. anencephaly, trigonocephaly, Dandy–Walker malformation, spina bifida, and myelomeningocele).

Differential diagnosis

The differential diagnosis of a sacrococcygeal teratoma is mainly meningocele or myelomeningocele. However, sacrococcygeal teratoma can be distinguished on the basis of its more completely cystic nature and its less abundant internal component. In addition, pressure on a myelomeningocele will often be noticeably transmitted to the anterior fontanelle. Less common differentials include lipomeningocele, hemangioma, lymphangioma, chordoma (50 percent occur in the sacrococcygeal region), pelvic neuroblastoma, sarcoma, hamartoma, cystic duplication of the rectum, neuroenteric cysts, dermoid cysts, meconium pseudocysts, and perirectal abscess.

Investigations

Aids to diagnosis include plain x-rays, which may demonstrate calcifications in the tumor in 60 percent of cases or identify spinal defects. Ultrasound will identify the lesion and any intra-abdominal or intrapelvic extensions. Detailed preoperative assessment of the lesion, any abdominal or pelvic extension, and its relationship to the adjacent structures, is made by computed tomography (CT) and/or magnetic resonance imaging (MRI).

In addition, markers such as alfa-fetoprotein (AFP) and beta-human chorionic gonadotropin (β-hCG) may be useful for the assessment of disease progression. Serum AFP is normally elevated significantly at birth and remains high for up to four months, decreasing to adult levels only at 6–12 months. However, most yolk-sac tumors and some embryonal carcinomas also secrete AFP.

Since malignant elements of sacrococcygeal tumors almost exclusively arise from one of these two sources, AFP measurement is a useful marker for malignant degeneration of benign lesions, or for the presence of residual or recurrent malignant disease. It can be measured in the serum and demonstrated in the cells by immunohistochemistry. Persistently high levels may be an indication for further surgery or chemotherapy. β-hCG is another marker that may be elevated. It is produced by choriocarcinomas and, rarely, carcinoembryonic antigen, and may be measured in plasma.

PRENATAL MANAGEMENT

Following intrauterine diagnosis of the tumor, management is based on fetal lung maturity and the presence or absence of placentomegaly and hydrops fetalis (the latter conditions being associated with almost 100 percent mortality). Upon fetal lung maturity without placentomegaly and/or hydrops fetalis, early elective delivery by Cesarean section is indicated.

Antenatal (fetal) intervention

Fetal interventions like amniodrainage, cyst aspiration, and relief of bladder outflow obstruction can be performed in those cases were hydrops and prematurity is present.

Consideration of open fetal surgery for debulking of SCTs is only considered in very selective cases.

Indications for surgery

The mainstay of the treatment of benign sacrococcygeal teratomas is early and en-bloc excision of the lesion within a few weeks of life, given that:

- the risk of malignant change in benign lesions increases with (a) age and (b) incompletely excised residual lesions; and
- the tumor's rich vascularity makes it vulnerable to spontaneous ulceration and hemorrhage if left unexcised.

PREOPERATIVE PREPARATION AND ANESTHESIA

1. Appropriate imaging (ultrasonography/CT/MRI) to delineate the anatomy and extent of the lesion, as the surgical approach will be dictated by whether the lesion has intra-abdominal or intrapelvic extension.
2. Serum assays of tumor markers (AFP/β-hCG) for postoperative comparisons.
3. Adequate intravenous access and blood products should be secured before starting the operation, especially with large tumors, where there may be brisk intraoperative blood loss. Other vascular access, including an arterial line for blood pressure monitoring, and central venous line monitoring are beneficial.

4. General anesthesia is mandatory. High-output cardiac failure secondary to arteriovenous channels in the tumor may limit the use of inhalation agents, which have known cardiodepressant effects.
5. Broad-spectrum antibiotics should be given at the induction of anesthesia.
6. The stomach is emptied with a nasogastric tube and an indwelling bladder catheter is inserted.

Prevention of blood loss

In infants with sacrococcygeal teratomas with large feeding vessels or highly vascularized tumors, preoperative embolization of the feeding vessels or laparoscopic interruption of the median sacral artery can be used prior to resection. The aim is to decrease intraoperative blood loss and therefore minimize intra- and postoperative morbidity.

OPERATION

Position of patient and preparation

3 In the majority of cases, where the major component of the tumor is extrapelvic, the procedure is performed with the infant in the prone jack-knife position. This is achieved by supporting the pelvis and shoulders with rolled towels, thus also allowing free respiratory movements of the chest and abdomen during ventilation.

The rectum may be prepared for digital manipulation during the course of the dissection, using an enema (e.g. 1 percent solution of povidone-iodine). Alternatively, for those who prefer to exclude the anus from the operative field, the rectum should be packed with gauze impregnated with vaseline, liquid paraffin, or povidone-iodine solution. Vaseline packing in the rectum facilitates its identification throughout the procedure.

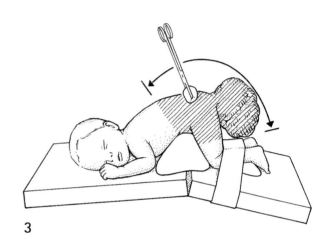

3

Incision

4 The traditional chevron incision is modified as this may leave protuberant 'dog ears' and extend across and below the infragluteal creases down onto the posterior thighs, causing undesirable buttock deformity. The incision is made as illustrated in figure 4 to minimizing redundant skin, restoring normal buttock contour, and avoiding scars crossing the infragluteal crease.

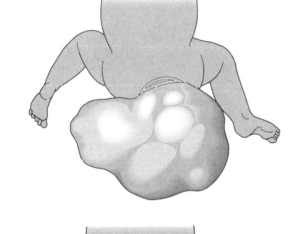

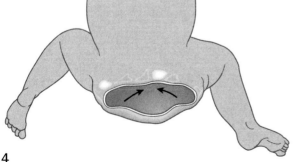

4

Removal of tumor and coccyx en bloc and ligation of sacral vessels

5 The tumor is dissected from the inferior and medial aspects of the gluteus maximus. The sacrum and coccyx are identified, and the coccyx is transected at the sacrococcygeal joint by cautery, taking the coccyx en bloc with the tumor. Failure to remove the coccyx is associated with a 30–40 percent incidence of recurrence, with more than 50 percent of cases becoming malignant.

The median and lateral sacral vessels are identified at this landmark, and coagulated or ligated in continuity with the tumor/coccyx. (With an extensive intra-abdominal tumor component, an initial transabdominal approach will be required to achieve vascular isolation of collateral vessels from the lateral sacral vessels.)

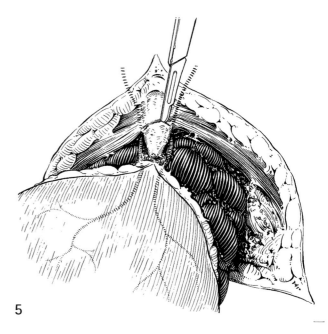

5

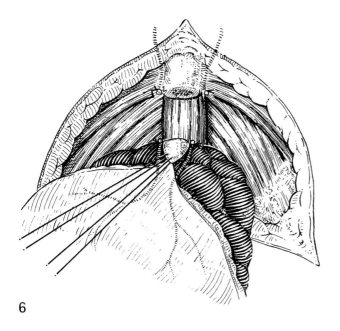

6

6 Using gentle traction, the coccyx and tumor are retracted and dissected free from the gluteus maximus and surrounding tissues, to the pelvic floor. The pelvic floor muscles are preserved and the proximal rectum identified. The tumor must be dissected and freed completely from the rectal wall and anorectal sphincter complex.

7 This dissection can be facilitated if necessary by placing a finger in the rectum. Rarely, the tumor completely surrounds the rectum, making total excision very difficult.

The excised tumor is sent for histological examination to identify the presence of any malignant components as well as to ensure tumor-free margins.

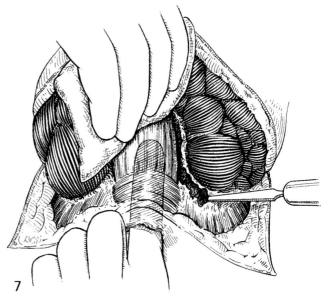

7

Pelvic floor reconstruction

8 The pelvic floor is reconstructed by suturing the superior and posterior portions of the levator muscles to the presacral fascia, behind the rectum. This allows the anus to assume a near-normal configuration and therefore the best possibility of achieving good fecal continence.

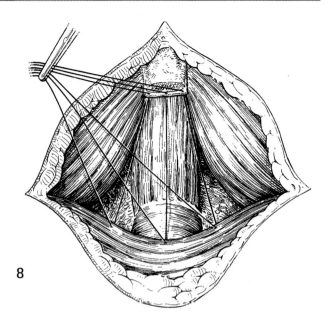

8

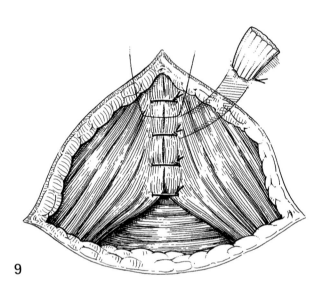

9

10, 11 After resection of massive sacrococcygeal teratoma a medial mobilization of redundant skin flaps is performed. Redundancy of flaps is resected medially to avoid scars below the infragluteal clefts.

Closure

9 The gluteus maximus muscles are apposed in the midline using interrupted sutures. A drain may be left in place in the perirectal space prior to this closure, and brought out through a separate stab incision.

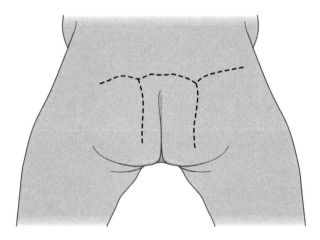

10

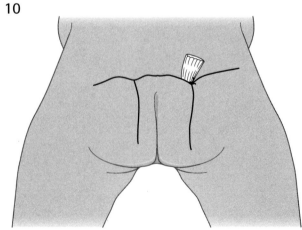

11

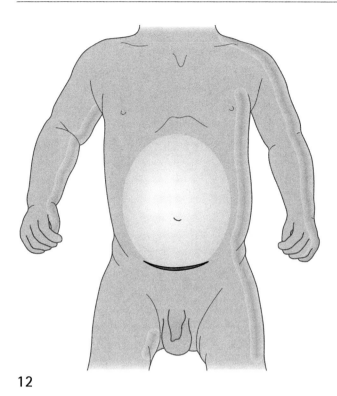

12

Modifications for extensive or intra-abdominal tumors

12 In type III tumors where there is significant intra-abdominal involvement, the pelvic excision must be preceded by a laparotomy. In these cases, the operation commences with the patient in a supine position, with a rolled gauze pad under the buttocks, thus raising the pelvic floor. A lower midline or transverse lower abdominal incision approach is used, depending on the extent of the intra-abdominal component of the tumor. The tumor is dissected free from the lower abdominal and pelvic viscera, and the sacral vessels can be controlled through this approach. The abdominal wall is then closed, and the patient is turned prone to complete the operation as described above.

Laparoscopic approach

Laparoscopy can be used for the resection or mobilization of intra-abdominal or pelvic portions of the SCT. This is combined with the external resection of the tumor and for litigation of the sacral vessels.

POSTOPERATIVE CARE

Immediate postoperative period

The child is kept in a prone position for 3 days to prevent soiling the wound with urine or feces. The urinary catheter is removed after 24 hours, and the drain after 48 hours. Oral feeding may be commenced when nasogastric aspirates are minimal, and the nasogastric tube may be removed thereafter. A pelvic neuropraxia may occur in the early postoperative period and may cause a poorly contracting, neurogenic bladder. This is generally temporary, but the patient will require intermittent catheterization until it resolves.

Chemotherapy

Malignant lesions respond poorly with surgery alone, with a 10 percent salvage rate. Adjuvant chemotherapy, particularly platinum-containing regimens, e.g. cisplatin, bleomycin, vinblastine, and/or VP-16 (etoposide), addressing the specific malignant element, has improved survival with such lesions. This regimen may shrink

the tumor, making it amenable to secondary resection. Resected tumors should also be examined for malignant elements, which may require subsequent chemotherapy.

Follow up

Beyond the immediate postoperative care period, careful monitoring is required as malignant germ-cell tumors can recur either from missed malignant elements in the original tumor or from malignant conversion of benign residual tissue. Follow up, including rectal examinations, should be performed at monthly intervals for the first year, at three-month intervals for at least three years (as most recurrences occur within the first three years), and then annually. Monitoring of serum AFP levels may also help detect the presence of malignant recurrence. Recurrent tumors should be excised, with preoperative chemotherapy for more extensive disease.

PROGNOSIS

The prognosis for patients with sacrococcygeal teratoma is dependent on the following:

- Antenatal/obstetric factors: hydrops or placentomegaly is associated with almost 100 percent mortality, whilst dystocia or tumor rupture during delivery may be associated with exsanguinating hemorrhage.
- Age at diagnosis: as the risk of malignant transformation in a benign lesion increases with age.

- Tumor histology and stage: up to 95 percent of benign tumors can be cured with excision surgery alone. Prognoses of malignant tumors are dependent on tumor type, stage, and location. Survival with malignant tumors can be achieved in up to 90 percent of cases using a combination of surgery and adjuvant chemotherapy, although the risk of late recurrences or second malignancies persists. Following surgical excision, mature teratomas are associated with an 11 percent risk of recurrence within five years.
- Associated anomalies.
- Surgical factors: recurrence is more likely with incompletely excised lesions or in the absence of coccygectomy. Failure to remove the coccyx is associated with a 30–40 percent incidence of recurrence, with more than 50 percent of cases being malignant.

In addition to tumor recurrence, long-term complications associated with sacrococcygeal teratomas are common: 40 percent will encounter mild bowel dysfunction (incontinence or constipation), while 10 percent will have urinary incontinence or neuropathic bladders, often associated with similar bowel symptoms. These patients required treatment and constant vigilance to prevent further problems.

FURTHER READING

Altman RP, Randolph JG, Lilly JR. Sacrococcygeal teratoma: American Academy of Pediatrics Surgical Section Survey, 1973. *Journal of Pediatric Surgery* 1974; **9**: 389–98.

Draper H, Chitayat D, Ein SH, Langer JC. Long-term functional results following resection of neonatal sacrococcygeal teratoma. *Pediatric Surgery International* 2009; **25**: 243–6.

Fishman SJ, Jennings RW, Johnson SM, and Kim HB. Contouring Buttock Reconstruction After Sacrococcygeal Teratoma Resection. *Journal of Pediatric Surgery* 2004; **39**: 439–441

Flake AW. Fetal sacrococcygeal teratoma. *Seminars in Pediatric Surgery* 1993; **2**: 113–20.

Lee LD, Alam S, Lim FY *et al.* Prenatal and postnatal urological complications of sacrococcygeal teratomas. *Journal of Pediatric Surgery* 2011; **46**: 1186–90.

Rescorla FJ, Sawin RS, Coran AG *et al.* Long-term outcome for infants and children with sacrococcygeal teratoma: a report from the Children's Cancer Group. *Journal of Pediatric Surgery* 1998; **33**: 171–6.

Skinner MA. Germ cell tumors. In: Oldham KT, Colombani PM, Foglia RP (eds). *Surgery of Infants and Children: Scientific Principles and Practice*. Philadelphia: Lippincott-Raven, 1997: 653–62.

SECTION VII

Endocrine

78

Thyroidectomy in children

TOM R KURZAWINSKI and PAOLO DE COPPI

INDICATIONS

Thyroid surgery in children is an uncommon operation and should be only performed where appropriate expertise and facilities are available to diagnose and treat thyroid problems. To avoid inappropriate or unnecessary surgery, each case should be discussed within the multidisciplinary team, which should include pediatric endocrinologist, pediatric or general surgeon with an expertise in pediatric and thyroid surgery, pediatric oncologist, nuclear physician, radiologist, pathologist, and clinical geneticist.

Indications for thyroid surgery in children include:

- Benign disease:
  - thyrotoxicosis (Graves' disease, toxic adenoma)
  - symptomatic multinodular goiter causing dysphagia, stridor, pain, or discomfort.
- Malignant disease:
  - solitary nodules suspected of being malignant
  - thyroid cancer (papillary, follicular, medullary)
  - prophylactic thyroidectomy for MEN type 2.

The approach to thyroid operations has changed in the last few decades and partial and subtotal thyroidectomy has been abandoned. Leaving residual thyroid tissue behind increases the risk of recurrence, and reoperations carry a much higher risks of complications.

Recommended types of surgery are:

- **Lobectomy and isthmusectomy.** Performed for solitary thyroid nodules, which are either causing compression symptoms and/or thyrotoxicosis, or are suspicious of being malignant.
- **Near-total thyroidectomy.** Operation of choice in thyrotoxicosis and large bilateral multinodular goiter. In this case, almost all thyroid tissue is removed; a small fragment of thyroid with capsule (2–3 mm^3) is left to preserve attached parathyroid.
- **Total thyroidectomy.** Indicated for treating thyroid cancer and as a prophylactic measure in children with MEN 2.

LYMPH NODE SURGERY FOR THYROID CANCER

Central lymphadenectomy aims to remove lymph nodes adjacent to thyroid (level VI) and should be performed for papillary cancers larger than 1 cm.

Unilateral or bilateral modified neck dissection with preservation of non-lymphatic structures is performed in children with thyroid cancer and metastases to the lymph nodes in the carotid chain (levels II, III, IV and V).

Preoperative

Clinical examination of the neck is always required to assess the size of the goiter, its retrosternal extension, nodularity, and presence of lymphadenopathy. Thyroid function tests (T3 and T4) (TSH), are essential to confirm normal function (with or without thyroxine, antithyroid drugs, etc.). Serum calcitonin is helpful in screening of children with MEN2, establishing diagnosis of medullary cancer and predicting volume of disease. Serum calcium and vitamin D levels should be measured and corrected if deficient.

Thyroid, particularly in children, can be easily imaged using neck ultrasound. Ultrasound, in particular, is invaluable in assessing thyroid nodules and lymph nodes (size, cystic or solid nature, number, blood flow, microcalcifications) and guiding the biopsy needle. Ultrasound characteristics suggestive of malignancy include microcalcifications, indistinct margins, and a variable echotexture. Ultrasonographic appearance alone, however, cannot reliably distinguish between benign and malignant lesions. Nuclear scans provide information about thyroid function (e.g. radioactive iodine) and expression of specific receptors (e.g. octreotide scan to stage medullary cancer). Positron emission tomography, computed tomography (CT) and/or magnetic resonance image (MRI) may be helpful in imaging malignant disease.

Fine needle aspiration cytology is pivotal in assessing potentially malignant thyroid nodules or enlarged lymph nodes. Older children can tolerate it without anesthesia. Solitary thyroid nodules in children carry a much higher risk of cancer, compared to the adult population, and negative cytology should not always obviate the need for surgical excision allowing for histological assessment if a high level of clinical suspicion exists.

Preoperative laryngoscopy is indicated for all children who report voice change or who have had previous neck surgery.

Thyroid surgery carries a risk of potential morbidity and is a significant source of litigation. Consent for the operation should be obtained by the senior surgeon, documented in the notes and include clear information about risks such as bleeding (1 percent), infection (<1 percent), recurrent laryngeal nerve injury (1 percent), hypocalcaemia (2–5 percent), and poor cosmesis (keloid).

Positioning of patient

The child should be positioned supine on the operating table with a sandbag between shoulders and head ring. Extending the neck improves the access and the head up tilt reduces venous pressure.

Incision

Skin crease incision is carried between sternomastoid muscles between the lower third and the upper two-thirds of the distance between the chin and the manubrium of the sternum. This level should give adequate access to the whole thyroid gland, especially to the vessels of the upper poles. The length of the incision depends on the size of the goiter and can be extended during the procedure. A 15-blade knife should be used to cut through the skin, subcutaneous fat, and platysma. Dissection of upper and lower flaps by developing a subplatysma plane should be performed using scissors, avoiding damage to the anterior jugular veins and cutaneous nerves. The upper flap should be raised to the level of thyroid cartilage. Bipolar diathermy should be used to control bleeding.

Exposure and dissection

1 Insert Joll's self-retaining retractor to retract skin flaps and identify the bloodless midline plane between strap muscles (raphe). It should be divided longitudinally, the strap muscles separated from the thyroid and retracted laterally with Langenbeck retractor. It should be borne in mind that in younger children, the thymus could be still large and can extend from the mediastinum upwards to the neck. When necessary, the thymus should be mobilized and retracted downwards to allow safe dissection of the thyroid and surrounding structures.

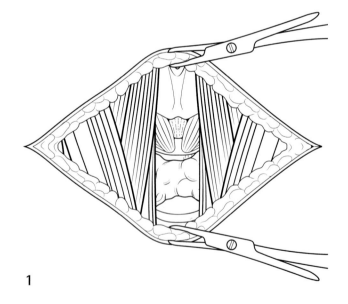

1

2 The surgeon should stand opposite the lobe which he aims to dissect. The controlateral side of the thyroid should be pulled by the surgeon towards himself and gently dissected laterally towards carotid artery, which should be retracted by the assistant using Langenbeck retractor. The smaller vessels should be divided with diathermy and the middle thyroid vein between ties using 4/0 or 3/0 absorbable sutures.

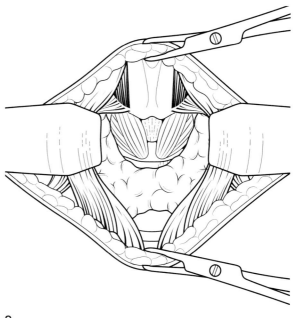

2

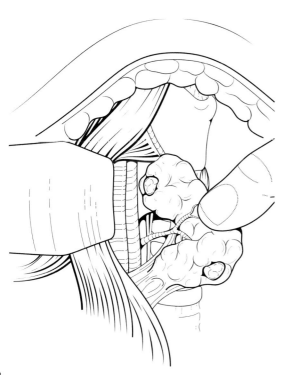

3

3 The sternothyroid muscle can be divided to provide better access to upper pole vessels, which should be carefully dissected and divided between ties. Identify and avoid damaging external branch of the laryngeal nerve, which lies close to the upper pole vessels.

4 The thyroid should be pulled upwards and to the middle, the strap muscles and carotid artery retracted laterally and branches of inferior thyroid artery and recurrent laryngeal nerve identified. This part of the operation should be performed gently avoiding unnecessary stretching and diathermy close to the nerve. The recurrent laryngeal nerve usually lies in the tracheoesophageal groove, either behind, between or in front of branches of inferior thyroid artery. It is usually easy to recognize by its white color and has vessels running on its surface. It should be remembered that sometimes (17 percent), the nerve bifurcates early before entering the cricopharyngeal muscle and it is important to identify this variant and preserve all branches. On the right side, the laryngeal nerve could be non-recurrent with a medial to lateral rather than vertical course.

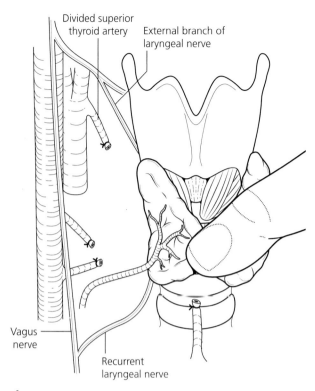

4

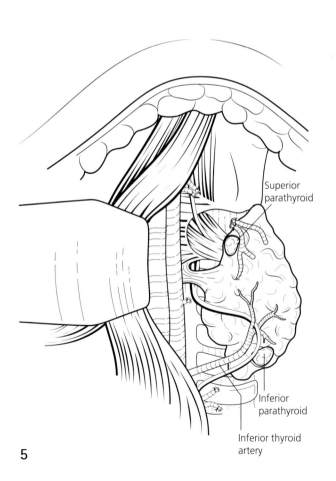

5

5 Before proceeding with further dissection, it is of paramount importance to trace the whole length of the nerve all the way behind the thyroid to its entry into the larynx behind the cricothyroid joint. The superior and inferior parathyroid glands should be identified and the small arterial branches of inferior thyroid artery divided between ties preserving the blood supply to the superior parathyroid gland. The blood vessels to the lower pole should be divided, preserving the inferior parathyroid on its vascular pedicle. Anatomical positions of parathyroids are variable but they should always be identified and dissected gently from the thyroid capsule using bipolar diathermy. Disruption of tiny blood vessels, which supply the parathyroid gland, will result in their color changing to dark blue or black and necessitate their autografting. In this scenario, the parathyroid should be preserved in gauze embedded in ice-cold saline until the thyroidectomy has been completed. The parathyroid should then be cut up into small pieces and implanted into small pockets in the sternomastoid muscle.

6 The recurrent laryngeal nerve at its entry into the larynx is covered by fibers of lateral thyroid (Berry) ligament which should be dissected by creating a tunnel parallel to the nerve with artery clips, and it should be divided between ties. Almost always there is a small arterial vessel, which can cause troublesome bleeding retracting behind the nerve. The use of bipolar diathermy should be avoided at any cost during this part of the dissection.

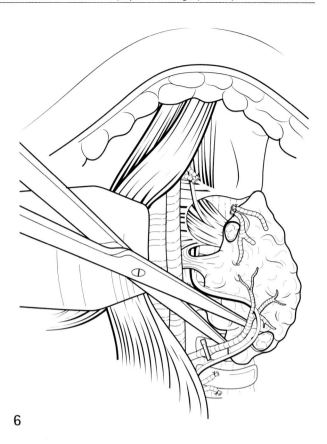

6

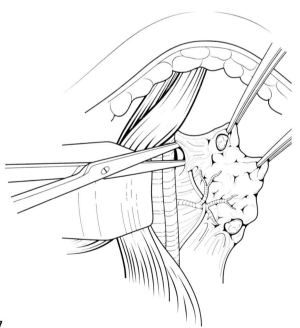

7

7 Once the nerve is isolated and dissected from the gland, the thyroid lobe can be detached from the trachea with sharp dissection and diathermy. It is important to dissect and remove the pyramidal lobe. If hemithyroidectomy is to be performed, the thyroid should be divided at the isthmus and the capsule of the contralateral lobe oversewn using 3/0 absorbable sutures.

If total thyroidectomy is planned, the procedure should continue as described above on the opposite side. The surgeon should also move to the other side of the patient to maintain good vision to the operative field.

8 Drains after thyroid surgery are not mandatory and seldom necessary. A small Surgicel patch can be placed in the thyroid bed. Before closing the wound, the surgeon should check for hemostasis, parathyroid viability, and integrity of the nerve. All bleeding points should be stopped by a combination of bipolar diathermy and 5/0 absorbable sutures. Closure of the wound starts with approximation of the strap muscles using absorbable stitches, leaving a small gap at the bottom to allow blood to escape into the superficial space to prevent compression in case of postoperative bleeding. The platysma and subcuticular layer should be closed with absorbable stitches and skin with subcuticular 5/0 Monocryl. Surgeon should be present during extubation and make sure that patient is breathing normally and there is no stridor.

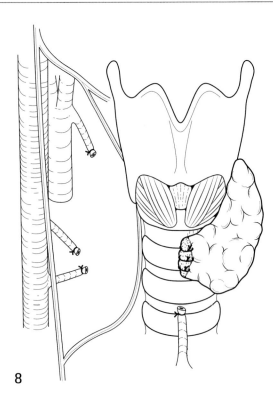

8

POSTOPERATIVE CARE

Follow up and surveillance

Immediately after surgery, children should be nursed in a semi-sitting position with routine observations (blood pressure, pulse, and respiratory rate) checked frequently. Neck swelling or excessive drain discharge must be reported urgently to the surgical team.

All children after thyroid surgery, especially for thyroid cancer, will require life-long surveillance. Pediatric thyroid cancer is a rare and treatable disease with an excellent prognosis. In children less than ten years of age, the incidence of differentiated thyroid cancer is one per million. Treatment with radioactive iodine is recommended for most children after total thyroidectomy for papillary and follicular cancer. Radioiodine ablation should be carried about 4 weeks after surgery with diagnostic scan six months later. Regular review should include neck palpation, serum thyroglobulin, and ultrasound with cytology if necessary. In case of a cancer, follow-up ultrasound and TSH-suppressed Tg level assessment is performed six months after initial therapy and at least annually thereafter, although following patients every six months for at least five years after diagnosis may be preferred for patients with more advanced initial or metastatic cancer. TSH-stimulated Tg levels are assessed six months after initial therapy, and 6–12 months thereafter, based on the suspicion of residual disease. Assessment of free T4, T3, and TSH levels is indicated every six months and between one and two months after dosage changes. The aim of thyroxine replacement in patients with thyroid cancer is not only to maintain euthyroid stage but also to suppress

TSH levels. Calcitonin is a marker of recurrent disease in medullary cancer.

Management of complications

- **Dyspnea or stridor.** Potentially life-threatening and may be due to recurrent laryngeal nerve injury or bleeding into the neck (approximately 1 percent). Immediate intervention at the bedside is required. If there is obvious neck swelling with stridor, the wound should be opened by cutting the skin and deeper stitches, the hematoma should be evacuated and the patient transferred to the operating room for further management. Emergency intubation is difficult and if necessary, should be performed by a senior anesthetist.
- **Hypocalcemia.** Occurs as a result of parathyroid damage. Temporary hypocalcemia after hemithyroidectomy is rare but common if total thyroidectomy and lymph node surgery is performed. Permanent hypocalcemia occurs in 1–3 percent of cases. Serum calcium levels should be checked 12-hourly postoperatively and symptomatic hypocalcemia (tingling, cramps, tetany-positive, Chvostek-positive, Trousseau signs) should be treated urgently with i.v. calcium infusion (1.7 mL/kg calcium gluconate 10 percent). Prolonged hypocalcemia requires treatment with oral calcium and vitamin D3.
- **Hypothyroidism.** Thyroxine replacement is often necessary. Lobectomy causes hypothyroidism in about 10–20 percent of children. Maintaining normal thyroid function depends on the volume of remaining thyroid tissue and its functional capacity. The decision to start thyroxine should be based on symptoms and

TSH levels during follow up. Patients after near-total thyroidectomy for benign disease should start thyroxine before discharge from the hospital. Initial dose depends on patient age and weight and should be titrated to achieve a euthyroid state. After total thyroidectomy for cancer, the initial replacement is with short-acting liothyronine (T3). It reduces the time of withdrawal necessary to render the patient hypothyroid before treatment with radioactive iodine. Once treatment with radioactive iodine is completed, liothyronine is replaced with lifelong thyroxine (T4) with an aim to suppress the TSH to undetectable levels. TSH can stimulate tumor growth and its suppression is very important.

- **Voice change.** This is caused by injury to the recurrent or superior laryngeal nerves and can be temporary (neuropraxia) or permanent. The risk of injuring a single recurrent laryngeal nerve is approximately 1 percent and causes a hoarse/croaky voice. Injury to both nerves is extremely rare and may require tracheostomy and laryngeal surgery. Injury to the external branch of the superior laryngeal nerve occurs in 2–5 percent of thyroidectomies and causes voice fatigue and weakness. Patients with abnormal sounding voice after surgery should be reassured that these changes are usually temporary. Laryngoscopy should be performed if changes persist.

FURTHER READING

Canadian Pediatric Thyroid Nodule (CaPTN) Study Group. The Canadian Pediatric Thyroid Nodule Study. An evaluation of current management practices. *Journal of Pediatric Surgery* 2008; **43**: 826–30.

Cooper DS, Doherty GM, Haugen BR *et al.* Revised American Thyroid Association management guidelines for patients with thyroid nodules and differentiated thyroid cancer. *Thyroid* 2009; **19**: 1167–214.

Hogan AR, Zhuge Y, Perez EA *et al.* Pediatric thyroid carcinoma: incidence and outcomes in 1753 patients. *Journal of Surgical Research* 2009; **156**: 167–72.

La Quaglia MP, Black T, Holcomb GW 3rd *et al.* Differentiated thyroid cancer: clinical characteristics, treatment, and outcome in patients under 21 years of age who present with distant metastases. A report from the Surgical Discipline Committee of the Children's Cancer Group. *Journal of Pediatric Surgery* 2000; **35**: 955–9.

Rivkees SA, Mazzaferri EL, Verburg FA *et al.* The treatment of differentiated thyroid cancer in children: emphasis on surgical approach and radioactive iodine therapy. *Endocrine Reviews* 2011; **32**: 798.

79

Pancreatic resection

LEWIS SPITZ and AGOSTINO PIERRO

HISTORY

Hyperinsulinemic hypoglycemia was previously known as 'nesidioblastosis' – a term coined by Laidlaw in 1938 to describe diffuse proliferation of islet cells. Nesidioblasts were defined as 'cells that differentiate out of the duct epithelium to build islets'.

PRINCIPLES AND JUSTIFICATION

Hypoglycemia in the neonatal period is defined as a blood glucose concentration of less than 2.6 mmol/L. The hypoglycemia may be transient, as in the 'stressed neonate' or the infant of a diabetic mother or in Beckwith–Wiedemann syndrome, or persistent. In persistent hypoglycemia, it is important to exclude leucin sensitivity and other endocrine disorders (e.g. hypopituitarism, cortisol deficiency) or inborn errors of metabolism (e.g. glycogen storage disease).

Congenital hyperinsulinism (CHI) is the most frequent cause of persistent hypoglycemia in infants, and it is associated with a high risk of neurological complications. Histologically, two subtypes of CHI have been described, focal and diffuse. Both forms share a similar clinical presentation, but result from different pathophysiological mechanisms and are managed differently.

The **diffuse form**, which affects the whole pancreas, is medically treated and surgery (near-total pancreatectomy) is required only when medical therapy is unsuccessful. Conversely, the **focal form** (40–50 percent of cases) which is localized to one region of the pancreas, can be completely cured by partial pancreatectomy including the focal lesion, which minimizes the risk of diabetes mellitus or exocrine insufficiency. Due to these differences, the preoperative identification of those children with a focal form is critical.

To distinguish between diffuse and focal subtypes, genetic analysis is performed. Typically, children with diffuse CHI have homozygous recessive or compound heterozygote mutations in the *ABCC8* and *KCNJ11* genes (which encode the SUR1 and KIR6.2 proteins of the pancreatic beta-cell). Focal CHI is associated with loss of heterozygosity for paternally inherited mutations in the K^+_{ATP} genes.

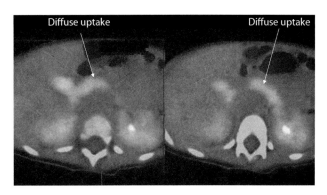

1

1-3 A major advance in the diagnosis and treatment of CHI is the ^{18}F *L*-3,4-dihydroxyphenylalanine positron emission tomography combined with computed tomography scan (^{18}F-DOPA-PET-CT scan). The PET-CT scan is useful in children without the characteristic genetic mutations of diffuse CHI as it can distinguish between diffuse and focal disease, where diffuse CHI exhibits a diffuse uptake on the PET-CT scan. In focal disease, the scan assists in localizing the site of the focal lesion, allowing a more directed pancreatic resection.

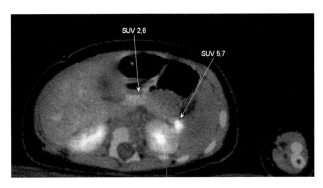

2 Focal lesion in the tail of the pancreas

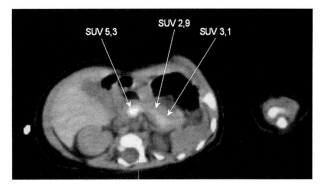

3 Focal lesion in the head of the pancreas

Diagnosis

The diagnosis of hyperinsulinism is based on the following criteria:

- inappropriately raised plasma insulin levels for blood glucose concentration;
- glucose infusion rate greater than 6–8 mg/kg per minute to maintain a blood glucose level above 2.6 mmol/L;
- low free fatty acids and blood ketone bodies during hypoglycemia;
- glycemic response to glucagon despite hypoglycemia.

Medical treatment consists of providing sufficient glucose to prevent hypoglycemia, which usually requires an intravenous infusion of 15 percent glucose solution. Diazoxide is the mainstay of medical management. It inhibits glucose-stimulated insulin secretion, and dosages of up to 25 mg/kg per day may be necessary. Its action is potentiated by the diuretic chlorothiazide. The somatostatin analog ostreotride infusion may be useful as a therapeutic adjunct in refractory cases.

Surgical treatment is indicated if the patient remains dependent on intravenous glucose despite full dosages of diazoxide and chlorothiazide.

Special investigations, such as ultrasonography, computed tomography, nuclear magnetic imaging, and selective arteriography, are of little value in the diagnosis of hyperinsulinism in infancy. In the older infant or child, they may be helpful in the localization of a focal adenoma.

Aim of surgery

The operative procedure consists of a near-total pancreatectomy for diffuse disease. For focal lesions, local resection should prove curative.

PREOPERATIVE PREPARATION

A central venous catheter is essential to monitor blood glucose levels at regular intervals, preoperatively, intraoperatively, and postoperatively. Prophylactic antibiotics (flucloxacillin and gentamicin) are advisable to prevent wound sepsis, as there is a high level of circulating blood glucose and an excessive amount of subcutaneous fat deposition.

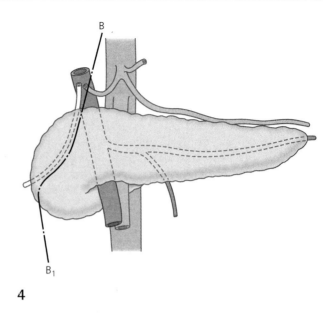

4

OPERATION

4 The operative procedure consists of a near-total pancreatectomy for diffuse involvement or limited resection for focal lesions.

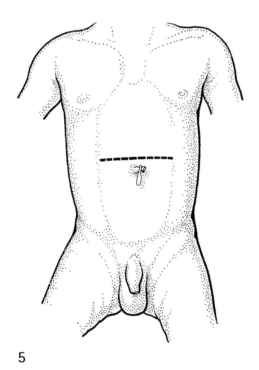

5

NEAR TOTAL PANCREATECTOMY

Incision

5 A laparotomy is performed via a generous supraumbilical transverse muscle-cutting incision, extending through both rectus abdominus muscles. A thorough search is made for sites of ectopic pancreatic tissue.

Exposure

6 The anterior surface of the pancreas is exposed by entering the lesser peritoneal sac via the gastrocolic omentum. Vessels in the greater omentum are ligated and divided or coagulated using bipolar diathermy, preserving the gastroepiploic and short gastric vessels.

The hepatic flexure of the colon is reflected medially and the duodenum Kocherized to expose the head of the pancreas. The entire pancreas is carefully inspected for the presence of an adenoma, which appears as a reddish-brown nodule on the surface of the grayish pancreas. Suspicious nodules should be excised and submitted for frozen-section histologic examination.

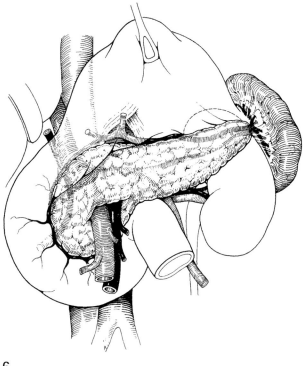

6

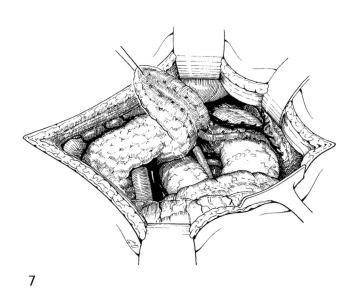

7

Mobilization of the body and tail of the pancreas

7 The tail of the pancreas is carefully dissected out of the hilum of the spleen. The short pancreatic vessels arising from the splenic artery and vein are coagulated with bipolar diathermy and divided. The dissection of the pancreas proceeds medially from the tail toward the neck of the pancreas, which lies just to the right of the superior mesenteric vessels. It is essential for future immunological competence to preserve the spleen. This is accomplished by carefully exposing the short pancreatic vessels passing from the splenic vessels to the pancreas. These vessels, especially the veins, are extremely friable, but with meticulous dissection they can be individually coagulated and divided without traumatizing the main vessels. Should hemorrhage occur from damage to the splenic vein, direct repair of the vein should be attempted. In the event of failure to achieve hemostasis, the main splenic vein can be ligated in the expectation that splenic integrity will be preserved by collateral supply from the short gastric vessels. When the dissection has progressed to the right of the superior mesenteric vessels, attention is directed to the head of the pancreas and, in particular, the uncinate process.

Mobilization of the uncinate process

8 The uncinate process, which can comprise up to 30 percent of the pancreatic weight, lies behind the superior mesenteric artery and vein. These vessels need to be retracted to the left, and the whole of the uncinate process should be carefully and meticulously mobilized, coagulating numerous short feeding vessels. Failure to resect the uncinate process exposes the patient to the risk of recurrent hypoglycemia.

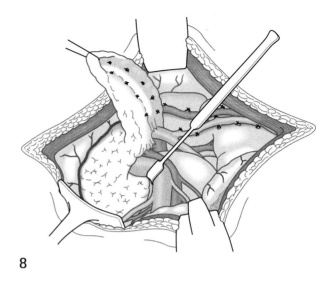

8

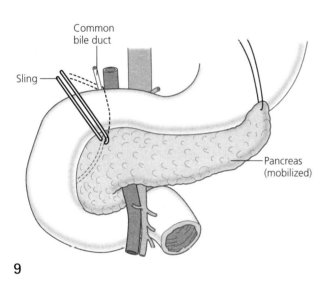

9

Exposure of the head of the pancreas

9 It is essential to define the course of the common bile duct accurately, which may pass through the head of the pancreas or lie posteriorly, either on the posterior surface or in a groove between the pancreas and duodenum. This is best achieved by identifying the common bile duct above the first part of the duodenum and passing a sling around the duct at this point. A blunt forceps is now passed from the undersurface of the first part of the duodenum, within the concavity of the C-loop of the duodenum, behind the duodenum, and then the sling is grasped and passed into the operative field above the head of the pancreas. This will allow the course of the common bile duct to be kept in view during the dissection of the head of the pancreas.

The head of the pancreas can now be mobilized with safety without injuring the common bile duct. The superior and inferior pancreaticoduodenal vessels are ligated and divided to ensure hemostasis when completing the pancreatic resection.

10 The head of the pancreas to the left of the common duct and in the concavity of the duodenal loop is excised, leaving a sliver of pancreatic tissue on the surface of the duodenum and on the left wall of the common duct. The pancreatic duct is identified and ligated with a non-absorbable ligature. Hemostasis is carefully and meticulously achieved. The remaining pancreatic tissue consists of that part of the gland between the duodenum and the common bile duct, and the sliver of tissue on the medial wall of the second part of the duodenum. This represents approximately 5 percent of the total volume of the pancreas. A suction drain introduced via a separate stab incision may be left in the pancreatic bed.

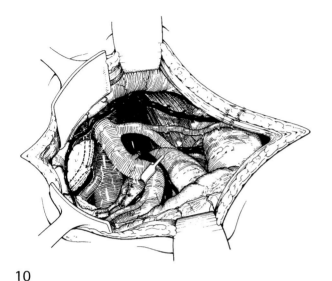

10

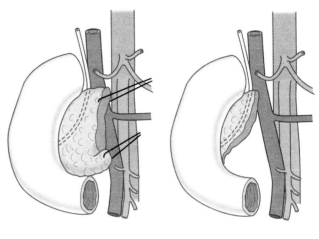

Closure

The wound is closed in layers or with an en-masse interrupted 3/0 polyglycolic acid suture. The subcutaneous fatty layer is closed separately with a running 4/0 absorbable suture. The skin edges are approximated with a 5/0 subcuticular suture.

Focal lesions

A focal lesion located in the body or in the tail of the pancreas is managed by resection of the distal pancreas. A lesion in the head of the pancreas requires resection of the head of the pancreas preserving the common bile duct and restoring pancreatic drainage by means of a Roux Y pancreato-jejunostomy(see laparoscopic section).

LAPAROSCOPIC PANCREATECTOMY

Diffuse CHI: laparoscopic near-total pancreatectomy

11 A 10-mm Hasson port is inserted at the umbilicus by an open technique; this large port allows the retrieval of the pancreas after excision. A 5-mm 30° optic is introduced and the following ports inserted under direct vision: a 5-mm port is positioned into the left lower quadrant, a Nathanson retractor is inserted into the epigastrium, and a further working port (3 mm) is inserted in the right flank.

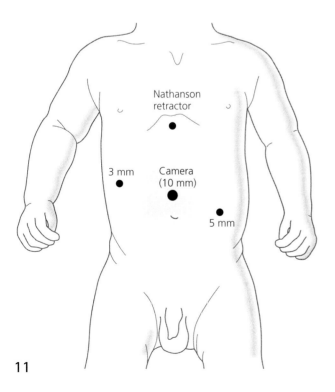

11

12 The gastrocolic omentum is divided using hook diathermy. The lesser sac is entered and the Nathanson retractor is used to retract the stomach cephalad and enable visualization of the pancreas. The head of the patient is elevated to help visualization of the pancreas as this provides gravitational traction on the intestine. A stay suture is inserted into the tail of the pancreas which is used to retract the pancreas superiorly since direct handling of the pancreas results in fracture of this friable organ. The pancreas is dissected from its attachment to the splenic vessels, beginning at the end of the tail with the dissection proceeding towards the body and the head.

The splenic artery and vein are connected to the pancreas via several short vessels. These are divided using a 3-mm hook diathermy at very high coagulation settings and the spleen is preserved. Meticulous dissection and coagulation of these vessels is aided by the magnification provided by the laparoscope and is essential as these vessels are the most common source of intraoperative hemorrhage. When there is hemorrhage from these vessels, gentle pressure to the area can be applied with an atraumatic bowel grasper (e.g. a Johan forceps) and hemostasis can be achieved. The pancreatic tail is resected using the Harmonic Scalpel® (Ethicon Endosurgery, Cincinnati, OH, USA), which avoids bleeding and deep histological damage at the cut surface. The pancreatic tail is removed via the umbilical 10-mm port and sent to the pathologist for intraoperative frozen section to confirm the diagnosis of diffuse CHI. No further resection takes place until this confirmation has been obtained.

Further excision of the pancreas is facilitated by the insertion of a stay suture at the cut surface of the remaining pancreas to allow visualization of the vessels and dissection of the pancreas. The pancreas is resected in segments of approximately 2 cm. Each segment is retrieved through the umbilical port and a new stay suture is inserted in the cut surface of the pancreas as described above. The dissection of the pancreas from the portal vein is facilitated by (1) the anatomical absence of vascular tributaries between pancreas and portal vein and (2) the presence of more space between portal vein and pancreatic parenchyma.

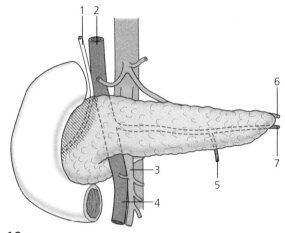

12a

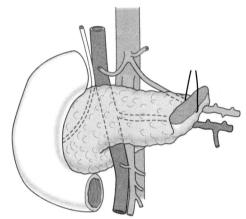

12b

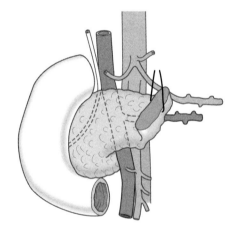

12c

13 To facilitate near-total excision of the head, a stay suture is inserted in the uncinate process and a second one in the remaining head of the pancreas.

14 Both sutures are retracted superiorly and a near-total pancreatectomy is performed by leaving a small rim of pancreas along the medial border of the duodenum where the common bile duct is expected. No abdominal drain is left and port sites are closed using absorbable sutures. A nasogastric tube is left in place; the patient is extubated and returned to the surgical ward.

Focal CHI

In patients with focal CHI, a localized resection of the focal lesion is curative. Prior to surgery, the diagnosis of focal CHI is confirmed using a combination of genetic analysis and findings on ^{18}F-DOPA-PET-CT scan (see illustrations 2 and 3). The site of the lesion seen on PET-CT scan allows preoperative planning of the anticipated procedure. However, it should be noted that the accuracy of localization in PET-CT scan is approximately 70 percent. In proximal lesions in the head and neck of the pancreas, a resection of the lesion with a rim of surrounding normal

pancreatic tissue is carried out and pancreaticojejunostomy is performed to allow drainage of the distal pancreas. In distal lesions, a distal pancreatectomy is performed.

LAPAROSCOPIC RESECTION FOR FOCAL CHI

The open procedure is similar to this operation.

The abdomen is accessed laparoscopically as described earlier. The pancreas is inspected for a nodular area indicating the site of the focal lesion, but this is very rarely present (<10 percent of cases in the authors' experience). In focal CHI, the lesion is often deep within the parenchyma of the pancreas and may not be visually evident. An intraoperative biopsy is performed for frozen section histological examination. Histology may reveal the following: (1) the presence of the focal lesion completely resected (normal pancreas at the resection margin); (2) focal lesion not completely resected; (3) the presence of normal pancreas excluding the presence of diffuse CHI and indicating that the focal lesion has not yet been excised.

FOCAL LESION IN HEAD OR NECK OF PANCREAS

Superficial lesions may be enucleated laparoscopically. When the focal lesion is deep in the head or neck of the pancreas, part of the head and neck are excised and a distal pancreaticojejunostomy is performed.

15 The pancreas is transected distal to the area containing the focal lesion on ^{18}F-DOPA-PET-CT scan. To transect the pancreas, a hook diathermy 3 mm is used and care is taken to avoid an injury to the splenic vein and artery. Once the pancreas is transected, a stay suture is inserted in the proximal pancreas to elevate it and facilitate its dissection from the splenic, superior mesenteric, and portal veins and from the splenic artery. Complete resection of the focal lesion is ascertained by frozen section histology. If necessary, the head of the pancreas is dissected in the direction of the duodenum, carefully avoiding the common bile duct. The head of the pancreas is resected using hook diathermy or Harmonic Scalpel.

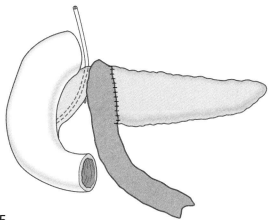

15

16 A pancreaticojejunostomy is then constructed to allow drainage of the distal pancreas. The distal pancreas is dissected free from the splenic vein and artery for approximately 0.5 cm. The first loop of jejunum is brought through the mesocolon and sutured to the inferior border of the transacted distal pancreas using interrupted sutures of Prolene 5/0. The jejunum is opened using monopolar diathermy and the posterior margin of the pancreas is sutured to the jejunum using interrupted Prolene 5/0 and intracorporeal knots. The anterior margin is also sutured to the jejunum using the same material. The laparoscopic magnification and the position of the instruments allow good visualization and anastomosis.

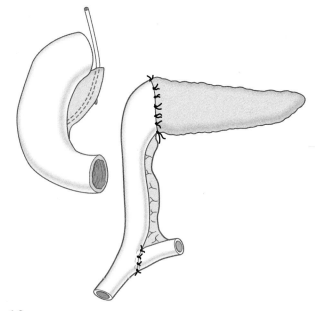

16

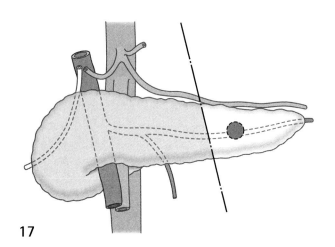

17

FOCAL LESION IN THE BODY OR TAIL OF THE PANCREAS

17 In more distal lesions, a laparoscopic distal pancreatectomy is performed using the same technique for pancreatic dissection as described previously: the dissection is started at the tail of the pancreas and progresses proximally to include the whole focal lesion. An adequate resection margin is confirmed by further frozen section analysis. The pancreas is transected using Harmonic Scalpel. There is no need for drains.

POSTOPERATIVE CARE

Nasogastric decompression and intravenous fluids are continued during the period of postoperative ileus. Blood glucose levels are closely monitored postoperatively, and soluble insulin is administered as required on a sliding scale. Rebound transient hyperglycemia is common in the early postoperative period. Occasionally, more prolonged use of small amounts of insulin is required, but adaptation usually occurs within 3–6 months. In the long term, refractory diabetes mellitus may occur, the control of which may be extremely difficult.

Complications

- Trauma to the common bile duct (10 percent incidence). The defect may be amenable to direct repair. If the duct has been transected, end-to-side anastomosis to the first part of the duodenum should be performed. Late strictures can develop as a result of ischemia.
- Inadequate resection. This will become evident within 48–72 hours of surgery and it is advisable to carry out a further resection at this early stage rather than later, when fibrosis can render the procedure extremely difficult.
- Wound sepsis and adhesion intestinal obstruction.

Note. Careful long-term follow up is necessary to assess the adequacy of pancreatic exocrine function.

FURTHER READING

Al-Shanafey S, Habib Z, Al Nassar S. Laparoscopic pancreatectomy for persistent hyperinsulinemic hypoglycemia of infancy. *Journal of Pediatric Surgery* 2009; **44**: 134–8.

Aynsley-Green A, Polak JM, Bloom SR *et al.* Nesidioblastosis of the pancreas: definition of the syndrome and the management of the severe neonatal hyperinsulinaemic hypoglycaemia. *Archives of Disease in Childhood* 1981; **56**: 496–508.

Cretolle C, Nihoul Fekete C, Jan D *et al.* Partial elective pancreatectomy is curative in focal form of permanent hyperinsulinemic hypoglycemia in infancy; a report of 45 cases from 1983 to 2000. *Journal of Pediatric Surgery* 2002; **37**: 155–8.

Lindley KJ, Spitz L. Surgery of persistent hyperinsulinaemic hypoglycaemia. *Seminars in Neonatology* 2003; **8**: 259–65.

McAndrew HF, Smith V, Spitz L. Surgical complications of pancreatectomy for persistent hyperinsulinaemic hypoglycaemia of infancy. *Journal of Pediatric Surgery* 2003; **38**: 13–16.

Pierro A, Nah SA. Surgical management of congenital hyperinsulinism of infancy. *Seminars in Pediatric Surgery* 2011; **20**: 50–3.

Zani A, Nah SA, Ron O *et al.* The predictive value of preoperative fluorine-18-L-3,4-dihydroxyphenylalanine positron emission tomography-computed tomography scans in children with congenital hyperinsulinism of infancy. *Journal of Pediatric Surgery* 2011; **46**: 204–8.

80

Adrenalectomy

PETER KIM and EMILY CHRISTISON-LAGAY

HISTORY

The first recorded adrenalectomy involved the en bloc removal of a 20-lb tumor from a 36-year-old woman with hirsutism and virilizing features (most probably a malignant adrenocortical carcinoma) by Thornton in 1889. Nevertheless malignant adrenocortical disease is very rare, accounting for less than 0.2 percent of all pediatric tumors and only 6 percent of adrenal tumors. Neuroblastoma is the most common adrenal lesion, accounting for a 50-fold greater number of adrenal tumors than the second most common tumor, pheochromocytoma.

EMBYROLOGY

The adrenal gland is composed of two endocrine tissues of differing embryonic origin, the medulla and the cortex. The chromaffin cells of the adrenal medulla are derived from the neuroectoderm, whereas the cells of the adrenal cortex are derived from the mesoderm. As gonadal tissues may also be traced back to a mesodermal origin and are similarly involved in the synthesis of steroid hormones, inborn enzymatic defects in one tissue are frequently present in the other. This common origin can therefore result in both medical and surgical presentations which involve multiple systems and which may require a multidisciplinary approach to treatment.

The adrenal cortex may be divided into three zones: (1) the zona glomerulosa, the outermost zone of the cortex responsible for the synthesis of aldosterone; (2) the zona fasciculata, the largest of the zones of the cortex, the cells of which produce cortisol; and (3) the zona reticularis, the innermost and smallest of the zones and the producer of adrenal androgens, dihydroepiandrosterone and androstenedione. The adrenal medulla is comprised of neuroendocrine (chromaffin) and glial cells.

Development of the adrenal gland begins between 3 and 4 weeks of gestation just cephalad to the developing mesonephros. At this point, the gonadal ridge has yet to form and there is no distinction between adrenal and gonadal tissue. By 5–6 weeks, however, steroidogenic gonadal cells begin their caudal migration, while those cells that will eventually comprise the zona reticularis migrate dorsally into the retroperitoneum. Over the next several weeks, there is a rapid enlargement of the inner cortex to form the fetal zone (the outer subcapsular rim remains as the definitive zone) and, simultaneously, migrating cells of the neuroectoderm also follow tropic signals to populate the adrenal medulla. These cells will subsequently be responsible for making and storing catecholamines. The fetal adrenal gland is proportionally much larger than that in the adult. At 8 weeks of gestation, the adrenals are larger than the kidneys, at term they are approximately one-third the size of the kidney, with the fetal cortex comprising most of the mass. Within several days of birth, the fetal cortex begins a rapid involution and is half its immediate postnatal size by one month and an eighth of its size by one year. During this time, the medulla begins a slow period of growth. The relative size of the neonatal adrenal gland is thought to contribute to perinatal adrenal hemorrhage (reported incidence 3/100 000 live births). Occasionally, hemorrhage can cause exsanguination and death or present as an abdominal mass, anemia, or scrotal hematoma.

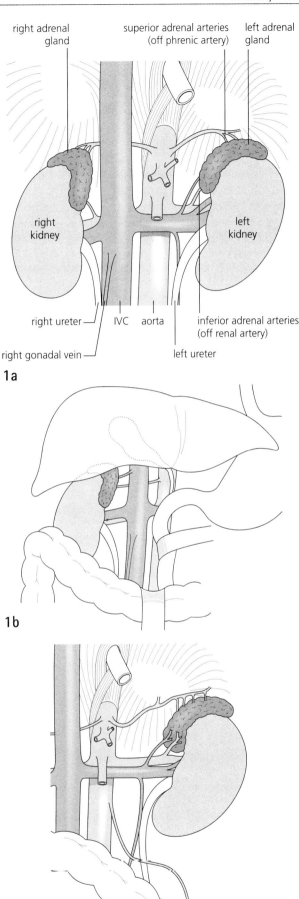

right adrenal gland   superior adrenal arteries (off phrenic artery)   left adrenal gland

right kidney   left kidney

right ureter — IVC aorta — inferior adrenal arteries (off renal artery)

right gonadal vein —   left ureter

1a

1b

1c

ANATOMY

1a–c The adrenal glands are paired but not identical structures that sit superomedially to the kidneys at the level of the 11th thoracic vertebrae. Posteriorly, both glands abut the posterior aspect of their respective hemidiaphragms. The posterior right lobe of the liver serves as the superior surface of the right adrenal and the inferior vena cava (IVC) provides its medial border. The right gland is triangular in shape and slightly smaller and more cephalad than the left. The left adrenal gland is an elongated and flat structure that lies posterior to the splenic vessels and the tail of the pancreas.

The adrenals take their arterial supply from three principle sources: branches of the phrenic artery off the celiac access, direct aortic perforators, and small perforators off the renal artery. As such, there is rarely a distinct adrenal artery, rather the adrenal is supplied by an end vascular arcade from these three sources. During surgical resection, caution must be used to cauterize these arterial sources to minimize intraoperative and postoperative blood loss. On the other hand, venous drainage of the adrenal occurs through a dominant vein. On the right side, this vein empties directly into the posterolateral IVC 3–4 cm above the right renal vein. There may be a smaller accessory right adrenal vein. The left adrenal vein drains into the left renal vein.

During embryogenesis, primordial adrenal cells may migrate caudally with other cells of the gonadal ridge. This migration accounts for the presence of accessory adrenal tissue in the retroperitoneum along the course of descent of the ovaries and testes.

Adrenalectomy

Indications for adrenalectomy include both benign and malignant disease. Benign indications include enlarging or endocrinologically active adrenal adenomas and hormone- or catecholamine-secreting neoplasms, including pheochromocytoma and aldosteroninoma. Malignant indications include neuroblastoma, ganglioneuroblastoma, adrenocortical carcinoma (ACC), and metastatic lesions. A variety of operative approaches exist; selection of any given approach must be individualized according to the adrenal pathology, patient body habitus and previous operative intervention, and surgeon comfort. Traditional approaches to adrenal surgery have included anterior, posterior, and thoracoabdominal techniques. The transabdominal approach is appropriate for large or bilateral tumors, tumors encasing central vascular structures (e.g. neuroblastoma) or for tumors like pheochromocytoma which may also be found in extra-adrenal locations. A complete abdominal exploration may be performed via this approach. The posterior approach is appropriate for resection of small adenomas or aldosterinomas or in patients in whom previous abdominal surgery has rendered the abdomen hostile to further operative approaches. It has the additional advantage of preventing the development of future adhesions and reduces the likelihood of postoperative small bowel obstruction. It is also associated with a shorter functional recovery and shorter hospital stay. Disadvantages include the impossibility of examining the abdominal viscera or contralateral adrenal and the relatively limited exposure in the event of vascular injury. Over the last decade, increasing experience has accumulated with laparoscopic adrenalectomy such that it accounts for greater than 75 percent of adrenal resections in some centers. Ideal candidates for a laparoscopic approach are those patients with a small, well-circumscribed, benign-appearing tumor. Although some authors have reported the successful laparoscopic removal of adrenocortical carcinoma, most surgical oncology authorities consider ACC a contraindication to the minimally invasive approach. Not only does the tumor have the tendency to invade nearby structures but, moreover, rupture of its capsule upstages the disease.

ANTERIOR APPROACH

The anterior approach provides excellent bilateral exposure to the structures of the upper abdomen and is frequently the approach of choice for large, malignant, or bilateral lesions. In a very large or obese patient, intra-abdominal fat and the position of the adrenals high under the dome of the diaphragm may make a thoracoabdominal approach more suitable. Postoperative morbidity is greater than with a posterior or laparoscopic approach with an increased risk of ileus, atelectasis, and incisional discomfort.

RIGHT ADRENAL

2a–e The child should be positioned supine on the operating room table with a roll under the right lower costal margin. A subcostal incision is typically employed and can be extended across the midline (chevron incision) for better exposure, however a midline incision may also be used. Upon entering the abdomen, the hepatic flexure of the colon is reflected inferomedially and a wide Kocher maneuver is performed, exposing the inferior vena cava. An external retractor (Buchwalter, Thompson, or Omni) is helpful to maintain exposure. The right lobe of the liver should be gently retracted cephalad to expose the superior surface of the adrenal gland that should be palpable superomedial to the kidney and lateral to the IVC. Occasionally, a tongue of adrenal can extend posterior to the IVC. The peritoneum overlying the adrenal should be excised to expose it more fully. The lateral border can be mobilized by the application of serial clamps and ties or by electrocautery. As the arterial supply to the adrenal comes from small perforators off the phrenic artery, aorta, and renal artery, the lateral border is relatively avascular. The medial border should then be dissected off of the IVC. Often, this will require a near-complete mobilization of the posterior surface of the IVC, allowing it to be retracted gently to the left. The right adrenal vein is a short, wide vessel that drains directly into the posterolateral IVC. The vein can be easily avulsed resulting in significant bleeding and gentle, careful dissection should be used during its dissection. Once the vein is skeletonized, it should be ligated and divided. Many surgeons place a clip behind the tie on the IVC for additional security. Inadvertent holes in the IVC should be repaired with 5/0 Prolene sutures. Control of the IVC can be obtained if necessary by the judicious use of sponge sticks or by a side-biting Satinsky clamp. The inferior and posterior surfaces of the adrenal are relatively avascular and dissection off the kidney and retroperitoneum can be accomplished by the use of electrocautery. The adrenal tissue itself can be quite friable and vascular and care should be taken during its dissection to avoid too much traction on the tissue which can result in organ fragmentation and bleeding.

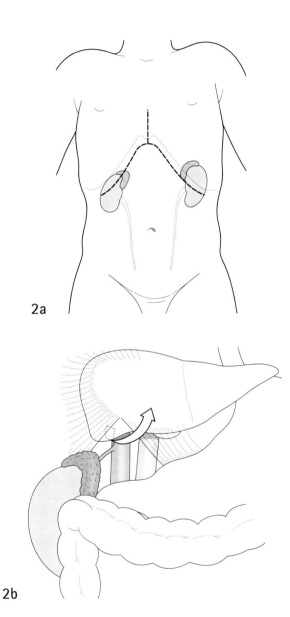

2a

2b

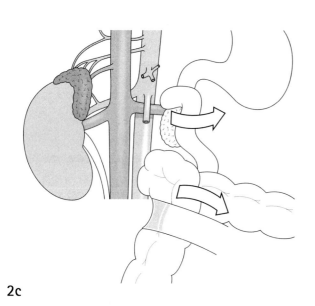

2c

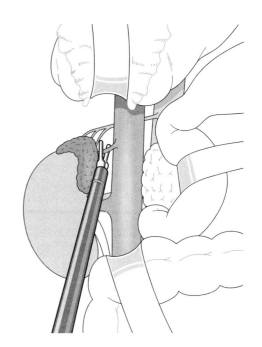

2d

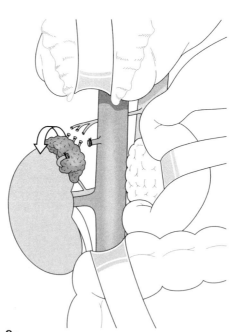

2e

LEFT ADRENAL

3a–c The patient is positioned in a similar fashion to the right adrenal with a roll under the lower left costal margin. Again, the operation is most frequently carried out via a left subcostal incision. Access to the adrenal may be obtained either through reflection of the left colon and splenic flexure or via the lesser sac. In this approach, the gastrocolic omentum is widely divided, taking care to preserve the gastroepiploic arcade supplying the greater curvature of the stomach. Upon entry into the lesser sac, the stomach is reflected superiorly and the peritoneal surface overlying the inferior border of the distal pancreas is incised, allowing the pancreas to be gently retracted cephalad. Downward retraction of the transverse colon typically allows visualization of the left renal vein which may be traced laterally to identify the medial border of the kidney and adrenal. The lienorenal ligament should be divided. Often, this approach requires more complete mobilization of the splenic flexure. Gerota's fascia overlying the superomedial border of the kidney should be incised to expose the adrenal gland which has a bright yellow, bosselated, and slightly grainy appearance. The anterior surface of the left renal vein should be dissected. The gonadal vein which enters the inferior edge of the renal vein is a helpful landmark. The adrenal vein enters the renal vein opposite the gonadal on the superior surface, typically about a centimeter closer to the renal hilum. Mobilization of the adrenal begins by the division of small arterial branches (chiefly supplied by the left phrenic artery) of the medial and superior surface with clips, ties, or the harmonic scalpel. The adrenal vein can now be divided and the stump used for traction to dissect the relatively avascular posterior and inferior surfaces.

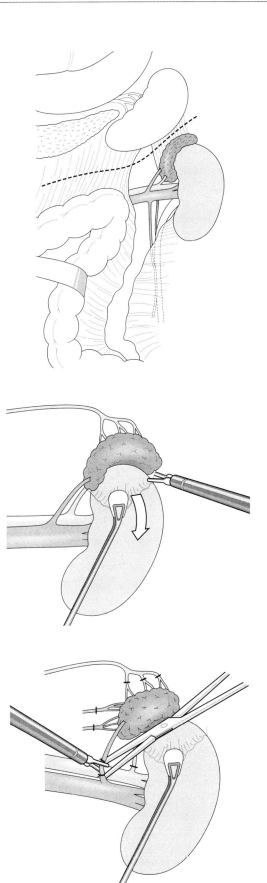

3a

3b

3c

EXPLORATION OF THE RETROPERITONEUM

Given the frequency of extra-adrenal disease associated with some adrenal tumors (i.e. pheochromcytoma), the remainder of the retroperitoneum should be palpated when performing an adrenalectomy. This includes palpation of the para-aortic chain and the organ of Zuckerkandl at the aortic bifurcation. Additionally, the bladder should also be checked for masses.

POSTERIOR ADRENALECTOMY

4a–h The posterior approach to adrenalectomy was described by Young in 1936. The patient is positioned prone on the operating room table with rolls underneath both the chest and hips sufficient to elevate the abdominal wall off the table and allowing the vena cava to fall forward away from the retroperitoneal organs and making the dissection more facile. The table should be angulated (jack-knifed) slightly at the midway point between the anterior superior iliac spine (ASIS) and the costal margin to straighten the curvature of the spine. The earliest surgical description featured a 'hockey stick' incision that extended vertically downward from the tenth rib, paralleling the spine, before curving gently toward the ASIS approximately 2 cm below the costal margin. This incision was then carried through the fascia and the inferior fibers of the trapezius and latissimus dorsi muscle. The attachments of the erector spinae muscle to the 12th rib were divided, the rib resected and the lumbodorsal fascia is divided longitudinally along the lateral margin of the quadratus lumborum to expose the diaphragm. Division of the diaphragm exposed Gerota's fascia.

This incision has been modified and largely replaced by an incision over the bed of the tenth or 11th rib on the right or the 11th or 12th rib on the left. The rib is then resected in the subperiosteal plane as far medial as possible to allow maximal visualization of the adrenal. The supraspinatus muscle defines the medial border of the resection and further visualization may be achieved by medial retraction of the muscle. The underlying pleura is divided in the direction of the rib bed and the lung is then retracted medially with a sponge or padded retractor. Next, the diaphragm is divided exposing the retroperitoneal space and Gerota's fascia is opened superiorly bringing the adrenal into view. Gentle downward traction on the kidney using a sponge stick improves exposure and the placement of a Finochetto retractor frees the assistant's hands for help with dissection.

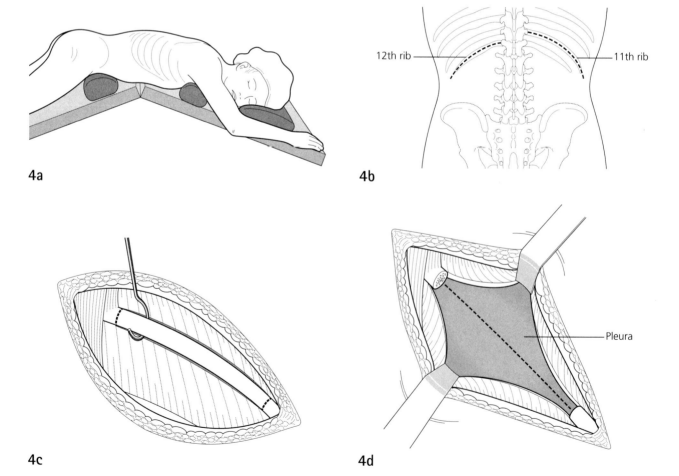

4a

4b

12th rib   11th rib

4c

4d

Pleura

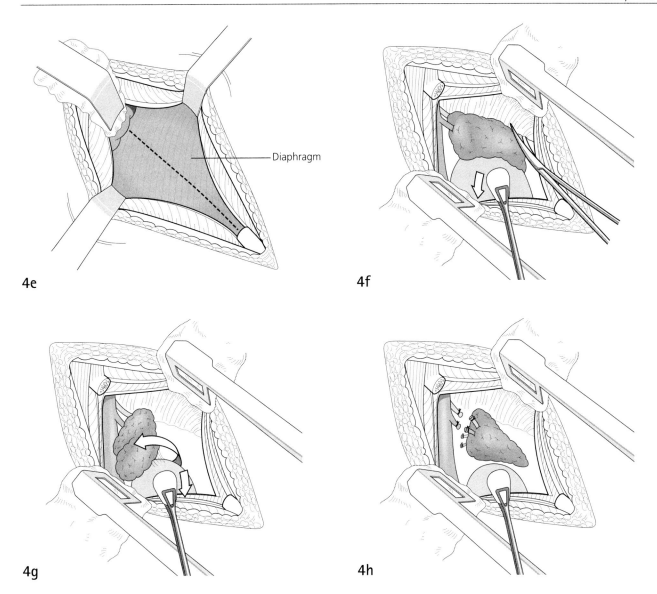

4e

Diaphragm

4f

4g

4h

On the right side, the liver is gently retracted superiorly. Loose adventitial tissue between the adrenal and liver can be carefully dissected. The superior edge of the adrenal is supplied by perforators off the aorta and phrenic artery travelling in an ill-defined vascular 'ligament'. This may be divided by a series of clips and electrocautery or by such tools as the harmonic scalpel. The lateral and inferior aspects of the adrenal are relatively avascular and can often be mobilized with monopolar electrocautery alone. The gland is then rotated medially to expose its anatomic anterior surface and facilitate dissection to its medial caval border. It is then returned to the standard position to expose the medial vascular attachments, most notably the adrenal vein. This is ligated and divided prior to completing the dissection of arterial perforators.

On the left side, dissection also begins with dissection of the superior vascular perforators and may require gentle upward retraction of the pancreatic tail. The lateral borders are next freed (these are largely avascular)

and the gland rotated medially to allow dissection of its anterior (avascular) surface. The adrenal vein can now be found travelling anterior and medial to the upper pole of the kidney where it joins the renal vein. This is suture-ligated and divided, typically exposing the inferior adrenal artery that is also controlled and divided. The final step involves division of the middle adrenal arteries as they enter the medial surface of the adrenal.

A modification of the posterior approach involves a flank approach through the bed of the 11th or 12th rib. In this event, the patient is not positioned prone, but in the lateral decubitus with the hips elevated and the shoulder and hip rotated anteriorly. Subperiosteal resection of the 11th rib allows for a blunt extrapleural dissection in the posterior rib bed. The diaphragm should be divided as far as its insertions at the lumbocostal arch. The peritoneum is visualized and reflected anteromedially exposing the kidney and adrenal. This approach allows excellent exposure of the inferior vena cava and the insertion of the adrenal vein on its posteromedial aspect.

Laparoscopic adrenalectomy

5a–f Laparoscopic adrenalectomy has largely supplanted the open approach for resection of both benign and malignant lesions. Advantages include improved visualization with a magnified view of the operative field, less postoperative pain, and a shorter hospital course. Disadvantages include the need for repositioning for bilateral tumors and the requirement for advanced laparoscopic skills on the part of the surgeon. While the exclusion criteria for laparoscopic adrenalectomy are ever decreasing, it is still relatively contraindicated for large malignant neoplasms or malignancies with potential lymph node involvement.

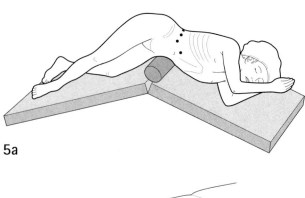

5a

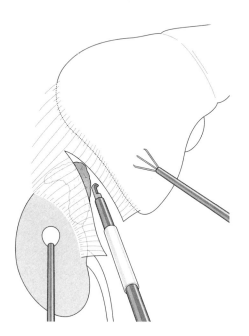

5b

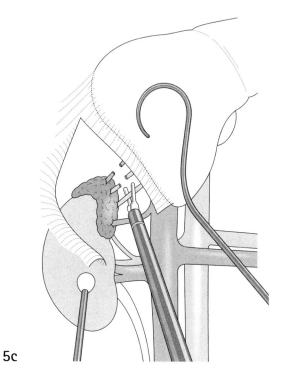

5c

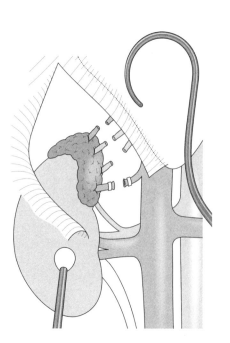

5d

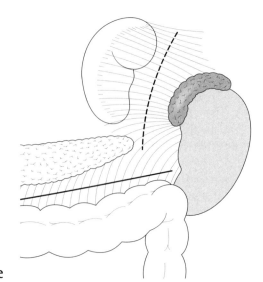

5e

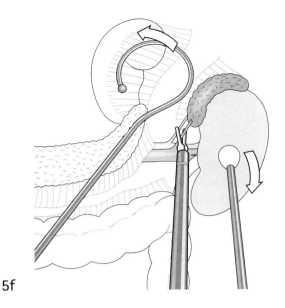

5f

As in open procedures, both transperitoneal and retroperitoneal approaches for laparoscopic adrenalectomy have been described. This chapter will describe the transperitoneal approach.

The patient is placed on a beanbag in the lateral decubitus position. Use of a kidney rest and table flexion at a point halfway between the ASIS and the costal margin opens the space between the iliac crest and the 12th rib. An axillary roll is also put in place. Either the true lateral decubitus or a gentle 15° rotation posteriorly off the true decubitus has been described. The beanbag is inflated. The ipsilateral arm should be supported on a mobile arm rest. The patient can be secured in this position with tape. There is no need for a urinary catheter.

RIGHT

The surgeon stands at the patient's back opposite the surgical assistant. A second assistant (camera holder) may stand adjacent to the surgeon. Typically, four trocars are used for a transperitoneal approach. Position of the trocars may vary slightly based upon patient body habitus. The first trocar (the optical trocar for a 5-mm, 30° scope) is inserted approximately halfway between umbilicus and the iliac crest. A second, operating trocar is placed about 5 cm anteromedial from the optical trocar, in the anterior axillary line. Another operating trochar is placed in the posterior axillary line at the same level. Occasionally, it is necessary to mobilize the right colon prior to placing this port. The fourth trocar is used for liver retraction and is placed medial and cephalad to the optical trocar. In larger patients, this may be placed 8–10 cm caudad to the xiphoid; in smaller patients, a supraumbilical site may be more useful. A triangular or curved liver retractor is placed through this port and secured to a self-retaining instrument holder.

Dissection begins through the lateral ports. Division of the right triangular ligament with L-hook electrocautery or the harmonic scalpel allows for better visualization of the adrenal. The liver retractor is now positioned to allow the right lobe to be retracted superomedially. Division of the lateral duodenal attachments (Kocher maneuver) allows visualization of the IVC. The vena cava is dissected superiorly and inferiorly exposing the right renal vein. The renal vein marks the inferior point of caval dissection. The harmonic scalpel is then used to dissect the peritonealized surface of the adrenal gland laterally, superiorly, and inferiorly. As this dissection progresses, it should be possible to identify the adrenal vein which can be visualized from its point of origin on the posterolateral wall of the vena cava. It should be skeletonized for approximately 1 cm, doubly clipped, and divided. The

lateral positioning of the patient facilitates this dissection. After the adrenal vein is divided, the adrenal should be gently retracted caudally. The gland itself is very friable and retraction should be done by gentle grasp of its peritonealized surface or by the use of laparoscopic Kitners. Occasionally (3–10 percent of cases), an accessory adrenal vein can also be visualized. After transection of the main adrenal vein, dissection should continue along the inferior aspect of the liver (superomedial aspect of the adrenal) to look for an accessory vein. This should be dissected, clipped, and divided. The adrenal is then gently retracted caudally and to the right and dissected along its medial side. Arterial feeders may be clipped and divided or divided. The laparoscopic harmonic scalpel is particularly good for this task. Once the upper pole of the adrenal is free, any remaining superior and lateral attachments of the adrenal may be dissected using hook electrocautery or the harmonic scalpel. The adjacent pole of the inferior medial attachments may contain the arterial supply off the renal artery. These attachments should be dissected carefully and any vessel of moderate size should be clipped prior to division or carefully cauterized using the harmonic scalpel. At this point, the adrenal gland is attached only by loose posterior fibroareolar tissue. Once it is separated from this, it may be placed into an extraction bag and removed from the abdomen. Typically, this will involve increasing one of the port sizes from 5 to 12 mm.

LEFT

The patient is positioned as in a right-sided approach, except with the left side elevated. Again it may be advantageous for the surgeon to work laterally to medially and thus stand at the patient's back. Trocar positioning is also similar with the most medial port located along the linea alba and the most lateral port located at the mid to posterior axillary line. The dissection begins by reflection of the descending colon and splenic flexure off the white line of Toldt and subsequent division of the lienophrenic and lienorenal ligaments. Dissection of the posterior spleen should be carried as far cephalad as the left diaphragmatic crus. The posterior surface of the pancreas may also be lifted off the splenic vein, permitting the spleen, pancreatic tail, and left colon to fall forward and medially. The retracting port can be used to assist in medial retraction of the spleen. The renal vein should now come into view. Gerota's fascia should be opened vertically beginning at the midpole of the kidney and moving superiorly. If the adrenal vein has been clearly visualized draining into the left renal vein, it may be dissected, skeletonized, doubly clipped, and divided at this time. Early division of the vein is especially useful when operating on pheochromocytoma as it disrupts the release of catecholaminergic agents and facilitates better blood pressure control. If it is not visible, dissection along the superior aspect of the perinephric fat at the superomedial edge of the kidney should uncover yellow-orange tissue of the adrenal gland. The adrenal can be dissected along its superior border. This dissection is greatly facilitated by the use of the harmonic scalpel that is able to cauterize small arterial branches from the left phrenic artery and aorta. Gentle antero-inferior retraction of the adrenal with a laparoscopic Kittner permits dissection of its lateral edge. If the adrenal vein has not been yet identified and divided, this should now occur. The final step in the dissection is to free the remaining tissue at the inferior and medial border of the adrenal. Occasionally, two to three small arterial perforators are present at this level supplied by the superior branch of the renal artery. This tissue may be divided by the harmonic scalpel. The free adrenal may now be placed into an extraction bag and removed from the abdomen through an enlarged port site.

CONCLUSION

Many adrenal disorders require adrenalectomy. No one approach is superior to another, but the choice of resection must be tailored to the specific pathologic process at hand, patient anatomy, and surgeon comfort. Laparoscopic adrenalectomy has been shown to be a safe and cost-effective approach to the resection of benign lesions, however, its applicability has not yet been widely broadened to include the resection of malignant lesions other than small neuroblastomas or the rare malignant pheochromocytoma.

FURTHER READING

Guz BV, Straffon RA, Novick AC. Operative approaches to the adrenal gland. *Urologic Clinics of North America* 1989; **16**: 527–34.

Mirallie E, Leclair MD, de Lagausie P *et al*. Laparoscopic adrenalectomy in children. *Surgical Endoscopy* 2001; **15**:156–60.

Rescorla FJ. Malignant adrenal tumors. *Seminars in Pediatric Surgery* 2006; **15**: 48–56.

Romano P, Avolio L, Martucciello G *et al*. Adrenal masses in children: the role of minimally invasive surgery. *Surgical Laparoscopy, Endoscopy and Percutaneous Techniques* 2007; **17**: 504–7.

Skarsgard ED, Albanese CT. The safety and efficacy of laparoscopic adrenalectomy in children. *Archives of Surgery* 2005; **140**: 905–8.

Stewart JN, Flageole H, Kavan P. A surgical approach to adrenocortical tumors in children: the mainstay of treatment. *Journal of Pediatric Surgery* 2004; **39**: 759–63.

Urology

81

Cystourethroscopy

JOHN M PARK

SET UP

One advantage of modern endoscopic procedures is the ability to transmit a clear, magnified image onto a video system (**Figure 81.1**). A high intensity light source, such as halogen and xenon, is necessary for proper illumination. Extreme care must be taken to avoid direct contact between the lighted cable and the patient or surgical drapes because of the intense heat generated. Hazardous fires and burn injuries can result. The patient is placed into a dorsal lithotomy position. In infants, the legs may be simply 'frog-legged'.

CYSTOURETHROSCOPE

The advancement of fiberoptic technology has led to the development of small caliber pediatric endoscopes. The outer sizes vary between 6 and 12 Fr (**Figure 81.2**). Infant resectoscopes have an outside diameter of 8.5 Fr. A variety of electrodes can be fitted for both cutting and coagulative procedures. The male neonatal urethra at full term can usually accommodate an 8.5-Fr instrument. The size is often dictated by the caliber of the urethral meatus. Gentle dilation or meatotomy may facilitate the insertion of scopes. The female urethra can, in general, accommodate between two and four Fr sizes larger than the male urethra.

WORKING INSTRUMENTS

Guidewires are commonly used in endourology. Passage of catheters across ureteric orifices, urethral strictures, and false passages is accomplished over guidewires using the Seldinger technique. There are different diameters, ranging from 0.018 to 0.038 inches (0.64–0.97 mm). The distal tip may be straight or angled. The flexible tip varies in length from 1 to 15 cm. Some have a moveable core wire, which offers varying lengths of distal flexibility. There are several types of coating, the most common being Teflon®.

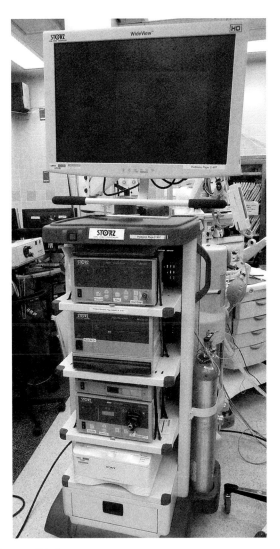

Figure 81.1 Modern video tower fitted with monitor, light source, image processor, and recording device.

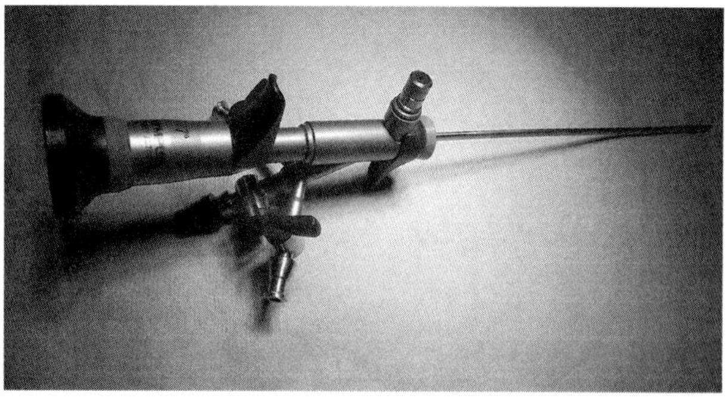

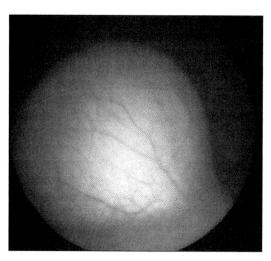

Figure 81.2 7.9 French integrated fiberoptic infant cystoscope.

Hydrophilic polymer coatings (called 'glide wires') decrease the friction of wires, making them useful for negotiating tortuous or narrow lumens. The slippery coating is activated by wetting with water or saline, and it should not be used with lubricant, which increases the friction.

Several cutting and fulgurating electrodes are available, ranging in size from 2 to 5 Fr. The electrical current is dispersed when using saline solution, and thus the irrigant should be either water or other osmotic solution, such as glycine.

CLINICAL APPLICATIONS

Ureterocele

Ureterocele is a congenital obstructive cystic dilation of the submucosal portion of the distal ureter. An intravesical (or orthotopic) ureterocele is contained entirely within the bladder (**Figure 81.3**), whereas an ectopic ureterocele's distal portion is located within the bladder neck or the urethra. Ectopic ureteroceles represent approximately 60 percent of all ureteroceles, are more prevalent in females, and are commonly associated with ureteral duplication. In

ureteral duplication, the ureteroceles belong to the upper pole segment. The management of ureterocele depends on many factors, including the degree of associated ureteral dilatation and obstruction, the function of the associated renal moiety, and lower pole ureter reflux. In many cases, endoscopic decompression using cystoscopy is an appropriate initial approach, especially in infants with urosepsis due to obstruction. Endoscopic decompression can result in secondary reflux, which may require subsequent intervention.

The visualization of a ureterocele is optimal when the bladder is not overly distended. With a full bladder, the ureterocele can efface and flatten, making it difficult to incise effectively. If there is a deficiency of bladder muscle backing at the site of the ureterocele, it will evert, making it look like a diverticulum. If the child is ill with urosepsis, a large transverse incision for definitive decompression is the primary goal, even if it results in secondary reflux. In the absence of clinical infection, a more limited incision or multiple punctures (like a 'watering can') can lead to effective decompression while minimizing the risk of secondary reflux.

Duplication anomalies

Although the true incidence of ureteral duplication is unknown, it is estimated to be approximately 1 in 125. According to the Weigert-Meyer rule of ureteral embryology, the two orifices of a complete duplication seen via cystoscopy are characteristically inverted in relation to the collecting systems they drain (**Figure 81.4**). The orifice to the lower pole ureter occupies the more cranial and lateral position, and that of the upper pole ureter has a caudal and medial position. In general, the lower pole

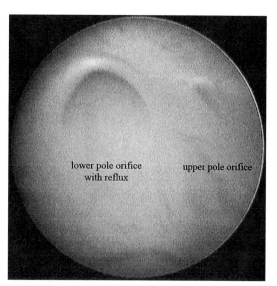

Figure 81.4 Duplicated orifices on the right with refluxing lower pole orifice situated more laterally compared to more medially located upper pole orifice.

Figure 81.3 Intravesical ureterocele.

orifice tends to be associated with vesicoureteral reflux, while the upper pole ureter tends to be ectopic, closer to the bladder neck and proximal urethra.

Posterior urethral valves

Posterior urethral valves (PUV) are the most common congenital urethral obstruction in male newborns. It is often detected *in utero* based on prenatal sonography. Severe obstruction can lead to multiple perinatal issues due to renal failure and oligohydramnios, leading to respiratory and orthopedic problems. A voiding cystourethrogram (VCUG) will confirm the diagnosis, based on the appearance of a severely trabeculated bladder, thickened bladder neck, dilated posterior urethra, and an obstructive lumen change between the posterior and membranous urethra (**Figure 81.5**). Three types of valves have been described classically, although type II is no longer considered valid. Type I valves arise from the verumontanum with a 'spinnaker' appearance to the leaflet (**Figure 81.6**). The visualization of type I valves is best accomplished by filling the bladder to its maximal capacity, positioning the scope near the distal portion of the posterior urethra at the verumontanum, and observing for the obstructing leaflets while the antegrade flow is induced with suprapubic pressure. Type III valves are located distal to the verumontanum and are diaphragmatic in appearance.

Unless the newborn is extremely premature, the standard infant resectoscope with an 8.5-Fr sheath may be used for direct vision valve ablation. The hook blade is well suited for engaging the leaflet of the valves. An optical cold knife, electrosurgical incision, and laser ablation will all work well. The valve leaflets are ablated at the 5 and 7 o'clock

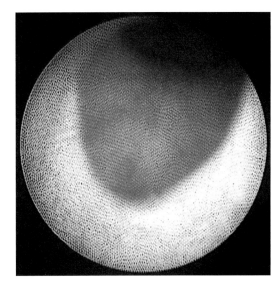

Figure 81.6 Obstructing leaflets of the posterior urethral valves.

positions. Sometimes there are residual obstructing valve remnants anteriorly, which may need additional ablation. For type III diaphragmatic valve obstruction, multiple, stellate incisions are most effective. It is important to avoid injury to the external urethral sphincter located distal to the valves. Although the bladder neck appears obstructive, it should not be incised since it may cause excessive bleeding, urinary incontinence, and future retrograde ejaculation.

Bladder stones

The term 'lithotomy' was coined in BC276 by the Greek surgeon Ammonious of Alexandria. The original Hippocratic oath used to contain a warning to leave the lithotomy procedure ('cutting for stone') to the specialists in this art, making the urologist the first surgical subspecialist. Because of diet poor in animal protein, endemic bladder stones were common until the time of the industrial revolution. Open cystolithotomy was the most common pediatric surgical procedure in the Great Ormond Street Hospital for Children in the 1900s. In modern pediatric urology and surgery practices, bladder stones occur in children with bladder outlet obstruction or neurogenic bladder dysfunction (**Figure 81.7**). In children undergoing enterocystoplasty for augmentation, the lifetime risk of bladder stone formation exceeds 30 percent. They are caused by urinary stasis, mucus production, and bacteriuria. Chronic bladder irritation by stone fragments can lead to future problems such as recurrent infections, hematuria, and malignancy. The removal of all stone fragments is essential to prevent a nidus for stone recurrence.

The cystoscopic removal of bladder calculi is limited by the small caliber of the urethra in young children,

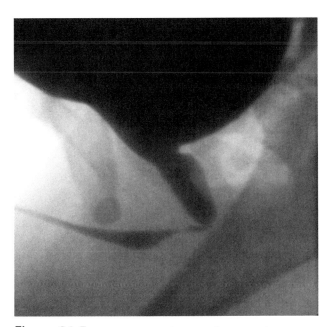

Figure 81.5 Voiding cystourethrogram demonstrating posterior urethral valves.

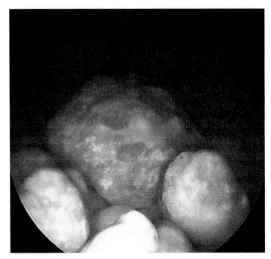

Figure 81.7 Bladder stones in the neurogenic bladder augmented previously with ileum.

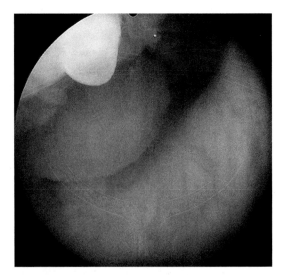

Figure 81.8 Botryoid-type of bladder neck rhabdomyosarcoma.

especially boys. Various forms of intracorporeal lithotripsy have proven to be effective in fragmenting stones. The electrohydraulic lithotripsy (EHL) involves generation of an electrical spark that produces a shock wave and a cavitation bubble for stone fragmentation. Other lithotripsy devices include ultrasonic, ballistic, and various forms of laser. It is important to take extreme caution and avoid direct contact with the bladder wall, as these techniques can lead to iatrogenic perforation. For large or multiple bladder stones, retrieval of numerous stone fragments after lithotripsy can be quite difficult, and thus open cystolithotomy may be preferred. Percutaneous removal of bladder stones has also been described, especially in reconstructed bladders where the urethra has been closed.

Bladder tumor

Approximately 15–20 percent of all pediatric rhabdomyosarcoma arise from the genitourinary system. The most common sites are prostate, bladder, and paratesticular. The rhabdomyosarcoma of bladder and prostate can present with urinary retention and hematuria. Imaging studies and cystoscopy will show a botryoid-type of sarcoma (**Figure 81.8**). In most cases, a cold-cup biopsy through the working channel of the cystoscope will yield the necessary tissue for diagnosis. If the child's urethra is large enough to accommodate the instrument, partial transurethral resection with a loop electrode will provide a generous tissue sample, deep enough for proper examination, as well as relieve obstruction.

Vesicoureteral reflux

Vesicoureteral reflux (VUR) results from a combination of multiple factors, including the functional integrity of ureter, the anatomic status of the ureterovesical junction

(UVJ), and the bladder storage/emptying. In children without bladder outlet obstruction and neuropathic conditions (such as spina bifida and urethral valves), VUR is thought to represent a congenital defect of the UVJ. The abnormal ureter length to diameter ratio of the intramural ureter leads to a failure of the 'flap-valve' mechanism. VUR diagnosis is made by VCUG, which provides a reproducible classification of grading, as well as other pertinent anatomic details that can help in the management decisions. The cystoscopic evaluation of children with VUR is no longer considered a routine part of the diagnostic work up. In the past, the characterization of the endoscopic appearance of the ureteric orifices was incorrectly thought to help in assessing the prognosis. In the modern VUR management, cystoscopy plays a major therapeutic role via subureteric injection. Various materials have been injected, including polytetrafluoroethylene paste, polymimethylsiloxane, and bovine collagen, with varying degrees of success and risk. Currently, the dextranomer-hyaluronic acid copolymer (Deflux®) is the only agent approved by the Food and Drug Administration for endoscopic VUR treatment. The success rate varies in direct proportion to the grade of reflux. Some have reported a short-term success rate of 90 percent in low-grade VUR after a single Deflux injection. The ureteric orifice is hydrodistended with the irrigant aimed at it. The orifice associated with high-grade reflux tends to distend widely, and in these situations, it is recommended to position the needle and inject into the floor of the intramural ureter, followed by a classic subureteric injection to elevate the lower lip of the orifice, causing a 'volcano'-shaped opening (**Figure 81.9**).

Incontinence

Incontinence secondary to anatomic abnormalities, such as congenital neuropathic conditions (spina bifida, sacral

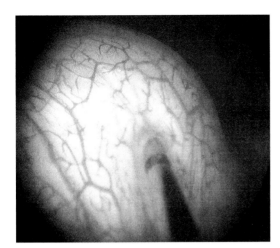

Figure 81.9 Deflux injection.

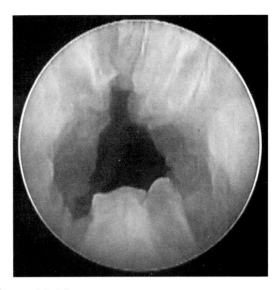

Figure 81.10 Open bladder neck causing incontinence.

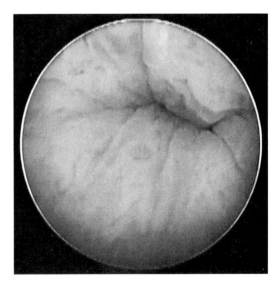

Figure 81.11 Bulging mucosa at the bladder neck after Deflux injection.

agenesis), exstrophy–epispadias complex and bilateral ectopic ureters, requires intervention. Endoscopic implantation of bulking agents is a simple and logical attempt to increase outlet resistance with minimal morbidity. The treatment strategy for incontinence must be developed within the physiological framework of normal bladder function. The hallmarks of a normal lower urinary tract include safe storage pressures, ample capacity, effective outlet resistance that can withstand intra-abdominal pressures, and finally, complete emptying of urine. Incontinence is rarely an isolated matter of inadequate outlet resistance alone. Most of the endoscopic treatment strategies for incontinence have focused on improving the quality of bladder outlet closure mechanism by implanting various bulking agents.

Injection of a bulking agent into the submucosal space of the urethra and bladder neck can be accomplished by two approaches. (1) In the transurethral approach, the injection needle is passed through the working channel of the cystoscope, and the needle is positioned into the submucosa of the bladder neck and proximal urethra under direct vision. The substance is injected slowly, while observing the bulging of the mucosa into the lumen (**Figures 81.10** and **81.11**). In females, the bulking agent may be placed either transurethrally or periurethrally. (2) In the periurethral approach, the injection needle (typically a long 25-gauge) is passed through the anterior vaginal wall to the appropriate submucosal location at the bladder neck, and the injection is performed under direct cystoscopic vision. The general principle is that the closer the injection occurs to the bladder neck and proximal urethra, the more effective the outlet mechanism becomes against stress urinary incontinence.

Recently, endoscopic treatment has been used in selected patients in whom the primary abnormality is one of detrusor dysfunction. In these situations, therapy is aimed at modification of detrusor function to improve bladder storage or emptying. Botulinum toxin A induces a muscle paralysis by blocking the fusion of acetylcholine-containing vesicles with the cell membrane, thereby impeding the release of acetylcholine into the synaptic space. The most common urologic indication has been the injection of botulinum toxin into the external urethral sphincter for the treatment of detrusor–sphincter dyssynergia, primarily in patients with spinal cord injury. More recently, some surgeons have injected botulinum toxin directly into the detrusor muscle to decrease contractility and increase functional capacity.

Urogenital sinus abnormalities and cloacal malformation

Urogenital sinus (UGS) abnormalities are most often seen in intersex cases, now referred as 'disorders of sex development' (DSD). In repairing the UGS abnormalities, certain critical details of the anatomy, including the length of the common UGS channel, the location of the vaginal confluence, its proximity to the bladder neck, the size/number of vaginas, and the presence of a cervix, must be defined (**Figure 81.12**). In patients with CAH (congenital adrenal hyperplasia), endoscopy is usually performed at the time of reconstruction. Some of these female patients will demonstrate a male-like external urethral sphincter with the vagina entering proximal to it in a verumontanum-like structure. As with UGS abnormalities, endoscopy is mandatory to define the anatomy of a cloacal malformation. The goals of endoscopy must include

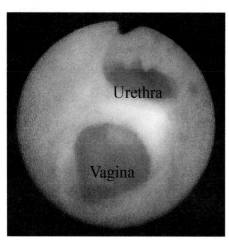

Figure 81.12 Vaginal confluence in a congenital adrenal hyperplasia patient with urogenital sinus abnormality.

identification of the rectal and vaginal confluence. The length of the urethra and its communication with the cloaca are important for reconstructive purposes. Vaginal duplication is frequently seen. The rectal confluence is most commonly located at the level of vaginal confluence.

FURTHER READING

Arndt C, Rodeberg D, Breitfeld PP *et al*. Does bladder preservation (as a surgical principle) lead to retaining bladder function in bladder/prostate rhabdomyosarcoma? Results from the Intergroup Rhabdomyosarcoma Study Group IV. *Journal of Urology* 2004; **171**: 2396–403.

Chertin B, deCaluwe D, Puri P. Is primary endoscopic puncture of ureterocele a long-term effective procedure? *Journal of Pediatric Surgery* 2003; **38**: 116–19.

Dinneen MD, Duffy PG. Posterior urethral valves. *British Journal of Urology* 1996; **78**: 275–81.

Kirsch AJ, Perez-Brayfield MR, Scherz HC. Minimally invasive treatment of vesicoureteral reflux with endoscopic injection of dextranomer/hyaluronic acid copolymer: the Children's Hospitals of Atlanta experience. *Journal of Urology* 2003; **170**: 211–15.

Pena A, Levitt MA, Hong A, Midulla P. Surgical management of cloacal malformation: A review of 339 patients. *Journal of Pediatric Surgery* 2004; **39**: 470–9.

82

Pelviureteric junction obstruction

DAVID A BLOOM, NICHOLAS SY CHAO, HOCK LIM TAN and JULIAN WAN

OPEN PELVIURETERIC JUNCTION OBSTRUCTION

DAVID A BLOOM and JULIAN WAN

PRINCIPLES AND JUSTIFICATION

The pelviureteric junction (PUJ) is the most common site of obstruction in the pediatric upper urinary tract. The PUJ is formed during the fifth week of embryogenesis. Urine flows across it from the kidney and down the length of the ureter by the twelfth week. Flow occurs when renal pelvic pressure exceeds upper ureteral pressure. The pressure gradient is created partly by the hydrostatic force of the filtered urine, but principally by the peristaltic contractions originating in the region of the renal pelvis called the pacemaker and progressing across the PUJ and down the ureter. Hydronephrosis develops either when the PUJ is obstructed or when the normal peristaltic waves are impeded.

Obstruction most commonly results from an intrinsic defect in the smooth muscle layer of the PUJ. External compression and blockage by aberrant renal vessels and adhesive bands occur in one-third of cases, and often a combination of external compression and intrinsic pathology exists. Light microscopy demonstrates that abnormal smooth muscle architecture and increased fibrosis are present in obstructed PUJs. Electron microscopy further shows disruption of the intercellular junctions needed to coordinate the transmission of peristaltic waves.

Incidence, signs, and symptoms

The incidence of obstruction of the PUJ is 1:1000 to 1:2000 live births and it is more common in boys than in girls. The left side is affected in 60 percent of cases, and 5–10 percent of cases are bilateral. In duplex systems, the lower pole moiety is more likely to be obstructed, although both systems can be involved.

Before the use of antenatal ultrasonography became widespread in the 1970s, the common signs and symptoms of PUJ obstruction were abdominal mass, gross hematuria, urinary tract infection, and pain. Antenatal ultrasonography now allows PUJ obstruction to be identified before becoming symptomatic and has increased the detection of asymptomatic obstruction five-fold, whereas the incidence of symptomatic obstruction has remained the same.

Older children and adolescents may have protean manifestations, including failure to thrive, vague sporadic flank and abdominal pain (especially with diuresis), nausea, vomiting, hypertension, and recurrent urinary tract infections. Hematuria or renal parenchymal injury may ensue from only minor trauma.

Particular attention should be paid to infants with other congenital anomalies. Conditions associated with PUJ obstruction include the VACTERL association (vertebral defects, imperforate anus, cardiac anomalies, tracheoesophageal fistula, radial anomalies, and renal dysplasia), contralateral multicystic kidney, and vesicoureteral reflux.

PREOPERATIVE

Imaging studies

Clinically suspected PUJ obstruction should be confirmed by imaging studies. Ultrasonography is non-invasive, radiation free, and well tolerated. Characteristically, the PUJ produces a central lucency, which is the renal pelvis surrounded by communicating dilated calyces. A voiding cystourethrogram is advisable for all patients suspected of obstruction to rule out vesicoureteral reflux and other lower tract causes of hydronephrosis, such as posterior urethral valves. Intravenous pyelography or urography provides excellent anatomic detail, and delayed films will best visualize the PUJ. The low glomerular filtration rate of neonates precludes the use of intravenous pyelography.

Diuretic renal scintigraphy is particularly helpful in diagnosing and quantifying the severity of obstruction. The most common radionuclides are DTPA (^{99m}Tc-diethylenetriamine penta-acetic acid) and MAG-3 (^{99m}Tc-mercaptoacetyltriglycine). A bladder catheter should be inserted in all patients undergoing a renal scan when evaluating obstruction. A full bladder can exert backpressure on the ureters and obscure the results. The scan produces two important results.

1. It determines the percentage of total renal effort contributed by each kidney. A poor or non-functional kidney should be considered for removal rather than repair.
2. The time it takes for half the radionuclide to wash out of the kidneys after administration of diuretic ($t_{1/2}$) is calculated. A $t_{1/2}$ of more than 20 minutes is most commonly associated with obstructed systems. Recent studies in infants with antenatally detected hydronephrosis suggest that an elevated half-time alone may not always be associated with clinically significant PUJ obstruction.

Advances in digital imaging algorithms allow computed tomography and magnetic resonance imaging to produce excellent images in the sagittal and coronal planes in addition to the traditional transverse images. These allow excellent visualization of renal anomalies, such as horseshoe kidney, although their cost limits their widespread use. Computed tomography involves sizable doses of radiation and for children magnetic resonance urography (MRU) is an attractive alternative. Dynamic gadolinium control enhanced MRU has been shown to be promising. It offers the same data of renal scintigraphy (percent function and $t_{1/2}$), as well as a clear depiction of the kidney, pelvis, and ureter. MRU is more expensive and requires young patients to be anesthetized to avoid motion artifact. Poor renal function further restricts the use of gadolinium.

Alternatives to pyeloplasty

The aims of surgery are to improve drainage of the PUJ, relieve symptoms, improve the hydronephrosis, and prevent renal deterioration. For these reasons, significant obstructions are best repaired promptly.

The management of PUJ obstructions detected by antenatal ultrasonography, but remaining asymptomatic in the infant and young child, has evolved over the past several decades. Many newborn kidneys continue to grow and develop normally, despite imaging studies consistent with mild PUJ obstruction.

Our understanding of PUJ obstruction and the methods used to identify it remain imperfect. In the presence of active symptoms and signs, such as urinary tract infection, nausea, vomiting, stone formation, or declining renal function, surgical treatment is an obvious choice.

Endourological techniques used for the treatment of ureteral calculi have been adapted to the treatment of PUJ obstruction. The obstructed segment is incised and dilated through either a percutaneous or retrograde approach, and is left to heal over an indwelling stent. Reports suggest that this method may be useful in older children after previous failed pyeloplasty, but we believe it has proven to be unsuitable for infants and children perhaps due to the smaller diameter of the ureter and the relatively larger size of the instruments currently available. Other constraints include large redundant pelves and crossing vessels.

Laparoscopic pyeloplasty has proven its worth in adults and has been applied to children and infants. The techniques are evolving and are discussed in Chapter 82b.

OPEN OPERATION

The technique described is dismembered pyeloplasty. Unlike methods using flaps and advancements, it excises the pathologic segment and may be applied to a variety of anatomic configurations.

Anesthesia

General anesthesia with endotracheal intubation is required and epidural catheterization is helpful, reducing the total amount of general anesthesia used and providing pain relief postoperatively. The epidural catheter should run along the back away from the ipsilateral side. Postoperatively, care must be taken to check regularly on the site for signs of infection and to be sure that the patient is adequately turned and repositioned regularly, as decreased sensation may favor pressure effects on the skin.

Instruments and equipment

In addition to a pediatric major surgery tray, fine forceps, magnifying loupes, 5- and 8-Fr feeding tubes, hooked and pointed scalpel blades, needle point electrocautery, and 3/0 to 6/0 synthetic or biologic absorbable suture with atraumatic needles should be available. While the choice of suture varies greatly among surgeons, permanent synthetic or biologic sutures (e.g. silk or Ethibond™ polyester suture; Ethicon Inc.) should not be used because they can become nidi of infection and stone formation.

Cystoscopy and intraoperative retrograde pyelography ensures there are no other regions of ureteral narrowing. This step can be skipped if a previous imaging study has cleared the length of the ureter.

Position of the patient

1 After intubation, a Foley catheter is placed and the patient is positioned. With the patient in the lateral decubitus position, the surgeon should stand facing the patient's back, with the assistant opposite. Padding and support should be placed under all pressure points. A kidney roll and axillary roll are also placed. The kidney rest is elevated and the table flexed. In small children, a modified anterior approach can be employed, with a small roll under the ipsilateral shoulder and thoracic side.

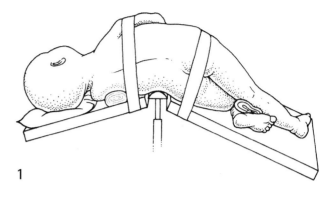

1

Incision

2 A supracostal, extrapleural flank approach is preferred. The skin incision is made astride the distal 12th rib and extended anteriorly following the natural skin creases towards, but short of the umbilicus. The external oblique and internal oblique, the latissimus dorsi, and the anterior edge of the serratus posterior muscles are divided until the periosteum of the rib is exposed. Other approaches include dorsal lumbotomy, anterolateral muscle splitting, and anterior transperitoneal. Lumbotomy allows direct access to the renal pelvis, but creates a scar that crosses normal skin folds, and there is limited mobility of the kidney should further maneuvers be necessary. The muscle-splitting approach is suitable in infants and young children, with a modified anterior position. A supine transperitoneal approach is useful when access to the abdominal contents or the contralateral kidney is required. It is also useful when the PUJ obstruction is only one part of a larger urinary tract reconstruction (e.g. augmentation cystoplasty and PUJ obstruction repair). When performing a reoperative pyeloplasty consideration should be given to either an alternative approach or extending the incision anteriorly beyond the current scar to allow entry into a pristine area so the subsequent dissection will be easier.

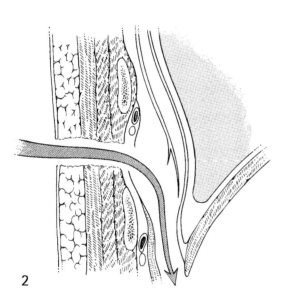

2

Releasing the diaphragm

3 Entry into the retroperitoneum is made at the rib tip and extended posteriorly along the superior edge of the rib. The intercostal muscles should be carefully taken off the rib, keeping above the rib to avoid the nerves and vessels. The diaphragmatic fibers are freed from their attachment to the rib using sharp dissection. The translucent pleura falls away as the diaphragmatic fibers are released. The assistant on the ventral side of the patient often has a better view. Patience and gentle dissection allow the fibers to move away naturally. The peritoneum anteriorly is carefully peeled away from Gerota's fascia and retracted to allow for more working room.

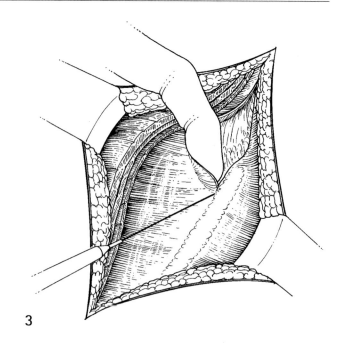

3

Kidney mobilization

A self-retaining retractor may aid exposure. Gerota's fascia is opened longitudinally and the overlying fat dissected away, taking care not to strip the renal capsule, which may be adherent. Patients who may have had renal leak or a decompressive nephrostomy tube also have an inflamed, scarred layer of fat. If possible, the dissected fat as a single layer should be maintained, as it will be useful at the end of the case. Small blood vessels are coagulated. Branches and tributaries of the renal vessels around the anterior hilum should be sought. It is rarely necessary to skeletonize the vessels. The kidney should be mobilized sufficiently to expose the renal pelvis. The kidney can be held either by a well-padded retractor or by an assistant's hand. Displacing the kidney out of the depths of the incision may improve exposure, but exaggerated positions should be avoided because of the stretch imposed on the renal vessels and the risk of thrombosis. In reoperative cases, approaching along the posterior aspect may be the safest way to begin mobilization; the hilum will be directly anterior with no major vessels to encounter before the pelvis.

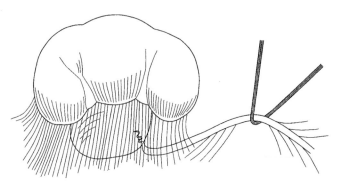

4

Identifying the ureter

4 The ureter is identified and traced toward the kidney. Care should be taken to avoid stripping away the supporting adventitial vessels. One should be careful on the left side not to confuse the gonadal vessels, which can have a similar course. Fine stay sutures and vessel loops are used to manipulate the ureter gently; the authors avoid grasping the pediatric ureter with forceps. Aberrant vessels, particularly those near the lower pole of the kidney, should be identified, teased away, but not divided.

Preparing the renal pelvis and dividing the PUJ

5 The PUJ is identified and the overlying fat and other attachments cleared away. The type of PUJ (for example, high insertion) encountered, presence of crossing vessels, or other findings causally related to the obstruction should be carefully observed and documented. The ureter is divided just below the PUJ and controlled by a stay suture. If cystoscopy and retrograde pyelography were not performed prior to surgery, the ureter should be intubated to ensure no distal narrowing. The ureter should be gently moved to check that adequate length has been mobilized. If insufficient length is available, further mobilization is necessary. Stay sutures are next placed on the renal pelvis at points lateral, medial, inferior, and superior to the PUJ to define the extent of the pyeloplasty.

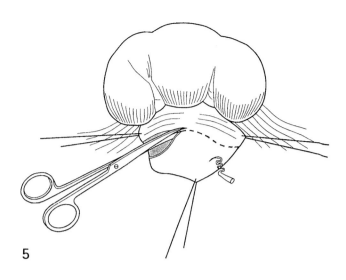

5

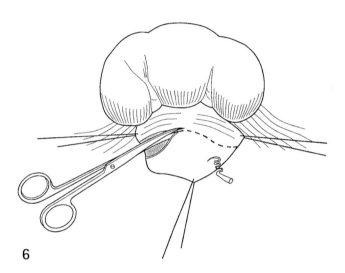

6

Excision of the PUJ and spatulation of the ureter

6 Traction is applied to the stay sutures to splay the decompressed renal pelvis flat. One smooth cut is made using sharp tissue scissors; repeated cuts tend to result in saw-tooth, jagged edges. A sharp hooked or pointed scalpel may be used instead of scissors. Irregular tags should be carefully trimmed. It should be borne in mind that if the patient has had a history of pyelonephritis or an indwelling nephrostomy catheter or stent, the wall of the pelvis might be thick. Additional pelvis may be excised if needed to reconfigure it easily into a funnel-shaped pyeloplasty. Debris or calculi are irrigated from the kidney. The course of the ureter is studied and noted. It is spatulated along the side that will be most likely to fit the lower extent of the pelvis without resulting in a twist or torsion of the ureter.

7 At this point, the authors consider a nephrostomy tube and ureteral stent. Neither is necessary for uncomplicated pyeloplasty, but intubation is a useful reassurance in difficult cases, floppy kidneys, revisions, or very redundant pelves. These can be ready made or adapted from feeding tubes and small-caliber (10–12 Fr) Malecot catheters.

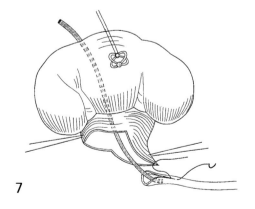

7

Anastomosis

8 The anastomosis should begin at the caudal end, where the lower lip of the renal pelvis meets the spatulated apex of the ureter. The first suture (6/0 or 5/0 in older children and adolescents) is placed at the apex and the next two sutures are positioned closely on either side. The length of the anastomosis should be ideally at least 1 cm; it can be longer in older children. For infants and small children, the practical limits of the slack on the ureter and the reach of the pelvis often determines how long the anastomosis can be. A running or interrupted technique completes the process. Sutures should advance up the posterior wall and then up the anterior wall, keeping each bite even so that the tissue is equally distributed and bunching does not occur. When the end of the ureter has been reached, suturing continues until the pelvis is closed.

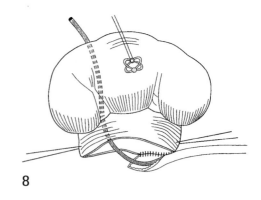

8

Fat wrap

A tongue of fat freed from Gerota's fascia is carefully but loosely wrapped around the anastomosis and secured by stitching it to itself. A small open drain should be placed in the region of the repair. Tubes are brought out through a separate stab incision. If no stents and nephrostomy tubes are used, a drain is mandatory.

Wound closure

The incision is closed in layers, with care taken to reapproximate the muscles. Local anesthetic can be infiltrated along the intercostal nerves for postoperative comfort. All tubes and drains should be securely sewn to the skin.

Postoperative care

The patient should take no solids overnight. Ice chips and sips of clear liquids may be possible if there are bowel sounds. The bladder catheter is removed the following morning and the diet advanced slowly. If the flank remains dry, the drain may be removed in the next day or so. If the repair is intubated, the tube should be left in place for 3 weeks, after which the stent may be removed and a nephrostogram performed if a nephrostomy had been placed. If no drainage is seen flowing down the ureter, the tube should be left to drainage for a further 2 weeks and the test repeated. If contrast flows across the repair, the tube may be removed. Follow-up renal scans and ultrasonography or intravenous pyelography are arranged three to six months after surgery.

COMPLICATIONS

The principal complication is stenosis of the anastomosis. Fortunately, this is rare and 90–95 percent of cases are successful. Although the repaired kidney may never look

normal on ultrasound scan or intravenous pyelogram, due to persisting hydronephrotic distortion, it should function and drain normally on follow-up diuretic renal scan.

Special situations

COMBINED PUJ AND VESICOURETERAL REFLUX

Patients who present with both vesicoureteral reflux and ipsilateral PUJ obstruction can be confusing. High-grade vesicoureteral reflux can distort the appearance of the PUJ. One should ask is the dilation of the renal pelvis due to the reflux or is it a separate concern? In these cases, the surgeon should first determine if it is truly an obstruction. Diuretic renal scintigraphy will rule out most cases of pseudo-PUJ obstruction. When obstruction has been established, the PUJ obstruction should be repaired first, and the reflux addressed later. Repairing the reflux first risks making the obstruction worse and jeopardizes the kidney.

DUPLEX SYSTEMS

Obstruction is most commonly found in the lower pole moiety of duplex systems. The open pyeloplasty technique described above may be used, but the surgeon must be careful to identify and isolate the appropriate ureter. If a particularly long obstruction is found, ureteropyelostomy or a pyelopyelostomy may be advantageous.

Horseshoe kidneys

In horseshoe kidneys, the ureter often inserts high into the renal pelvis; a longer, more caudally placed anastomosis is needed. Division of the isthmus is usually not necessary. A Y–V flap advancement style of pyeloplasty may be useful in some anatomic configurations but a dismembered pyeloplasty can usually be done.

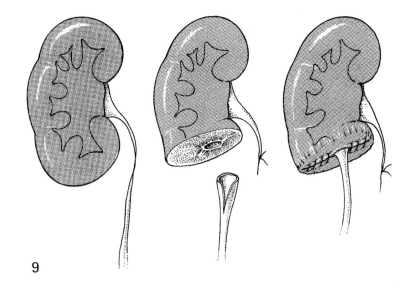

URETEROCALYCOSTOMY

9 If the renal pelvis is too small, intrarenal, or too fibrotic to achieve dependent drainage, an ureterocalycostomy may be necessary. The principal features of this rare procedure are the selection of the most dependent calyx and a thorough amputation of the lower pole of the kidney to prevent postoperative compression.

9

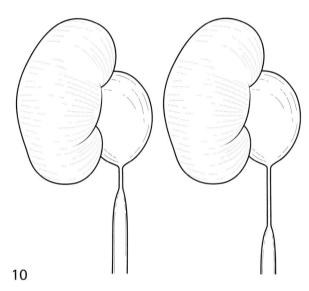

10

FLAP PYELOPLASTY

10 Usually the area of stenosis is short and the pelvis and normal ureter are in very close approximation. If there is a long stenotic ureter segment, before disconnecting the ureter the surgeon should be sure that an anastomosis can be done without tension. If the stenotic segment is 2 cm or longer attempts should be made to fully mobilize the kidney and ureter. If an anastomosis cannot be done without tension, a flap pyeloplasty should be considered.

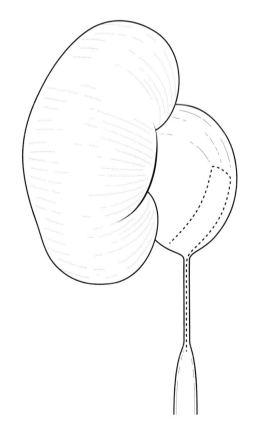

11 The stenotic segment and the flap should be carefully measured and marked out so that they will closely match. The incision should completely open up the stenotic portion. The flap should be equal to the length of the segment. The flap can be straight or curve around the contour of the pelvis as needed. Stay sutures should be used to help orient and control the flap and ureter. They will also help obviate the need to pick up the ureter and flap with forceps. For clarity, these are not shown in the accompanying illustrations but are very helpful in determining proper orientation and length. The width of the flap should be about the circumference of the normal ureter.

11

12 Incise the flap using a fresh hooked (a No. 12 scalpel) or pointed blade. Rotate the flap down and carefully sew the lateral edge to the incised ureter. Interrupted or running 6/0 sutures can be used. If a running stitch is used, consideration should be given to placing an interrupted suture at the distal end. This will help line up the edges to prevent bunching and spiraling of the running stitch.

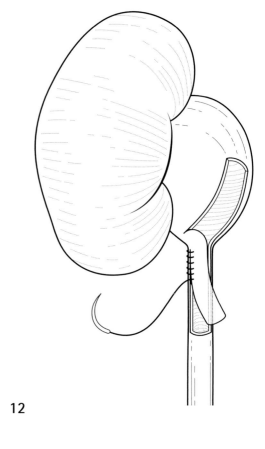

12

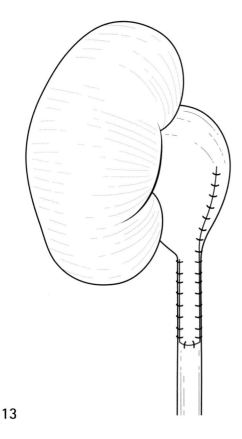

13

13 The anterior edge of the flap should be closed with a similar stitch. A stent and nephrostomy tube are advisable in addition to the usual Penrose drain. The stent should be left in for 1–2 weeks.

ILEAL URETER

In some situations, the gap is too long to bridge by mobilizing the kidney and distal ureter. This is usually observed in patients who have already undergone extensive surgery or trauma resulting in a long atretic ureter. In such patients, an interposition of a piece of prepared ileum is an option. On the right side, an appendiceal interposition may prove to be very useful. This interposition should be placed so that the normal peristaltic course is directed toward the bladder.

LAPAROSCOPIC DISMEMBERED PYELOPLASTY

HOCK LIM TAN and NICHOLAS SY CHAO

INTRODUCTION

There are two groups of patients that present with ureteropelvic junction (UPJ) obstruction. Those that present in the older age will usually require surgical intervention, whereas the prenatally diagnosed hydronephrosis, which constitutes the larger proportion of patients, may not require surgery. The challenge for pediatric urologists is to identify those that warrant early surgical intervention against the majority of congenital hydronephrosis which resolve and can be safely observed.

In general, there are very few indications to perform a pyeloplasty in a newborn given that the condition has existed antenatally. It is best to wait a few weeks until the newborn kidney has developed the ability to concentrate urine, at around 44 weeks' gestation, as early functional evaluation may lead to misleading results on the MAG3 scan.

Laparoscopic Anderson Hynes dismembered pyeloplasty is one of the most technically challenging of operations and requires meticulous attention to every detail.

PATIENT SELECTION

In infants, significant impairment of renal function with gross delay in excretion and severe hydronephrosis are indications for pyeloplasty. Increasing hydronephrosis with evidence of progressive deterioration of renal function is an indication.

Older patients usually present with clinical symptoms of obstructive uropathy and may include recurrent abdominal pain with vomiting.

CONTRAINDICATIONS

Laparoscopic Anderson Hynes dismembered pyeloplasty can be successfully performed with good functional results in the very young. However, this operation is recommended in smaller babies only if the surgeon (1) is very adept at laparoscopic suturing and (2) has appropriately sized ureteric stent and appropriate laparoscopic 'needlescopic' instruments.

Laparoscopic pyeloplasty can also be performed on horseshoe kidneys. Pelvic ectopic kidneys cannot be approached laparoscopically, as the ureteropelvic junction is completely obscured from view.

Children presenting with intermittent obstruction with an intrarenal pelvis which only distends when obstructed presents a special challenge because the renal pelvis will retract into the renal sinus once opened, unless the surgeon ensures that the pelvis is transfixed with a 'hitch stitch' before the renal pelvis is opened.

APPROACH

Transperitoneal versus retroperitoneal

The retroperitoneal approach is popular for performing nephrectomies and heminephrectomies having the supposed advantage of avoiding intraperitoneal adhesions. There is no statistical difference in the outcome of the intraperitoneal versus extraperitoneal route. The authors prefer the transperitoneal route for pyeloplasty as it provides a much larger working space and better ergonomics, especially for fine intracorporeal suturing.

Small incision combined with laparoscopic/retroperitoneoscopic assisted mobilization

While conventional open pyeloplasty via small lateral or posterolateral incision is often feasible in small infants because of their normally lower-lying kidneys, a 'small incision' approach may be modified for older infants and children using combined laparoscopic or retroperitoneoscopic mobilization.

Laparoscopic mobilization of the renal pelvis may be performed using a single- or two-port technique, either transperitoneally or retroperitoneally. The renal pelvis may then be exteriorized via an extended small incision, and open Anderson-Hynes dismembered pyeloplasty can be performed in the standard fashion. Comparable functional and cosmetic outcomes have been reported.

THE TRANSPERITONEAL LAPAROSCOPIC PYELOPLASTY

Instrumentation and telescopes

It is not necessary to have an extensive range of laparoscopic instruments. It is preferable to use a few, selected, good instruments. A short 5-mm 30 degree telescope provides adequate illumination and resolution to allow one to perform very delicate suturing. The authors use 3-mm, 20-cm 'needlescopic' instruments for infants and young children. While finer needlescopic 2-mm instruments are widely available, the authors' experience with these is that they have limited tissue grip, provide insufficient leverage, and are easily bent. Avoid using long instruments in young children. The limited internal working space in a child results in long instruments protruding excessively, leading to exaggerated movements with instrument clash.

Preoperative preparation and general considerations

Informed consent should be obtained for transperitoneal or conventional dismembered pyeloplasty. An enema to evacuate stool from the left colon should be administered, especially for left-sided pelviureteric junction obstruction (UPJO). While some authors advocate the insertion of a stent preoperatively, it has not always been found to be helpful as it only leads to complete decompression of the renal pelvis, making it more difficult to mobilize the pelvis and ureteropelvic junction. The stent may also become entangled with the suture, making an already challenging task more difficult. It is the authors' preference to insert an antegrade stent as an intraoperative procedure, after completion of the posterior anastomosis. A transurethral Foley catheter should be inserted before the patient is positioned.

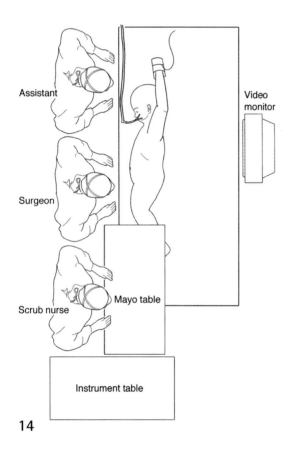

14 The patient, surgeon, assistant, and scrub nurse should be positioned as per floor plan. This is the most ergonomic position.

14

Patient positioning

15 The patient should be positioned at the edge of the table tilted at about 45° lateral decubitus. It is important to ensure that the hips are not flexed, otherwise the legs will impede the manipulation of instruments. The patient should be secured to the table.

A circumumbilical incision is then made in the periumbilical skin crease down to the linea alba about 1 cm cephalic to the umbilical cicatrix, and the linea alba grasped between two hemostats and incised. The peritoneum can be easily identified deep to this and opened. A purse string is placed around the linea alba and a 7-mm Hasson port inserted and secured by tightening the purse string around it.

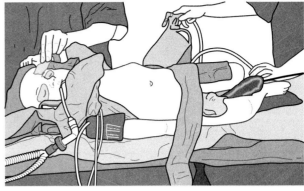

15

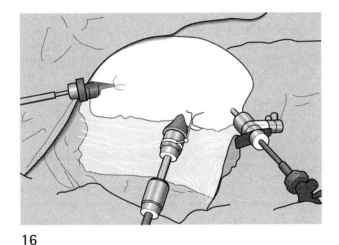

16

16 Port positions are critical for pyeloplasty. It is not possible to perform a satisfactory intracorporeal anastomosis if the needle driver is not in line with the intended line of anastomosis. This means that the suturing port should be placed as close to the mid-line as possible.

Only two instrument ports are used for the procedure, a 3.5- and a 6-mm port, which is necessary to pass the laparoscopic suture into the abdomen. The 6-mm instrument trocar should be the right-handed port, unless the surgeon is left handed in which case port placement should be reversed.

In infants less than 7 kg, it is possible to perform the operation without the use of instrument ports by passing the instruments through the abdominal wall.

17a The first step of the operation is to detach the colon from the kidney and Gerota's fascia. It is important to identify the correct tissue plane. The renal capsule is covered by a thin film of loose adventitia and it is important to be deep to this plane, keeping absolutely snug on the renal capsule. The plane is developed medially into the sinus where the renal pelvis should then be easily identified. The renal vein may be exposed during this maneuver.

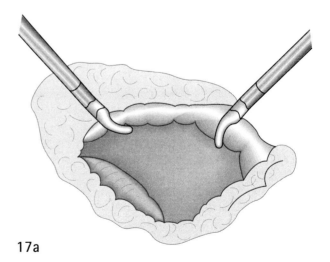

17a

17b The ureteropelvic junction can usually be identified at this point.

The gonadal vessels are usually located near the ureteropelvic junction. Once the UPJ is identified, the ureter should be mobilized gently by lifting it out of its bed to develop a small window to hold it up. Minimal mobilization of proximal ureter is performed to preserve the vascular supply. The renal pelvis is mobilized more extensively, sweeping the renal vessels towards the upper pole. This is usually a bloodless procedure if you are in the correct plane. Clear about 2 m of renal pelvis above the upper limits of your intended pyelotomy.

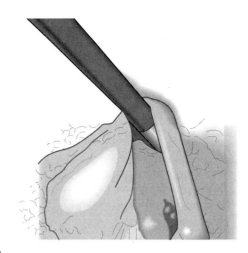

17b

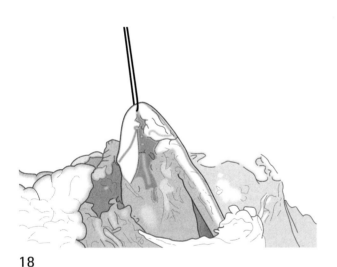

18

18 At this point, a 4/0 monofilament suture on a straight needle is then passed through the anterior abdominal wall at the mid- or posterior axillary line just below the costal margin and grasped from the inside with a laparoscopic needle holder. The renal pelvis should be transfixed about 1–2 cm above the intended upper limits of the pyelotomy and the needle then passed through the abdominal wall near its insertion point. The renal pelvis can then be lifted out of its bed by this hitch stitch, displaying the ureteropelvic junction in full view. A pair of hemostats is applied to both ends of the hitch stitch on the outside to stabilize the renal pelvis for the duration of the pyeloplasty.

It is important to leave a good length of the suture on the outside, as it may be necessary to loosen the hitch stitch, if the anastomosis is under tension. A second hitch stitch should not be placed on the proximal ureter as this makes for a more difficult anastomosis because of suture clash and may even distract the ureter from the renal pelvis.

It is important at this stage to spend a few minutes to clear the renal pelvis and proximal ureter of any loose connective tissue before dividing the UPJ, otherwise the ureter will retract within the sleeve of connective tissue making for a difficult anastomosis. It is also important at this point of the operation to follow the proximal ureter down to ensure that the obstruction is not caused by a crossing lower pole vessel.

19 With the ureteropelvic junction now stabilized by the hitch stitch, the most dependent part of the pelvis is identified and opened. Only the anterior wall of the renal pelvis is then divided along the entire length of the intended pyelotomy. The posterior wall of the pyelotomy, especially the superior portion, should be left intact at this point.

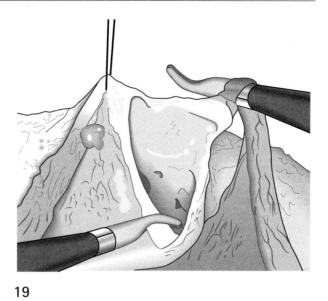

19

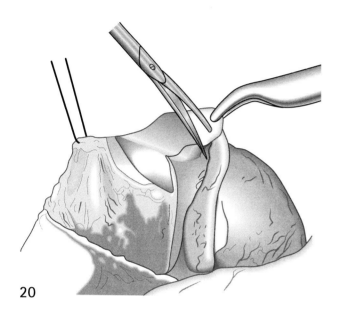

20

20 The UPJ should not be completely dismembered, as the attached posterior wall makes it much easier to spatulate the ureter, as the ureter can be stabilized by applying countertraction between the partially divided pelvis.

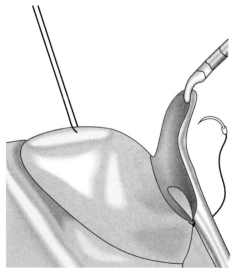

21a

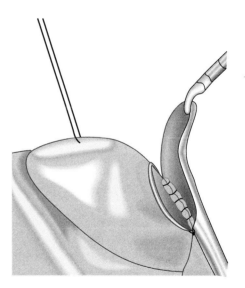

21b

21a,b The first suture should be placed at the angle of the spatulated ureter which is then attached to the most dependent part of the renal pelvis as in open pyeloplasty. The posterior wall of the renal pelvis is only dismembered after the ureter is reanastomosed to the renal pelvis.

The redundant pelvis still attached to the ureter should not be trimmed. This redundant pelvic tissue can be

grasped with impunity to manipulate the ureter during the anastomosis, without handling the mucosa. The posterior anastomosis is completed as a continuous suture. The anastomosis should then be inspected internally by opening up the ureter by applying countertraction on the redundant renal pelvis still attached.

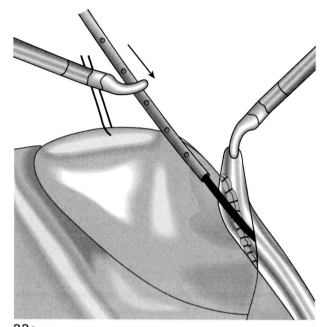

22a

22a–c The antegrade stent should then be inserted at this point. A 19 Fr Teflon sheathed needle is inserted through the anterior abdominal wall just in front of the hitch stitch and in line with the ureter, and the Teflon sheath passed down to the ureterovesical junction, over a guidewire. It is best to use a hydrophilic coated 'slippery wire'. The guidewire is removed when the Teflon sheath is positioned at the ureterovesical junction and 1–2 mL of sterile water soluble lubricant (KY jelly) is squirted into the distal ureter. The guidewire is then reinserted into the Teflon sheath and passed into the bladder. Some resistance will be felt when the guidewire passes through the uterovesical junction (UVJ). The Teflon sheath is then removed and a well-lubricated JJ stent is passed over the guidewire and introduced into the bladder. It is best to pass the entire length into the bladder leaving only a single loop proximally, to ensure that the distal end is in the bladder.

The previously inserted Foley catheter will prevent the stent from migrating into the urethra. It should be possible to express one or two drops of urine after withdrawal of the guidewire by suprapubic compression, to check that the distal end is in the bladder. The redundant renal pelvis can be grasped to exert countertraction on the pigtail when passing it through the UVJ, taking the tension off the posterior anastomosis. The proximal end of the pigtail catheter is then introduced into the renal pelvis, and the redundant renal pelvis is then trimmed and discarded.

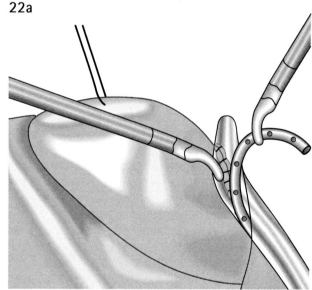

22b

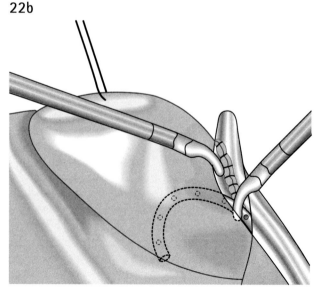

22c

23 The anterior anastomosis is completed with a 5/0 or 6/0 continuous PDS suture, starting at the top of the pyelotomy down to the angle of the spatulated ureter and tying the loose end of the previously completed posterior anastomosis. The anastomosis is then inspected after the hitch stitch is removed and the pelvis and ureter returned to its bed, ensuring that it is not kinked.

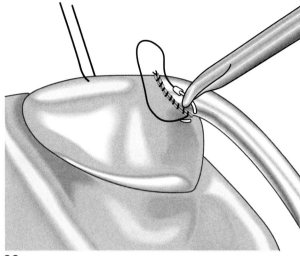

23

POINTS OF TECHNIQUE

Patients presenting with intermittent UPJ obstruction with predominantly intrarenal pelvis presents a special challenge as the intrarenal pelvis can severely restrict the surgeon's ability to manipulate the laparoscopic instruments. It requires the patient to have a fluid load and frusemide to produce maximum diuresis. The surgeon should wait for maximal distention of the renal pelvis before placing the hitch stitch to lift the renal pelvis away from the hilum. Under no circumstances should the ureteropelvic junction be divided before the renal pelvis is transfixed as this will result in the pelvis retracting into the depths of the hilum making suturing impossible.

Crossing lower polar vessels are easily identified laparoscopically without the need for computed tomography (CT) imaging. If the pathology is an aberrant lower pole vessel, it will be necessary to completely dismember the ureter from the pelvis in order to transpose the vessels, but spatulate the ureter before dismembering the UPJ.

On completion of pyeloplasty, tilt the patient's head up to allow the urine to drain into the bony pelvis where it can be aspirated. The patient is then tilted away from the surgeon, the bean bag supporting the back removed and the patient placed as supine as possible. The colon is then remanipulated into its original position. The peritoneal incision will then be completely covered by the colon, leaving no raw surfaces. There is no need for a perinephric drain.

LAPAROSCOPIC TRANSPOSITION OF LOWER POLE CROSSING VESSELS: THE 'VASCULAR HITCH'

Crossing lower pole renal vessels have been implicated in the etiology of UPJO in up to 30 percent of cases.

Conventional surgical treatment in these cases is standard dismembered pyeloplasty, Hellström's nephroplication, or transposition of lower pole crossing vessels may be performed laparoscopically in selected patients. This may be an attractive surgical alternative as it eliminates the need to violate the collecting system, thus avoiding the potential anastomotic complications, and is also less challenging than performing fine intracorporeal suturing.

The crossing lower pole vessels should be plicated to the renal pelvis cephalad from the UPJ by imbricating the redundant pelvis over the vessels with two or three absorbable sutures.

ROBOTIC PYELOPLASTY IN CHILDREN

Allowing seven degrees of freedom and stereoscopic field of vision, robotics overcomes some of the restrictions of laparoscopic surgery and has become popular for pyeloplasty. However, it suffers from lack of haptic feedback and the surgeon is completely dependent on visual cues. At present, the smallest robotic instruments are 5 mm and the minimum distance required between the robotic instruments required for the 'endowrist' to function adequately precludes robotic pyeloplasty from the younger age group.

Conventional laparoscopic pyeloplasty remains the preferred operation for the competent laparoscopists.

FURTHER READING

Anderson JC, Hynes W. Retrocaval ureter: a case diagnosed pre-operatively and treated successfully by a plastic operation. *British Journal of Urology* 1949; **21**: 209–14.

Bomalaski MD, Hirschl RB, Bloom DA. Vesicoureteral reflux and ureteropelvic junction obstruction:

association, treatment options and outcome. *Journal of Urology* 1997; **157**: 969–74.

Casale P. Robotic pyeloplasty in the pediatric population. *Current Opinion in Urology* 2009; **19**: 97–101.

Cascio S, Tien A, Chee W, Tan HL. Laparoscopic dismembered pyeloplasty in children younger than 2 years. *Journal of Urology* 2007; **177**: 335–8.

Culp OS, DeWeerd JH. A pelvic flap operation for certain types of ureteropelvic obstruction: observations after two years' experience. *Journal of Urology* 1954; **71**: 523–9.

Gundeti MS, Reynolds WS, Duffy PG, Mushtaq I. Further experience with the vascular hitch (laparoscopic transposition of lower pole crossing vessels): an alternate treatment for pediatric ureterovascular ureteropelvic junction obstruction. *Journal of Urology* 2008; **180**: 1804–32.

Hendren WH, Radhakrishnan J, Middleton AW Jr. Pediatric pyeloplasty. *Journal of Pediatric Surgery* 1980; **15**: 133–44.

Kavoussi LR, Meretyk S, Direks SM *et al.* Endopyelotomy for secondary ureteropelvic junction obstruction in children. *Journal of Urology* 1991; **145**: 345–9.

McDaniel BB, Jones RA, Scherz H *et al.* Dynamic contrast-enhanced MR urography in the evaluation of pediatric hydronephrosis. Part 2: anatomic and functional assessment of ureteropelvic junction obstruction. *American Journal of Roentgenology* 2005; **185**: 1608–14.

Rassweiler JJ, Teber D, Frede T. Complications of laparoscopic pyeloplasty. *World Journal of Urology* 2008; **26**: 539–47.

Scardino PL, Prince CL. Vertical flap ureteropelvioplasty. *Southern Medical Journal* 1953; **46**: 325–31.

Tan HL. Laparoscopic Anderson-Hynes dismembered pyeloplasty in children using needlescopic instrumentation. *Urologic Clinics of North America* 2001; **28**: 43–51.

Tan HL, Najmaldin A, Webb DR. Endopyelotomy for pelvi-ureteric junction obstruction in children. *European Urology* 1993; **24**(1): 84–8.

Valla JS, Breaud J, Griffin SJ *et al.* Retroperitoneoscopic vs open dismembered pyeloplasty for ureteropelvic junction obstruction in children. *Journal of Pediatric Urology* 2009; **5**: 368–73.

83

Nephrectomy and partial nephrectomy

IMRAN MUSHTAQ

OPEN NEPHRECTOMY

HISTORY

The first successful nephrectomy was performed by the German surgeon Gustav Simon on August 2, 1869 in Heidelberg. An account of the events leading up to the operation and this most extraordinary surgeon is provided by Moll and Rathert. The patient was a 46-year-old washerwoman who had undergone a hystero-oophorectomy for an ovarian cyst. Due to adhesions, she had suffered damage to the ureter and following multiple failed attempts to stem the flow of urine from the wound, Simon decided that the only remaining option would be to remove the kidney. In animal experiments, he proved that one healthy kidney could be sufficient for urine excretion. The operation was performed through a flank incision using the retroperitoneal approach. The operation was completed in 40 minutes, with only 50 mL blood loss. On August 8, Simon performed a second nephrectomy, this time for urolithiasis, which was also successful. Simon pioneered scientifically orientated thinking in urology and paved the way for future developments in reconstructive procedures.

Partial nephrectomy is designed to remove only diseased tissue from the kidney and leave intact the maximum amount of renal substance. Partial nephrectomy may be considered as a radical procedure (tumors) or may rank as conservative surgery (duplex renal systems) according to the disease process under treatment. In children, a partial nephrectomy is usually performed in the context of duplex renal anomalies where either the upper or lower renal moiety demonstrates diminished function in the presence of obstruction or reflux. Partial nephrectomy for childhood renal tumors is discussed elsewhere. Historically, the first partial nephrectomy is widely attributed to Czerny in 1889, but in 1884 Wells had performed a partial nephrectomy to remove a perirenal lipoma. Following these early reports,

the procedure languished until it was revived in the 1940s as a practical method for treating localized tuberculous disease of the kidney.

PRINCIPLES AND JUSTIFICATION

Approach

There are several approaches for renal surgery in children. The flank or lateral approach is derived from experience in adults, but most pediatric surgeons and urologists favor the anterior muscle-splitting extraperitoneal approach. This approach gives excellent exposure of the kidney through a relatively small skin incision, and is suitable for nephrectomy and partial nephrectomy for benign diseases. In addition, it gives a very acceptable cosmetic outcome.

The transperitoneal approach, favored for oncological procedures, should be considered in cases of xanthogranulomatous pyelonephritis or when it is anticipated there will be dense scarring around the kidney and renal hilum. This approach has the advantage of providing rapid access to the renal hilum and major vessels. Inevitably, the choice of approach will also be influenced by the surgeon's experience and training.

In this chapter, only the anterior muscle-splitting extraperitoneal approach will be discussed.

Indications

NEPHRECTOMY

The most common indications for nephrectomy or nephroureterectomy in modern pediatric practice include congenital poorly functioning dysplastic kidney, reflux-associated nephropathy and in some centers, multicystic dysplastic kidney. Less common indications include the following:

- pelviureteric junction obstruction with loss of function;
- congenital nephrotic syndrome causing intractable protein loss;
- pretransplant in children with focal segmental glomerulosclerosis.

PARTIAL NEPHRECTOMY

The most common indication for partial nephrectomy in a child is a poorly functioning upper moiety of a duplex kidney. In such instances, the upper pole may be dilated due to an obstructing ureterocele or there may be a small dysplastic upper moiety with ectopic insertion of the distal ureter into the urethra or vagina. Less frequently, a lower pole partial nephrectomy is required when there is reduced lower moiety function with significant vesicoureteric reflux and/or recurrent urinary infections.

PREOPERATIVE

The preoperative preparation always includes a detailed review of all relevant radiological investigations. This includes the most recent renal ultrasound, a DMSA and/or MAG3 scan and in most cases, a micturating cystourethrogram. The information gained from these investigations confirms the correct side for surgery and allows for planning the length of the incision, the extent of ureterectomy, and whether the ureter requires ligation or transection alone.

Preoperative blood tests should include serum creatinine, hemoglobin level, and a group and save of serum. Clotting parameters do not need to be checked routinely, unless there is a history of bleeding disorders.

All children should be administered a single dose of intravenous antibiotic, either prior to leaving the ward or at the induction of anesthesia.

OPERATION

Anesthesia

Endotracheal intubation is required in all cases for general anesthesia. Perioperative and postoperative analgesia is provided by pre-emptive local infiltration of the incision with 0.25 percent bupivocaine.

NEPHRECTOMY

Position of patient

1 The patient is positioned supine with the affected side raised with a cotton wool or gel-filled support. The ipsilateral arm is placed across the chest and the head is turned to the contralateral side. The incision for the anterior muscle-splitting approach extends medially from the tip of the 12th rib towards the umbilicus. The length of

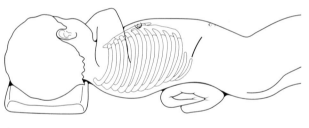

1

the incision ranges from 3 cm in infants to 5–6 cm in older children. The planned incision should be marked with an indelible surgical marker prior to skin preparation. The exposed anterior and lateral aspects of the abdomen are prepared and draped in a sterile manner.

Surgical access

2 The skin incision is made along the line previously marked. Monopolar diathermy is used to deepen the incision, dividing Scarpa's fascia and exposing the underlying external oblique muscle. Using Kilner cat's paw retractors to lift the edges of the skin and subcutaneous tissue, the wound is undermined in a circumferential manner to expose a broad area of the external oblique muscle, particularly in a posterior direction. Monopolar diathermy or scissors can be used for this dissection. This maneuver is essential for achieving good exposure of the kidney through a relatively small skin incision.

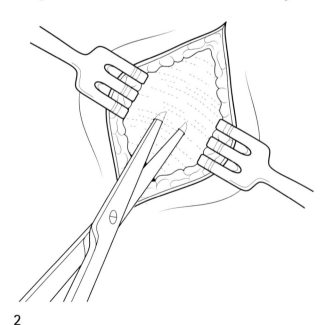

2

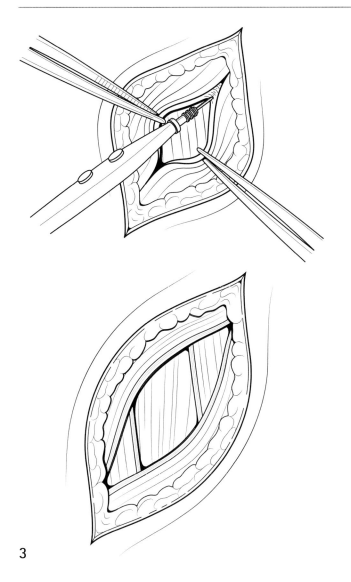

3 Monopolar diathermy is used to split the external and internal oblique muscle layers, along the line of the muscle fibers, to expose the underlying transversus abdominis muscle. Once again, the muscle layers are undermined to expose a broad area of muscle. Care is taken to identify and preserve the neurovascular bundles.

3

4 Commencing posteriorly to avoid entering the peritoneal cavity, the transversus abdominis muscle is split gently with scissors and retractors. Using the index fingers of both hands, the peritoneum is swept medially moving in a posterior direction until the vertebral column can be palpated. A self-retracting or hand-held retractor can be used to display the kidney beneath Gerota's fascia. Gerota's fascia is entered with scissors and the opening enlarged with the index fingers of both hands. The surface of the kidney should be easily identifiable beneath the perinephric fat.

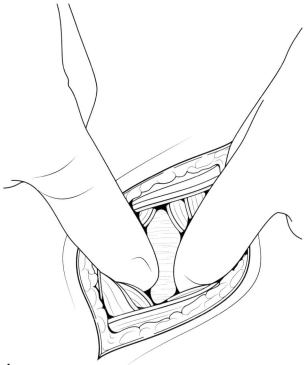

4

5 The perinephric fat is then dissected by both blunt dissection and bipolar diathermy to expose the hilar vessels and ureter. The vessels should be individually isolated, ligated, and divided. The arterial supply should be divided first. In the case of small dysplastic or multicystic dysplastic kidneys, the entire vascular pedicle can be ligated and divided together.

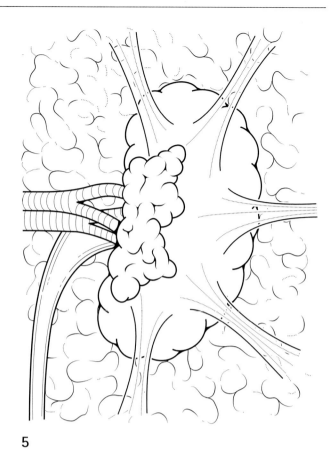

5

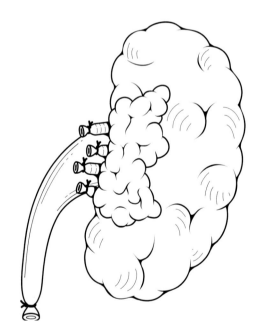

6

6 Once the vascular pedicle has been divided, the kidney is mobilized on all surfaces and delivered from the wound. The attached ureter is then traced distally as far as possible (usually the level of the pelvic brim) and divided. In the absence of ipsilateral vesicoureteric reflux, the distal ureter can be safely left open without postoperative bladder drainage Alternatively, the ureteric stump can be open and urethral catheter be left *in situ* for 48 hours.

7 The wound is inspected to ensure secure hemostasis and then closed in layers. A continuous absorbable suture is utilized for the three muscle layers, an interrupted suture for Scarpa's fascia and a continuous subcuticular suture for the skin. Local anesthetic infiltration of the wound is customary at the end of the procedure.

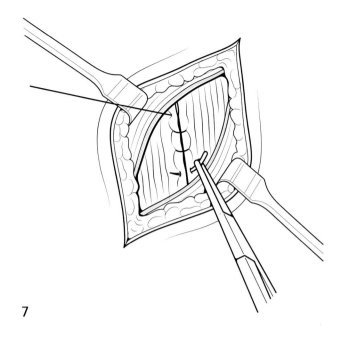

7

PARTIAL NEPHRECTOMY

The room set up, patient positioning, and the steps for surgical access are exactly the same for a partial nephrectomy as they are for a nephrectomy. In particular, the position of the patient and the incision site are identical. This applies whether an upper or lower pole partial nephrectomy is to be performed.

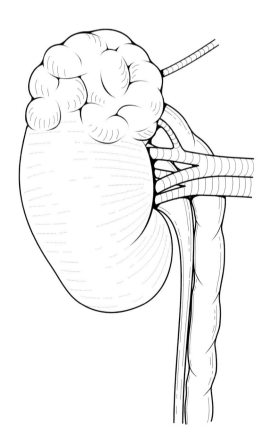

8 Once the wound has been opened and Gerota's fascia has been incised, the dissection proceeds to expose the anteromedial surface of the kidney and display renal hilum as for a nephrectomy. It is mandatory to visualize clearly both upper and lower moiety ureters from the outset, as this will confirm the anatomy and provide a guide to the vascular supply to both renal moieties. The vessels supplying the affected moiety are individually identified, ligated, and divided. Often, particularly in relation to the lower renal moiety, there are short segmental vessels originating from the main vessels close to the renal hilum.

8

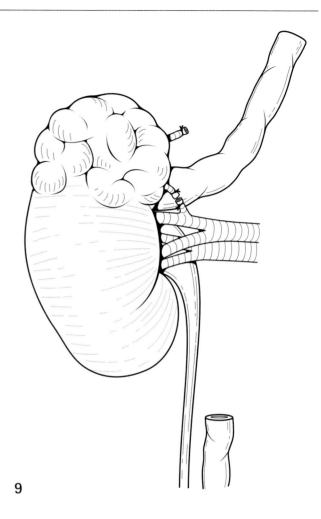

9 The ureter from the affected moiety is separated from the unaffected moiety ureter and divided just distal to the pelviureteric junction. The proximal stump of this ureter is lifted cranially, rotating it laterally to expose the posteromedial surface. There may be additional vessels supplying the affected moiety, which only become evident with this maneuver. These should be ligated and divided. Maintaining the dissection plane close to the wall of the transacted ureter allows access into the renal sinus between the two collecting systems.

9

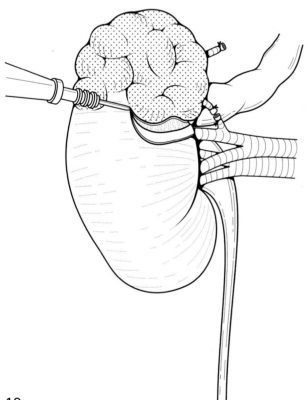

10 Once the vascular supply to the affected moiety has been divided, there will be purplish discoloration of the parenchyma indicating hypoperfusion. This will serve as a guide to the line of resection through the renal parenchyma. The renal capsule is scored with monopolar diathermy at the junction between the two moieties.

10

11a,b The affected moiety is excised with monopolar diathermy, and control of bleeding is achieved with a combination of gentle manual compression, cautery, and suture ligation. Mattress sutures of a 3/0 or 4/0 braided absorbable suture are placed to approximate the cut surfaces of the renal parenchyma. Pledgets of perirenal fat or Surgicel® (oxidized, regenerated cellulose) can be used to facilitate hemostasis and to prevent the suture cutting through the renal parenchyma.

The distal ureteric stump should be removed as far distally as possible. Care must be taken to clearly visualize the ureter from the unaffected moiety, especially in the pelvis where they lie within a joint vascular sheath. The ureter should be ligated in all cases with documented vesicoureteric reflux into the affected ureter.

The wound is closed in the same manner as for a nephrectomy. There is no need for the routine placement of a wound drain or urethral catheter.

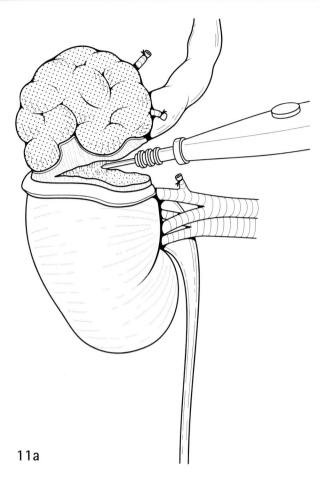

11a

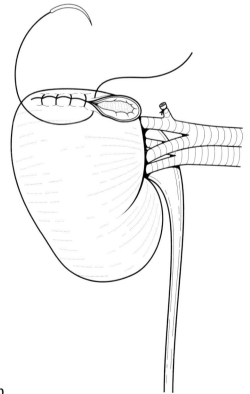

11b

POSTOPERATIVE CARE

In the immediate postoperative period, particular attention needs to be paid to the possibility of hemorrhage. The patient should be kept well hydrated and the blood pressure and pulse monitored closely. Oral fluids and milk/diet can be commenced on return from the operating room. Children undergoing partial nephrectomy are at risk of developing postoperative pyrexia and intravenous antibiotics may need to be given postoperatively if this occurs.

Most patients can be mobilized the day after surgery and discharged once they are stable and any pain is well controlled with oral analgesics.

Complications

URINE LEAK

A retroperitoneal urinoma can occur from the reflux of urine from the distal ureteric stump or from the cut surface of the kidney following partial nephrectomy. The risk can be minimized by careful attention to the possibility of entering the collecting system during transection of the renal parenchyma. When this occurs, the defect should be closed and if necessary a double-J stent could be left *in situ*. Most urinomas will, however, resolve with the placement of a urethral catheter for at least 48–72 hours. A persistent urine leak or an infected urinoma may require the placement of a percutaneous wound drain.

ATROPHY OF THE REMNANT RENAL MOIETY

This complication can occur as the result of vasospasm or a traction injury to the renal pedicle. In some cases, where there is documented fever in the postoperative period, loss of function can be the result of a pyelonephritic episode in the renal remnant. Prevention of this complication is the most important factor, as recognition is extremely difficult in the postoperative period. The loss of function will often go unrecognized until the child attends for routine follow-up investigations.

LAPAROSCOPIC NEPHRECTOMY

HISTORY

Laparoscopic procedures for the treatment of benign renal conditions in children are gradually replacing open procedures. Nephrectomy, heminephrectomy, and nephroureterectomy have now become standard procedures by laparoscopy in centers where expertise is available. The transperitoneal approach was initially popular due to the familiarity of surgeons with laparoscopic gastrointestinal surgery. After the landmark publication of Gaur describing the retroperitoneoscopic approach, it has found favor with many surgeons. Regardless of the approach utilized, the benefits to the child in terms of a faster postoperative recovery and improved cosmesis are without question.

Laparoscopy has also paved the way for novel techniques for managing children with end-stage renal disease who require bilateral native nephrectomy. These children can undergo retroperitoneoscopic nephrectomy, which maintains the integrity of the peritoneum and thereby allows for immediate postoperative peritoneal dialysis. Hemodialysis can therefore be avoided.

PRINCIPLES AND JUSTIFICATION

Approach

Every pediatric urologist should be familiar with the possible approaches for laparoscopic renal surgery in children. The choice is essentially between a transperitoneal and a retroperitoneoscopic approach, with each having its own merits. Although the transperitoneal approach was believed to be better for beginners, it has largely been replaced by the retroperitoneoscopic approach. The retroperitoneoscopic approach avoids colonic mobilization, the risk of injury to hollow viscera, and the potential risk of adhesion formation. However, it is believed to be more difficult to master, due to the reversed orientation of the kidney and hilum with the patient in a prone or semi-prone position. Another possible advantage of the retroperitoneoscopic approach is reduced postoperative pain due to the absence of peritoneal irritation by blood and/or urine.

Some surgeons still prefer the transperitoneal approach for operations such as pyeloplasty, as it provides for a larger working space, which facilitates intracorporeal suturing. It may also be preferable in children who have previously undergone surgery to the affected kidney, in whom fibrosis and scarring may prevent the creation of a retroperitoneal working space. Inevitably, the choice of approach will also be influenced by the surgeon's experience and training.

In this chapter, only the retroperitoneoscopic approach will be discussed, as this is the current technique of choice for laparoscopic nephrectomy and heminephrectomy.

Indications

NEPHRECTOMY

A laparoscopic nephrectomy or nephroureterectomy is indicated in the following cases:

- congenital non-functioning or poorly functioning dysplastic kidney;
- pelviureteric junction obstruction with loss of function;
- multicystic dysplastic kidney that has failed to involute or is associated with systemic hypertension;
- reflux-associated nephropathy;

- congenital nephrotic syndrome causing intractable protein loss;
- pretransplant in children with focal segmental glomerulosclerosis.

HEMINEPHRECTOMY

A laparoscopic heminephrectomy is indicated in children with complicated renal duplication anomalies. An upper pole heminephrectomy is performed most commonly, typically in the setting of hydroureteronephrosis of the upper moiety with reduced or poor function. In some girls, this surgery is performed for urinary incontinence when the upper moiety ureter drains ectopically into the vagina or into the urethra below the external urinary sphincter.

A lower pole heminephrectomy is performed when there is reflux-associated nephropathy of the lower moiety or in those rare cases of lower moiety pelviureteric junction obstruction with loss of function.

PREOPERATIVE

Nephrectomy

A recent renal ultrasound scan and MAG-3/DMSA scan must be available in the operating room on the day of surgery. In children with a history of vesicoureteric reflux, the micturating cystogram images must also be reviewed. The renal ultrasound will provide information about renal size and the degree of hydronephrosis, when present. In children with a multicystic dysplastic kidney, the size and number of cysts must be noted, as this will determine whether specimen removal will be facilitated by cyst aspiration.

In general, the child will require routine preoperative blood tests, which should include serum creatinine, hemoglobin level, and a group and save of serum. Clotting parameters do not need to be checked routinely, unless there is a history of bleeding disorders.

All children should be administered a single dose of intravenous antibiotic, either prior to leaving the ward or at the induction of anesthesia.

Heminephrectomy

All relevant imaging must be reviewed and present in the operating room for a laparoscopic heminephrectomy. A detailed knowledge of the degree of hydronephrosis and ureteric dilatation, presence of collecting system debris, presence of ureterocele, reflux status, and variation in function within the affected kidney is essential. If the child has undergone previous surgery, e.g. ureterocele puncture, this information must be available, as it may influence whether the affected ureter is ligated or left open.

Routine preoperative blood tests should be performed, including serum creatinine, hemoglobin level, and a blood crossmatch. Clotting parameters do not need to be checked routinely, unless there is a history of bleeding disorders. All children should be administered a single dose of intravenous antibiotic, either prior to leaving the ward or at the induction of anesthesia.

Anesthesia

Endotracheal intubation is required in all cases using either a cuffed or reinforced endotracheal tube, securely fastened. This is to prevent tube dislodgement when the child is positioned prone for the surgery. Perioperative and postoperative analgesia is provided by pre-emptive local infiltration of the planned incisions with 0.25 percent bupivacaine.

OPERATION

Retroperitoneoscopic nephrectomy

ROOM SET UP

12 As the patient is positioned prone for the operation, the laparoscopic stack system should be placed on the side opposite to the affected kidney, toward the head of the table, with the screen pointing toward the pelvis. The scrub nurse should be positioned adjacent to the laparoscopic stack, with both the operating surgeon and assistant on the side of the affected kidney.

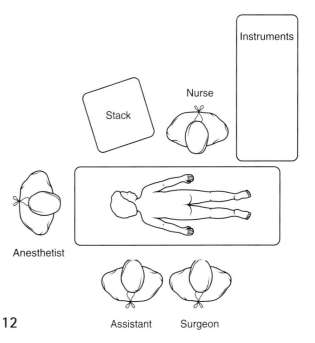

12

Surgical access

13 The patient is positioned fully prone under general anesthesia. The exposed dorsal and lateral aspects of the trunk are prepared and draped in a sterile manner. Topographic landmarks and anticipated port sites are marked as shown.

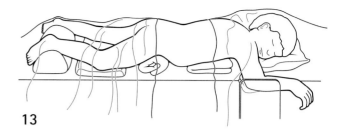

13

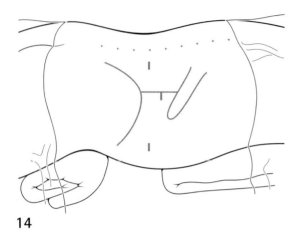

14

14 A 5-mm transverse incision is made midway between the iliac crest and the tip of the 12th rib, just lateral to the outer border of the sacrospinalis muscle.

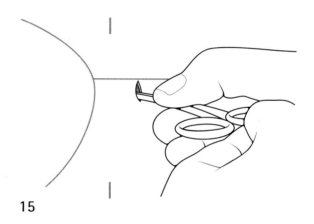

15

15 Through this incision, a small area of the retroperitoneum is dissected bluntly with artery forceps to allow insertion of the retroperitoneal dissecting device.

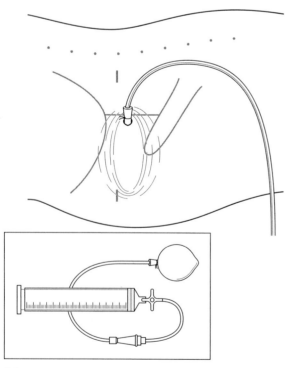

16 The retroperitoneal space is developed outside Gerota's fascia by a technique described by Gill. A dissecting balloon is made by securing the finger of a sterile surgical glove to the end of a 12 Fr Jacques catheter with a silk tie. The catheter is connected to a three-way tap and a 50-mL Luerlock syringe. Depending on the size of the patient, 100–250 mL of air is injected slowly to develop the retroperitoneal space. The balloon is left inflated for 2 minutes to promote hemostasis, and then deflated and withdrawn.

16

17 A 6-mm Hasson cannula is inserted into the port site, followed by insufflation of the retroperitoneum with carbon dioxide to a pressure of 10–12 mmHg. The Hasson port is secured by a suture to the skin. A 5-mm instrument port is placed under direct vision below the tip of the 11th rib and above the iliac crest. A 30° 5-mm laparoscope is recommended for all retroperitoneoscopic surgery, as it can be rotated along its longitudinal axis to alter and maximize the viewpoint for the surgeon.

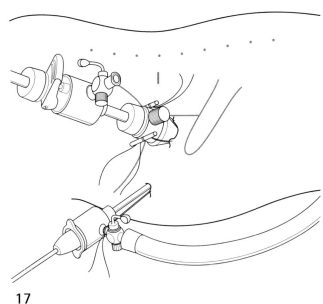

17

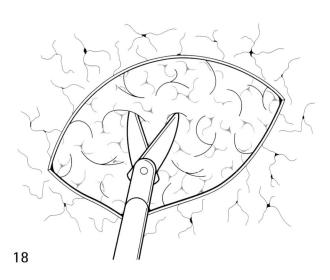

18

OPERATIVE TECHNIQUE

18 Gerota's fascia is incised longitudinally adjacent to the posterior abdominal wall using scissors. Bleeding points are meticulously controlled with monopolar diathermy. The loose areolar adventitial tissue can then be visualized through the window in Gerota's fascia. This tissue is dissected in a blunt manner to create a large perinephric working space, thereby exposing the posterolateral surface of the kidney.

19 In the author's experience, the entire operation can be performed safely through a single instrument port. However, for surgeons with limited experience, it is recommended that a second instrument should be placed. The second instrument will provide counter-traction for dissection and the application of hemoclips.

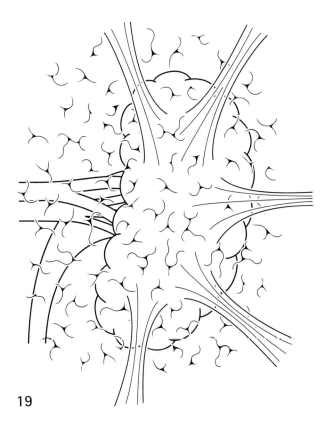

19

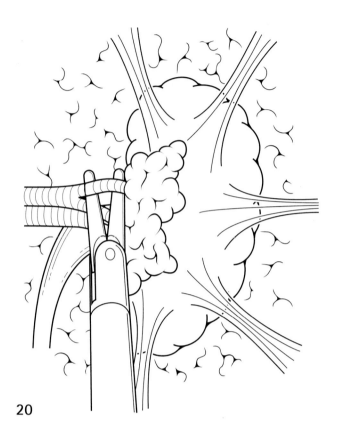

20 Dissection is started at the apex and continued along the medial aspect of the kidney, pushing it laterally and anteriorly to expose the posteromedial surface further, in particular, the renal hilum. The lateral and inferior attachments are maintained intact to facilitate exposure of the renal pedicle by gravity pull of the kidney on the vessels.

20

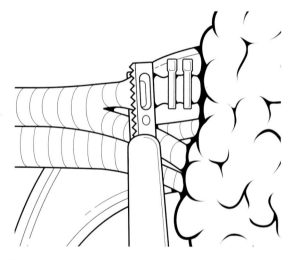

21

21 After adequate mobilization of the renal pedicle, the vessels are divided between hemoclips or with a Harmonic scalpel when the vessels are less than 3 mm in diameter. A minimum of three clips should be applied on all vessels, with at least two clips remaining behind on the proximal stump of the divided vessel. Care must be taken to identify and divide every possible vessel, particularly in the case of multicystic dysplastic kidneys, in which anomalous vessels are frequently found.

22 The ureter is dissected distally as far as required and divided/ligated. If a near-complete ureterectomy is intended, such as in cases with reflux-associated nephropathy, the retroperitoneoscopic approach will allow access into the pelvis to just below the level of the pelvic brim. In all cases of documented ipsilateral reflux, it is the author's practice to ligate the ureter with a 3/0 Vicryl endoloop suture. If this were not possible, an alternative would be to leave the ureteric stump open and to drain the bladder with an in-dwelling urethral catheter for 48 hours. In the absence of ipsilateral vesicoureteric reflux, the ureter can be safely left open without postoperative bladder drainage.

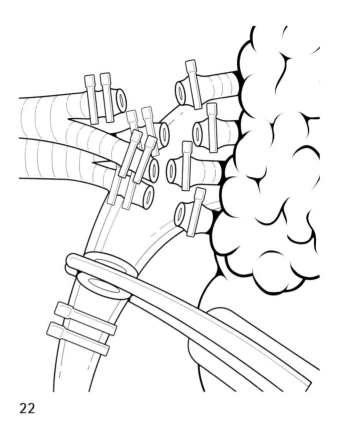

22

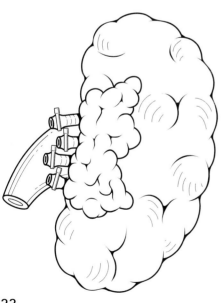

23

23 The remaining attachments of the kidney are divided using a combination of blunt dissection, monopolar diathermy, and/or the Harmonic scalpel. In the case of a large multicystic dysplastic kidney, complete intracorporeal mobilization can be technically difficult, time-consuming, and risks creating a tear in the closely attached peritoneum. In such cases, after all vessels have been divided and the cysts decompressed, the kidney can be withdrawn via the camera port incision and the remainder of the dissection completed in an extracorporeal manner.

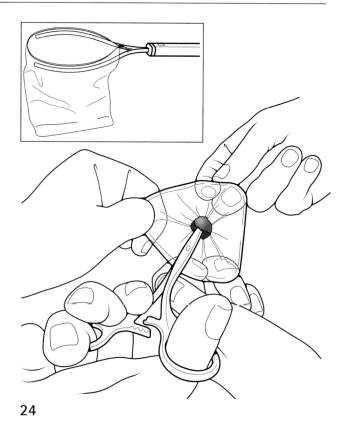

24 The specimen can be extracted directly through the camera port incision in the case of a multicystic dysplastic kidney, grossly hydronephrotic kidney, or a small dysplastic kidney. Larger specimens are extracted with the use of a 10-mm Endopouch specimen retrieval device. The specimen is entrapped within the endobag and removed piecemeal with the use of sponge-holding forceps. The wound is closed in layers, without the use of a drain.

24

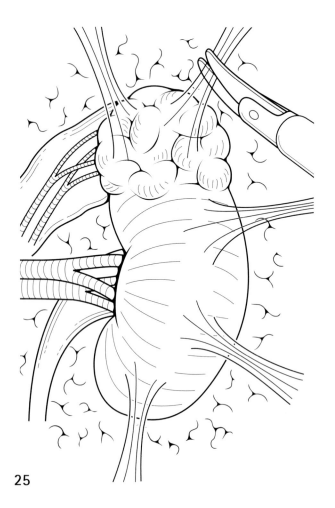

25

Retroperitoneoscopic heminephrectomy

25 Once the retroperitoneoscopic space has been created and Gerota's fascia has been incised, the dissection proceeds to expose the posterolateral surface of the kidney and display renal hilum as for a nephrectomy. It is mandatory to visualize clearly both upper and lower moiety ureters from the outset, as this will confirm the anatomy and provide a guide to the vascular supply to both renal moieties.

The room set up, patient positioning, and steps for surgical access are the same for a retroperitoneoscopic heminephrectomy as they are for a retroperitoneoscopic nephrectomy. In particular, the position of the patient and the port sites are identical. This applies whether an upper or lower pole heminephrectomy is to be performed.

26 The vessels supplying the affected moiety are selectively identified and divided between clips or with a Harmonic scalpel. In some cases, the polar vessels will be clearly evident, whereas in other cases there will be short segmental vessels originating from the main vessels close to the renal hilum. The latter scenario is seen more frequently when the affected renal moiety is small and dysplastic.

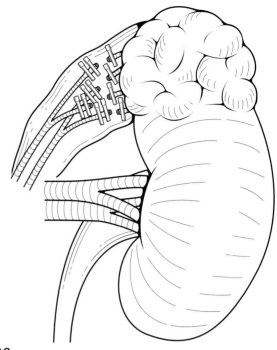

26

27 The ureter from the affected moiety is separated from the non-diseased ureter and divided just distal to the pelviureteric junction. The proximal stump of this ureter is used to lift the kidney, rotating it laterally to expose the anteromedial surface. There may be additional vessels supplying the affected moiety, which only become evident with this maneuver. These should be secured and divided.

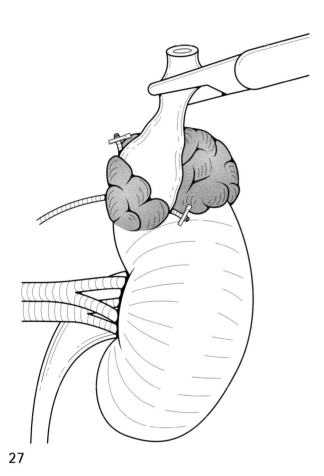

27

28 Once all the vessels to the affected moiety have been secured, there will be blanching of the parenchyma, indicating hypoperfusion. This will provide a guide to the portion of renal parenchyma to be resected. The renal capsule is scored with monopolar diathermy at the junction between the two moieties.

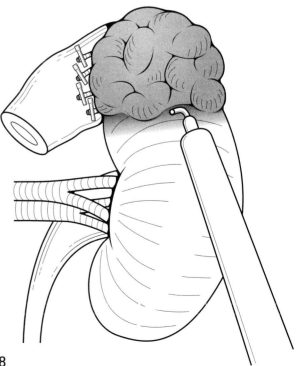

28

29 A 3/0 Vicryl endoloop suture is placed over the affected moiety, using the proximal end of the divided ureter as counter-traction to facilitate this sometimes difficult step. The ligature is firmly tightened at the junction between the renal moieties, providing secure hemostasis and minimizing the risk of urine leak. The parenchyma is transected with hook scissors 5–10 mm distal to the ligature. The cut surface is carefully inspected to detect any remaining arterial bleeding points, which are rare with the endoloop technique, but would need to be secured with diathermy or a further endoloop suture.

The distal ureteric stump should be removed as far distally as possible. Care must be taken to visualize clearly the ureter from the unaffected moiety, especially in the pelvis, where both ureters lie within a common sheath. The ureter should be ligated in all cases with documented vesicoureteric reflux into the affected ureter.

The specimen can be extracted directly through the camera port incision in the majority of cases. Larger specimens are extracted with the use of a 10-mm endopouch specimen retrieval device. The wound is closed in layers, without the use of a drain.

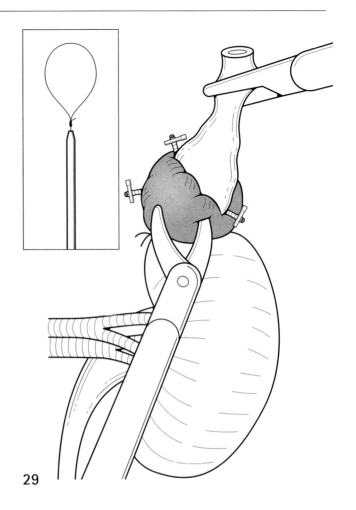

29

POSTOPERATIVE CARE

In the immediate postoperative period, particular attention needs to be paid to the possibility of hemorrhage. The patient should be kept well hydrated and the blood pressure and pulse monitored closely. Oral fluids and milk/diet can be commenced on return from the operating room. Children undergoing heminephrectomy are at risk of developing postoperative pyrexia, and intravenous antibiotics may need to be given if this occurs.

Most patients can be mobilized the day after surgery and allowed home provided they are stable and pain is well controlled.

Complications

PERITONEAL TEAR

The posterior prone approach minimizes the risk of a peritoneal tear as compared to other approaches for retroperitoneoscopic surgery. Peritoneal tear can occur when the dissecting balloon is inflated too rapidly, when the balloon is too small for the size of the patient, in adolescent children, and in children on peritoneal dialysis.

BALLOON RUPTURE

Rupture of the dissecting balloon can occur when the balloon is inflated too rapidly, with over-inflation of the balloon, or when excessive external pressure is applied over the balloon. When it occurs, the ruptured balloon must be carefully examined for lost fragments, which should be sought and removed from the retroperitoneal space.

INTRAOPERATIVE BLEEDING

Intraoperative bleeding is most likely to be due to slipping of hemoclips from a renal vein or to inadvertent damage to a renal vein or vena cava by a laparoscopic instrument. In most cases, hemorrhage can be controlled by the prompt application of hemoclips to the affected vessel or side wall of the vena cava. Uncontrollable hemorrhage will require conversion to an open approach to ligate or oversew the bleeding vessel.

URINE LEAK

A retroperitoneal urinoma can occur from the reflux of urine from the distal ureteric stump or from the cut surface of the kidney following heminephrectomy. The risk can be kept to a minimum by the use of an endoloop suture on the renal parenchyma and by endoloop ligation of refluxing ureters as opposed to the use of hemoclips or the Harmonic scalpel to seal the ureter. Most urinomas will resolve with the placement of a urethral catheter for at least 48–72 hours. A persistent urine leak or an infected urinoma may require the placement of a percutaneous wound drain.

FURTHER READING

Gundeti MS, Ransley PG, Duffy PG et al. Renal outcome following heminephrectomy for duplex kidney. *Journal of Urology* 2005; **173**: 1743–4.

Hidalgo-Tamola J, Shnorhavorian M, Koyle MA. 'Open' minimally invasive surgery in pediatric urology. *Journal of Pediatric Urology* 2009; **5**: 221–7.

Keating MA. Ureteral duplication anomalies: ectopic ureters and ureteroceles. In: Docimo SG, Canning DA, Khoury AE (eds). *Clinical Pediatric Urology*. London: Informa Healthcare, 2007: 593–647.

Mushtaq I. Nephrectomy and heminephrectomy. In: Godbole PP (ed.). *Pediatric Endourology Techniques*. London: Springer, 2007: 13–18.

Singh RR, Wagener S, Chandran H. Laparoscopic management and outcomes in non-functioning moieties of duplex kidneys in children. *Journal of Pediatric Urology* 2010; **6**: 66–9.

Skinner A, Maoate K, Beasley S. Retroperitoneal laparoscopic nephrectomy: the effect of the learning curve, and concentrating expertise, on operating times. *Journal of Laparoendoscopic and Advanced Surgical Techniques* 2010; **20**: 383–5.

Subramanium R, Dickson AP. Subcostal muscle-split incision in paediatric urology. *Pediatric Surgery International* 1998; **15**: 565–6.

Tam YH, Sihoe JD, Cheung ST et al. Single-incision laparoscopic nephrectomy and heminephroureterectomy in young children using conventional instruments: first report of initial experience. *Urology* 2011; **77**: 711–15.

Traxel EJ, Minevich EA, Noh PH. A review: the application of minimally invasive surgery to pediatric urology: upper urinary tract procedures. *Urology*. 2010; **76**: 122–33.

84

Vesicoureteric reflux

DELPHINE DEMÈDE, MICHEL FRANÇOIS, PIERRE MOURIQUAND, and PREM PURI

VESICOURETERIC REFLUX – OPEN AND LAPAROSCOPIC

DELPHINE DEMÈDE, MICHEL FRANÇOIS, and PIERRE MOURIQUAND

INTRODUCTION

Definition

Vesicoureteric reflux (VUR) may be defined as a permanent or intermittent intrusion of bladder urine into the upper urinary tract due to a defective ureterovesical junction. The defect in the ureterovesical junction may be a primary disorder or may arise secondary to bladder dysfunction (neuropathic bladder, dyssynergic bladder) or bladder outlet obstruction (posterior urethral valve). The refluxing urine can fill the upper excretory system (ureters and renal pelvis) between and/or during micturition, and can sometimes penetrate into the renal substance (intrarenal reflux). The volume of refluxing urine can vary in the same patient at different times. Attempts to classify the degree of reflux are therefore of limited practical interest, as reflux may change in intensity in individual patients.

PATHOPHYSIOLOGY AND PRESENTATIONS OF VESICOURETERIC REFLUX

The pathophysiology of VUR remains unclear, but there is a general consensus that intrarenal reflux of infected urine can cause renal damage (reflux nephropathy). It is also likely that other disorders, such as immune reactions, associated renal dysplasia, change of urine biochemistry, etc., can also be responsible for renal deterioration. The difficulty is that there is no investigation able to distinguish acquired or congenital renal lesions.

There are essentially two different types of clinical presentation of VUR.

1. **Primary malformative VUR.** Major VUR associated with dilated upper urinary tracts on prenatal and postnatal ultrasound scans, abnormal dimercaptosuccinate (DMSA) in more than 50 percent of cases, and a low spontaneous regression rate. This type occurs mainly in boys (90 percent) and is due to a congenital malposition of the emergence of the ureteric bud resulting in a morphological abnormality at the level of the vesicoureteric function.
2. **Secondary VUR.** Vesicoureteric reflux secondary to lower urinary tract dysfunction and abnormal bladder urodynamics is more common than primary reflux. The reflux does not cause upper tract dilatation, is not detectable prenatally, is not associated with an abnormal DMSA scan, and usually occurs in girls with poor bladder and bowel function. The resolution rate is around 80 percent with bladder training. Radical treatment is seldom required.

Indications

As a consequence of the failure to reach a consensus on the precise indications for surgery, it is difficult to select the ideal treatment for each patient. However, during the last decade, several studies have shown the importance of the couple 'kidney–bladder' and it is now accepted by many that VUR with normal kidneys (DMSA) at an early stage of life will resolve spontaneously with maturation of the bladder. It is therefore logical that children with recurrent urinary tract infections (RUTIs) should undergo initial evaluation of their kidneys (DMSA) and only those children with abnormal DMSA would require a cystography (top-down approach). A common policy in refluxers is to prescribe prophylactic antibiotic treatment for prolonged periods (12–36 months) in expectation of spontaneous maturation of the ureterovesical junction and a resolution of the VUR. The long-term side effects of prophylactic treatment are unknown, and there are reservations regarding its effectiveness in preventing infection. If the child suffers from recurrent breakthrough infections or if there are signs of continued deterioration of the renal substance, more radical treatment should be considered. Surgery consists of reimplanting the ureters into the bladder; endoscopic treatment consists of injecting a substance behind the intramural ureter to create an effective posterior backing, which helps to restore the antireflux mechanisms. The aim of these modalities of treatment is to stop the reflux. This does not necessarily mean that the progression of renal damage is halted or that further urinary tract infections are prevented. In cases where VUR has caused severe damage to the kidney (relative function less than 10 percent), a nephroureterectomy may be the best option. The choice between surgical, laparoscopic, and endoscopic correction of reflux is an individual matter, each technique having its own protagonists. The best result with endoscopic treatment is with low-grade refluxes, where spontaneous resolution is high and where underlying bladder dysfunction is common. Although simple and less invasive, the place of endoscopic treatment is therefore unclear and one should remain cautious about the current trend to extend its indications (see **Table 84.1**).

Table 84.1 Reflux symptom (bladder dysfunction) and reflux disease.

	Reflux – symptom	Reflux – disease
Presentation	Recurrent urinary tract infections	Prenatal diagnosis
Ultrasound	Normal	Dilatation
Cystography	Grades I–III	Grades III–V
DMSA scan	Normal	Abnormal
Resolution	>80%	<50%
Etiology	Bladder dysfunction	Abnormal vesicoureteric junction + renal dysplasia
Treatment	Training	Surgery

DMSA, dimercaptosuccinate.

PREOPERATIVE ASSESSMENT

Before VUR correction, several investigations are commonly performed:

- Cystography. Micturating cystography is the standard method to identify and grade VUR. Its indications have certainly decreased with the 'top-down approach', but remains mandatory prior to surgery.
- Direct contrast micturating cystography with bladder catheterization is the most common. Indirect radioisotope cystography is less reliable, but may be used in the follow up of VUR patients. Direct isotopic micturating cystography has the advantage of a considerably reduced radiation dose, but is not widely available.
- DMSA or ^{99m}Tc-labeled mercaptoacetyl triglycine (MAG-3) renal scanning. This assesses the presence of renal scars and provides a measure of the relative function of each individual kidney.
- Urodynamic study. This is important for detecting an underlying bladder dysfunction.
- Ultrasonographic scanning of the urinary tract. Although a poor investigation to detect reflux, this can be useful for assessing the size, shape, and echogenicity of each kidney, the degree of dilatation of the ureter and bladder wall thickness.
- Cystoscopy. Evaluation of the shape of the ureteric orifice or the length of the submucosal portion of the ureter is often subjective and will rarely alter the therapeutic decision. It is, however, recommended if the VUR is associated with a contralateral or ipsilateral ureterocele or if the reflux has occurred secondary to bladder dysfunction or bladder outlet obstruction.

Anesthesia

General endotracheal anesthesia is complemented by caudal anesthesia.

OPERATIONS

Transhiatal reimplantation of the ureter (Cohen's or Glenn–Anderson's procedure), suprahiatal reimplantation of the ureter and extravesical reimplantation are the three main surgical options. The aim is to mobilize the distal segment of the ureter(s) (transmural ureter) and place it under a tunnel of bladder mucosa in order to restore the flap valve mechanism that is designed to prevent VUR.

Transhiatal reimplantation of the ureter

This is mainly represented by Cohen's procedure.

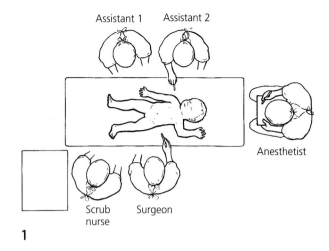

POSITION OF PATIENT

1 The patient lies supine on the operating table. A right-handed surgeon should stand on the left side of the patient, with the scrub nurse on his or her left. The assistant(s) should stand on the right side of the patient.

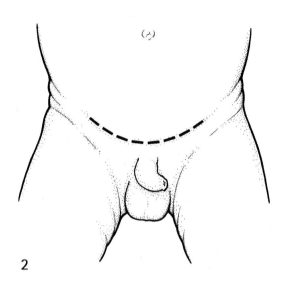

INCISION

2 A transverse suprapubic incision is made 2 cm above the pubic symphysis, in the low abdominal crease.

3 The subcutaneous tissues are incised, exposing the rectus sheath, which is opened vertically in the midline. Both recti are separated and the peritoneum is gently pushed upwards, superiorly, providing good exposure of the bladder.

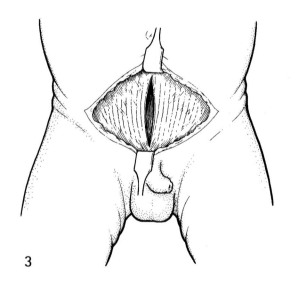

4 A Denis Browne retractor is inserted.

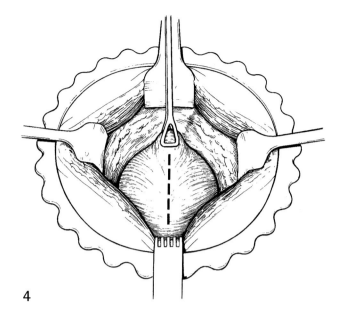

4

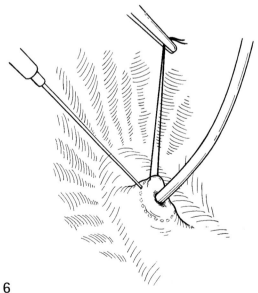

5

EXPOSURE OF THE TRIGONE

5 The anterior wall of the bladder is incised vertically and two stay sutures suspend each edge of the vesicotomy. Swabs are put inside the bladder and retracted upwards with a Deaver retractor in order to expose the trigone. A 3/0 or 4/0 absorbable suture is placed at the lowest point of the vesicotomy to prevent splitting of the incision downwards into the urethra.

The trigone is exposed and an infant feeding tube (3, 4, 6, or 8 Fr) is inserted into each ureter. A stay suture (5/0) is placed around each ureteric orifice. The assistant holds this stay suture with mild traction.

TRANSHIATAL DISSECTION OF THE URETER

6 The ureteric orifice is circumcised with diathermy (cutting and coagulation should be very low) and mobilization of the distal 2 cm of ureter can be performed with diathermy alone (these 2 cm will be excised later).

6

7 It is essential to enter the correct plane between the bladder and the transparietal ureter, commencing below the orifice. Sharp scissors should be avoided, and Reynolds scissors make this procedure much easier. The tip of the Reynolds scissors elevates the muscle fibers that attach the ureter to the bladder musculature. These fibers are grasped with fine forceps, coagulated, and divided. The dissection continues progressively, circumferentially until the ureter is completely free. Coagulation of the fibers should be carried out some distance from the ureter to avoid damaging its blood supply. The peritoneum is visible at the end of this dissection and should be teased away from the ureter. In boys, the vas deferens may lie close to the ureter at this point and care must be taken to avoid damaging it. A similar procedure can be used for the opposite ureter. In cases of ureteric duplication, both ureters are dissected together and should not be separated, thus avoiding damage to their blood supply.

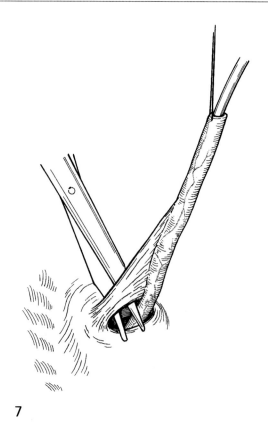

7

COHEN OR TRIGONAL REIMPLANTATION OF THE URETER

In some cases, the ureteric hiatus is wide and should be narrowed by one or two absorbable sutures. This is done to prevent the formation of a diverticulum. These sutures should narrow the hiatus, but still allow the free movement of the ureter and not restrict or constrict it.

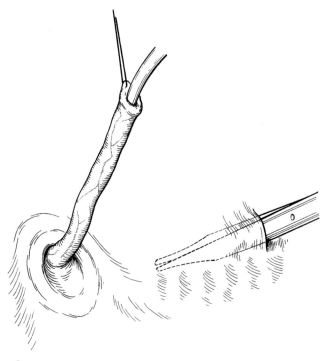

8 The submucosal tunnel is then constructed. It is usually a horizontal tunnel, crossing the midline of the posterior surface of the bladder, just above the trigone. Its length should be at least five times the ureteric diameter (Paquin's rule) and if this condition cannot be fulfilled, trimming or remodeling of the ureter should be considered (see below). The site of the new ureteric orifice is selected and the bladder mucosa is lifted from the underlying bladder muscles with a pair of Reynolds scissors, starting either from the hiatus or from the new ureteric orifice. The tunnel should be wide enough to allow easy insertion of the ureter without constriction.

8

9 A similar procedure can be carried out for the opposite ureter in cases of bilateral reimplantation. The construction of the lowest tunnel that crosses the trigone can cause bleeding and the lifting of the mucosa is slightly less easy. A pair of artery forceps or right-angled forceps is inserted through the tunnel, the stay suture is grasped and gently pulled to draw the ureter into place, taking care not to twist or kink it in the process.

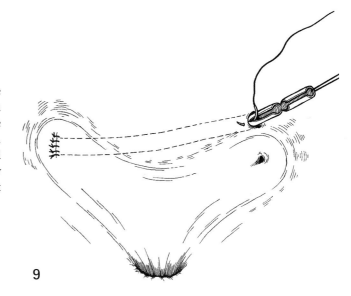

9

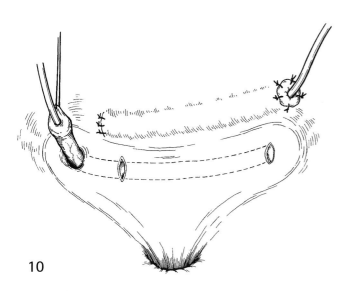

10

10 The last 2 cm of ureter are excised and the ureteric opening is spatulated with a pair of angulated Potts scissors. The 5/0 absorbable suture anchors the ureter to the bladder muscles and the ureterovesicostomy is completed with interrupted 6/0 absorbable sutures.

CLOSURE AND DRAINAGE

11 An infant feeding tube or a modified JJ stent (multipurpose Blue stent™; Bard, Angiomed, UK) is inserted into the reimplanted ureter and exteriorized through the bladder wall, the rectus muscle, and the skin. The feeding tube is left in position for 2 days, or for 10–15 days if the ureter has been remodeled. Alternatively, a retrievable JJ stent can be used. There is no consensus on the efficacy of drainage of the reimplanted ureter and some authors do not leave a drain.

The bladder is drained either by a transurethral catheter, which is left *in situ* for 5 days, or by a suprapubic catheter. The bladder is closed with a 3/0 or 4/0 suture (interrupted or continuous). The prevesical and subcutaneous spaces are drained by a suction drain. The abdominal wall, the subcutaneous tissues, and the skin are then closed.

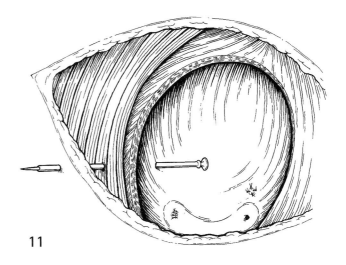

11

Suprahiatal reimplantation of the ureter

Megaureters are the principal indication for this technique, which should be performed by an experienced pediatric urologist. It is a difficult procedure, which carries a significant complication rate.

The approach to the bladder, the retraction with the Denis-Browne retractor, and the exposure of the bladder mucosa are as in the transhiatal procedure. The extravesical approach to the ureter is the main step in this procedure.

12 The peritoneum covering the dome and the lateral face of the bladder should be pushed upwards, which involves ligation of the obliterated hypogastric ligament. It is then easy to mobilize the peritoneum upwards and to expose the full length of the iliac vessels. The vas deferens and its pedicle are easily located and should also be freed before the ureteric reimplantation.

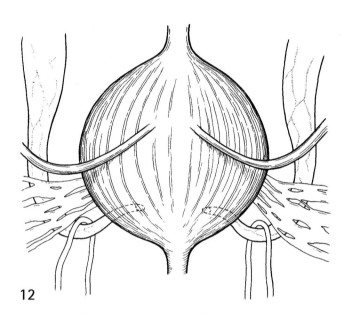

12

IDENTIFICATION OF THE URETER

The ureter is now identified passing over the iliac vessels close to their division into the external iliac and hypogastric arteries. The ureter is progressively mobilized from this point down to the bladder, preserving its blood supply and the blood supply of the bladder. There is, in fact, a plethora of small vessels and nerves arising from the pelvic pedicles to the bladder, which cross the distal part of the extravesical ureter and should be preserved. In severe megaureters, the ureter is grossly dilated and kinked, and its dissection should be very meticulous to straighten it and maintain enough tissue around it to preserve its blood supply and innervation. The ureter is divided at its entrance into the bladder and a stay suture facilitates its mobilization. The ureter, which normally passes under the vas deferens, should be redirected over it to straighten it out.

EXCISION OF THE DISTAL SEGMENT OF URETER AND REMODELING

The distal segment of the ureter is usually narrowed and its excision allows urine to flow out freely. The ureteric diameter rapidly contracts and it is then possible to decide whether ureteric reimplantation can be achieved with or without remodeling or trimming. This decision is dictated by Paquin's rule: the length of the submucosal tunnel should represent at least five times the ureteric diameter.

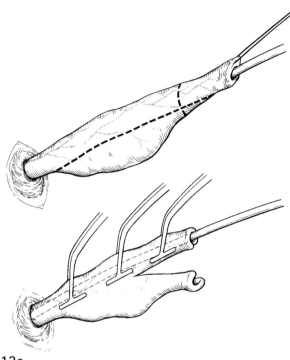

13 If the ureter remains too large after excision of its distal end, its caliber should be reduced, either by excising a strip of ureter (Hendren's technique) or by infolding the ureter (Kalicinski's technique).

Excision of a strip of ureter may threaten the ureteric blood supply, whereas ureter infolding can create a certain degree of obstruction. Whichever technique is chosen, the length of the remodeled or trimmed segment of ureter should not exceed the length of the submucosal tunnel.

13a

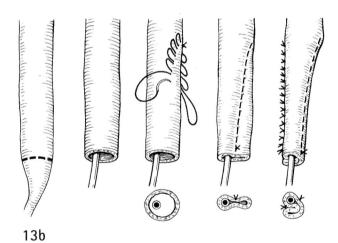

13b

REIMPLANTATION OF THE URETER CREATING A NEW HIATUS OF ENTRANCE

14 The hiatus of entrance of the ureter into the bladder should be medial and high at the top of the posterior surface of the bladder. The ureter should not be constricted at this level, and it is necessary to excise a disk of bladder to allow free passage of the ureter. The submucosal tunnel is fashioned, as described above, and should be vertical. Its distal end should open on the trigone. The passage of the freed ureter through the tunnel is the most difficult step of this procedure. The ureter should not be twisted or kinked, especially at the entrance into the bladder, and its pelvic course should be smooth. A few absorbable sutures are placed at its entrance into the bladder and sometimes the bladder itself is tacked down on the psoas muscle to maintain the smooth course of the ureter. The ureterovesicostomy is as described above. A bilateral procedure may be performed, although a bilateral extravesical approach of the ureters may affect bladder innervations and cause transient bladder dysfunction. Some authors prefer to perform a transureteroureterostomy to avoid bilateral suprahiatal reimplantation.

CLOSURE

Closure and drainage are as described above, except that the ureteric stent is maintained for at least 10 days if the ureter has been remodeled.

POSTOPERATIVE CARE

The child is usually hospitalized for 5 days. The ureteric stent is removed after 2 days (or 10 days if the ureter has been remodeled). The bladder catheter is removed on the fifth postoperative day. Both suction drains are usually removed on the second day. Bladder spasms are common, and administration of oxybutinin can be useful to reduce the discomfort. Antibiotic prophylaxis is a possible option

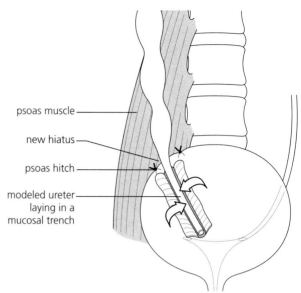

14

psoas muscle

new hiatus

psoas hitch

modeled ureter laying in a mucosal trench

with trimethoprim with or without sulphamethoxazole (co-trimoxazole).

Pain is controlled with diclofenac suppositories (12.5 mg). The child should stay away from school for 8–15 days and avoid sport for one month. An ultrasound scan of the urinary tract is recommended three months after surgery to ensure that there is no increased dilatation of the ureters. If the child is clinically well, control of absence of VUR is no longer necessary after surgery as micturating cystogram is a rather unpleasant investigation with significant radiations and a risk of secondary urinary tract infection (UTI). If the kidney was damaged at the time of diagnosis, a repeated DMSA scan a few months after surgery might be useful.

EXTRAVESICAL REIMPLANTATION OF THE URETER (GREGOIR LICH TECHNIQUE)

15 An alternative technique consists of creating a submucosal tunnel by incising obliquely the detrusor muscle from the ureteric entry for 4 or 5 cm. The ureter is then laid inside the muscular trench and the muscular edges are sutured over it. This technique, which can be performed either open or laparoscopically and implies a dissection of the posterolateral aspect of the bladder which, when performed bilaterally, may cause transient bladder dysfunction. The main advantage of this technique is that it avoids the opening of the bladder and reduces postoperative bladder spasms.

(a)   (b)   (c)

15

OUTCOME

It is essential to reiterate that these procedures only aim at stopping VUR. Their effects on the renal damage and on the recurrence of urinary tract infections are questionable. Transhiatal procedures resolve VUR in more than 95 percent of cases. Suprahiatal procedures are more difficult and have a significant incidence of complications (around 10 percent), including persistent reflux, secondary dilatation of the upper tract, and stenosis. Extravesical reimplantation has a less good score in term of stopping VUR, although still quite good.

LAPAROSCOPIC PROCEDURES

The Lich Gregoir procedure

16 Set up and instruments: The patient is supine with the arms lying along the body. The surgeon stands at the head of the patient and the two assistants on each side. The screen and insufflator stand at the feet of the patient. A bladder catheter is placed and should be accessible during the procedure. 3-mm instruments are used: blunt grasper, bipolar forceps, hook, needle holder, scissors, and a 5-mm 30° optic.

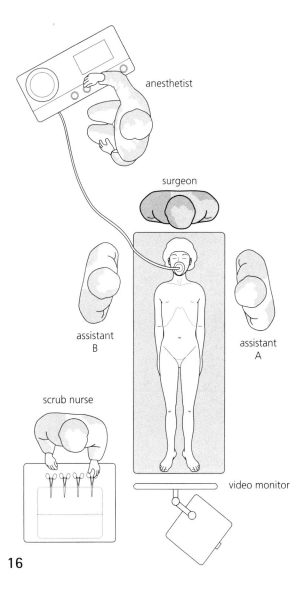

16

TECHNIQUE

A transperitoneal approach is used. A 5-mm port is inserted with the open laparoscopy technique to avoid visceral damage. One 3-mm trocar is inserted in the left and one in the right flank.

Ureteral dissection

With the bladder empty, the ureter is easily identified where it crosses the external iliac vessels. The peritoneum is opened down to the ureterovesical junction. In boys, the vas deferens is teased away from the ureter. In girls, the dissection is pursued through the broad ligament with preservation of the uterine artery. A 4- to 5-cm length mobilization of the ureter is needed.

The bladder dome is suspended to the anterior abdominal with a transcutaneous stay suture in order to expose the ureterovesical junction.

Detrusorotomy and exposure of the bladder mucosa

17 The direction and length of the muscular incision is outlined with the unipolar coagulation following the Paquin's rule. A, bladder suspension; B, suspension of the distal end of the detrusorotomy; C, vas deferens; D, ureter; E, incision line of the detrusor.

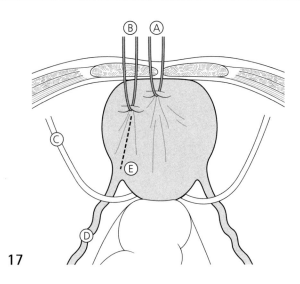

17

18 A second stay suture is placed at the tip of the incision. The bladder is filled to create a bulging out of the mucosa. The muscular fibers are divided with the scissors (see illustration 20). In case of mucosal tear, we favor the endoloop blinding, rather than direct suture. A, bladder suspension; B, suspension of the distal end of the detrusorotomy; C, vas deferens; D, ureter; E, detrusorotomy.

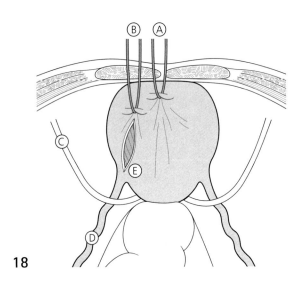

18

Detrusororrhaphy

19 The ureter is laid between the two edges of muscular trench and kept in this position with a third stay suture. A, bladder suspension; B, suspension of the distal end of the detrusorotomy; C, vas deferens; D, ureter; E, ureteric suspension.

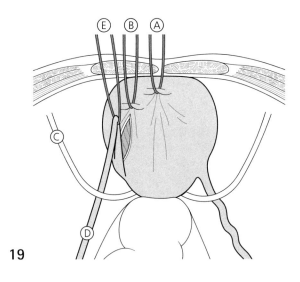

19

20 The detrusor is then sutured over the ureter with three to four stitches of 3/0 or 4/0 non-resorbable suture. Particular attention should be given to avoid narrowing the entry of the ureter into the trench. A, bladder suspension; B, suspension of the distal end of the detrusorotomy; C, vas deferens; D, ureter; E, ureteric suspension.

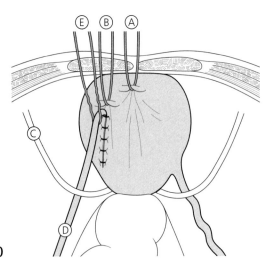

20

Closure

The peritoneum is sutured, the trocars removed, their orifices stitched and the bladder catheter removed. No drainage is left.

The same procedure can be done on both sides with the same approach. In case of ureteral duplication, both ureters are dissected and laid into the trench together.

POSTOPERATIVE CARE

The patient can go home the next day with standard pain killers and no antibiotics. We usually keep the child off school for 8 days with no sport for one month. An ultrasound scan is performed at one month following the operation.

This technique significantly reduces postoperative bladder spasms and adverse effects of bladder opening. Its success rate is comparable to all extravesical ureteric reimplantation. The risk of transient bladder dysfunction following bilateral laparoscopic ureteral reimplantation seems to be less than with open procedures.

Vesicoscopic Cohen reimplantation of the ureters

SET UP AND INSTRUMENTS

21 The patient is in a cystoscopy position with access to the urethral meatus. In children under five years of age, the position of the surgeon is the same as described for the laparoscopic Gregoir Lich technique. In older children, the surgeon stands on one side with the screen at the foot of the patient. Intravenous antibiotic is administered at the start of the procedure. Instruments are similar to those used in the previous technique.

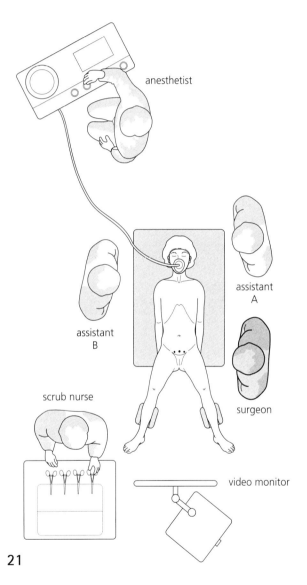

21

OPERATIVE PROCEDURE

22 A cystoscopy is performed to monitor the placement of the 5-mm trocar inserted through a midline suprapubic incision. The bladder is filled and the dome is suspended to the anterior abdominal wall as described before. Two 3- or 5-mm trocars are inserted through each side of the bladder with a concomitant endoscopic control. The cystoscope is then removed and the CO_2 insufflation is started with the median trocar with a pressure of 8–12 mmHg. A, C, operating ports; B, optical port.

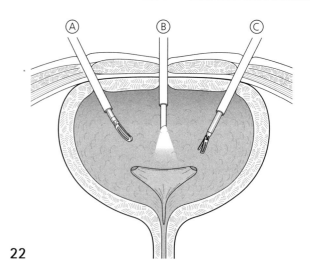

22

- **Transhiatal ureteral dissection**. A 4-cm ureteral stent is inserted into each ureter and stitched to the ureteral meatus with a 5/0 PDS. The ureteral dissection follows the Cohen technique using the hook and a pledget. The ureteral hiatus is narrowed with several stitches to avoid CO_2 leaked outside the bladder. The ureter is stitched to the detrusor muscle to avoid its retraction as with the open procedure.
- **Ureteral reimplantation**. Subcutaneous tunnels are fashioned with the scissors and each ureter is pulled under the bladder mucosa using a stay suture and/or a ureteral stent. The extremity of each ureter is excised, spatulated, and stitched to the detrusor with 5/0 and 6/0 PDS. The mucosa is stitched as with the open procedure.

CLOSURE

The trocar orifices are closed under endoscopic control. The gas is removed via a transurethral catheter and left in place for 48 hours.

POSTOPERATIVE CARE

The child can go home 48 hours after surgery with the same advice as those given before.

The success rate is equivalent to the open Cohen procedure with much less postoperative discomfort. However, this technique is more challenging and the learning curve is longer.

VESICOURETERAL REFLUX – ENDOSCOPIC

PREM PURI

INTRODUCTION

Primary vesicoureteral reflux (VUR) is the most common urological anomaly in children and has been reported in 1–2 percent of the pediatric population and in 30–50 percent of children, who present with urinary tract infection (UTI). The familial nature of VUR is well established with a reported prevalence of between 27 and 51 percent in siblings of index patients with VUR. The association of VUR, UTI, and renal parenchymal damage is well known. Reflux nephropathy is recognized as a major cause of end-stage renal failure in children and young adults. Primary vesicoureteral reflux is caused by congenital absence or deficiency of the longitudinal muscle of the submucosal ureters. This results in upward and lateral displacement of the ureteric orifice during micturition, thereby reducing the length and obliquity of the submucosal ureter. There has been no consensus regarding when medical or surgical therapy should be used. A number of prospective studies have shown low probability of spontaneous resolution of high-grade reflux during conservative follow up. Furthermore, all of these studies revealed that observation therapy does carry an ongoing risk of renal scarring.

Since the United States of America's Food and Drug Administration (FDA) approval in 2001 of dextranomer/hyaluronic acid copolymer (Deflux®) as a tissue-augmenting substance for subureteral injection, endoscopic treatment has become a widely accepted minimally invasive alternative to long-term prophylaxis and open surgical treatment in the management of VUR. It has been reported that Deflux is biodegradable, has no immunogenic properties, and has no potential for malignant transformation.

PRINCIPLES AND JUSTIFICATION

Indications

The indications for endoscopic correction of vesicoureteric reflux are the same as for open antireflux operations.

It is generally agreed that lesser grades of reflux (grade I or II international classification) can be managed conservatively. Grade II reflux is conservatively managed unless there are 'breakthrough infections' while on antimicrobial therapy, or poor compliance on medical management. Children with grade III–V vesicoureteric reflux are generally considered candidates for endoscopic treatment. In addition to primary VUR, the endoscopic procedure has been used successfully to treat VUR in Duplex systems, VUR secondary to neuropathic bladder and posterior urethral valves, VUR in failed reimplanted bladders, and VUR in refluxing ureteral stumps.

PREOPERATIVE

Material

Currently, the tissue-augmenting substance most commonly used for subureteral injection is dextranomer/ hyaluronic acid copolymer (Deflux). Dextranomer microspheres in sodium hyaluronic acid solution consists of microspheres of dextranomers mixed in a 1 percent high molecular weight sodium hyaluronan solution. Each milliliter of Deflux contains 0.5-mL sodium hyaluronan and 0.5 mL of microspheres.

Instruments

23 The disposable Puri catheter for Deflux injection (Storz) is a 4-Fr nylon catheter onto which is swaged a 21-gauge needle with 1 cm of the needle protruding from the catheter. Alternatively, a rigid needle can be used.

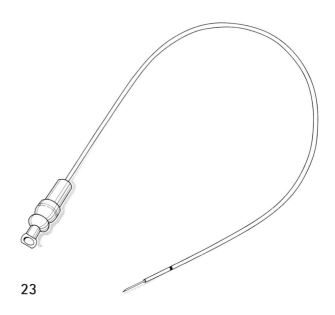

23

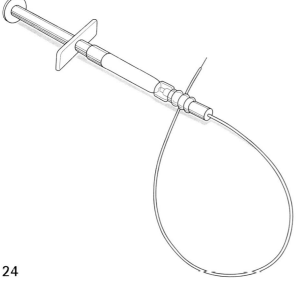

24 A 1-mL syringe prefilled with Deflux is attached to the injection catheter.

24

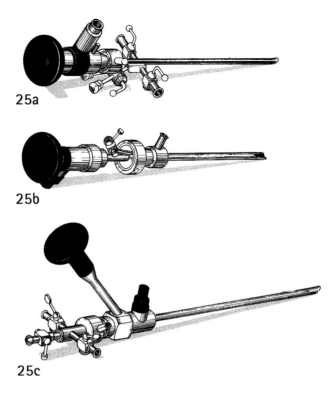

25a

25b

25c

25a–c All cystoscopes available for infants and children can be used for this procedure. The injection catheter is introduced through the cystoscope. An angled cystoscope allows for a straight route for the needle through the cystoscope, which is particularly helpful when using a rigid needle.

OPERATION

Injection technique

The patient should be placed in a lithotomy position. The cystoscope is passed and the bladder wall, the trigone, bladder neck, and both ureteric orifices inspected. The bladder should be almost empty before proceeding with injection, since this helps to keep the ureteric orifice flat rather than away in a lateral part of the field.

26 The injection of Deflux should not begin until the operator has a clear view all around the ureteric orifice. Under direct vision through the cystoscope, the needle is introduced under the bladder mucosa 2–3 mm below the affected ureteric orifice at the 6 o'clock position. In children with grade IV and V reflux with wide ureteric orifices, the needle should be inserted not below, but directly into the affected ureteral orifice. It is important to introduce the needle with pinpoint accuracy.

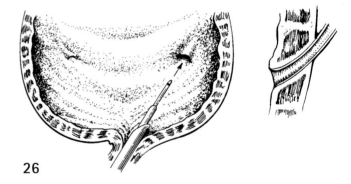

26

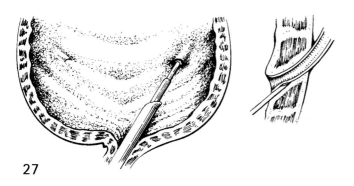

27

27 The needle is advanced about 4–5 mm into the lamina propria in the submucosal portion of the ureters and the injection started slowly. As the paste is injected, a bulge appears in the floor of the submucosal ureters. During injection, the needle is slowly withdrawn until a 'volcanic' bulge of paste is seen. Most refluxing ureters require 0.4–1.0 mL Deflux to correct reflux.

28 A correctly placed injection creates the appearance of a nipple on the top of which is a slit-like or inverted crescentic orifice. If the bulge appears in an incorrect place, e.g. at the side of the ureter or proximal to it, the needle should not be withdrawn, but should be moved so that the point is in a more favorable position. The non-injected ureteric roof retains its compliance while preventing reflux.

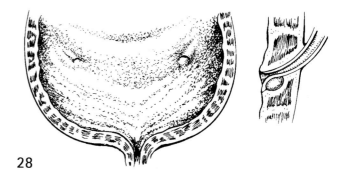

28

POSTOPERATIVE CARE

Postoperative urethral catheterization is not necessary. The majority of patients are treated as day cases. Co-trimoxazole is prescribed in prophylactic doses for 6–12 weeks after the procedure. Micturating cystography and renal ultrasonography are performed 6–12 weeks after discharge. A follow-up renal and bladder ultrasonographic scan is obtained 12 months after endoscopic correction of reflux.

Complications

Procedure-related complications are rare. The only significant complication with this procedure has been failure. This may be initial failure, i.e. the reflux is not abolished by the injection, or recurrence, where initial correction is not maintained. About 15 percent of refluxing ureters require more than one endoscopic injection of paste to correct the condition. Between 2001 and 2010, the author treated 1551 children with intermediate- and high-grade VUR by endoscopic injection of Deflux. VUR was unilateral in 761 children and bilateral in 790. Renal scarring was detected in 469 (30.2 percent) of children. Reflux grade in 2341 ureters was grade II–V in 98 (4.2 percent), 1340 (57.3 percent), 818 (34.9 percent), and 85 (3.6 percent), respectively. VUR resolved after the first, second, and third injection in 2039 (87.1 percent), 264 (11.3 percent), and 38 (1.6 percent) ureters, respectively. Sixty-nine (4.4 percent) patients developed febrile UTIs during a mean follow up of 6.2 years. None of the patients in the series needed reimplantation of ureters or developed any significant complications, confirming the efficacy and safety of this 15-minute outpatient procedure in the management of intermediate and high-grade VUR.

FURTHER READING

Cohen SJ. Ureterozystoneostomie: eine neue antirefluxtechnik. *Aktuel Urology* 1975; **6**: 1–8.

Grégoir W, Van Regemorter G. Le reflux vésico-urétéral congenital. *Urology International* 1964; **18**:122.

Hendren WH. Operative repair of megaureter in children. *Journal of Urology* 1969; **101**: 491–507.

Lopez M, Varlet F. Laparoscopic extravesical transperitoneal approach following the Lich–Gregoir technique in the treatment of vesicoureteral reflux in children. *Journal of Pediatric Surgery* 2010; **45**: 806–10.

Menezes M, Puri P. The role of endoscopic treatment in the management of grade V primary vesicoureteral reflux. *European Urology* 2007; **52**: 1501–9.

Puri P, Kutasy B, Colhoun E, Hunziker M. Single centre experience with endoscopic subureteral dextranomer/hyaluronic acid injection as first line of treatment in 1551 children with high-grade vesicoureteral reflux. *Journal of Urology* 2012; **188**: 1485–9.

Puri P, Menezes M. Endoscopic treatment of vesicoureteral reflux. In: Gearhart JP, Rink RC, Mouriquand PDE (eds). *Pediatric Urology*. Philadelphia, PA: Saunders Elsevier, 2010: 322–9.

Puri P, Mohanan N, Menezes M, Colhoun E. Endoscopic treatment of moderate and high-grade vesicoureteral reflux in infants using dextranomer/hyaluronic acid. *Journal of Urology* 2007; **178**: 1714–16.

Puri P, Pirker M, Mohanan N et al. Subureteral dextranomer/hyaluronic acid injection as first line treatment in the management of high-grade vesicoureteral reflux. *Journal of Urology* 2006; **176**: 1856–60.

Valla JS, Steyaert H, Griffin SJ et al. Transvesicoscopic Cohen ureteric reimplantation for vesicoureteral reflux in children: a single centre 5 year experience. *Journal of Pediatric Urology* 2009; **5**: 466–71.

Yeung CK, Sihoe JD, Borzi PA. Endoscopic cross-trigonal ureteral reimplantation under carbon bladder insufflations: a novel technique. *Journal of Endourology* 2005; **19**: 295–9.

85

Ureteric duplication

GARRETT D POHLMAN and DUNCAN T WILCOX

HISTORY

Ureteric duplication occurs with duplications of the kidney. Post-mortem studies have demonstrated upper tract duplication in 0.8 percent of the population. There is not a predilection to a particular side as the left and right kidneys are affected equally, and bilateral duplication occurs in approximately 40 percent of cases. It can be inherited as an autosomal dominant trait with incomplete penetrance. The incidence of duplication among members of affected families is 8 percent.

An understanding of the embryology of normal renal development is critical to an appreciation of the anatomy of ureteral abnormalities and how these conditions develop. At the end of the fourth week of gestation, epithelial out-pouchings from the distal mesonephric duct grow laterally (normally one ureteric bud on each side) into the metanephric blastema. A process of reciprocal induction between the metanephros and the ureteric bud cause nephrogenesis to occur. The metanephros gives rise to the glomerulus, the convoluted tubules and loop of Henlé, whereas the ureteric bud undergoes several generations of bifurcation, and is the origin of the collecting ducts, calyces, renal pelvis, and ureter. During development, the ureteral orifice migrates within the bladder in a cranial and lateral direction.

Incomplete duplication occurs when a ureteric bud bifurcates early just after its origin from the mesonephric duct. This duplication ultimately creates two separate collecting systems which join into one common ureter with a single ureteral orifice in the normal location of the trigone. Complete duplication occurs when two ureteric buds arise from the mesonephric duct resulting in two separate collecting systems, ureters, and ureteral orifices. The ureteral orifices are inverted in relation to the collecting system they drain and have been termed the Weigert–Meyer rule (see below). This rule is important to keep in mind from a clinical standpoint as the lower (distally placed) orifice is the orifice to the upper pole and the higher (more cranial orifice) is the lower pole orifice.

Ureteric buds arising proximally or distally to the normal site of origin on the mesonephric duct can induce nephrogenesis in a less competent part of the metanephros producing a dysplastic pole of the kidney. The part of the mesonephric duct distal to the ureteric bud(s) (also called the excretory duct, common mesonephric duct) becomes incorporated into the posterior wall of the developing bladder (which develops from the cranial part of the urogenital sinus) in a cranial to caudal direction, forming the trigone. Stephen's hypothesis describes how distal ureteric buds drain the lower poles of Duplex kidneys and become incorporated into the bladder earlier which allows it to travel more laterally and cranially than usual. The resultant position in the bladder gives a shorter intramural tunnel and is more prone to vesicoureteral reflux (VUR) to the lower pole of the kidney. On the other hand, proximal ureteric buds drain the upper poles and become incorporated into the trigone later and more distally. In extremely proximal cases, the part of the mesonephric duct to which the upper pole ureter is attached never becomes incorporated into the trigone or urethra, giving rise to an ectopic ureter to a mesonephric duct derivative. In the male, these derivatives include the vas, seminal vesicles, epididymis, and prostate, which are all suprasphincteric so urinary incontinence is uncommon. In the female, they include epoophoron, oophoron, or Gartner's duct which may be above the sphincter mechanism (suprasphincteric), or below it (infrasphincteric) to the introitus or vagina. The ectopic ureter in females is commonly infrasphincteric giving a clinical picture of constant wetting from the ectopic ureter.

The terminology describing the spectrum of abnormalities is reviewed here:

- **Duplex kidney** has two, separate pelvicalyceal systems, and consequently an upper and a lower pole. Duplication may be partial or complete. In incomplete duplication, the ureters may join at any point: a bifid system joins at the ureteropelvic junction (UPJ); bifid ureters join at some point proximal to the bladder. Complete duplication occurs with double ureters, which drain their respective poles and empty separately into the genitourinary tract.

- **Ectopic ureter** drains into the urethra below the bladder neck or outside the urinary tract.
- **Weigert–Meyer rule** states that the lower pole ureter enters the bladder lateral and cephalad to the upper pole ureter. The lower pole ureter therefore has a deficient antireflux mechanism compared to the upper pole ureter, so the lower pole ureter often refluxes, whereas the upper pole ureter does not.
- **Ureterocele** is a cystic dilatation of the terminal part of the ureter (upper pole ureter if associated with a Duplex system). A ureterocele may be intravesical (also called orthotopic, or simple), entirely contained within the bladder, or ectopic, if any part of it extends to the bladder neck or distally to the urethra. The orifice can be described as stenotic, sphincteric (orifice distal to the bladder neck), sphincterostenotic (tight and distal to the bladder neck), or cecoureterocele (intravesical orifice, but with an extension submucosally into the urethra, most severe type, and occurs in girls).

PRINCIPLES AND JUSTIFICATION

The vast majority of duplications are partial, and not clinically significant. Upper tract duplication has been demonstrated to be 0.8 percent in an autopsy population, and the incidence is even higher at 2–4 percent in patients with urinary symptoms. These present during childhood, and more than 50 percent are now detected antenatally because of dilatation related to reflux, obstruction, or dysmorphism.

Duplex system ureteroceles

Duplex system ureteroceles are related to the upper pole ureters and are present in 0.02 percent of the population (80 percent female). These may have other associations and consequences: obstruction of upper pole ureter itself; VUR to the ipsilateral lower pole (50 percent); bladder outflow obstruction by ectopic ureterocele; compromise of contralateral kidney by bladder outflow obstruction; incidental contralateral reflux (25 percent); and urethral prolapse of ureterocele in girls. Sixty percent are antenatally detected, otherwise they present in infancy with urinary tract infection (UTI) or urosepsis. Occasionally, they present with urinary retention. Baby girls may present with prolapse of the ureterocele. Surgical intervention for Duplex ureteroceles should be considered: (1) if symptomatic; (2) for bladder outflow obstruction; and (3) for ureterocele prolapse.

Ectopic ureters

Ectopic ureters are detected antenatally if the upper pole ureter or upper pole of the kidney is dilated. Postnatally, suprasphincteric ectopic ureters present with UTI (epididymo-orchitis in boys). Infrasphincteric ectopic ureters occur in girls and present with a history of continuous dribbling of urine, but with a normal pattern of micturition.

PREOPERATIVE ASSESSMENT AND PREPARATION

Every case of duplicated ureter should be assessed and a specific management plan made that is tailored to the individual. The overall aims of treatment are preservation of renal function, urinary continence, reduction of infection risk by removal of obstruction, and treatment of VUR. All patients with antenatally diagnosed ureteroceles should receive prophylactic antibiotics postnatally. These investigations may be useful:

- **Ultrasound** will detect lower pole dilatation (may be secondary to VUR or UPJ obstruction), and upper pole dilatation (ureterocele or ectopic ureter). Dilatation affecting both upper and lower poles is usually secondary to a Duplex system ureterocele. Occasionally, girls may have a 'cryptic duplication' that is small and dysplastic, associated with an undilated ectopic ureter.
- **Dimercaptosuccinnic acid (DMSA) scintigraphy** will allow assessment of function of the renal units and may reveal a 'cryptic' Duplex kidney.
- **Micturating cystourethrography (MCUG)** will allow detection of lower pole VUR. Reflux, if present in both moieties, suggests incomplete duplication.
- **Intravenous urography (IVU)** is rarely required, but may be useful in identifying a poorly functioning, undilated 'cryptic' upper pole. The signs include missing calyces, lateral and downward displacement of the lower moiety ('drooping lily' sign), and a scalloped, tortuous lower moiety ureter, and laterally displaced lower moiety ureter.
- **Cystoscopy** is useful to allow determination of the site of the orifice of a ureterocele, and the number and sites of any other ureteric orifices. Endoscopic puncture can be performed at the same time.
- **Magnetic resonance imaging (MRI)** can be utilized for select patients with complex forms of duplication to provide higher quality images and further definition of anatomy.

OPERATIONS FOR DUPLEX URETEROCELE

There are now endoscopic, laparoscopic, robotic, and open surgical techniques to correct and address the many clinical problems presented by a ureteric duplication. Choosing the correct approach can be a difficult problem.

Endoscopic puncture of ureterocele

1a,b Endoscopic puncture of a ureterocele is a minimally invasive approach and is best utilized for either an intravesical ureterocele or a ureterocele associated with a functioning upper pole. The ureterocele should be punctured at its base, proximal to the bladder neck, at the most medial aspect of the ureterocele to allow for a long tunnel. Puncture can be done using a Bugbee electrode or an endoscopic cold knife. The opening created should ideally be intravesical in location to avoid obstruction by the bladder neck, particularly when the bladder is empty. The endoscopic puncture technique helps prevent VUR as the roof of the ureterocele collapses onto the floor of the bladder, acting as a flap valve. Large incisions of ureteroceles run the risk of allowing reflux to occur.

Following endoscopic puncture in intravesical ureteroceles, more than 90 percent will decompress and more than 95 percent will have maintained upper pole function; the risk of creating reflux occurs in 18 percent and 7 percent will require further surgery. For ectopic ureteroceles, the outcome is not as good: 75 percent result in upper tract decompression, upper pole function is preserved in less than 50 percent, reflux occurs in nearly 50 percent, and second procedures are needed in 50 percent.

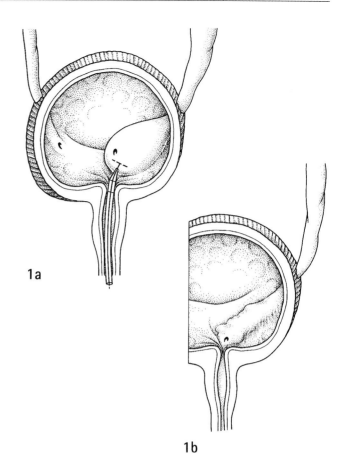

1a

1b

Upper pole heminephrectomy

2a–c The indication for this procedure is a poorly functioning upper pole. The procedure can be performed by an open approach, through an anterior muscle-splitting incision or flank incision, or by a laparoscopic approach (either transperitoneal or retroperitoneal). The procedure involves transection of the upper pole ureter, allowing traction. Ligation of the upper pole vessels allows demarcation to occur, enabling preservation of the normal renal parenchyma. The upper pole capsule can be stripped off in continuity and used to cover the cut edge at the end of the procedure. A varying length of the upper pole ureter is removed and the ureteric stump is left *in situ*. While dissecting and removing the upper pole ureter, care should be taken to not damage the blood supply to the lower pole ureter. The ureterocele should be aspirated through the upper pole ureter at the end of the procedure. With this procedure, the excised upper pole moiety and ureter can be removed through the same incision. Eight percent of patients will require further surgery if only a high approach is used. The risk of the need for further intervention is increased by ectopic ureterocele (reoperation risk of 65 percent) and high-grade reflux into another moiety (50–70 percent reoperation rate).

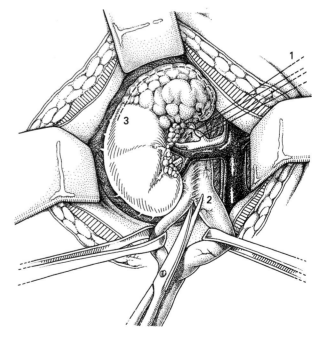

2a

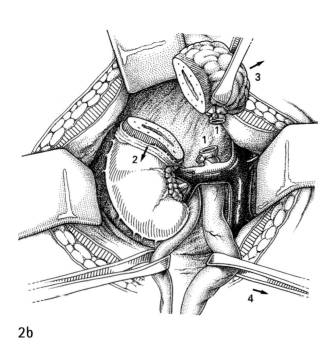

2b

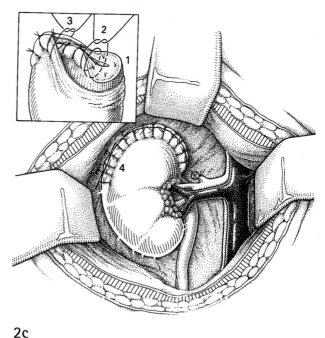

2c

Upper pole heminephrectomy, ureterectomy, and excision of ureterocele

This is indicated for prolapsing ureterocele, ectopic ureterocele, and high-grade reflux (≥grade 3) to the lower pole. This approach requires two incisions, the upper one as described and the lower one, a Pfannenstiel. The first part of the procedure is described above, the second below. There is a ≤15 percent risk of requiring reoperation, but also a risk of damage to the sphincter mechanism when an ectopic ureterocele is enucleated.

Ureteropyeloplasty

3a–c This allows preservation of a functioning upper pole in association with obstructed Duplex ureterocele (rare). An open approach, through an anterior muscle-splitting incision or flank incision, or a laparoscopic approach, either transperitoneal or retroperitoneal, is made. Ureteropyeloplasty is performed. The ureterocele must be aspirated through the upper pole ureter, followed by placement of a ureteric stent which is left in place for approximately 5 days. There is a reoperation rate for continuing reflux into the lower pole ureter, or into the upper pole stump. The risk of further surgery is increased, as described above.

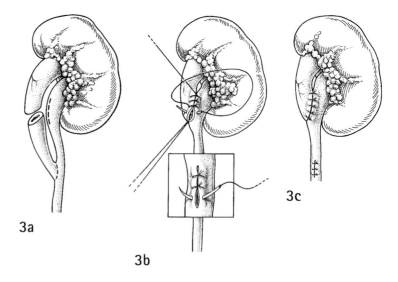

3a

3b

3c

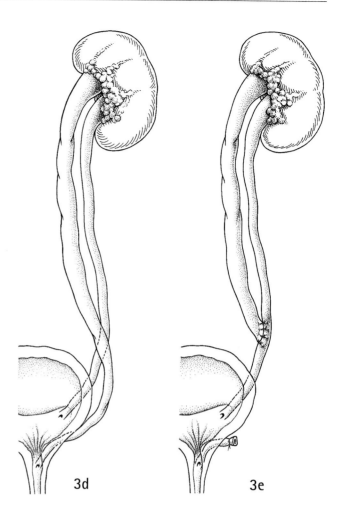

3d,e Increasingly, this operation is being replaced as ureteroureterostomy is more commonly being utilized now by surgeons. Ureteroureterostomy is an option for patients that do not have lower pole VUR. This procedure is performed through a small inguinal incision and muscle-splitting approach allowing access to the retroperitoneal space. Both ureters are identified, the upper pole ureter is transected and the remaining distal upper pole ureter removed to the level of the sphincter. The lower pole ureter is incised and then ureteroureterostomy performed without leaving a ureteral stent or drain in place postoperatively.

3d

3e

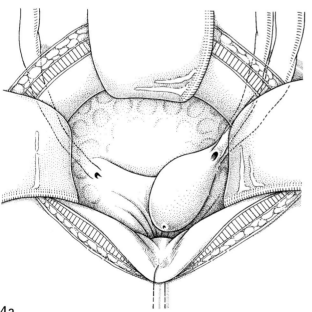

4a

Removal of intravesical ureterocele and reimplantation of the ureter

4a–d This is indicated when there is still useable lower pole function in the setting of continuing reflux, infection, or obstruction of the upper pole ureter. A Pfannenstiel approach is used. The ureterocele is excised carefully, because the common sheath of double ureters means that the blood supply is common to both. Common sheath reimplantation is performed, reimplanting the two ureters submucosally, with tapering as needed for a significantly dilated upper pole ureter.

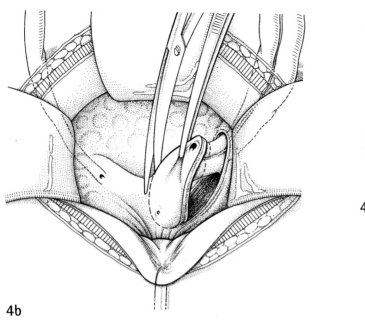

4b

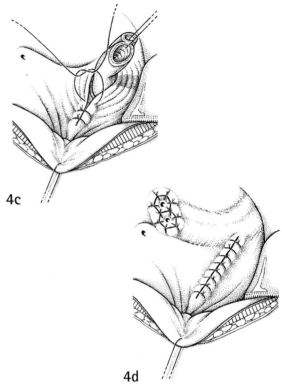

4c

4d

Removal of extravesical ureterocele and reimplantation

5a–f The approach and procedure are as described above, but plication of the posterior bladder wall may be needed if the ureterocele is prolapsed and the posterior wall is deficient. Care must be taken with extravesical extension, as this can lead to damage of the sphincter mechanism. Occasionally, with a cecoureterocele, the posterior portion of the bladder neck and urethra has been damaged resulting in urinary incontinence. This requires more extensive dissection and a formal bladder neck reconstruction (discussed in **Chapter 86**).

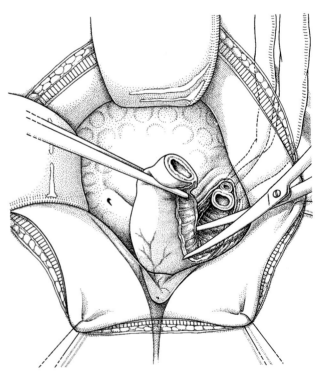

5a

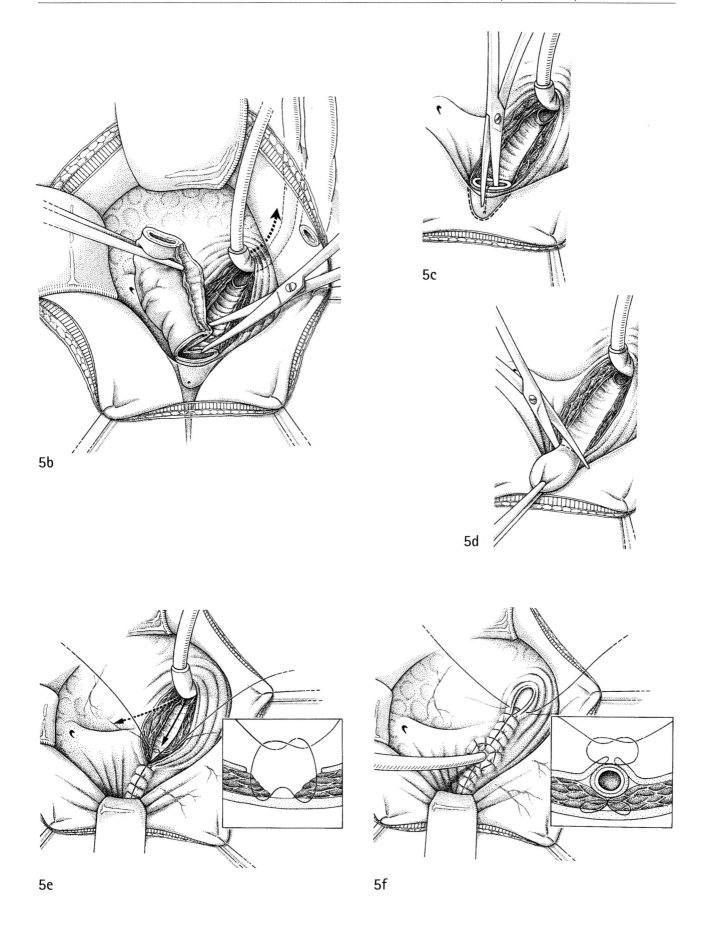

5b

5c

5d

5e

5f

Nephrectomy

This is described in Chapters 83a and 83b.

OPERATIONS FOR ECTOPIC URETER

Suprasphincteric ectopic ureter

The indications depend on the symptoms from recurrent UTIs.

- **Upper pole heminephrectomy** (see illustration 2). In most cases, this is indicated by lack of function in the upper pole moiety. This can be achieved through either an open or laparoscopic approach.
- **Ureteric reimplantation** (see illustration 6). This is only possible when there is a well-functioning upper pole. An en-bloc reimplantation is performed because both upper and lower pole ureters share a common sheath and blood supply.
- **Ureteroureterostomy** (see illustration 3d,e). This procedure, described above, is performed using an extraperitoneal groin incision.

Infrasphincteric ectopic ureter

The main problem is diagnostic: identifying 'cryptic' upper pole, 10 percent of cases which will have a coexistent and detectable contralateral Duplex kidney. For poorly functioning moieties (the majority), upper pole nephrectomy will be curative (see illustration 2). Good function is very rare; if reimplantation is needed, both ureters on the affected side will need to be reimplanted because of the presence of the common ureteric sheath distally (see illustration 6 below).

OPERATIONS FOR VESICOURETERAL REFLUX ASSOCIATED WITH DUPLEX SYSTEM

Ureteric reimplantation

6a,b   The indication of ureteric reimplantation is persistent VUR with breakthrough infections once voiding dysfunction and constipation have been corrected.

A Pfannenstiel approach is used for a Cohen cross-trigonal reimplantation. Care must be taken to reimplant double ureters en bloc, otherwise the shared blood supply associated with the common sheath will be impaired. At some institutions, either sub- or intraureteric injection of a bulking agent (see **Chapter 84**) is being used instead of a ureteric reimplantation.

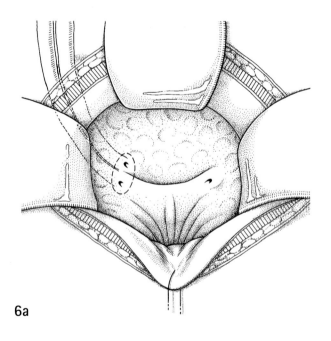
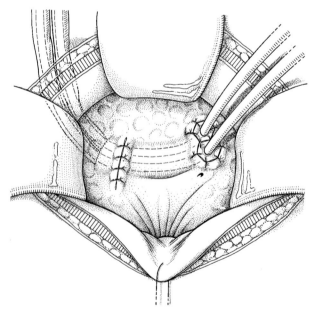

6a

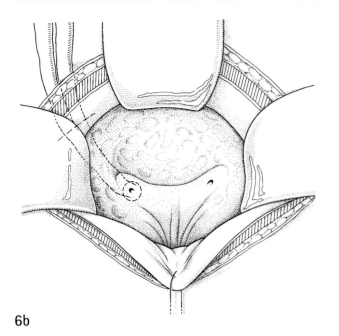

6b

Lower pole heminephrectomy

7a–e The indication for this is a poor/non-functional lower pole, with recurrent UTIs. The procedure may be done with an open approach or laparoscopically. If performed laparoscopically, the kidney may be approached transperitoneally or retroperitoneally. The kidney is visualized and the blood vessels are ligated with clips and divided. The ureter is divided. An endoloop is placed at the point where demarcation occurs and tightened. The lower pole is then excised and removed.

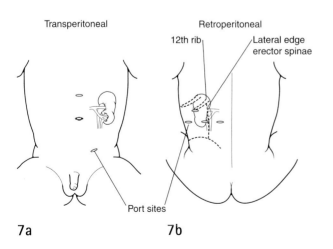

Transperitoneal   Retroperitoneal

12th rib

Lateral edge
erector spinae

Port sites

7a   **7b**

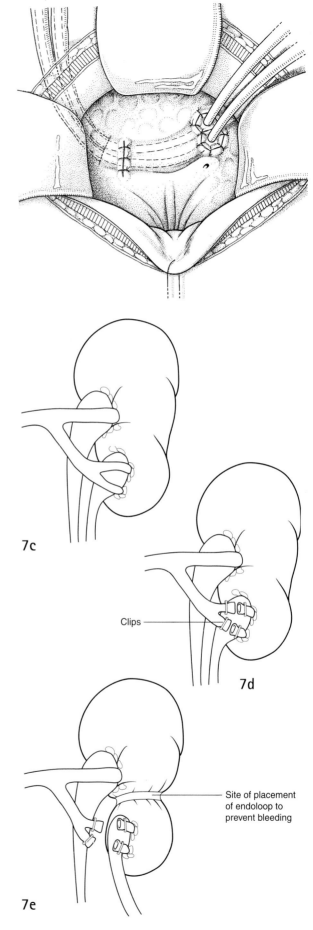

7c

Clips

7d

Site of placement
of endoloop to
prevent bleeding

7e

POSTOPERATIVE CARE

Intravenous fluids and adequate analgesia (which may include a morphine infusion) are continued until patients are drinking adequately. No stents or drains are needed for nephrectomies or partial nephrectomies, whereas bladder drainage is appropriate if cystotomy has been performed to allow excision of a ureterocele or ureteric reimplantation.

FURTHER READING

Mackie CG, Stephens FD. Duplex kidneys: a correlation with renal dysplasia with position of the ureteric orifice. *Journal of Urology* 1975; **114**: 274.

Nepple KG, Cooper CS, Synder HM. Ureteral duplication, ectopy and ureteroceles. In: Gearhart JP, Rink RC, Mouriquand PDE (eds). *Pediatric Urology*, 2nd edn. Philadelphia: Saunders, 2010: 337–52.

Rickwood AMK, Madden NP, Boddy SM. Duplication anomalies, ureteroceles and ectopic ureters. In: Thomas DFM, Rickwood AMK, Duffy PD (eds). *Essentials of Paediatric Urology*, 2nd edn. London: Martin Dunitz, 2008, 93–108.

Schlussel RN, Retik AB. Ectopic ureter, ureterocele, and other anomalies of the ureter. In: Wein AJ, Kavoussi LR, Novick AC *et al.* (eds). *Campbell's Urology*, 9th edn, vol. 4. Philadelphia: Saunders, 2002: 3383–422.

86

Urinary diversion in children

PRASAD GODBOLE and DUNCAN T WILCOX

PRINCIPLES AND JUSTIFICATION

Urinary diversion, although uncommon in children, is a useful tool in the armamentarium of the pediatric urologist. The primary aim of urinary diversion is to ensure adequate drainage of the urinary tract and thereby preserve renal function. The secondary aim is to achieve continence for social reasons. Urinary diversions may be incontinent or continent. Incontinent diversions entail cutaneous drainage of urine into a pad, nappy, or stoma bag. A continent diversion aims to create a low-pressure, compliant, and capacious reservoir and a catheterizable conduit for drainage of the reservoir where the urethra is found to be unsuitable.

The majority of urinary diversions are performed for congenital anomalies of the urinary tract and their consequences, e.g. neuropathic bladder due to spinal dysraphism, the exstrophy epispadias complex, posterior urethral valves, functional bladder disorders such as the Hinman bladder, or bladder malignancy. The choice of diversion depends on the child's diagnosis, body habitus, manual dexterity, compliance, and social circumstances. For example, a child with a neuropathic bladder, severe developmental delay, difficult social circumstances, and deteriorating upper tracts may be better off with a vesicostomy rather than a bladder augmentation and a Mitrofanoff conduit.

PREOPERATIVE ASSESSMENT AND PREPARATION

The assessment and preparation of children for surgery consist of three components:

1. overall assessment
2. renal assessment
3. assessment and preparation for the specific procedure.

Overall assessment

This entails assessment of the overall fitness of the child for the surgery involved. For example, a child with severe kyphoscoliosis may have decreased respiratory reserve and may require a chest x-ray. Attention should also be directed toward the nutritional status, cardiovascular status, and neurological status of the child. Assessment by the anesthetist well in advance of surgery may be advisable in complicated cases.

Renal assessment

All children should have baseline biochemistry and hematology. Those children with chronic renal failure require input from the nephrologists preoperatively and postoperatively. All children for diversion should also have a baseline ultrasound scan and functional imaging – either a mercaptoacetyl triglycine (MAG-3) or dimercaptosuccinic acid (DMSA) scan. Additional investigations depend on individual patients, e.g. videourodynamics, micturating cystourethrogram.

Assessment and preparation for the specific procedure

This forms a very important component of the assessment process. Before a decision can be made regarding the appropriate procedure for a particular child, the capabilities, compliance, and circumstances of the child and carers must be taken into consideration. In the authors' institute, this is conducted in part by the clinicians in outpatient consultations, but mainly by a dedicated team of clinical urology nurse specialists. Once a decision regarding the type of procedure has been made, the child and carers are prepared for the surgery by being given leaflets with information about the procedure, as well as other visual aids such as videos, and the child is allowed to interact with other children who have had a similar procedure. Surgery is carried out once the child and carers are deemed 'ready' for the procedure. Attention must be paid to the need for bowel preparation, e.g. in colocystoplasty. However, where the ileum is used, routine bowel preparation may not be necessary. In the authors' practice, clear fluids for 24 hours preoperatively is sufficient in these cases. In general, for most urological procedures, we use a broad-spectrum urinary antiseptic based on local hospital guidance, such as amikacin alone or a combination of amikacin, benzylpenicillin, and metronidazole, at induction and for up to 48 hours postoperatively. Further need for antibiotics depends on the clinical situation.

Anesthesia

All procedures are performed under general anesthesia with endotracheal intubation and full muscle relaxation. Concomitant regional analgesia, such as an epidural catheter or caudal block, may also be used. Children deemed unsuitable for these regional techniques may receive postoperative nurse-controlled analgesia or patient-controlled analgesia.

OPERATIONS

The following operations are described:

- Incontinent diversions:
  - open or button vesicostomy;
  - ureterostomy and pyelostomy;
  - conduit diversion: ileal conduit, colonic conduit.
- Continent diversions:
  - surgery of the reservoir: ileocystoplasty, colocystoplasty;
  - the continent catheterizable conduit – the Mitrofanoff principle and its variants: appendicovesicostomy, ileovesicostomy (Yang–Monti), continent tube vesicostomy;
  - stoma: the VQZ plasty.

INCONTINENT URINARY DIVERSION

Vesicostomy

A vesicostomy may be performed as a temporary measure for urinary diversion in selected cases such as posterior urethral valves, gross vesicoureteric reflux, or neuropathic bladder. In cases of posterior urethral valves, although primary fulguration is the ideal method of treatment, we have found there to be no difference in the outcome for boys with posterior urethral valves who had an initial vesicostomy and delayed ablation as compared to primary fulguration. Vesicostomy has a high incidence of stomal stenosis and prolapse in the long term and should not be considered as a permanent option.

An alternative to vesicostomy is the use of a suprapubic MicKey button inserted via an open technique. This allows intermittent drainage of urine in a 'continent' manner.

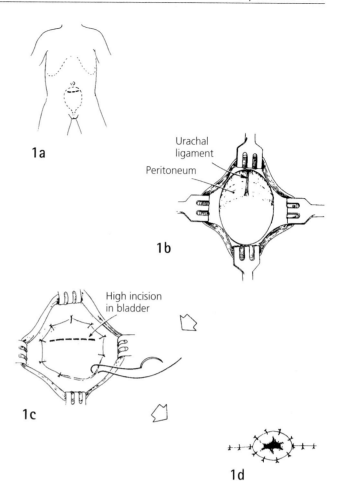

TECHNIQUE

Position

1a The patient is placed in the supine position.

Incision

1b,c A short transverse incision a few centimeters in length is made above the pubic symphysis in an area that will drain into the pad/nappy.

Procedure

1d The bladder is mobilized extraperitoneally and the dome is identified by the urachal remnant, which is ligated with an absorbable suture. The dome is sutured circumferentially with interrupted 4/0 absorbable sutures to the fascia. The dome is then opened and the mucocutaneous anastomosis is performed with circumferential 4/0 absorbable, interrupted sutures.

POSTOPERATIVE CARE

A 12 Fr catheter is left *in situ* for 24 hours and then removed. Subsequently, the vesicostomy is allowed to drain into the nappy.

COMPLICATIONS

1e If the vesicostomy is made too low, prolapse of the posterior wall may occur. Stomal stenosis may occur in the long term.

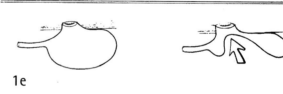

Ureterostomy/pyelostomy

A cutaneous ureterostomy is used as a temporary measure in carefully selected cases for decompression of the upper tracts. Debate still exists as to its role in posterior urethral valves with deteriorating upper tracts either as a primary procedure or even after valve fulguration. We have used this method in selected children under one year of age with solitary kidneys and a ureterovesical junction obstruction with deteriorating renal function. A ureterostomy may also be performed where malignancy necessitates large pelvic resections. In selected cases of posterior urethral valves with gross unilateral vesicoureteric reflux, a 'refluxing' ureterostomy may be performed on the side of reflux concomitant to valve resection to act as a pop-off mechanism and thereby protect the upper tracts. The ureterostomy may be created distally or proximally. The description below is of a distal ureterostomy.

TECHNIQUE

Position

The patient is placed in a supine position; a more oblique position is required for a higher diversion.

Incision

2a A short inguinal groin crease incision is made on the affected side. The site of the incision is modified depending on the site of the intended diversion; however, the approach to the ureter remains extraperitoneal.

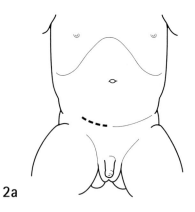

2a

Procedure

2b A flap of skin is raised superiorly to gain access to the extraperitoneal space via a muscle split. The peritoneum is reflected medially. The ureter is identified by dividing the obliterated umbilical artery (illustration b). In cases of end ureterostomy, the ureter is detached close to the bladder and the bladder end is oversewn with 4/0 absorbable suture – either polyglactic acid (Vicryl) or polydioxanone (PDS).

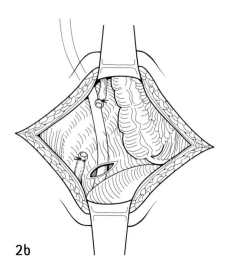

2b

2c The ureter is brought out of the groin crease incision and the mucocutaneous anastomosis creating a small everted nipple is performed with interrupted 6/0 absorbable sutures.

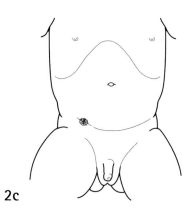

2c

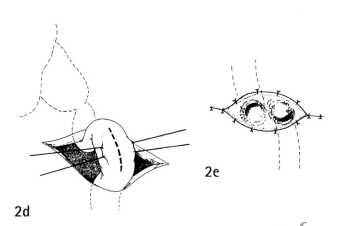

2d

2e

2d,e If a loop ureterostomy is performed, the ureter is opened longitudinally and mucocutaneous anastomosis of both limbs is performed with interrupted 6/0 absorbable sutures.

2f,g A pyelostomy is performed using a similar technique.

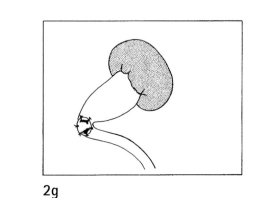

2f

2g

POSTOPERATIVE CARE

The ureterostomy is allowed to drain freely into the nappy.

COMPLICATIONS

Stomal stenosis or stomal prolapse may occur. In cases of dilated tortuous and adynamic upper tracts, good drainage may not be achieved with a ureterostomy and an indwelling catheter or intermittent catheterization of the stoma may be necessary.

Ileal conduit

Because of the high incidence of complications, an ileal conduit diversion is very uncommon nowadays in children.

However, in very carefully selected cases, this may be a useful option, for example in children with neuropathic bladder or pelvic malignancy who, along with their carers, may prefer this to major urinary tract reconstruction and continent diversion in the short to medium term.

TECHNIQUE

Position

The patient is placed in a supine position.

Incision

The ileum can be approached through the same incision as that for the primary procedure if the diversion is being performed concomitantly. If being performed in isolation, a lower midline incision may be preferable.

Procedure

3a–f A short, 6–10 cm, segment of ileum on its mesentery is isolated and the proximal end is oversewn with a 4/0 or 5/0 PDS extramucosal, single-layer, interrupted or continuous suture. Intestinal continuity is restored with 5/0 PDS extramucosal, single-layer interrupted or continuous suture. The ureters are spatulated (illustration a) and implanted in the conduit in a submucosal tunnel, and the anastomosis is completed with 6/0 PDS interrupted sutures (illustration b). The distal end of the ileal loop is brought out at a suitable premarked position in the right iliac fossa and everted to create a nipple (illustration c). The mucocutaneous anastomosis is completed with interrupted 5/0 or 6/0 PDS sutures. Two 4- or 6-Fr feeding tubes are left indwelling within the implanted ureters and exiting via the stoma. If the ureters are dilated, the spatulated ends may be anastomosed with 6/0 PDS to form a common channel (illustration d), which is in turn anastomosed to the proximal end of the conduit with 4/0 or 5/0 PDS sutures (illustrations e and f).

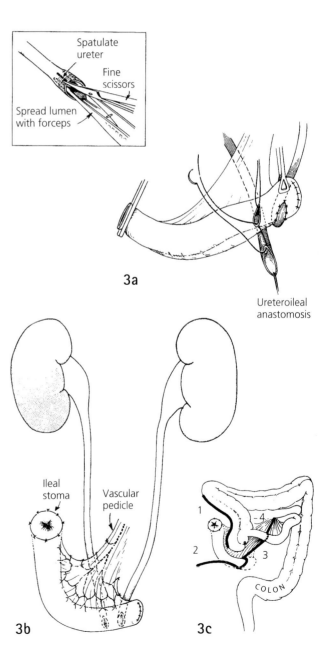

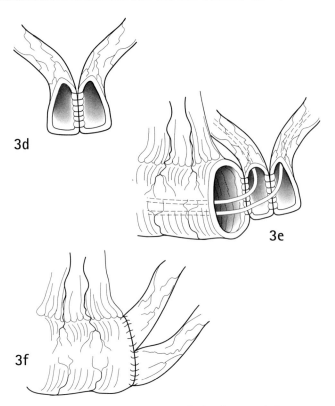

3d

3e

3f

POSTOPERATIVE CARE

The feeding tubes are removed 10 days to 2 weeks after surgery. Close monitoring of the upper tracts is essential.

COMPLICATIONS

Problems with ureteral stenosis or vesicoureteric reflux may occur along with deterioration of renal function. Therefore, close follow up is mandatory.

Procedure

4a–d A suitable segment of colon, preferably the sigmoid colon, is isolated on its mesentery and intestinal continuity is restored with 5/0 PDS sutures (illustrations a and b). The distal end is oversewn and the ureters are spatulated and implanted in the conduit in a non-refluxing manner (illustration c). The distal end of the conduit is brought out as a stoma at a predetermined, premarked site on the abdominal wall and everted. Mucocutaneous anastomosis is performed with absorbable sutures of 5/0 Vicryl or 5/0 PDS sutures (illustration d).

Colonic conduit

TECHNIQUE
Position

The patient is placed in a supine position.

Incision

A lower midline incision is preferred.

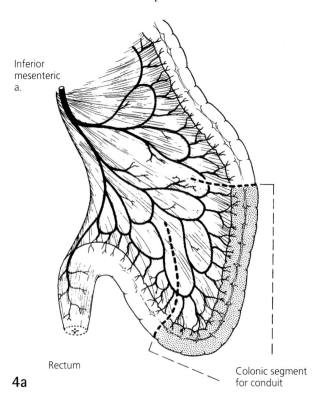

Inferior mesenteric a.

Rectum

Colonic segment for conduit

4a

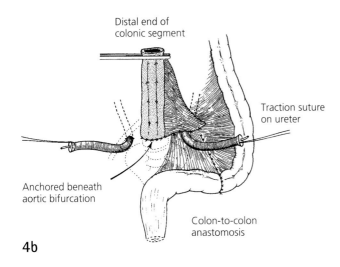

Distal end of
colonic segment

Traction suture
on ureter

Anchored beneath
aortic bifurcation

Colon-to-colon
anastomosis

4b

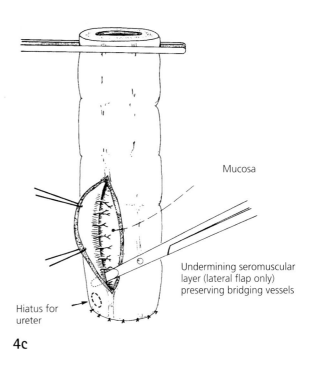

Mucosa

Undermining seromuscular
layer (lateral flap only)
preserving bridging vessels

Hiatus for
ureter

4c

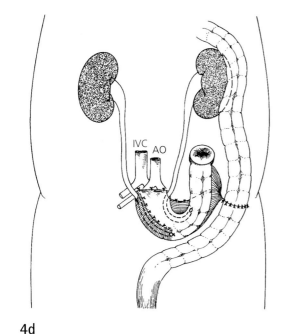

IVC   AO

4d

POSTOPERATIVE CARE

As with the ileal conduit, careful monitoring of the upper tracts is essential.

COMPLICATIONS

These are similar to those of an ileal conduit and include ureteral stenosis and kinking and deterioration of the upper tracts.

CONTINENT URINARY DIVERSION

While in the majority of cases, surgery for continent urinary diversion is performed by the open route (described here), there have been increasing reports of these interventions carried out by minimally invasive (laparoscopic or robotic) instrumentation. The full impact of these techniques are yet to be fully evaluated.

Surgery of the reservoir

ILEOCYSTOPLASTY

A detubularized segment of ileum is usually used for bladder augmentation. In cases where the mesentery is too short to reach the pelvis, e.g. gross kyphosis, colon may be used. A bladder outlet procedure may be performed simultaneously to increase outlet resistance. We do not routinely advocate preoperative bowel preparation for an ileocystoplasty, as the contents of the ileum are fluid and, in our opinion, do not need mechanical cleansing.

TECHNIQUE
Position

The patient is placed in a supine position.

Incision

A Pfannenstiel or midline incision is preferred.

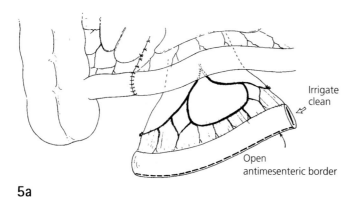

5a

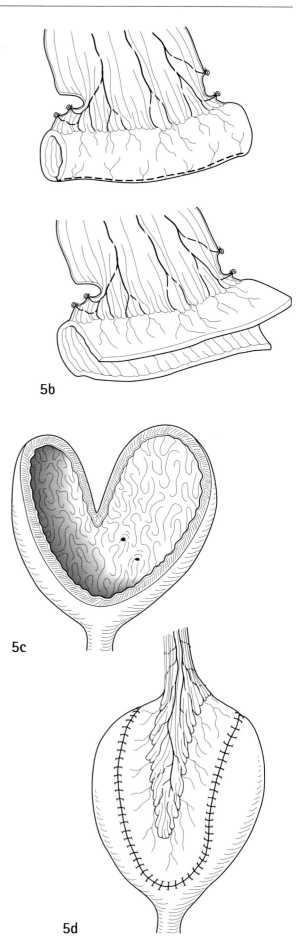

5b

5c

5d

Procedure

5a–g Initial extraperitoneal mobilization of the bladder is carried out circumferentially down to the region of the bladder neck. A small opening is made in the posterior aspect of the reflected peritoneum and the cecum and terminal ileum are delivered. If an appendicovesicostomy is to be performed, mobilization of the appendix and mesentery can be performed at this stage. A suitable segment of ileum approximately 25 cm long and 20 cm from the ileocecal junction is isolated on its mesentery and intestinal continuity is restored with 5/0 PDS sutures (illustration a). The ileum is detubularized along its antimesenteric border (illustration b). The peritoneum is closed, thereby extraperitonealizing the segment of ileum and bladder. The bladder is opened from one ureteric orifice to the other in either the coronal or sagittal plane (illustration c). The appendix is reimplanted in the bladder at this stage and a clam cystoplasty is performed with continuous 3/0 absorbable suture (illustration d). Just before completion of the anastomosis, a large-bore 16- or 18-Fr Foley catheter is inserted suprapubically. If an appendicovesicostomy has been created, an indwelling catheter is left within this conduit. If the bladder is very small, thick-walled, and contracted, it may be excised, leaving only the bladder plate comprising the trigone and the ureteric orifices. In this case, the ileal patch may be reconfigured as a pouch (illustrations e–g), which can be sutured to the bladder remnant.

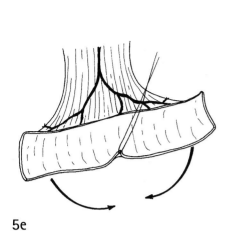

5e

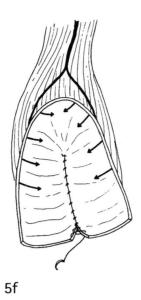

5f

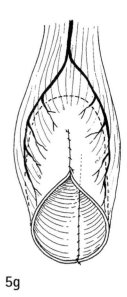

5g

POSTOPERATIVE CARE

The suprapubic catheter is left on free drainage for 3 weeks with bladder washouts as required. A regime of clamp and release is then instituted prior to commencing clean intermittent catheterization either urethrally or via the Mitrofanoff channel. All patients should have periodic renal ultrasound scans and regular estimation of biochemical parameters, including acid–base status.

COMPLICATIONS

The patient and carers must be warned of the potential risks of this procedure. These include mucus blockage, urinary infections, the development of bladder calculi, persistence of a high-pressure neoreservoir, metabolic and acid–base disturbances, and the possibility in the long term of the development of adenocarcinoma.

COLOCYSTOPLASTY

The segment used may be detubularized sigmoid colon, the transverse colon, or the ileocecal and ascending colon. The principles of the technique are similar to those described above, as are the postoperative care and complications.

The Mitrofanoff principle

In 1911, Coffey described the flap valve technique of ureteral reimplantation in ureterosigmoidostomy. This principle was utilized by Mitrofanoff in 1980 to create a continent, catheterizable appendicovesicostomy. The main components of the Mitrofanoff technique are:

- a narrow, supple conduit brought to the skin as a catheterizable stoma;
- an antirefluxing connection between the conduit and the reservoir (flap valve);
- a large, low-pressure urinary reservoir;
- an antirefluxing mechanism between the upper urinary tract and the reservoir;
- intermittent catheterization to allow effective, regular, low-pressure emptying of the reservoir.

Appendicovesicostomy

TECHNIQUE

Position

The patient is placed in a supine position.

Incision

A Pfannenstiel or lower midline incision is used.

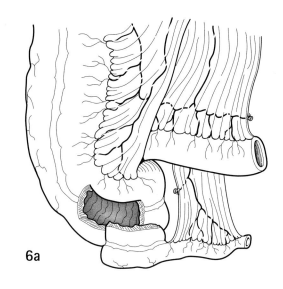

6a

Procedure

6a,b Assessment is made of the length of the appendix and its suitability as a conduit. The appendix is mobilized with its mesentery and detached from the cecum, which is closed with absorbable sutures. A cuff of cecum may be mobilized with the appendix and tubularized to gain additional length, if necessary (illustration a). The tip of the appendix is incised and a 12-Fr feeding tube is inserted to confirm patency and diameter of the lumen. The lumen is irrigated with dilute betadine solution. The distal end of the appendix is then tunneled into the bladder in a submucosal tunnel for 3–4 cm to maintain a 5:1 ratio and ensure a competent flap-valve mechanism (illustration b). This is then anchored to the muscle and mucosa of the bladder using absorbable suture. The rest of the circumference of the appendix is sutured to the bladder mucosa using absorbable sutures. The appendix is also anchored at its entry into the bladder by a few interrupted sutures.

The proximal end of the appendix is brought out as a stoma by the shortest and straightest route possible to enable easy catheterization. The site of the stoma will therefore be variable. The umbilicus may be used to site the stoma in certain children for easy access, or a VQZ stoma technique for abdominal Mitrofanoff stomas can be used.

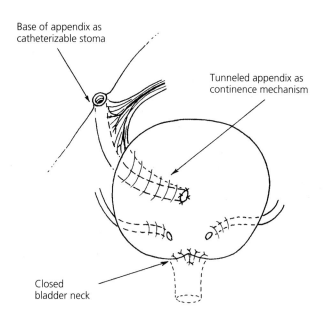

Base of appendix as catheterizable stoma

Tunneled appendix as continence mechanism

Closed bladder neck

6b

POSTOPERATIVE CARE

An indwelling 10- or 12-Fr Jacques catheter is left for 3 weeks and is followed by clamp and release and clean intermittent catheterization under nursing supervision.

COMPLICATIONS

Problems with the conduit include stomal stenosis, difficulty in catheterization leading to the creation of a false passage, and the development of calculi.

Ileovesicostomy

Where the appendix is absent or not suitable, a segment of ileum can be utilized to create a transverse ileal tube. This is the preferred second-line option for creating the Mitrofanoff channel, especially when ileum is used for bladder augmentation.

TECHNIQUE

Procedure

7a–c A segment of ileum approximately 1.5–2 cm in width adjacent to that used for the cystoplasty is isolated on its mesentery and opened longitudinally on its antimesenteric border. The position of the mesentery along the tube can be moved depending on the position of the longitudinal opening. This tube is then tubularized transversely over a 12-Fr catheter (a). In patients with a long distance between the reservoir and the abdominal wall or the umbilicus, two adjacent segments can be isolated, tubularized, and anastomosed (Full Monti, illustration b). A similar technique has been described by Casale using a single piece of bowel to gain additional length (illustration c). The tube is then tunneled into the reservoir as described above to create the Mitrofanoff flap valve.

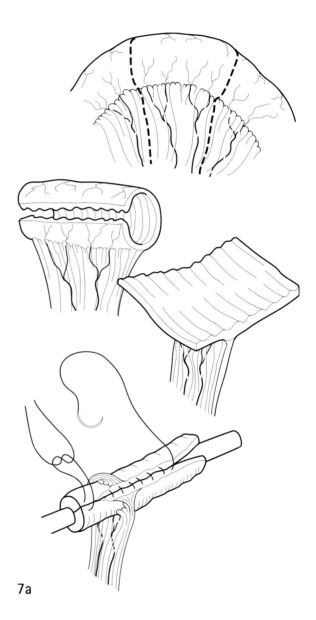

7a

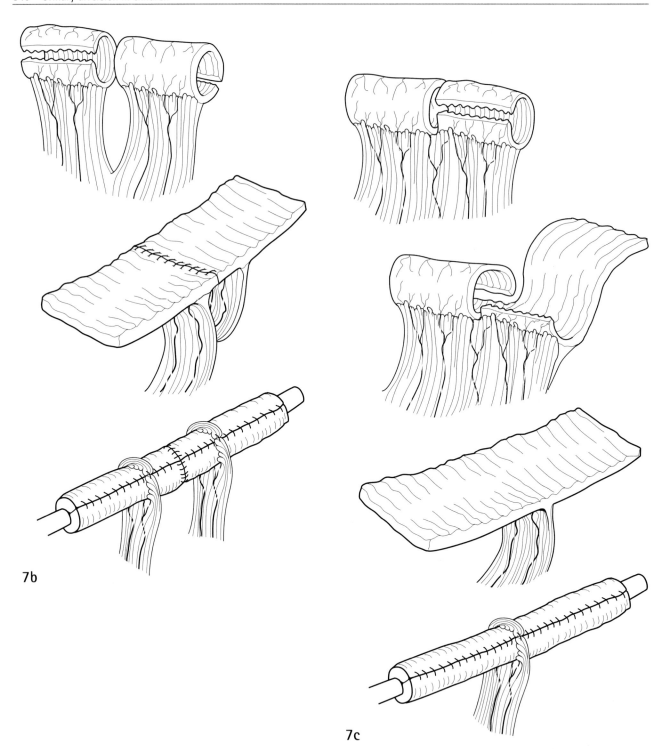

7b

7c

POSTOPERATIVE CARE

As with the appendicovesicostomy, an indwelling catheter is left *in situ* for 3 weeks before instituting clamp and release and clean intermittent catheterization.

COMPLICATIONS

Due to the elasticity of the ileum, more problems may be encountered with catheterization than with the appendicovesicostomy.

Detrusor tube vesicostomy

This technique involves a segment of tubularized bladder with an antireflux flap valve constructed primarily of mucosa. Patients must have a large bladder capacity to be considered suitable.

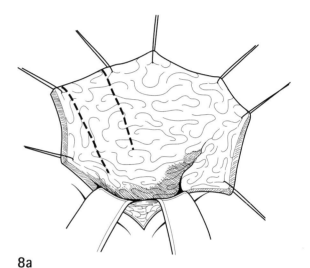

8a

TECHNIQUE

Procedure

8a–f A broad-based rectangular flap (approximately 3 cm × 7 mm) of full-thickness detrusor muscle and mucosa is raised on its vascular supply from the superior vesical pedicle. This is tubularized in two layers (mucosa and muscle) over a 12-Fr catheter. The proximal mucosal end is further tubularized within the bladder for about 2 cm and covered by laterally raised adjacent mucosal flaps.

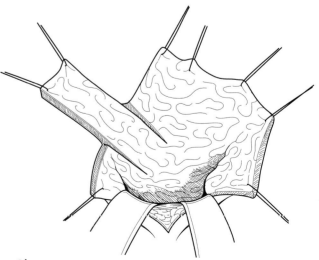

8b

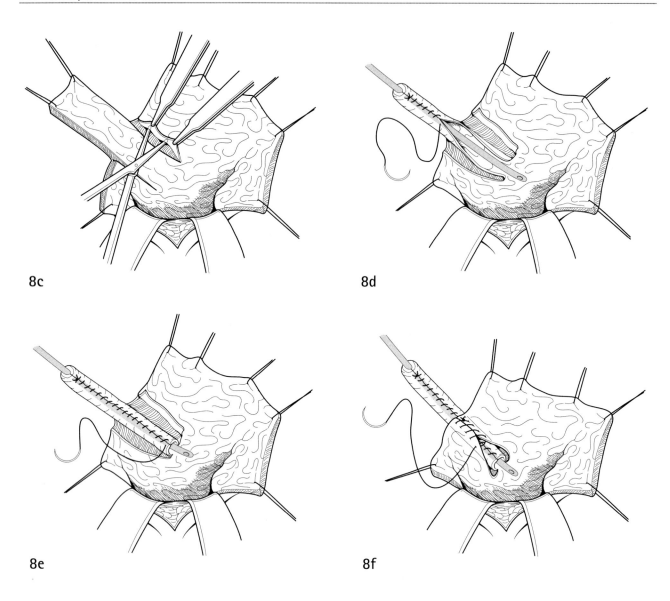

8c

8d

8e

8f

POSTOPERATIVE CARE

Postoperative care is similar to that for appendicovesicostomy.

COMPLICATIONS

Stomal stenosis is the main complicating factor.

The VQZ stoma

The VQZ plasty for the cutaneous opening into a Mitrofanoff conduit has several advantages over the standard V flap or flush stoma in that it is discrete and there is no exposed mucosa and hence less likelihood of contact bleeding.

TECHNIQUE

Position

The patient is placed in a supine position.

Incision and procedure

9a–k A V flap is raised with its base in the region of the exiting appendix (illustration a). A generous opening is made into the layers of the anterior abdominal wall and the appendix is delivered. The abdominal incision is then closed. The appendix is incised along its antimesenteric border and the flap is sutured in place with 5/0 PDS along its entire length up to its angle on its superior border, but stopping 5–10 mm short on its inferior border (illustrations b–d). The Q flap is then raised and rotated, and sutured into place along the rest of the appendicular margin and the remaining inferior border of the V flap (illustrations e–g). The mucosa is therefore entirely covered. A standard Z plasty is performed to rotate the adjacent skin to cover the defect (illustrations h–k). Subcutaneous 3/0 PDS sutures may be required at the angles of the Z plasty, which will be under some tension. The rest of the skin is closed with 5/0 or 6/0 PDS sutures.

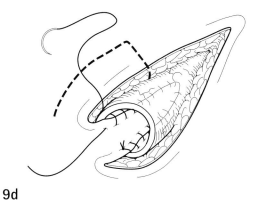

9d

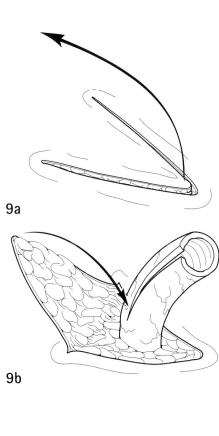

9a

9b

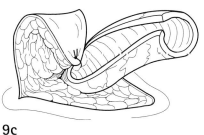

9c

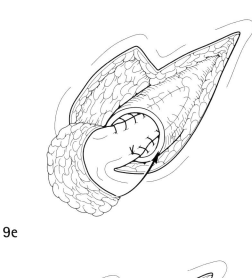

9e

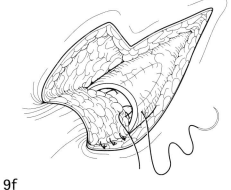

9f

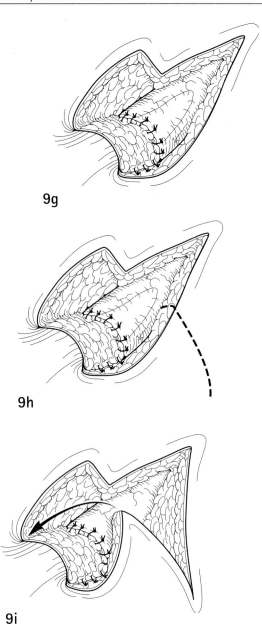

9g

9h

9i

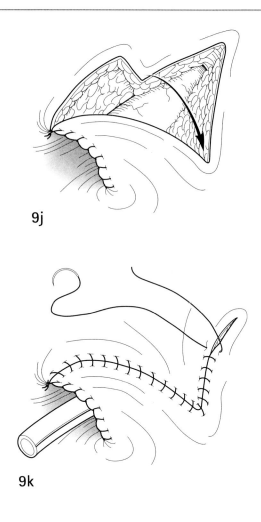

9j

9k

POSTOPERATIVE CARE

The wound should be left open to allow regular inspection of the stoma site.

COMPLICATIONS

Wound infection and wound dehiscence may occur. Stomal stenosis may require further skin-level revisions.

CONCLUSION

Numerous techniques are available for urinary diversion in children. The choice depends on careful patient selection and requires a close working relationship between multidisciplinary teams, including urologists,

nurse specialists, physiotherapists, psychologists, and nephrologists. The ultimate goal remains the preservation of renal function by any technique that is appropriate for, and acceptable to, the individual child and his or her carers.

FURTHER READING

Adams MC, Rink RC. Augmentation cystoplasty. In: Gearhart J, Mouriquand P, Rink R (eds). *Pediatric Urology.* Philadelphia, PA: WB Saunders, 2010: 748–61.

Farrugia MK, Malone PS. Educational article: the Mitrofanoff procedure. *Journal of Pediatric Urology* 2010; **6**: 330–7.

Godbole PP. Augmentation cystoplasty. In: Wilcox DT, Godbole PP, Koyle MA (eds). *Pediatric Urology, Surgical Complications and Management*. London: Wiley-Blackwell, 2008: 307–15.

Leslie JA, Dussinger AM, Meldrum KK. Creation of continence mechanisms (Mitrofanoff) without appendix: the Monti and spiral Monti procedures. *Urologic Oncology* 2007; **25**: 148–53.

Metcalfe PD, Cain MP. Incontinent and continent urinary diversion. In: Gearhart J, Mouriquand P, Rink R (eds). *Pediatric Urology*. Philadelphia, PA: WB Saunders, 2010: 737–48.

Traxel EJ, Minevich EA, Noh PH. A review: the application of minimally invasive surgery to pediatric urology: lower urinary tract reconstructive procedures. *Urology* 2010; **76**: 115–20.

87

Renal calculi

NAIMA SMEULDERS

EPIDEMIOLOGY

Stone formation in the urinary tract affects approximately 5–10 percent of the population. Children account for just 1–3 percent of all stone patients. The incidence of urolithiasis shows marked geographical variation: while very rare in Greenland and Japan, a 'stone belt' extends from the Balkans across Turkey, Pakistan, and northern India.

Overall, boys are twice as often affected as girls and tend to present at a younger age, with an average age at presentation of 36 months for boys and 48 months for girls. Presenting features are macroscopic hematuria, urinary tract infection, or abdominal pain; some children (17 percent) appear to be asymptomatic. Obstruction related to calculi may result in pyonephrosis, perinephric abscess, or progressive pyelonephritis, and renal loss.

ETIOLOGY

In the past, the majority of renal calculi in children were considered infective in origin. The organisms most commonly associated with infective calculi are the urea-splitting *Proteus* and *Escherichia coli*. Infective calculi are usually soft, containing organic matrix, and may be poorly opacified. They usually consist of calcium magnesium and ammonium phosphate.

Today, a metabolic abnormality is detected in 44 percent of children with urolithiasis in the UK. Hypercalciuria (57 percent) is the most common metabolic abnormality, followed by cystinuria (23 percent), hyperoxaluria (17 percent), hyperuricosuria (2 percent), and unclassified hypercalcemia (2 percent).

PREOPERATIVE

Radiology

In children, the main imaging modality is ultrasound. It can detect stones throughout the urinary tract, although stones in the mid- or distal ureter may be obscured by bowel gas, especially if the bladder is empty. The ultrasound should give an assessment of the size, shape, number, and location of calculi. Dilatation proximal to an obstructing stone will also be demonstrated, and the presence of debris will raise the suspicion of infection and the need to relieve the obstruction urgently.

A plain abdominal x-ray of the whole urinary tract may be a useful adjunct. In children, however, bowel gas may make interpretation difficult. Uric acid and cystine calculi are mildly radio-opaque. Xanthine and dihydroxyadenine stones are radiolucent.

For the majority of children, a detailed ultrasound provides sufficient anatomical information to plan their treatment. Rarely, additional information may be sought from a non-contrast enhanced computed tomography or intravenous pyelogram.

A dimercaptosuccinyl acid (DMSA) scan or mercaptoacetyl-triglycine (Mag3) will provide functional information of the kidneys.

Urinalysis

Microscopy and urine culture are performed. Stones are analyzed for chemical composition. Urine is sent for determination of pH, calcium, urate, oxalate, cystine, and creatinine. These investigations may be performed before surgery or much later when the child is stone free.

Plasma

Creatinine, urea, potassium, sodium, chloride, bicarbonate, magnesium, calcium, phosphate, alkaline phosphatase, albumin, and urate tests are performed.

The findings of nephrocalcinosis, bilateral calculi, or recurrent calculi suggest a metabolic abnormality. Nephrocalcinosis may be associated with renal tubular acidosis, hyperoxaluria, and hypercalcemia.

OPERATIONS

As a result of the dramatic advances in technology over the last decades, the less invasive techniques of extracorporeal shock-wave lithotripsy (ESWL), percutaneous nephrolithotomy (PCNL), and ureterorenoscopy (URS) have also superseded the more traditional forms of open surgery for renal calculi in children. The aim of treatment is to render the child stone free with preservation of maximum renal function and minimal complications. In order to reduce the risk of sepsis, urinary infection must be sought preoperatively and treated, as well as appropriate intravenous antibiotics administered on induction of anesthesia in all. The treatment modality/modalities chosen will depend on the stone burden and etiology, pelvicalyceal location and anatomy, the symptoms and complications caused by the stone(s), as well as co-morbidities.

Extracorporeal shock-wave lithotripsy

1 First performed in 1980, the principle of shock-wave lithotripsy is to shatter a stone into smaller fragments, which can pass spontaneously through the urinary tract. Pulses of externally generated shock waves are focussed by an external parabolic dish onto the stone in question, resulting in fragmentation of the stone. The shock wave was originally generated by an electric spark, but other methods of inducing shock waves including rapid vibration of piezoelectric crystals or electromagnetic diaphragms have since evolved. The newer second-generation machines employ a water cushion rather than a large water bath for coupling, and are combined with more accurate ultrasound- and fluoroscopy-guided targeting systems in the third-generation lithotripters. These improvements have resulted in less discomfort, and pediatric patients may be treated under simple analgesia. In practice, however, it is difficult to maintain the child in one position during treatment (typically 45 minutes), and general anesthesia continues to be utilized in young children and babies.

Success rates are in the order of 80 percent, although repeat procedures are needed in about a third. Side effects of transient hematuria, bruising, and renal pain are common. Complications of hematoma, sepsis, and stone fragment ureteric obstruction (steinstrasse) occur in approximately 5 percent. The long-term effects of ESWL on the developing kidney is unknown.

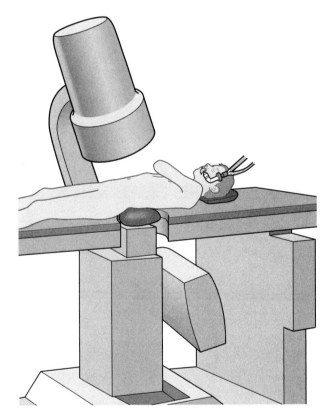

1

Percutaneous nephrolithotomy

Percutaneous nephrolithotomy involves needle puncture of the kidney under ultrasound or x-ray guidance and dilatation of the tract to allow direct visualization, fragmentation, and removal of renal stones. It is utilized to disintegrate and remove (1) multiple, large, or staghorn calculi, (2) calculi in patients with gross spinal deformities where focusing the shock waves onto the stone is difficult, and (3) moderate-sized calculi without disintegration and risk of residual fragments (e.g. above a long narrow infundibular neck or in a calyceal diverticulum, or in a horseshoe kidney).

The risks are sepsis, bleeding, hypothermia, residual calculi, renal injury. A blood 'group and save' is mandatory and a cross-match may be required for some. Hypothermia is a significant risk and all facilities to prevent this should be employed: such as, warming of the operating room, warming of intravenous and of irrigation fluid, forced-air warming systems, and the careful application of plastic sticky drapes to prevent the pooling of irrigation fluid around the child.

For the procedure, the child is fully anesthetized. In order for the head to be turned to the same side as the kidney to be operated on in the prone position, the anesthetist should be asked to secure the endotracheal tube to the side of the affected kidney.

2 By cystoscopy, a guidewire is passed retrograde into the ipsilateral ureter. A ureteric catheter is screened to just below the ureteropelvic junction and the guidewire removed. The ureteric catheter is secured to a urethral catheter (e.g. balloon catheter), and both are taped to the leg of the child. The purposes of the ureteric catheter are, first, to enable contrast to be instilled into the pelvicalyceal system and, second, for stone fragments that threaten to migrate down the ureter during the PCNL to be flushed back into the pelvis for extraction. The child is then turned prone and supported by gel-pads as demonstrated, and a bolster placed under the relevant pole of the kidney to elevate it.

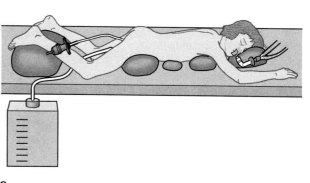

2

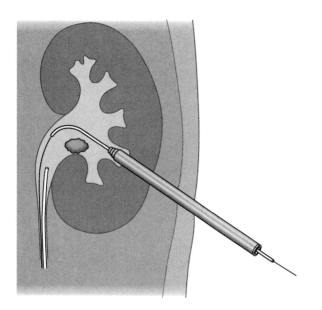

3 Under ultrasound and/or fluoroscopy guidance, an appropriate calyx is punctured and a guidewire advanced down the ureter. The needle is removed over the guidewire and the tract dilated.

3

4 An Amplatz sheath is placed over the dilator. The size of the sheath chosen will depend on the size of the child, the locations and volume of the stones, and the telescope to be used. By nephroscopy, a small stone can be removed through the sheath with graspers.

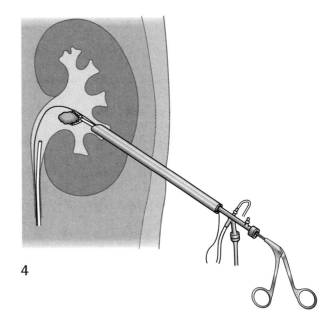

4

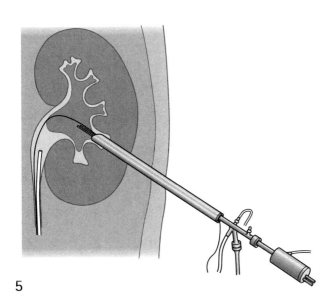

5

5 A staghorn calculus can be disintegrated under direct vision using an ultrasound and/or lithoclast probe. For complex stones, multiple tracts into different calyces may be required, although the number of tracts can be reduced through the additional use of flexible operating telescopes. Although the working channels of the current flexible telescopes are small, stones may be fragmented by laser, or, using a basket, repositioned in line with the primary tract for prompt extraction.

POSTOPERATIVE

Nephrostomy drainage is advised for all except simple 'lift out' PCNLs for 24–48 hours. The average hospital stay is 4 days. Stone-free rates are 90–100 percent.

Ureterorenoscopy

Small (4.5–7.5 Fr) rigid or flexible telescopes can be passed through the bladder into the ureter and kidney, enabling fragmentation and extraction of ureteric and small renal stones. By cystoscopy, a guidewire is inserted into the ureter and placed into the renal pelvis under fluoroscopy guidance. A retrograde ureteropyelogram helps to delineate the ureter and pelvicalyceal system. Especially at the point of impaction of ureteric calculi, care must be taken to ensure the guidewire does not undermine the urothelium and perforate the ureter. The guidewire may need to be advanced past an impacted stone under direct vision by ureteroscopy.

6 For ureteroscopy, the ureteric orifice is intubated. Insertion under the guidewire is facilitated by rotating the ureteroscope so as to allow the bulky end of the telescope to pass along the floor of the ureteric orifice. For a difficult ureteric orifice, the hydrostatic pressure may be temporarily increased (after emptying the bladder), the ureteroscope can be passed over a second guidewire or the ureteric orifice may be predilated by placement of a JJ stent for 10–14 days. For repetitive access to the proximal ureter or renal pelvis, deployment of a ureteric access sheath (internal diameter at least 2 Fr larger than the ureteroscope) can be considered in older children, although ureteric ischemia due to excessive stretch remains a concern.

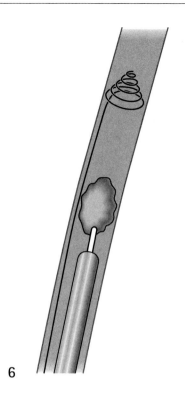

6

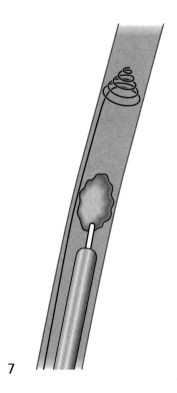

7

7 The ureteroscope is carefully advanced while maintaining the ureteric lumen in the center of the field of view and only in the absence of resistance. Holmium laser stone fragmentation within the pediatric ureter has a good safety profile and trauma to the urothelium can be minimized by placement of the laser fiber onto the stone surface. Slow irrigation or placement of a stone cone above the calculus will prevent retropulsion. In the absence of ureteric or vesicoureteric junction edema, stone fragments can then be cleared under direct vision with a basket and sent for stone analysis. If a basket cannot be withdrawn, traction must stop immediately. Flushing with a syringe may help to distend the ureter enabling the basket to be opened to release its contents. If this fails, the handle of the basket may be detached, and the ureteroscope removed over the basket wire leaving the basket and stone *in situ*. The ureteroscope can then be repassed alongside the basket wire and its contents laser-fragmented. As a final resort, a JJ stent may be placed alongside the trapped basket and a repeat ureteroscopy performed 4–7 days later or the stone fragmented by ESWL. Small stone fragments may be left to pass spontaneously. Placement of a JJ stent at the end of the procedure is advised in the presence of ureteric edema (e.g. at the site of stone impaction), injury, or dilatation (e.g. after use of an access sheath), residual fragments, after recent infection, and in those with impaired renal function or a solitary or transplant kidney.

8 With continuing advances in flexible telescopes, renal stones are now accessible endoscopically in children. The current flexible ureteroscopes are still significantly larger than their rigid counterparts and many children will require prestenting. The flexible scope is best inserted over a second soft-tipped guidewire under fluoroscopy. To prevent damage to these expensive scopes laser fibers and baskets must be inserted in the undeflected state. Lower pole stones are best repositioned to an upper or interpolar calyx rather than lasered *in situ*.

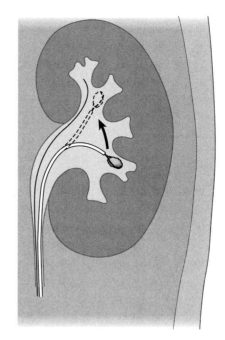

8

Laparoscopy

Depending on surgeon experience, laparoscopic stone removal can be considered for stones, for instance, located in a hydronephrotic renal pelvis needing pyeloplasty or in an abnormally located kidney.

Open surgery

Although it remains an essential tool for large bladder stones, for ureteric and renal stones, open surgery is now rarely employed. Open surgery is indicated when stone extraction is to be combined with, for example, pyeloplasty, or in patients in whom a percutaneous approach is impossible. The patient is positioned and the kidney exposed as for pyeloplasty, nephrectomy, or heminephrectomy (see Chapters 82, 83, or 85). The ureter is identified and secured with a sling.

Renal pelvic stones

9 The surface of the pelvis is freed of adventitia and the parenchyma retracted. Formal dissection of the renal sinus is not usually required in children. With a large extrarenal pelvis, a vertical incision may be employed. If the pelvis is small, an oblique incision extending up toward the infundibulum of the upper calyx gives better access and may be continued into the lower calyx to raise a triangular flap. Stay sutures are applied to the margins of the incision.

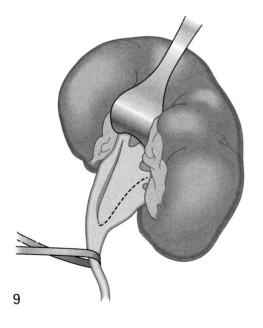

9

10 A stone in the renal pelvis will now be visible and can be lifted out gently with stone forceps.

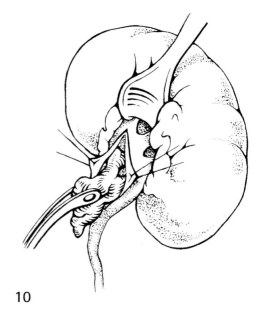

10

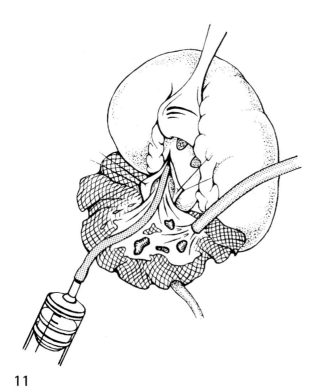

11

11 For irrigation of the pelvicalyceal system, gauze swabs are now placed around the pelvis to catch small stones and debris to allow suction without fatty tissue occluding the sucker. A soft catheter with an end hole rather than side holes is introduced and the calyces are irrigated systematically with normal saline. Stones and debris are carefully removed and any lost into the wound must be retrieved to prevent confusion on later x-rays and sinus tract formation. A radiograph of the exposed kidney is then taken to confirm complete clearance. A marker should be included in the film to assist orientation. Intraoperative ultrasound may aid in the detection of residual calculi.

Calyceal stones

12 Calyceal stones may be removed via the renal pelvis with curved stone forceps. A calyceal stone can be identified using stone forceps, palpation, or ultrasound probe. Alternatively, a nephrotomy incision directly onto the stone permits easy removal.

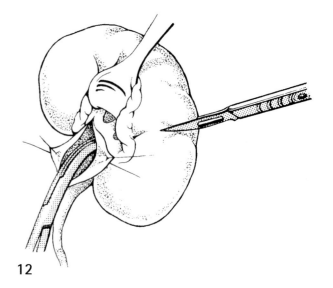

12

13 Large staghorn stones may require the exposure of several calyces. A bulldog clip is applied to the renal artery or the whole renal pedicle is occluded with a soft sling. The longitudinal incision of the posterior surface parallel to the lateral margin of the kidney gives good access. Following removal of the stones, the clamps are released intermittently to allow identification and under-running of major vessels. The calyces are approximated with interrupted 4/0 or 5/0 absorbable sutures and the kidney parenchyma is opposed with loosely tied horizontal mattress sutures through the capsule. The kidney swells on removal of the clamps and if these sutures are too tight they will cut out.

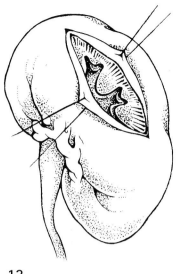

13

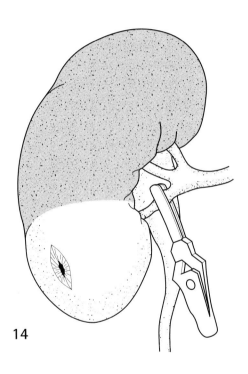

14

Lower pole calculi

14 The lower branch of the renal artery is readily identifiable and may be occluded with a bulldog clip. Intravenous methylene blue following occlusion may aid demarcation. Simple incision into the lower pole calyx may then be performed.

Closure

Following radiographic confirmation of complete clearance, the incision in the renal pelvis is closed with interrupted 5/0 or 6/0 absorbable sutures. A drain may be positioned adjacent to the renal pelvis and Gerota's fascia is reconstructed over this area. The wound is closed in layers with absorbable sutures. The stones are sent for analysis.

POSTOPERATIVE FOLLOW UP

In general, children are maintained on low-dose antibiotics until investigations are complete. Follow-up investigations include ultrasound and Mag3 or DMSA, to confirm complete absence of calculi. In children with no metabolic abnormality whose kidneys have been completely cleared of calculi, review is required only for a period of two years. Provided the urine remains sterile, recurrences are rare. Surgery may occasionally be required to correct vesicoureteric reflux or an obstructive etiology.

FURTHER READING

Bogris S, Papatsoris AG. Status quo of percutaneous nephrolithotomy in children. *Urology Research* 2010; **38**: 1–5.

Choong S, Whitfield H, Duffy P *et al*. The management of paediatric urolithiasis. *BJU International* 2000; **86**: 857–60.

Coward RJM, Peters CJ, Duffy PG *et al*. Epidemiology of paediatric renal stone disease in the UK. *Archives of Disease in Childhood* 2003; **88**: 962–5.

Nelson CP. Extracorporeal shock wave lithotripsy in the pediatric population. *Urology Research* 2010; **38**: 327–31.

Straub M, Gschwend J, Zorn C. Pediatric urolithiasis: the current surgical management. *Pediatric Nephrology* 2010; **25**: 1239–44.

Thomas JC. How effective is ureteroscopy in the treatment of pediatric stone disease? *Urology Research* 2010; **38**: 333–5.

88

Posterior urethral valve

IAN A AARONSON

PRINCIPLES AND JUSTIFICATION

1 A posterior urethral valve is a single structure that originates from the inferior margin of the verumontanum. Although its embryology is uncertain, it lies in the position of the infracollicular folds, which can often be discerned in the normal posterior urethra running downwards from the verumontanum toward the bulb on either side of the midline.

1

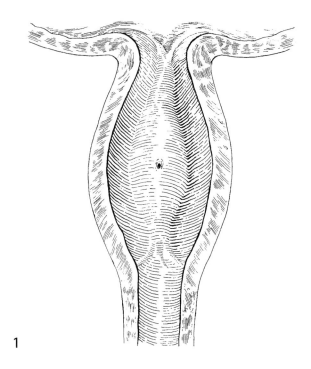

2a–c When exposed at autopsy through the anterior urethral wall, a posterior urethral valve appears as two separate leaflets. Above the valve, back pressure effects are nearly always present, namely a widely dilated posterior urethra, a thick-walled and usually trabeculated bladder, widely dilated tortuous ureters, and bilateral symmetrical hydronephrosis. Vesicoureteral reflux is common and often associated with dysplasia of the affected kidney.

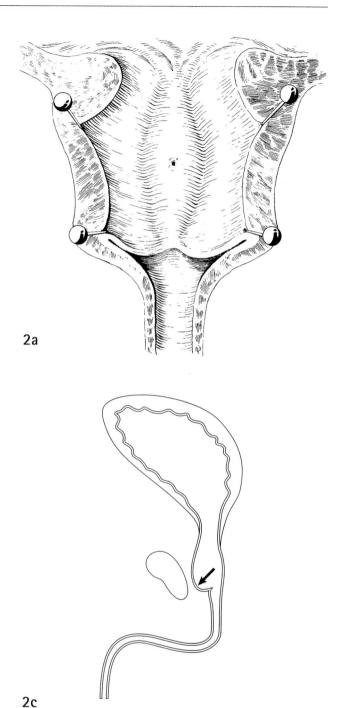

2a

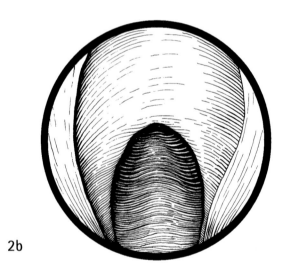

2b

2c

Nowadays, the diagnosis is usually made either before birth as a result of antenatal ultrasonography, or immediately afterwards because of a persistently palpable bladder. Urinary ascites is an occasional presentation in the first weeks of life.

Infants in whom the diagnosis has been missed usually present with urinary infection and acute or chronic renal failure. This is generally accompanied by hyperkalemia and a severe metabolic acidosis, which may lead to respiratory arrest. Water and sodium balance is often also profoundly disturbed. Septicemia is common and may be complicated by a consumptive coagulopathy. Older boys may also present with urinary infection, but often the main complaint is of a poor stream with straining or urinary incontinence.

The diagnosis is usually suspected on clinical grounds and supported by the ultrasonographic findings of a widened posterior urethra, distended bladder, and dilated upper urinary tract.

PREOPERATIVE

On suspicion of the diagnosis, an 8-Fr plastic infant feeding tube should be passed transurethrally and secured for continuous bladder drainage. Self-retaining catheters should be avoided, as the hypertrophied bladder tends to clamp down around the balloon and obstruct the ureters.

It is essential that the bladder drains well, and failure to do so is usually because the catheter has curled up in the dilated posterior urethra. Withdrawing the catheter for a few centimeters and repassing it with a finger in the rectum will usually ensure its passage through the hypertrophied bladderneck. Persistent difficulty can usually be resolved by injecting a few milliliters of contrast medium through the catheter and manipulating it under fluoroscopic control.

A full blood count including platelets, plasma electrolytes, creatinine, and acid–base status should be determined, and severe derangements, particularly hyperkalemia or a severe metabolic acidosis, should be corrected as a matter of urgency. An assessment should also be made of the infant's state of hydration. In difficult cases, the aid of a pediatric nephrologist should be sought.

When the urine appears to be infected, both a blood sample and a urine sample should be sent for culture, following which ampicillin and an aminoglycoside or a third-generation cephalosporin should be started intravenously. When septicemia is suspected, blood coagulation studies should also be carried out.

All infants with any respiratory distress should undergo chest radiography to exclude a pneumothorax secondary to pulmonary hypoplasia.

In most cases, the above actions will result in a rapid improvement in the infant's metabolic state and general condition. Those infants who remain in a toxic state or whose plasma creatinine does not begin to fall within 24 hours, despite correction of other metabolic abnormalities, should be considered for percutaneous drainage of both kidneys.

3a,b The presence of a posterior urethral valve should be confirmed by micturating cystourethrography, but this should be delayed until urinary infection has been brought completely under control and metabolic disturbances have been corrected. A voiding film taken in the steep oblique projection during full micturition is necessary to demonstrate the valve, when a thin stream will be seen emerging from the posterior margin of the obstruction (illustration a). Dilatation of the urethra proximal to the valve is essential to the diagnosis, and signs of bladder wall hypertrophy are usually also present. A very lax valve may occasionally prolapse down as far as the bulbar urethra (illustration b). Here, the posterior run-off may not be readily apparent, but the filling defect caused by the valve leaflets can usually be made out running down from the verumontanum.

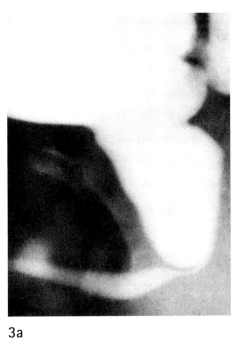

3a

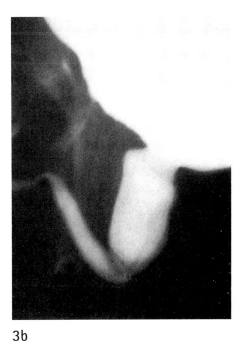

3b

Most valves are thin, filmy structures that balloon downwards during voiding, but a few are thicker and more rigid, forming a transverse obstruction in the mid-posterior urethra. As all true valves originate from the inferior aspect of the verumontanum, Young's classification should be regarded as only of historic interest.

Minor degrees of valves are sometimes encountered, in which the two leaflets blend with the lateral urethral wall. They are more properly regarded as prominent infracollicular folds. It is unlikely they ever cause symptoms or obstruction and, therefore, do not require treatment.

A variety of other conditions may masquerade as a posterior urethral valve on the cystogram, and failure to recognize them often leads to inappropriate treatment. Among these are prominent infracollicular folds, which can sometimes be made out on a good-quality study in normal children.

Hesitant voiding in a normal baby may cause an abrupt change in caliber of the posterior urethra, while extrinsic compression by the pelvic floor may cause one or more concentric indentations in the urethral contour. Neither of these is associated with evidence of obstruction above the lesion, however, and both should be regarded as normal variants.

A neuropathic bladder may closely simulate a posterior urethral valve, but the thin stream below the obstruction will be seen emerging from the center of the external urethral sphincter rather than from the posterior margin, as seen with a valve. In such cases, the spine should be carefully examined and other evidence sought of a neurologic deficit in the perineum or lower limbs.

A posterior urethral stricture may cause a similar appearance, but this will usually be associated with a history of urethral or pelvic trauma.

The prune-belly syndrome may closely mimic a posterior urethral valve, but the correct diagnosis should be suspected from the appearance of the bladder, which lies horizontally and is invariably smooth walled, and the dog-leg configuration of the posterior urethra, which often bears a utriculus masculinus.

A distended, non-visualized ectopic ureter opening into the ejaculatory duct may distort and partially obstruct the posterior urethra and thus simulate a valve, while dilatation of the posterior urethra may also be caused by a prolapsed ectopic ureterocele or posterior urethral polyp. Careful examination of these films, however, will usually reveal a filling defect, leading to the correct diagnosis.

OPERATION

Resection in full-term infants and children

Under endotracheal anesthesia, the intubated infant is placed supine with the buttocks brought well down to the end of the operating table. The legs should be well protected with cotton wool and fixed with crepe bandages, either to pediatric stirrups or in the frog-leg position, taking care to provide ample support to the thighs. The skin is prepared and drapes applied, taking care to exclude the anus from the operative field. Fixing the posterior towel to the perineal skin with three staples or 4/0 nylon sutures will ensure that the anus does not become exposed during subsequent manipulations.

The caliber of the penile urethra should first be checked with a well-lubricated 8-Fr sound, which should be introduced only for 1–2 cm. If necessary, a meatotomy can be performed, but no attempt should be made to dilate the urethra. The diagnosis is then confirmed using a well-lubricated 6.5- or 9.5-Fr cystoscope introduced under vision.

4 Resection of the valve is undertaken using a pediatric resectoscope fitted with a hooked ball electrode (Storz; Wolf). The instrument is first assembled and the alignment of the working parts checked using the 0° telescope. The sheath is then dried and thoroughly coated with a water-soluble lubricant, and with its introducer in place is gently inserted through the meatus. The introducer is removed and the instrument reassembled and gently advanced under vision towards the bladder neck. It is usually necessary to angle the eyepiece end of the instrument downwards to allow the beak to move anteriorly and pass through the bladder neck. Once in the bladder, the shape and position of the ureteric orifices are noted and the presence of any paraureteral diverticulum recorded.

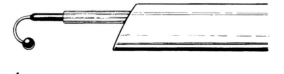

4

5a–c The instrument is now rotated through 180° (illustration a), and with the irrigation fluid flowing in under low pressure, it is progressively withdrawn. Once through the bladderneck, the ball is run down along the anterior wall of the posterior urethra (illustration b) until, just beyond the verumontanum, the valve suddenly snaps across the anterior portion of the field of view like a curtain. Further withdrawal of the instrument and manipulation of the trigger will cause the ball to engage the valve in the 12 o'clock position. A short burst of cutting current is then applied (illustration c).

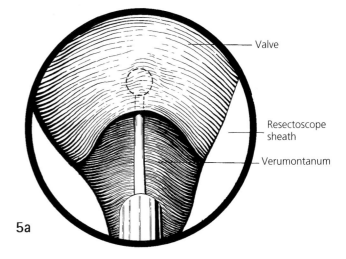

Valve

Resectoscope sheath

Verumontanum

5a

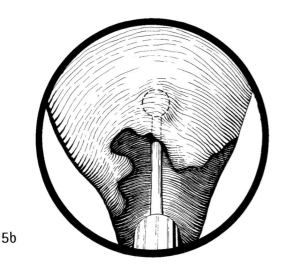

5b

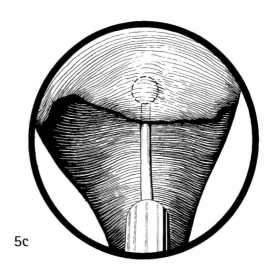

5c

The instrument is returned to the normal position and advanced under vision back into the bladder. It is again rotated 180° and withdrawn into the posterior urethra to engage the now partially disrupted valve in the 12 o'clock position, where it is further disrupted. This maneuver should be repeated until it is certain that the anterior portion of the valve has been completely ablated.

The instrument is again returned to the bladder and is rotated to engage residual valve tissue in the 10 o'clock, 2 o'clock, 8 o'clock, and finally the 4 o'clock positions. Any remaining freely floating tags do not require treatment.

The resectoscope is removed and the presence of an unobstructed urethra confirmed by manual expression of the bladder. Finally, an 8-Fr feeding tube is passed, placing a double-gloved finger in the rectum, if necessary, to ensure that it is not curled up in the dilated posterior urethra. This is retained in place with a 4/0 nylon suture passed through the prepuce or distal shaft skin and connected to a sealed drainage bag. The tube is removed after 48 hours.

If any significant bleeding occurs, attempts at valve ablation should be immediately discontinued and the situation reassessed after 2–3 days of catheter drainage.

Resection in preterm infants

It is inadvisable to attempt to pass a 9.5-Fr resectoscope in infants weighing less than 2.5 kg. In such cases, a few days of bladder drainage, using initially a 6-Fr urethral feeding tube, will have the effect of gently dilating the urethra so that a 6.5-Fr or even a 9.5-Fr resectoscope can be safely used. Alternatively, a very small cystoscope may be employed, introducing through the working channel a 3-Fr Bugbee electrode to coagulate the valve in a circumferential fashion.

Other techniques are also available for resecting the valve in a very small infant, but all have some disadvantages. The Whitaker hook electrode is a slender, insulated metal instrument that can be introduced through the urethra under fluoroscopic control and withdrawn to engage the valve. Short bursts of cutting current may relieve the obstruction, but the procedure is essentially blind and carries the risk of urethral trauma.

A Fogarty catheter with the balloon inflated with 0.1–0.3 mL of water has also been used to disrupt the valve (1), but carries the risk of avulsion of the urethra. Laser resection of the valve (2), and cold knife valvulotomy (3) have also been described.

Access to the valve with the pediatric resectoscope sheath can usually be achieved via a perineal urethrotomy. The small caliber of the urethra and the friable nature of the urothelium, however, render the operation difficult in the neonate and it may be complicated by bleeding, a persistent urinary fistula, urethral diverticulum, or stricture.

An alternative approach is to create a suprapubic cystotomy through which the valve can be resected in an antegrade fashion. Using a 10-Fr sheath and the hooked ball electrode, the valve is first engaged in the 12 o'clock position and coagulated. However, the hypertrophied bladderneck sometimes closes across the telescope lens so that the procedure has to be carried out blindly.

Vesicostomy

In very small infants, it is the author's preference to carry out a vesicostomy rather than attempt to disrupt the valve by the above methods. A few months later, when the infant has reached an adequate size, the valve is coagulated through the urethra using the hooked ball electrode in the standard fashion. The vesicostomy is closed at the same time and the urethral catheter removed 10 days later.

Upper tract drainage

Following relief of the urethral obstruction, correction of metabolic derangements, and eradication of infection, the plasma creatinine will in most cases rapidly fall to within the normal range for the patient's age. When it remains elevated, the possibility of obstruction of the dilated flaccid ureters as they pass through the hypertrophied bladder wall must be considered. In most cases, this phenomenon is transient and, provided that the infant remains well and the plasma creatinine is showing some improvement, an expectant policy may be adopted.

A persistently elevated or rising serum creatinine following successful valve ablation may be the result of infection, hyponatremia, or aminoglycoside toxicity. However, when these causes have been excluded, percutaneous nephrostomies should be carried out. A subsequent fall in the serum creatinine will confirm the diagnosis of obstruction at the ureterovesical junctions. After 2 weeks, the tubes are clamped. If the serum creatinine remains low, they are removed. When this results in a rise of the serum creatinine, Sober Y cutaneous ureterostomies should be carried out to provide optimal tube-free upper tract drainage. The cutaneous limb can then be tied off when the infant is ready to come out of diapers. Alternatively, the ureters may be remodeled and reimplanted, but this operation is rendered difficult by the thickness of the bladder wall and trabeculation, and in inexperienced hands complications are common.

Failure of the serum creatinine to fall after placement of bilateral percutaneous nephrostomies is indicative of irreversible renal dysplasia.

POSTOPERATIVE CARE

Following removal of the urethral catheter, adequate emptying of the bladder should be confirmed clinically or by ultrasonography. Postoperative antibiotic prophylaxis, usually with trimethoprim-sulphamethoxozole, is continued for one month to guard against infection in the healing posterior urethra. In infants in whom preoperative cystography revealed the presence of vesicoureteric reflux, this should be continued for six months. Sodium bicarbonate supplements are also often necessary to correct a persistent metabolic acidosis, and these may need to be given for one year or more. Polyuria is also common, and the parents should be advised to give supplementary clear feeds early in the event of a diarrheal illness.

7 At six months, micturating cystourethrography is repeated to confirm adequate resection of the valve and the absence of any stricture of the urethra, and to determine whether any previously noted vesicoureteric reflux is still present. In about one-third of cases, it will be found to have disappeared. When reflux is persistent and unilateral, renal scanning using ^{99m}Tc-DMSA (dimercaptosuccinic acid) is carried out to determine the contribution of the kidney on the refluxing side to total renal function. When this is negligible, nephroureterectomy should be carried out through two incisions to ensure safe ligation of the ureteric stump. Ureteral reimplantation should be considered if the reflux persists and the kidney is useful, particularly when urinary infections supervene.

At three months, the glomerular filtration rate of each kidney may be measured by the slope clearance method using ^{99m}Tc-DTPA (diethylenetriaminepenta-acetate), and intravenous urography is carried out. Both of these will serve as a baseline for any future studies. A blood sample is also taken to check the plasma creatinine, electrolytes, and acid–base status.

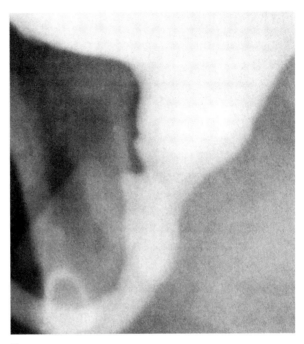

7

Urinary infections occurring during childhood after successful valve ablation are often due to incomplete bladder emptying. Double or triple micturition should be tried before instituting clean intermittent catheterizations.

All infants and those older children with impaired renal function at presentation will require close supervision until adult life is reached. A progressive rise in plasma creatinine is often seen during childhood, and in the most severe cases, renal transplantation may be required before puberty. Persistent urinary incontinence is an indication for cystometrography. Bladders showing severe hyperreflexia or very poor compliance generally require augmentation, which should be carried out before transplantation.

FURTHER READING

Chertin B, Cozzi D, Puri P. Long-term results of primary avulsion of posterior urethral valves using a Fogarty balloon catheter. *Journal of Urology* 2002; **168**: 1841–3.

Clifton MS, Harrison MR, Ball R, Lee H. Fetoscopic transuterine release of posterior urethral valves: a new technique. *Fetal Diagnosis and Therapy* 2008; **23**: 89–94.

Ghanem MA, Nijman RJ. Long-term follow up of bilateral high (Sober) urinary diversion in patients with posterior urethral valves and its effect on bladder function. *Journal of Urology* 2005; **173**: 1721–4.

Heikkila J, Rintala R, Taskinen S. Vesicoureteral reflux in conjunction with posterior urethral valves. *Journal of Urology* 2009; **184**: 1555–60.

Kousidis G, Thomas DF, Morgan H *et al.* Long term outcome of prenatally diagnosed posterior urethral valves: a 10- to 23-year follow-up study. *BJU International* 2008; **102**: 1020–4.

Stuhldreier G, Schweitzer P, Hacker HW, Barthlen W. Laser resection of posterior urethral valves. *Pediatric Surgery International* 2001; **17**: 16–20.

89

Dialysis

MARCUS D JARBOE and RONALD B HIRSCHL

PRINCIPLES AND JUSTIFICATIONS

There are numerous options for chronic dialysis including peritoneal dialysis (PD), intravenous catheter-based dialysis, and arteriovenous fistulas (AVF). The choice of dialysis depends on many factors, such as patient age, social situation, opportunities for kidney transplantation, and options for venous access. With the promotion of the Fistula First National Vascular Access Improvement Initiative (www.fistulafirst.org), however, there have been increased efforts to create arteriovenous fistulas as primary hemodialysis access in children.

The management of access for dialysis begins from the moment there is recognition of renal insufficiency. In many cases, access for acute dialysis is required early in a hospital course while in others the progression of renal failure is insidious with requirement for dialysis identified well in advance of its need. Procedures for such access should be performed with the recognition that peripheral venous fistula formation may be required in the future. Our protocol calls for immediate bilateral upper extremity venous evaluation in order to identify the preferred arm for a future fistula. Central venous access for acute dialysis is preferably performed in the upper extremity least favorable for fistula formation and almost always via the internal jugular rather than the subclavian vein. Intravenous catheters and peripheral intravenous central catheters (PICC) are avoided in candidate veins for fistula formation, such as the cephalic and basilica veins.

PERITONEAL DIALYSIS

Preoperative

Age is not a limiting factor for PD; in fact, the authors have successfully placed catheters in patients as young as a few days old. However, the presence of sufficient peritoneal surface area for dialysis is a factor which determines success.

In fact, adequate dialysis may be difficult to achieve in patients with numerous adhesions due to prior abdominal procedures. In patients of adequate size and in whom adhesions do not present sufficient risk, a laparoscopic approach may be entertained. Plans should be made to excise the omentum since it is frequently associated with catheter occlusion. Studies have demonstrated that catheter infections are reduced when a double cuff catheter is used and when the catheter exits from the abdomen in a downward direction. As such, swan neck catheters of the following size should be used:

- infants 5–10 kg: infant, double-cuff, swan-neck, coiled catheter (38.9 cm) (Covidien, Mansfield, MA, USA);
- Pediatric patients 10–30 kg: pediatric double-cuff, swan-neck, coiled catheter (42 cm);
- pediatric patients 30–45 kg: small adult, double-cuff, swan-neck, coiled catheter (57 cm);
- pediatric patients greater than 45 kg: adult, double-cuff, swan-neck, coiled catheter (62.2 cm).

Operation

OPEN PERITONEAL DIALYSIS CATHETER PLACEMENT
Position

The patient should be placed supine with both arms tucked and secured well to bed.

Preparation of skin

Preparation of the skin is with a cholorahexidine/alcohol preparation, extending from the nipples to the pubic ramus.

Anesthesia

Anesthesia is general via an endotracheal tube.

Antibiotics

Antibiotic therapy using cefazolin should be instituted.

Procedure

From an infectious standpoint, the catheter should be positioned so that both the intraperitoneal end of the catheter and the exit site are facing downward or caudal (in infants the exit may be lateral) (**Figure 89.1a**). In order to determine the exact locations of the incisions, the catheter should be placed on the abdomen and the positions of the internal cuff, tunnel cuff, and exit site should be marked on the skin with the catheter lying naturally. The position of the tunnel cuff or exit site should avoid the belt line in children and teenagers. The distance from tunnel cuff to exit site should be at least 1.5 cm to reduce the risk of extrusion.

A transverse incision is made in the upper quadrant with a No. 15 scalpel. The rectus fascia and peritoneum are incised. As noted above, an omentectomy should always be performed. The omentum is delivered through the incision and excised using 3-0 polyglactin ties. The peritoneal end of the swan neck peritoneal dialysis catheter is placed into the peritoneal cavity with the curled end in the pelvis. The peritoneum/posterior rectus fascia is closed with a running polypropylene suture (2-0 for <10 years of age and 0 polypropylene suture for ≥10 years of age) with the cuff maintained just external to the posterior fascia so that it sits within the rectus sheath. The fascial suture should be placed such that it tightens the fascia around the catheter. In the open setting, a purse-string suture can be placed through the cuff and the posterior rectus fascia, further sealing and securing the cuff to the posterior rectus fascia. These maneuvers help to seal the space where the catheter traverses the posterior rectus fascia and thus reduce the risk of leakage once dialysis is started. The external aspect of the catheter is tunneled 1–2 cm superiorly in the rectus sheath and exits through a separate incision in the anterior rectus sheath. A minimal incision is made for the catheter skin exit site lower in the abdomen and a tendon passer used to create a subcutaneous tunnel. Again, it is important that the swan-neck catheter be tunneled caudally so that the exit site is in the lower abdomen with the exit site facing downward. The second cuff lies in the subcutaneous tunnel. This configuration is demonstrated in **Figure 89.1a,b**.

The function of the catheter is now tested. The titanium Luer lock adapter is placed into the end of the catheter. The transfer set is placed on the end of the Luer lock adapter (**Figure 89.2**). The function of the peritoneal dialysis catheter is tested by infusing 30 mL/kg of saline from an intravenous set up with sterile connectors and then draining some of the infused saline by dropping the intravenous bag below the patient. A sterile betadine minicap is then placed on the end of the transfer set.

The skin is closed with running 4-0 absorbable monofilament suture. No sutures are placed at the exit site. Mastisol (Ferndale Laboratories, Ferndale, MI, USA) and 0.5-inch Steristrips (3M Healthcare, St Paul, MN, USA) are placed to reinforce the incision, and Tegaderm with a pad (3M Healthcare) is used at the catheter exit site.

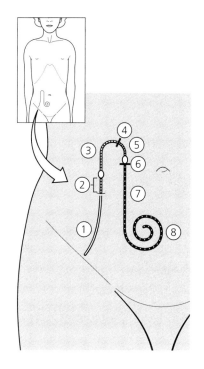

a

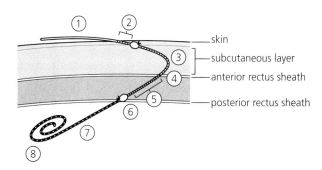

① catheter outside skin and must point in caudal direction

② 1.5 cm or greater from cuff to skin exit site

③ subcutaneous catheter

④ catheter trangresses anterior rectus sheath

⑤ catheter tunnels obliquely between posterior and anterior rectus sheaths (1–2 cm long)

⑥ inside cuff pursestring to posterior rectus sheath at incision site

⑦ intraperitoneal portion

⑧ curl in pelvis

b

Figure 89.1 Peritoneal dialysis catheter position with landmarks. (a) Anterior/posterior view of catheter layout with both ends in the caudal direction (b) sagittal view of catheter showing relationships with the anterior and posterior rectus sheath.

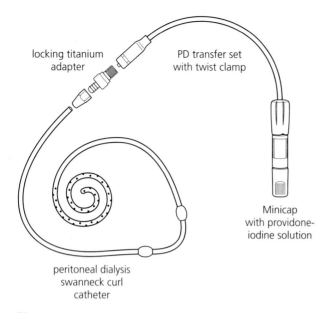

Figure 89.2 Peritoneal dialysis catheter set up.

LAPAROSCOPIC PERITONEAL DIALYSIS CATHETER PLACEMENT
Position

The patient is placed supine with both arms tucked in (if only one arm can be tucked in, it should be the left arm) and secured well to the bed. The monitor position is as shown in **Figure 89.3**.

Preparation of skin

Skin preparation is with a cholorahexidine/alcohol preparation, and extends from the nipples to the pubic ramus.

Anesthesia

General anesthesia is via endotracheal tube.

Antibiotics

Antibiotic therapy using cefazolin should be instituted.

Procedure

The catheter should be positioned and marked in a similar fashion as described for the open procedure. A periumbilical incision is made with a scalpel. The fascia is incised and a Veress needle and sheath are placed into the peritoneal cavity. The abdomen is insufflated with CO_2. Except in infants, a 12-mm umbilical port is placed followed by a 5 mm, 30° scope. An additional 5-mm port is placed at the intended peritoneal entry site of the catheter (**Figure 89.4**).

As with the open technique, an omentectomy should always be performed. The scope is placed through the 5-mm port and a grasper is used to grab the omentum through the 12-mm port. The omentum is delivered through the port site as the port is removed. The omentum is ligated with 3/0 polyglactin ties or an energy source. The port is then replaced. This is done repeatedly until the omentum

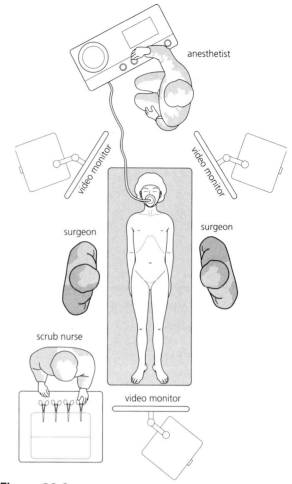

Figure 89.3 Laparascopic peritoneal dialysis catheter placement room set up .

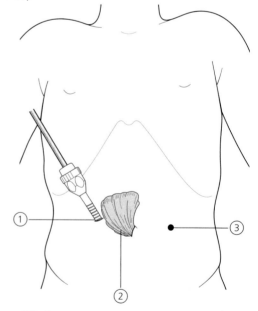

Figure 89.4 Laparoscopic port position for peritoneal dialysis catheter placement (1) 5 mm port to the right of the umbilicus should be where the catheter will traverse the anterior rectus sheath (position 4 of Figure 89.1). (2) 12 mm port at the umbilicus where bring out omentum. (3) Port site on left is optional-only used if intracorporeal omentectomy is performed.

is completely excised (**Figure 89.4**). Alternatively, a third port (5 mm) can be placed in the left side of the abdomen and a surgical energy device can be used to perform the omentectomy intracorporeally and then the specimen can be removed through the umbilical site.

The scope is then placed through the 12-mm port and the 5-mm port is removed. Under direct vision, the catheter can be placed through the port site into the pelvis. Alternatively, a 16 Fr peel-away sheath can be placed through the 5-mm port site incision and angled inferiorly so that a tangential passage is created through the rectus sheath. This can be facilitated by 18- or 19-gauge needle and 0.035-inch guidewire (**Figure 89.5a,b**). The peritoneal end of the swan-neck peritoneal dialysis catheter is placed through the sheath and directed into the pelvis. The peel-away sheath is removed. These steps are performed under direct visualization with the camera.

A small incision is made for the catheter skin exit site lower in the abdomen and a tendon passer used to create the subcutaneous tunnel. Again, it is important that the swan-neck catheter be tunneled caudally so that the exit site is in the lower abdomen with the exit site facing downward (Figure 89.1). One cuff is located just above the rectus fascia. The second cuff resides in the subcutaneous tunnel (~1.5 cm away from exit site). The fascia is closed at the umbilicus with 2-0 or 0 polyglactin on a UR-6 needle.

The function of the catheter is now tested and wounds are closed and dressed as delineated in the open section above.

Postoperative

If it is necessary to perform peritoneal dialysis immediately, then low volumes (10 mL/kg per dialysate infusion exchange) are used increasing by 10 mL/kg every 2 weeks until full volume peritoneal dialysis at 40 mL/kg per exchange is achieved. If the patient's situation allows, the catheter is not used for 4 weeks after which peritoneal dialysis is performed with 20 mL/kg exchanges, increasing by 10 mL/kg every 2 weeks until full peritoneal dialysis (40 mL/kg) is achieved. Antibiotics are administered in the operating room, but not postoperatively.

The most frequent complication in the first month is outflow failure. This is usually caused by omentum or remnant portions of the omentum obstructing the catheter. If there are inflow problems as well, it may be due to malposition. Laparoscopic exploration, repositioning and cleaning out the catheter can be successful, but replacement is necessary in most cases. Leakage is also common immediately after placement. This can be treated with decreasing the amount of dialysate and increasing the number of exchanges. Nearly all these leaks will seal with conservative management unless the inner cuff has been dislodged. Intra-abdominal bleeding postoperatively can also be a problem. If the hematocrit of the effluent is <2 or the red cell count is less than 60 000/cm³, then the bleeding is insignificant. Peritonitis is a common late complication of peritoneal dialysis. It is also

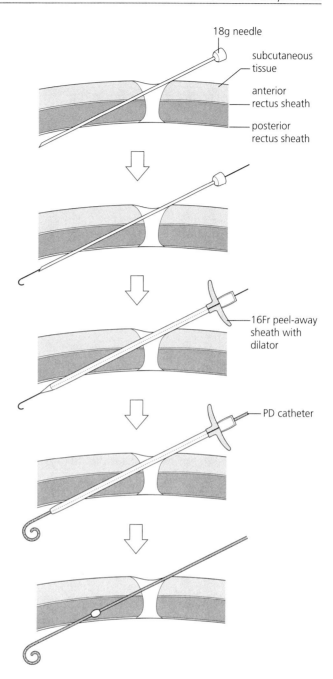

Figure 89.5 Using a needle, guidewire and peel-away sheath to make an oblique tunnel between anterior and posterior rectus sheath (sagittal view)

a major source of morbidity associated with the catheters. Peritonitis will likely be clinically evident on examination. The effluent may have a cloudy characteristic and will have a white cell count greater than 100/cm³ with a neutrophil predominance. The most common organism is coagulase-negative *Staphylococcus*. Catheter infections can sometimes be treated with antibiotics placed through the catheter. If this fails, then removal of the catheter may be necessary. Infections of the tunneled portion of the catheter can also cause peritonitis.

CENTRAL VENOUS DIALYSIS CATHETER PLACEMENT

PREOPERATIVE

It is important to perform ultrasound evaluation of central vein patency in those patients in whom numerous access devices have previously been placed. All anticoagulants should be discontinued and the platelet count and clotting factors should be normalized.

OPERATION

Position

The patient should be placed supine with a neck roll and in the Trendelenberg position as needed.

Preparation of skin

Preparation of the skin is with chloroprep unless <2 months of age, extending from the neck and chest or groin, as appropriate

Anesthesia

General anesthesia should be instituted.

Antibiotics

Antibiotic therapy is with cefazolin.

PROCEDURE

An ultrasound is used to identify the vein. Access to the internal jugular vein is performed via a low (just above the clavicle) and posterior approach behind the sternocleidomastoid muscle (**Figure 89.6**). The needle should go in at a longitudinal orientation to the ultrasound probe to allow for continuous guidance of the needle with the ultrasound (**Figure 89.7**). This approach allows for a smooth curve to the catheter which is critical for optimal dialysis flow, as well as for avoidance of carotid artery puncture and pneumothorax. For children <5 years of age, a 21-g needle is used to gain access with an 0.018-inch guidewire. Once the 0.018-inch wire is in place, it should be exchanged for an 0.035-inch guidewire using a 3/4 exchange dilator. The standard 18–19-gauge needle is used for patients >5 years of age to access the vein followed by placement of the 0.035-inch guidewire through the needle.

Using a No. 11 scalpel, a small incision is made in the skin enlarging the wire's insertion site. The catheter is placed on the skin and lined up with the wire in the superior vena cava with fluoroscopy in order to determine the appropriate location of the exit site incision. This site is placed in a position that leaves a gentle curve in the catheter and allows the tip of the catheter to set at the junction of the superior vena cava and the right atrium. This junction can best be estimated at fluoroscopy as a distance of 1.5–2

vertebral bodies below the level of the carina (**Figure 89.8**). Please note if the hemodialysis catheter has a split/staggered tip with one lumen shorter than the other, the short tip should be placed at the cavoatrial junction while the longer tip should sit slightly deeper into the atrium but still well away from the tricuspid valve.

A tendon passer is used to pass the catheter between incisions. Marcaine (0.25 percent) is infiltrated into the tissues surrounding the tunnel before the catheter is pulled through. A dilator and peel-away sheath are placed over the wire under fluoroscopic guidance followed by placement of the catheter into the peel-away

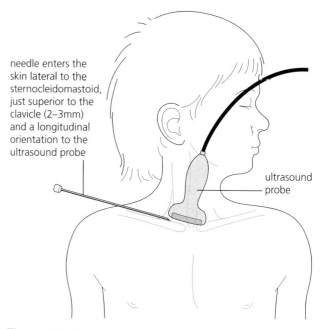

Figure 89.6 Probe position and needle entry site for tunneled hemodialysis catheter.

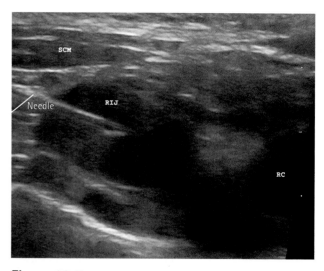

Figure 89.7 Ultrasound view of needle entering lateral (from the left side of screen) into the right internal jugular (RIJ) vein under the sternocleidomastoid muscle (SCM) with the right carotid (RC) artery on the right of the screen.

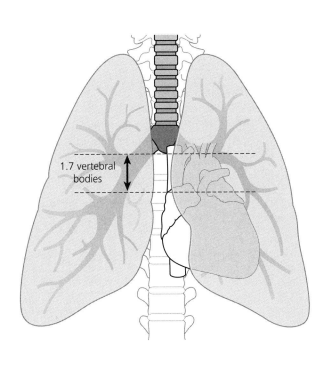

Figure 89.8 Estimating the junction of the right atrium and the superior vena cava. Junction is best estimated as 1.7 vertebral bodies below the level of the carina (1.5 to 2 vertebral bodies).

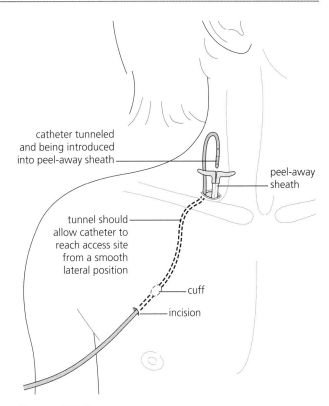

Figure 89.9 Tunnel path taken for catheter and demonstration of peel-away sheath used to place catheter into vein.

sheath with forceps (**Figure 89.9**). The peel-away is removed and fluoroscopy used to document placement. The catheter is flushed with heparinized saline, 10 units/mL (note that most nephrologists use 1000 units/mL heparin for catheters after dialysis, however, in the perioperative period the author's group only uses 10 units/mL heparin) and the neck incision is closed with an absorbable suture or skin glue. The catheter is anchored with a 2/0 nylon suture and a sterile dressing is placed over the exit site.

POSTOPERATIVE

A postoperative chest radiograph is obtained to confirm catheter placement. Bleeding is a rare, but important complication. If ultrasound guidance is used for the lateral/posterior approach, as described above, pneumothorax is extremely rare.

ARTERIOVENOUS FISTULAS

Preoperative

ARTERIOVENOUS FISTULA PLACEMENT

Ultrasound evaluation of both arms for venous and arterial patency with assessment of cephalic and basilic vein diameter is critical. In general, contrast or CO_2 venography is required because of previous line placements and potential areas of stricture. An Allen's test should be performed when a radiocephalic AVF is planned. The non-dominant arm should be used first if there are no contraindications.

In concept, the approach to fistula construction is to perform the most distal access first and to utilize autogenous rather than synthetic material. Thus, a typical order for access would be the following:

- radiocephalic (Brescia-Cimino) followed by brachiobasilic in the non-dominant arm first and then the dominant arm;
- brachiocephalic graft followed by brachioaxillary graft in the non-dominant arm first followed by the dominant arm.

The author's group has successfully performed brachiobasilic vein AVF procedures in patients as young as two years. However, performance of an AVF in a vein that is less than 2 mm is unlikely to be successful. As a result, we often prefer a brachiobasilic AVF as the first option in young children. The multi-incision technique initially used with subcutaneous tunneling of the basilic vein between the two incisions has been further modified to a two-staged procedure. The two stages allow arterialization of the vein before transferring it to a superficial location. The authors prefer the two-stage elevation technique because the creation of the arteriovenous anastomosis without dissection of the proximal vein at the first stage minimizes trauma to the small-caliber vein that might predispose it to spasm, kinking, and subsequent thrombosis.

Operation

RADIOCEPHALIC (BRESCIA–CIMINO) ARTERIOVENOUS FISTULA FORMATION

1 The radial artery and the cephalic vein are identified and an incision is made between the two. The radial artery and the cephalic vein are dissected free and surrounded with vessel loops with care taken to avoid injury to the superficial branch of the radial nerve. Intravenous heparin 100 units/kg is administered and the artery and vein clamped proximally and distally with Heifitz or small bulldog clamps.

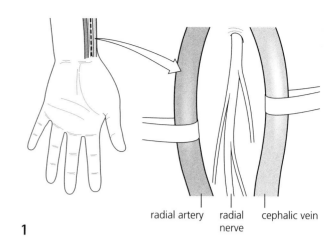

radial artery　radial nerve　cephalic vein

1

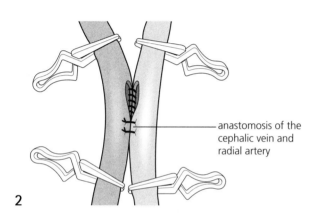

anastomosis of the cephalic vein and radial artery

2

2 An approximately 1-cm anastomosis is performed between the radial artery and the cephalic vein with 6-0 polypropylene suture. The anastomosis is initiated at the proximal aspect of the venotomy and the arteriotomy. First, the suture is run on the posterior aspect of the anastomosis, continuing three-quarters of the way around the anastomosis onto the anterior aspect. The other end of the suture is then run to meet the previous suture and complete the anterior aspect of the anastomosis. In small children, who will have significant growth in the size of the vessels, the anastomosis is completed with one or two interrupted sutures to allow for growth (although in most small children, the fistula is formed with the basilic vein for reasons of size). The anastomosis is flushed just prior to completion. The clamps are removed and the fistula checked for Doppler presence of flow and a palpable thrill. The incision is closed with interrupted 3-0 polyglactin for the subcutaneous tissues and 5-0 absorbable monofilament suture for skin.

BASILIC VEIN TRANSPOSITION

3 Basilic vein transposition (BVT) fistulas may be created using a single stage or two-stage transposition technique. In the former, an incision is performed just proximal to the antecubital fossa and a second incision is made in the mid-upper arm. Through the lower incision, the basilic vein and brachial artery are identified and dissected, with all venous side branches tied off. The vein is transected as distally as possible, delivered into the upper incision, and the anterior surface is marked (with a surgical marker pen) to monitor and avoid twisting as it is pulled through a gently curved subcutaneous tunnel. An end-to-side anastomosis between the basilica vein and the brachial artery is then performed.

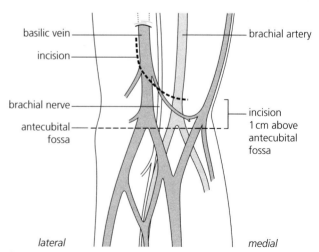

basilic vein　brachial artery

incision

brachial nerve

antecubital fossa

incision 1 cm above antecubital fossa

lateral　*medial*

3

4 Our preference is to perform a two-stage BVT fistula in children. The first stage entails the identification of the basilic vein just proximal to the antecubital fossa with division of the vein as distally as possible. Care is taken to avoid injury to the median antebrachial cutaneous nerve which surrounds the basilic vein. The brachial artery is found in the middle of the arm, lateral to the median nerve, usually surrounded by the brachial veins. The artery and vein are controlled with vessel loops. Intravenous heparin 100 units/kg is administered by the anesthetist. A Heifitz clamp or a small bulldog is placed proximally on the vein, although the presence of a valve may prevent back bleeding and preclude the need for a clamp. In most cases, ligation of the basilic vein is performed just distal to a branched vein. The branches are opened to provide a spatulated hood for an end-to-side anastomosis (see inset illustration 4). Before division, the vein is marked with ink on the anterior surface to prevent twisting. The basilic vein is dissected proximally only enough to allow a smooth curve to the brachial artery. Care should be taken to make the vein short enough to avoid kinking. Some additional venous branches may occasionally need to be ligated. The artery is occluded with proximal and distal Heifitz or small bulldog clamps. An arteriotomy approximately 1 cm in length is made and an arteriovenous anastomosis performed with 6-0 or 7-0 polypropylene. The anastomosis is initiated at the heel of the vein and the proximal aspect of the arteriotomy. Next, the suture is run on the posterior aspect of the anastomosis, continuing three-quarters of the way around the anastomosis onto the anterior aspect.

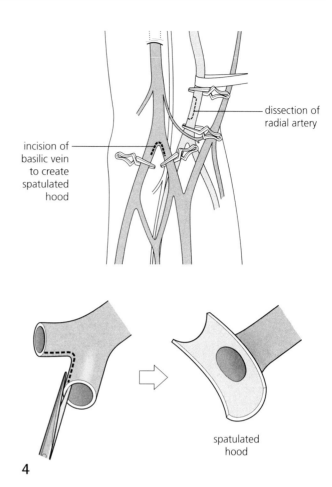

incision of basilic vein to create spatulated hood

dissection of radial artery

spatulated hood

4

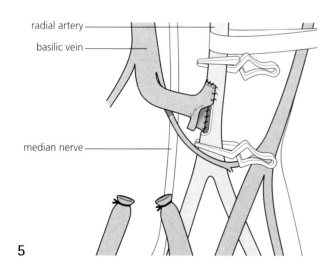

radial artery

basilic vein

median nerve

5

5 The other end of the suture is then run to meet the previous suture and complete the anterior aspect of the anastomosis. In small children, the anastomosis is completed with one or two interrupted sutures to allow for growth. Visual magnification is also used in small children, as well as a microvascular instrument set. The anastomosis is flushed just prior to completion. The clamps are removed and the fistula checked for Doppler presence of flow and a palpable thrill. The incision is closed with interrupted 3-0 polyglactin suture for the subcutaneous tissues and 5-0 absorbable, monofilament suture for the skin.

6 Over the ensuing weeks, the vein is examined by serial ultrasound studies until it is confirmed that the caliber has increased to greater than 0.6 cm. Once sufficient vein size is confirmed, fistula elevation is undertaken.

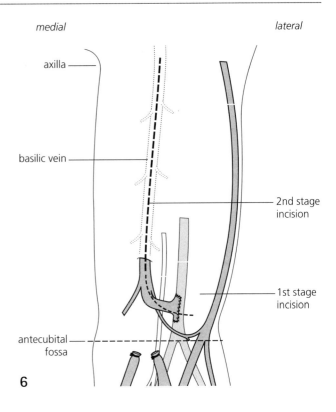

6

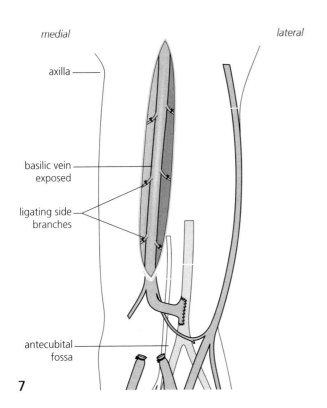

7

7 The second stage involves an incision along the medial upper arm over the basilic vein. Heparin 100 units/kg is administered and the vein dissected free up into the axilla. All side branches are ligated with suture ligatures.

8 The brachial fascia and subcutaneous tissues are closed deep to the vein. Subcutaneous flaps are developed and the incision closed directly over the vein.

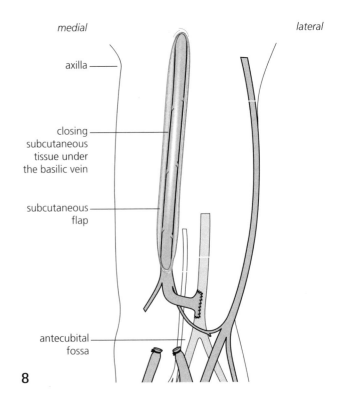

8

Postoperative

Postoperatively, the author's group uses a thromboprophylaxis protocol for all pediatric patients undergoing an AVF. In essence, a continuous infusion of heparin at 10 units/hour is administered starting in the operating room when the anastomosis is complete, followed by low-molecular weight heparin (full anticoagulation dosing) on postoperative day 1. The low-molecular weight heparin is continued until maturation is documented approximately 2–3 weeks after the second-stage procedure.

Fistula failure occurs in 7 percent of the two-stage BVT group compared with 59 percent in the other AVF approaches. Other complications include thrombosis (33 percent), bleeding (10 percent), hematoma formation (14 percent), cellulitis (5 percent), development of stenosis (12 percent), and steal (2 percent). The use of a two-stage BVT in children results in a higher rate of success in creating an AVF which is used for dialysis (87 versus 48 percent). Overall, mean patency (or duration of use) of AVF in children has been reported to be as low as six months and as high as 30 months.

Thrombosis is the most common postoperative complication with fistulas. Early thrombosis (within the first three months) is usually secondary to technical errors in fistula construction, such as twisting of the vein, small-sized anastomosis, or low flow secondary to compression or hypotension. Late thrombosis is usually caused by stenosis secondary to intimal hyperplasia or repeated access punctures. Physical examination, ultrasound, and angiography are all useful in evaluating potential problems. Interventions include thrombectomy, angioplasty, and revision of the fistula.

FURTHER READING

Baskin KM, Jimenez RM, Cahill AM *et al.* Cavoatrial junction and central venous anatomy: implications for central venous access tip position. *Journal of Vascular and Interventional Radiology* 2008; **19**(3): 359–65.

Chand DH, Valentini RP. International pediatric fistula first initiative: a call to action. *American Journal of Kidney Disease* 2008; **51**: 1016–24.

Clinical Practice Guidelines for Vascular Access. *American Journal of Kidney Diseases.* 2006): **48**(Suppl 1); S248–S276 [No authors listed].

Davis JB, Howell CG, Humphries AL. Hemodialysis access: elevated basilic vein arteriovenous fistula. *Journal of Pediatric Surgery* 1986; **21**: 1182–3.

Dix FP, Khan Y, Al-Khaffaf H. The brachial artery-basilic vein arterio-venous fistula in vascular access for haemodialysis – a review paper. *European Journal of Vascular and Endovascular Surgery* 2006; **31**: 70–9.

Gradman WS, Lerner G, Mentser M *et al.* Experience with autogenous arteriovenous access for hemodialysis in children and adolescents. *Annals of Vascular Surgery* 2005; **19**: 609–12.

Haricharan RN, Aprahamian CJ, Morgan TL *et al.* Intermediate-term patency of upper arm arteriovenous fistulae for hemodialysis access in children. *Journal of Pediatric Surgery* 2008; **43**: 147–51.

Kim AC, McLean S, Swearingen AM *et al.* Two-stage basilic vein transposition-a new approach for pediatric dialysis access. *Journal of Pediatric Surgery* 2010; **45**: 177–84.

Pasch AR. A two-staged technique for basilic vein transposition. *Journal of Vascular Access* 2007; **8**: 225–7.

Sharathkumar A, Hirschl R, Pipe S *et al.* Primary thromboprophylaxis with heparin for arteriovenous fistula failure in pediatric patients. *Journal of Vascular Access* 2007; **8**: 235–44.

Tannuri U, Tannuri AC, Watanabe A. Arteriovenous fistula for chronic hemodialysis in pediatric candidates for renal transplantation: technical details and refinements. *Pediatric Transplantation* 2009; 13: 360–4.

Wolford HY, Hsu J, Rhodes JM *et al.* Outcome after autogenous brachial-basilic upper arm transpositions in the post-National Kidney Foundation Dialysis Outcomes Quality Initiative era. *Journal of Vascular Surgery* 2005; **42**: 951–6.

90

Hypospadias

JOHN M PARK and DAVID A BLOOM

INTRODUCTION

1 Hypospadias is classically defined as an association of three congenital anatomic anomalies of the penis: (1) an abnormal ventral opening of the urethral meatus, (2) an abnormal ventral curvature of the penis (called 'chordee'), and (3) an abnormal dorsal 'hood' distribution of the foreskin with ventral deficiency. The diagnosis of hypospadias is evident on newborn examination, but in some instances of mild hypospadias such as the megameatus-intact prepuce (MIP) variant, in which the foreskin is normal, detection of hypospadias might not occur until the foreskin is retracted. The most common classification system employs anatomic description of meatal position.

Glanular, coronal, and subcoronal positions constitute the majority of cases (approximately 70 percent), but hypospadias can occur in more severe forms with the urethral meatus opening near the scrotum and perineum (**Figures 90.1, 90.2, and 90.3**).

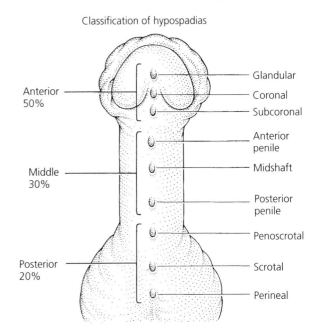

Classification of hypospadias

Anterior 50%
Middle 30%
Posterior 20%

Glandular
Coronal
Subcoronal
Anterior penile
Midshaft
Posterior penile
Penoscrotal
Scrotal
Perineal

1

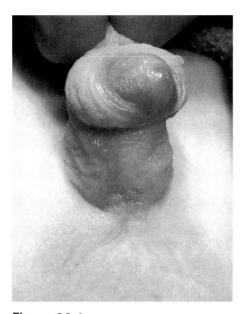

Figure 90.1 Mild hypospadias in which the urethral meatus is distally located and the penile shaft is associated with mild chordee and ventrally deficient prepuce.

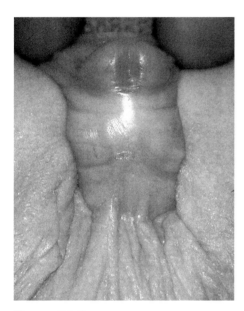

Figure 90.2 Moderate hypospadias in which the urethral meatus is subcoronal. There is a deep glanular groove distal to meatus (called urethral plate), and the prepuce is deficient ventrally.

INCIDENCE AND ASSOCIATED CONDITIONS

Hypospadias has been reported to occur approximately in one out of 100–300 live male births. In a case controlled study by Sweet *et al.*, hypospadias was present once in every 122 births. The great majority (87 percent) were mild – coronal or glanular. Interestingly, the rate of severe

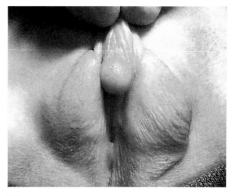

Figure 90.3 Severe hypospadias with the urethral opening in the perineum.

hypospadias seems to have increased three- to five-fold over the last two decades. This trend could reflect more frequent reporting and earlier diagnosis, or it may reflect other undefined biological factors, such as environmental endocrine disruptors during pregnancy. Hypospadias is most likely an inherited congenital defect, as it occurs in 6–8 percent of fathers of affected boys and 14 percent of male siblings.

Associated anomalies include cryptorchidism (8–9 percent) and inguinal hernia/hydrocele (9–16 percent). The rate of associated genital anomalies increases in patients with more severe proximal defects. An intersex condition, or disorders of sex development (DSD), should be considered in patients with concomitant hypospadias and cryptorchidism. Patients with severe hypospadias may also have a significantly enlarged utricle, which may serve as a nidus for urinary tract infections and cause voiding difficulties.

Chordee (congenital penile curvature)

Early on, the ventral curvature was thought to be caused primarily by fibrous tissues encasing the hypospadiac urethra, thereby tethering and bowing the penis, and this led to the proposal that the most important part of the chordee correction was aggressive excision of so-called 'chordee tissues'. Penile embryology and anatomic studies have shown that the etiology of chordee is much more complex, and it includes (1) abnormal development of the urethral plate (the mucosa-lined longitudinal groove between urethral meatus and glans), (2) abnormal, fibrous tissue at the urethral meatus, and (3) corporal disproportion between dorsal and ventral cavernosal tissues. The concept of corporal disproportion is particularly important in that a routine division and lifting of the urethral plate should no longer be considered as the principal maneuver in chordee correction. Indeed, the preservation of the urethral plate for neourethra reconstruction along with corporal repair for chordee correction constitutes a fundamental approach in modern hypospadias repair techniques.

2 Although chordee is commonly seen in association with hypospadias, it can occur in isolation with orthotopically located urethral meatus. In some cases, this is caused by a simple skin tethering, representing a simple surgical problem. In other instances the chordee is a 'form fruste' of hypospadias in that more extensive anatomic abnormalities coexist such as thin, dysplastic urethra and disproportionate corpora, which may require a significant reconstruction.

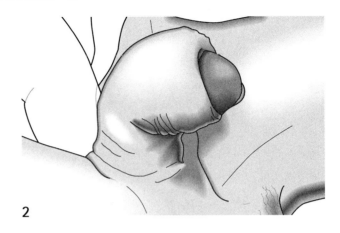

2

Megameatus-intact prepuce

In this situation, the prepuce is circumferentially formed and the hypospadiac urethral meatus is not evident until the foreskin is fully retracted (i.e. at the time of circumcision). Typically, distal to the coronal or glandular meatus, there is a wide and deep groove that can be tubularized into the neourethra. In most situations, MIP is not associated with significant chordee.

PREOPERATIVE ASSESSMENT AND PREPARATION

Preoperative evaluations

In general, the literature does not support routine evaluation of the urinary tract with either ultrasonography or other imaging modalities for hypospadias patients. In patients with a severe defect, such as perineal hypospadias, lower urinary tract evaluation with either endoscopy (at the time of repair) or voiding cystourethrography may define the utricle size and reveal concurrent anomalies. Routine endocrinologic and genetic evaluation of patients with isolated hypospadias is probably unnecessary, unless the defect is severe or associated with cryptorchidism.

Hormonal manipulations

There is considerable disagreement regarding the use of hormonal stimulation prior to hypospadias repair for the purpose of penile enlargement. Suggestions were made that preoperative human chorionic gonadotropin treatment may decrease the severity of hypospadias and increase the vascularity and thickness of proximal corpus spongiosum, thereby allowing more simple repairs. Preoperative testosterone was shown to increase penile size, along with improved skin availability and local vascularity. Hormonal supplementation may be useful in children with microphallus and with previously failed repairs, in which local tissues are deficient. Testosterone

may be given as either intramuscular depo-testosterone injection or topical cream applied around the genital area several weeks prior to the surgery.

Timing of the surgery

A report by the American Academy of Pediatrics suggested that the best time for hypospadias surgery may be between 6 and 12 months of age. This recommendation was made based on a number of factors, including the psychological effects of the genital surgery in children, improved technical aspects of hypospadias surgery, and advances in pediatric anesthesia. Postoperative management issues such as the care of neourethral catheter and wound dressings are significantly easier and safer in infants as well.

Anesthesia

In young children, general anesthesia with endotracheal intubation is the most reliable approach. Adjunctive regional analgesia using long-acting injectable nerve-blocking agents, such as bupivacaine, delivered via either caudal route or penile block, is safe and efficacious.

SURGICAL PRINCIPLES

Routine perioperative antibiotics are not necessary, unless the urethra and bladder are intubated postoperatively. Hemostasis must be accomplished with precision, applying judicious cauterization, since ischemic tissue necrosis will lead to the breakdown of repair, infection, and urethrocutaneous fistula. Careful use of vasoconstrictive agent (epinephrine diluted to 1:200 000) around the region of the corona and glans will also reduce the amount of bleeding intraoperatively. A tourniquet may be applied to the base of the penis during certain parts of the surgery, but it must not be used excessively for a prolonged time. Most surgeons rely on optical magnification to enhance surgical precision.

Orthoplasty (chordee correction)

The degree of ventral curvature influences the type of hypospadias repair. Even if the urethral opening is not severely ectopic, the penis may require an extensive reconstruction (even a staged one) in order to accomplish adequate straightening of the phallus. Preoperatively, gentle retraction of the penile base allows a reasonable assessment of the location and the severity of overall chordee.

3 Intraoperative evaluation of chordee using an artificial erection test is critical. After the degloving of the penile shaft, injection of one of the corpus cavernosum is performed directly using 5–10 mL of saline solution with a small 23-gauge butterfly needle. Alternatively, the needle may be passed through the glans and into the tip of a corpus in order to minimize hematoma beneath the Buck's fascia.

At times, release of tethering ventral skin may be all that is required for orthoplasty. In this situation, some of the dorsal prepuce and penile skin may need to be transposed ventrally to make up for the skin deficiency.

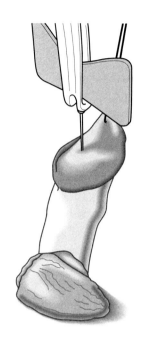

3

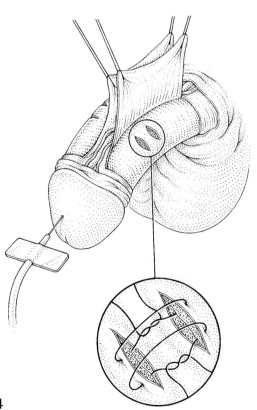

4

4 One of the most reliable techniques of orthoplasty is dorsal corporal plication, as described by Nesbit. His original description involved mobilization of dorsal midline neurovascular bundle, followed by making an elliptical excision of dorsal tunica albuginea vertically and approximating these defects horizontally (the Heineke–Mikulicz principle). This concept was extended further by Baskin and Duckett, in which two parallel lines of incision are made in the tunica albuginea transversely on the dorsolateral aspects of each corpus cavernosum at the point of maximal curvature, and the outer edges of the incisions are approximated using buried sutures.

5a–c In patients with severe curvature or with short phallic length, dorsal plication technique may not be optimal because of potential shortening, and ventral transverse incision of tunica albuginea and patch grafting may be more suitable. The corporal defect created after the incision is then covered with de-epithelialized dermis harvested from the lower abdominal wall, tunica vaginalis, or a synthetic graft in older patients.

Hypospadiac penis may be associated with counterclockwise penile torsion. In mild cases, this may be corrected simply by rotating the penile skin coverage, but in more severe cases, additional correction may be required, such as corporal plication and dorsal dartos flap rotation.

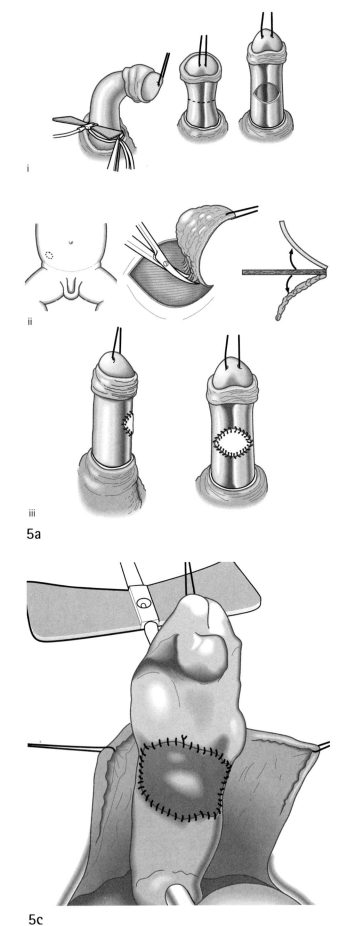

5a

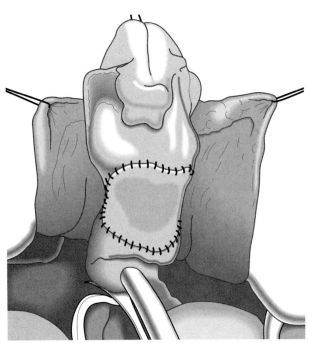

5b

5c

Urethroplasty

An important surgical principle in neourethra formation is meticulous tissue transfer. In urethroplasty, the tissue source may be adjacent tissue, local tissue flaps, or free grafts of either genital or extragenital tissue origin.

The neourethra may be created by tubularization of the native urethral plate, especially if there is a deep glanular groove. Biologically speaking, the urethral plate contains an epithelial lining with urethral mucosal differentiation and will likely perform best as neourethra, provided that tubularization can occur without suture line tension and meatal stenosis. Local tissue flaps employed for urethral reconstruction must be thin, non-hair-bearing, and easy to handle. They are often derived from distal penile shaft skin or prepuce, and they are called 'fasciocutaneous flaps' because of their reliance upon the dartos fascia serving

as the conduit for vascular supply and drainage. The term 'graft' implies that tissue has been excised from one location and transferred to another site, where a new blood supply develops.

Neourethral coverage

It is critical to establish multiple layer coverage of the urethroplasty suture line prior to skin closure in order to decrease the risk of urethrocutaneous fistula formation. Not only does it provide additional protection during the healing of reconstructed urethra, but also the ventrally mobilized flap improves the overall functional and cosmetic outcome. Various vascularized flaps may be used for this purpose, including penile/preputial dartos, tunica vaginalis, and periurethral corpus spongiosum.

6a,b   The dorsal prepuce is unfolded, and the subcutaneous dartos flap is sharply dissected off the undersurface of the penile skin down to the base. To prevent penile twisting, the flap may be divided down the middle, preserving the vessels, brought around the shaft

to the ventral area, and secured over the neourethra as a double crossover flap. For a tunica vaginalis flap, a testicle is delivered and its tunica vaginalis is dissected off the spermatic cord. The flap must be adequately mobilized to avoid ventral tethering.

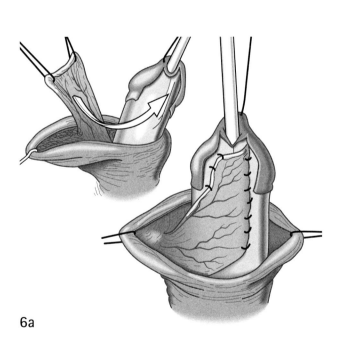

6a

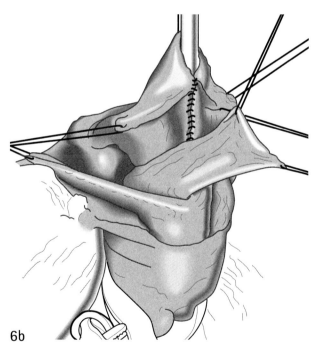

6b

7 In most cases of hypospadias, the corpus spongiosum becomes flat distal to the meatus and fans out around the urethral plate. After the urethroplasty, this layer of tissue can be mobilized and approximated over the midline as the second layer coverage. Unlike dartos and tunica vaginalis flaps, the corpus spongiosum used in this way is less likely to cause ventral tethering and penile twisting.

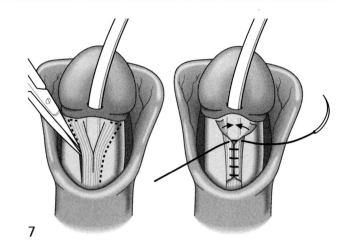

7

Meatoplasty and glanuloplasty

All attempts at neourethral reconstruction will be for naught if careful attention is not given to this phase of the hypospadias repair. Glans wings (the lateral flaps of glans tissue that are brought around and approximated over the middle) must be loose with minimal tension, with enough space to accommodate both the neourethra and the coverage flaps. If the glanuloplasty is performed with tension, it can lead to either a troublesome meatal stenosis or breakdown of the distal repair, resulting in a recurrence of coronal hypospadias or a 'blow-out' type of urethrocutaneous fistula, most often at the subcoronal location. In all techniques of hypospadias repair, the final meatal caliber must be ample (8 Fr for infants and at least 10 Fr for children older than three years) with a generous spatulation. It is best to avoid a circumferential suture line around the meatus, which predisposes to meatal stenosis.

INTRAOPERATIVE DECISION-MAKING: USING THE RIGHT TISSUES AND CHOOSING THE RIGHT PROCEDURE

Decision-making begins with assessment of meatal location, penile size, curvature, and the quality of ventral skin over the native urethra. In most patients, hypospadias is repairable using well-vascularized local tissues. In mild glanular hypospadias, simple meatal advancement and glanuloplasty (MAGPI) may be all that is required. In other situations, consideration is given to neourethral reconstruction using either flap technique or urethral plate tubularization. If the urethral plate is healthy with decent width and vascularity, it may be tubularized, either with or without the help of vertical midline incision technique (TIP/Snodgrass). If it is too narrow or too shallow for effective, tension-free tubularization, then a preputial (onlay urethroplasty) or perimeatal-based proximal skin (Mathieu procedure) fasciocutaneous flap is approximated onto the urethral plate as the ventral portion of the neourethra. In some situations, the actual meatal location is distal, but the quality of distal urethra leading up to the meatus is thin and dysplastic, along with near absent penile skin ventrally. This type of hypospadias should be treated as a more severe proximal defect.

The choice of urethroplasty technique may depend upon the degree of chordee. The penile shaft is degloved after making a subcoronal incision, preserving the urethral plate of 8–10 mm width, except for severe hypospadias such as scrotal and perineal variety in which urethral plate preservation is unlikely from the outset. The penis is evaluated for curvature with an artificial erection test. If the curvature is severe (greater than 90°), along with short phallic length, correcting chordee by aggressive dorsal corporal plication may not be the best option, since it may lead to shortening of the phallus. In this situation, consideration must be given to division of the urethral plate, excision of ventral fibrous chordee tissues, and placement of a corporal patch after a relaxing transverse incision of tunica albuginea. The neourethra may be then created later using transposed dorsal preputial skin (staged operation), or immediately with island pedicle flap (transverse island tube urethroplasty), or free graft (oral mucosa graft urethroplasty).

SPECIFIC OPERATIONS

There is no single, universally applicable technique of hypospadias repair. A surgeon attempting an effective hypospadias reconstruction must be familiar with several different techniques, understanding their pros and cons, along with their indications for specific anatomic configurations. It is unwise to rigidly apply one or two 'favorite' techniques to all situations. Instead, a given anatomic situation must dictate the procedure to be employed, and the surgeon must maintain flexibility and versatility. It is not possible within the scope of this chapter to discuss all reported techniques of hypospadias repair. The authors will present several of their own preferred techniques.

Meatal advancement and glanuloplasty

8a–j For the glanular and some of the coronal hypospadias without significant chordee, MAGPI is a simple, yet elegant, procedure with an excellent functional and cosmetic outcome. In many cases of distal hypospadias, there is a transverse glanular tissue ridge that separates the true meatus from a distal blind-ending groove. In the first step of MAGPI, this tissue ridge is incised deeply in a vertical direction, creating a diamond-shaped defect, which is then closed in a transverse direction (the Heineke–Mikulicz principle). This maneuver widens, advances, and flattens the urethral meatus. A circumferential incision is then made in the subcoronal region, and the penis is degloved. After addressing any chordee, the glanuloplasty is performed. After ventrolateral de-epithelialization and mobilization of the glans tissue proximal to the urethral meatus, glanuloplasty is performed in two layers, while gently retracting the lower lip of the urethral meatus upward. By avoiding an urethroplasty suture line, there is little to no risk of urethrocutaneous fistula formation, but a meatal retraction back to the hypospadiac position may occur postoperatively if the glanuloplasty is done under tension without adequate mobilization of the glanular wings.

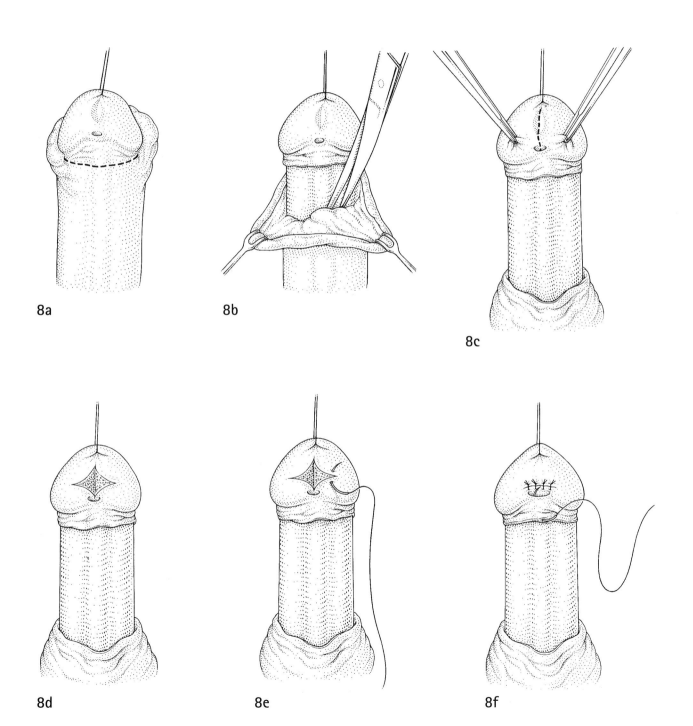

8a

8b

8c

8d

8e

8f

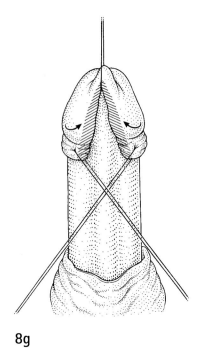

8g

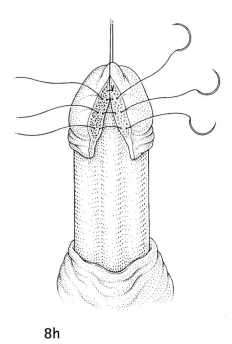

8h

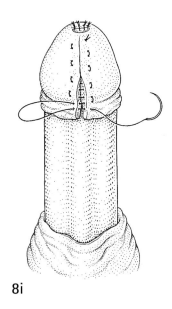

8i

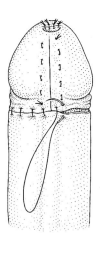

8j

Tubularized incised plate urethroplasty (TIP or Snodgrass) repair

9 Thiersch and Duplay were the first to describe the technique of urethral plate tubularization in repairing hypospadias. Additional modifications were described by King and Zaontz (GAP procedure). These techniques all result in excellent cosmetic and functional outcome in patients with hypospadiac penis associated with a deep glanular groove. However, urethral tubularization techniques were not deemed suitable for penis associated with a flat urethral plate, with the fear that there would be an excessive tension of the neourethral suture line along with the risk of meatal stenosis. Snodgrass combined the vertical distal urethral plate incision technique to relax its tension with the Thiersch–Duplay tubularization technique, to propose the tubularized incised plate (TIP) repair technique. Many reports from various institutions have reported excellent outcomes with this procedure. Unlike the traditional urethral plate tubularization techniques, TIP repair is versatile for many different anatomical presentations, including proximal and the previously failed cases.

The urethral plate is marked out 8–10 mm wide distal to the urethral meatus, and incisions are made along the lateral borders of the urethral plate. The distal limit of this incision must be carefully planned, so that at the end of neourethral tubularization, one does not end up with a circumferentially sutured urethral meatus, which may contract and stenose. An incision is made subcoronally and is completed ventrally proximal to the urethral meatus. The penis is carefully degloved down to the base. Ventrally, the skin can be quite thin and adherent to the urethra, and a sharp iris scissor dissection using carefully placed skin hooks for upward counter-traction provides an optimal visualization of the surgical dissection planes to avoid buttonholing into a thin native urethra. After addressing any chordee, glanular wings are adequately developed lateral to the urethral plate, so that the subsequent glanuloplasty can be performed without tension. The urethral plate is gently wrapped around an 8 Fr (10 Fr in older children) tube to check for any areas of tension. While providing a symmetrical traction and counter-traction, a deep midline vertical incision is made with a knife in the urethral plate. The adequacy of hinging is confirmed by again wrapping the urethral plate margins around the tube. The neourethra is then reconstructed using multiple interrupted or running sutures. Again, care is taken to ensure that the newly reconstructed meatus is wide in caliber and without circumferential suture line. A second layer coverage is then sought with either mobilized dorsal dartos, tunica vaginalis, or fanned out Y-shaped distal spongiosal tissues. Skin coverage of the phallic shaft and glanuloplasty complete the procedure.

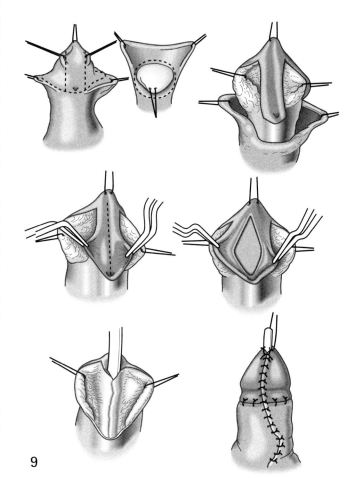

9

Perimeatal–based flap urethroplasty (Mathieu)

10 Among the more commonly used local flap techniques for coronal and subcoronal hypospadias is the perimeatal-based flap technique of Mathieu. This requires ample penile ventral skin proximal to the hypospadiac meatus. It is begun by measuring the length of the defect from the urethral meatus to the glans. An equal distance flap is then measured from the meatus toward the base of the penis on the proximal shaft skin. The urethral plate and the matching proximal shaft skin flap are incised to be approximately 7–8 mm wide, and the penis is degloved after subcoronal circumferential incision. Glanular wings are developed deeply in order to perform a tension-free glanuloplasty. If the urethral plate is very flat distally, or if the distal limit of urethral plate is too ventral, the Barcat balanic groove technique may be employed. In this modification, the urethral plate is dissected off the glans tissue, and after incising the dorsal glans tissue in the midline, the urethral plate is advanced further posteriorly to achieve a more distal neourethral opening. After correcting the chordee, the premeasured proximal shaft skin flap is mobilized carefully and transposed upward toward the urethral plate. This flap is folded over the urethral meatus, and both edges are approximated with precisely placed fine absorbable sutures. After maturing a wide caliber meatus, a second layer coverage is performed as described previously. Glanuloplasty and skin coverage complete the procedure.

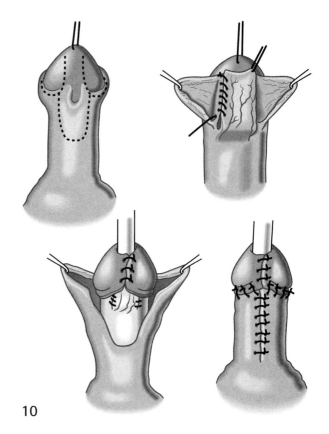

10

Preputial island pedicle flap urethroplasty

11a–f, 12a–f Duckett, Asopa, and Standoli described preputial onlay urethroplasties nearly simultaneously, although the Duckett variant became the popular choice. The penis is prepared by means of degloving, and orthoplasty is performed as described above, preserving the urethral plate similar to the TIP repair. The hood of foreskin is laid out and a rectangular portion is marked on the inner surface with a marking pen to outline the graft for the intended neourethra. In general, this should be at least 8–10 mm wide to produce a reasonable caliber, and a length of 3–4 cm is not an unreasonable expectation for infant hypospadias repairs. The use of gentle fine traction sutures to display the foreskin minimizes the trauma to the flap by repetitive forcep grasping. Injecting dilute (1:200 000) epinephrine solution subcutaneously is useful for hemostasis and for separating the inner and outer layers of prepuce. A rectangular flap is developed using sharp knife and iris scissor dissections, leaving it attached to a broad dartos vascular pedicle. This island pedicle flap must be mobilized adequately down to the penile base in order to swing it away from the remainder of the foreskin and bring it around the penile shaft ventrally without twisting the shaft. The native urethral meatus is prepared to assure that it is vascular, ample, and spatulated. The island flap is then sutured onto the urethral plate using fine absorbable sutures (onlay technique). If the urethral plate is not available or unsuitable for onlay urethroplasty, the flap is then tubularized over an 8 to 10 Fr catheter to fashion a tubular neourethra. The neourethral suture line should be positioned dorsally against the corporal bodies to minimize the chance of fistula. A spatulated anastomosis is performed between native urethral meatus and the neourethra. The neourethra is then secured to the penile shaft ventrum with several interrupted fine absorbable sutures to stabilize it. In general, the onlay technique is associated with a lower incidence of proximal anastomotic stricture as compared to the tubular neourethra, but at times, urethral plate may need to be divided from the native urethral meatus in order to perform an effective correction of severe ventral chordee, necessitating the use of a tubular neourethra. The glanuloplasty is performed either by splitting the glans and creating lateral glanular wings to bring over the distal neourethra, or by a tunneling technique to bore an ample core through the glans. In either case, the distal meatus is secured to the glans with fine interrupted absorbable sutures, and the new urethral meatus must be spatulated and fashioned wide to prevent stenosis. A critical next step is to provide a supporting vascular tissue to cover the neourethra before skin closure using either the remaining penile dartos or tunica vaginalis. Lastly, ventral skin approximation is accomplished using the dorsal remnants of prepuce.

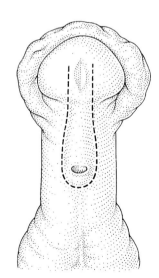

11a

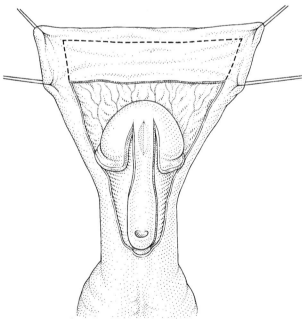

11b

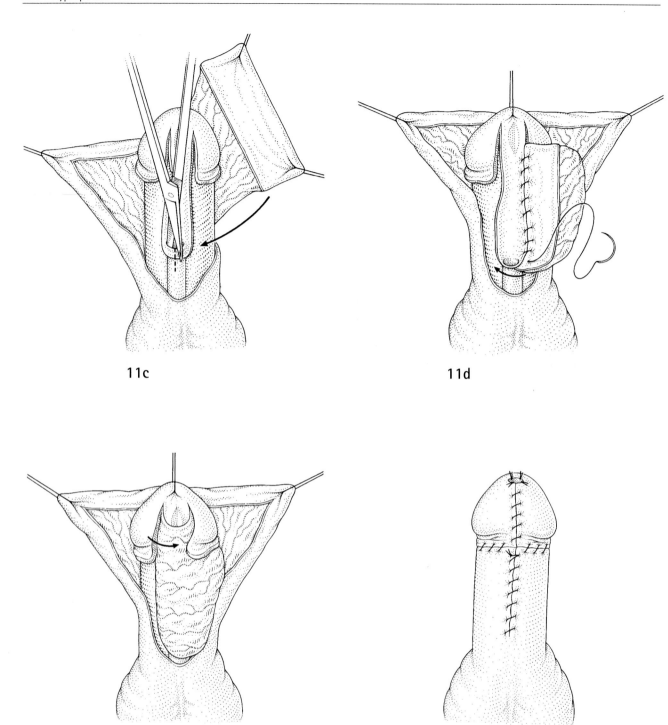

11c

11d

11e

11f

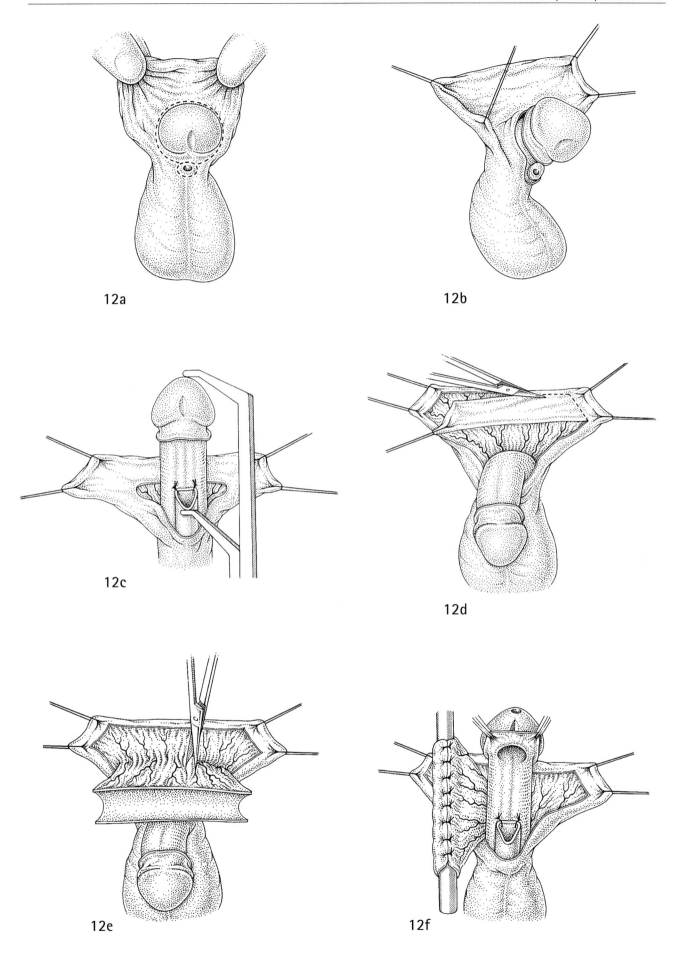

12a

12b

12c

12d

12e

12f

Staged repair

13 Staged repair was once preferred for most instances of hypospadias. Accumulated expertise in hypospadiology relegated staged repairs to the more difficult instances of hypospadias, and some even favored complex single repairs for all instances of hypospadias. Pendulums, however, do swing, and many surgeons prefer to manage patients with complex hypospadias via several dependable, if less heroic, steps. The principles of staged repair are to correct any chordee and other scrotal anomalies (such as penoscrotal transposition) during the first repair, followed by subsequent urethroplasty at another setting. Some patients present with extreme chordee (>90°) along with severe hypospadias. In this scenario, even after straightening the penis perfectly at the time of surgery as proven by an artificial erection test, some recurrence of chordee becomes evident after a number of months. Thus, for the first stage, an initial orthoplasty is performed along with ventral resurfacing with dorsal preputial skin. At least six months later, the patient is brought back for the second stage. Here the residual chordee (which is invariably much less than at the initial procedure) can be corrected definitively, and the neourethra can then be fashioned either by tubularization of the previously transposed preputial tissue or by free graft (which we now favor from an oral mucosal source).

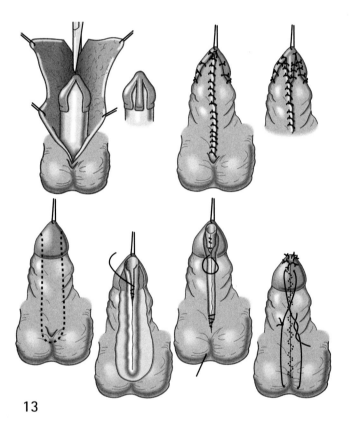

13

Oral mucosa graft urethroplasty

14a–f Humby reported this technique in 1941 in a single case, but somehow the best hypospadiologists remained ignorant of this innovative technique for more than 40 years until it was rediscovered and resurrected in Italy and France. The next set of papers appeared in the early 1990s, and the use of oral mucosa increased steadily over the next decade in the reconstruction of hypospadias and other urethral problems. This procedure was first applied for hypospadiac 'cripples' who had failed multiple operations and were left with no viable local penile tissues for adequate repair, but its use has now expanded satisfactorily to primary repairs in severe hypospadias. It may be used as a single stage or a staged repair depending on the anatomic situation. The oral mucosa graft may be obtained from either the inner lining of the lower lip or inner cheek, and sometimes a contiguous combination of both is useful when a longer graft is needed. An 8–10 cm long graft can be achieved with this technique. In case of shorter grafts, inner cheek is preferable, and during the harvesting, one must be careful to avoid injury to the Stensen's duct, which is opposite the second upper molar in most patients. The graft harvest site is marked out with a marking pen, retracting the mouth with a combination of retractors and fine traction sutures. Subcutaneous injection of dilute (1:200 000) epinephrine solution is useful for purposes of hemostasis and facilitating the dissection of the oral mucosa. A sharp dissection is performed using knife and iris scissors, leaving muscle bundles in the mouth. Handling the graft with fine traction sutures minimizes

the trauma from repetitive forcep grasping. Once the graft is harvested, it is rinsed multiple times and placed in saline solution to minimize desiccation. Bleeders in the graft bed are managed with a combination of direct pressure, pinpoint coagulation, or fine suture ligatures. The harvest site may be closed with fine absorbable sutures (such as 4/0 chromic), or it may be left open. No clear-cut advantage has been demonstrated for either strategy, and postoperative morbidity in terms of pain and dietary issues has been negligible. Most patients can resume a normal diet in 24–36 hours. The underside of the graft is then carefully trimmed to remove any extraneous adipose and muscle tissues, leaving behind the whitish-colored dermal layer only. Once the graft is prepared, it is rinsed several times and then kept in a saline bath. During the entire oral procedure, the initial operative field over the penis and the surgical instruments are segregated before the mouth is prepared and draped. After completing the graft harvest and preparation, the surgeons reglove and gown and return to the original operative field and instruments. The graft is then employed for creating neourethra via either onlay (if an adequate urethral plate is present) or tubular neourethra technique. Stabilizing the graft and finding a healthy vascular supporting tissue for graft coverage are critical for graft take. Distal glanular urethra and neourethral meatus must be fashioned widely to avoid stenosis. After penile skin coverage, the dressing must be applied loosely, and the patient's activity must be restricted for 24–48 hours to encourage vascular ingrowth into the graft. In general, the neourethra is intubated with an appropriately sized catheter for 10–14 days.

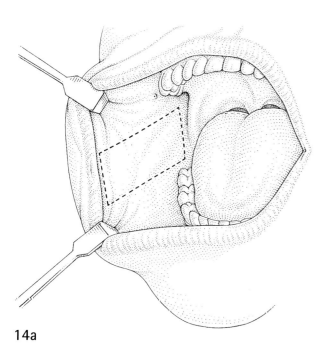

14a

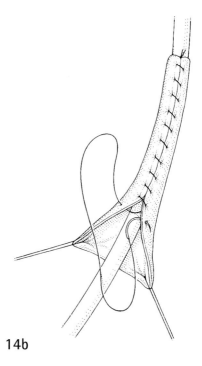

14b

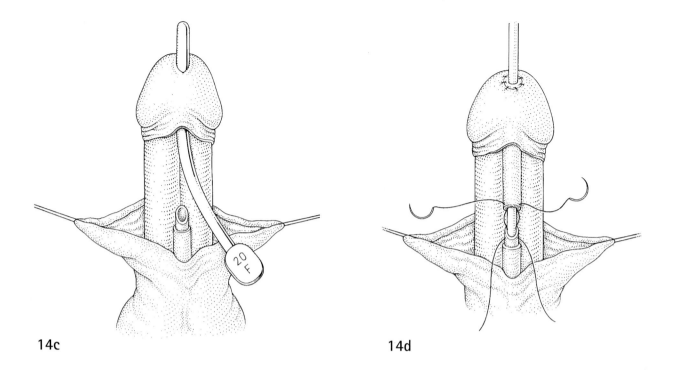

14c

14d

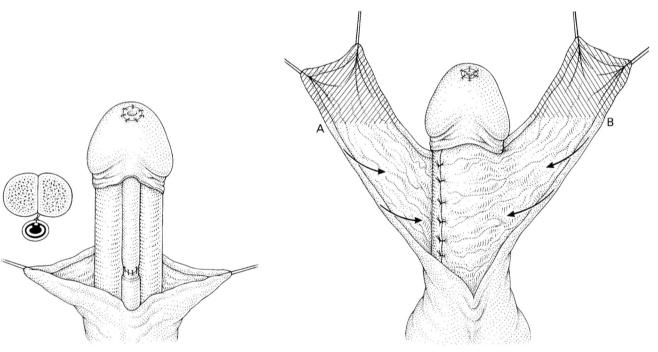

14e

14f

POSTOPERATIVE CARE

Urethral catheter

Intuitively, a newly reconstructed urethra with a long suture line is likely to be better protected during healing with the use of diverting urethral catheter. It is routine among many surgeons to leave an indwelling urethral catheter postoperatively for 7–10 days. However, recent studies have not proven the benefit of urethral catheter. In a multicenter report, excellent results were obtained in 96.7 percent of over 300 patients undergoing mild to moderate hypospadias repair with the Mathieu technique, and the complication rate was not affected by the catheterization status. Others have speculated that the routine use of urethral catheter may at times increase the chance of complications. Based on these observations, a routine use of urethral catheter may not offer any significant advantage in mild to moderate cases of hypospadias with a straightforward neourethra reconstruction. If the authors were to use a catheter, a soft, silastic tube of 8–10 Fr caliber without retention balloon is preferred, secured at the meatus using sutures. Urine is usually drained via a double diaper technique in infants, in which the catheter is brought through a ventral hole in the inner diaper and is allowed to continuously drain into the outer diaper. With this set up, fecal material is kept away from the catheter opening, and the double diaper provides a secure, additional padding over the genitalia without the worry of drainage bag pulling on the reconstructed urethra.

Dressing

An ideal penile dressing after hypospadias repair should be nonadherent, absorbant, and compressive, while being soft and elastic enough to accommodate postoperative swelling. Several variations have been reported in the literature. A careful application of secure penile dressing can prevent postoperative complications, such as hematoma and edema, and may additionally reduce parental anxiety. It is critical to keep the reconstructed meatus moist and free of dried up secretions by generously applying a petroleum-based ointment for several weeks.

COMPLICATIONS

Bleeding

In most hypospadias repairs, electrocautery must be used very sparsely, applying precise pinpoint cauterizations. Bleeding from the exposed spongiosal tissues, either from glans, corpus spongiosum, or corpus cavernosum, should not be managed with aggressive cauterization, not only because of ineffectiveness in stopping the bleeding

but also because of excessive tissue ischemia and injury following such maneuvers. Dilute epinephrine solution, direct pressure, or fine suture ligatures are appropriate for most intraoperative bleeding. Pressure dressings are useful for hypospadias repairs with the caveat that they should not be too tight to cause ischemia. Occasionally, a patient will return to the emergency room a day or so after hypospadias repair because of unanticipated bleeding, and in these instances, we will simply reapply a pressure dressing. It may be necessary on rare occasions to return to the operating room to evacuate a clot and control a bleeding source. Late bleeding, more than a week postoperatively, is unusual and may occur from trauma. Large expanding hematomas are best evacuated under anesthesia, with control of active bleeding sites and reapplication of a pressure dressing.

Meatal stenosis

A wide distal anastomosis without a circumferential suture line, while preserving good vascularity to all the involved tissues, should minimize subsequent meatal stenosis. In the initial few postoperative months, it is critical to keep the distal meatus continuously moist with petroleum-based ointment. When we see the patients back in clinic, we have a low threshold for passing a small caliber feeding tube to assure patency. When meatal stenosis is suspected, we will often ask the families or the patients to pass a tube on a regular basis to keep it open. Topical vitamin E or corticosteroids may help soften up an incipient stricture. A late stricture may require an anesthetic for aggressive dilation or urethrotomy. It is important to distinguish true meatal stenosis from distal urethral stenosis, which would require more aggressive management and even redo urethroplasty.

Urethrocutaneous fistula

A very distal fistula in the glans or corona can be corrected by simply incising the intervening glanular tissue to create a more ample meatus, even if it becomes slightly hypospadiac, as long as there is no chordee. More proximal fistulas are corrected by generous incision to expose the defect and multiple layers of closure, usually using some type of de-epithelialized skin edges to create vascular coverage layers. Some fistulas represent only the tip of an iceberg, as it were, and are indicative of unhealthy tissue over a portion of the neourethra or distal urethral stricture. In these instances, one must consider doing a complete revision of neourethra with alternative tissue sources, such as the oral mucosa. Not appreciating the poor quality of neourethra as the true cause of fistulas will likely lead to their recurrence. In many instances, the *sine qua non* for a successful fistula repair is 'Make it a big operation to fix a little hole'.

Infection

True skin infections with cellulitis are uncommon after hypospadias repair. When they are suspected, however, an aggressive antibiotic treatment with broadened coverage should be initiated, and the child brought back into hospital for several days of intravenous antibiotic coverage. When the children are sent home with a catheter in place, they are routinely given a low-dose prophylactic antibiotic coverage daily to minimize colonization and reduce the risk of urinary tract infection until the catheter is removed.

Urethral diverticulum

This complication occurs as the result of either distal urethral stenosis and/or insufficient ventral tissue coverage of the neourethra. A small diverticulum may be left alone if a patient is willing to support the sacculed area manually while voiding; however, more substantial urethral diverticuli are best managed surgically, first by ensuring no distal stenosis and second by exposing the diverticulum, removing excess tissue, and reclosing the urethra. The critical step is finding adequate tissue (either dartos or tunica vaginalis) to support the area of the resected diverticulum before closing the skin. Again, if a significant portion of urethra is unhealthy or ischemic, it is better to perform a revision urethroplasty using an oral mucosa graft.

Stricture

Urethral stricture may occur at the meatus (meatal stenosis), in the glanular portion of the urethra, or at a proximal anastomotic site. Strictures within the middle portion of the neourethra are less common. Early strictures are best managed by gentle dilation and intermittent catheterization. More severe strictures, particularly along the course of the urethra, may be corrected by a dilation technique or internal urethrotomy using either endoscopic knife or laser. Generally speaking, if the strictured segment is long and is surrounded by dense periurethral fibrosis, the above-mentioned minimally invasive techniques are ineffective, and the stricture is prone to recur. It is advised that in these situations, one should consider a revision urethroplasty using oral mucosa. Placing an oral mucosa graft dorsally against corpora cavernosal bodies will minimize the risk of fistula formation.

Reoperative hypospadias repair

Some patients present with difficult constellation of failed hypospadias repair, residual chordee, recurrent stricture, fistula, or other functional residua after multiple attempts at repair. These patients have been called 'hypospadiac cripples'. The fundamental principle of management is thorough assessment of the relevant symptoms and anatomic features of the patient. Most often, this is best done by examination under anesthesia with cystourethroscopy. The first principle is to properly inform the patient and family about the problems and likely etiologies, plan for correction, and potential complications. Establishing realistic expectations is critical. The second principle is to recognize any related anatomic features, such as penoscrotal transposition and chordee, as well as any available viable tissues not only for neourethra formation and penile skin coverage but also vascular supporting tissues for covering the neourethra. At times, planning a staged approach, correcting chordee, and debriding unhealthy local tissues before proceeding with neourethra reconstruction, may be prudent. Third, the neourethra must be reconstructed from robust, mucosa-lined tissues with an excellent potential for neovascularity (most likely this will be oral mucosa). Stubbornly insisting on using the remnant of fibrotic preputial and penile skin will lead to an inevitable failure and poor long-term outcome. Finally, a period of postoperative catheterization, early reassessment with calibration of the neourethra, and even a confirmation endoscopic examination when appropriate, will be essential.

FURTHER READING

Baskin LS, Duckett JW Jr. Dorsal tunica albuginea plication for hypospadias curvature. *Journal of Urology* 1994; **151**: 895–9.

Duckett JW Jr. Transverse preputial island flap technique for repair of severe hypospadias. *Journal of Urology* 1980; **167**: 1179–82.

Duckett JW Jr, Coplen D, Ewalt D *et al.* Buccal mucosal urethral replacement. *Journal of Urology* 1995; **153**: 1660–3.

Park JM, Faerber GJ, Bloom DA. Long-term outcome evaluation of patients undergoing the meatal advancement and glanuloplasty procedure. *Journal of Urology* 1995; **153**: 1655–6.

Snodgrass W. Tubularized, incised plate urethroplasty for distal hypospadias. *Journal of Urology* 1994; **151**: 464–5.

91

Orchidopexy

JOHN M HUTSON

PRINCIPLES AND JUSTIFICATION

Undescended testis is a common abnormality, affecting 3–5 percent of males. In preterm infants, the incidence may be 20 percent or more. Many testes not in the scrotum at birth descend by 12 weeks after birth, so that by three months of age the incidence of congenital undescended testes is approximately 1–2 percent. Some testes that descend late into the scrotum may reascend later in childhood, producing an acquired variant of maldescent, known as ascending testes.

Embryology

The urogenital ridge forms on the posterior abdominal wall and contains the mesonephros, its draining duct and the developing gonads. Primitive germ cells migrate from the yolk sac in the sixth week of gestation, as the gonad in the male develops into a testis. By 7–8 weeks, the testis is producing hormones that control its subsequent descent.

Descent of the testes

Descent of the testes occurs in two morphologically and hormonally distinct phases. The key structure in controlling the process is the gubernaculum, which is the embryonic ligament anchoring the testis and urogenital ridge to the inguinal region. The gubernaculum enlarges in the first phase to anchor the testis near the inguinal region as the embryo enlarges between 10 and 15 weeks of gestation. In the second phase, which occurs between 28 and 35 weeks of gestation, the gubernaculum migrates through the inguinal canal, across the pubic region, and into the scrotum. The processus vaginalis develops as a peritoneal diverticulum within the elongating gubernaculum, creating an intraperitoneal space into which the testis can descend.

The main hormone controlling the first phase is the homolog of insulin and relaxin, known as insulin-like hormone 3 (Insl3). This hormone is produced by Leydig cells, and stimulates distal gubernaculum, with some augmentation of its effect by Müllerian inhibiting substance (MIS) and possibly testosterone. In the second phase, testosterone acts apparently indirectly via the genitofemoral nerve, which supplies the gubernaculum and scrotum. Calcitonin gene-related peptide (CGRP) has been identified within sensory branches of the genitofemoral nerve and has been postulated to modulate androgenic control of descent. Androgens probably cause masculinization of the sensory branches of the genitofemoral nerve between 15 and 25 weeks of gestation, and the masculinized nerve then controls the direction of gubernacular migration by the release of CGRP in the periphery.

Some undescended testes in humans may be caused by physiologic or anatomic abnormalities of the genitofemoral nerve or its neurotransmitter, CGRP. The common cause of maldescent is failed gubernacular migration, leaving the testes in the groin, or so-called 'superficial inguinal pouch,' caused by primarily anatomic or secondary abnormal hormone development. Rarely, undescended testes are caused by recognized anomalies in the hypothalamic–pituitary–gonadal axis or in the secretion or action of Insl3 and MIS. Recognizable hormonal syndromes, however, are rare causes of cryptorchidism in clinical practice.

Undescended testes

Failed gubernacular migration leads to arrest of gubernacular migration along the normal pathway or aberrant migration to an ectopic location in the perineal, prepubic, or femoral region. Many undescended testes are located in the superficial inguinal pouch, the subcutaneous space arrest just above and lateral to the external inguinal ring containing the processus vaginalis (with its contained testis). This is the most common position for an undescended testis and is not categorized as ectopic.

There is controversy about whether 'ascending' testes are abnormal. These testes are located in the scrotum by 12 weeks of age, but later in childhood retract out of the scrotum, and often have an exaggerated cremaster reflex. It may be acquired maldescent, with the testis becoming relatively higher as the child gets older. Actually, in most cases, the spermatic cord fails to elongate normally, while the distance between the inguinal canal and scrotum doubles with growth during the first decade. Surgical intervention is not indicated unless the testis is no longer residing spontaneously in the scrotum. If the testis is near the top of the scrotum, regular follow up is required to make sure that it does not ascend out of the scrotum with time. This often leads to orchidopexy being recommended in 5–11-year-old boys.

Indications

Surgery is recommended for three common reasons: abnormal fertility, a risk of testicular tumors in adult life, and the obvious cosmetic abnormalities. Although many undescended testes have patent processus vaginalis, this is an uncommon presentation for an inguinal hernia. If an infant presents with an inguinal hernia, however, orchidopexy with associated herniotomy is performed immediately. Trauma and torsion in undescended testes are more common than when the testis is descended, although these are unlikely indications for surgery.

Germ-cell development in cryptorchidism is normal in the first six months, but then becomes abnormal subsequently due to secondary degeneration. This is caused by the testes residing at a higher temperature (35–37°C) than when in the scrotum (33°C). In some instances, there may be an intrinsic anomaly of testicular function.

The risk of malignancy in young adults with undescended testes is approximately five- to ten-fold that of young men with descended testes. These risk calculations are not based on current practice, however, but on results when children had orchidopexy at approximately ten years of age. With the current practice of recommending surgery at a much younger age, it is hoped that the cancer risk in the next generation will be lower, although this is unproven. The risk of malignancy affects not only the unilateral undescended testis, but also the contralateral descended testis in some patients. Evidence is now emerging that acquired cryptorchidism has a much lower risk of subsequent malignancy.

Recommended age for orchidopexy

To prevent secondary testicular degeneration with loss of germ cells and increasing risk of malignancy, orchidopexy is best performed in infancy. Although it is not proven for humans, it is clear in animal experiments that early surgery is better than a delayed operation. Operation can be performed at any time between three and six months and one year of age, depending on the surgeon's experience. Those with less experience would be wise to delay surgery to the older end of the range, rather than to attempt orchidopexy in a young infant, to avoid testicular atrophy. Magnification should be mandatory for surgery in babies less than one year of age.

PREOPERATIVE

Secondary preoperative preparation

In older boys with possible ascending testes, a course of gonadatrophins may be appropriate, although this is controversial. In bilateral impalpable testes, a human chorionic gonadotrophin (hCG) stimulation test should be performed to determine whether testicular tissue is present at all. Serum levels of MIS/anti-Müllerian hormone will reflect the presence of Sertoli cells. If hCG stimulation shows the presence of Leydig cells, laparoscopy is indicated at the beginning of the operation to determine the exact site and nature of the intra-abdominal testes.

Anesthesia

As orchidopexy is now a day-case procedure, the type of general anesthesia reflects the need for early mobilization. No premedication is usually required, although an oral preparation would be preferable to intramuscular injections. On admission to the day surgical unit, anesthetic cream containing lidocaine (lignocaine) and prilocaine is applied to the back of the hand so that intravenous access can be obtained without pain. An ilioinguinal nerve block, local anesthesia, or caudal anesthesia is provided to control pain for the first 4–6 hours after operation.

OPERATION: STANDARD ORCHIDOPEXY

Skin preparation and position of patient

The patient is placed supine on the operating table with the legs slightly apart. Povidone-iodine, or other appropriate antiseptic, is painted on the skin from the umbilicus to below the scrotum and perineum.

Standard orchidopexy for a palpable testis (which occurs in approximately 80–90 percent of cases) involves an inguinal incision, full exposure of the inguinal canal, separation of the processus vaginalis, and mobilization of the testis and spermatic cord. The second part of the operation is the orchidopexy itself, or fixation of the testis in the scrotum.

Mobilization of the testis

1 A transverse skin crease incision is made over the inguinal canal. This incision is usually about one finger's breadth above the base of the penis in an infant. The medial end of the incision is level with the pubic tubercle, while the lateral end is at the mid-inguinal point.

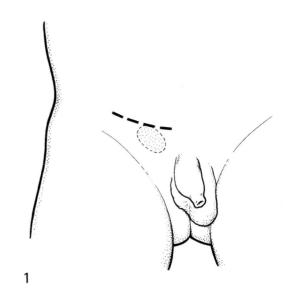

1

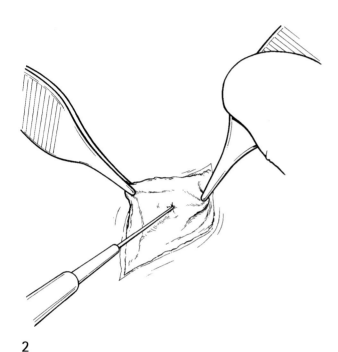

2

2 The incision is deepened through the subcutaneous fatty tissue with scissors or diathermy. The superficial fascia is in two layers: a more superficial fatty layer and a deeper, well-developed fibrous layer known as Scarpa's fascia. The superficial inferior epigastric vein may be seen in the subcutaneous tissue running obliquely across the incision. Sometimes square-ended retractors can pull the vessel out of the way, and at other times it is best coagulated by diathermy and divided.

3 Once Scarpa's fascia has been divided, the external oblique aponeurosis can be distinguished deep to Scarpa's fascia by the oblique orientation of its fibers, which are absent in Scarpa's fascia. The surface of the external oblique muscle is cleared by placing square retractors under Scarpa's fascia to expose the lower border of the external oblique muscle where the inguinal ligament lies. A sweeping motion with closed scissors parallel to the external oblique fibers will expose the rolled edge of the inguinal ligament and the site of the external inguinal ring, where the spermatic cord is seen bulging.

The inguinal canal is opened with a scalpel incision in the external oblique muscle, with extension with scissors in line with the external ring. The incision can be extended with scissors by cutting the fibers toward the external ring. The edges of the external oblique muscle are best stabilized with small artery forceps so that they can be identified easily later in the operation. The ilioinguinal nerve will run parallel to the incision, just under the external oblique aponeurosis, and should be identified and carefully avoided. Accidental transection of the nerve

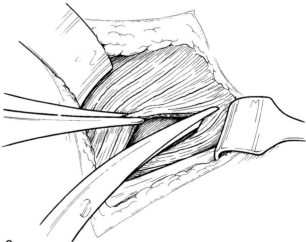

3

will produce a sensory deficit in the region of the anterior scrotum. Blunt dissection is used to mobilize the inner layer of the external oblique aponeurosis off the surface of the spermatic cord, and the external ring is opened with scissors if this has not already been done.

4 The testis and attached spermatic cord are mobilized with blunt dissection and delivered out of the wound. This should identify the abnormal attachment of the gubernaculum, which causes dimpling of the skin above and lateral to the neck of the scrotum. The gubernacular attachment is divided carefully with scissors or diathermy, taking care to avoid any structures within the processus vaginalis, such as the vas deferens, which may extend below the lower pole of the testis. The gubernaculum at this level is usually transparent, with an occasional fine vessel and some fat, and is easy to divide without risk to other structures.

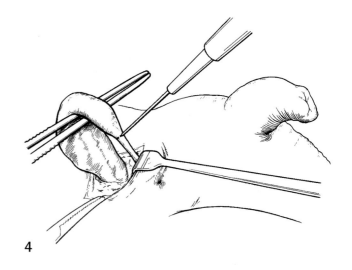

4

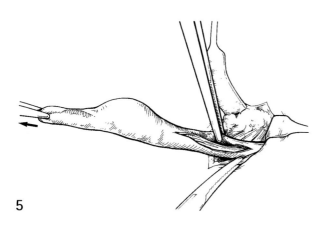

5

5 Small artery forceps are placed on the gubernacular attachment to the testis and the tunica vaginalis and this is placed on tension. This enables any remaining cremaster fibers surrounding the outside of the spermatic cord to be stripped off with blunt-ended forceps.

Dissection of the hernial sac

The processus vaginalis is commonly widely patent in the undescended testis. Careful separation of the patent processus vaginalis or obvious hernial sac from the vas deferens and the testicular vessels is an important part of the procedure, as this increases the effective length of the spermatic cord. The hernial sac may be stretched over the index finger while round-ended, non-toothed dissecting forceps gently sweep off the other cord structures, carefully avoiding direct application of the forceps on the vas deferens or vessels. Alternatively, the sac can be held with small artery forceps while the vas deferens and testicular vessels are isolated en masse off the sac. It is best to attempt to separate the hernial sac completely without opening it, as an unrecognized tear may extend through the internal ring into the peritoneum, making closure of the hernial sac difficult. It is absolutely essential that the testicular vessels, and particularly the vas deferens, are visualized clearly before the sac is divided. It is important to note that the vas deferens is closely adherent to the posterior surface of the sac before dissection.

6 With the cord on traction, the testicular vessels and vas deferens are separated from the hernial sac with a small retractor and adequately identified before clamping the hernial sac with artery forceps and dividing it with scissors immediately distal to the artery forceps.

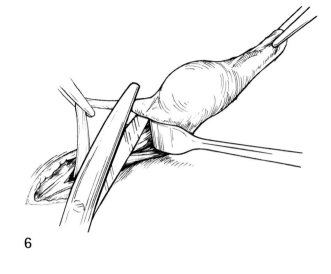

6

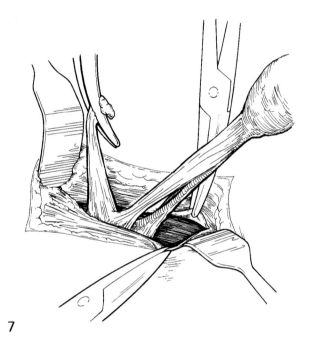

7

7 The divided processus vaginalis is pulled cranially to put the membrane under tension, and the testicular vessels and vas deferens are separated with blunt dissection from the posterior surface of the sac right up to the internal ring. At the junction between the processus vaginalis and the peritoneum proper, the translucent processus vaginalis becomes an opaque, white membrane with a triangular widening of the base. At this level, the vas deferens curves medially around the edge of the transversalis fascia, adjacent to the inferior epigastric vessels. By contrast, the testicular vessels pass cranially on the lateral side of the internal ring and disappear into the retroperitoneal space.

8 If the spermatic cord is not long enough to reach the scrotum, the retroperitoneal plane behind the processus vaginalis above the internal ring is developed, and a Langenbeck's retractor is inserted to pull the peritoneal membrane anteriorly. This reveals the testicular vessels passing cranially in the retroperitoneum. The vessels tend to follow a gentle convex curve laterally, and there are a number of lateral fibrous bands attached to the vessels. These should be divided by sharp or blunt dissection once the testicular vessels themselves have been identified. Continuous, gentle traction on the testis allows the testicular vessels to be seen and preserved.

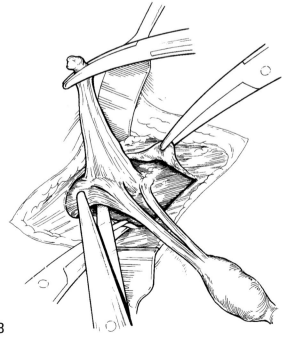

8

9 There should now be adequate length of vas deferens and vessels to allow the testis to reach the scrotum. The processus vaginalis is now twisted up to the internal ring to make sure that it contains no intraperitoneal contents, and it is transfixed and ligated at this level. At this point, if the length of the vas deferens is a limiting factor in the position of the testis, the inferior epigastric vessels can be divided electively to gain an extra 0.5–1 cm.

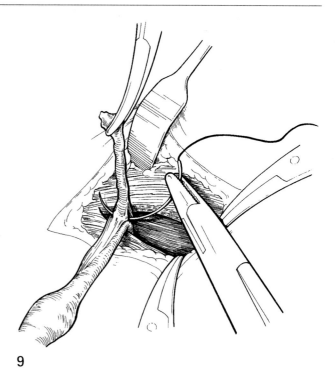

9

10 Traction on the testis is now stopped and a finger is introduced through the incision and down to the scrotum, breaking down any fascial layers near the neck of the scrotum so that the tip of the index finger can reach the mid-scrotum. The scrotal skin is immobilized between the index finger internally and the thumb externally. A scrotal incision is then made, going just through the skin but not through the deeper tissues. This incision can be either horizontal (the author's preference) or midline in the scrotal septum. Horizontal incisions are associated with less bleeding.

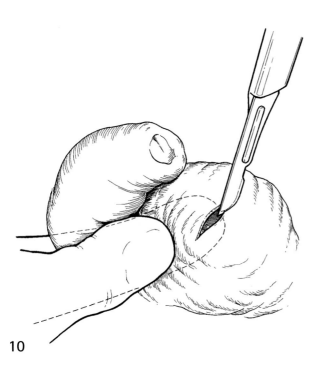

10

11 While the index finger is still inside the scrotum and the thumb is immobilizing the scrotal skin, fine artery forceps or scissors are used to develop a subcutaneous pouch, just deep to the dartos muscle. This should be developed inferiorly more than superiorly, so that the external incision is placed near the cranial end of this subcutaneous pouch. Any bleeding is controlled by diathermy before proceeding further. This is an important step, as a scrotal hematoma will inevitably become infected and lead to wound breakdown.

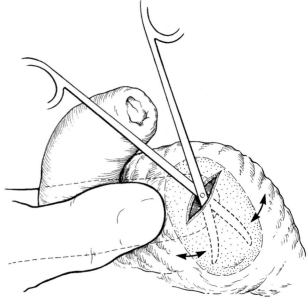

11

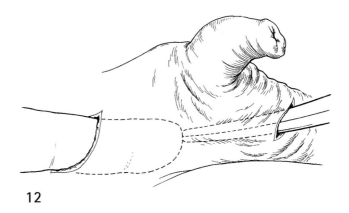

12 Fine artery forceps are placed through the incision in the scrotum and pressed against the index finger internally. The index finger then guides the artery forceps back to the inguinal incision where the tip of the artery forceps is pushed through any residual fascial plane.

12

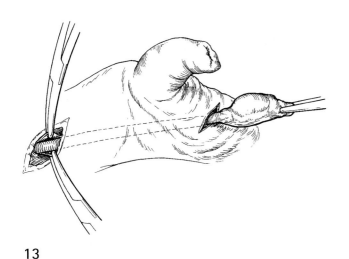

13

13 The artery forceps, which have been pushed up through the scrotal incision to the inguinal incision, then grasps the gubernacular attachments of the testis, making sure that the cord structures are not twisted. The testis and attached structures are then drawn gently down through the track made by blunt dissection and pulled through the 'buttonhole' in the subdartos fascia and delivered through the scrotal incision.

14 If the hole through the fascial planes between the two incisions is not too large, the testis will sit comfortably in the scrotal pouch like a button through a buttonhole. If there is any concern that the testis may retract through a larger defect, it can be anchored to the midline scrotal septum with a 3/0 absorbable suture through the tunica albuginea, but not through the body of the testis. Many surgeons deliberately open the tunica vaginalis so that the anatomy of the testis can be defined precisely and any testicular appendages can be excised at this time. The testis, epididymis, and adjacent coverings can then be placed in the subcutaneous scrotal pouch using blunt forceps. The scrotal incision is closed with a 4/0 subcuticular absorbable suture.

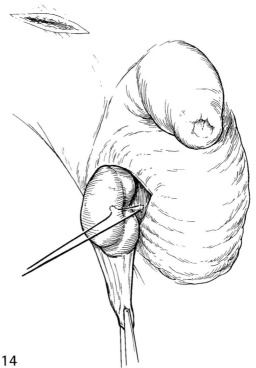

14

The surgeon now returns to the inguinal incision, where the external oblique aponeurosis is reconstituted with one to three interrupted sutures or a short continuous suture of 3/0 absorbable material.

The retractors are removed from the wound, and the fibrous subcutaneous (Scarpa's) fascia is identified and closed with one or two interrupted sutures. The skin is approximated with a 4/0 subcuticular suture. The inguinal incision can be covered with a sterile, semipermeable, adhesive film dressing, which provides a waterproof and childproof covering for the wound for the first 7–10 days. A similar dressing can be applied to the scrotal incision, or alternatively this can be sprayed with a plastic skin spray. Depending on the anesthesia used, local anesthetic infiltration to both the inguinal and scrotal wounds can be performed near the end of the procedure.

OPERATION: SCROTAL ORCHIDOPEXY

Where the testis can be manipulated into the scrotum and held there by the assistant, an upper scrotal incision can be made to deliver the testis. The rest of the operation is similar to standard orchidopexy, except the external spermatic fascia needs to be stripped off the cord first. Mobilization up to the canal is often sufficient without opening it, especially for acquired cryptorchidism. If there is inadequate length, an inguinal incision with canalicular mobilization can be done as described above.

OPERATION: LAPAROSCOPIC ORCHIDOPEXY

Diagnostic laparoscopy (as described in Chapter 41, Abdominal surgery: general principles of access) is carried out for impalpable testes. This will identify the vanishing testis, where the internal inguinal ring (IIR) is closed and the proximal spermatic vessels appear from beneath the colon but are then blind-ending. The vas deferens may also be blind-ending, or exit through the closed inguinal ring. Some surgeons may then open the scrotum to remove the atrophic testicular nubbin (following perinatal torsion), but this is controversial.

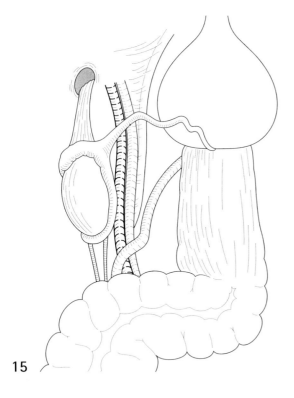

15

15, 16 When the testis is intra-abdominal, it is usually close to the IIR. One-stage orchidopexy is straightforward if the testis can be dragged to the opposite IIR with graspers, indicating adequate length of cord structures.

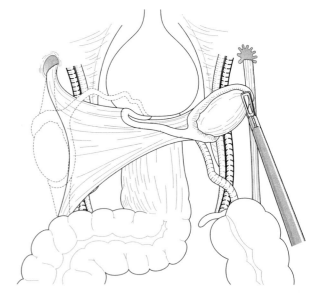

16

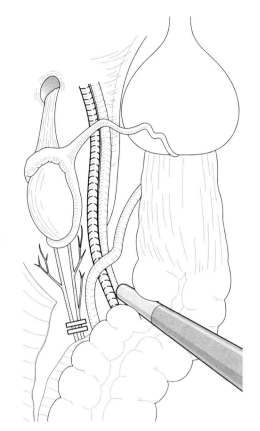

17 For high intra-abdominal testes, the colon is mobilized to expose the proximal gonadal vessels far enough away from the testis to preserve any collateral vessels. The spermatic vessels are then clipped or ligated, as part of the first stage of a Fowler–Stephens operation.

17

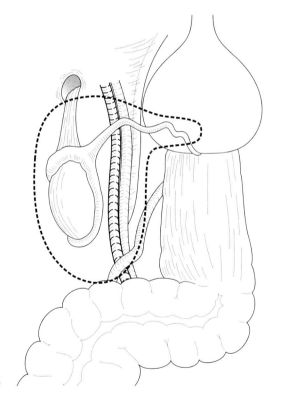

18

18 Six months later, after spermatic vessel clipping, or at the first laparoscopy if length is adequate, the peritoneum is divided in a tennis-racquet shape around the testis and vas deferens to mobilize the testis on its blood supply.

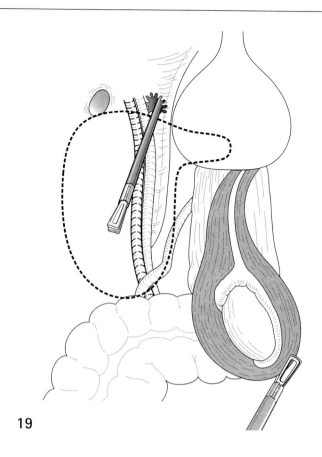

19 The scrotum is opened through a small incision and a grasper is pushed up into the abdomen through the external inguinal ring (and usually between the inferior epigastric vessels laterally and the obliterated umbilical artery medially. It is important to ensure the tunnel created is stretched up enough to allow the testis to be pulled down. This is now grasped and pulled gently down to the scrotum, ensuring no twisting of the spermatic vessels. The operation is concluded by scrotal fixation and closure as for standard orchidopexy and the laparoscopic port sites are closed in the usual way.

19

POSTOPERATIVE CARE

The patient is discharged from hospital the same day, unless an overnight stay is necessary, such as may be the case with bilateral impalpable testes. Most boys return to normal activities within 2–3 days, although they may need to refrain from active sport for 1–2 weeks.

The dressing is removed and the position of the testis checked after 1–2 weeks and again at six months after surgery.

Complications

Wound infection and hematoma are the two most common complications. Hematoma can be avoided by meticulous hemostasis with diathermy at the time of surgery. Wound sepsis can be avoided by the placement of waterproof dressings on both incisions, which remain in place for at least 1 week. The risk of testicular atrophy, which is determined at six months after surgery, should be less than 5 percent; in most series, it is 1–2 percent. There is a small risk of retraction of the testis into the groin, particularly if there is significant sepsis or hematoma, or postoperative trauma.

FURTHER READING

Fowler R, Stephens FD. The role of testicular vascular anatomy in the salvage of high undescended testes. *Australia and New Zealand Journal of Surgery* 1959; **29**: 92–106.

Hutson JM, Balic A, Nation T, Southwell B. Cryptorchidism. *Seminars in Pediatric Surgery* 2010; **19**: 215–24.

Hvistendahl GM, Poulsen EU. Laparoscopy for the impalpable testes: experience with 80 intra-abdominal testes. *Journal of Pediatric Urology* 2009; **5**: 389.

Kravarusic D, Freud E. The impact of laparoscopy in the management of non-palpable testes. *Pediatric Endocrinology Reviews* 2009; **7**: 44.

Ritzen EM, Kollin C. Management of undescended testes: how and when? *Pediatric Endocrinology Reviews* 2009; **7**: 32–7.

92

Testicular torsion

SU-ANNA M BODDY and FEILIM L MURPHY

INTRODUCTION

Torsion of the testis must be the first consideration in any child or adolescent with scrotal pain. There are two peaks in the incidence, in the perinatal period and between 11 and 25 years.

Torsion of the testis

1 If the tunica vaginalis invests the whole of the epididymis and the distal part of the spermatic cord, the testis is in effect suspended in the scrotal cavity like a bell clapper and therefore is free to rotate within the tunica vaginalis in an intravaginal fashion.

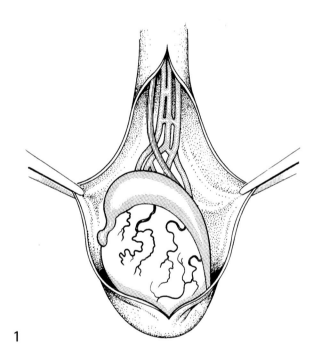

1

Neonatal torsion

Neonatal torsion accounts for up to 12 percent of all cases of childhood torsion. Neonatal torsion is classically described as 'extravaginal' implying that the torsion occurs due to failure of the tunica vaginalis to attach to surrounding structures. However, this concept of neonatal torsion always being extravaginal has recently been questioned. The management of neonatal torsion has also been complicated by the concept of pre- and postnatal torsion. Due to the reports of synchronous and asynchronous contralateral torsion and salvage of the postnatal torted testis, urgent exploration with contralateral fixation is highly recommended.

DIFFERENTIAL DIAGNOSIS

Torsion of the testicular appendage

Torsion of a testicular appendage presents at 3–11 years. Careful palpation will reveal an exquisitely tender nodule which is usually associated with the upper pole of the testis with the body of the testis not tender. On transillumination, a dark nodule (dot) may appear. If the diagnosis of a torted appendix testis is made clinically, hospital observation, radiology, or surgery are not mandatory.

Acute epididymo-orchitis

Unilateral epididymo-orchitis is rare in children in whom it may be associated with urinary tract infections and anomalies of the urinary tract.

Mumps

This rarely occurs before puberty, is usually bilateral and appears within 3–7 days after the onset of parotitis.

Idiopathic scrotal edema

In this condition, erythema and swelling of the scrotal skin spread into the groin, perineum and/or the base of the penis. The skin may be tender, but the patients being usually between the ages of 3 and 6 years, do not complain of pain. The underlying testis and cord are normal. The diagnosis can normally be made clinically and reassurance is usually all that is required.

Recurrent torsion

There can be a history of episodic testicular pain, with or without swelling of the testis. The testis may lie more transversely in the scrotum, but more commonly is entirely normal. One should have an extremely low threshold for exploratory surgery in patients with recurrent scrotal pain.

OPERATION

Timing

In most cases, the diagnosis of acute testicular torsion can be made clinically. Any delay in operation once the diagnosis is suspected will prejudice the survival of the testis.

2 The testis is easily delivered from the scrotum through an incision over its longitudinal axis, or obliquely in the line of scrotal rugae or through the midline raphe.

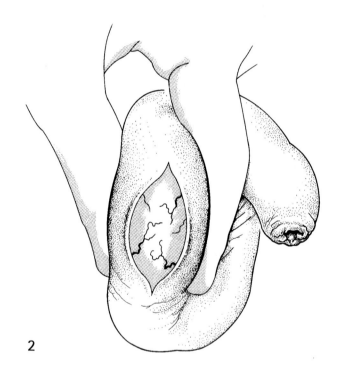

2

3 The testis is delivered from the tunica vaginalis and the cord is untwisted in the appropriate direction.

The tunica albuginea can be incised to assess viability and it may release the pressure within the underlying tubules.

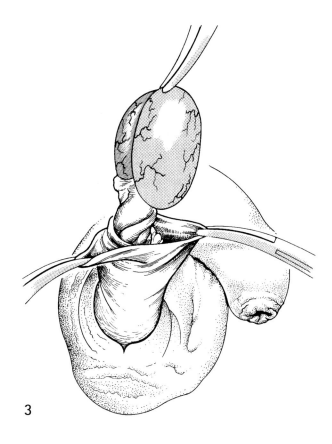

3

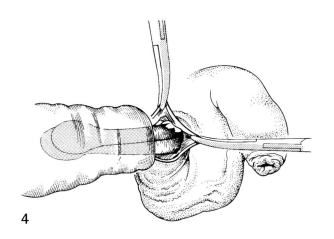

4

4 The untwisted testis should be wrapped in moist warm swabs and its color observed intermittently. While waiting to confirm whether perfusion has been re-established, the contralateral testis can be fixed.

Conservation or removal of the testis

If the testis is completely black, necrotic and non-viable, it should be removed. The spermatic cord is ligated within the scrotum with an absorbable suture and the testis excised. If there is any question that some perfusion might be re-established, the testis should be conserved. The contralateral testis must always be fixed.

Fixation of the testis

5 Two methods of fixation of the testis are commonly used: (1) The testis can be everted from the tunica vaginalis and fixed with three 6/0 monofilament sutures placed between the tunica albuginea and the lateral wall of the scrotum at the upper and lower poles as well as at the equator. There is concern that the use of absorbable sutures may allow torsion to occur at a future date while non-absorbable can be associate with chronic pain in the prepuberal group. (2) Fixation of the testis in a scrotal pouch may cause less damage to the testis and, more importantly, offer better fixation, preventing subsequent torsion.

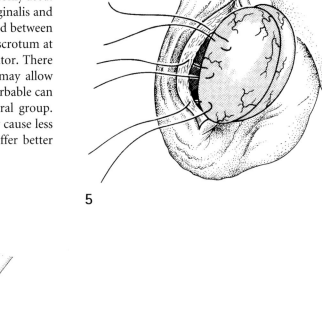

5

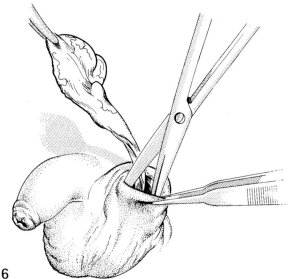

6

6 The testis is delivered through the horizontal or oblique incision and the tunica vaginalis is everted. The testis is retracted superiorly on to the lower abdominal wall. Fine-tooth forceps lift the inferior edge of the wound and with blunt dissection an adequate scrotal pouch is formed. The testis, which is still everted from the tunica vaginalis, is placed in the newly formed scrotal pouch.

7 The wound can be closed continuously or interruptedly with 4/0 to 6/0 sutures depending on the age of the child. Short-lasting absorbable sutures, such as Vicryl rapide or monocryl, should be used. If an incision is made in the midline, then a layer closure to recreate the septum is advisable.

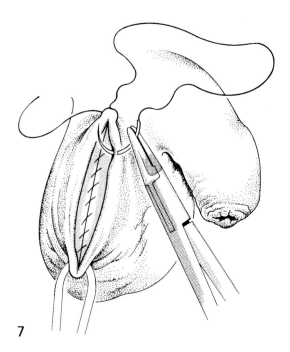

7

FURTHER READING

Frank JD, O'Brien M. Fixation of the testis. *British Journal of Urology* 2002; **89**: 331–3.

Kyriaziz ID, Dimopoulos J, Sakellaris G *et al.* Extravaginal testicular torsion: a clinical entity with unspecified surgical anatomy. *International Brazilian Journal of Urology* 2008; **34**: 617–23.

Soccorso G, Ninan GK, Rajimwale A, Nour S. Acute scrotum: is the scrotal exploration the best management? *European Journal of Pediatric Surgery* 2010; **20**: 313–15.

93

Circumcision, meatotomy, and meatoplasty

IMRAN MUSHTAQ

PRINCIPLES AND JUSTIFICATION

Indications

1 Most circumcisions are performed for non-medical reasons, namely for religious beliefs or cultural practices. Jewish boys are circumcised on the eighth day of life, and Muslim boys are usually circumcised during childhood. In addition, many boys are circumcised in the neonatal period, particularly in the United States.

The only true medical indication for circumcision is a pathological phimosis, which is usually related to balanitis xerotica obliterans (BXO). Other indications include recurrent balanoposthitis and in boys at risk of recurrent urinary tract infections due to an abnormal urinary tract (e.g. vesicoureteric reflux and posterior urethral valves).

Contraindications for circumcision include hypospadias and buried penis. Meatal stenosis can arise following circumcision in between 0 and 11 percent of cases, particularly in boys with BXO. The majority of these patients can be treated by a simple meatotomy, but recurrent meatal stenosis may require meatoplasty.

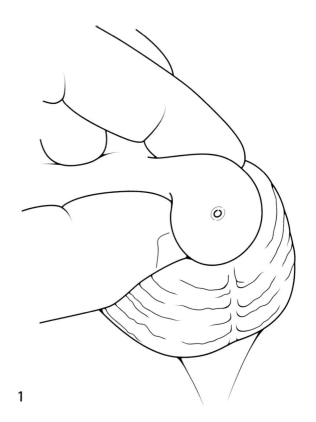

1

PREOPERATIVE

Anesthesia

Neonatal circumcision is usually performed under local anesthesia using a penile block. Older boys require general anesthesia with the addition of caudal anesthesia for postoperative pain relief.

OPERATIONS

Sleeve circumcision

2a–c The phimotic foreskin is dilated with artery forceps and completely retracted. Congenital preputial adhesions are divided and the glans is cleaned with antiseptic solution. A surgical pen is used to mark the line of circumferential incision just proximal to the coronal sulcus, leaving a cuff of inner preputial skin below the glans.

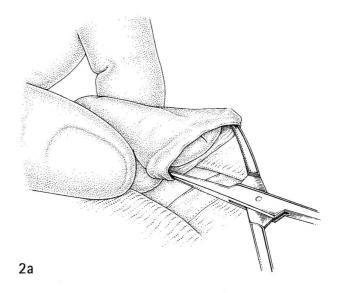

2a

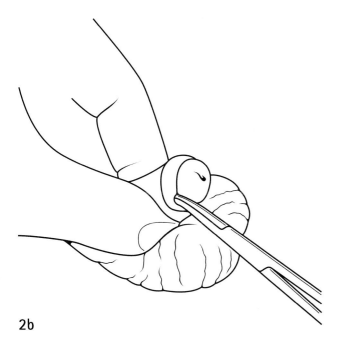

2b

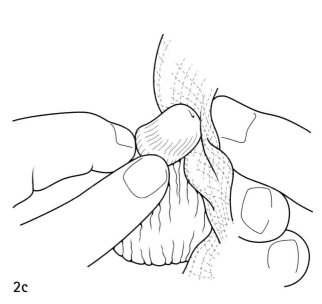

2c

3a–f The incision is then made with a scalpel knife to sufficient depth to allow the penile skin to be retracted proximally. The foreskin is elevated by placing one artery forceps ventrally and one dorsally. A circumferential line of incision on the penile shaft skin is marked with a surgical pen, allowing sufficient skin to cover the full length of the penis without tension. The skin is incised along the line with a scalpel knife. The excess foreskin is removed by dividing the subcutaneous layer between the inner and outer skin layers with bipolar diathermy.

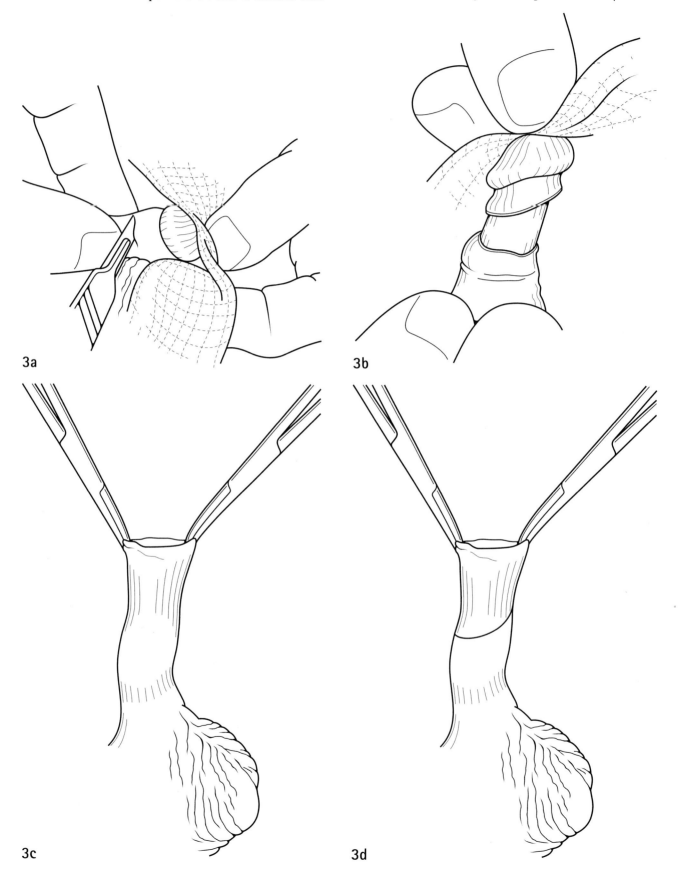

3a

3b

3c

3d

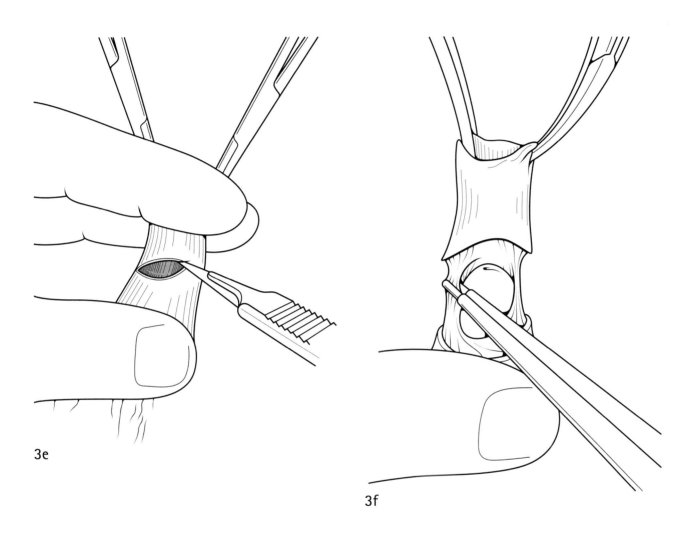

3e

3f

4a–c The outer skin is retracted and any bleeding points are coagulated with bipolar diathermy. The wound is closed with an interrupted absorbable suture, such as 6/0 Vicryl rapide or monocryl. The application of chloramphenicol ointment twice daily for 7 days may help to prevent infection and stops undergarments adhering to the penis.

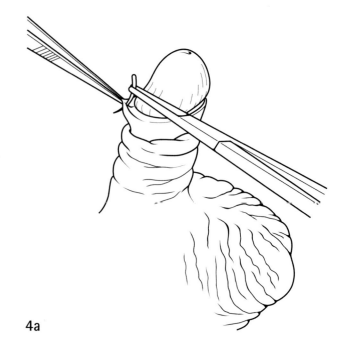

4a

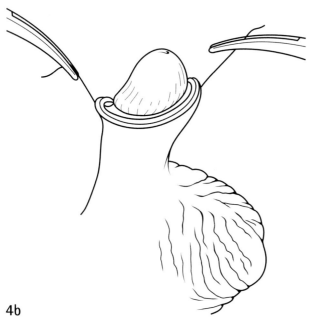

4b

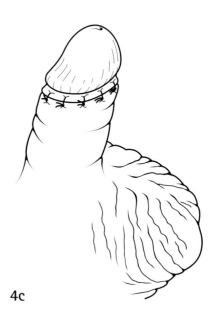

4c

Plastibell circumcision

5a The Plastibell device is a development from metallic devices used as templates for ischemic necrosis of redundant foreskin in circumcision. It is well established as a quick and safe method in neonates and is widely practiced.

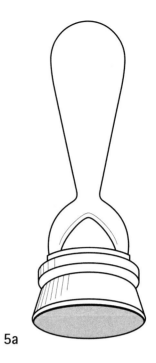

5a

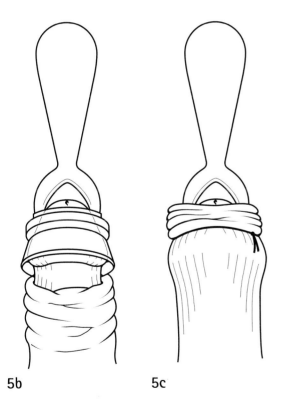

5b   5c

5b,c The preputial opening is dilated and the adhesions between the prepuce and the glans are freed with a probe. The prepuce is fully retracted to expose the coronal sulcus, which should be cleaned of smegma. An appropriate-sized bell is placed over the glans as far as the preputial reflection. A correctly sized bell should stay in position comfortably and without pressure on the glans. A suture is tied around the prepuce onto the outer ridge of the bell as tightly as possible.

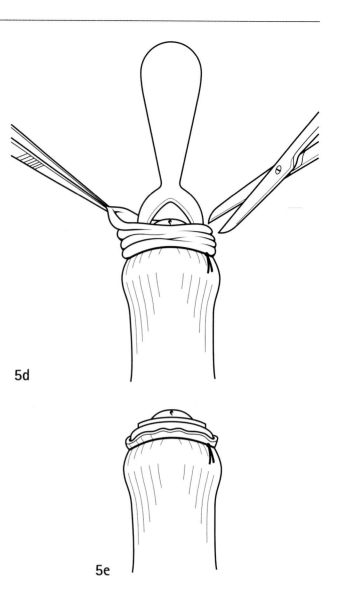

5d

5e

5d,e After about a minute, the preputial skin becomes insensitive and is trimmed off immediately distal to the ligature with iris scissors. The handle is snapped off, leaving the bell in position. Skin necrosis will occur at the site of the suture and will allow the bell to separate and fall off, after a mean of 9 days. In the meantime, the child voids through the open end of the bell.

COMPLICATIONS

Circumcision is often regarded as a minor surgical procedure, usually delegated to junior surgical staff. However, there are probably more complications associated with this operation than with more complex urological procedures.

Hemorrhage

Careful attention to hemostasis using bipolar diathermy during surgery will prevent primary postoperative hemorrhage. If postoperative hemorrhage does occur, a pressure dressing may arrest the bleeding in the first instance. If in doubt, it is best to return the child to the operating room and deal with the bleeding point under general anesthesia.

Infection

Infections after circumcision are not uncommon, with an incidence of around 5 percent. These infections generally respond well to oral antibiotics and regular bathing.

Urethrocutaneous fistulas

Fistula formation is a rare complication of circumcision and is usually seen at the level of the coronal sulcus. The two most common causes are overzealous use of diathermy and a suture placed too deeply to stop bleeding from the frenulum. Surgical repair should be performed six months after the original circumcision.

Removal of too much or too little skin

Removal of too little skin can cause annular scarring at the line of excision and recurrence of the phimosis. In such cases, a further circumcision is required. Removal of too much skin may give the appearance of a buried penis, but only rarely is skin grafting required to achieve a satisfactory appearance.

Meatal stenosis

Meatal stenosis is the most significant complication, reported in up to 11 percent of cases. In neonates, it may be the result of ammoniacal dermatitis due to contact with wet nappies. In older children, it is usually the result of the BXO, which affects the prepuce causing the original phimosis. Such cases are troublesome to treat, but usually respond to meatotomy and/or meatoplasty.

Meatotomy

6a–c The meatus is calibrated with a lacrimal probe to determine the severity of the stenosis. An artery forceps is used to crush the tissue ventrally through the meatus for a period of 1 minute. The artery forceps is removed and the crushed tissue is divided with iris scissors. Bleeding is rare with this technique, but if it does occur, it can be readily controlled with bipolar diathermy.

The main complication of this procedure is recurrence of the meatal stenosis, which may require a more formal meatoplasty.

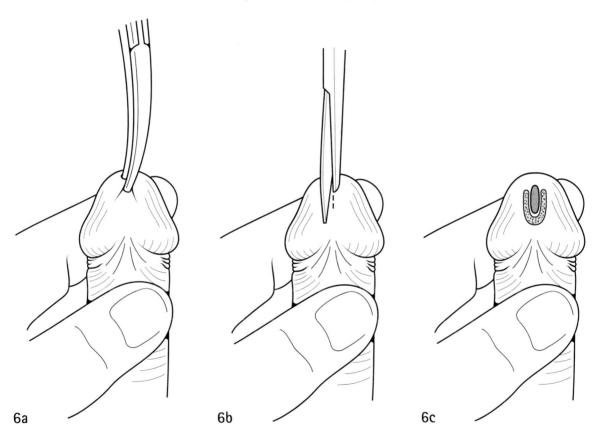

6a   6b   6c

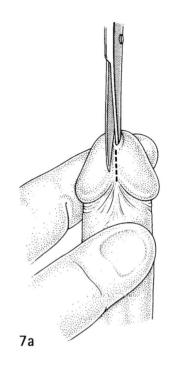

Meatoplasty

7a–c A pair of iris scissors is used to make a generous ventral incision through the meatus. The edges of the urethral mucosa are approximated to the adjacent skin with 7/0 or 6/0 absorbable sutures.

This procedure creates a large meatus with the appearance of a glanular hypospadias. This may cause some deviation of the urinary stream, but it is unlikely to cause functional difficulties.

7a

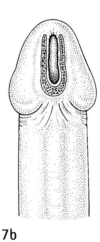

7b

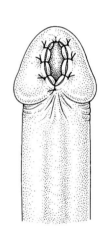

7c

FURTHER READING

Cartwright PC, Masterson TA, Snow BA. Office paediatric urology. In: Docimo SG, Canning DA, Khoury AE (eds). *Clinical Pediatric Urology*. London: Informa Healthcare, 2007: 199–213.

MacDonald MF, Barthold JS, Kass EJ. Abnormalities of the penis and foreskin. In: Docimo SG, Canning DA, Khoury AE (eds). *Clinical Pediatric Urology*. London: Informa Healthcare, 2007: 1239–70.

Rickwood AMK. Medical indications for circumcision. *British Journal of Urology International* 1999; **83** (Suppl. 1): 45–51.

94

Varicocele

HOCK LIM TAN and JOSELITO TANTOCO

INTRODUCTION

Varicoceles are common with an estimated incidence of 15 percent in teenagers. Most varicoceles (80–90 percent) occur on the left side. Isolated right-sided varicoceles are rare; these patients usually present with bilateral disease. Bilateral varicoceles may be caused by factors that cause increase in central venous pressure, such as congenital heart disease.

Varicoceles are thought to cause infertility, as 35 percent of males presenting to infertility clinics have varicoceles. This may be due to increased testicular temperature resulting from the venous back pressure from the incompetent valve(s) in the left gonadal vein which drains directly into the left renal vein. Varicoceles usually appear in boys around the onset of puberty. It is important to exclude a left renal lesion if a varicocele is diagnosed in a young child.

DIAGNOSIS

The classical description of varicoceleis is as a 'bag of worms' best noticed when the child is standing. The grading of varicocele should be performed with the child standing, as follows:

- Grade 0: not visible nor palpable and identified only by ultrasound.
- Grade I: not visible but palpable in upright position with valsalva.
- Grade II: not visible but palpable in upright position without valsava.
- Grade III: visible and palpable without valsalva.

Volumetric evaluation of the testis with Prader orchidometer or ultrasonography should be performed to exclude testicular growth arrest.

Differential diagnosis includes an inguinal hernia, hydrocele, paratesticular tumors, renal vein thrombosis, and renal tumor.

SURGICAL TREATMENT

Indications

There is no clear correlation between varicocele in an adolescent and male infertility. The indication for treatment includes evidence of testicular atrophy or clinical symptoms. A reasonable guide for intervention is where there is 2–3 cc volume difference or 20 percent volume loss in the affected testis. A relative indication is if the varicocele is particularly large and the child is self-conscious and has issues with self-esteem.

Surgical options

The basic principle for management of varicoceles is to interrupt the venous return through the internal spermatic vein. There are principally three methods of achieving this. Radiological percutaneous embolization of the gonadal vein is gaining in popularity. The two surgical methods are open or laparoscopic ablation of the internal spermatic veins. The recurrence rate of varicocele after simple ablation of the internal spermatic or gonadal vein is 11 percent. This has resulted in the alternative of dividing the internal spermatic veins and internal spermatic artery, the so-called 'Palomo' procedure which has a significantly lower recurrence rate of 1.5 percent. There have not been any reports of testicular atrophy following this procedure as collateral vessels from the vas appear to provide an adequate blood supply to the subservient testis. However, the incidence of postoperative variocele is 10 percent, a result of this technique, presumably due to interruption of lymphatic drainage. This has led to a relatively new 'lymphatic-sparing' procedure which preserves the lymphatic drainage and is our preferred approach.

PREOPERATIVE PREPARATION

A preoperative ultrasound should be performed to exclude a pre-existing hydrocele.

Anesthesia

1 The procedure is performed under general anesthesia with full relaxation. Following the induction of anesthesia, 2 mL of methylene blue is injected into the space between the tunica vaginalis and tunica albuginea, and the scrotum is massaged for a few minutes to promote drainage of the methylene blue into the testicular lymphatics.

Position of patient

The patient is positioned supine with the video monitor at the end of the bed. The table should be tilted to 20–30° in the Trendelenberg position.

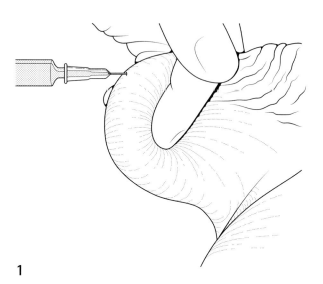

2

Laparoscopic instrumentation

Very few instruments are required:

- 0° 5-mm telescope;
- 7-mm Hasson cannula;
- Two 5-mm instrument ports;
- 5-mm tissue dissector (Maryland);
- 5-mm atraumatic grasper (De Bakey);
- 5-mm pointed scissors;
- 5-mm monopolar hook diathermy;
- 5-mm multiclip applicator.

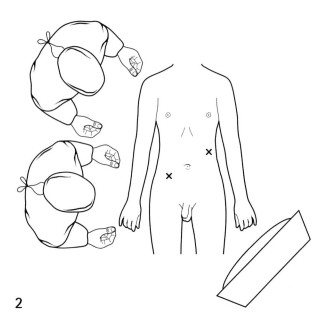

1

Port placements

2 The 7-mm Hasson port is placed in the umbilicus by open technique and the instrument ports for the left hand is inserted in the left paracolic gutter just above the umbilicus. The right instrument port is inserted in the right lower quadrant taking care to avoid the inferior epigastric artery.

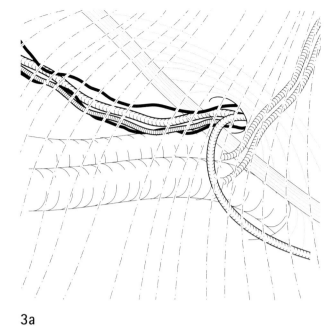

3a

Exposure of the internal spermatic vessels

3a,b The peritoneal overlying the internal spermatic vessels is opened 2–3 cm proximal to the internal ring, and the vascular bundle identified, with its brightly stained lymphatic vessels.

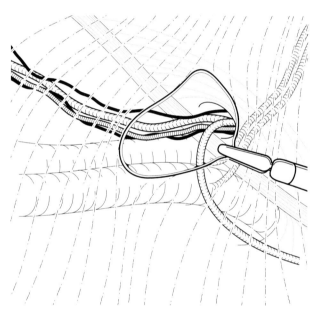

3b

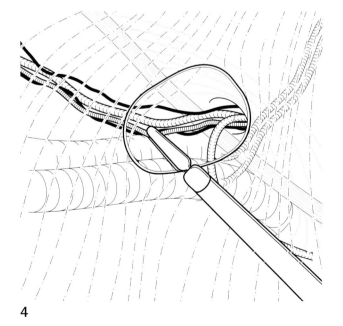

4

4 The entire internal spermatic vascular bundle is lifted out of its bed and the lymphatic vessels are 'cherry picked', from the rest of artery and vein. The major lymphatic vessels are easily separable, but there will be some lymphatic vessels somewhat like 'vasa vasorum' which are intimately attached to the artery and veins that cannot be spared.

Division of the spermatic vessels

5 The lymphatic channels are separated for a distance of about 2 cm, and two 5-mm clips are applied on the separated vascular bundle which is then divided. The bed with its preserved lymphatic vessels is inspected to ensure that there are no collaterals that may need to be divided.

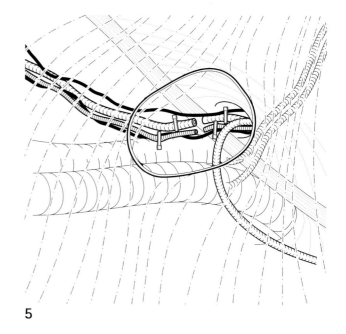

5

Closure

The abdomen should then be desufflated and the fascial layer of the instrument ports closed with a single absorbable suture. The Hasson cannula port is closed with the purse string suture previously inserted to secure the port. The skin is accurately opposed with a pair of fine forceps and cyanoacrylate glue applied. The port sites are infiltrated with local anesthetic.

POSTOPERATIVE CARE

The procedure is usually performed as a day case. It is not uncommon for the varicocele to appear engorged immediately after the operation, although this is less after a non-artery-sparing Palomo procedure. A testicular ultrasound is performed six months following surgery to ensure that a secondary hydrocele has not developed.

Open retroperitoneal varicocele ligation

The preferred option is to perform a high retroperitoneal ligation of the internal spermatic bundle as this avoids disturbing the complex pampiniform plexus and the collaterals, if the inguinal approach is used.

The patient is positioned supine and 2 mL of methylene blue injected into the scrotum as in the laparoscopic approach and the testis massaged, before draping the patient.

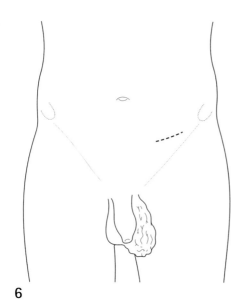

6 A 2–3-cm incision is made just above and medial to the anterior superior iliac spine and a muscle-splitting incision is made down to the preperitoneal fascia just deep to the transversalis fascia.

6

Using blunt finger dissection, the peritoneum is freed from the lateral wall of the abdomen to reach the retroperitoneal plane. This should be a relatively easy tissue plane to enter as the fatty properitoneal plane forms a distinct layer separating the peritoneum from the musculature.

7 The leash of spermatic vessels is identified and lifted out of the incision, together with the accompanying lymphatics, easily identified by its brightly colored appearance. The lymphatic vessels are cherry picked off the internal spermatic artery and vein, which at this level, is usually a single channel. These vessels are ligated and divided.

The abdominal wall is closed with absorbable sutures and the incision closed.

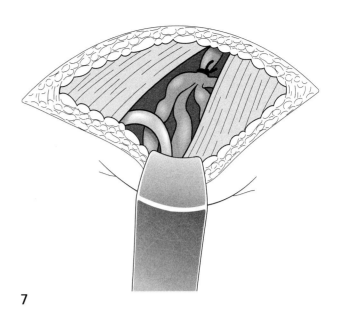

7

POSTOPERATIVE CARE

Postoperative care is as for the laparoscopic procedure.

FURTHER READING

Hutson JM, O'Brien M, Woodward AA, Beasley SW (eds). Undescended testis and varicocele. *Jones' Clinical Paediatric Surgery: Diagnosis and Management.* Oxford: Wiley-Blackwell, 2009: 168–71.

Oldham KT, Colombani PM, Foglia RP, Skinner MA (eds). Male genital tract. In: *Principles and Practice of Paediatric Surgery*, 4th edn. Philadelphia, PA: Lippincott Williams and Wilkins, 2004: 1608.

Tan HL, Tecson B, Ee M, Tantoco J. Lymphatic sparing laparoscopic varicocelectomy: a new surgical technique. *Pediatric Surgery International* 2004; **20**: 797–8.

Zelkovic P, Kogan SJ. The pediatric varicocele. In: Gearheart JP, Rink RC, Mouriquand PDE (eds). *Pediatric Urology*, 2nd edn. Philadelphia, PA: Saunders Elsevier, 2010: 585–94.

95

Bladder exstrophy closure and epispadias

PETER CUCKOW and PEDRO-JOSÉ LOPEZ

PRINCIPLES AND JUSTIFICATION

Bladder exstrophy has an incidence of 1 in 30 000 live births, with a preponderance of males (males:females, 3:1). Primary epispadias has a similar male bias but is much less common, with an incidence of 1 in 120 000. In the UK, there are between 15 and 20 cases of primary bladder exstrophy and four to six cases of primary epispadias presenting per year. The surgical management of this rare group of anomalies tends to be focused on major surgical centers and this has enabled the refinement of different surgical approaches. The aims of exstrophy and epispadias repair are:

- to place the bladder within the abdomen and ultimately to achieve urinary continence;
- to create satisfactory genital appearance and near-normal function;
- to preserve or enable fertility.

1, 2 Bladder exstrophy presents at birth with a low-set umbilicus and a split rectus abdominis muscle attached on either side to separated pubic rami. The bladder fills this low abdominal wall defect as an open plate with the ureters draining directly onto its surface. It is continuous with the open urethral plate, which runs down the dorsum of the penile corpora in the male to an open glans. In the female, the urethral plate is shorter and runs between a divided clitoris and the labia minora to the anterior rim of the vaginal orifice. Inguinal hernias are a common association. Nearly 80 percent of boys have a patent processus vaginalis, and during the primary exstrophy closure, it is routine practice to perform bilateral herniotomies. This is less common in girls (incidence of 15 percent) and so the need to perform routine herniotomy is debatable. The perineum appears foreshortened due to lack of anterior structures, principally the anterior pelvic ring. The anus is anteriorly placed, principally because of this lack of anterior structures, although it may be more anteriorly placed relative to the back.

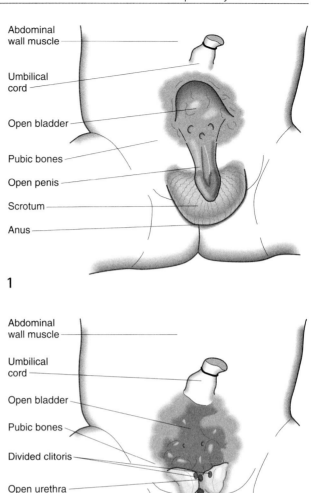

1

2

3 Separation of the pubic bones (referred to as the diastasis) varies considerably. In primary epispadias, where only the urethra is open, the recti may be together and the symphysis may actually be joined, whereas in the most severe forms of exstrophy the diastasis in newborns may be greater than 5 cm. The defect in the abdominal wall and the degree of difficulty in closure of the abdomen are directly related to the extent of the diastasis. The proximal ends of the penile corpora are attached on either side to the inferior pubic rams. While they may be shorter than normal corporal bodies, the separation of the pubic symphysis results in a Y-shaped penis and further limitation of the penile length. The urethra in the male is an open plate on the dorsum of the corpora and it has no relation to any sphincter muscles at birth. A normal sphincter complex is present in the perineum, however, and can be demonstrated by direct stimulation in the area of the prostate gland between the proximal penile corporal attachments.

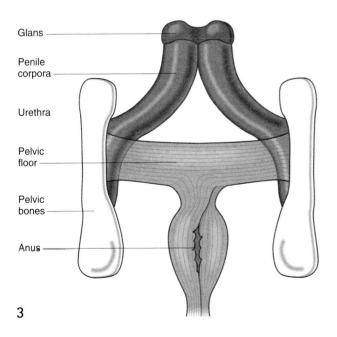

3

The inadequacy of the penis has led some in the past to opt for female sex of rearing. Current reconstructive procedures, however, with detachment of the penile corpora, produce greater penile length. As a result, sexual reassignment is never required in cases of primary bladder exstrophy and may now be avoided in many cases of cloacal exstrophy.

Isolated male epispadias varies considerably in severity from that which simply involves the glans of the penis, to a much more severe abnormality involving the entire urethra, bladderneck, and sphincter complex. In all but the least severe cases, patients have stress incontinence, and many bladders fail to achieve capacity.

4 In females with primary bladder exstrophy, there is a similar anatomical arrangement to this. The divided clitoral corpora are attached to the pubic rami with muscle present, running between them. The urethral plate is anterior to the vagina and not associated with this muscle complex bladders fail to achieve capacity.

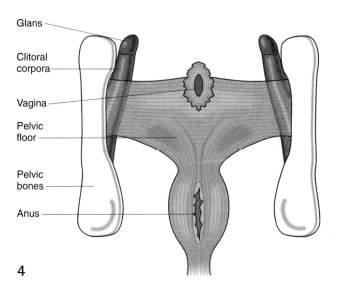

Glans
Clitoral corpora
Vagina
Pelvic floor
Pelvic bones
Anus

4

For the majority of these cases, a reconstructive procedure is required, not only for the penis, but also for continence, and for this we have used the Kelly soft tissue reconstruction (see below). In females, the rare anomaly of isolated epispadias includes a bifid clitoris, a short patulous urethra, and a variably open bladderneck resulting in a range of incontinence.

The current surgical approach is to close the exstrophy bladder shortly after birth, returning it to the lower abdomen and reconstructing the abdominal wall. The resulting bladder cannot adequately store urine and continence is only rarely achieved, the child characteristically dribbling continuously and requiring another procedure. A successful primary closure, however, does form a sound basis for the subsequent continence procedure in the form of soft-tissue reconstruction or Kelly's procedure. Through a complete mobilization of the pelvic soft tissues, including the penile corpora, pelvic floor, and bladder, the bladder outlet, proximal urethra, and sphincter mechanism can be reconstructed. The new bladder outlet resistance is a stimulus to its growth and an increase in capacity. These two factors combine to provide continence.

In addition, by mobilizing the penis in boys, greater penile protrusion is possible. In girls, a united clitoris and improved perineal cosmesis are achieved. In males, even greater penile length may be achieved by completely detaching the urethral plate from the dorsum of the corpora and creating a hypospadiac meatus. A subsequent

urethroplasty is required to create the distal urethra and a terminal meatus. This procedure has been successful in cases where penile length is significantly impaired and may be a primary indication for the Kelly procedure in patients who have already had a continent urinary diversion. An alternative approach to the penis is to combine the soft-tissue mobilization with a Cantwell–Ransley epispadias repair. The decision to do this is made at the time of operation and depends on penile and urethral length.

As historically patients have not normally been continent following exstrophy repair, bladderneck resistance procedures such as the Young Dees Ledbetter bladderneck reconstruction have been required. In the majority of patients, an additional bladder augmentation cystoplasty (usually an ileocystoplasty) to increase capacity and an appendicovesicostomy (Mitrofanoff channel) has provided a continent conduit for bladder emptying by intermittent catheterization. This will remain the ultimate management strategy in a number of patients, but currently the soft-tissue mobilization allows some (at least 50 percent) to void spontaneously per urethra with an adequate native bladder for storage.

As with many conditions in pediatric urology, lack of standardized assessment and nomenclature has led to much confusion about the results of treatment of bladder exstrophy. Our group has proposed a standardized definition of levels of incontinence in bladder exstrophy by which all interventions should be assessed (**Table 95.1**).

Table 95.1 Levels of continence in exstrophy.

0	Dribbles urine all the time with no control
1	Able to retain urine with a 'dry interval'. Some control, but still wearing protection
2	Sufficient dry intervals by day. In underwear and not needing protection. Wet at night
3	Dry by day and night, no protection or accidents. 'Normal' as peers

SURGICAL STEPS TO CLOSURE

The surgical steps may be summarized as follows:

1. Closure of the bladder in the neonatal period within the first 24–48 hours may proceed with approximation of the pubic bones without the need for osteotomy. After 48 hours, osteotomy is advised and a modified Salter anterior iliac osteotomy is currently recommended. Postoperative immobilization of the lower limbs with a frog plaster or a mermaid dressing is recommended whether or not osteotomy has been performed. This immobilizes the baby and greatly facilitates nursing care. In complex cases, restricted handling and continuous suction of bladder urine with a Replogle tube postoperatively are also advised.

2. Late closure usually requires osteotomy, as does reclosure after dehiscence. In these cases, external fixation of the pelvis is recommended.

3. Radical soft-tissue reconstruction (Kelly procedure) is proposed between six and nine months after primary closure, although it can be performed at any age. Bilateral ureteric reimplantation is usually performed at this time, to avoid the compromise to the upper urinary tract that a combination of increased outlet resistance and ureteric reflux may bring.

4. Completion of the urethroplasty in boys is performed in the third year of life or 18 months after the Kelly procedure. This is usually performed in two stages, with skin grafting to create a neourethral plate and glans groove on the penis, followed by urethral closure 12 months later.

5. Primary male epispadias is treated by the Kelly procedure if there is incontinence or poor penile length, or both. The timing of this procedure varies, but it may be performed after six months of age. Less severe cases (those that are continent) are treated by the Cantwell–Ransley epispadias repair.

6. Primary female epispadias is usually incontinent and so a Kelly soft-tissue mobilization is used.

7. Bladderneck reconstruction, augmentation cystoplasty, and appendicovesicostomy are available for patients in whom spontaneous voiding continence is not achieved by the above procedures. Continence may develop slowly after the Kelly procedure, so this salvage surgery is usually not performed before the fifth year of life.

The aim of this chapter is to show the basic steps of bladder closure, radical soft-tissue reconstruction, and epispadias repair; however, a detailed guide to the management of the patient with bladder exstrophy can be found in the further reading recommendations.

PREOPERATIVE

In these days of antenatal diagnostic ultrasound, many exstrophy cases are diagnosed *in utero* with characteristic non-visualization of the bladder, a low insertion of the umbilical cord, a short, thick phallus, and an irregular lower abdominal wall. Families should be counseled during pregnancy so they understand the implications of the diagnosis and the postnatal surgical strategy.

After birth, the bladder is covered with plastic wrap and the baby is transferred to the surgical center. Surgery may be delayed for up to 24–48 hours to allow the mother to recover from the delivery and for a preliminary work up of the baby, to include renal ultrasound and a blood crossmatch. Premature babies may require a longer period of medical stabilization before closure, which can be delayed for several weeks if this is medically indicated.

Vitamin K is given to neonates if it was omitted at birth, and they are started on oral clotrimazole suspension to help prevent fungal colonization of the urinary tract. Referring hospitals and doctors looking after preoperative neonates should be encouraged to use the lower limbs for blood sampling and cannulae. These veins will not be available postoperatively, when the surgical team will need good access via the upper limb veins.

General anesthesia is required with the usual neonatal precautions. A caudal anesthetic is helpful or, preferably, an epidural catheter is inserted to provide excellent peroperative and postoperative pain control in both babies and older children having the Kelly procedure. In some difficult neonatal cases and where abdominal closure has been tight, a period of postoperative ventilation in an intensive care unit is required.

BLADDER EXSTROPHY CLOSURE

Operation

POSITION OF PATIENT

The patient is positioned flat and supine. Total lower body preparation with individual wrapping of the legs allows maximum maneuverability at the time of the surgery and access for the orthopedic surgeons to perform osteotomies if required. Amikacin (7.5 mg/kg), metronidazole (7.5 mg/kg), and ampicillin (6 mg/kg) are given intravenously in the anesthetic room and continued postoperatively for at least 48 hours.

SKIN INCISION

5 The umbilicus is ligated and trimmed but retained. A stay suture is placed through the end of the glans penis to aid its retraction (4/0 monofilament with a round-bodied needle). Incisions are made beginning in the midline above the umbilicus, extending around the margins of the bladder, and forward onto the root of the penis, on either side of the urethral plate as far as the distal limit of the veru montanum. The incisions are deepened with diathermy but the distal incisions may be left superficial at this stage.

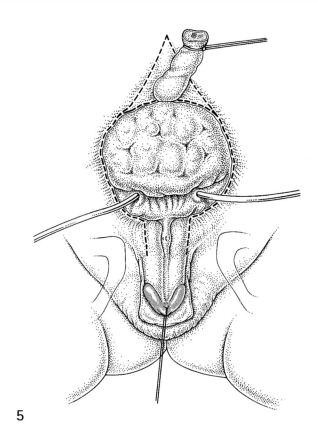

5

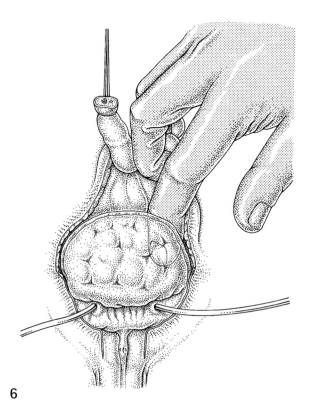

6

BLADDER MOBILIZATION

6 Working from above the umbilicus, the incision is deepened through the midline to expose the umbilical vein, without opening the peritoneum. As dissection continues distally, the umbilical arteries serve as a guide on each side to the extraperitoneal plane. Both are divided, allowing the umbilicus to move upward to a more anatomical position. Careful blunt dissection opens up a plane behind the rectus muscles on each side, in front of the ureters (stent in position for palpation), and down to the pelvic floor at the bladderneck.

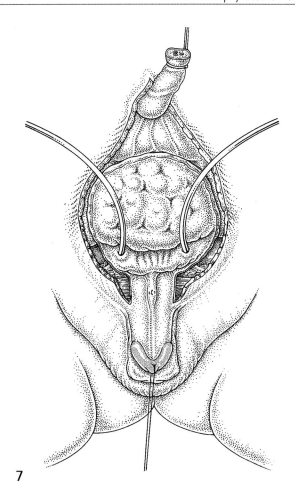

7

COMPLETION OF DISTAL INCISION

7 With a finger in position behind the abdominal wall, the distal incisions may be completed with diathermy to create freedom of the bladder on each side. The intrapubic bar tissue fusing with the bladderneck is now visible and is an important landmark.

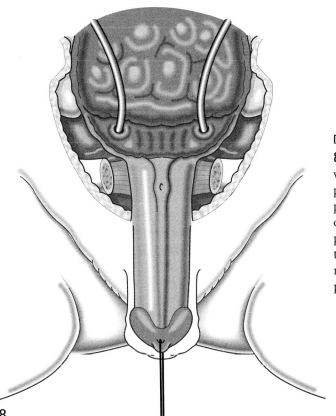

8

DISSECTION OF PROXIMAL URETHRA

8 The intrapubic bar tissue is divided lateral to the veru montanum to release the bladderneck and allow its placement inside the pelvis. The ends of this tissue and the pubic bones are then available to bring together in front of the bladderneck. Radical corporal mobilization is not performed at this stage, although the incisions may need to be extended distally to facilitate the closure of the pelvic ring. It is preferable to stay above the corporal bodies in patients subsequently having a Kelly procedure.

BLADDER CLOSURE

9 The bladder and proximal urethra are now sufficiently free to drop back into the pelvis. An 8 Fr feeding tube catheter with opposed eyes to avoid obstruction is sutured to the bladder wall with 6/0 monocryl. Bladder closure begins from the apex using interrupted 4/0 monocryl sutures after trimming the bladder edges. The two ureteric feeding tubes (which have also been secured with 6/0 monocryl sutures) are brought out between sutures. Closure is continued to the proximal urethra, although the lower sutures may be left untied until pelvic approximation is achieved.

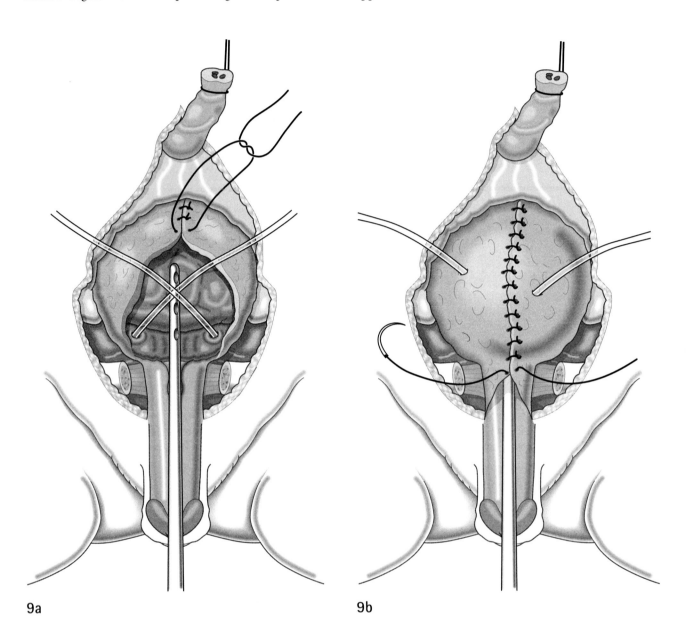

9a   9b

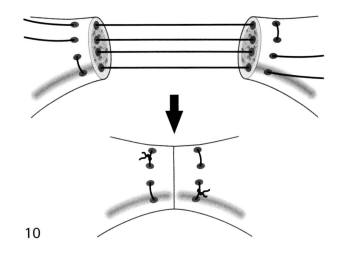

APPROXIMATION OF PUBIC BONES

10 One or two mattress (0 or 1) polydioxanone sutures (PDS) are laid in position in the pubic bones before abdominal wall closure and are tied once rectus muscle approximation is complete. This helps to prevent a bowstring effect cutting back into the urethra if the bones separate a little postoperatively.

10

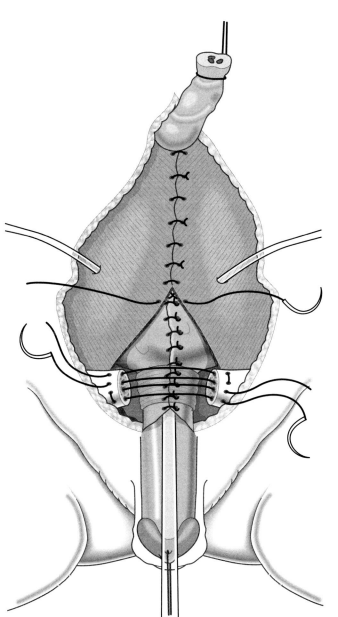

TRANSPOSITIONAL OMPHALOPLASTY AND WOUND CLOSURE

11 The umbilicus, suspended on the umbilical vein, is displaced to the apex of the abdominal incision. Closure of the abdominal wound begins by bringing the rectus muscles together, starting from above and proceeding downwards. The aim is to even out the tension of closure throughout the whole length of the wound so that the strain of closure is not taken by the symphysial sutures alone. Interrupted figure-of-eight sutures of 3/0 PDS are used proximally, increasing to 2/0 PDS as the closure proceeds distally. The ureteric stents are brought out on either side of the abdominal wall by cutting off their connectors and threading them through large intravenous cannulae, passed from the outside. Finally, the pubic bones are approximated by tying their sutures. During this maneuver, internal rotation of the hips by the assistant and compression of the pelvis may be helpful.

11

SKIN CLOSURE

12 The skin is closed in two layers of interrupted 4/0 Vicryl sutures.

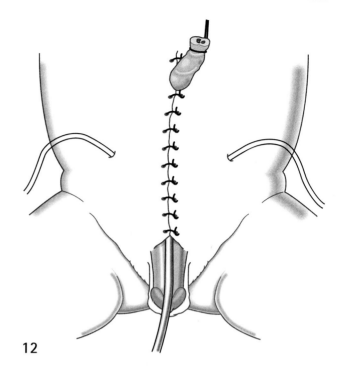

12

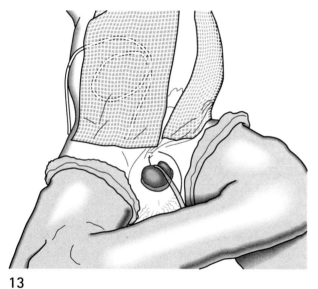

13

IMMOBILIZATION

13 Either a frog plaster, with internal rotation of the hips and slight adduction with flexion of the knees, or a mermaid bandage is used to immobilize the lower limbs. This is kept in place for 3–6 weeks.

Radical soft-tissue reconstruction (Kelly procedure)

This operation reopens and dissects the bladder, mobilizes the urethral plate completely from the penile corpora, releases the pelvic floor muscle, and detaches the penis from the pubic rami, preserving its neurovascular bundle (the pudendal pedicle). It allows radical reconstruction of the bladderneck and urethra and recreates a muscular sphincter. Another major benefit is the improvement in penile length that is achieved. In respect of the penis, there are two choices. Combining the operation with a Cantwell–Ransley epispadias repair leaves the urethral plate attached distally to the glans and enables a single-stage procedure, but at the expense of some penile length.

Alternatively, completely detaching the urethral plate frees the penis for more length, but leaves a hypospadiac meatus and the need for a later distal urethroplasty.

Deconstruction/dissection

POSITION OF PATIENT

The patient is prepared as for primary closure and is supine on the table with a full lower body preparation and legs wrapped in sterile drapes and in the field to permit full mobility. In addition, a purse-string suture of 0/0 PDS is placed around the anus to prevent fecal spillage during the procedure, which is removed immediately after the operation.

SKIN INCISION

14 A stay suture is placed in the glans as before to retract the penis. The old incision is reopened, excising any hypertrophic scar, and deepened through the muscle to expose the bladder. The epispadiac meatus is opened to the bladder above, taking care to keep in the midline and avoid damage to the urethral plate.

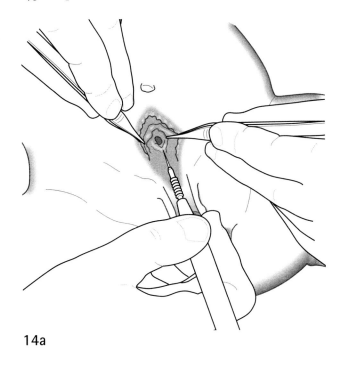

14a

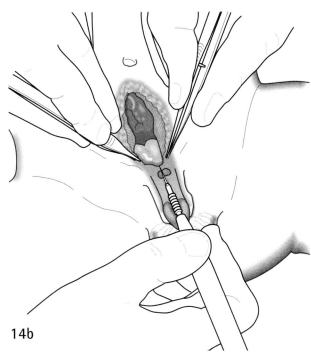

14b

BLADDER MOBILIZATION

15a,b The lateral edges of the bladder are freed from the abdominal wall on either side and the bladder is reopened anteriorly in the midline. The lateral edges of the bladder are dissected free to the level of the veru montanum, as in primary repair.

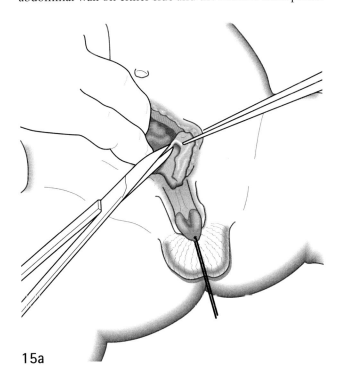

15a

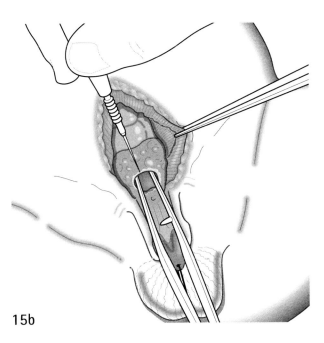

15b

URETERIC REIMPLANTATION

16a–c A small Finochetto retractor is used to separate the pubic rami. Two 6 Fr feeding tubes are placed as ureteric stents and the ureters fully dissected through the bladder, keeping close to the ureters. A Cohen-type ureteric reimplantation is completed using a transverse tunnel.

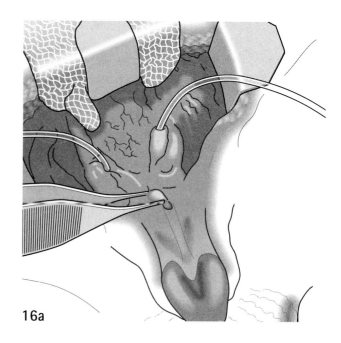

16a

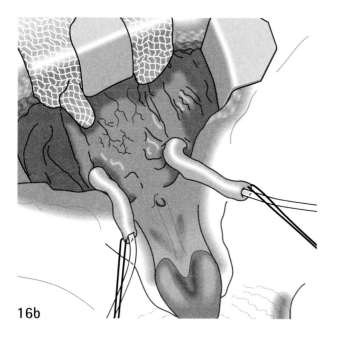

16b

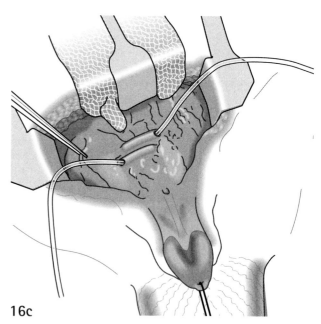

16c

URETHRAL AND PENILE SKIN DISSECTION

17a–c The urethral plate is marked out from either side of the veru, distally to the edge of the corpora, and incised. Ventrally, the penile skin is marked and incised to leave a cuff beneath the glans. The skin is lifted off the ventrum and sides of the penis and dissected proximally to expose the undersurfaces of the corporal bodies.

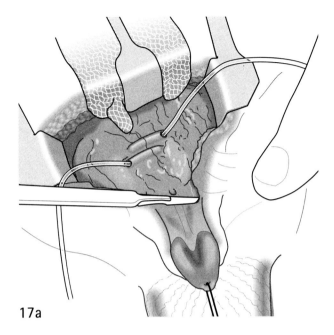

17a

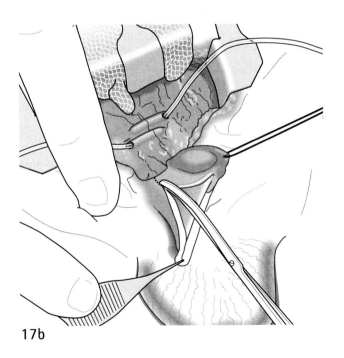

17b

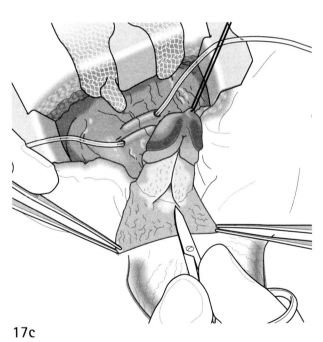

17c

DISSECTING THE PENIS

18a–c Dissection continues proximally along the corporal bodies. The separation of the corpora and the prostate gland in between them are identified. Laterally, each corpus is traced until its point of attachment to the inferior pubic ramus can be seen and palpated. The perineal muscle can be identified with the muscle stimulator, running between the bases of the corpora.

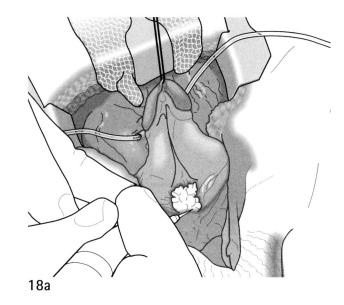

18a

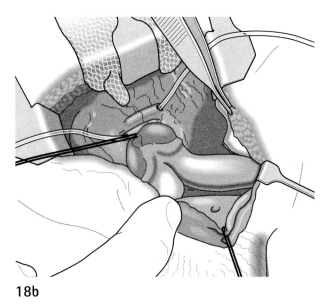

18b

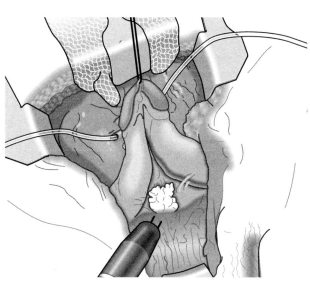

18c

DISSECTING THE URETHRAL PLATE

19a−c The urethral plate is dissected from above and below the penis. The tissue below the plate is separated from the corporal bodies by dissecting the bloodless plane between them on both sides, keeping close to the corpora. Dissection is completed anteriorly on either side of the plate, and vessel loops are passed around each corpus. Separation of the plate is completed, distally to the edge of the glans and proximally to the level of the prostate.

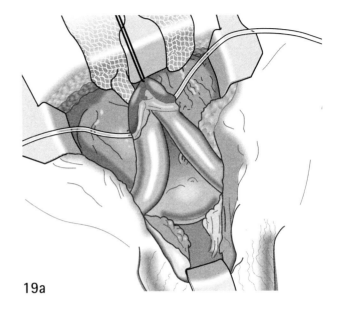

19a

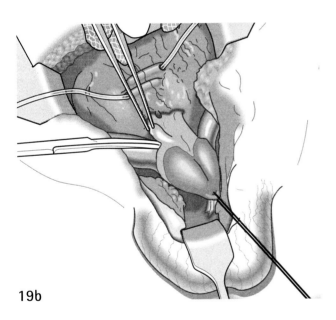

19b

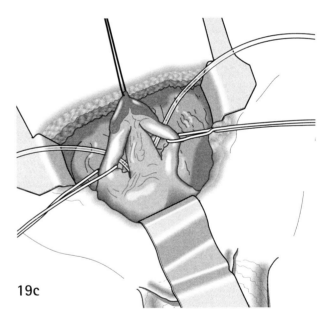

19c

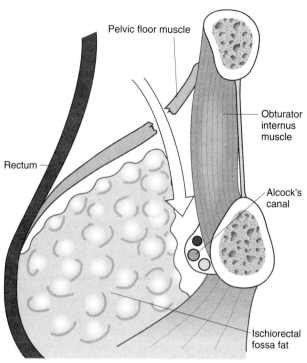

20a

RELEASING THE PELVIC FLOOR FROM ABOVE

20a–c To mobilize the base of the corpora, their neurovascular supply (the pudendal artery, veins, and nerve) must be freed along their course from behind the spine of the ischium from where they run forward in Alcock's canal. This is a fascial channel that runs forward on the surface of the internal obturator fascia, lateral to the ischiorectal fossa, below the pelvic floor. A retroperitoneal plane lateral to the bladder is developed by forefinger dissection behind the lower rectus toward the pelvic floor. Medial retraction of the bladder and rectum behind it reveals the pelvic floor muscles and a muscle stimulator helps to define their attachment to the obturator fascia (the so-called white line). The muscle fibers are divided about 0.5 cm medial to the white line with bipolar diathermy. This exposes the ischiorectal fat, which can be pushed downwards and medially to expose the fascia over the internal obturator muscle.

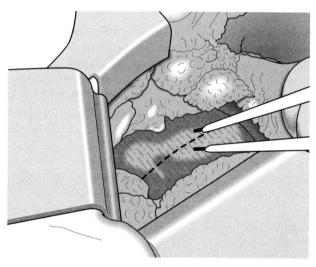

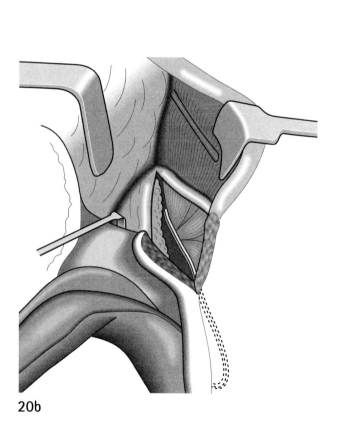

20b

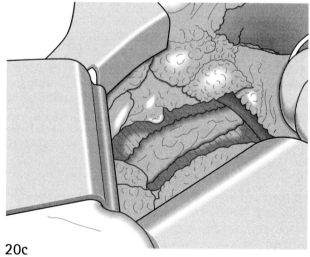

20c

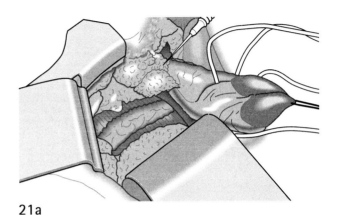

21a

RELEASING THE BASE OF THE PENIS AND EXPOSING THE PEDICLE

21 This dissection is continued anteriorly toward the pubic ramus, where the muscle is often thicker. The corporal body is now released from the bone by first incising along the inferior pubic ramus, lateral to its attachment. A combination of blunt and bipolar dissection peels the periosteal attachment of the corpus off the bone. By careful dissection from above and below, the corpus is freed and the pedicle can be demonstrated running from behind and along it. Once it is seen, any fascial attachments lateral to the pedicle are divided, exposing fat and releasing the neurovascular bundle and the corpus medially.

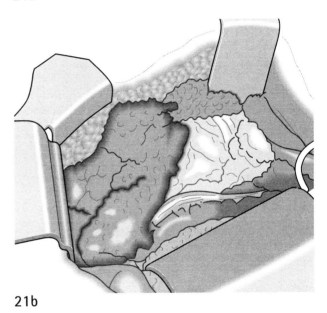

21b

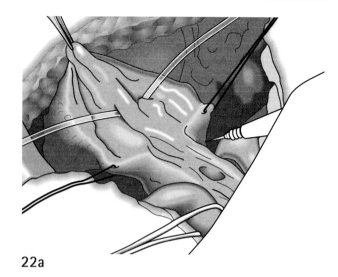

22a

Reconstruction

BLADDERNECK, BLADDER, AND PROXIMAL URETHRAL CLOSURE

22 The veru montanum is identified proximally on the urethral plate. The urethral plate is continued proximally and the area of the bladderneck is identified by marking and excising two triangles of bladder mucosa on either side. The bladderneck is reconstructed around a 10 Fr silicone stent whose proximal end is secured to the bladder mucosa with a fine, absorbable suture. Two layers of interrupted 4/0 monocryl sutures are used and these are continued proximally in a single layer to close the bladder. A 12 Fr Malecot catheter is inserted into the bladder to be used for suprapubic drainage and the two stents are brought out through the midline closure. The closure is continued anteriorly along the urethral plate.

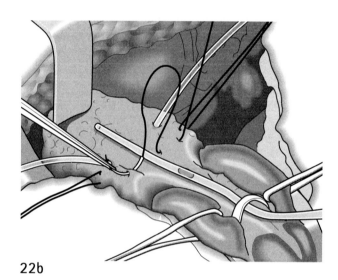

22b

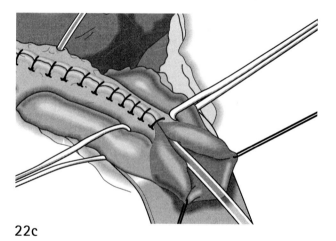

22c

CLOSURE OF URETHRA AND EPISPADIAS REPAIR

Alternative 1: Cantwell–Ransley type of repair

If the penis is a good length and protrudes well, a decision may be made at this stage to perform a one-stage repair, including complete repair of the epispadias. It is important to note that most experience has been gained with the second alternative (creation of a hypospadias) and the long-term results (especially for continence) are still to be evaluated.

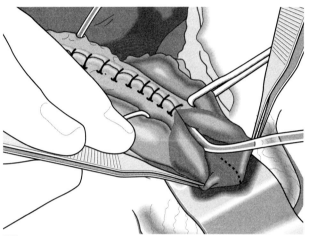

23a

'IPGAM' MANEUVER

23 The distal urethral plate at the tip of the glans is incised longitudinally and the incision is closed transversely with fine, absorbable sutures. This 'IPGAM' maneuver brings the urethral meatus more ventrally on the glans.

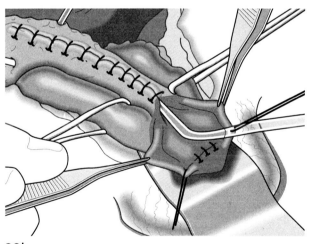

23b

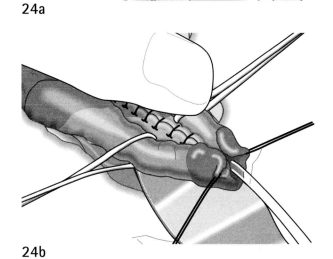

24a

CLOSURE OF THE URETHRA AND GLANS

24 Two triangles of mucosa are marked and excised from either side of the glans, preserving the central strip of urethral plate. Proximally, the plate is lifted from the corpora to provide greater mobility, which will allow the urethra's displacement ventral to the corpora and closure of the glans behind it. The plate is then closed with interrupted 5/0 PDS sutures. The gland is reconstructed dorsal to it with two layers of interrupted, subcuticular, 5/0 PDS.

24b

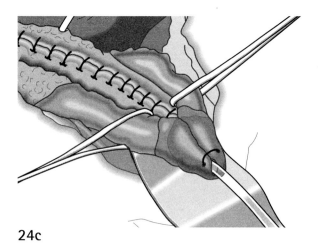

24c

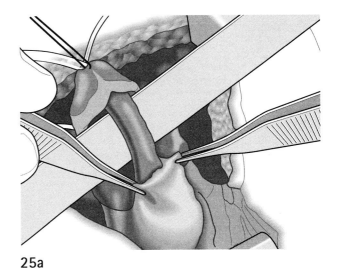

25a

CREATION OF THE SPHINCTER

25 The urethra is now free to bring ventral to the corpora, and this can be demonstrated by inserting a copper retractor. The muscle between the corpora, at and below the level of the prostate, is again identified with the muscle stimulator. A sling of this muscle is wrapped around the urethra by passing two 4/0 monocryl sutures on either side from behind. The wrap is not circumferential and the sutures should be tied dorsally, so as to be snug but not tight. The two corporal bodies are now sutured together in the midline with 4/0 monocryl. External rotation of each at this time will help correct the dorsal chordee.

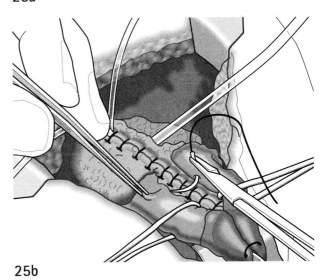

25b

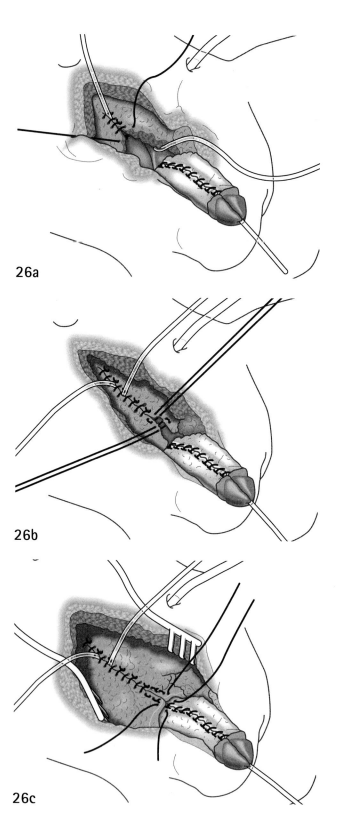

26a

26b

26c

CLOSURE

26 The abdominal wall is closed from above with serial figure-of-eight sutures of 2/0 PDS, as for primary closure. The stents are brought out through the wound, while the Malekot is tunneled and brought out to the left of the midline. Two 0/0 or 1/0 PDS sutures are placed at the lower end of the wound to reclose the symphyseal area. The base of each corpus (corresponding to the area previously separated from the bone) is sutured to the lower end of the abdominal closure with 3/0 PDS sutures. Care must be taken to avoid damaging the pedicle at this point.

PENILE SKIN COVER AND SKIN CLOSURE

27   The penile skin flap is now lifted and flattened. It is incised in the midline and the apex of this incision is sutured to the frenular area of the skin cuff with 6/0 monocryl sutures. The penis is wrapped and the skin closed dorsally in the midline or with z-plasties. The edges are trimmed before the circumcision wound is closed with 6/0 monocryl. The abdominal wall subcutaneous layers and skin are closed with layers of absorbable sutures.

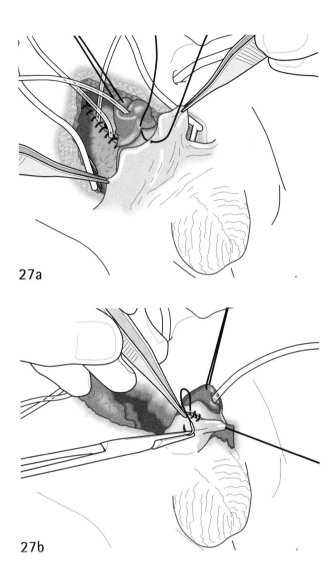

27a

27b

Alternative 2: creation of hypospadias

Where the penile length is compromised (as is often the case) and in particular when the urethral plate seems to limit its length, this alternative approach is used. In practice, surgeons have more experience with this approach and the published data on continence are principally from these patients. Subsequent procedures are required to create the distal urethra, with or without skin grafting.

LIFTING OF THE URETHRAL PLATE FROM THE CORPORA AND GLANS

28 The urethral plate is separated completely from the corpora, including its glanular portion. This is tubularized throughout its length using interrupted 5/0 monocryl sutures. The neourethra is then dropped between the two corporal bodies. From the ventral aspect, the perineal muscle is identified and wrapped around the urethra using interrupted 4/0 monocryl sutures. The wrap may not be complete and the sutures are snug, but not tight. The corpora are joined dorsally and the penile shaft reconstruction is completed as above, with corporal rotation to correct the chordee. The glans halves are joined in layers of 5/0 PDS. The urethral opening is secured to the ventral shaft with 5/0 PDS. When the shaft shin is reconstructed, a midline opening is made to accommodate the hypospadiac meatus, which is secured around its circumference with absorbable sutures.

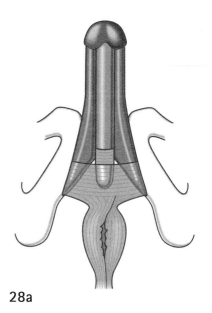

28a

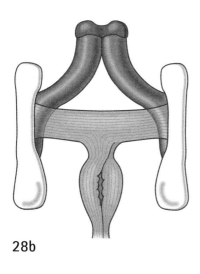

28b

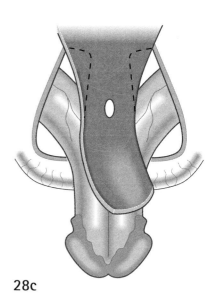

28c

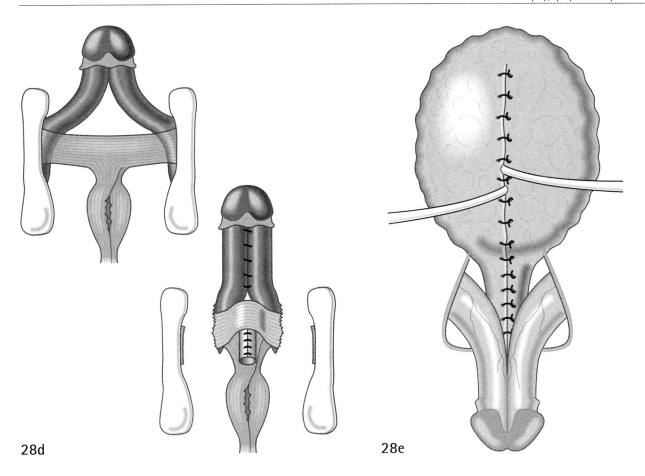

28d

28e

FEMALE EXSTROPHY/EPISPADIAS REPAIR

29 In females after successful primary closure in exstrophy or primary epispadias, soft-tissue reconstruction is used to create continence and also to improve genital appearance. The clitoral corpora are dissected as for the penile corpora, with the labia minora skin flaps left attached around the glans for subsequent reconstruction. The pelvic floor and pudendal pedicles are dissected in the same way and the muscle is identified below and lateral to the vagina – attached to the base of the corpora on either side. At the time of bladder outlet reconstruction, this muscle is brought around the dorsum of the proximal urethra and effectively wraps both the urethra and vagina. At closure, the hemiclitori can be brought together and the labia minora replaced lateral to the neourethral orifice and the vagina. The mons is reconstructed by mobilizing subcutaneous fat from either side.

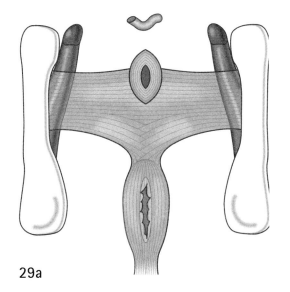

29a

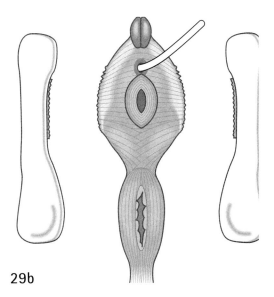

29b

Postoperative care

After radical soft-tissue reconstruction and epispadias repair, the penis is enclosed in a foam dressing for 1 week. The ureteric stents are left on drainage and removed after 1 week, and the bladder remains on free drainage for 3 further weeks. At this time, the urethral stent is removed and the suprapubic Malekot catheter is clamped intermittently. When this is possible for 3 hours and the child has voided urethrally (checked by ultrasound), the suprapubic catheter is removed. Continence and bladder capacity will evolve with time, and regular evaluations at approximately three-month intervals are required. Cystoscopic evaluation of the bladder outlet is performed with a fine cystoscope (8 Fr) at between three and six months.

FURTHER READING

Gearhart JP. The bladder exstrophy–epispadia–cloacal exstrophy complex. In: Gearhart JP, Rink RC, Moriquand P (eds). *Pediatric Urology*. Philadelphia, PA: Saunders, 2001: 511–46.

Kelly JH. Exstrophy and epispadias: Kelly's method of repair. In: O'Neill JA, Rowe MI, Grosfeld JL *et al.* (eds). *Pediatric Surgery*, 5th edn. St Louis, MO: Mosby, 1998: 1732–59.

Woodhouse CR, Fisch MM, Peppas DS, Reiner WG. Failed bladder exstrophy closure. *Dialogues in Pediatric Urology* 1999; **22**.

96

Surgical treatment of disorders of sexual development

RAFAEL V PIERETTI and PATRICIA K DONAHOE

INTRODUCTION AND PRINCIPLES

A child born with disorders of sexual development (DSD) must be evaluated immediately at birth by a well-organized and experienced medical team. Many syndromes can affect later sexual development, but only four result in DSD at birth: 46,XX DSD (formerly known as female pseudohermaphroditism), ovotesticular DSD (true hermaphroditism), 46,XY DSD (previously known as male pseudohermaphroditism and undervirilization or undermasculinization of an XY male), and mixed gonadal dysgenesis (MGD) 45,X/46,XY. A child with pure gonadal dysgenesis, although having a 46,XY karyotype, is phenotypically female. The gender, which is appropriate to the anatomy of the infant, must be decided as early as possible, since new parents are asked about the sex of the child as soon as the birth is known. They must be able to give an answer that is commensurate with the gender assignment that will eventually provide the most satisfying functional result. However, it is important that parents be reassured and to work closely with a team of DSD experts who will help the family make a decision with which all will be most comfortable.

Two practical screening criteria, gonadal symmetry or asymmetry and the presence of a Y chromosome can be used to help in the diagnosis of the infant as having one of the four DSD disorders. Probes for SRY can be used to sequence or genotype the *SRY* gene. Gonadal symmetry is determined by the position of one gonad relative to the other, either above or below the external inguinal ring. If both gonads are symmetrical, then a diffuse biochemical cause underlies the abnormality, as in 46,XX DSD or 46,XY DSD, which are biochemical anomalies that influence both gonads equally. Asymmetry occurs in MGD or ovotesticular DSD (true hermaphroditism), which are chromosomal abnormalities in which a predominant testis descends and a predominant ovary remains above

the external ring. The karyotype is always 46,XX in cases of 46,XX DSD (female pseudohermaphroditism with adrenogenital syndrome) and is most often the case in patients with ovotesticular DSD (true hermaphroditism). Patients with 46,XY DSD (male pseudohermaphroditism) or MGD always have a Y chromosome in their karyotype (see studies from MacLaughlin and Donahoe in 2004 and Donahoe and colleagues in 2005).

Following this initial evaluation, rapid analysis for 17 hydroxyprogesterone to detect CYP21 disorders must be carried out in patients with 46,XX with symmetrical undescended gonads. A detailed history and physical examination can be coupled with polymerase chain reaction (PCR), fluorescent *in situ* hybridization (FISH), or direct sequencing to detect mutations or deletions known to cause defects in the four major categories, and to define these disorders more fully and guide sex assignment.

Genetic females, no matter how severely virilized, should be raised as females. In genetic males, the gender assignment must be based on the infant's anatomy, that is, the size of the phallus, and not on the 46XY karyotype. If the phallus is inadequate, one should strongly consider assignment to the female gender. The average penile length at 30 weeks' gestation is 2.5 ± 0.4 cm, increasing to 3.5 ± 0.4 cm at term, with a width of 1–1.5 cm. A term size below 2×0.9 cm should cause concern. Failure to respond to a trial of exogenous testosterone is an important criterion in some cases. Exceptions, however, must always be made if the patient presents late, and has become fully committed to the male role, or in the event of a diagnosis of 5-α-reductase deficiency.

Female pseudohermaphroditism occurs when a genetic female (46XX) is exposed *in utero* to androgens, either exogenous or endogenous as in the congenital adrenal hyperplasia syndromes. The phenotype can vary from clitoral enlargement alone to complete labioscrotal fusion and formation of an entirely normal male penis with a closed urethra formed to its tip. Cortisol deficiency can lead to salt wasting, which can be life-threatening unless replacement is instituted. All masculinized females have normal child-bearing potential and should be raised as females.

Male pseudohermaphroditism occurs in 46XY genetic males with deficient masculinization of the external genitalia due to insufficient testosterone production, conversion, or inadequate target organ response. Many patients with male pseudohermaphroditism have been raised as males. However, if the female gender is chosen, then gonadectomy should be done at the time of perineal reconstruction. The patient with absent or rudimentary vagina usually requires only a clitoroplasty and labioscrotal reduction. The labioscrotal folds should be partially reduced during the first procedure and dilatation or a substitute vaginoplasty planned for the late adolescent or early adult years. Patients with testicular feminization in whom an introitus is often present may have this dilated with bougies at a later age to form a functional vagina.

True hermaphrodites have well-developed, non-dysgenetic male and female gonadal tissue in many combinations, i.e. a testis on one side and an ovary on the other, two ovotestes, or a normal gonad on one side and an ovotestis on the other. Although 80 percent of these patients have a 46,XX karyotype, testicular tissue is present. The patient with a small phallus should be raised as a female. However, the final decision should be taken following adequate discussion with the parents or guardians about full options and choices of how their child can be reared. The patient with a large phallus already committed as a male should be raised as a male. Gonads should be bivalved and biopsied longitudinally. The gonadal tissue commensurate with the sex of rearing (ovary tissue is peripheral, testicular is central) should be salvaged. Perineal reconstruction should be accompanied by removal of Wolffian structures if the female sex is chosen. If the phallus is adequate for male gender assignment, ovarian and Müllerian structures can be removed, followed by hypospadias repair. Testicular prostheses can be inserted later, should the testicular tissue be inadequate.

Mixed gonadal dysgenesis patients have dysgenetic gonads, retained Müllerian structures, internal and external asymmetry, and a mosaic karyotype, often 45X/46XY. The dysgenetic gonads can develop neoplasms such as gonadoblastoma or seminoma-dysgerminoma; therefore, in cases of asymmetric gonadal phenotype, the intra-abdominal or streak gonad should be removed. In general, the assignment of gender in children with mixed gonadal dysgenesis is controversial, and deserves careful consultation. In some cases, consideration should be given to raise the child as a female with removal of the gonads, perineal reconstruction with flap vaginoplasty, with estrogen and progesterone replacement at adolescence. Alternatively, patients may undergo complex repair of their severe hypospadias and be reared as a male. In either case, long-term follow up will be needed, as gender reassignment has occurred regardless of initial gender designation.

If the patient is already committed to the male role, then hypospadias repair will be required. The gonads must be carefully observed for tumor development, which may occur as early as the newborn period.

SURGICAL TREATMENT OF UROGENITAL SINUS ANOMALIES AND DISORDERS OF SEX DEVELOPMENT

Patients with DSD and urogenital sinus (UGS) abnormalities are a source of great emotional stress for parents and patients, and present challenges for the medical team involved in their treatment.

There has been significant recent progress resulting from studies on clitoral innervation, most importantly the introduction of new nerve-sparing clitoroplasty techniques and the more widespread use of UGS mobilization procedures. However, there is a lack of sufficient long-term results regarding sexual function and acceptance of genital appearance in most patients, because most of the published studies have analyzed patients who have been reconstructed by operative techniques, which have been more recently modified.

PREOPERATIVE EVALUATION

Imaging evaluation

1a,b, 2 A retrograde genitography is performed by occluding the opening of the urogenital sinus with the inflated balloon of a size 8 Fr Foley catheter placed outside the meatus and secured in place with tape; lateral and oblique images are required. The catheter should be then advanced into the bladder for a voiding cystourethogram (VCUG). In approximately 80 percent of the cases, the level of confluence of the urogenital sinus in relation to the bladderneck and external sphincter can be identified, thus facilitating the planning of the surgical procedure

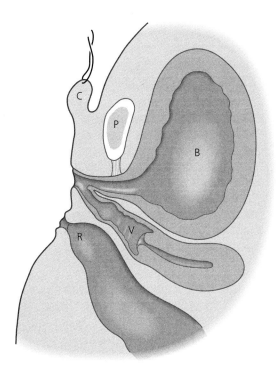

1a Low confluence

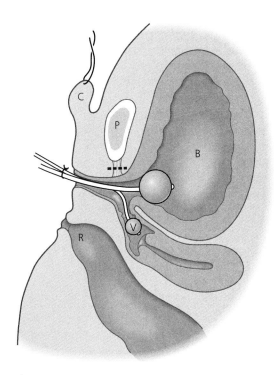

1b High confluence

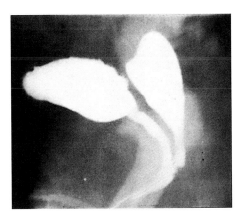

2 Low confluence

3, 4 Ultrasonography gives important information about the urinary tract and the uterus, vagina, and gonads can be visualized. In those cases in which the anatomy is not well demonstrated, magnetic resonance imaging (MRI) of the pelvis, can clearly define the anatomy of the pelvic organs.

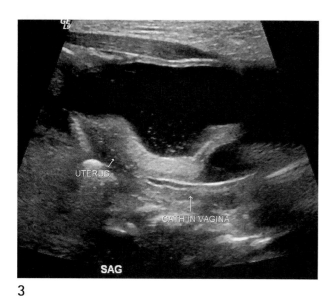

3

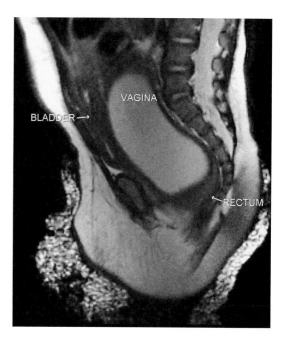

4

Laparoscopy

Laparoscopy allows excellent visualization of the pelvic organs; it can be used to perform a gonadal biopsy or gonadectomy, and can be very helpful for identification or removal of Müllerian structures. In addition, laparoscopy can be used to perform other procedures, such as a laparoscopic-assisted sigmoid vaginoplasty, and for the removal of an enlarged and symptomatic Müllerian duct remnant.

RECONSTRUCTION FOR FEMALE GENDER ASSIGNMENT

All 46,XX DSD newborns should be assigned to the female gender, regardless of the extent of masculinization, and should undergo surgical reconstruction concordant with the female gender assignment. Similar repairs can be used for selected patients who are not severely masculinized because of 46,XY DSD, MGD, or ovotesticular DSD. The key steps of a feminizing genitoplasty are clitoroplasty, labioplasty, and vaginoplasty. Surgical procedures must preserve clitoral sensation and result in normal looking external genitalia, with a well-lubricated vagina, which will allow satisfactory and painless sexual intercourse. Due to some concerns regarding the benefits of clitoroplasty, it should be undertaken only after extensive discussions with the family, because another option is for deferral until the patient is capable of making her own decision.

Preoperative preparation

The bowel must be prepared before repair. For low repairs, magnesium citrate should be given starting 2 days before repair. For high repairs, a polyethylene glycol isotonic solution (Golytely; Braintree Laboratories, Braintree, MA, USA) is administered by mouth beginning 3 days before surgery for 2 consecutive days, followed by magnesium citrate 1 day before surgery. If needed, ondansetron may be indicated to prevent nausea, or Golytely can be administered through a small nasogastric tube. The use of Golytely should be discontinued at least 24 hours before surgery to avoid leakage during the procedure. Magnesium citrate, which shrinks the bowel, is given on the last day to prevent leakage. Oral administration of neomycin plus erythromycin can be prescribed to reduce bacterial concentration.

Hormonal management of the 46,XX patient with adrenogenital syndrome is coordinated with experienced pediatric endocrinologists. Stress doses of steroids are given at the time of anesthetic induction. Steroids are continued during surgery and for 2–3 days after surgery at double the usual oral dose, followed by a tapering of the dosage. Patients on dexamethasone are asked to omit this medication, but children on prednisone take the usual morning dose on the day of surgery.

Surgical reconstruction

PLANNING AND TIMING THE SURGICAL RECONSTRUCTION

The magnitude and timing of surgical reconstruction is the subject of significant controversy. Some groups advocate delaying sex assignment to an age in which each patient can make his or her own decisions; however, as mentioned earlier, most of these studies have been based on analysis of the outcomes of older surgical procedures. The authors believe that newer techniques result in an improved cosmetic appearance, a reduced complication rate, and are more likely to preserve sensation.

All available treatment alternatives are discussed with the parents, and recommend that the different steps of the surgical reconstruction should be incorporated into a single surgical procedure, and be performed at an early age in order to take advantage of all available tissues, with the objective of achieving the best possible functional and cosmetic results. Patients with a low confluence urogenital sinus can be operated once their metabolic management is well controlled; in most cases, the authors undertake an elective reconstruction at between three and six months of age, but repair can be done in the newborn period if the social situation so warrants. Patients with a mid-level or high confluence can be electively repaired at 9–12 months of age. Adequate and controlled hormonal treatment is needed to prevent clitoral hypertrophy after correction.

Planning of the surgical reconstruction should incorporate the three components of a feminizing genitoplasty, in which the prepuce is used to create labia minora, if needed the clitoris is reduced, and the labiosacrotal swellings are used to fashion female-appearing labia majora and to enhance the vaginoplasty.

To improve surgical exposure, the authors use a hyperextended lithotomy position with the buttocks lying over and slightly beyond several folded towels. All procedures must begin with a panendoscopy.

Panendoscopy

5a,b All reconstructive procedures must begin with a panendoscopy using a pediatric cystoscope with 0° and 30° optics. High flow irrigation of the urogenital sinus facilitates finding a very small vaginal orifice in the back wall of the UGS; in some cases, there may be only a pinpoint orifice, which can usually be found by probing with a 3 Fr ureteral catheter. For surgical planning, one must precisely find the location of the confluence point between the vagina and urethra in relation with the bladderneck and the external sphincter. Those anomalies with the confluence point at or above the veru montanum/external sphincter are considered high, and those below are considered low. Patients with 46,XX DSD, MGD, and ovotesticular DSD, as well as those with 46,XY or 45,X/46,XY MGD have a cervix at the most proximal part of the vagina. Patients with 46,XY DSD have either a small prostatic utricle or a deeper, more generous cavity that has no proximal cervix. The prostatic utricle is characteristically found in the center of a flattened veru montanum, but has no surrounding prostatic tissue. In those patients with a mid-level and high confluence, a Fogarty catheter with a stopcock valve is passed into the vagina and the balloon is inflated; a small Foley catheter is also placed in the bladder, and both are labeled and tied together (see also illustration 1a,b).

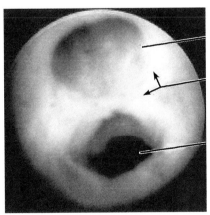

Urethra

External sphincter

Vaginal orifice

5a

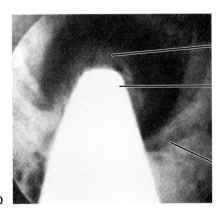

Verumontanum

Proximal vagina

External sphincter

5b

CLITOROPLASTY

6 Clitoral resection and recession are of historical interest and no longer recommended. The goal of current techniques is to preserve sensation for future orgasms, provide an acceptable cosmesis, and avoid painful erections. A subtunical excision of the erectile tissue has been used extensively and led to newer nerve-sparing techniques. In 1999, Baskin *et al.* found that distribution of the sensory nerves of the clitoris, similar to the sensory nerves of the penis, is found on the dorsal aspect of the clitoris coursing under the pubis. Circumferential branches from the dorsal neurovascular bundle encircle the clitoral shaft toward the ventrum, thus making a ventral approach to the corpora most likely to avoid nerve injury. In Baskin's technique, corporal tissue proximal to the bifurcation is left intact. In cases with severe masculinization, the clitoris is too large resembling a penis; in such cases, the authors discuss the anatomical characteristics with the parents and advise a clitoroplasty.

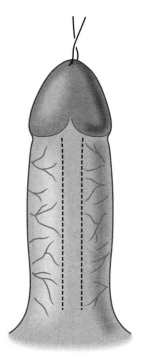

6

7, 8 A 5/0 Prolene stay suture is placed in the glans. Two vertical incisions are outlined with a marking pen on each side of the urethral plate, and the meatus is circumscribed as for hypospadias surgery, taking care to leave a redundant segment of dorsal inner foreskin to fashion a hooded prepuce, thus preserving an important source of sensation. Prior infiltration of incisions with 0.25 percent marcaine/1:200 000 epinephrine prevents excess blood loss. The vaginoplasty is incorporated into the surgical reconstruction outlining a wide base inverted 'U'-shaped perineal flap based on the anus and using the ischial tuberosities as a landmark; the apex of this flap is advanced and placed at the estimated final location of the widened vagina. The clitoris is degloved; the ventral strip of the urethral plate should initially be kept intact. Following degloving of the dorsal skin, the distal portion of the UGS (urethral plate) is divided below the glans clitoris. The urethral plate (UGS) is mobilized off the ventral aspect of the clitoral shaft downward to below the bifurcation of the corporal bodies. Next, clitoral reduction is carried out; the authors do not use a tourniquet as it has been observed that bleeding from the erectile tissues is not significant, particularly in infants, although it can be considerable in the older child. Longitudinal ventral incisions are made; the erectile tissue is dissected within the bodies. The body of the glans is sutured to the corporal body stumps with absorbable sutures. The redundant dorsal tunica albuginea and neurovascular bundle are placed in a subcutaneous pocket above the pubic bone, taking care not to impair the neurovascular elements. The reduced clitoral shaft is covered with surrounding fat tissue, thus fashioning a normal-looking mons pubis. In most cases, the authors try to avoid reduction of the glans clitoris, but in patients with severe enlargement, a wedge of glans tissue can be excised from the ventral aspect of the glans with careful reapproximation of the glans tissue with interrupted sutures of 6/0 PDS. The dorsal mucosal collar should cover the glans partially, giving it a hooded appearance. The remainder of the dorsal prepuce is divided in the midline (Byars technique) and reattached to the mucosal collar as with hypospadias repair. The preputial skin wings are rotated inferiorly and incorporated lateral to the urethral plate to create labia minora.

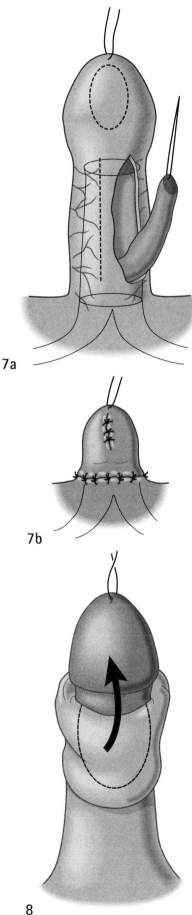

7a

7b

8

LABIOPLASTY

9, 10 Most girls with 46,XX DSD have labioscrotal swellings that are anterior in relation to the vagina than normal labia majora. Significant skin rugation may be present as well. To move this labioscrotal skin posteriorly, 'Y'-shaped incisions are outlined with an extension posterior to the swellings. The scrotal flaps are cautiously defatted and moved posteriorly, besides the introitus, as bilateral Y–V advancements. The medial aspects of these skin flaps are then sutured to the lateral edges of the prepucial skin flaps mobilized during clitoroplasty (now labia minora). The result is an anatomically correct positioning of the labia minora and majora posteriorly, beside the introitus, rather than anterior-laterally.

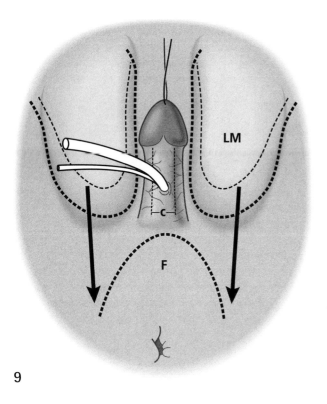

9

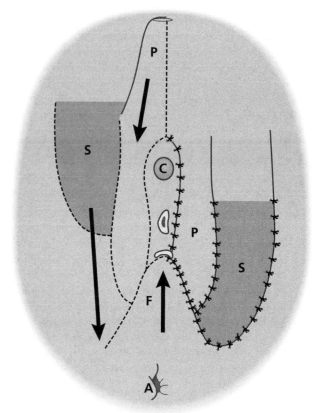

10

VAGINOPLASTY

The type of vaginoplasty is dictated by the anatomic location of the UGS confluence. There are six types of vaginoplasty: cut-back, flap, pull-through, total and partial urogenital sinus mobilization (TUM and PUM), and vaginal replacement.

Low confluence flap vaginoplasty

11a–c Flap vaginoplasty should only be used in cases with a very low confluence UGS, as otherwise it does not bring the merging point of the vagina with the urethra any closer to the perineum. The authors use a thick inverted perineal skin 'U' flap, based on the anus, which is outlined with a marking pen, when advanced it should reach the edge of the sinus. The posterior wall of the vagina is dissected with care not to injure the rectum. Next, the posterior wall of the sinus must be opened longitudinally into normal caliber vagina to avoid a vaginal stricture. The apex of the flap is inserted into the apex of the vaginal wall, and secured in place beginning with three interrupted, full-thickness sutures of 4/0 Vicryl, which should be tied carefully to prevent tearing the fragile vaginal wall; the rest of the sutures are placed in a sequential manner. In low confluence vaginoplasty, there is no need to insert a finger in the rectum, but a roll of Vaseline gauze can be inserted in the rectum to avoid rectal injury. In low vaginoplasty, there is no need to mobilize the UGS. Once the urogenital sinus is dissected off the corpora, its ventral wall is opened longitudinally down to the vaginal opening to create a wet introitus. Later during labioplasty, the medial edge of the prepuce (labia minora) will be sutured to the outer edge of the opened, non-mobilized urethral plate/UGS.

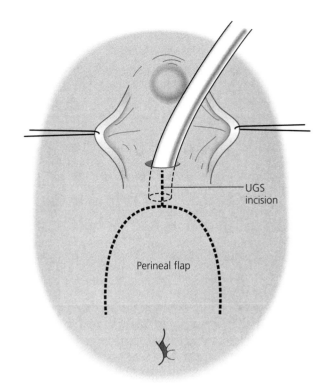

11a

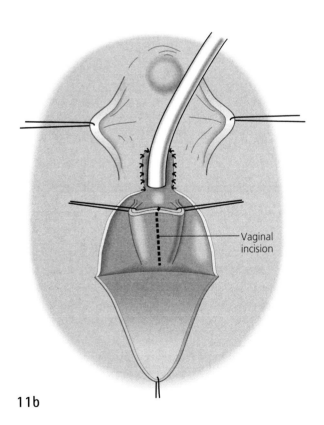

11b

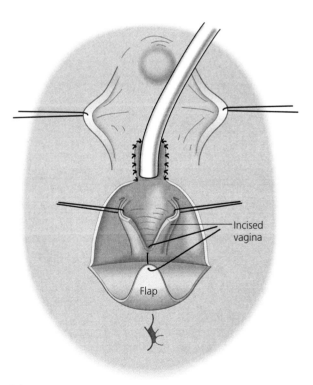

11c

Vaginoplasty using urogenital mobilization

12a Total urogenital sinus mobilization (TUM) was described in 1997 by Alberto Peña as a technique to repair the UGS component of cloacal malformations. Currently, most surgeons for UGS repair are using this procedure, or a modification thereof. Urogenital sinus mobilization has the advantage of better visualization of the merging point and it obviates the need for vaginal separation, thus reducing the difficulty of the procedure. The Fogarty balloon, placed in the vagina during the panendoscopy, allows the identification of the confluence. In addition, in those cases where vaginal separation is required, it can be less extensive. In this technique, since the confluence is brought closer to the perineum, the mobilization of skin flaps is minimized. The posterior dissection is similar to that done for a pull-through or flap procedures, with careful, midline, mobilization of the UGS off the rectum. The circumferential dissection in cases requiring a total urogenital sinus mobilization is done past the puburethral ligament, under the pubis, resulting in significant mobilization of the sinus, which in high cases permits the confluence to be brought more easily to the perineum.

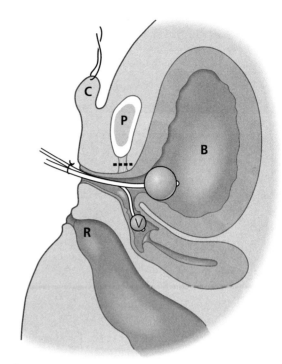

12a High confluence

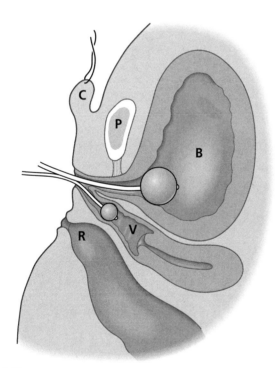

12b Low confluence

12b In response to concerns for possible complications of urinary incontinence, resulting from the dissection of the UGS beyond the puburethral ligament, Rink *et al.* (2006) proposed the use of a partial urogenital mobilization (PUM). In this technique, the anterior dissection stops at the puburethral ligament aiming to avoid compromising the innervation to the bladder outlet and clitoris. Circumferential, partial mobilization of the UGS allows the mid-level vaginal confluence to be brought down to the perineum without tension, avoiding the need for separation of the vagina from the urethra as in the classical pull-through vaginoplasty. This procedure is adequate in most cases except for patients with a very high confluence in whom additional mobilization past the puburethral ligament may be needed.

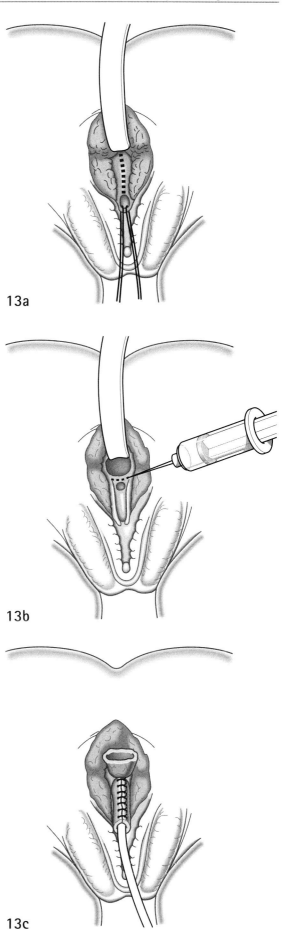

13a

13a–c In high confluence cases, if the perineum cannot be reached without tension, the vagina must be sharply dissected from the back wall of the bladder before the anastomosis to the inverted perineal 'U' flap can be attempted. In these cases, the use of a prone position can facilitate the dissection of the vagina off the bladder.

In both total and partial urogenital sinus mobilization, as previously described for low confluence vaginoplasty, the distal segment of the vagina can be quite narrow; hence its posterior wall must be incised up to normal caliber vagina to avoid a vaginal stricture. The apex of the inverted perineal 'U' flap is inserted into the apex of the vagina wall, and secured in with interrupted full thickness sutures of 4/0 Vicryl as previously described for a low vaginoplasty (see illustration 11a-c).

13b

13c

Splitting the urogenital sinus

14a–d The common urogenital sinus can be split to enhance the vaginoplasty in one of the following manners. (1) In very low confluence cases, the authors do not mobilize the urogenital sinus, and incise it longitudinally on its ventral aspect down to the confluence point; the lateral aspects of the opened sinus are then sutured to the medial aspects of the prepuce wings, thus resulting in a more normal anatomical configuration. (2) Split the sinus ventrally to fashion a mucosa-lined vestibule. (3) Split the sinus dorsally to create a flap which will enhance the anterior aspect of the vagina. (4) The sinus can be split laterally to create and rotate a flap to elongate the vagina.

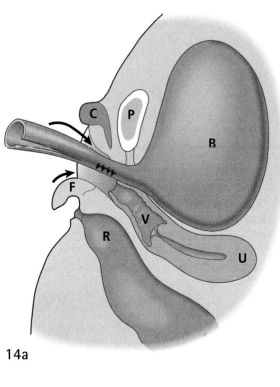

14a

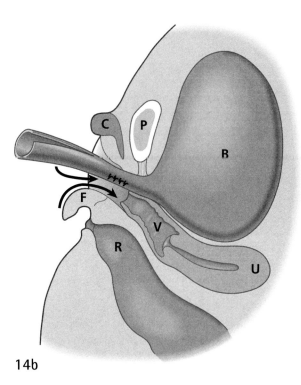

14b

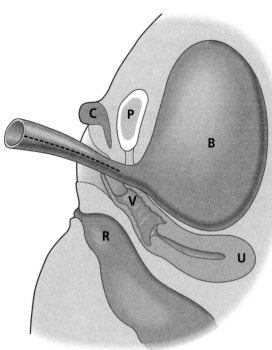

14c

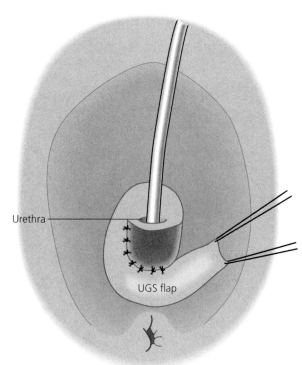

14d

Pull-through vaginoplasty for mid- and high-level vaginal confluence

15a–h Before the advent of the urogenital sinus mobilization procedures, the majority of girls were reconstructed using a pull-through vaginoplasty; however, now the urogenital sinus mobilization techniques are preferred. All patients undergo a total lower body preparation from nipples to toes, the legs are wrapped, and the lower body is passed through the aperture in the drapes, which allows the patient to be rotated either supine or prone during the procedure. The initial aspects of the dissection are similar to the description previously mentioned for lower confluences. The operation begins with a panendoscopy during which the confluence is localized, and a Fogarty catheter connected to a stopcock valve is maneuvered into the vagina, where the balloon is inflated and the valve closed. A Foley catheter is passed into the bladder; both catheters are secured together with a silk suture. An inverted perineal 'U' flap is made, the urogenital sinus is exposed, and the balloon of the Fogarty catheter is palpated. Intermittent insertion of a finger inside the rectum, to flatten out its anterior wall, reassures the surgeon that the rectum has not been injured. The vagina is mobilized circumferentially and meticulously separated off the bladder anteriorly. The UGS is closed with interrupted stitches of a 6/0 PDS. A labial flap or an anterior island flap, which for this procedure must be fashioned in the midline, can now easily reach the anterior vagina. In patients with a very high confluence, the authors have found that rotating to the prone position improves visualization and surgical field, allowing the vagina to be safely mobilized off the urogenital sinus and bladder. The placement of a small malleable retractor into the vagina combined with slight upward traction facilitates the surgical dissection. The opening in the UGS is then closed with interrupted stitches of 6/0 PDS. The vagina is then mobilized circumferentially and brought to the perineum where it is sutured to the perineal skin flap as described for vaginoplasty.

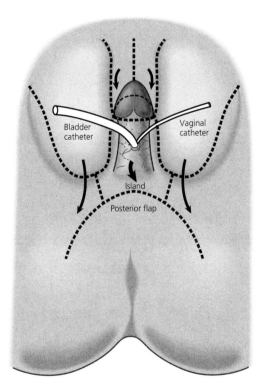

15a

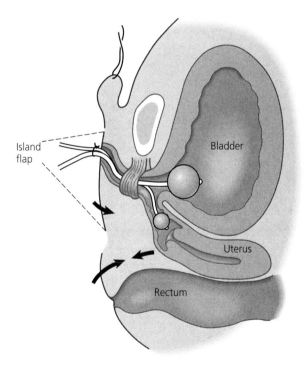

15b

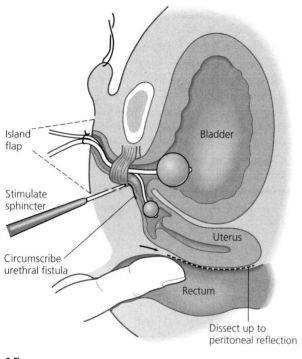

Island flap

Stimulate sphincter

Circumscribe urethral fistula

Bladder

Uterus

Rectum

Dissect up to peritoneal reflection

15c

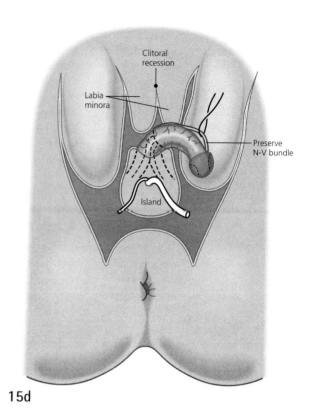

Clitoral recession

Labia minora

Preserve N-V bundle

Island

15d

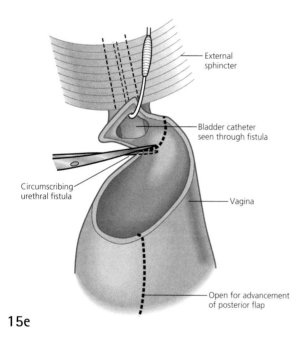

External sphincter

Bladder catheter seen through fistula

Circumscribing urethral fistula

Vagina

Open for advancement of posterior flap

15e

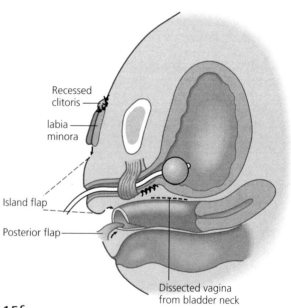

Recessed clitoris

labia minora

Island flap

Posterior flap

Dissected vagina from bladder neck

15f

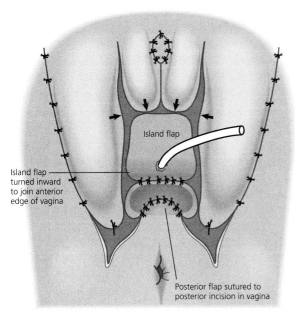

15g

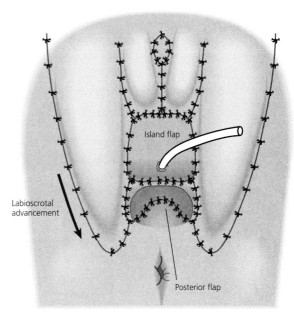

15h

Postoperative care of the female patient

A size 8 Fr Foley catheter is left indwelling for 3–4 days. Immobilization with a mermaid dressing, in which the lower extremities are wrapped with stockinet and an elastic bandage to prevent abduction, reduces tension on the suture lines. A soft foam or cotton is placed between the knees and ankles, and the anus is left exposed. This dressing is kept in place for 4–5 days. A broad-spectrum antibiotic is used during the first 2 postoperative days. Hormonal replacement appropriate to the patient's diagnosis is given.

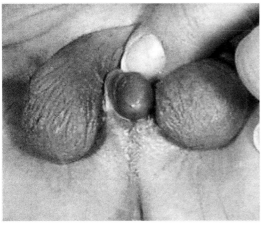

16

RECONSTRUCTION FOR MALE GENDER ASSIGNMENT

16 The treatment strategy is similar for all patients assigned to the male gender. Most of these patients have a small penis with a penoscrotal, scrotal, or a perineal hypospadias; a severe ventral curvature; and a partial or complete prepenile scrotum. Preoperative treatment with testosterone is helpful in those cases with a small penis.

17 The authors' preferred approach is to perform a one-stage hypospadias repair, but if necessary, the procedure can be staged. In patients with an adequate urethral plate, the authors use the extended applications of the tubularized incised plate urethroplasty. In this technique, the urethral plate is preserved; aggressive and meticulous degloving of the foreskin is carried out beyond the hypospadiac meatus into the scrotum, thus, achieving in many cases, significant correction of the ventral curvature. Then, an artificial erection is induced and, if needed, additional ventral penile curvature correction is accomplished with a dorsal plication, placing one or two 5/0 Prolene stitches at the 12 o'clock position dorsally, at the point of maximum angulation. In patients with a persistent, greater than 30° ventral penile curvature, the urethral plate can be dissected and elevated from the corpora cavernosa up to normal urethra, and if needed the correction can be enhanced with three transverse corporotomies, placing the first one at the point of maximal bending. The authors perform the urethroplasty in two layers, the first with interrupted subcuticular stitches of 7/0 PDS, followed by a second running layer of the same material. The suture line should be covered with a well-vascularized dartos flap harvested from the dorsal prepuce, or with a tunica vaginalis flap.

If the urethral plate cannot be preserved, a multistage repair is indicated. A dermal graft is harvested from a non-hair bearing donor site, defatted and placed in normal saline solution. A transverse corporotomy is made at the point of maximal concavity and the dermal graft is sutured to the edges of the defect. The second stage, composite repair, is performed between six and nine months later, using an anterior tubularized incised plate urethroplasty combined with a posterior Thiersch–Duplay procedure (tubularization of local skin to fashion the neourethra). Also, the use of a buccal mucosa graft or an onlay island flap gives satisfactory results at this stage.

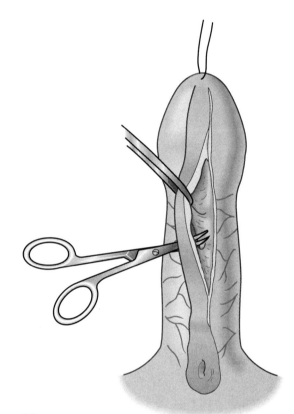

17

Penoscrotal transposition

18, 19a–f Partial or complete penoscrotal transposition is often found in cases with penoscrotal and perineal hypospadias. The least severe forms are known as bifid scrotum, prepenile scrotum, and shawl scrotum. The scrotoplasty should be delayed until after the hypospadias repair is completed, because the base of the flaps needed for the hypospadias repair must be divided and displaced during correction of the prepenile scrotum. Six months or more should elapse between the urethroplasty and repositioning of the scrotum. This anomaly is repaired by displacing scrotal skin posteriorly and the penis anteriorly. The base of the penis is advanced forward onto the anterior abdominal wall by creating a square, distally based flap, which circumscribes the base of the penis. The flap is dropped distally to restore normal scrotal length. The abdominal wall is then undermined and swung around the base of the penis to join ventrally in the midline. It is important to mobilize the anterior abdominal wall flaps sufficiently so that midline separation does not occur.

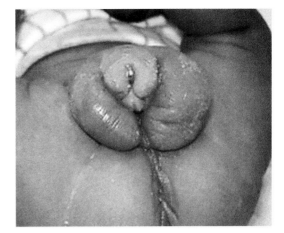

18

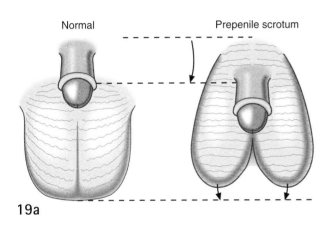

19a

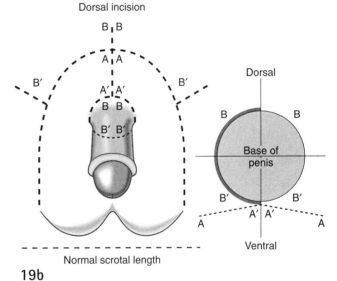

19b

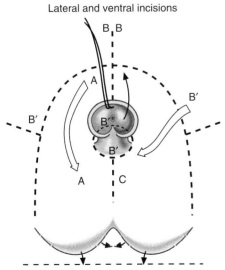

Scrotum to be lengthened and bifid scrotum to be corrected

19c

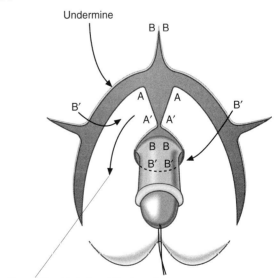

Prepenile skin to be shifted caudad

19d

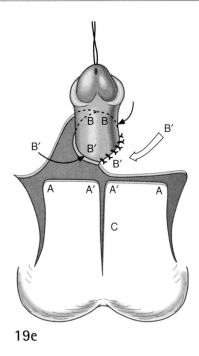

19e

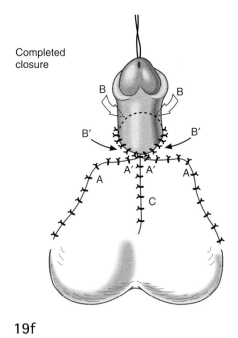

Completed
closure

19f

Removal of retained Müllerian ducts and creation of neoseminal vesicle

20   In patients with severe hypospadias, ovotesticular disease, or mixed gonadal dysgenesis who have been assigned the male gender, the retained Müllerian ducts can become quite enlarged leading to recurrent urinary tract infections, epididymo-orchitis, urinary retention, secondary incontinence due to urine trapping, and infertility. Also, malignant transformation has been reported. In cases with these complications, the Müllerian duct remnant may have been removed.

Surgical treatment of Müllerian duct remnants is challenging, because of their close proximity to the ejaculatory ducts, pelvic nerves, rectum, vas deferens, and ureters. A number of surgical approaches have been described, including transperitoneal, posterior with rectal retraction, anterior and posterior saggital transrectal, transtrigonal, perineal, transurethral fulguration, laparoscopic and robotic. The authors have successfully used the transtrigonal technique; however, the laparoscopic or robotic-assisted procedures are less invasive and minimize possible damage to adjacent anatomical structures. The case corresponding to illustration 20 was successfully operated by a robotic-assisted laparoscopic procedure.

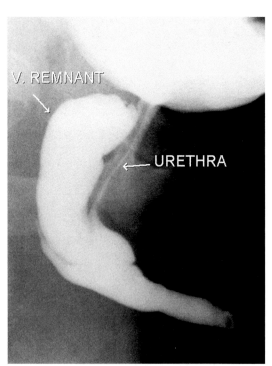

20

21a–c In males with retained Müllerian ducts, the vas deferens often lies within the sidewall of the dilated vagina; its course, however, cannot usually be palpated in the thickened vaginal wall, therefore a strip of vagina surrounding the predicted course of the vas from its entrance to its termination with the urethra is preserved while the uterus and the remainder of the vagina are resected. The vaginal strip is turned in and tubularized from the proximal vas to the point of union with the urethra using interrupted sutures of 5/0 Vicryl. If the vas courses in the wall of the uterus, it is not possible to perform this procedure.

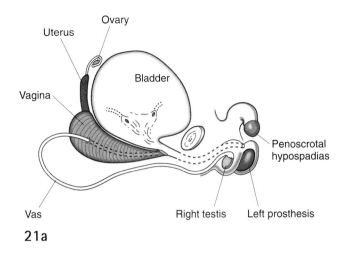

21a

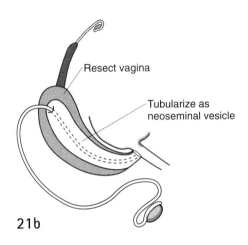

21b

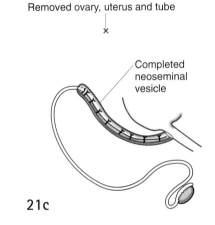

21c

Penile agenesis

22 Penile agenesis occurs in 1 in 30 million births. It appears to be the result of a development failure of the genital tubercle during the fourth week of embryogenesis; the scrotum appears normal and contains normal testicles. Patients can present with an imperforate anus and a rectourethral fistula, with a normal anus and a rectourethral fistula, or with the urethra located in the perineum inside a skin tag resembling a foreskin. Patients are otherwise normal 46,XY males.

In the past, gender reassignment was the most frequent choice for these patients. Initial surgical treatment of female assigned patients requires bilateral orchiectomy. Cases with an associated imperforate anus and rectourethral fistula need an urgent colostomy and a vesicostomy. Children assigned to the female sex require the creation of a neovagina, which is most frequently performed with a sleeve of sigmoid colon. However, some patients have been unhappy with the assigned female sex, and prefer to be males.

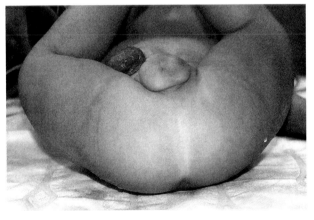

22

23 The diagnostic evaluation of patients with penile agenesis includes a renal ultrasound, pelvic MRI, retrograde urethrogram, and in cases associated with an imperforate anus, a distal colonogram through the mucous fistula, using hydrosoluble contrast material. The colonogram can be combined with an antegrade VCUG via the cutaneous vesicostomy. An experienced medical team must evaluate newborns with penile agenesis. Families must be given all available information regarding sex assignment, surgical procedures, and immediate and long-term results so they can make a decision, which is in the best interest of their child.

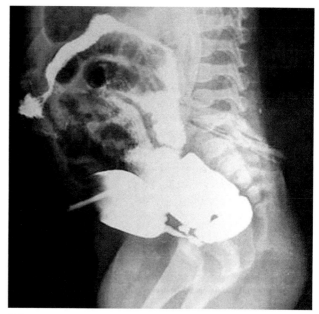

23

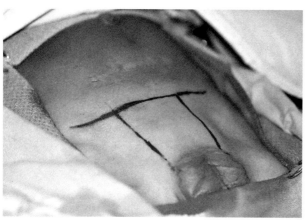

24a

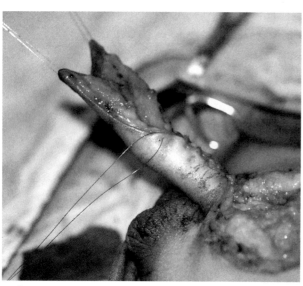

24b

24a–c In adolescents and adults, the most frequently used phalloplasty procedure is the radial forearm flap, which is a complex and rare operation, performed only in highly specialized centers. The description by De Castro of a phalloplasty technique and complete urethroplasty using a quadrangle lower abdominal flap can bridge the interval between childhood and adolescence until a more definitive procedure can be performed. The quadrangle of lower abdominal flap fashioned to create the new penis is 4 × 5 cm for babies, and slightly larger in an older child to fashion the new penis. De Castro recommends the use of oral or bladder mucosa for the urethroplasty, although the single stage buccal mucosa urethroplasty has had a high complication rate.

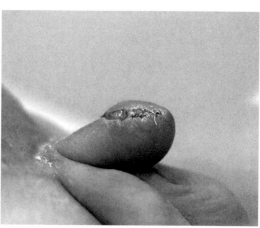

24c

The authors are in favor of staging the surgical reconstruction. As mentioned before, cases with an imperforate anus and a rectourethral fistula require an urgent colostomy with a mucous fistula and a vesicostomy, followed a few months later by a posterior saggital rectourethral pull-through, with subsequent closure of both the vesicostomy and colostomy. Patients born with a normal anus and a rectourethral fistula can be operated through a transperineal approach using a hyperextended position. The authors have used the quadrangle lower abdominal flap to fashion the neopenis in three patients, but prefer a two-stage buccal mucosa urethroplasty to avoid or minimize complications.

Vaginal agenesis

Vaginal agenesis is known as the Mayer–Rokitansky–Kuster–Hauser syndrome, it is a rare abnormality affecting approximately 1 in 5000–10 000 females. In this condition, there is absence of the proximal portion of the vagina, resulting from failure of the sinovaginal bulbs to develop and form the vaginal plate.

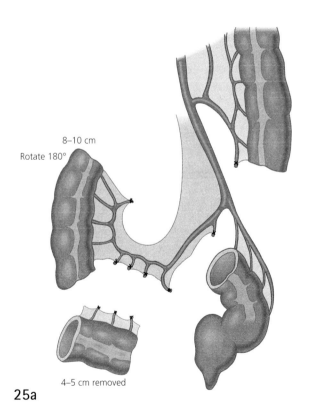

8–10 cm

Rotate 180°

4–5 cm removed

25a

This condition can be discovered at birth when the examination does not reveal a vaginal opening, but most cases present with primary amenorrhea. A small group of patients with imperforate anus will have vaginal agenesis, and each of the females requires inspection of the vaginal orifice prior to proceeding with definitive pull-through. Few patients complain of dyspareunia or failed intercourse. Physical examination reveals an absent vagina, but the hymen and a distal vaginal dimple or even an introitus are present, because these structures are derived from the urogenital sinus. The diagnosis can be confirmed by pelvic ultrasound and MRI.

SURGICAL TREATMENT OF VAGINAL AGENESIS

Vaginal dilatation is an alternative in patients with a generous vaginal dimple or introitus. A program of daily, graduated, dilatations over several months, using Hegar or similar sounds can result in a good-size vagina to allow intercourse. Once a satisfactory vaginal size is obtained, regular sexual intercourse maintains an adequate vaginal cavity.

25a–b Different techniques for vaginal construction in patients with vaginal agenesis have been used, including the construction of a skin neovagina, and the creation of an intestinal neovagina using sigmoid, cecum, and small intestine. Our preferred technique for vaginal replacement is the use of a 10-cm segment of distal sigmoid colon based on the left colic or superior hemorrhoidal vessels. Mechanical and antibiotic bowel preparation must be done before the procedure. A lower transverse abdominal incision gives adequate exposure. A supine position with legs spread and the knees slightly bent, using Allen stirrups is recommended. The sleeve of sigmoid is selected between non-crushing clamps; a short distal sigmoid segment can be discarded to increase the length on the mesenteric vasculature for the neovagina. The sigmoid sleeve can be rotated 180° to allow placement in the perineum. The proximal end is closed with two layers of absorbable suture material. Either a cruciate or H-shaped large perineal opening is made; the rectovesical space is dissected to create a large tunnel that will allow the easy introduction of two fingers in the perineum. The sigmoid segment is pulled through the perineal channel and anastomosed directly to the perineum with absorbable sutures. Two-point fixation between the proximal end of the neovagina and the presacral fascia prevents prolapse of the bowel. The authors do not elevate the proximal vaginal dimple into the cul-de-sac to perform the anastomosis, because in our experience, it results in a higher frequency of strictures. Alternatively, a laparoscopic-assisted procedure can be done with a satisfactory outcome.

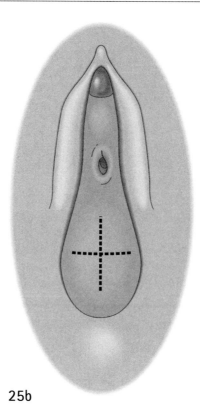

25b

The creation of a sigmoid neovagina has several advantages, such as natural lubrication without excessive mucous production; long-term use of a stent is avoided, stenosis is infrequent, and most patients have normal sexual intercourse.

SUMMARY

The surgical treatment of disorders of sex development should be undertaken by experienced surgeons who must be familiar with all the available techniques, so satisfactory repairs can be performed either to support the male or female gender. The treatment plan must be thoroughly discussed with parents, with the goal of giving the child, thereafter, the most satisfactory quality of life possible. However, long-term studies are needed to assess the functional and sensory outcomes of newer surgical techniques.

ACKNOWLEDGMENTS

The authors would like to acknowledge that they received written authorization from Elsevier to reproduce the following figures from Chapter 123 (Disorders of sexual development, by Rafael V Pieretti and Patricia K Donahoe) in *Pediatric Surgery* (2011): Figure 123.4a,b; Figure 123.6a,b; Figure 123.7; Figure 123.8; Figure 123.9; Figure 123.10a,b; Figure 123.11; Figure 123.12; Figure 123.13; Figure 123.14a–c; Figure 123.15a,b; Figure 123.16a–c; Figure 123.17a–h; Figure 123.19; Figure 123.22a–c;

Figure 123.25a–c; Figure 123.24; Figure 123.26a,b; Figure 123.27. In addition, the authors obtained authorization to use, modify, and adapt some paragraphs from the basic science and the surgical treatment sections of Chapter 123.

FURTHER READING

Baskin LS, Erol A, Li YW *et al.* Anatomical studies of the human clitoris. *Journal of Urology* 1999; **162**: 1015–20.

De Castro R, Merlini E, Rigamonti W, Macedo A Jr. Phalloplasty and urethroplasty in children with penile agenesis: preliminary report. *Journal of Urology* 2007; **177**: 1112–16; discussion 1117.

Donahoe PK, Schnitzer JJ, Pieretti RV. Ambiguous genitalia in the newborn. In: O'Neill JA, Rowe ML, Grosfeld JL *et al.* (eds). *Pediatric Surgery*, 6th edn. St Louis: Mosby-Year Book, 2005: 1911–34.

Ludwikowski B, Oesch Hayward I, Gonzalez R. Total urogenital sinus mobilization: expanded applications. *BJU International*1999; **83**: 820–2.

MacLaughlin DT, Donahoe PK. Sex determination and differentiation. *New England Journal of Medicine* 2004; **350**: 367–78.

Peña A. Total urogenital mobilization-an easier way to repair cloacas. *Journal of Pediatric Surgery* 1997; **32**: 263–7; discussion 267–8.

Rink RC, Metcalfe PD, Kaefer MA *et al.* Partial urogenital mobilization: a limited proximal dissection. *Journal of Pediatric Urology* 2006; **2**: 351–6.

97

Ovarian cyst and tumors

BRYAN J DICKEN and DEBORAH F BILLMIRE

PRINCIPLES

Ovarian cysts are relatively common and should be regarded as a separate entity from cystic ovarian neoplasms when considering surgical management. Follicular cysts are not neoplastic and are sensitive to hormonal stimulation. For clarity, ovarian cysts and neoplasms will be discussed separately.

NON-NEOPLASTIC CYSTS

Neonatal ovarian cysts

Neonatal ovarian cysts arise from maternal estrogen or human gonadotropin. The majority are of no clinical significance and will resolve spontaneously within three to four months. The risks of torsion and/or hemorrhage cannot be predicted on the basis of size.

Simple cysts are completely anechoic with a thin wall on ultrasound. They may be followed with serial ultrasound unless symptomatic due to large size. Cyst aspiration is associated with high recurrence rates and carries the risk of inducing hemorrhage. Surgical management by open or laparoscopic technique is preferred for symptomatic cases, and consists of fenestration or unroofing.

1a,b Complex ovarian cysts have undergone hemorrhage and are heterogeneous with internal septa and fluid-debris levels. Most are asymptomatic and resolve spontaneously with preserved ovarian function. As with simple cysts, surgical treatment should emphasize preservation of ovarian parenchyma. Open or laparoscopic detorsion, if present, with unroofing or fenestration of the cyst wall is indicated.

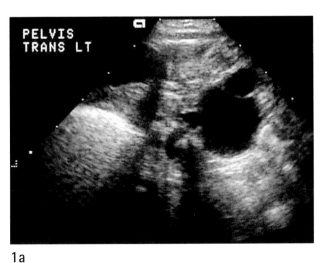

1a

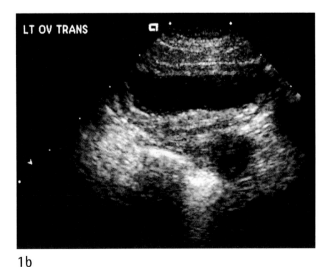

1b

Ovarian cysts beyond the neonatal period

Beyond the neonatal period, follicular cysts are detected most often after puberty.

Females presenting with precocious puberty, vaginal bleeding, and an ovarian cyst should prompt a pediatric endocrinology consultation to exclude McCune–Albright syndrome. This is a sporadic disorder associated with autonomous estrogen-producing ovarian cysts that resolve spontaneously. Children usually present between one and five years of age with vaginal bleeding. This disorder is most frequently confused with an ovarian tumor, such as a juvenile granulosa cell tumor, resulting in unnecessary surgery.

Follicular cysts may be asymptomatic or present with pain due to large size, hemorrhage, or torsion. Most simple cysts will resolve spontaneously within three to four menstrual cycles. Indications for surgical intervention include persistent symptoms, pain, or evidence of torsion. As with neonatal non-neoplastic cysts, emphasis should be placed on ovarian parenchyma-preserving procedures.

Preoperative assessment

Ultrasound is the preferred initial modality for characterizing ovarian lesions. Simple cysts can be distinguished from neoplastic cysts and blood flow to the ovary can be determined. Serial examinations can be done for asymptomatic cysts. With precocious puberty, estrogen levels should be measured. Ultrasound findings suggestive of neoplasm require further work up as described within the ovarian neoplasm section.

OPERATIVE PROCEDURES FOR NON-NEOPLASTIC OVARIAN CYSTS

Anesthesia

General endotracheal anesthesia with muscle relaxation is required. For both open and laparoscopic procedures, decompression of the bladder with a Foley catheter is recommended to provide optimal access to the pelvis. For laparoscopic procedures, orogastric decompression is also recommended.

Laparotomy for non-neoplastic ovarian cysts

2 A low transverse incision on the side of the lesion is convenient. The cyst is delivered through the incision. A tense cyst may be needle aspirated to facilitate grasping and delivery through a smaller incision. The ovary is inspected to locate the normal parenchyma and pedicle. The cyst may be enucleated if a plane is easily developed without injury to the ovarian parenchyma.

Alternatively, the free margin of the cyst wall is excised with cautery. The ovary is returned to the peritoneal cavity after confirming hemostasis. The fascia is closed, followed by subcuticular skin closure.

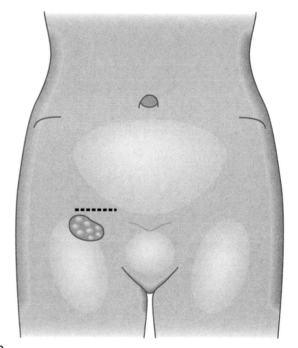

2

Laparoscopy for non-neoplastic cysts

3 For laparoscopic cases, a 5-mm umbilical port is placed for insufflation and inspection with the camera. This may be upsized to a 10- or 12-mm port if necessary to facilitate utilization of a retrieval bag. Two additional 5-mm trocars are placed for grasping and manipulation. Placement of the working ports is best dictated by the ability to triangulate the lesion. In general, this involves a suprapubic port and a contralateral lower quadrant port. Transabdominal aspiration under direct vision with a long 18-gauge spinal needle may allow the cyst to be grasped more securely. A portion of the cyst wall is excised with hook cautery to create an adequate fenestration.

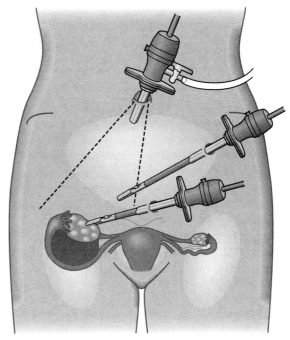

3

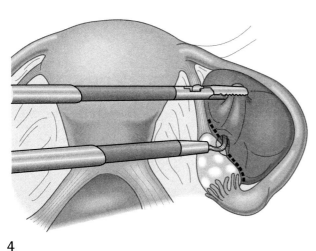

4

4 When the cyst is clearly demarcated from the ovarian parenchyma, cyst enucleation is the best option. This can be done with a hook cautery or Ligasure (Covidien, Mansfield, MA, USA). The peritoneum is incised circumferentially to demarcate the cyst attachment to the underlying parenchyma. The cyst is then easily enucleated. Occasionally, laparoscopy for presumed ovarian pathology reveals a paratubal cyst. These are remnants of the paramesonephric duct. They may lie within the leaves of the mesosalpinx or as a pedunculated cyst near the fimbria, and may have evidence of torsion. These lesions may be resected, enucleated, or unroofed.

Surgical therapy for ovarian torsion

5 Ovarian torsion may occur with a normal ovary, ovarian cyst, or ovarian tumor. Ultrasound frequently demonstrates multiple small peripherally located, uniform cysts in the involved ovary. This appearance arises secondary to displaced follicles, due to venous congestion and edema. Color Doppler may reveal absence of arterial flow. A twisted pedicle may also be seen. In cases involving simple cysts, management of the cyst with ovarian preservation is the goal of therapy. Since it is not possible to differentiate benign from malignant lesions in the acute setting of torsion, the principles of ovarian preservation are still valid. If a neoplasm is present, management should be as directed in the section on ovarian neoplasm below. In the absence of evidence of neoplasm, it is preferable to untwist the ovary, and consider oophoropexy to allow resolution of inflammation and edema. This can be accomplished by detorsion, then fixation of the ovary with absorbable suture through the tunica of the ovarian pole to the adjacent utero-ovarian ligament, or to the psoas tendon. Care must be exercised to identify the ureter prior to suture fixation. Patients should be followed by close postoperative surveillance of the ovary with ultrasound in 6–8 weeks.

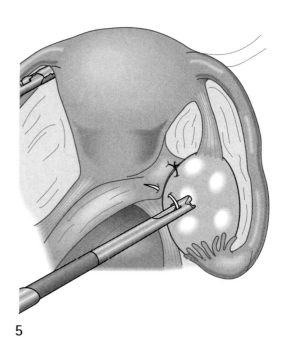

5

OVARIAN NEOPLASMS

Ovarian neoplasms often have a cystic component. The overall risk of malignancy for ovarian neoplasms in children and adolescents is approximately 20 percent. Pelvic ultrasound, although useful in confirming the presence of neoplasm, is not helpful in determining pathologic nature. There are no gross characteristics that clearly distinguish benign from malignant neoplasms and therefore it is best to approach all ovarian neoplasms as if malignancy may be present.

Ultrasound findings suspicious for neoplasm should also be evaluated by computed tomography (CT) scan to assess for adenopathy, hepatic involvement, and presence of tumor elsewhere within the peritoneal cavity. Tumor markers alfa fetoprotein (AFP) and beta-human chorionic gonadotropin (β-HCG) should be determined preoperatively. AFP is elevated in tumors that contain the malignant germ cell element endodermal sinus tumor and β-HCG is elevated in tumors that contain the malignant element choriocarcinoma.

Although elevated tumor markers are associated with malignancy, they may be normal in up to 45 percent of malignant pediatric ovarian masses. Epithelial-based tumors may have elevation of CA125.

OPERATION FOR OVARIAN NEOPLASM

At present, there is insufficient evidence to support laparoscopic management of ovarian tumors with features to suggest malignancy. The available data, primarily from the adult literature, suggest the incidence of tumor rupture is unacceptably higher in the laparoscopy (65–100 percent) group versus the laparotomy (5–10 percent) group, for both oophorectomy and for enucleation. The risk of malignancy in pediatric ovarian neoplasms and the ability to complete a full staging procedure make an open approach preferable in most cases.

Laparotomy for ovarian neoplasms

The choice of incision depends on the size of the lesion and the surgeon's preference. In general, a lesion with a diameter less than the span of the iliac crests may be successfully approached by a transverse incision in the lowest skin crease, or a muscle-sparing Pfannenstiel incision. Lesions exceeding this size will best be approached by a midline incision. The procedure should then follow a systematic assessment, as follows.

PERITONEAL CYTOLOGY

Immediately upon entering the peritoneal cavity, any fluid in the pelvis should be aspirated for ascitic cytology. If no fluid is present, pelvic washing should be done with normal saline.

INSPECTION OF THE OVARY

The involved ovary should be inspected for resectability.

COMPLETE ABDOMINOPELVIC EVALUATION

The remaining staging maneuvers should then be completed for all neoplastic lesions. These include:

- Inspection and palpation of the omentum, with removal of any abnormal areas.

- Inspection and palpation of the retroperitoneal lymph nodes from the iliac chains up along the aorta and vena cava, at least as far as the renal pedicle. Any enlarged or firm nodes should be biopsied.
- Inspection of the pelvic and visceral peritoneal surfaces with biopsy of any abnormal areas.
- Inspection and palpation of the contralateral ovary with enucleation of any abnormal masses. It is not necessary or recommended to bisect a normal appearing contralateral ovary.
- In the context of epithelial (mucinous) tumors, an appendectomy should be considered at the time of surgery.

Management of the ovarian mass

ENUCLEATION OF OVARIAN MASS

6 Enucleation of ovarian neoplasms may be considered for smaller masses with normal markers and a clear dissection plane from normal ovarian tissue, or in patients with bilateral suspected neoplasms with visible residual normal parenchyma. If no visible dissection plane is seen on the capsule, but a focal mass lesion can be felt, the ovarian cortex is incised to expose the border between the parenchyma and the mass. Dissection should remain outside the capsule of the neoplasm with care not to rupture it. The ovarian capsule edges may be reapproximated with absorbable suture to minimize raw surface area.

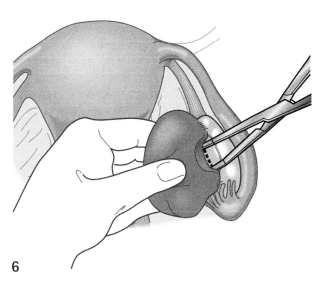

6

OOPHERECTOMY

If the tumor markers are elevated or there is no demarcation between normal ovary and neoplasm, oophorectomy should be undertaken. In most cases, the Fallopian tube is not involved and may be spared.

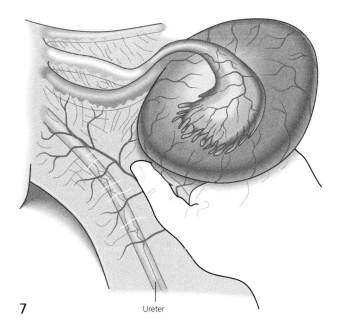

7   Ureter

7 With large tumors, the leaves of the mesovarium are widely splayed and the Fallopian tube may be draped over the mass. The peritoneum of the mesovarium is incised in an avascular plane between the tube and ovary with cautery dissection. This maneuver will expose the vascular pedicle of the ovary. If the tumor is large, the venous plexus is often engorged and the pedicle may need to be taken in stepwise fashion with pairs of clamps, division of the tissue, and ligation. The assistant should maintain manual compression of the pedicle as the dissection proceeds. If the tube is adherent, it may be taken in continuity with the ovary. Caution should be taken to clearly identify the ureter before proceeding with division of the mesosalpinx.

BIOPSY

If the lesion is invading the uterus or adjacent pelvic structures, it should not be resected at the primary operation. A biopsy for tissue diagnosis should be done with a plan for later resection after chemotherapy. Chemotherapy is highly successful in producing shrinkage of tumors to allow later resection without sacrifice of uterus or other pelvic structures.

POSTOPERATIVE CARE

Regardless of approach chosen, the Foley catheter can generally be removed immediately after the procedure for small- to moderate-sized lesions and rapid advancement of diet is tolerated. For large lesions requiring a generous incision, it may be more comfortable for the patient to leave the Foley catheter in place for 24 hours. If a large tumor requiring a generous incision is present, supplemental epidural catheter for postoperative pain management should be considered.

OUTCOME

Fenestration for non-neoplastic cysts has excellent outcome with minimal long-term consequences. Malignant germ cell tumors are treated with platinum-based multiagent chemotherapy. Survival with current regimens is greater than 90 percent at five years.

All neoplastic lesions, whether benign or malignant, have some risk of contralateral recurrence. These patients should undergo periodic ultrasound surveillance to allow detection of new lesions at an early stage so that an ovary-sparing procedure may be undertaken with greater chance of success in preserving endocrine function and fertility. Tumors with positive markers should be followed with postoperative serum markers to help detect recurrence. Epithelial malignant neoplasms should adhere to adult treatment and follow-up protocols due to the rare nature of these tumors.

FURTHER READING

Billmire D, Vinocur C, Rescorla F *et al.* Outcome and staging evaluation in malignant germ cell tumors of the ovary in children and adolescents: an intergroup study. *Journal of Pediatric Surgery* 2004; **39**: 424–9.

Brandt ML, Helmrath MA. Ovarian cysts in infants and children. *Seminars in Pediatric Surgery* 2005; **14**: 78–85.

Chang HC, Bhatt S, Dogra VS. Pearls and pitfalls in diagnosis of ovarian torsion. *Radiographics* 2008; **28**: 1355–68.

Morowitz M, Huff S, von Allmen D. Epithelial ovarian tumors in children: a retrospective analysis. *Journal of Pediatric Surgery* 2003; **38**: 331–5.

Nabhan ZM, West KW, Eugster EA. Oopherectomy in McCune–Albright syndrome: a case of mistaken identity. *Journal of Pediatric Surgery* 2007; **42**: 1578–83.

Song T, Choi CH, Lee Y-Y *et al.* Pediatric borderline ovarian tumors: a retrospective analysis. *Journal of Pediatric Surgery* 2010; **45**: 1955–9.

98

Myelomeningocele

KARIN M MURASZKO and SHAWN L HERVEY-JUMPER

PRINCIPLES AND JUSTIFICATION

Myelomeningocele is the most severe of the spinal dysraphic states and still the most common, although its incidence is decreasing with improved prenatal maternal nutrition and through the availability of prenatal screening mechanisms. Myelomeningocele is a central nervous system fusion defect. Neural tube defects affect both men and woman and have a slight female preponderance. There have been clusters of increased incidence of myelomeningocele in certain populations, such as the Irish, British, Sikhs, Guatemalans, and the Egyptians of Alexandria. Siblings of an affected child have an increased risk of neural tube defects when compared with the general population. The rate of recurrence ranges from about 1 percent to nearly 10 percent in different series. A clear correlation between maternal diet and neural tube defects has been determined. A seven-fold reduction in neural tube defects has been achieved with folate and vitamin supplementation before and during pregnancy.

Embryology

The central nervous system begins as a focal proliferation of ectoderm. The central groove develops and forms two folds of neural tissue. At approximately gestational day 20–28, the lips of this fold touch and the neural tube fuses. Starting at the center, the fusion of this fold eventually becomes the craniovertebral junction. This fusion proceeds in a caudal and cephalic direction. The caudal section is the last to close. A plane develops between the neural ectoderm that has fused the overlying superficial ectoderm. Between these layers migrate mesenchymal cells, which give rise to the arch of the vertebrae and the paraspinal muscles. Myelomeningocele represents a failure of fusion of the neural fold, leaving the vertebral arches open and the unfused spinal cord or neural placode either exposed or covered by a thin membrane. It is important to distinguish a myelomeningocele from less severe defects such as meningoceles, which consist only of a spinal fluid-filled sac with meningeal and cutaneous coverings. Meningoceles contain no spinal elements, but can occasionally contain some nerve roots. True meningoceles are rare. Lipomyelomeningoceles are usually covered by well-developed dermal elements and fat, and consist of spina bifida with associated abnormalities of the spinal cord and extension of fat into the spinal canal.

Associated problems

Like most congenital anomalies, spina bifida is a spectrum of disorders. Myelomeningocele represents the most severe of these spinal dysraphic states and includes anomalies of the brain such as the Chiari II malformation and hydrocephalus. It has implications for other organs, such as those of the genitourinary and musculoskeletal systems. Most children with myelomeningocele have some degree of weakness of their lower extremities and many have significant orthopedic problems. As a result of denervation, muscle imbalance ensues and can result in abnormalities at the hip, knee, and foot. Anesthesia of various portions of the skin can lead to pressure sores, particularly later in life. Anorectal neuropathy may cause a variety of defecatory dysfunctions.

Urologic abnormalities are common in children with myelomeningocele and are best managed with intermittent catheterization. Careful follow up with evaluation of the kidney and bladder function is extremely important.

The cornerstone of the management of children with myelomeningocele is a multidisciplinary team that treats and assesses the various needs of both the child and the family. The development of cerebrospinal fluid (CSF) diversionary devices (shunts) in the 1950s has allowed these children to be successfully managed and has dramatically changed the outlook for them. More recently, endoscopic techniques have been developed that allow more physiologic diversionary procedures of the CSF (third ventriculostomy) and these have also been used successfully in children with myelomeningocele. Such physiological diversionary procedures may be particularly important in that they eliminate the need for a mechanical device.

Selection criteria

The controversial discussion about the selection of children for myelomeningocele repair has largely subsided, as more effective means of diagnosis and treatment have been developed. Before the development of successful methods of treating hydrocephalus, selection of candidates for non-treatment was commonly practiced. With shunting devices available, the cognitive outcome for these children has significantly improved and, in most cases, children with myelomeningocele receive early repair. Although discussion among various groups, including ethicists, clerics, jurists, administrators, legislators, and physicians, still continues, most children now receive repair of their myelomeningocele and are treated by a team with a variety of specialists. At best, selection criteria related to which children should not be repaired are inconsistent. Studies that discuss the outcome of such unrepaired children must be viewed cautiously, as many who were initially not treated received later repair, and not all who were left unrepaired died, as had been anticipated. The ease of care of children with myelomeningocele is greatly improved following repair, and thus even chronic care facilities often will not accept children with open defects. Unless associated additional central nervous system defects or other congenital anomalies are of such magnitude as to suggest that meaningful survival is unlikely, repair of myelomeningocele in children is now considered a standard of practice.

PREOPERATIVE

Assessment

The principles involved in the repair of myelomeningocele in children consist initially of a complete evaluation of the child, including detailed physical and neurologic examination. Ultrasonographic imaging of the head, spine above and below the area of the defect, and kidneys can be an important adjuvant to constructing a surgical plan for an individual child. If there are many associated intracranial or spinal anomalies on ultrasonic examination, computed tomography (CT) scanning or magnetic resonance imaging (MRI) should be performed to evaluate these abnormalities more carefully. Radiographs of the spine can identify additional anomalies such as diastematomyelia, which may require repair at the time of the initial surgery. Blood should be crossmatched and available. Consideration of

the timing of surgery must also include assessment of underlying medical issues. The decision as to whether a diversionary procedure for the CSF is necessary at the time of the initial repair must also be made.

Preparation

Infants born with myelomeningocele require the skilled services of a multidisciplinary team. After initial determination of cardiorespiratory stability, and any underlying infections, the child may be transferred to an appropriate institution. The lesion itself should be covered with moist, sterile gauze dressings surrounded by a protective plastic sheet. The use of sponges impregnated with bacitracin ointment covered by a thin plastic layer is recommended to prevent additional skin breakdown. Alternatively, sterile saline-soaked sponges may also be appropriately applied to the myelomeningocele placode.

Emergency operative intervention is seldom necessary in neonates with myelomeningocele; the repair can be safely carried out within the first 48–72 hours after delivery. Delaying closure for more prolonged periods may increase the risk of central nervous system infection and may decrease motor function by increasing the trauma to the exposed neural placode. In one study, deterioration of motor function occurred in children left untreated, and a 37 percent incidence of ventriculitis was found in children in whom repair was delayed, while other studies have found no difference in ventriculitis among newborns based on the time of back closure. The use of broad-spectrum prophylactic antibiotics before back closure has also been an area of debate. Though there is currently no standard among all treating physicians, some studies suggest that prophylactic broad-spectrum antibiotic treatment is effective at minimizing the risk of ventriculitis in newborns undergoing surgery after 48 hours.

Most myelomeningoceles are in the lumbosacral region, although they can occur anywhere along the spinal cord. Assessment with good spinal ultrasonography can help alert the surgeon to associated abnormalities such as diastematomyelia, arachnoid cysts, and intradural masses such as dermoids, which may complicate the repair of the myelomeningocele.

If significant hydrocephalus is found in the preoperative cranial ultrasound, either shunting or a diversionary procedure of CSF, such as endoscopic third ventriculostomy, should be considered. If ventriculomegaly is mild to moderate, such a diversionary procedure may not be performed at the same time as the myelomeningocele repair, but may be delayed. A significant proportion of children with myelomeningocele will require shunting in the first days of life. This number has ranged from 60 to 80 percent of children with myelomeningocele. It should also be noted that there may be an increased risk of leakage from the repair site in those children in whom shunting is delayed.

Anesthesia

General endotracheal anesthesia with overhead warming lights is appropriate. Occasionally, intraoperative use of a nerve stimulator is necessary to distinguish functional nerve roots; so paralytic agents must be used appropriately and no longer be present when stimulation is planned.

Intravenous lines must be of sufficient size to accommodate blood transfusion. Careful assessment of blood loss is necessary, as blood loss can be significant, particularly when rotational flaps are employed. A Foley catheter is generally used for bladder drainage and proves to be a useful adjunct in keeping the repair site clean and dry during the postoperative period.

OPERATION

Position of the patient

1 Repair of the myelomeningocele is performed with the child in the prone position. Careful attention to the position of the neck is important, as almost all children with myelomeningocele have a Chiari II malformation and most will also have some aspect of hydrocephalus. Head size may occasionally be quite large in such children. Positioning of the head must therefore be done in such a way as to avoid kinking of the internal jugular veins and undue extension or flexion of the cervical spine. The abdomen must be hanging free so that intra-abdominal pressure is not increased. Increases in intra-abdominal pressure lead to compression of Batson's venous plexus and result in increased engorgement and bleeding from epidural veins. The author has found that a foam-rubber donut that has been cut out at the top and the bottom acts as an excellent bolster. Various bolsters and rolls have been employed, with the goal always to allow the abdomen to be hanging free. Careful attention to positioning of the upper extremities to avoid brachial plexus stretching injury is also necessary. The lower extremities also require careful positioning and padding, as congenital dislocations of the hips and multiple orthopedic anomalies may be present and they make such positioning quite difficult.

The central neural placode and membranous areas are cleansed with sterile saline. The surrounding areas of skin are cleansed with an iodinated solution; iodinated solutions should not be applied directly to the neural placode. Most surgeons find magnifying loupes useful in further repair of such myelomeningoceles. Occasionally, the operating microscope can also be of benefit. Bipolar electrocoagulation should be available, as it is employed throughout the procedure to control bleeding.

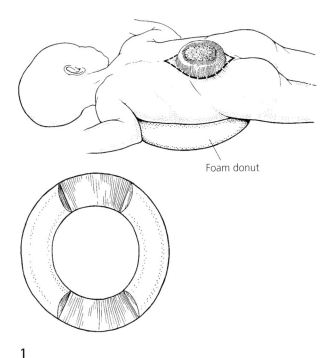

Foam donut

1

Freeing the neural placode

2 Dissection of the neural placode begins at the lateral aspect of the placode at the junction of the zona epitheliosa and the edge of the hemangiomatous skin (zona cutanea). This can be done with sharp iris scissors or tenotomy scissors. A significant amount of yellowish CSF will egress when the sack is opened, which deflates the cystic portion of the myelomeningocele sac. At this point, careful inspection of the interior of the sac is necessary.

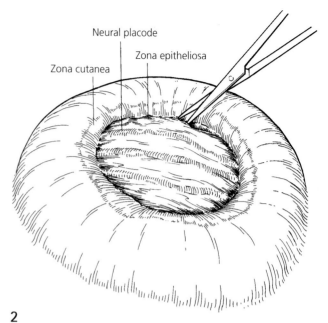

2

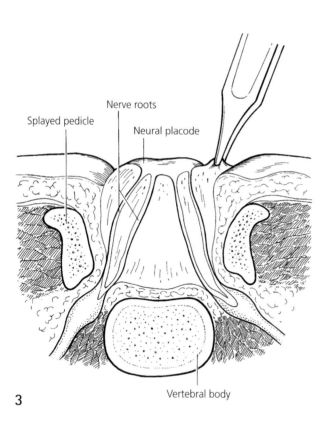

3

3 Examination of the contents of the sac demonstrates that the floor of the sac is formed by the glistening white dura, which is adherent to the surrounding fat and mesodermal elements. Medially, nerve roots can be seen passing from the neural placode down to the spinal canal, which is also flattened relative to a normal canal.

The sharp dissection is carried out on either side and then completed at the cephalic and caudal ends. It should be noted that at the upper end the placode is nearly a normal spinal cord and is invested by normal arachnoid and dura and has the typical cylindrical shape of the spinal cord.

At the upper end of the neural placode, filamentous adhesions may bind the cord/placode to the dura. These should be carefully divided. Dissection of the placode from the zona epitheliosa and the hemangiomatous skin edges is important and it is here that magnification proves to be particularly useful.

Dissection is most difficult at the cephalic and caudal portions of the placode, as there are usually multiple adhesions to both the dura and the surrounding skin. Occasionally, additional laminectomies and dural opening are necessary to achieve adequate exposure of the spinal cord to free adhesions. An important goal of myelomeningocele closure is the untethering of the neural placode, as well as repair of the skin and dural defects. Freeing of these adhesions allows the cord to slide more gently within the dural sac. Particularly at the most distal portion of the placode, there may be a very prominent fibrous band, which is a form of filum terminale.

Inspection of the internal contents should include a check for fibrocartilaginous or bony spurs near the level of the first intact lamina. Such spurs, often seen on preoperative radiographs, suggest a narrowed intervertebral space if a vertebral body anomaly is seen or if a midline septum is seen on ultrasonographic examination. A laminectomy at one or two levels above this level may be necessary to visualize and deal with such septae adequately. Adhesion of the terminal portion of the placode can be quite dense. Where there are significant fibrous bands, use of a nerve stimulator can often help to distinguish these bands from functioning neural tissue.

Placement of the neural placode back into the spinal canal

4 The edges of the neural placode should be carefully inspected to be certain that there are no dermal elements included in the placode. Pieces of the membranous tissue of the zona epitheliosa and thin parchment skin from the zona cutanea should be sharply debrided from the edges of the placode. The placode, if completely freed of adhesions, should rest within the spinal canal.

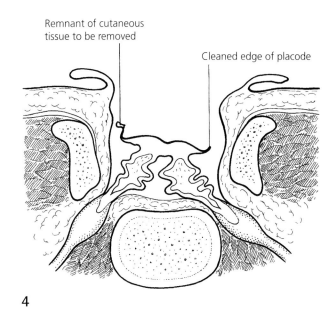

Remnant of cutaneous tissue to be removed

Cleaned edge of placode

4

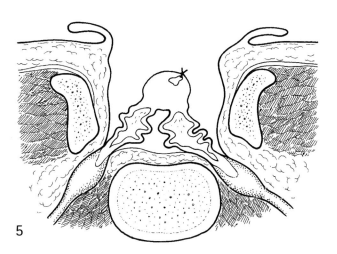

5

Reconstitution of the neural tube

5 Controversy exists as to whether reconstitution of the neural tube is beneficial. If the neural placode is very thin, the edges may be brought together to reconstitute the neural tube. A few sutures of 10/0 polypropylene (Prolene) can be placed into the arachnoid elements at the edge of the placode to reconstitute the tube. It is hoped that the maneuver will decrease tethering and prevent adherence to the surrounding dura. Care must be taken not to place these sutures through neural elements, and reconstitution of the tube should not be performed if the edges of the placode do not easily come together. If such a maneuver will cause undue strangulation or pressure on the placode, it should not be performed.

Identification of the dural edges

6 One of the most important aspects of the repair of myelomeningocele in a child is the achievement of a watertight dural closure. The dura (a glistening white structure) is adherent to the edges of the myelomeningocele sac. It is most easily identified by carefully examining the upper end of the sac near where the neural placode is reconstituted into a normal spinal cord. It may not be reconstituted at the lower end, depending on the level and extent of the myelomeningocele defect. The dura is dissected initially at the upper end of the paraspinous fascia. Care must be taken to go high enough up along the walls of the sac to provide sufficient dura to close over the placode and to obtain a watertight closure. It is important that the dural closure is sufficiently capacious to prevent strangulation or vascular compression of the neural placode.

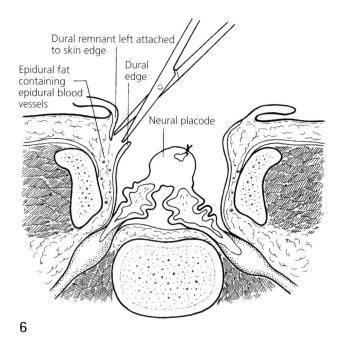

6

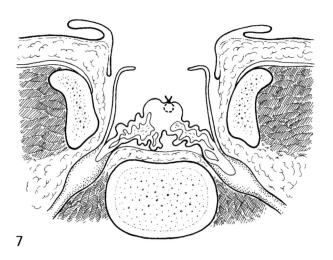

7

Dissecting of the dural edges

7 A cuff of residual dura is left along the edges and can be used to anchor subcutaneous stitches to assist in the closure of the skin edges. An important landmark in identifying the plane of dissection to free the dura from the surrounding tissue is identification of the epidural fat. The epidural fat is more loosely developed than subcutaneous fat and has within it a rich blood supply including significant epidural veins. These epidural veins can be quite large and should be coagulated where necessary.

Closing the dura

8 The dural edges should be brought together using a running stitch of either 4/0 or 5/0 polypropylene or braided non-absorbable nylon sutures. If insufficient dura is available, a piece of paraspinous fascia may be used as a patch graft to complete the repair. Dura substitutes, such as bovine pericardium, may also be used for a patch graft if insufficient fascia is available.

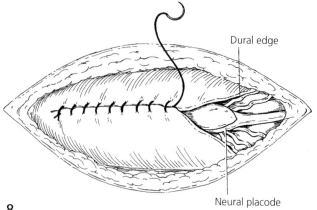

8

Closing the fascia

9 Where possible, the fascia should be closed over the dura. However, this is not possible in many areas, due to insufficient fascia. In addition, as the pedicles of the spine are widely bifid, the fascia usually ends up lateral to the dura. Splitting of the fascia into superficial and deep layers laterally can provide a sufficient amount of fascia to allow closure over the midline. Here again, closure of the fascia should not cause strangulation of the placode. A complete fascial closure should be attempted, but again, only if it is not likely to cause injury to the placode itself.

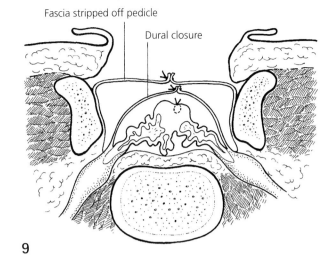

Fascia stripped off pedicle

Dural closure

9

Skin closure

Closure of the skin defect is among the most difficult elements of a myelomeningocele repair. Serious consideration must be given to employing the talents of a pediatric plastic surgeon when dealing with large defects. Important factors that contribute to the breakdown of the skin repair are the use of poor quality skin, placing the skin under undue tension at the suture line, and inadequate dural closure or hydrocephalus resulting in leakage of CSF.

10 All of the skin surrounding the area should be employed, and thin, transitional skin should not be used as it will break down. If the defect in the skin is less than half the width of the back, primary closure can be achieved by carefully undermining the skin. The direction of the closure is not as important as avoidance of pressure and stretching of the skin elements. Undermining the skin edges using blunt finger dissection is useful. Division of the tight fibrous bands tethering the subcutaneous tissue and skin near the iliac crest can be particularly helpful in mobilizing the skin of the lower lumbosacral area.

Occasionally, especially if there is a significant kyphotic deformity, resecting a portion of the pedicles associated with the deformity can be helpful in approximating the skin edges. In more severe cases, kyphectomy may have to be performed to achieve skin closure. This can be done in collaboration with an orthopedic surgeon.

The skin should be closed in two layers, making use of the residual dural cuff that is still attached to the skin edges. Interrupted 3/0 absorbable suture works well in the subcutaneous tissues. Vertical mattress sutures or running baseball-type nylon stitches may also be used on the skin edges. Intravenous fluorescein can demonstrate the blood supply to the skin and may be helpful in identifying any non-viable areas.

Adequate closure may not be possible in a large defect, and the various rotational flaps may be considered. In addition, relaxing incisions may allow closure of the undermined skin.

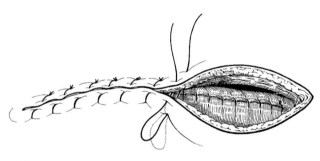

10

POSTOPERATIVE CARE

The mortality rates for repair of myelomeningoceles range from 2 to 19 percent, but postoperative deaths are exceedingly rare. The early postoperative death rate is about 2 percent and is associated with respiratory failure or severe infection such as meningitis.

The repair site is covered with a light, non-compressive dressing. Plastic drapes should be used to prevent fecal matter from contaminating the wound. Maintenance of a clear dressing is crucial. The child should be kept off the repair site and can be nursed in a lateral position. The use of a Foley catheter or intermittent catheterization is necessary to prevent stasis and avoid urinary tract infections. Because neonatal ureteric peristalsis may be weak, hydronephrosis may develop, and therefore should be looked for. Ultrasonic examination of the kidneys can be helpful in identifying such problems.

Wound care must be meticulous and the wound must be inspected regularly for areas of breakdown. Bacitracin or silver sulfadiazine (Silvadene) ointment may be useful in keeping the wound moist and clean. Small areas of wound breakdown will usually respond to local wound management and will eventually granulate in. Wound care is particularly important when lateral releasing incisions have been employed. In most cases, however, rotational flaps created with the assistance of the plastic surgeon should avoid the need for such relaxing incisions.

Leakage of CSF, if present, is usually the result of progressive hydrocephalus. Such diversionary procedures are often necessary within the first days to weeks of life. In those children in whom shunting or CSF diversionary procedures have not been performed, follow up is mandatory.

Repeated cranial ultrasounds and careful head measurements can identify such progressive hydrocephalus. A ventriculoperitoneal shunt is most commonly employed to relieve such hydrocephalus, but endoscopic third ventriculostomy has also now become more widely used. Recent studies do not suggest any increased risk of infection if the shunt or diversionary procedure is performed at the same time as the repair. However, children with myelomeningoceles are still at increased risk of shunt infections, and physicians must be on the alert for these in the first few weeks after repair.

Occasionally, the Chiari II malformation may become symptomatic during the first few months of life. The Chiari II malformation is characterized by downward displacement of the vermis into the cervical canal, causing compression of the underlying brainstem and spinal cord. It is part of a complex of various congenital anomalies of the brain that can occur in children with myelomeningocele. Symptoms include apnea, stridor, high-pitched cry, and lower cranial nerve paresis. Initial evaluation must be directed toward evaluation of the shunt and treatment of the hydrocephalus. However, if such evaluation proves negative, consideration must be given to early decompression of the Chiari II malformation. It is important to remember that despite adequate decompression of the Chiari II malformation and adequate CSF diversion, a small percentage of children still have intrinsic developmental anomalies of the brainstem that result in brainstem dysfunction necessitating tracheostomy and insertion of a feeding tube.

OUTCOME

Counseling and education of the parents and caregivers of children with myelomeningocele must be considered a vital part of the postoperative care. Multidisciplinary management of these children permits most to lead productive and fulfilling lives. As the technical ability to treat these children and the radiographic capacity to image their associated abnormalities both *in utero* and postpartum are improved, and, most importantly, as we

learn from long-term follow up with these children, it is clear that the outcome for most is quite good.

Survival for children with myelomeningocele is improving. Most tertiary care centers find that 98 percent of these children survive with aggressive medical management. Associated abnormalities of the central nervous system, particularly complications related to the Chiari II malformation and other systemic anomalies, account for mortality in many of the present-day non-survivors. Shunt failure or acute hydrocephalus also can result in significant morbidity and mortality in these children. Antibiotic therapy has greatly decreased the mortality associated with ventriculitis. Ventriculoperitoneal shunting has successfully managed hydrocephalus, but such shunts can have variable failure, which must be quickly and appropriately diagnosed. McLone has shown that intellectual function is significantly lower in children in whom meningitis has developed in the postoperative period. Some form of learning disability will be present in 70–80 percent of cases, and special education or special programs will be required while in school. Routine evaluation with ultrasound, MRI scan, or CT scans of the head in the first few years of life can be helpful in identifying indolent shunt malfunction. Excessive CT scanning should be avoided, as even the low doses of radiation associated with CT scans may have long-term cognitive consequences for these children. As the children grow older, school performance can be used to follow intellectual function.

Some 80–90 percent of children with myelomeningocele have neurogenic bladder dysfunction. Among the lifelong risks associated with this dysfunction are urinary stasis and infection, trabeculation and diverticula of the bladder, ureteric reflux, hydronephrosis, and renal failure. The use of intermittent catheterization has reduced the incidence of hydronephrosis and urinary tract infections. It has also improved continence such that 90 percent of affected children can now achieve continence with regular catheterization.

Improvement in urologic management means that urine diversionary procedures are now infrequently employed. Control of defecation can be achieved in 50–75 percent of patients with the assistance of careful dietary management, the use of dietary supplements, and the occasional use of suppositories and enemas. Anterior continence enema procedures have been described as a safe and effective option for the treatment of children with chronic defecation when maximal medical therapies have failed. The surgical procedure involves creating a pathway proximal to the anus through which enemas can be given to facilitate fecal evacuation. This is often achieved by creating a connection between the abdominal wall and appendix or cecum.

Multiple orthopedic problems can occur. Scoliosis occurs in 65–75 percent of patients and may require surgical correction. Significant kyphoscoliosis is seen in 5–10 percent of patients and may require surgical correction if respiratory function is impeded. Many lower extremity deformities can occur and often require surgical correction or bracing. The use of orthotic devices in these children requires the specialized attention of a pediatric orthotist familiar with children who have significant sensory deficits, and therefore may have a greatly increased chance of skin breakdown. Functional outcome can be significantly improved in children for whom multidisciplinary care has been achieved, and a significant number of children may, in fact, become ambulatory.

Careful neurologic monitoring is necessary. Delayed neurologic complications in these children can occur as a result of several problems. Indolent shunt malfunction must always be considered when there is clinical deterioration of any type in a child with myelomeningocele. Chiari II malformation may cause bulbar compression and result in lower cranial nerve dysfunction. It may also result in syringomyelia or cervical cord dysfunction, which may become manifest as upper extremity weakness or numbness. Magnetic resonance imaging has greatly improved our understanding of the Chiari II malformation by allowing us an excellent view of the malformation and the subsequent problems that it may cause. It should be noted that many children with myelomeningocele have significant syringomyelia, which is of no clinical significance, and therefore does not require intervention. However, it must be monitored carefully, as ascending syringomyelia may cause cord dysfunction, and therefore upper extremity dysfunction. Particularly for non-ambulators who are restricted to a wheelchair, loss of upper extremity function can be devastating.

Changes in segmental motor or sensory deficits, evidence of increased spasticity, change in bowel or bladder function, progressive neuromusculoskeletal deformity at the ankle or leg, and progressive scoliosis may occur secondary to tethering of the spinal cord. Because all children with myelomeningocele have some evidence of a tethered cord on MRI, careful clinical evaluation must be employed to determine if such tethering is clinically significant and warrants further surgery to untether the spinal cord. It must be remembered that all children with myelomeningocele will have radiographic evidence of a low-lying cord, and this does not equate with clinical dysfunction. In addition, less common causes of progressive deficit may include dermoid cyst formation, diastematomyelia with septae, and arachnoid cyst formation.

It cannot be overemphasized that shunt malfunction is the most common cause of clinical deterioration in children with myelomeningocele. It must always be considered, and shunt function must be carefully evaluated before such deterioration is attributed to other causes, such as Chiari II malformation or tethered cord.

IN UTERO REPAIR OF MYELOMENINGOCELE/ FETAL SURGERY

Because of the improved nature of *in utero* ultrasound screening, amniocentesis, and the emergence of prenatal MRI scanning, early first-trimester detection of neural tube defects is increasing. Until ten years ago, treatment of myelomeningocele included surgical closure at birth followed by supportive care and surveillance for future spinal cord tethering. The development of surgical techniques applicable to the fetus and the emergence of drugs for the prevention of premature labor have, over the past 13 years, provided for *in utero* correction of myelomeningocele. The goal of *in utero* correction is to limit trauma and amniotic fluid exposure to unprotected neural tissues throughout gestation. The first reported case of *in utero* myelomeningocele repair occurred in 1997 by Tulipan and Bruner. Since this original report, surgical technique has evolved from endoscopic coverage of the fetal neural placode during late gestation to open surgical repair in early gestation (between weeks 19 and 25).

The concern must largely lie with the safety of the mother, but a significant secondary goal is the safety of and outcome for the fetus. Avoidance of preterm labor is crucial to this outcome. Because of the technical difficulty and fragility of the tissues, the surgery is generally limited to after 18 weeks of gestation, and because premature labor increases dramatically after 30 weeks, it is usually not recommended after 30 weeks. In this mid-gestational repair, the uterus is exposed through a low transverse abdominal incision and the fetus and placenta are positioned in such a way as to provide an optimal view of the myelomeningocele placode. Hysterotomy is performed and the fetus is exposed in as limited a fashion as possible. The goal is to maintain intrauterine volume to prevent placental separation, contraction, and expulsion of the fetus. This is generally accomplished by high-volume profusion of the amniotic cavity with warm Ringer's lactate.

The myelomeningocele closure is really quite similar to that in the already born fetus. The fringe of the full thickness at the region of the zona epitheliosa is incised and a dural as well as fascial closure is performed. Skin closure can be accomplished using absorbable suture. In cases where the defect may be too large to be closed, an acellular human dermal graft can be used to complete the closure, in which case, a secondary closure may be necessary after delivery.

It is estimated that over 400 fetal operations have been performed for myelomeningocele worldwide, however the results are still being interpreted. Due to the risks associated with prenatal intervention, intrauterine repair was initially offered only to mothers of children with Arnold Chiari II malformations, ventriculomegaly, large thoracolumbar defects, normal leg movements without clubbing of the feet, normal karyotype, and no severe associated abnormalities. Because of promising results in these early patients, surgery for smaller defects was considered. Several single institution series between 1998 and 2003 have shown reversal of hindbrain herniation (associated with Arnold Chiari II malformations) in patients repaired *in utero*. Hindbrain herniation was present in 95 percent of patients repaired postnatally.

After *in utero* repair, less than 38 percent demonstrated cerebellar herniation. Review of the data from the Children's Hospital in Philadelphia suggests that the overall ventricular shunting rate was 84 percent in children who had their myelomeningoceles postnatally repaired. When these results were compared with a combined series from the Children's Hospital of Philadelphia and Vanderbilt, looking at shunting rates for children who had had *in utero* repair of their myelomeningoceles, the overall ventricular shunting rate was found to be 46 percent. Neurological motor outcome in children after prenatal repair revealed that 66 percent of toddlers were able to ambulate independently, although they were limited by coordination and balance dysfunction characteristic of all children with spina bifida.

These preliminary institutional studies suggest that prenatal surgery for myelomeningocele may have certain clear advantages. Although preliminary beneficial results may be due in part to selection bias and changing management indications, there seems to be a reversal or improvement of hindbrain herniation, a decrease in the need for shunting, and at least preservation of lower extremity function, which is somewhat dependent on the gestational age at the time of repair. There is clear evidence of selection bias in each of these studies, and obviously significant risks to both the mother and the fetus with *in utero* surgery. It is because of this that the first randomized prospective trial for intrauterine myelomeningocele repair (the Management of Myelomeningocele or MOMS trial) was started in 2003 and completed with published data in March 2011. This study was sponsored by the National Institutes of Health involving three centers in the United States: the Children's Hospital of Philadelphia, Vanderbilt University, and the University of California in San Francisco, with an independent data and study coordinating center at George Washington University Biostatistics Center. With the goal of 100 fetal repairs and 100 postnatal repairs, this trial was stopped after the recruitment of 183 patients. The primary objective of this trial is to determine if intrauterine repair of fetal myelomeningocele at 19–25 weeks of gestation improves primary and secondary outcomes, including the need for shunting, hindbrain herniation, and developmental motor function. Intrauterine myelomeningocele repair reduces the need for shunting by 50 percent and offers improvements in hindbrain herniation by 12 months and ambulation by 30 months. Prenatal surgery is, however, associated with risks to both mother and fetus, including preterm delivery and uterine dehiscence at the time of delivery.

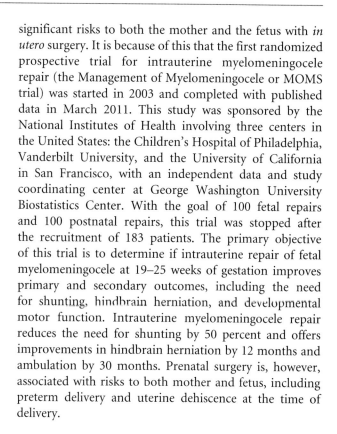

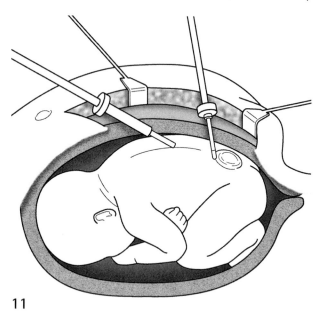

11

11 In the operating room the fetus is positioned with myelomeningocele visible through the uterine incision. Examination of the contents of the dural sac reveals a placode, dura, and soft tissue which are slowly mobilized from the surrounding skin. Native dura is closed primarily or covered with collagen material.

FURTHER READING

Adzick NS, Thom EA, Spong CY *et al.* A randomized trial of prenatal versus postnatal repair of myelomeningocele. *New England Journal of Medicine* 2011; **364**: 993–1004.

Adzick NS. Fetal myelomeningocele: natural history, pathophysiology, and *in-utero* intervention. *Seminars in Fetal and Neonatal Medicine* 2010; **15**: 9–14.

Brock DJ, Sutcliffe RG. Alpha-fetoprotein in the antenatal diagnosis of anencephaly and spina bifida. *Lancet* 1972; **2**: 197–9.

Charney E, Weller SC, Sutton LN *et al.* Management of the newborn with myelomeningocele: time for a decision making process. *Pediatrics* 1985; **75**: 58–64.

Hirose S, Farmer DL. Fetal surgery for myelomeningocele. *Clinical Perinatology* 2009; **36**: 431–8.

McLone DG, Naidich TP. Myelomeningocele: outcome and late complications. In: McLaurin RL, Schut L, Venes JL, Epstein F (eds). *Pediatric Neurosurgery – Surgery of the Developing Nervous System*, 2nd edn. Philadelphia, PA: WB Saunders, 1989: 53–70.

Sutton LN, Adzick NS. Fetal surgery for myelomeningocele. *Clinics in Neurosurgery* 2004; **51**: 155–62.

99

Ventricular shunting procedure

DOMINIC NP THOMPSON and JESSICA TERNIER

HISTORY

It is not until the sixteenth century that we have the first references to the condition that we would recognize as hydrocephalus (Versalius, 1514–1564). Robert Wytt's essay on dropsy of the ventricles of the brain (1768) provides a clear clinical description of the condition. The surgical treatment of hydrocephalus has included ventricular puncture, extirpation of the choroid plexus, and cerebrospinal fluid (CSF) diversion to a variety of body cavities. Drainage of the CSF to the jugular vein via a simple valve housed in rubber tubing was described by Nulsen and Spitz in 1952 and was a major landmark in hydrocephalus treatment, but it was the introduction of valved tubing made from durable, biocompatible material (Silastic®) that heralded the modern era of shunt technology and hydrocephalus treatment. Endoscopic third ventriculostomy entails perforating the floor of the third ventricle via an endoscope introduced via the lateral ventricle and is now an established technique in the neurosurgical treatment of hydrocephalus.

PRINCIPLES AND JUSTIFICATION

Hydrocephalus is the accumulation of CSF that results when there is obstruction to its normal circulation and absorption. As a consequence, the cerebral ventricles enlarge, intracranial pressure increases, and cerebral function may be impaired. There are numerous etiologies, both congenital and acquired, but the principles of treatment remain the same – namely, to divert CSF from proximal to the point of obstruction to some distal site where absorption can take place.

PREOPERATIVE ASSESSMENT AND PREPARATION

Diagnosis

It is mandatory that the results of neuroimaging be interpreted in the light of clinical features before the diagnosis of hydrocephalus can be made and the decision to place a shunt taken. Dilatation of the ventricular system that is static and not associated with raised intracranial pressure may occur in a number of settings, and intervention is not indicated (e.g. parenchymal brain damage, central nervous system (CNS) malformations, post-irradiation, arrested hydrocephalus). Indeed, shunt placement in such circumstances may be harmful and result in symptoms of over-drainage and subdural hematoma formation.

The classical symptoms of raised intracranial pressure, namely headache, vomiting, and drowsiness are often not present, particularly in the neonate or infant, in whom head circumference, anterior fontanelle tension, and general neurodevelopmental progress may be more useful indices of progressive hydrocephalus. Provided there is no overt clinical urgency, a period of observation and sequential imaging may help distinguish between active hydrocephalus and simple ventriculomegaly.

Serial head circumference measurements accurately measured and plotted on a head circumference chart are an essential adjunct to the brain imaging in assessing the necessity for shunt placement in a neonate with post-hemorrhagic hydrocephalus or following closure of a myelomeningocele.

Radiological features

1   Axial imaging, either computed tomography (CT) scan or magnetic resonance imaging (MRI), should be performed prior to shunt placement. This provides clear visualization of the ventricular anatomy, may indicate the underlying etiology, and can be used to plan shunt placement. Ultrasonography is a useful modality with which to monitor ventricular size, but is restricted to infants with a sufficiently patent fontanelle and may not allow adequate visualization of the entire intracranial contents.

Once the indication for treatment has been confirmed, the surgeon must decide, first, what type of CSF diversion procedure to perform, and second, what type of device to use.

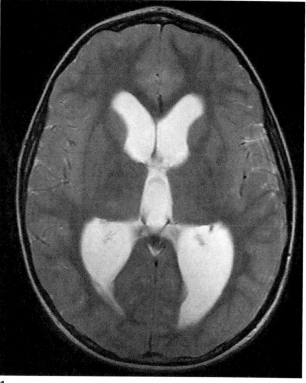

1

Surgical treatments for hydrocephalus

VENTRICULOPERITONEAL SHUNT

Drainage is directly to the peritoneal cavity. This remains the most common technique. In most instances, it is quick, effective, and relatively simple to perform.

VENTRICULOATRIAL SHUNT

The distal tubing is placed in the right atrium via a major neck vein. This is a technically more demanding procedure (particularly at revision) and there are well-recognized long-term complications. This technique has therefore become very much second- or third-line treatment.

VENTRICULOPLEURAL SHUNT

The pleural cavity provides an effective absorptive surface; however, the risks of symptomatic pleural effusion and a higher rate of blockage mean that it is not recommended as a primary treatment.

ENDOSCOPIC THIRD VENTRICULOSTOMY

Endoscopic third ventriculostomy (ETV) entails making an opening in the floor of the third ventricle permitting the flow of CSF from the intraventricular compartment to the basal subarachnoid cisterns from where it can be absorbed in the usual manner (see below).

Choice of shunt device

2   There are numerous shunt devices on the market; none has any proven advantage. It is strongly recommended that the surgeon becomes familiar with a particular shunt type for regular use, reserving more novel devices (such as programmable shunts) for exceptional circumstances. Shunts comprise three components: a ventricular catheter, a valve, and a distal catheter. A reservoir chamber is often included and positioned at the burr hole site or integral to the valve. The reservoir can be punctured percutaneously to obtain CSF in cases of suspected infection or blockage.

Antibiotic impregnated shunt tubing is now available. This can be used in association with most valve types. The current literature suggests that this may be effective in reducing the incidence of shunt infection.

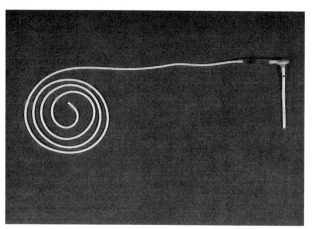

2

Contraindications to surgery

Intercurrent sepsis, particularly CNS infection, should be regarded as a contraindication to surgery. Blood or high levels of protein in the CSF should be considered relative contraindications to shunt placement, as these may increase the likelihood of early shunt failure due to blockage.

Anesthesia

The procedure is performed using a balanced anesthetic technique requiring endotracheal intubation and intermittent positive pressure ventilation (IPPV). Particular attention is paid to the control of PCO_2 in view of the presence of raised intracranial pressure (ICP). The proposed shunt position should be discussed with the anesthetist to ensure that vascular access (e.g. intravenous neck lines) and endotracheal tube strapping do not obscure the shunt trajectory. Prophylactic antibiotics are administered at the time of induction of anesthesia.

OPERATION

Positioning and draping

3a,b The importance of positioning the child for ventriculoperitoneal (VP) shunt cannot be over-emphasized. The head needs to be rotated and the neck extended by placing a sand bag beneath the shoulders to ensure that there is a level trajectory for subcutaneous tunneling between the cranial and abdominal incisions. This position opens out the neck skin creases and reduces the risk of 'buttonholing' the skin during tunneling. Skin preparation should cover the entire area from cranial to abdominal incision; the preparation fluid should be allowed to dry before drapes are applied. An adhesive plastic drape is placed to cover the entire operative field.

The shunt should be assembled at the beginning of the procedure. This reduces both operating time and the tendency for clumsy manipulations of the shunt *in situ*. Methods of assembly and testing of the shunt vary for different types of shunt and therefore the manufacturer's recommendations should be followed.

The required ventricular catheter length can be estimated from imaging – the tip of the catheter should sit well into the body of the ventricle.

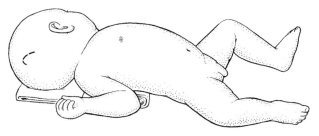

3a

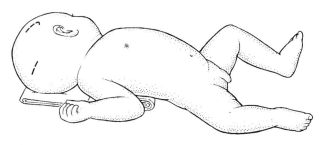

3b

Incisions

Shunt infection is one of the major complications of shunt surgery. Commensal skin organisms are the most common pathogens. The following precautions are recommended to reduce the risk of contamination.

- The cranial incision is semicircular and large enough to ensure that the wound does not overlie the shunt tubing.

- Instruments used in skin opening should be put aside until the time of closure.
- Tissue handling should be kept to a minimum and the wound edges lined with betadine-soaked cottonoid strips.
- The use of the diathermy needs to be kept to a minimum. In the infant, it is very easy to inflict burns at the skin edges.
- A no-touch technique should be maintained throughout the procedure.

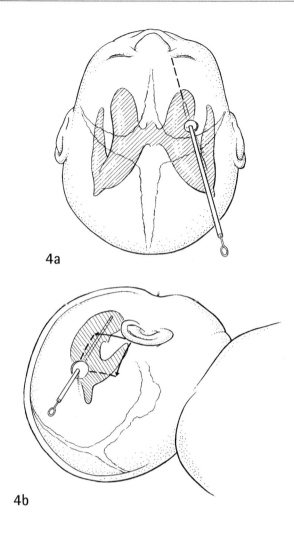

4a

4b

4a,b The cranial incision may be frontal or parieto-occipital; there is no clear advantage of one over the other. A frontal shunt will require an additional incision behind the ear to facilitate tunneling to the abdomen. The burr hole for a frontal shunt should be just anterior to the coronal suture and in the line of the pupil. A parieto-occipital burr hole is made approximately 3 cm above and behind the top of the pinna.

The burr hole is made in the standard manner, using a power drill or perforator; care is required in the infant due to the thin calvarium. Once the bone is breeched, the burr hole can be enlarged using bone rongeurs. The dural opening should be small, sufficient only to pass the ventricular catheter. Larger openings increase the risk of subcutaneous CSF collections.

Ventricles may be asymmetric and vary considerably in size, particularly in children; the precise site of the burr hole will therefore often be dictated by the underlying ventricular configuration.

Subcutaneous tunneling

The subcutaneous tunneling device may be passed in either direction. The tunneling is performed deep to the subcutaneous fat, but superficial to the deep fascia. Care should be taken to avoid perforating the skin; with one hand holding the device, the other hand can be used to palpate the course of the tunneling device as it advances to the abdomen. Care should be taken to avoid damaging the breast bud in female patients.

Once in position, the shunt tubing can be threaded down the tunneling device, which is then removed.

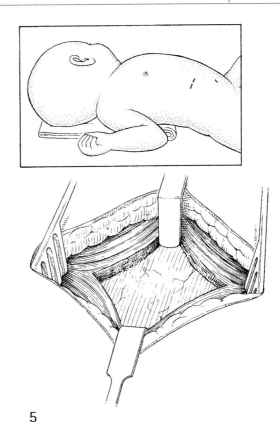

Peritoneal exposure

5 The peritoneal end of the shunt is usually placed via a minilaparotomy below the costal margin over the rectus abdominis. The rectus sheath is opened, and a longitudinal muscle-splitting technique is used to expose the peritoneum. The peritoneum is then opened; it is important to be quite certain that the peritoneal cavity has been entered to avoid extraperitoneal placement. It is also important to be sure that there is a good flow of CSF from the distal catheter before this is internalized. The entire distal tubing is then fed under direct vision into the peritoneal cavity. A good length of distal tubing reduces the likelihood of the tubing migrating out of the peritoneal cavity as the child grows.

5

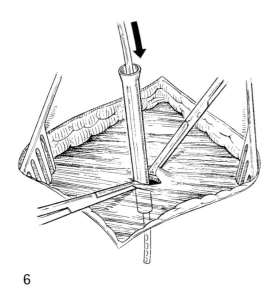

6

6 An alternative method of inserting the peritoneal catheter is by means of a Trocar. This is quicker and requires a much smaller incision, but damage to the abdominal contents is a reported complication of this technique.

In current practice, the distal end of the shunt is increasingly being inserted into the peritoneal cavity by laparoscopy and where required by thoracoscopy for intrapleural placement.

Catheter placement

The ventricular catheter mounted on a stilette is then placed through the dural opening and slowly advanced into the lateral ventricle. As soon as the ventricle is entered, the stilette is stabilized and the catheter is advanced into position.

Particularly when the ventricles are small or very asymmetric, it is useful to have rehearsed the catheter placement, predetermining the desired trajectory before perforating the brain substance. For a standard frontal approach, the catheter is passed perpendicular to the skull surface, aiming toward the medial canthus of the ipsilateral eye. In a posterior approach, the catheter is aimed at the midpoint of the forehead. Brisk flow of CSF along the catheter needs to be confirmed before proceeding. If there is no CSF flow or flow is sluggish, the catheter must be resited.

If the ventricular catheter is not already attached to the rest of the shunt, this is now done. The distal tubing, now draining CSF, is placed in the peritoneal cavity. The catheter should thread easily. The entire length of distal tubing is placed to allow for subsequent growth of the child.

Wound closure

Meticulous attention must be paid to wound closure. The wounds are closed in layers; an absorbable suture is used to close the skin. Wound infection or CSF leakage invariably results in infection of the shunt.

POSTOPERATIVE CARE

The wound dressings are left undisturbed and the child nursed off the wounds. In a small infant with large ventricles, it is wise to elevate the child slowly over 24–48 hours in an attempt to avoid too rapid decompression of the ventricular system.

ADDITIONAL SHUNT PROCEDURES

Occasionally, drainage into the peritoneum is precluded, most commonly because of adhesions or repeated lower end failure. In this situation, an alternative site for distal drainage must be sought. In each case, the details relating to proximal placement are as described above.

Ventriculopleural shunt

It is important that the upper end of the shunt procedure has been completed and that CSF flow from the distal catheter has been established before the pleura is opened. A bulldog clip is placed on the tubing while the distal site is prepared. The lower incision is made at the level of the fifth rib in the anterior axillary line. The intercostal muscles are split just above the rib to prevent injury to the neurovascular bundle. The pleura is exposed and incised; the distal shunt, having been cut to an appropriate length, is then gently threaded into the pleural cavity, avoiding direct trauma to the lung. The anesthetist is requested to induce Valsalva's manuever in an attempt to reduce the risk of pneumothorax. The muscle layer is then closed around the tubing.

Ventriculoatrial shunt

7 Again, it is important to have completed the upper end of the shunt insertion before the venous system is opened. The neck incision is sited over the anterior border of the sternomastoid muscle. The carotid sheath and internal jugular vein lie just deep to this muscle. It is generally advised that the common facial vein be exposed, mobilized, and divided. The tubing is passed along this tributary into the internal jugular vein and thence into the right atrium. In small children, it is often necessary to insert the tubing directly in the jugular vein. A purse-string suture is placed in the vein wall before the venotomy; the purse string is then tied to seal the opening around the shunt tubing. The tip of the catheter must be in the right atrium and this is confirmed with fluoroscopy. The tubing is then connected to the rest of the shunt by means of a straight connector.

A simpler and more elegant method of placement of the atrial catheter is by a percutaneous technique using ultrasound guidance (see **Chapter 4**).

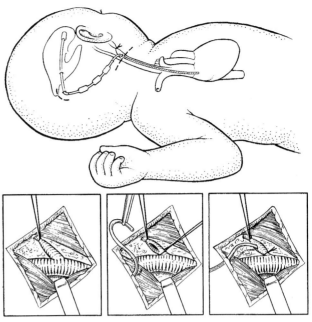

7

ENDOSCOPIC THIRD VENTRICULOSTOMY (VENTRICULOCISTERNOSTOMY)

The aim of this procedure is to create a communication between the third ventricle and the subarachnoid spaces beneath the brain in front of the brainstem (the prepontine cistern). It is essential that the pathways to absorb CSF back into the venous system are functional and so this technique is reserved for cases of obstructive hydrocephalus, for example aqueduct stenosis and hydrocephalus due to a posterior fossa tumor. Where the cause of hydrocephalus is deemed to be in the extracerebral circulation or absorption of CSF, then a shunting procedure would be more appropriate.

Additionally, neuroendoscopy can be of benefit in the treatment of congenital cysts and multicompartmental hydrocephalus, although this will not be dealt with here.

Preoperative assessment and preparation

DIAGNOSIS

MRI is highly recommended before proceeding to an endoscopic third ventriculostomy to confirm the obstructive origin of the hydrocephalus. MRI features suggesting an obstructive hydrocephalus include depression of the floor of the third ventricle and dilatation of the supraoptic and pineal recesses. Anatomical variants that might preclude endoscopic access and safe ventriculostomy will be better visualized on MRI. The width of the third ventricle must be at least 3 mm to allow endoscopic access and note must be made of the position of the basilar artery.

CHOICE OF ENDOSCOPE

A designated pediatric endoscope is recommended as the diameter is smaller and the risk of cortical injury therefore reduced.

Different categories of neuroendoscope are available:

- rigid neuroscope (camera and light are remote from the working area) 0° optic;
- rigid neuroendoscope (camera within the working area) 0 or 30° angulated optic.
- flexible endoscope (fiberscope).

Light source, camera, viewing monitor, and irrigation pump must be available.

Apart from the flexible endoscope which should be reserved for the experienced neurosurgeon, the choice of endoscope will depend on the surgeon's preference.

Additionally, the following should be available:

- operating sheath (provided with the endoscope or single use peel-away catheter);
- small balloon catheter (Fogarty or figure of eight);
- blunt monopolar probe;
- grasping forceps.

Prior to skin incision, the endoscope needs to be focused, orientated, and the zoom adapted. The irrigation system should be connected (warmed saline or Ringer's lactate) and the Fogarty balloon catheter must be tested to confirm it is functional and assess balloon size.

Operation

POSITIONING AND DRAPING

8, 9 The patient is place in the supine position with the head in slight flexion such that there is a vertical alignment of the external canthus and the external auditory canal. Draping should permit exposure of the entire frontal region, including the midline.

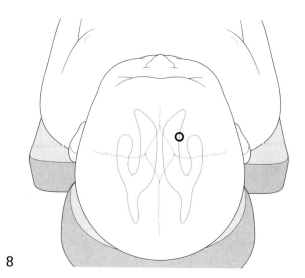

8

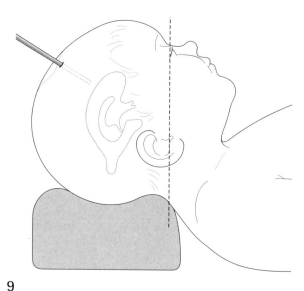

9

INCISIONS

The skin incision can be longitudinal or semi-circular. The semi-circular skin incision allows the surgeon to elevate a periosteum flap which will reduce the risk of CSF leak. The skin incision is centered by an entry point situated 1 cm in front of the coronal suture and 2–2.5 cm laterally to the midline. The burr hole is performed in a standard manner also using the power drill. The burr hole size must be appropriate to the diameter of the operative sheath.

The dural opening must remain small and the cortex must be coagulated to avoid cortical bleeding at the operative sheath insertion.

The sheath with Trocar is placed perpendicular to the bone and advanced into the lateral ventricle. The operative sheath can be fixed to a rigid arm or more commonly clipped to the drape if a peel-away catheter is used. The endoscope is introduced along the sheath to the ventricular cavity under endoscopic vision.

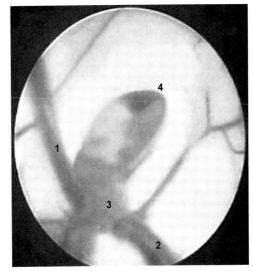

10 On entering the lateral ventricle cavity, three anatomical landmarks need to be recognized and identified before proceeding: these landmarks surround the foramen of Monro and comprise:

- veins: thalamostriate vein (2) and septal vein (1) which converge on the foramen of Monro,
- the choroid plexus (3) at the inferior margin,
- the fornix (4) at the superior edge.

10

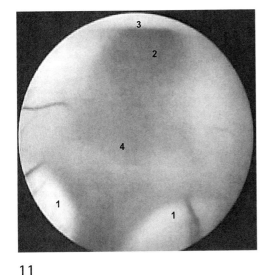

11 The endoscope is then gently passed through the foramen into the third ventricle cavity. At this stage, three further anatomical landmarks must be identified before going any further:

- mammillary bodies (1);
- tuber cinereum (2);
- optic chiasm (3).

The floor (4) of the third ventricle is the membrane lying between the mammillary bodies and the tuber cinereum.

11

The floor of the third ventricle is now perforated using the blunt monopolar electrode (without current). The site of entry is at the anterior two-thirds of the line from the mammillary bodies and the tuber cinereum. If the basilar artery is visualized and bulges at this location, it is recommended to use a more anterior entry point.

Cautery is usually not required, but if the floor is thick cautery might be necessary. The authors advise a very low setting for the monopolar electrode.

The dilatation of the stoma is carried out with the balloon catheter and will allow the endoscope to pass through the stoma. The Lillequist membrane may need some further perforation and will be performed in the same manner.

The pulsatility of the floor of the third ventricle is stopped after irrigation and is usually a sign of adequate flow of CSF through the stoma. The endoscope is withdrawn keeping the same trajectory of entry avoiding any forniceal or choroid plexus injury. Hemostasis needs to be confirmed prior to removal of the endoscope. Areas of mild bleeding usually come under control with patience and prolonged irrigation.

In the event of severe blood staining of the CSF or an inability to locate the anatomical landmarks due to technical or anatomical factors, the procedure should be abandoned and an external drainage left in place pending clarification of the CSF and re-evaluation of the surgical procedure.

CLOSURE

The dura should be sealed with artificial dura or a 'cork' of a hemostatic material such as Surgicel®.

The periosteal flap is stitched over the burr hole. Attention to the skin closure after an endoscopic surgery must be as meticulous as in a shunt surgery to avoid CSF leak or CSF infection which can compromise the outcome of the ventriculostomy.

Postoperative care

Close postoperative neurological observations are essential. A postoperative MRI scan is recommended either immediately or at the time of outpatient follow up to assess ventricular size and patency of the ventriculostomy stoma.

Early or late reclosure are recognized complications of ETV. In this event, the procedure may be repeated or consideration given to the placement of VP shunt.

OUTCOME

Shunt placement results in prompt and sustained control of intracranial pressure in the majority of cases. The two most common shunt complications are infection and blockage.

Shunt infection

Shunt infection occurs in up to 8 percent of cases. Seventy percent of shunt infections will have declared themselves within two months of shunt surgery. A raised temperature, irritability, abdominal pain, and any evidence of a wound problem should raise the possibility of a shunt infection.

Cerebrospinal fluid needs to be obtained and can be sampled from the reservoir. If infection is confirmed, the shunt should be removed and replaced with an external ventricular drain while the infection is treated.

Shunt blockage

Approximately half of the shunts inserted will have become blocked on at least one occasion in the ten years following insertion. Shunt blockage is a surgical emergency. The following points should be borne in mind in planning and performing shunt revision surgery:

- Aspiration of CSF from the shunt reservoir via a butterfly needle may be a useful temporizing measure in an obtunded child with a blocked shunt. Clearly, this will not be possible if the proximal catheter is the site of the blockage.
- An apparently normal or small ventricular system on CT scan does not exclude shunt malfunction.
- At surgery, the child is prepared as for a shunt insertion; access to the entire shunt must be possible.
- If in any doubt, the entire shunt should be replaced.
- Exploration of the proximal shunt is performed first. The ventricular catheter is disconnected to see whether there is proximal CSF flow. A saline-primed manometer is connected to the distal system to assess distal run off.
- Extreme caution should be exercised when removing blocked ventricular catheters. Choroid plexus may be stuck to the shunt and is easily avulsed, resulting in intraventricular hemorrhage. If the catheter cannot be removed easily, a stilette passed down the catheter can be diathermized using monopolar diathermy. This will often shrink away the choroid plexus and make removal easier.
- If bleeding is encountered, the CSF should be allowed to drain freely from the end of the catheter until it clears. If it remains blood-stained, it is safer to leave an external ventricular drain in position for a day or two until the CSF returns to normal.

FURTHER READING

Drake JM, Sainte-Rose C. *The Shunt Book*. Oxford: Blackwell Science, 1994.

Thompson DNP. Hydrocephalus and shunts. In: Moore A, Newell D (eds). *Springer Specialist Surgical Series*. New York: Springer Verlag, 2004.

Trauma

100

Soft tissue trauma

MICHAEL E HÖLLWARTH

INTRODUCTION

Major soft tissue injuries including the skin, the subcutaneous and muscle layers, and occasionally involving additional damage to nerves, vessels, and bones, are a therapeutic challenge at pediatric trauma centers. Owing to the variety of anatomical structures involved, these injuries frequently require multidisciplinary management. Soft tissue wounds occur at a similar frequency in all children, but a marked rise in the incidence is noted when adolescents start to use motorcycles. Boys are more frequently affected than girls, the male female ratio being 3:2. The predominant causes of these injuries are falls with a major crush of the body on a hard surface, e.g. after skateboard, bicycle, motorcycle or car accidents. Extensive soft tissue damage may occur after accidents with a lawn mower, or when using other equipment with fast-spinning parts (such as those used in farming) and after gunshots. Another cause of extensive soft tissue injury is avulsions, which may occur when a child is run over by a car, or bitten by a dog.

Soft tissue wounds are generally more problematic than surgical wounds. The reasons are many: (1) the extent of the injury may only become evident after 2 or 3 days; (2) the possibility of additional injury to nerves, vessels, and bones; (3) the wound may be heavily contaminated; and (4) devitalized tissue is prone to bacterial contamination.

PATHOPHYSIOLOGY

The extent of soft tissue injury is one of the factors responsible for significant metabolic reactions to such injuries. Macrophages and inflammatory cytokines are activated and cause additional soft tissue edema. A rise in pressure within muscle and/or fascia may lead to a compartment syndrome. Local ischemic processes, reduced oxygenation in parts of the tissue, and necrotic areas are responsible for tissue acidosis thus aggravating the local and systemic inflammatory response, as well as the likelihood of infection.

EVALUATION AND INITIAL TREATMENT

The first step is to evaluate the cause, location, and extent of the soft tissue trauma, the child's general condition, and the presence of any additional injuries especially in cases of multiple trauma. The clinical investigation includes active and passive mobility, the neurological status including the presence or loss of sensitivity, and control of peripheral circulation, as well as the capillary refilling time (Table 100.1). Photographic documentation is another important aspect of the initial steps.

Table 100.1 Primary clinical investigation, followed by laboratory and imaging procedures.

Causes and circumstances of the trauma
General status of the patient (Glasgow Coma Scale)
Which parts of the body are injured – local injury or polytrauma
Location and extent of soft tissue injury
Additional local injuries – bones, major arteries, or veins and nerves
Local sensitivity, possibility of active or passive motion
Peripheral circulation, capillary refilling time

As open wounds are frequently contaminated by a variety of bacteria, swabs should be taken for bacteriological cultures. Broad-spectrum antibiotics may be given as initial treatment before the results of bacteriological cultures become available. Once available, the most appropriate therapy may be selected. The use of topical antibiotics, such as neomycin or a combination of bacitracin and polymyxin B, is recommended.

The two essential strategies in the treatment of major soft tissue injuries are (1) to avoid infection and (2) to achieve clean wounds, which may be subjected to primary or secondary closure. Soft tissue wounds with a minimal crush component and minimal contamination, that require minor debridement, can be closed immediately if the tissue is free of tension, or may even be subjected to definite primary coverage. Injuries with a significantly crushed soft tissue structure or exposure of nerves, vessels, tendons, or bones require stepwise treatment. Heavily contaminated wounds can be effectively cleaned by high pressure irrigation, which will significantly reduce infection rates. After the cleaning procedure, we recommend renewed antiseptic preparation and draping, as well as a change of instruments. Local treatment with antiseptics, such as betadine or hydrogen peroxide, is recommended. It may be initially difficult to establish the true extent of damaged tissue that requires debridement. Therefore, second-look surgery with subsequent inspection and further debridement sessions after 24 and 48 hours may be necessary. It is essential to remove all necrotic tissue, including muscles and dislocated bone fragments, in order to achieve an entirely clean wound. The debridement of muscles is based on the observation of the so-called four C's: color, consistency, capillary bleeding, and contractility. Care must be taken to avoid additional damage to intact structures, such as nerves, vessels, and tendons.

1 Vacuum-assisted sterile dressings (VAC) are optimal as primary dressing or between planned debridement procedures. These special dressings can be used to remove the wound exudate and are a very effective means of preventing the development of infection. Additionally, the VAC dressing induces the development of clean, thick, and solid granulation tissue which provides an optimal base for secondary wound closure techniques with temporary dermal regeneration templates, skin grafts, local or distant vascularized flaps.

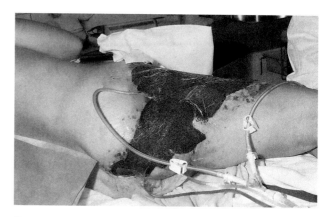

1

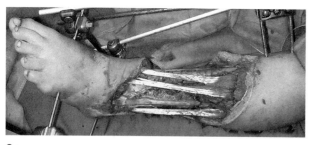

2a

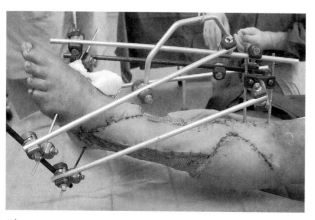

2b

2a,b Extensive soft tissue injuries are frequently complicated by open fractures. The latter are classified into different grades depending on the size of the wound, the type of fracture, the quality of soft tissue, the grade of contamination, and the presence of injuries to nerves and vessels. Appropriate stabilization of fractures is an essential aspect of initial therapy. The use of a fixateur externe (external stabilization) is the treatment of choice (illustration a). It reduces pain and makes it much easier for the surgeon to carry out the next steps in the treatment of the soft tissue injury. Once the wound is clean and the bone has been adequately covered, the fixateur externe may be replaced by plates or intramedullary nailing.

SECONDARY TREATMENT

3 A large number of soft tissue wounds cannot be closed primarily. The preliminary steps consist of adequate debridement, prevention of infection, and preparation of the wound so that secondary closure can be performed. Intermediate-sized defects (provided enough skin is available) may be closed in a stepwise manner with elastic bands, e.g. vessel loops, which allow the size of the defect to reduce in 1 or 2 weeks. Definite closure can be performed after this. Skin grafts may be used when no vital structures are exposed. Major soft tissue defects will require local or distant flaps.

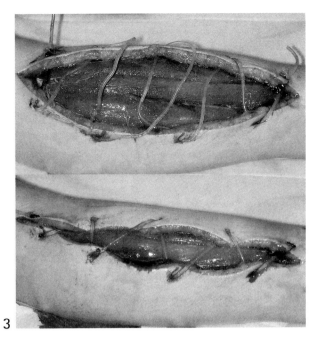

3

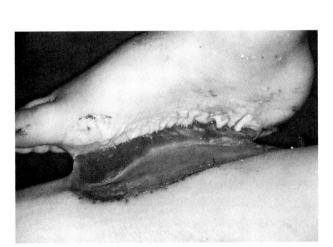

4a

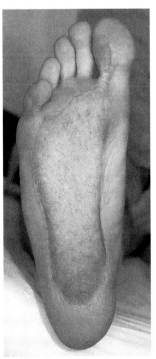

4b

Small defects with relatively intact tissue can be covered with a full thickness graft. The skin may be taken from the groin, dorsal site of the ear, the neck, or the inside of the upper arm. The advantages of full-thickness grafts are their favorable appearance and the fact that they are prone to very little contraction. Full-thickness grafts are therefore commonly used in cases of small defects on the face or hands. Split thickness skin grafts are used to cover larger defects. Their size can be increased significantly by meshing the skin. Meshed grafts allow wound secretion to escape and are significantly less vulnerable than full-thickness skin grafts. As soon as skin grafts are stable, physiotherapy, pressure garments, and other scar prevention programs, e.g. laser therapy, are needed to optimize late results.

4a,b Many patients require flaps. Local flaps are connected to their original blood supply, but are detached from the adjacent structures and either rotated, advanced, or transposed in order to cover the defect. They may consist of skin with subcutaneous tissue or may be fasciocutaneous, myocutaneous, or isolated muscle flaps. Cross flaps are taken from neighboring structures such as arms, legs digits, or abdominal skin. Their original site can be closed either directly or by the use of skin grafts. In contrast to local flaps, free flaps become completely detached from their origin. Their major artery and vein must be reconnected to suitable vessels in the recipient region. Whether local or free flaps are indicated depends on the quantity of tissue that is needed, as well as the location of the wound. Smaller defects on the hands, feet, or face can usually be closed with local flaps or full-thickness skin grafts. Large defects on the trunk, upper arm, or leg may require local myocutaneous flaps, while large defects on the forearm or lower leg usually need free myocutaneous flaps or even composite flaps (usually a fibular free flap) that cover bone segments and are used to bridge osseous defects.

SPECIFIC PROBLEMS

The compartment syndrome is a critical complication of soft tissue injuries of the extremities, usually in the lower leg, foot, forearm, or hand. Any significant bleeding or post-ischemic swelling or edema in a muscle compartment that is closed in circular fashion by a fascia can cause rapid and significant increase in local tissue pressure, leading primarily to venous occlusion and subsequently to complete circulatory arrest in the compartment, followed by irreversible damage to muscles and nerves. Clinical signs include a tense and swollen compartment, severe local pain, characteristic inability to achieve active motion of the fingers or toes, and extreme pain on passive stretching. Early recognition is essential.

5 Intracompartmental pressure can be measured with a pressure recording system. A pressure difference of less than 20 mmHg compared with the mean diastolic pressure or less than 40 mmHg compared with mean systemic arterial pressure indicates that tissue perfusion has been disrupted. Immediate longitudinal incision of the skin and the fascia of the compartment (dermatofasciotomy) is necessary to avoid complete necrosis of the intracompartmental structures. Decompression surgery of the hand can be performed by making several longitudinal incisions. Volar forearm decompression should include the superficial and deep compartment, as well as the carpal tunnel. The dorsal compartment should be incised from the lateral humeral epicondyle to the wrist. On the leg, the compartments are incised according to their anatomical limits and margins. On the lower leg, it is advisable to open compartments by a parafibular approach. In the event of a compartment syndrome of the foot, dorsal and medial incisions are needed to free the interosseous and flexor muscles. A VAC dressing is very useful to cover the defect. As soon as tissue edema has been resolved, the skin can be closed either directly or stepwise with elastic bands or by the use of a split-skin graft. Complete closure of the fascia is not usually achieved.

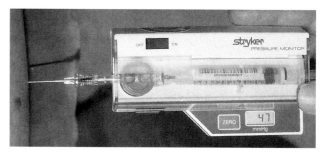

5

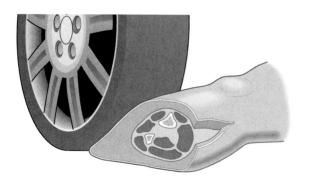

6

6 Degloving injuries occur when a tangential force grips the skin which commonly occurs in rollover accidents involving a car or truck. The term 'Morel–Lavaleé trauma' notes an extensive degloving injury. The skin and subcutaneous layers remain intact, but are detached from the underlying fascia. Any part of the body may be injured, but the lower extremities are most frequently affected. The skin is markedly crushed and may become necrotic in its central portion. A large hematoma with partly necrotic subcutaneous fatty tissue is found under the skin. The extent of the injury can be estimated by ultrasonography. Surgical treatment consists of debridement and resection of necrotic tissue. If the skin is intact it should be opened surgically at its center and the necrotic areas should be removed. Devascularized but otherwise intact skin may be resutured as with a full-thickness skin graft. A local VAC dressing permits removal of all exudates and allows second-look sessions until the wound can be closed again.

Accidents caused by rotating parts of machines such as a lawn-mower, a manure spreader, or other commonly used equipment on farms cause the most complex injuries. The affected parts most frequently involved are the extremities. The injuries may even result in traumatic amputation. The basic aspects of initial therapy are the same: cleaning the wounds, removing necrotic tissues, re-establishing any disrupted arteries or veins, stabilizing fractured bones, and open wound treatment with a VAC dressing. Local flaps or free flaps may be needed to cover the injured area. Nerves may be repaired primarily when the wound is clean or can be reanastomosed after 6–12 weeks under sterile conditions. Surgical repair of extensive injury is more successful in children than in adults. In exceptional cases, amputation may be necessary. Growth plates should be preserved as far as possible, especially in the distal femoral epiphyseal zone. Excessive growth of distal bone might cause problems in children. We would recommend that the level of amputation be carried out as far distally as possible as a longer stump helps to position the prosthesis. Replantation procedures can be successful provided that the warm ischemic time is no longer than 6 hours or the cold ischemic time less than 18 hours. However, the child's parents should be informed that their child may require secondary amputation and that long-term function might be limited.

7 Animal bites in childhood involving significant soft tissue injuries are commonly dog and occasionally horse bites. The breed of dogs most frequently responsible is the German Shepherd. Dog bites in infants and younger children are often located on the face. The risk of bacterial contamination after an animal bite is significant and the wound must be carefully cleaned with antiseptic solution. Treatment with appropriate broad-spectrum antibiotics is also essential. Large defects should be left open or treated with a VAC dressing to avoid early infection. Wounds on the face are preferably subjected to primary closure, including a small suction drain. Follow-up observations at frequent intervals will be required to identify local infectious complications at an early stage. Parents or caregivers should be informed that the patient may need secondary scar revision to improve the cosmetic result.

Many accidents can be prevented or at least the extent of the injury markedly reduced by wearing protective devices or taking suitable measures. The use of protective devices for inline skating, bicycling, or skiing, and appropriate clothes for motorcyclists can prevent or reduce injury. Children should not be permitted to enter the vicinity of machines with fast-moving rotational parts. Appropriate training of dogs and education of children (such as not to disturb the dog during its meal) may also reduce the high prevalence of these injuries.

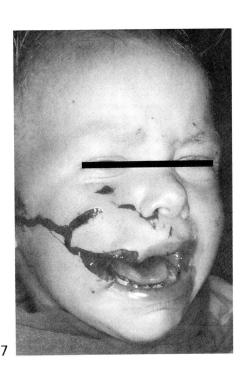

7

FURTHER READING

Halvorson EG, Disa JJ. Breast, skin and soft tissue. In: *Principles of Wound Management and Soft Tissue Repair*. ACS Surgery: Principles and Practice, vol. 3. Hamilton, Ontario: BC Decker, 2009: 1–19.

Hierner R, Nast-Kolb D, Stoel AM *et al.* Degloving injuries of the lower limb. *Unfallheilkunde* 2009; **112**: 55–63.

Levin LS. Principles of definite soft tissue coverage with flaps. *Journal of Orthopaedic Trauma* 2008; **22** (Suppl.): S161–S166.

Schalamon J, Ainoedhofer H, Singer G *et al.* Analysis of dog bites in children who are younger than 17 years. *Pediatrics* 2006; **117**: e374–9.

Tu YK, Tong GO, Wu CH *et al.* Soft-tissue injury in orthopedic trauma. *Injury* 2008; **39** (S4): S3–S17.

101

Thermal injuries

HEINZ RODE and DAVID M HEIMBACH

HISTORY

Burns are among the most serious injuries that can occur and, although many problems are still unresolved, substantial progress has been made since Neanderthal man treated burns with plant extract. In ancient Egypt, remedies were mainly fatty or oily substances of animal or vegetable sources and dry powder. During the thirteenth century, burns were divided into three degrees, characterized by redness, blisters, and crusts indicating reversible changes and, if left untreated, could extend into deeper tissues.

However, in the nineteenth century, remedies became less complicated and there was a gradual change from the practice of earlier times to more targeted methods with the use of carron oil, silver nitrate, hydrotherapy, and raw cotton dressings. The Indian tilemaker caste is credited with the earliest recorded method of skin grafting and George Pollock of London performed the first skin graft for a burn in 1870. In 1874, Thiersch used more extensive pieces of skin and, in 1875, Wolfe utilized a free full-thickness graft to repair a defect on the lower eyelid. Lustgarten described a technique of early excision and grafting of small burns in 1891. Brown of St Louis established the practical aspects of biological skin dressings as life-saving procedures in extensively burnt patients.

The prognosis of burnt patients did not improve substantially during the nineteenth century. The causes of death were speculative and treatment rudimentary until the middle period of the twentieth century. The modern treatment of burns has become a logical exercise in resuscitation, infection control, surgical wound care, pain control, nutrition, and psychological and physical rehabilitation. A combination of early eschar excision and autografting or allografting (cadaver skin), biological and synthetic skin substitutes have substantially transformed burn care management with a 50 percent predicted survival for a burn of 70 percent total body surface area (TBSA) in otherwise healthy adults and children.

PRINCIPLES AND JUSTIFICATION

- Burns in infants are not superficial.
- Burns often have a different geographical depth distribution being superficial in one area and deeper in another.
- Burns are dynamic, often deepen over the following 2–3 days and do not become more superficial.
- Hot water scald burns in children are best left for 2 weeks to assess the need for operative intervention, thereby reducing the area for excision by two-thirds.
- Hot water burns above the clavicle in toddlers may have an inhalational component.
- Surgery is an elective procedure in a stable patient.
- Early excision and grafting should be considered the treatment of choice for all deep burns. Inadequate excision leads to skin graft loss. Exceptions are burns on the ears, palms, soles of the feet, and genitalia.
- Once the burn wound has been excised, immediate wound closure with autografts, allografts, or biological alternatives is required.
- Surgical excision may safely be undertaken in the presence of inhalational injury, although operative time and blood loss must be kept to a minimum.
- Surgery should be delayed in burns which are more than 24 hours old on admission. Beta-hemolytic *Streptococcus* infection is a contraindication to surgical excision and grafting.
- Non-life threatening burns in patients with severe concomitant diseases or injuries should only be excised when the patients are stable and the life-threatening processes have been controlled.

BURN SEVERITY

The severity of a burn is determined by its depth and size, the anatomic site, concomitant disease or injury, and the age and physiologic status of the patient. Skin does not reach adult thickness until puberty; hence, the younger the child, the deeper the burn.

Burn depth

1 No objective clinical methods are available to determine the depth of thermal injury and no standardized method has been adopted. Most burns are a combination of superficial and deeper burns and the best assessment can be made 2–3 days after the injury when wound evolution has been completed.

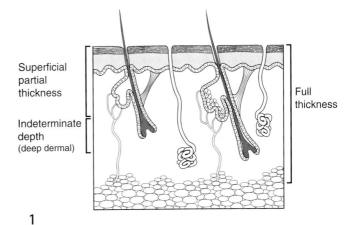

1

SUPERFICIAL PARTIAL THICKNESS: DESTRUCTION OF ONLY SUPERFICIAL LAYERS OF THE SKIN

These wounds will epithelialize spontaneously within 3 weeks; excision is contraindicated and the wounds rarely cause functional or cosmetic defects or hypertrophic scars. They characteristically have an erythematous, moist homogeneous surface with blister formation, are painful and hypersensitive to touch, blanch readily, and have a normal to firm texture on palpation.

INDETERMINATE DEPTH (DEEP DERMAL BURN): DESTRUCTION OF EPIDERMIS AND VARYING AMOUNTS OF DERMIS

These wounds are difficult to assess during the first 3 days after injury due to the ongoing evolution within the burn wound, which can be modulated by infection and dehydration. These wounds present with a reticulated red, white dry surface and may blister. Capillary circulation may be sluggish or absent when pressure is applied to

the wound. The healing time for these wounds may be variable and may require several weeks leading to severe hypertrophic scarring.

UNEQUIVOCALLY FULL THICKNESS: TOTAL IRREVERSIBLE DESTRUCTION OF ALL ELEMENTS OF THE SKIN WITH OR WITHOUT EXTENSION INTO THE DEEPER TISSUES AND STRUCTURES

These wounds will not heal spontaneously within 3 weeks and have unsatisfactory functional and cosmetic results. The best treatment entails early eschar excision and immediate grafting. These wounds may mimic the appearance of an indeterminate burn and are usually mottled, white, red, or charred and dry in appearance, insensitive to pain, and leathery to palpation. Blisters are unusual and, if present, are thin walled and do not enlarge. Clotted superficial vessels may be visible. The appearance of the burn remains static with little change over the ensuing days.

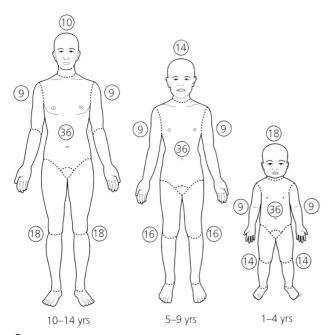

10–14 yrs   5–9 yrs   1–4 yrs

Estimating the extent of the burn

2 The extent of the burn is expressed as a percentage of the TBSA involved. Two methods of assessment are used. The palmar surface of the open hand of a patient amounts to approximately 1 percent of the TBSA and is used to estimate the size of small burns. Difference age-related values are used to calculate the percentage area burned in larger burns, because body proportions change with age. The 'pediatric rule of nine' can be modified for different ages, but at the age of ten years, the general rule of nine can be used as for adults. Surface area reaches adult proportions at ten years

2

MANAGEMENT

Emergency management

- At the scene of the injury, smoldering or hot clothing should be removed and the adequacy and patency of the airway ensured. Further onsite assessment entails a primary survey to identify and treat life-threatening conditions followed by a secondary head-to-toe survey and management if required.
- Hydrotherapy: Small burns (<25 percent TBSA) are immersed in cold or running water (15–18°C) or covered with cold, wet compresses for at least 30 minutes to relieve pain and discomfort. Cold water should be used cautiously for larger burns to prevent hypothermia.
- Copious irrigation of the wound with water is indicated for chemical burns (for at least 30 minutes); neutralizing agents should not be used.
- Burn wounds should be covered with a clean plastic sheet.
- In electrical burns, the patient's circulation and ventilation must be evaluated and maintained.
- For suspected inhalation injury, 100 percent oxygen is given by face mask. Progressive airway obstruction may occur over the first hours after the burn. It is safest to intubate early, before extensive head or laryngeal swelling occurs and airway obstruction becomes imminent.
- Oral fluids should be withheld initially.
- The patient must be stabilized before transportation is undertaken.

Definitive treatment

MINOR BURNS

Initial therapy of minor burns should include administration of analgesics, cleaning the wound with bland soap and water or detergent, removal of topically applied agents, and shaving hair where necessary. Dead tissue should be debrided and any tar removed with soft paraffin in a water base. Topical antibacterial agents and occlusive dressings or an adhesive polyurethane sheet should be used to dress the wound and tetanus toxoid should be administered. The patient should be encouraged to move the affected area. Local topical therapy is applied on a regular basis until the wounds have healed. Prophylactic antibiotics are not required.

Fluid resuscitation proportional to burn size

The patient should be assessed for shock and if present, a crystalloid fluid volume of 20 mL/kg of Ringer's lactate solution should be given immediately. This should be repeated until the hypovolemic stage has been corrected. Fluid therapy thereafter consists of two components, namely ongoing fluid loss replacement at 3 mL/kg per percentage burn TBSA for the first day and standard maintenance fluid given intravenously at 100 mL/kg up to 10 kg + 50 mL/kg from 10 to 20 kg + 20 mg/kg for each kg over 20 kg in weight. Enteral feeding should be started as soon as possible. These formulations are only a guide and are used to maintain hemodynamic stability and urine output at 1 mL/kg per hour. Glucose-containing intravenous fluid must be given to children under two years of age.

MAJOR BURNS

Management of major burns is a particularly time- and energy-intensive process and the requirement of a coherent multidisciplinary team cannot be underestimated. Primary skin grafting for superficial wounds will not decrease morbidity or improve the functional outcome. On the other hand, deep or full thickness burns should be excised and grafted. Many burns, however, cannot be easily categorized and the decision to excise and graft is therefore crucial.

Other factors that will require ongoing management include treatment of inhalational injuries, nutrition, pain control, prevention and treatment of infection, physical and psychological rehabilitation.

SURGICAL GUIDELINES

The process of excision, grafting, and burn wound coverage must follow a predetermined progression. Flexibility will be needed. Burns represent a unique challenge due to the nature of the operation and the concomitant physiological responses to injury.

The operating room procedure follows a set program:

- Administer anaesthesia. Important components are maintenance of an adequate and secured airway, especially in the presence of inhalational injury and facial burns, choice of anesthetic agents, maintenance of anesthesia, temperature, and hemodynamic stability, regional anesthesia and the use of pharmacological agents, the position of the patient during surgery, the site of surgery (eschar and donor area) and continual monitoring.
- Clean the wound with bland soap and water or detergent.
- Remove any topically applied agents.
- Joint and burn mobilization by allied therapists.
- The depth and extent of the burn wound will determine the surgical approach.
- Excise and graft as per treatment plan.
- The amount to be excised at each procedure depends on the stability of the patient, the burn size, availability of auto- and allograft, the volume of blood loss incurred during the procedure and the adequacy of anesthesia.
- Dress the wound with topical antibacterial agents, occlusive dressings, a non-adhesive polyurethane sheet or temporary skin substitutes.
- Routine intraoperative antibiotics are usually not administered, but may be given when the burn wounds are infected or with large excisions.

Intraoperative considerations

VASCULAR ACCESS

Normal anatomical landmarks may be distorted and the use of ultrasound guidance may be required. Adequate and secure vascular access is critical. A large bore venous cannula is usually placed in either the subclavian, internal jugular, or femoral veins (not a preferred site) or another suitable surface vessel. Additional arterial access is established for major burns and when large blood losses are expected.

TEMPERATURE CONTROL

Hypothermia is a significant problem and preventable measures include an ambient operating room temperature of 28–32°C, warmed anesthetic gases, and intravenous fluids at 37°C. Radiant heaters can be used and the patient lies on a plastic-covered warming blanket. Exposed areas may be covered with sterile plastic drapes. Body temperature should be at or above 37°C.

MONITORING

Electrocardiogram electrodes may be difficult to site and any accessible area will suffice as the configuration is irrelevant. The electrodes can be secured with surgical clips. A urinary catheter is inserted. Non-invasive blood pressure monitoring with pulse oximetry, a central temperature probe, and urine output at 1 mL/kg per hour are essential. Postoperatively, the child is kept in the recovery area and constantly monitored until fully awake with satisfactory vital signs and is normothermic. Adequate postoperative analgesia and sedation is required.

FLUID REQUIREMENTS

Maintenance fluid is given as isotonic crystalloids at 4 mL/kg per hour and blood loss is replaced volume/volume to maintain the hematocrit above 30 percent. Weighing surgical swabs is a satisfactory measure of blood loss determination. Blood loss of between 0.4 and 0.74 mL/cm^2 of tissue excised can be expected.

Decompression escharotomy

Decompression escharotomies are emergency procedures done at the time of first assessment of the patient to avoid irreversible ischemic and hypoxic damage to tissue. Releasing incisions must be done where a circumferential deep burn is impeding circulation to more distal parts, especially round the arms, legs, or chest where respiration may be impaired.

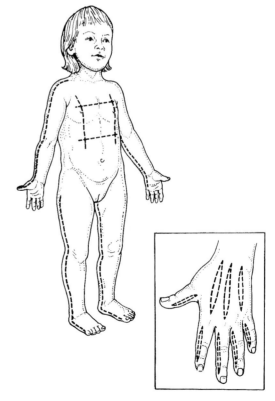

3 The incision must traverse the dead tissue as far into the subcutaneous layer as necessary to encounter viable tissue, and must extend from non-viable through to viable tissue. Bleeding may be a problem, especially if the incisions are too deep or performed across major vessels. Vital structures (e.g. nerves, blood vessels) may be damaged if the incisions are incorrectly sited. Transverse incisions in the limbs should not be made.

PRACTICAL APPROACH TO SURGICAL EXCISION

- Superficial partial thickness burns: conservative therapy.
- Deep partial and full thickness burns: excision and autografting.
- Indeterminate depth: wait for 10–14 days with regular assessment and definitive surgical treatment if the burn wound would not be epithelialized by 3 weeks.
- Burns <10 percent TBSA: excision and autografting are performed using meshed 1.5:1 or 2:1 or sheet grafts. Sheet grafts are placed on all vital and visual areas (face, neck, chest, hands) and all small grafted areas.
- Burns 10–30 percent TBSA: excision and autografting.
- Burns 30–40 percent TBSA: sufficient donor sites are usually available to graft the excised bed despite the fact that about 30 percent TBSA is unavailable for donation (face, neck, hands, and feet). The grafts should be meshed at 1.5:1 or 2:1, or temporary allografts or a synthetic skin substitute applied.
- Burns >40 percent TBSA: donor sites are limited and it is impossible to primarily cover all the excised wounds with autografts. The preferred method is to perform total or sequential (20 percent TBSA every alternate day) excisions. Skin cover should then be applied (autograft 1.5:1, 2:1, or 3:1 and/or autograft 3:1 with allograft 2:1 overlay, and/or synthetic skin substitutes).

Timing and extent of excision

In general terms, excision is carried out as soon after injury as possible, i.e. as soon as the cardiovascular system is stable and resuscitation completed, metabolic and physiologic balance restored, and vital signs, urine output, hematocrit and albumin levels are satisfactory. This time may vary from a few hours to several days, but a good timing goal is day 3. Excision is therefore an elective procedure in a stable patient. The order of priority of areas for major excision are the posterior trunk, anterior trunk, and clavicular area, one lower extremity, second lower extremity, both upper extremities and hands, and all unhealed areas on the face, neck, and head.

The amount to be excised at each procedure depends on the stability of the patient, the burn size, availability of auto- and allografts, and the volume of blood loss incurred during the procedure. Most deep burns of less than 40 percent TBSA should be excised and grafted within the first few days as adequate donor sites are usually available. In large burns, the principle is to reduce the burn surface area expeditiously.

METHODS OF REMOVING ESCHAR

Three different methods of removing eschar are used: (1) tangential or sequential excision, (2) fascial excision, and (3) delayed escharectomy.

Tangential or sequential excision

4 This method entails the sequential excision of thin layers of burn eschar until a viable bed is encountered. If done correctly, the minimum amount of living tissue is sacrificed; dermal elements are retained with satisfactory functional and cosmetic results. Tangential excision is best done within the first 1–5 days before hypervascularity and wound infection becomes established. Excision is best performed by using a hand-held Humby or Watson knife, held at a tangent to the wound surface. Excision over uneven surfaces or bony prominences can be aided by subeschar injection of saline. The appropriate level of excision or end-point is characterized by a shiny white surface with brisk arteriolar or punctuate bleeding or viable yellow, non-hemorrhagic subcutaneous fat globules with briskly bleeding vessels in all areas. Clotted vessels, dullness, punctate hemorrhages, dark pink-brown hemorrhagic fat represent non-viable areas and must be removed as residual necrotic areas will jeopardize graft take. Tissue staining with hemoglobin from lysed red cells indicates inadequate excision.

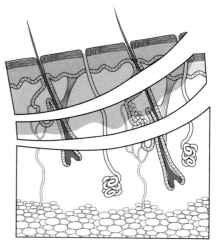

4

Dissection may become difficult once the level of excision has gone beyond the dermis. It is important to preserve subdermal fat over bony prominences for esthetic reasons, but grafting onto subdermal fat results in a lower success rate. Most extremity burns can be excised under tourniquet control, but experience is necessary since the sign of a bleeding bed is no longer available. Blood loss may be substantial and effective control of hemorrhage must be established. It is advisable to limit excision to 25–100 cm², control hemorrhage, and then to proceed with further excision. A maximum of ±20 percent TBSA should be excised at any one time. Alternatively, extremity excisions could be done under subeschar clysis where adrenalin and a local anesthetic are deposited in the subcutaneous tissue prior to surgical excision.

Once excised to the appropriate level and hemostasis secured, an immediate split-thickness skin graft (autograft) is performed. Sheet grafts are placed on important cosmetic and functional areas. To prevent desiccation of exposed and viable tissue, mesh grafts should not be expanded more than 1.5:1–2:1. If greater expansion is needed, temporary skin substitutes (cadaver or Biobrane™) should overlay the autograft. The latter method is also used for all excised and non-grafted areas.

Fascial excision

5 This method is generally reserved for very large life-threatening or deep full-thickness burns and burns in the elderly. The excision is performed using a combination of sharp dissection, traction, and hemorrhage control. The amount excised at each procedure is determined by the stability of the child, blood loss, and the availability of autografts or skin substitutes. Fascial excision assures a viable bed for skin grafting with moderate blood loss, especially if done under tourniquet control. An excellent graft take may be expected if done within the first few days after injury. By incising at the periphery of the eschar vertically downward to the level of the deep investing fascia, a flap of eschar is raised and the dissection extended until all the dead tissue down to fascia level has been excised. The skin edges should be sutured to the excised bed to limit movement. It is preferable to leave a thin layer of fat over the subcutaneous bony prominences and tendon sheaths. Complete hemostasis with electrocoagulation should minimize blood loss substantially, but bleeding often occurs from the skin edges. Topical vasoconstrictive agents could be applied to the fascia as the dissection proceeds. At completion, the extremity is wrapped with a pressure bandage and elevated for 10 minutes. The excised area is covered with an expanded split-thickness skin graft. If the ratio exceeds 2:1, the autograft should be covered with a 1.5:1 meshed cadaveric allograft or consider VAC or other temporary skin substitutes. The major disadvantage of this method is that it causes damage to lymphatics and cutaneous nerves, loss of subcutaneous fat, long-term cosmetic deformity, and distal edema.

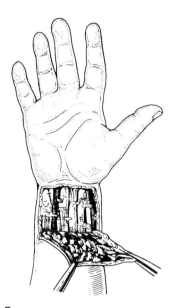

5

Delayed escharectomy

Delayed escharectomy after 7 days, or following spontaneous eschar separation, allows for the formulation of a bed of granulation tissue. Daily debridement by means of hydrotherapy (showering or bathing), or coarse mesh gauze dressings will hasten eschar separation. The burn wound is ready for split skin grafting when there is a shiny, slightly granular pinkish/red uniform bed of granulation tissue with no debris or evidence of infection. This method is most often used for old, neglected burn wounds. Enzymatic debriding agents are seldom used.

SKIN SUBSTITUTES

Allograft is the principal alternative wound closure material and can be used as a (1.5:1.3) meshed graft overlaying an expanded autograft, as a biological dressing, or as a temporary cover on excised wounds in the absence of available autografts for immediate wound closure. Allografts should be removed before rejection becomes evident. In practice, this means removal every 10–12 days and replacement with pool allografts or permanent replacement with autograft when available. If this procedure is followed, the likelihood of rejection and poor recipient bed is reduced. If allografts are left for more than 14 days, removal can only be achieved by excision. Alternative methods (xenografts, cultured keratinocytes, and other biological skin substitutes) are not reliable for routine use and at best function only as temporary skin cover.

Alternatively, the excised wounds can be covered with Biobrane (a fibroblast derived temporary skin substitute) or Integra (a permanent composite non-cellular dermal substitute) until epithelialization with a thin autograft can be achieved.

DONOR SKIN PROCUREMENT

6 Most unburned areas can serve as donor sites, although certain areas, i.e. face, hands, perineum, and cervical areas are unsuitable as donor sites. The preferred donor sites are the legs, buttocks, and back and best colour match between donor and recipient areas can be obtained from the 'blushing' area of the body for facial and neck burns. Donor skin thickness should be between 0.02 cm (0.008 inches thin) and 0.025 cm (0.010 inches thicker). Thicker grafts are more pliable and cause less scarring. Skin grafts are best procured with an electric dermatome. Subcutaneous injection of saline + adrenaline + bupivocane (marcaine) vasopressin will greatly facilitate graft procurement over bony or uneven prominences. Donor sites are usually ready for reuse after 14 days, but can only be used once full epithelialization has occurred. Grafts are usually meshed with a Tanner–Vandeput meshgraft dermatome at a ratio of 1.5:1, 2:1, or 3:1, or used as sheet grafts on vital or cosmetically important areas.

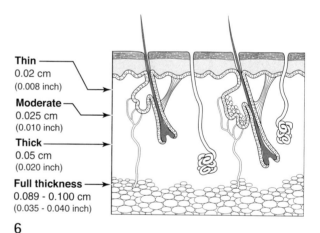

Thin
0.02 cm
(0.008 inch)

Moderate
0.025 cm
(0.010 inch)

Thick
0.05 cm
(0.020 inch)

Full thickness
0.089 - 0.100 cm
(0.035 - 0.040 inch)

6

HEMOSTATIC CONTROL

It is important to ensure that the excision is adequate before topical adrenalin is applied as vasoconstriction may change the cut surface to take on a uniform avascular appearance. Bleeding from excised areas should be minimized by limiting excisional procedures to 25–100 cm^2 at any one time, until hemostasis is ensured. Other methods employed are local pressure for 10 minutes, diathermy coagulation, suture ligation, calcium-enriched alginate dressings, and the topical application of sponges soaked in 1:10 000/1:30 000 epinephrine (adrenaline) solution to the excised bed for 10 minutes or pre-excisional subeschar injection (clysis or tumescence) of adrenaline. Topical adrenaline should not be used in patients with cardiac disease or arrythmias. Additionally, extremity exsanguinations and pneumatic tourniquet methods can be used.

SKIN GRAFT PLACEMENT

The procured skin is grafted onto the recipient area at the time of eschar excision, directly from the mesh board. Grafts are placed with the shiny or cut surface facing the prepared recipient bed, either longitudinally or transversely over joints. The edges should be approximated or slightly overlapping and secured with surgical clips, sutures, synthetic tissue glue with a fine mesh gauze overlay, or with a silicone nylon dressing to prevent dislodgement of the graft.

WOUND DRESSINGS

Recipient area

In general terms, the recipient area is covered with an occlusive dressing to prevent infection, avulsion, and desiccation of the graft, and to allow for graft vascularization (3–4 days if grafts are placed on dermis or fascia and 5–7 days if placed on fat). Both sheet and mesh grafts are covered with a layer of fine mesh gauze, impregnated with topical antibiotics, followed by an absorbable dressing and an elastic dressing and splinting in a functional position where indicated. Sheet grafts may be left exposed, especially on the face and neck areas. The outer dressings, down to the layer of fine gauze, are taken down the following day

to remove any blood clots or wound exudate. Thereafter, the dressings can be left for a few days or changed if there is strike-through bleeding or exudation or suspected infection. All dressings, clips, or sutures should be removed after 5–6 days and the wounds thereafter protected with Vaseline gauze and bandages until healed.

Donor sites

As all donor sites scar to some degree, it is preferable to procure skin from an area that can be hidden under most circumstances. The donor site needs to be treated as a partial thickness burn. Initial bleeding is stopped with epinephrine swab compression; the wound is then covered either with an antiseptic or occlusive dressing, such as Opsite™, Biobrane, Iaban, or Hypofix™. Discomfort is minimal and rapid healing is experienced. The dressing is either left intact until healing has occurred or removed after a few days.

FOLLOW UP

All wounds not healed within 3 weeks and all grafted areas would require pressure garments for 6–18 months. All burnt, grafted, and donor areas should be protected from direct sun exposure for at least 6–12 months. Topical application of a bland moisturising agent may improve skin texture and color.

Early reconstruction principles form an integral part of all surgical procedures and long-term problems can be circumvented or minimized by proper positioning, supportive splints, and pressure devices, judicious use of skeletal traction and suspension to maintain joint excursions and mobility.

FURTHER READING

Heimbach DM, Engrav LH. *Surgical Management of the Burn Wound*. New York: Raven Press, 1984.

Janzekovic Z. A new concept in the early excision and immediate grafting of burns. *Journal of Trauma* 1970; **10**: 1103–8.

Klasen HJ. *History of Burns*. Rotterdam: Erasmus Publishing, 2004.

102

Thoracic injuries

MICHAEL E HÖLLWARTH

INTRODUCTION

Severe injury to the chest wall or intrathoracic organs is a rare occurrence in children. The data of the National Pediatric Trauma Registry (United States) show that 86 percent causes of thoracic injuries were blunt (falls from a height, bicycle or motor vehicle accidents), while 14 percent were penetrating (gunshot or stab wounds). Boys are more commonly affected than girls (ratio 2:1). In the author's region, traffic accidents account for 43 percent, falls from heights for 24 percent, sports accidents for 13 percent, and accidents related to farming work for 8 percent of all thoracic injuries in children. In one third of the cases, significant additional injuries, mainly head injuries, were present. Mortality is high in cases of penetrating injuries, but much lower in blunt trauma, chiefly related to the concomitant cerebral injury.

The pattern of thoracic injuries in younger children differs from that in adults. The high elasticity of the chest wall in children permits enormous compression in a sagittal direction. Thus, rib fractures are not as common as they are in adults undergoing similar trauma. The frequency of hematopneumothorax is also lower, because rib fractures commonly occur within the periosteal sleeve. Severe injuries to parenchymal organs may occur without evidence of rib fractures on x-ray. Even a rollover injury from a car may occur without causing a rib fracture in a young child. The injury pattern in adolescents becomes increasingly similar to that in adults.

Resuscitation efforts in major chest trauma must take into account the smaller diameter of the upper airways, the higher normal ventilation frequency, and the normal inspiratory to expiratory time of 1:1.5 or 1:2 (**Table 102.1**). Supplementary oxygen by assisted ventilation, two large intravenous lines, a nasogastric tube, continuous monitoring of lung function and gas exchange, as well as control of blood counts, electrolytes, liver, heart, and kidney function are parts of the basic management. Plain films of the chest are a routine procedure in the emergency setting. However, significant lung contusions may not be visible during the first few hours after the injury. Therefore, computed tomography (CT) imaging with or without intravenous contrast injection is indicated. In cases of major trauma, the CT should include the head and the abdomen. Other investigations, such as echocardiography, tracheobronchoscopy, video-assisted thoracoscopy (VATS), or an isotope heart scan may be indicated in certain circumstances.

Table 102.1 Normal respiratory frequency in different age groups.

Age	Respiratory frequency per minute
Newborns	55
Infants	40
Until the age of three years	35
Until the age of seven years	25
Until the age of 12 years	15–20

INJURY TO THE CHEST WALL

1 Severe compression trauma of the chest in a young child causes an acute shift of blood from the intrathoracic vena cava to the neck and head. This sudden increase of volume and pressure in peripheral veins causes capillary extravasation with petechial bleeding on the skin of the face and neck (Perthes syndrome). Children may manifest cyanosis of the face or petechial bleedings in the eyes (subconjuctiva, retina, or vitreous). Capillary hemorrhage affecting the brain may cause disorientation, loss of consciousness and seizures. Perthes syndrome does not require any special treatment.

All significant soft tissue injuries of the chest wall are signs of additional injury in the skeleton or intrathoracic organs. Severe soft tissue injury may occur after a rollover accident with a car. The lateral skin and subcutaneous tissue of the chest is hit by the car tires, lifted from the chest wall, and severely compressed against the ground. The tread of the tire may be visible on the skin. Large skin defects may require plastic surgery.

A traumatic subcutaneous lung hernia may occur as a rare consequence of traumatic rupture of intercostal muscles. The condition is marked by a circumscript paradoxical movement on respiration and requires surgical repair of the ruptured muscle and fascia.

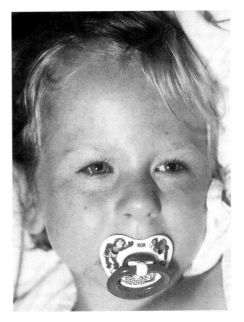

1

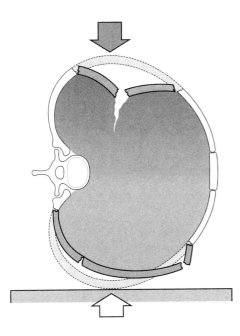

2

2 Rib fractures (single or serial) may result from circumscribed trauma at the site of impact or a widely acting force that leads to rib fractures along the ventral and dorsal circumference eventually causing a flail chest. Subcutaneous emphysema is common when extensive fractures occur in conjunction with lung lacerations. Fractures of the first and the second rib are a reliable sign of major trauma and may further indicate severe injury to organs or major vessels particularly if the chest radiograph shows abnormalities within the mediastinum.

3 Infants and young children experience rib fractures only when an enormous force is exerted on the thoracic cage. Therefore, any rib fracture in a young child is strongly indicative of physical abuse. A very special pattern of intraperiosteal rib fractures in abused small infants – often manifested as a secondary callus formation on the chest x-ray – occurs after forceful ventral to dorsal compression of the chest with both hands.

3

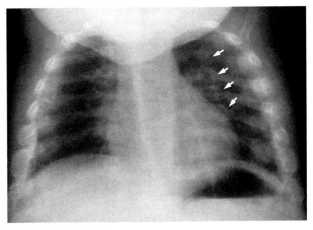

The treatment of uncomplicated rib fractures consists of rest and appropriate analgesia to maximize the child's well-being and prevent atelectasis or pneumonia as a result of superficial respiratory movements. In cases of serial rib fractures, pain relief is best achieved by epidural blockade and the administration of intravenous analgesics. In children with an unstable flail chest, first aid will consist of stabilizing the chest with the open hand or a sand bag. When respiratory insufficiency with paradoxical chest wall movements persists, the child may require temporary ventilation with appropriate PEEP (positive end-expiratory pressure) for 3–6 weeks depending on the child's age. Spontaneous healing occurs and the chest wall stability is restored.

Fractures of the sternum are usually located within the body of the sternum and may occur in rare instances following direct trauma after a fall on the sharp edge of a table, a chair, or other objects. Accompanying contusion of the heart should be ruled out. As a rule, dislocation is minimal and the fractures heal spontaneously after appropriate analgesic therapy.

INTRATHORACIC ORGANS

Lung contusions are a common finding after severe chest trauma. Due to the high elasticity of the chest wall, lung contusion may occur without a fracture of the chest wall. Significant compression of the lung leads to intraparenchymatous bleeding and tissue rupture, usually in the posterior portion of the lung. Typical signs of lung contusion on the x-ray are patchy, cloud-like, confluent shadows in a non-anatomic distribution. Serial x-rays may reveal progression of the lesion due to peripheral edema and atelectasis. In order to evaluate the true extent of the lesion and exclude further intrathoracic injuries, a chest CT scan should be performed. Most lung contusions can be treated conservatively with physiotherapy and appropriate antibiotics. Pneumonia is thus avoided in the majority of patients. Patients with respiratory insufficiency may require PEEP-driven ventilation. A central lung rupture may be present in the contused region. In rare cases, a cystic lesion, a so-called 'pneumatocele', develops in 2 or 3 weeks. The condition is managed conservatively except in those cases in which a large communication to a bronchus necessitates local resection.

4 Lung ruptures may also occur on the visceral surface after external compression, but more commonly lung lacerations result from fractured ribs injuring adjacent lung regions. Both injuries cause a pneumothorax, hematothorax, and most often a hematopneumothorax diagnosed by chest x-ray, and/or CT scan. A mediastinal emphysema indicates lung ruptures involving the mediastinal pleura – or may be a sign of injury to the trachea or bronchi. A pneumothorax is either asymptomatic or shows, in addition to chest pain, clinical signs of tachypnea, respiratory distress, decreased oxygen saturation and a typical hollow sound on percussion. An asymptomatic simple pneumothorax can be treated by observation alone. However, the treatment usually consists of a chest tube drain inserted into the fourth or fifth intercostal space in the mid-axillary line, connected to a suction device with an underwater seal. The skin incision should be performed 2–4 cm distal to the intercostal space, as this will permit perfect closure of the tissue in layers when the drain is being removed. Recommended tube sizes vary from 12 to 16 Fr for newborns, 16–18 Fr for infants, 18–24 Fr for school-age children, and 28–32 Fr for adolescents. As soon as the air leak stops, the tube should be clamped for 12 hours and removed when the x-ray confirms the absence of a recurrent pneumothorax.

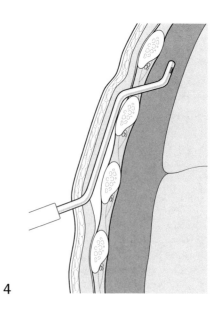

4

A tension pneumothorax after lung lacerations is characterized by a one-way valve-like mechanism. Air that reaches the pleural space cannot flow back during expiration. The resulting intrapleural pressure causes a total ipsilateral lung collapse and a shift of the mediastinal organs to the contralateral site, thus compressing the opposite lung. Increasing respiratory distress, reduced venous backflow with engorged neck veins, and finally life-threatening shock, are the typical clinical signs. These signs and a hyper-resonant percussion on the affected site distinguish the tension pneumothorax adequately from a pericardial tamponade, thus necessitating emergency intervention with a needle or catheter drainage without waiting for additional imaging procedures.

An open pneumothorax is rare in children. It is a life-threatening condition that causes complete collapse of the lung and flattening of the mediastinum, rapidly leading to severe respiratory distress. Emergency treatment consists of an occlusive dressing that serves as a flatter valve, and subsequently insertion of a pleural drainage.

5 A hematothorax is the most common finding after severe chest trauma. Intrapleural blood accumulates either due to a rib fracture or rupture of an intercostal or internal mammary vessel, or associated with an additional lung laceration which may lead to a hematopneumothorax. It should be noted that in young children even significant blood loss is accompanied by minimal clinical signs because the blood pressure in a child is maintained within the normal ranges for a longer period of time. This is due to efficient contraction of vessels. However, once the hypovolemic shock becomes clinically evident, one is confronted with a late emergency situation. Circulatory symptoms depend on the quantity of blood loss. Auscultation and percussion will reveal diminished respiratory sounds. The x-ray will show poor aeration of the lung with or without an additional pneumothorax. The treatment of a hematothorax consists of intercostal drainage. In contrast to the pneumothorax, blood should be evacuated as early as possible, and this is best achieved either by needle puncture or by the insertion of a thoracic drain in a lower intercostal space. Ultrasound-guided insertion is useful to select the most suitable position. In most cases, the bleeding soon stops, especially after lung lacerations, due to the low pressure of intrapulmonary blood flow. Thoracotomy is recommended only when the bleeding exceeds 5 percent of the estimated blood volume/hour, or when the initial blood loss exceeds 30 percent of the blood volume.

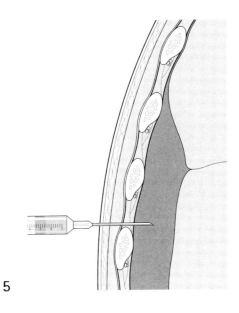

5

Tracheal injuries are uncommon in childhood, but some children may die of respiratory insufficiency before they reach the hospital. Ruptures of the membranous portion of the trachea usually occur 2–3 cm above the carina. They are preceded by a massive increase in intraluminal pressure and simultaneous closure of the glottis. Symptoms may vary from dyspnea to stridor, cyanosis, hemoptysis and massive mediastinal and subcutaneous emphysema. Initial treatment consists of endotracheal intubation as deep as needed to establish adequate ventilation. Flexible endoscopy through the endotracheal tube permits localization of the defect and its extent. Short and well-adapted defects, as well as longer defects which are adequately bridged over by the tube, usually respond to conservative treatment. Larger defects and continuous emphysema despite tracheal intubation requires surgical repair through a right-sided lateroposterior thoracotomy. In injuries involving the upper trachea, care must be taken to avoid damage to the recurrent laryngeal nerve.

Injuries in the main bronchi are rare in childhood, although more common than tracheal ruptures. Due to the high elasticity of the pediatric chest, ruptures of the bronchus occur more commonly in children. Massive sagittal compression of the chest in conjunction with hyperextension of the vertebral column is the mechanism that leads to partial bronchial rupture in the typical location 1–2 cm distal to the carina. After complete rupture, the lung collapses towards the angle between the diaphragm and the mediastinum ('the dropped lung'). Symptoms may not be evident initially, but are usually similar to those associated with tracheal ruptures, such as mediastinal and subcutaneous emphysema, uni- or bilateral pneumothorax, dyspnea, stridor, and hemoptysis. Bronchoscopy or a three-dimensional reconstructed CT scan is most appropriate for a detailed diagnostic study. Smaller ruptures may be treated conservatively. Major ruptures of the main right or left bronchus can be operated on by performing a right lateroposterior thoracotomy. More distal ruptures of the left main bronchus require a left-sided thoracotomy. Granulation tissue in missed bronchial ruptures may cause subtotal or complete closure of the airway with peripheral atelectasis, pneumonia, abscess formation, and bronchiectasis. Bronchoscopy will confirm the diagnosis. The airway can be reopened by local

dilatation and endoscopic laser therapy. In completely occluded bronchi, secondary reconstruction may be performed as long as the lung tissue is still functioning and the vessels are patent.

Esophagotracheal fistula is a rare injury after blunt thoracic trauma and is possibly subject to the same mechanism as that described for tracheal ruptures. The principal symptoms are retrosternal pain, mediastinal emphysema, and shock. Bradycardia is a symptom of irritation of the vagal nerve. Penetrating injuries may cause esophageal lacerations in the neck region. Diagnostic procedures consist of endoscopy and radiological investigation by the use of water-soluble contrast material. Initial surgery is useful when the condition is diagnosed within 12 hours. Delayed diagnosis is associated with mediastinal inflammation and requires local drainage, salivary diversion either with a Replogle tube or cervical esophagostomy, gastrostomy, and antibiotics. Local stabilization is followed by open repair.

6 Injuries of the heart, pericardium, and major thoracic vessels are rare in childhood. Sudden cardiac arrest, most often during exhausting sport activities, is defined as 'commotio cordis' when the autopsy shows no evidence of an organic injury. The underlying pathology is most likely ventricular fibrillation. Acceleration and deceleration mechanisms after car accidents or after a major fall from a height may cause contracoup contusion of the heart, atrial or ventricular septal defects, or traumatic rupture of major intrathoracic vessels. Contusion of the heart muscle secondary to blunt trauma may be observed after a rollover accident with a car or result from an inadequately restrained child seat during a frontal accident. Contusion injuries range from minimal bleeding to severe muscle damage. Echocardiography, CT scans of the heart and pathological heart enzymes (CKMB, troponin I and T) confirm the type and severity of the injury. Transmural ischemic damage may give rise to ventricular aneurysm, occasionally followed by muscle rupture 2–3 weeks later. Pericardial tamponade may be caused by a penetrating or blunt heart injury. As the elasticity of the pericardium is minimal, even 100–200 mL blood in the pericardial space may cause a tamponade, thus compressing the ventricle during the diastolic filling phase. Clinical signs are engorged neck veins, systemic hypotension, and muffled heart sounds (Beck's triad). Echocardiography confirms the diagnosis and should be followed immediately by needle puncture of the pericardium (pericardiocentesis) and catheter insertion. Thoracotomy and repair of the injury are indicated when bleeding persists.

6

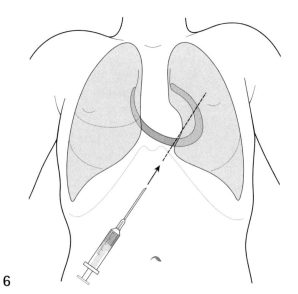

PENETRATING INJURIES

Penetrating injuries in children and adolescents, caused by knife wounds and gunshots, result in a variety of thoracic injuries comprising all of the intrathoracic organs. Most patients require urgent interventions and, frequently, surgery. The type of interventions is similar to that in the presence of blunt trauma.

FURTHER READING

Bliss D, Silen M. Pediatric thoracic trauma. *Critical Care Medicine* 2002; **30**: S409–S415.

Haxhija EQ, Nöres H, Schober P, Höllwarth ME. Lung contusion-lacerations after blunt thoracic trauma in children. *Pediatric Surgery International* 2004; **20**: 412–14.

Lofland GK, O'Brien JE. Thoracic Trauma in Children. In:Ashcraft KW, Holcomb GW, Murphy JP (eds). *Pediatric Surgery*, 4th edn. Philadelphia, PA: Elsevier Saunders, 2005: 185–200.

Sartorelli KH, Vane DW. The diagnosis and management of children with blunt injury of the chest. *Seminars in Pediatric Surgery* 2004; **13**: 98–105.

Tepas JJ. The national pediatric trauma registry: a legacy of commitment to control of childhood injury. *Seminars in Pediatric Surgery* 2004; **13**: 126–32.

Tovar JA. The lung and pediatric trauma. *Seminars in Pediatric Surgery* 2008; **17**: 53–9.

103

Abdominal trauma

STEVEN STYLIANOS and MARK V MAZZIOTTI

> If a disease were killing our children in the proportions that accidents are, people would be outraged and demand that this killer be stopped.
>
> C Everett Koop MD ScD

HISTORY

Who could have imagined the influence of James Simpson's publication in 1968 on the successful non-operative treatment of select children presumed to have splenic injury. Initially suggested in the early 1950s by Tim Warnsborough, then Chief of General Surgery at the Hospital for Sick Children in Toronto, it is remarkable to consider that the era of non-operative management for pediatric spleen injury began with the report of 12 children treated between 1956 and 1965. The diagnosis of splenic injury in this select group was made by clinical findings together with routine laboratory and plain x-ray findings. It should be borne in mind that the report predated ultrasound, computed tomography (CT), or isotope imaging.

Nearly half a century later, the standard treatment of hemodynamically stable children with splenic injury is non-operative and this concept has now been successfully applied to most blunt injuries of the liver, kidney, and pancreas as well. Surgical restraint has been the theme, based on an increased awareness of the anatomic patterns and physiologic responses characteristic of injured children. Our colleagues in adult trauma care have slowly acknowledged this success and applied many of the principles learned in pediatric trauma to their patients.

Few surgeons have extensive experience with massive abdominal solid organ injury requiring immediate surgery. It is imperative that surgeons familiarize themselves with current treatment algorithms for life-threatening abdominal trauma. Important contributions have been made to the diagnosis and treatment of children with abdominal injury by radiologists and endoscopists. The resolution and speed of CT, the screening capabilities of focused abdominal sonography for trauma (FAST), and the percutaneous, angiographic, and endoscopic interventions of non-surgeon members of the pediatric trauma team have all enhanced patient care and improved outcomes. This chapter focuses on the more common blunt injuries of the spleen, liver, duodenum, pancreas, and kidney.

RESUSCITATION

A multitrauma patient entering a medical facility should be treated by an organized team of surgeons, physicians, and nurses. The composition of the team will vary, but the senior surgeon should be the team leader. Preparation is mandatory and includes ensuring the availability of equipment appropriate to children of varying ages and the establishment of a resuscitation protocol. The 'checklist approach' is the surest way to accomplish the essential steps of diagnosis and treatment while individualizing care for each patient. The initial evaluation of the acutely injured child is similar to that of the adult. Plain radiographs of the C-spine (cervical spine), chest, and pelvis are obtained following the initial survey and evaluation of A (airway), B (breathing), and C (circulation). As imaging modalities have improved, treatment algorithms have changed significantly in children with a suspected intra-abdominal injury. Prompt identification of potentially life-threatening injuries is now possible in the vast majority of children.

Airway control, vascular access, spinal precautions, and temperature regulation must be assured throughout the initial evaluation and treatment of injured children. The reader is referred to the *Textbook of Pediatric Advanced Life Support* (American Academy of Pediatrics) and the *Textbook of Advanced Trauma Life Support* (American College of Surgeons) for specific details of airway management, pharmacologic therapy, and central venous access in injured children.

DIAGNOSIS OF BLUNT ABDOMINAL INJURIES

Recognition of significant abdominal injuries in children with blunt multisystem trauma can be difficult. Physical examination is inaccurate in more than 30 percent of cases, particularly in those patients seen soon after injury or with central nervous system injuries and an abnormal neurologic examination. It is no surprise that advances in diagnosis have paralleled the development of new imaging technology. Prompt and accurate recognition of abdominal injuries, now possible with CT, allows for focused treatment plans.

CT has become the imaging study of choice for the evaluation of injured children because of several advantages. It is now readily accessible in most healthcare facilities, is non-invasive, is a very accurate method of identifying and qualifying the extent of abdominal injury, and has reduced the incidence of non-therapeutic exploratory laparotomy. Controversy remains regarding the benefits of enteral contrast for diagnosis of gastrointestinal (GI) tract injuries. Many authors conclude that CT with enteral contrast does not improve diagnosis of GI injuries in the acute trauma setting and can lead to delays in diagnosis and aspiration.

1a,b The use of intravenous contrast is essential, and the utilization of 'dynamic' methods of scanning has optimized vascular and parenchymal enhancement. The impact on resource utilization and outcome of a contrast 'blush' on CT in children with blunt spleen and liver injury continues to be debated. Many emphasize that CT blush is worrisome, but that most patients can still be managed successfully without operation. The role and impact of angiographic embolization in adults is still debated and has yet to be determined in pediatric spleen injury. Initial retrospective studies have found angiographic embolization to be safe and effective in children, however, selection criteria remain undefined.

A head CT, if indicated, should be performed first without contrast, to avoid contrast concealing a hemorrhagic brain injury.

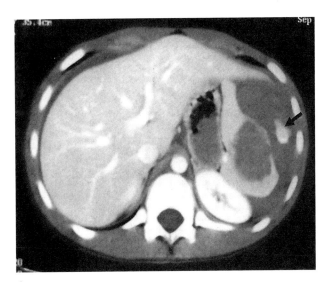

1a

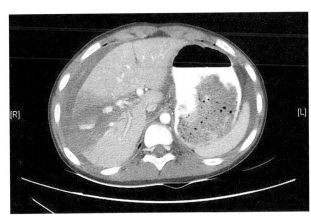

1b

Focused abdominal sonography for trauma

2 Clinician-performed sonography for the early evaluation of the injured child is currently being assessed to determine its optimal use. The standard four-view FAST examination includes Morrison's pouch, the left flank to include the perisplenic anatomy, and a subxiphoid view to visualize the pericardium and the pouch of Douglas/pelvis. This bedside examination may be useful as a rapid screening study, particularly in those patients too unstable to undergo an abdominal CT scan. Early reports have found FAST to be a useful screening tool in children, with a high specificity (95 percent), but a low sensitivity (33 percent) in identifying intestinal injury. A lack of identifiable free fluid does not exclude a significant injury. FAST may be very useful in decreasing the number of CT scans performed for 'low-likelihood' injuries. A recent meta-analysis of FAST in pediatric blunt trauma patients revealed modest sensitivity for hemoperitoneum. The authors concluded that a negative FAST may have questionable utility as the sole diagnostic test to rule out the presence of an intra-abdominal injury. A hemodynamically stable child with a positive FAST should undergo CT.

Recent literature has suggested that laparoscopy can both diagnose and, in some cases, allow definitive surgical management without laparotomy, further limiting the usefulness of diagnostic peritoneal lavage (DPL).

Large series using laparoscopy in adults have demonstrated increased diagnostic accuracy, definitive management of related injuries, decreased non-therapeutic laparotomy rates, and a significant decrease in hospital length of stay, with an attendant reduction in costs. As with elective abdominal surgery, the role of laparoscopy in trauma will increase substantially as trauma centers redirect their training of residents to this modality and as more pediatric centers report outcome studies for laparoscopic trauma management in children.

TREATMENT OF SPECIFIC ABDOMINAL INJURIES

Spleen and liver

The spleen and liver are the organs most commonly injured in blunt abdominal trauma, with each accounting for one-third of injuries. Non-operative treatment of isolated splenic and hepatic injuries in stable children is now standard practice. Although non-operative treatment of children with isolated blunt spleen or liver injury has been universally successful, there has been great variation in the management algorithms used by individual pediatric surgeons. Review of the National Pediatric Trauma Registry and recent surveys of the American Pediatric

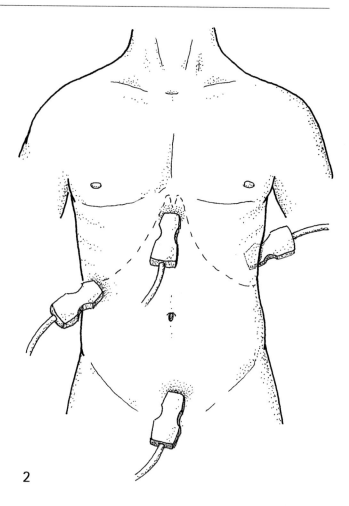

2

Surgical Association (APSA) membership confirm the wide disparity in practice.

The APSA Trauma Committee has defined consensus guidelines for resource utilization in hemodynamically stable children with isolated liver or spleen injury based on CT grading. Consensus guidelines on intensive care unit (ICU) stay, length of hospital stay, use of follow-up imaging, and physical activity restriction for clinically stable children with isolated spleen or liver injuries (grades I–IV) were defined by analysis of this database (**Table 103.1**).

Table 103.1 Proposed guidelines for resource utilization in children with isolated spleen or liver injury.

CT grade	I	II	III	IV
ICU days	None	None	None	1
Hospital stay (days)	2	3	4	5
Pre-discharge imaging	None	None	None	None
Post-discharge imaging	None	None	None	None
Activity restriction (weeks)[a]	3	4	5	6

[a]Return to full contact, competitive sports (i.e. football, wrestling, hockey, lacrosse, mountain climbing, etc.) should be at the discretion of the individual pediatric trauma surgeon. The proposed guidelines for return to unrestricted activity include 'normal' age-appropriate activities.
CT, computed tomography; ICU, intensive care unit.

The guidelines were then applied prospectively in 312 children. **It is imperative to emphasize that these proposed guidelines assume hemodynamic stability.** The extremely low rates of transfusion and operation document the stability of the study patients. Compared with the previously studied 832 patients, the 312 patients managed prospectively by the proposed guidelines had a significant reduction in ICU stay ($p < 0.0001$), hospital stay ($p < 0.0006$), follow-up imaging ($p < 0.0001$), and interval of physical activity restriction ($p < 0.04$) within each grade of injury. The pendulum continues to swing toward less hospitalization in stable children with solid liver or spleen injury. Retrospective and prospective studies suggest that the APSA guidelines for hospital length of stay can be reduced further.

Authors from the Arkansas Children's Hospital reported on an abbreviated protocol based on hemodynamics while 'throwing out' the CT grade of injury in 101 patients with isolated spleen or liver injury. Their protocol resulted in a significant reduction in length of stay (3.5 versus 1.9, $p < 0.001$) from that predicted by APSA guidelines.

Routine follow-up imaging studies have identified pseudocysts and pseudoaneurysms following splenic injury. Splenic pseudoaneurysms often cause no symptoms and appear to resolve with time. The true incidence of self-limited, post-traumatic splenic pseudoaneurysms is unknown, as routine follow-up imaging after successful non-operative treatment has been largely abandoned. Once identified, the actual risk of splenic pseudoaneurysm rupture is also unclear. These lesions can be treated successfully with angiographic embolization techniques, obviating the need for open surgery and loss of splenic parenchyma.

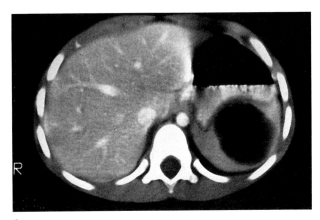

3a–c Splenic pseudocysts can achieve enormous size, leading to pain and gastrointestinal disturbance (illustration a). Simple percutaneous aspiration leads to a high recurrence rate. Laparoscopic excision and marsupialization is highly effective (illustrations b and c).

3a

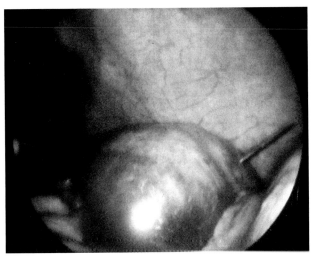

3b

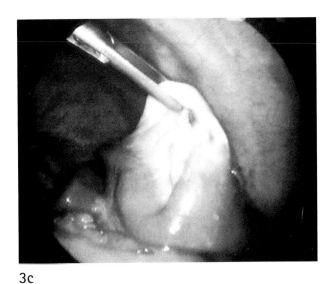

3c

4a,b Even the most severe solid organ injuries can be treated without surgery if there is prompt response to resuscitation. In contrast, emergency laparotomy and/or embolization are indicated in patients who are hemodynamically unstable, despite fluid and red blood cell transfusion (**Figure 103.1**). Most spleen and liver injuries requiring operation are amenable to simple methods of hemostasis using a combination of manual compression, direct suture, topical hemostatic agents, and woven polyglycolic mesh wrapping.

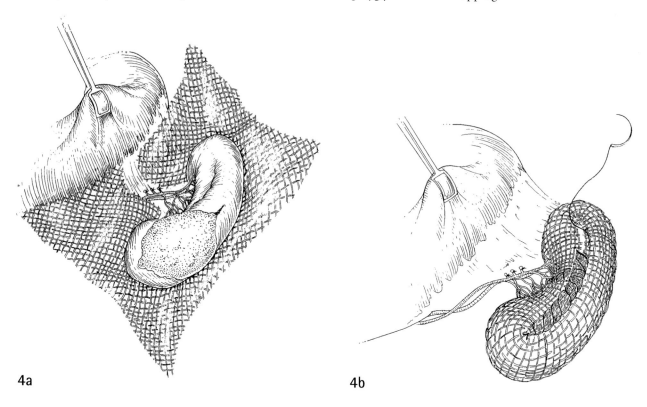

4a

4b

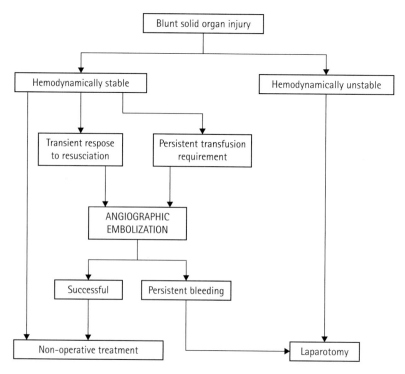

Figure 103.1 Algorithm for selected use of angiographic embolization in patients with blunt solid organ injury (modified from M Nance, CHOP, Philadelphia, PA, USA).

5 In young children with significant hepatic injury, the sternum can be divided rapidly to expose the suprahepatic or intrapericardial inferior vena cava, allowing for total hepatic vascular isolation with occlusion of the porta hepatis, suprahepatic, and infrahepatic inferior vena cava, and supraceliac aorta (optional). Children will tolerate periods of vascular isolation as long as their blood volume is replenished. With this exposure, the liver and major perihepatic veins can be isolated and the bleeding controlled to permit direct suture repair or ligation of the offending vessel. Although the cumbersome and dangerous technique of atriocaval shunting has been largely abandoned, newer endovascular balloon catheters can be useful for temporary vascular occlusion to allow access to the juxtahepatic vena cava.

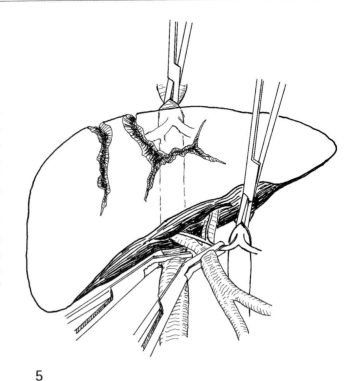

5

The early morbidity and mortality of severe hepatic injuries are related to the effects of massive blood loss and replacement with large volumes of cold blood products. The consequences of prolonged operations with massive blood product replacement include hypothermia, coagulopathy, and acidosis (**Figure 103.2**). Although the surgical team may keep pace with blood loss, life-threatening physiologic and metabolic consequences are inevitable, and many of these critically ill patients are unlikely to survive once their physiologic reserves have been exceeded. Maintenance of physiologic stability during the struggle for surgical control of severe bleeding is a formidable challenge even for the most experienced operative team, particularly when hypothermia, coagulopathy, and acidosis occur. This triad creates a vicious cycle in which each derangement exacerbates the others, and the physiologic and metabolic consequences of the triad often preclude completion of the procedure. Lethal coagulopathy from dilution, hypothermia, and acidosis can occur rapidly. The infusion of activated recombinant Factor VII in patients with massive hemorrhage has shown promising results.

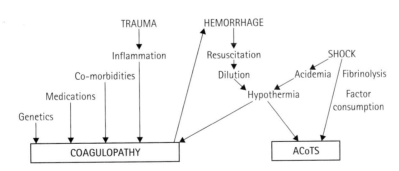

Figure 103.2 Acute coagulopathy of trauma and shock.

Increased emphasis on physiologic and metabolic stability in emergency abdominal operations has led to the development of staged, multidisciplinary treatment plans including abbreviated laparotomy, perihepatic packing, temporary abdominal closure, angiographic embolization, and endoscopic biliary stenting. Abbreviated laparotomy with packing for hemostasis allowing resuscitation prior to planned reoperation is an alternative in unstable patients where further blood loss would be untenable. This 'damage control' philosophy is a systematic, phased approach to the management of the exsanguinating trauma patient. The three phases of damage control are detailed in **Table 103.2**.

Once patients are rewarmed, coagulation factors replaced, and oxygen delivery optimized, they can be returned to the operating room for pack removal and definitive repair of injuries.

While the success of abdominal packing is encouraging, it may contribute to significant morbidity, such as intra-abdominal sepsis, organ failure, and increased intra-abdominal pressure. It is essential to emphasize that the success of the abbreviated laparotomy and planned reoperation depends on an early decision to employ this strategy prior to irreversible shock. Abdominal packing, when employed as a desperate, last-ditch resort after prolonged attempts at hemostasis have failed, has been uniformly unsuccessful.

Table 103.2 Damage control strategy in the exsanguinating trauma patient.

Phase 1	Abbreviated laparotomy for exploration
	Control of hemorrhage and contamination
	Packing and temporary abdominal wall closure
Phase 2	Aggressive ICU resuscitation
	Core rewarming
	Optimize volume and oxygen delivery
	Correction of coagulopathy
Phase 3	Planned reoperation(s) for packing change
	Definitive repair of injuries
	Abdominal wall closure

ICU, intensive care unit.

6a,b The obvious benefits of hemostasis provided by packing are also balanced against the potential deleterious effects of increased intra-abdominal pressure on ventilation, cardiac output, renal function, mesenteric circulation, and intracranial pressure. Timely alleviation of the secondary 'abdominal compartment syndrome' may be a critical salvage maneuver for patients. Temporary abdominal wall closure at the time of packing can prevent the occurrence of this life-threatening syndrome. We recommend temporary abdominal wall expansion in all patients requiring packing until the hemostasis is obtained and visceral edema subsides. Many materials have been suggested for use in temporary patch abdominoplasty, including silastic sheeting (illustration a), Goretex® patches, intravenous bags, cystoscopy bags, ostomy appliances, and various mesh materials. The vacuum-pack technique, used successfully in adults, has been an outstanding addition in children (illustration b). Use of the vacuum-pack technique at the first trauma laparotomy may limit the early benefits of the open abdomen which results in a lower volume reserve capacity.

A staged operative strategy for unstable trauma patients represents advanced surgical care and requires sound judgment and technical expertise. Intra-abdominal packing for the control of exsanguinating hemorrhage is a life-saving maneuver in highly selected patients in whom coagulopathy, hypothermia, and acidosis render further surgical procedures unduly hazardous. Early identification of patients likely to benefit from abbreviated laparotomy techniques is crucial for success.

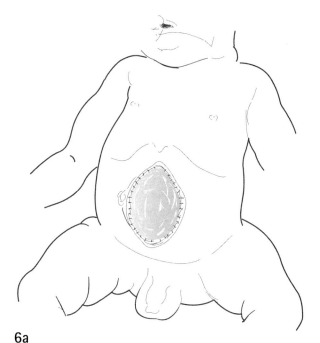

6a

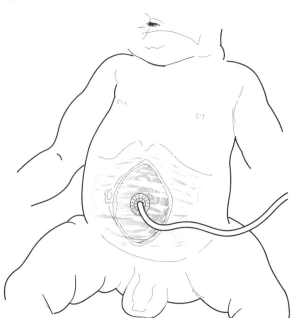

6b

Duodenum and pancreas

7 Patients sustaining duodenal perforation are treated operatively in a variety of ways depending on the severity of the injury and the surgeon's preference (**Box 103.1**). The authors recommend primary closure of the duodenal perforation (whenever possible). Extensive lateral duodenal injury should be treated by primary duodenal repair and pyloric exclusion consisting of temporary closure of the pylorus with an absorbable suture and gastrojejunostomy. Closed suction drainage of the repair is not depicted in this illustration. Feeding jejunostomy is often added to the procedure. When the duodenum is excluded, complete healing of the injury routinely occurs prior to the spontaneous reopening of the pyloric channel and spontaneous closure of the gastrojejunostomy.

> ### Box 103.1 Surgical options in duodenal trauma
>
> - Repair of the duodenum
> - Diversion of the gastrointestinal tract (pyloric exclusion or a duodenal diverticulization)
> - Gastric decompression (gastric tube insertion or gastrojejunostomy)
> - Gastrointestinal tract access for feeding (jejunostomy tube or gastrojejunal anastomosis)
> - Decompression of the duodenum (duodenostomy tube)
> - Biliary tube drainage
> - Wide drainage of the repaired area (lateral duodenal drains)

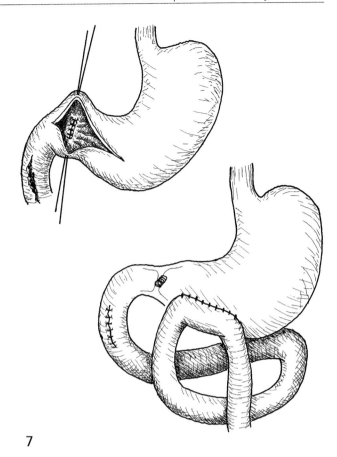

7

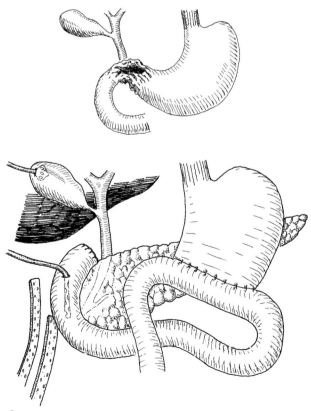

8

8 Duodenal diverticularization is an effective procedure for combined proximal duodenal and pancreatic injury. Resection and closure of the duodenal stump with decompressive tube duodenostomy, biliary drainage via tube cholecystectomy, gastrojejunostomy, and multiple closed suction drains are depicted. A feeding jejunostomy should be strongly considered (not depicted). No matter what repair the surgeon selects, a summary of the literature demonstrates that protecting the duodenal closure (drain and exclusion) and a route for enteral feeds (gastrojejunostomy ± or feeding jejunostomy) reduces morbidity and length of stay. A pancreaticoduodenectomy (Whipple procedure) should rarely be required. Although occasionally reported in the literature, pancreaticoduodenectomy should be reserved for the most severe injuries to the duodenum and pancreas when the common blood supply is destroyed and any possibility of reconstruction is impossible.

Injuries to the pancreas are slightly more common than duodenal injuries, with estimated ranges from 3 to 12 percent in children sustaining blunt abdominal trauma. A summary comparing the San Diego and Toronto protocols is depicted in **Figure 103.3**. The striking differences in these series are the 100 percent diagnostic sensitivity of CT scanning in Toronto versus 69 percent in San Diego,

and the 44 percent operative rate in San Diego versus 0 percent in Toronto. The Toronto group concludes that distal parenchymal atrophy or ductal recanalization occurs uniformly with no long-term morbidity in patients following the non-operative treatment of blunt pancreatic trauma.

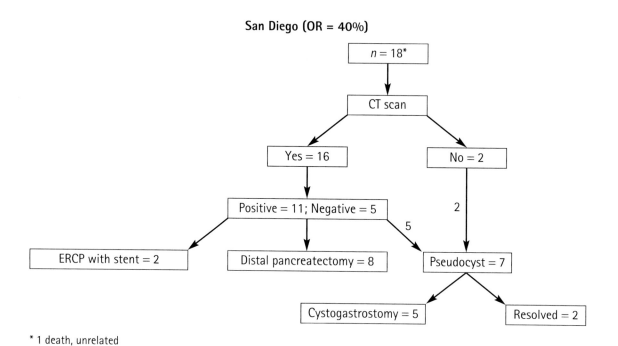

Figure 103.3 A comparison of protocols in the management of blunt pancreas injury in children. CT, computed tomography; ERCP, endoscopic retrograde cholangiopancreatography; OR, operation.

Reports from major pediatric trauma centers are clearly in conflict. Some favor and document the efficacy and safety of observational care for virtually all pancreatic traumas including ductal disruption, whereas others favor early distal pancreatectomy for transection to the left of the spine. It is clear that with simple transection of the pancreas at or to the left of the spine, spleen-sparing distal pancreatectomy can accomplish definitive care for this isolated injury with short hospitalization and acceptable morbidity. The procedure can be performed using minimally invasive techniques.

9 A recent report from Denver documents their experience with pediatric pancreas injury over an 11-year period. All ($n = 18$) with grade I injuries were treated non-operatively. Children with grades II–IV received operative treatment in 14 and non-operative in 11 cases. They concluded that children undergoing operative treatment had fewer pseudocysts but similar length of stay due to non-pancreatic complications.

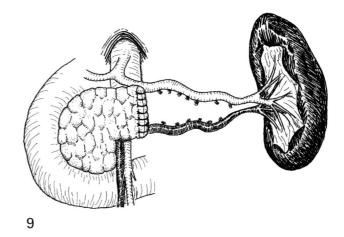

9

Kidney

Renal injuries in children are often caused by high-energy impact associated with motor vehicle accidents or other serious abdominal trauma. Hematuria is present in 41–68 percent of children following blunt abdominal trauma. Most authors report direct correlation between the amount of hematuria and the severity of genitourinary injury, but renovascular injuries may result in no hematuria. Historically, congenital abnormalities in injured kidneys have been reported to vary from 1 to 21 percent. More accurate recent reviews have shown that incidence rates are 1–5 percent. Renal abnormalities, particularly hydronephrotic kidneys, may be first diagnosed after minor blunt abdominal trauma. Usually, these patients present with hematuria following blunt trauma.

It is imperative to acknowledge that major renal injuries, such as ureteropelvic junction (UPJ) disruption or segmental arterial thrombosis, may occur without the presence of hematuria or hypotension. Therefore, a high index of suspicion is necessary to diagnose these injuries. Non-visualization of the injured kidney on intravenous pyelogram and failure to uptake contrast with a large associated perirenal hematoma on CT are hallmark findings for renal artery thrombosis. Ureteropelvic junction disruption is classically seen as perihilar extravasation of contrast with non-visualization of the distal ureter.

The majority of blunt renal injuries are treated without operation when uncontrolled hemorrhage or other indications for abdominal exploration are absent. This approach is safe and effective in 77–86 percent of children and most have excellent functional outcome without hypertension. Successful renal salvage at operation by partial nephrectomy or nephrorrhaphy depends on the severity of both the renal injury and associated injuries. Collecting system injuries should be repaired with absorbable sutures after evacuation of pelvic clots and debridement of devascularized parenchyma. Intravenous infusion of indigo carmine (a vital dye excreted in the urine) at operation may help identify sites of extravasation, and proximal control of the renal vessels prior to opening Gerota's fascia may facilitate retroperitoneal exploration. Early control of the vessels increases the rate of renal salvage. When proximal vascular control is performed before any renal exploration, nephrectomy is required in less than 12 percent of cases. When primary vascular control is not achieved and massive bleeding is encountered, the nephrectomy rate increases. Nephrectomy is recommended for major renal injuries in hemodynamically unstable patients with multiple injuries, and in those patients with avulsion injuries. Vascular repair can be attempted within 12 hours of injury and in the absence of multiple injuries.

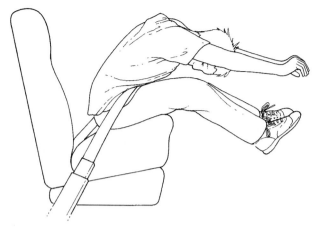

10a

The 'seat-belt syndrome'

10a–c A decrease in motor vehicle-related fatalities has occurred in association with mandatory seat-belt legislation. Concurrently, a pattern of injuries caused by lap-belt restraints has emerged. This 'seat-belt syndrome' includes abdominal wall contusion, injury to a hollow viscus, and vertebral fracture. The mechanism of injury is hyperflexion of the torso caused by deceleration forces with the lap-belt as a fulcrum (illustration a). Children are at particular risk for these injuries due to their higher center of gravity, thin abdominal wall, non-prominent iliac crest, and immature supporting structures of the vertebral bodies. Bowel injuries associated with lap-belt use can occur by several mechanisms: compression against the vertebral column with a crush injury, shearing of the bowel and mesentery at fixed points in the retroperitoneum, and immediate closed-loop burst injuries on the anti-mesenteric border when fluid-filled loops are subjected to sudden increases in intraluminal pressure. The crush and shearing mechanisms may lead to progressive ischemia with delayed perforation or stricture (illustration b). In recent reports from Philadelphia, a database created by the State Farm Insurance Company was used to review 147 985 children who were passengers in motor vehicle crashes. In that series, 1967 children (1.33 percent) had abdominal bruising from seat-belt restraints. Although abdominal wall bruising was infrequent, those with this finding were 232 times more likely to have a significant intra-abdominal injury than were those without a bruise. These data further revealed that one of nine children with an abdominal seat-belt sign had a significant intra-abdominal injury. Children with the 'seat-belt sign' across their lower abdomen should be admitted for serial examinations even if the initial examination and diagnostic tests are normal (illustration c).

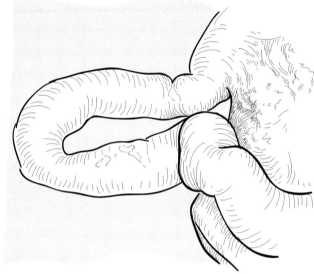

10b

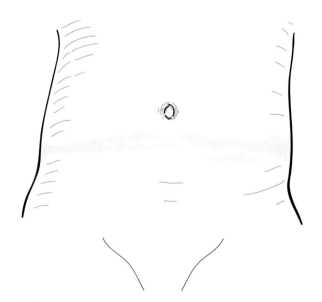

10c

CONCLUSIONS

The essential ingredient of pediatric trauma care is commitment to the special needs of injured children – personal, institutional, and community commitment. Recent advances in the delivery of trauma and critical care in children have resulted in improved outcome following major injuries. Incorporation of newer minimal access, endoscopy, and interventional radiology techniques is strongly urged. Although an increasing emphasis on non-operative treatment has occurred in the last two decades, the pediatric surgeon should remain the principal physician in the multidisciplinary care of these critically injured children.

The decision not to operate is always a surgical decision.

ACKNOWLEDGEMENT

Original illustrations 2, 5, 7, 8 and 9 by Mark Mazziotti, MD.

FURTHER READING

Holmes JF, Gladman A, Chang CH. Performance of abdominal ultrasonography in pediatric blunt trauma patients: a meta-analysis. *Journal of Pediatric Surgery* 2007; **42**: 1588–94.

Kiankhooy A, Sartorelli KH, Vane DW, Bhave AD. Angiographic embolization is safe and effective therapy for blunt abdominal solid organ injury in children. *Journal of Trauma* 2010; **68**: 526–31.

Lutz N, Nance ML, Kallan MJ *et al*. Incidence and clinical significance of abdominal wall bruising in restrained children involved in motor vehicle crashes. *Journal of Pediatric Surgery* 2004; **39**: 972–5.

Nikfarjam M, Rosen M, Ponsky T. Early management of traumatic pancreatic transection by spleen-preserving laparoscopic distal pancreatectomy. *Journal of Pediatric Surgery* 2009; **44**: 455–8.

Stylianos S and the APSA Trauma Study Group. Prospective validation of evidence-based guidelines for resource utilization in children with isolated spleen or liver injury. *Journal of Pediatric Surgery* 2002; **37**: 453–6.

Wood JH, Partrick DA, Bruny JL *et al*. Operative vs nonoperative management of blunt pancreatic trauma in children. *Journal of Pediatric Surgery* 2010; **45**: 401–6.

Special section

104

Vascular anomalies

STEVEN J FISHMAN

HISTORY

The terminology applied to vascular anomalies has been inconsistent and confusing. Thus, misdiagnosis and misunderstanding of the natural history and treatment options for afflicted patients is common. The International Society for the Study of Vascular Anomalies (ISSVA) has accepted the terminology proposed by Mulliken in 1982 that classifies lesions broadly into vascular tumors and vascular malformations.

Most of the vascular tumors are hemangioma of infancy. These common lesions, often referred to as 'strawberry hemangioma', become apparent within the first week or two after birth, proliferate for approximately ten months and then slowly involute. Involuted superficial lesions may leave behind a fibrofatty residuum or atrophic skin. Ulceration during the proliferative phase can destroy vital tissues and create severe scarring. Hepatic hemangioma may cause high output cardiac failure, abdominal compartment syndrome, or severe hypothyroidism. Rare gastrointestinal hemangioma can cause life-threatening hemorrhage. Most hemangiomas can be observed and allowed to involute spontaneously; proliferation of threatening lesions can be abated and involution accelerated by administration of corticosteroid or propranolol. Rare vascular tumors include Kaposiform hemangioendothelioma, rapidly involuting congenital hemangioma (RICH), non-involuting congenital hemangioma (NICH), and tufted angioma.

Vascular malformations result from morphogenic errors in development of blood vessels. They are classified by the type of vascular channel: capillary malformation, lymphatic malformation, venous malformation, arterial malformation. Combined malformations include arteriovenous and capillary lymphaticovenous. Vascular malformations are commonly mislabeled as hemangioma or with terms including 'hemangioma'. There is no such lesion as a 'cavernous hemangioma' (truly venous malformation) or 'lymphohemangioma' (truly lymphatic malformation with intralesional bleeding). Improper terminology often leads to inappropriate therapy. Vascular malformations have often also been given eponymous names, such as Klippel–Trenaunay syndrome (capillary lymphaticovenous malformation with overgrowth), Parkes Weber syndrome (capillary arteriolymphaticovenous malformation with overgrowth), Sturge–Weber syndrome (facial and leptomeningeal capillary malformation with glaucoma).

Vascular malformations do not involute spontaneously, nor do they respond to pharmacologic agents. Capillary malformations may lighten after pulsed dye laser photocoagulation. Venous malformations are generally sponge-like collections of relatively stagnant blood. Lymphatic malformations can have multiple large macrocystic collections of lymph fluid, many tiny honeycomb-like microcysts, or a combination of macrocystic and microcystic components. Venous malformations and predominantly macrocystic lymphatic malformations may often be successfully treated with cautious intralesional sclerotherapy. Sclerosants employed include ethanol, doxycycline, sodium tetradecyl sulfate, and OK-432 (an investigational agent). Sclerotherapy is best performed under fluoroscopic guidance. Sclerotherapy is not effective for microcystic components. Unlike slow-flow malformations, arteriovenous lesions are biologically aggressive in that they can steal flow and oxygen from distal and surrounding tissues resulting in ischemia, ulceration, and occasionally high-output cardiac failure. Arteriovenous malformations (AVMs) are very difficult to eradicate. They often involve multiple tissues making complete resection prohibitively morbid. Embolization by transarterial, transvenous, and direct puncture techniques can control an AVM temporarily and, occasionally for long periods, if not permanently. It is crucial that the nidus of the malformation be embolized rather than the feeding arteries. Embolization or ligation of feeding vessels will inevitably lead to recruitment of arterial inflow from collateral channels while eliminating the access route for proper transarterial embolization.

Surgical excision is warranted for many microcystic and mixed lymphatic malformations. Resection can also be employed for malformations of any channel type if very large or associated with soft tissue overgrowth such that sclerotherapy or embolization will not sufficiently reduce the excess bulk. Excision of a common lymphatic malformation is illustrated below. Similar principles and techniques can be employed from vascular malformations of other types and locations. However, intraoperative hemorrhage presents a significant risk in resecting venous and arteriovenous lesions. In all cases, appreciation and identification of the vital structures in the region is essential, particularly when hemorrhage mandates rapid dissection.

PRINCIPLES AND JUSTIFICATION

Cervical lymphatic malformations have traditionally been called 'cystic hygromas' or 'lymphangiomas'. Most commonly, those with large cysts have been termed 'hygromas' and those with more tissue parenchyma termed 'lymphangiomas'. Both terms are antiquated and should be abandoned. In modern medical parlance, the suffix '-oma' implies a tumor with active cellular proliferation.

Lymphatic malformations represent morphogenic errors in development of the lymphatic vessels. They are most commonly located in regions of confluence of major lymphatic channels, including the neck (75 percent), axilla (20 percent), mediastinum, retroperitoneum, pelvis, and groin. Cervical lesions may extend into the mediastinum and/or axilla. Malformations may be detected antenatally and are usually visible at birth. Occasionally, a mass may not become apparent for months or rarely years.

These vascular anomalies may become infected or sustain intralesional hemorrhage in addition to causing disfigurement. Very extensive cervical lesions may threaten the airway immediately at delivery. On occasion, *ex utero* intrapartum treatment (EXIT) procedures may be indicated to prevent neonatal asphyxiation.

Excision may result in a number of potential complications. Prolonged drainage is virtually assured and families should be informed that surgical drains will remain for weeks to months. Re-enlargement of residual lesion is not uncommon if an anatomic region is not adequately resected. Vesicle formation in and around surgical scars may occur if the malformation involves the dermis of the remaining skin. Malformations tend to invest normal structures. Thus injury to the thyroid, parathyroids, main and accessory thoracic ducts may occur. In particular, the vagus, phrenic, recurrent laryngeal, accessory, transverse cervical, and marginal mandibular nerves are at risk. A Horner's syndrome may result from stellate ganglion injury. Great care must be taken to avoid injury to the brachial plexus. Bleeding should be minimal, with blood transfusion rarely necessary. Mortality is not expected.

PREOPERATIVE ASSESSMENT AND PREPARATION

Physical examination

1 Physical examination is usually sufficient to make a diagnosis. The posterior triangle of the neck is the most common location. The lesion is usually ballotable and may transilluminate.

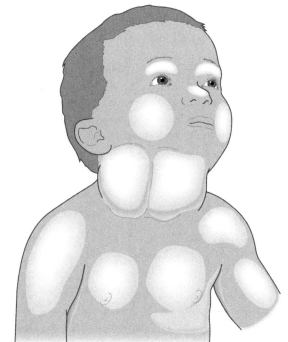

1

Imaging

2 Ultrasound can differentiate macrocystic from microcystic components. Magnetic resonance imaging (MRI) is most useful in establishing the anatomic extent of a lesion and its relationship to vital structures.

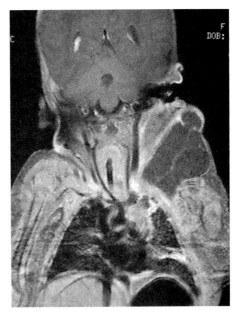

2

Timing and extent

Unless there is actual or threatened airway impairment, resection can be scheduled at between three and six months of age. On rare occasions, a lesion may deflate to become undetectable during this interval. Very extensive lesions often require staged procedures. An anatomic region with specific defined borders should be chosen and completed in each procedure to minimize the necessity to return to a scarred incompletely resected area. For example, a cervical lesion extending into the axilla should be resected down to the brachial plexus, with the intent to complete the infraplexus component at a separate sitting. Facial extension is often best left until the child is older, as they will often 'grow into' their lesion to achieve a better contour than might be achieved surgically. Bilateral lesions are generally best handled one side at a time. Since these lesions are histologically benign, the goal of resection is to be '99 percent' complete within the chosen region, while preserving all vital neurovascular structures. In order to achieve this degree of extirpation while preserving all vital structures, a lengthy meticulous dissection may be required for extensive lesions. It is crucial to avoid letting the clock determine the pace or end points of dissection. An inadequate resection will undoubtedly lead to a much more difficult secondary operation with greater risk of morbidity.

Laboratory studies

Hematologic and chemistry studies are not crucial. A specimen for blood crossmatch should be sent to the blood bank, although transfusion should not be frequently necessary.

Anesthesia

General anesthesia with endotracheal intubation is mandatory. Pharmacologic paralysis should be avoided to permit nerve stimulation during dissection. Direct laryngoscopy prior to incision may be elected to confirm preoperative vocal cord function.

OPERATION

Position and incision

3 The patient is supine with a roll under the shoulders to extend the neck. The head is turned away from the lesion. The exposure is through a supraclavicular incision parallel to the clavicle.

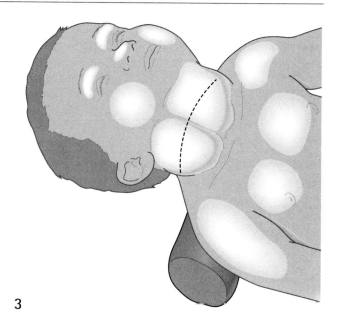

3

Exposure

4 Superior and inferior flaps are created deep to the platysma, extending superiorly, medially, and laterally to the extent of the superficial aspect of the malformation.

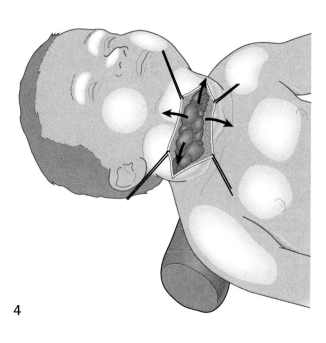

4

Deep posterior dissection

5 The malformation is meticulously dissected from the underlying and adjacent strap muscles, neurovascular structures, thyroid, trachea, and sometimes esophagus. The vagus, recurrent laryngeal and phrenic nerves should be identified and preserved, even if the malformation tissue must be split to free these structures. Successful dissection is facilitated by full cysts, so an attempt should be made to avoid deflating macrocystic components as long as possible.

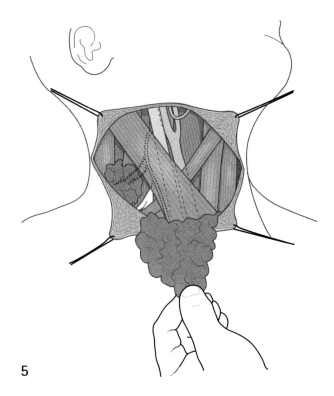

5

Root of neck

6 After deep neck structures are identified, the malformation is dissected off the underlying brachial plexus. Care must be taken to avoid injury to the subclavian vessels and the thoracic duct (left) or accessory thoracic duct (right). If the lesion extends into the mediastinum, the malformation may be lifted superiorly out of the thoracic inlet, facilitating at least partial separation from the thymus and removal. Sternotomy need not be performed in the absence of symptoms referable to the intrathoracic component.

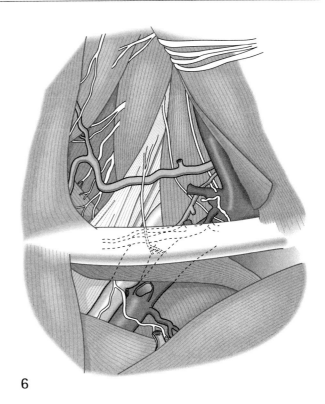

6

Closure

7 Excess skin is resected only if prominently redundant after removal of the underlying malformation tissue. A closed suction drain is placed in the wound and brought out through a reasonably long subcutaneous tunnel to avoid leakage around the drain. The platysma and subcutaneous tissues are closed with running braided absorbable suture. This skin is closed with a running subcuticular closure.

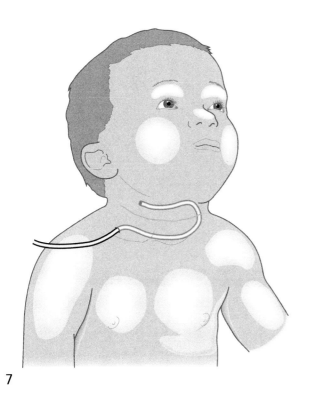

7

POSTOPERATIVE CARE

Long procedures with extensive dissections may require a period of postoperative intubation. Pain management is generally straightforward, as muscular disruption is minimal. An oral diet may be resumed as soon as tolerated. Closed suction drains may be required for weeks after hospital discharge. Parents should be taught to empty and record drain output. Postoperative infection is not uncommon and generally requires intravenous antibiotics.

OUTCOME

Though re-enlargement occasionally occurs, satisfaction is generally achieved. Contour is not always completely symmetric with the uninvolved side. Neurovascular injury can occur, but should be uncommon.

FURTHER READING

Alomari AI, Dubois J. Interventional management of vascular malformations. *Techniques in Vascular and Interventional Radiology* 2011; **14**: 22–31.

Mulliken JB, Fishman SJ, Burrow PE (eds). *Vascular Anomalies: Hemangiomas and Malformations.* New York: Oxford University Press, 2011.

Mulliken JB, Fishman SJ, Burrows PE. Vascular anomalies. *Current Problems in Surgery* 2000; **37**: 517–84.

Ogita S, Tsuto T, Nakamura K *et al.* OK-432 therapy in 64 patients with lymphangioma. *Journal of Pediatric Surgery* 1994; **29**: 784–5.

Padwa BL, Hayward PG, Ferraro NF, Mulliken JB. Cervicofacial lymphatic malformation: clinical course, surgical intervention, and pathogenesis of skeletal hypertrophy. *Plastic and Reconstructive Surgery* 1995; **95**: 951–60.

105

Fetal surgery

ALAN FLAKE

PRINCIPLES AND JUSTIFICATION

Maternal–fetal surgery is a specialty born of clinical necessity; a congenital defect alters normal development and causes irreversible organ damage before birth, leading to prenatal or neonatal death. The compelling rationale for maternal–fetal surgery is to restore normal development by correcting the defect before birth. Improvements in fetal imaging and serial clinical observation have allowed better definition of fetal pathophysiology, and better prediction of which fetuses might benefit from prenatal intervention. Because of the potential maternal risk, maternal–fetal surgery has historically been reserved for fetal disorders deemed to have a high probability of causing fetal or neonatal death. Recently, however, the success of the Management of Myelomeningocele Study (MOMS) in reducing the neurologic morbidity associated with myelomeningocele (MMC) has expanded the potential application of maternal–fetal surgery to non-lethal conditions.

The term 'maternal–fetal surgery' includes a procedural spectrum ranging from ultrasound-guided shunt placement to image-guided fetoscopic procedures, to the more invasive open fetal surgery and *ex utero* intrapartum treatment (EXIT) procedures (**Table 105.1**). Minimally invasive procedures have become feasible due to the development of fetoscopic equipment in recent years, and most can be performed entirely percutaneously with local anesthesia and less maternal morbidity than open surgery. The EXIT procedure, originally developed for use in fetuses undergoing tracheal occlusion for congenital diaphragmatic hernia (CDH), is now used in a variety of disorders in which difficulty obtaining an airway or achieving adequate ventilation is anticipated. Despite the progress in minimally invasive surgery, open fetal surgery continues to be required for correction of most fetal structural anomalies.

Table 105.1 Indications for EXIT.

Airway obstruction	Cervical teratoma
	Lymphangioma/lymphatic malformation
	CHAOS
	Tracheal/laryngeal atresia
	Laryngeal web
	Severe micrognathia/hypoplastic craniofacial syndrome
Chest masses	Congenital cystic adenomatoid malformation
	Bronchopulmonary sequestration
	Mediastinal/pericardial teratoma
Circulatory support	Congenital diaphragmatic hernia with associated cardiac malformation
	Congenital heart disease (hypoplastic left heart syndrome)
	Sacrococcygeal teratoma – debulking procedure

EXIT, *ex utero* intrapartum treatment.

There have been two recent randomized controlled multicenter clinical trials supporting fetal intervention. The MOMS trial demonstrated improvement in neurologic morbidity of MMC with prenatal closure and the European trial demonstrated efficacy of fetoscopic laser separation versus amnioreduction in twin-to-twin transfusion syndrome (TTTS). Further randomized trials are clearly needed prior to broad application of controversial procedures, such as fetoscopic balloon tracheal occlusion for CDH, however they would be impractical and potentially unethical in rare anomalies requiring fetal intervention such as congenital cystic adenomatoid malformation (CCAM), and sacrococcygeal teratoma (SCT), and in circumstances of clear rationale and demonstrated efficacy like the EXIT procedure for obstructive airway lesions.

PATIENT SELECTION

The prerequisites for fetal surgery formulated by Dr Michael Harrison three decades ago continue to apply with some minor modifications:

- accurate prenatal diagnosis;
- the absence of severe associated anomalies;
- a well-defined natural history;
- the presence of a correctable lesion which if uncorrected will lead to fetal death due to irreversible organ dysfunction;
- both maternal and fetal risk: benefit ratios must support fetal intervention.

PREOPERATIVE

Assessment and preparation

Patients suspected of carrying a fetus with a major anomaly should be referred to a fetal treatment center for comprehensive multidisciplinary evaluation. Evaluation should include detailed ultrasonographic characterization, fetal echocardiography, and often ultrafast magnetic resonance imaging (MRI). Parents should undergo detailed non-directive counseling based on the results of this work up. All available options for the pregnancy should be presented, along with the risks and benefits of each. If open fetal surgery is offered, the mother must be counseled regarding the need for Cesarean section in this and all future pregnancies, and care must be taken to 'allow' eligible families to choose non-surgical management, including termination or palliative care. A fetal karyotype or rapid fluorescent in situ hybridization (FISH) analysis for major chromosomal abnormalities should be performed. In general, significant associated anomalies, chromosomal abnormalities, or maternal risk factors such as heavy smoking, obesity, serious co-morbid conditions, placentomegaly, and the maternal mirror syndrome are considered to be contraindications to open maternal–fetal surgery.

Anesthesia and tocolysis (open maternal–fetal surgery)

Patients should be admitted prior to any planned open procedure for monitoring and initiation of tocolysis. Because any invasive fetal procedure involves the risk of preterm labor, separation/rupture of the membranes, and chorioamnionitis, a 50-mg indomethacin suppository should be given 6 hours preoperatively for tocolysis and intravenous cefazolin should be given prior to incision. Tocolysis should be continued postoperatively with an intravenous 6-g loading dose of magnesium sulfate, followed by a continuous infusion at 2–4 g/hour for 18–24 hours. Magnesium levels should be closely monitored, and patients should be assessed for any clinical signs of magnesium toxicity during this period. Indomethacin suppositories should be given every 6 hours for the 48 hours following the procedure. After this time, patients may be converted to an oral nifedipine regimen of 10–20 mg every 6 hours, continued until delivery.

In order to ensure adequate uterine relaxation, an epidural catheter should be placed preoperatively and deep inhalational general anesthesia should be induced. Maternal monitoring should include a radial arterial catheter and blood pressure cuff, bladder catheter, EKG leads, and pulse oximetry, while access should include multiple large-bore intravenous catheters. Sequential compression devices should be employed to prevent deep venous thromboses. Positioning should be supine with left lateral tilt, to minimize aortocaval compression from the gravid uterus. Fluid management strategies should be aimed at euvolemia, to prevent postoperative non-cardiac pulmonary edema in the pregnant patient.

Because the mother and fetus have separate, though codependent, anesthetic concerns, both an obstetric and a pediatric anesthesiologist are necessary. A sonographer/echocardiographer should be part of the surgery team, and a high-resolution ultrasound machine with color Doppler should be used to identify fetal and placental anatomy and to assess for potential hazards, such as velamentous cord insertion. During the procedure, continuous echocardiography should be used in combination with pulse oximetry to monitor fetal heart rate, cardiac function, and volume status.

FETAL SURGERY TECHNIQUES

Open fetal surgery

MATERNAL INCISION

1a,b In most patients, a low transverse skin incision may be used for cosmetic purposes. The placental location should be identified in order to determine the appropriate fascial incision. For a posterior placenta, skin flaps should be raised to allow exposure through a vertical midline fascial incision, as the uterus will remain in the abdomen during the procedure. In cases with an anterior placenta, the uterus must be tilted out of the abdomen, and division of the rectus muscles is required to prevent compression of the lateral uterine vessels with posterior hysterotomy.

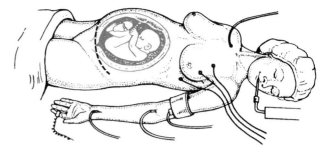

1a

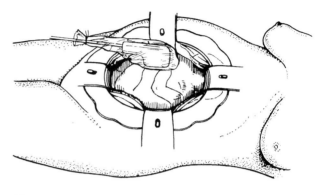

1b

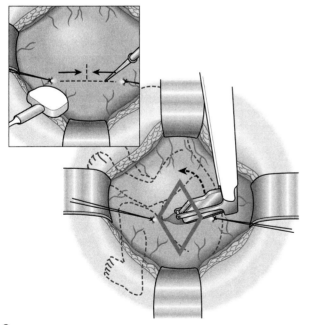

2

HYSTEROTOMY

2 Prior to hysterotomy, the uterus is palpated to determine whether sufficient relaxation has been achieved. Transuterine ultrasound confirms fetal and placental position, and electrocautery is used to map the placental margins on the surface of the uterus. The hysterotomy site should avoid uterine vasculature and be at least 6 cm from the placental edge. The lower segment of the uterus is avoided due to increased risk of amniotic fluid leak, chorioamnionitis, and preterm labor.

Once a site is chosen, opposing 0 PDS traction sutures are placed through the uterine wall and fetal membranes under ultrasound guidance. Using electrocautery, a 2-cm incision is made between the sutures. A specialized uterine stapler is then placed through the fetal membranes and fired once in either direction to compress the myometrium and minimize blood loss during hysterotomy, while maintaining membrane integrity for closure. Absorbable staples are used to avoid subsequent fertility issues. Using a rapid infuser, warmed lactated Ringer's solution is infused into the amniotic space via a catheter to maintain amniotic fluid volumes and fetal temperature, while preventing cord compression.

FETAL EXPOSURE

3 Following hysterotomy, the fetus is positioned within the uterus to expose the body part of interest. Continuous fetal echocardiography should be used to monitor cardiac function and ventricular rate. A fetal intravenous catheter is placed for infusion of fluids, blood, or medications, and intramuscular fetal anesthesia and paralysis is provided with fentanyl and vecuronium. A pulse oximeter should be wrapped around the fetal hand or foot and covered with aluminum foil and Tegaderm™. Operative repair should proceed in standard fashion, taking care to keep the fetus warm, buoyant, and as submerged as possible.

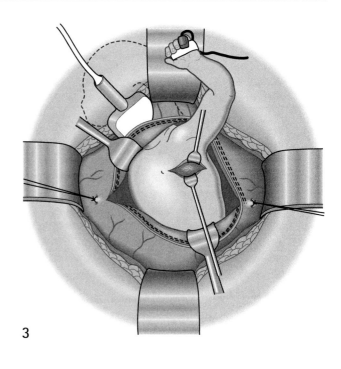

3

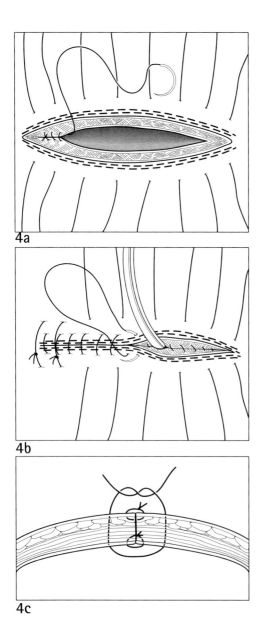

4a

4b

4c

UTERINE CLOSURE

4a–d The uterine closure must have adequate strength to prevent rupture and be watertight to prevent amniotic fluid leaks. A two-layer closure should be performed, using double-armed full thickness 0 PDS stay sutures approximately 1 cm apart and 2 cm back from the staple

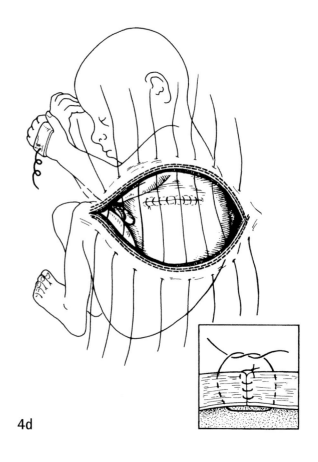

4d

line and a running 2/0 PDS suture through myometrium and membranes. Prior to completion of the running layer, approximately 400 mL of warmed lactated Ringer's solution containing 500 mg of oxacillin should be instilled into the amniotic cavity with ultrasound confirmation of adequate fluid volumes. An omental flap buttresses the uterine closure, and the maternal laparotomy should be closed in layers. A transparent Tegaderm dressing allows continued fetal monitoring postoperatively.

POSITIONING

5 The procedure can generally be performed percutaneously under local or regional anesthesia. The patient is placed in low lithotomy position and intraoperative ultrasound is used to define the position of the placenta and fetus(es).

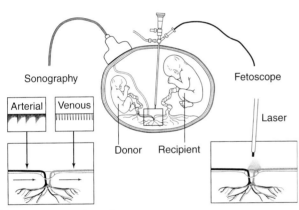

Artero-venous anastomosis

6

PROCEDURE

Laser fibers can be inserted through the side port of a fetoscopic operating sheath, allowing the use of a single trocar in TTTS. Under ultrasound guidance, unpaired vessels are coagulated. The introduction of more than one trocar increases the risks of preterm labor and membrane disruption and leak. The majority of currently performed fetoscopic procedures are performed through a single trocar and extensively utilize image guidance. The risk of amniotic fluid leak is low with trocar sizes of 3 mm or less, and closure of the amniotic sac or fascia is not required. While more complex procedures may one day be possible using multiple trocars or single port technology, the capabilities of fetoscopy currently remain limited.

Fetoscopy

Minimally invasive approaches may offer lower risk of preterm labor than open fetal surgery, potentially changing the risk–benefit ratio for fetal intervention. Currently, fetoscopic approaches are being investigated for several indications, although the most commonly performed procedure is fetoscopic photocoagulation of anomalous placental anastomoses in TTTS.

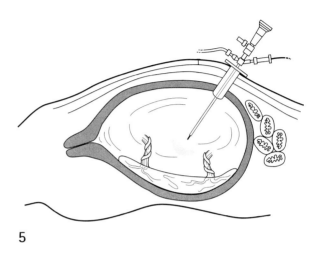

5

TROCAR INSERTION

6 A stab incision is made for ultrasound-guided placement of an external trocar, usually ranging in diameter from 2 to 4 mm. For complex fetal interventions, an irrigating fetoscope can be used to exchange turbid amniotic fluid.

EXIT procedure

The main goal of the procedure is to maintain uteroplacental blood flow, providing gas exchange for the fetus while establishing an airway, resecting a neck or chest mass, or cannulating for extracorporeal membrane oxygenation (ECMO). This requires complete uterine relaxation and maintenance of uterine volume to avoid placental abruption and interruption of blood flow. Unlike a standard Cesarean section, the procedure is performed under a deep inhalational anesthetic in order to promote uterine relaxation. Fetal anesthesia is supplemented with intramuscular fentanyl and vecuronium for more complex procedures requiring operative dissection and/or fetal immobilization.

SPECIFIC ANESTHETIC CONCERNS

During the procedure, uteroplacental blood flow must be maintained despite the vasodilatory effects of general anesthesia. Maternal blood pressure should be maintained within 10 percent of normal, and continuous fetal monitoring should assess for myocardial depression. As the fetus is delivered at the end of the procedure, tocolytics are not routinely required, but may be used synergistically with inhaled anesthetic for uterine relaxation. Prior to clamping the cord, measures should be taken to prevent excessive bleeding due to uterine atony, including discontinuation of inhaled anesthetic, administration of oxytocin, and uterine massage. Methergine and carboprost may also help to recover uterine tone in refractory cases.

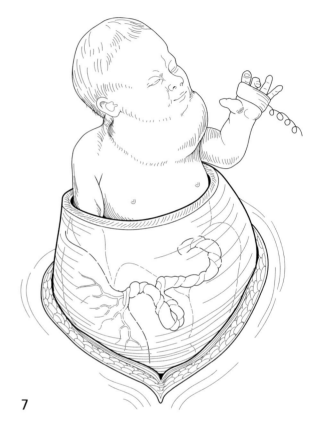

7

INCISION AND EXPOSURE

7 Maternal incision is carried out as described above. In cases with severe polyhydramnios or large cystic masses, amnioreduction or cyst aspiration may be required. Following ultrasound mapping of the placental edges, hemostatic hysterotomy is performed with the specialized uterine stapler used for open fetal surgery, and only the necessary fetal parts are exposed. Warm lactated Ringer's solution is infused and monitors are placed as described previously.

SECURING THE AIRWAY

8 Irrespective of the procedure, the fetal airway should be controlled as early as possible. Direct laryngoscopy and endotracheal intubation are preferred, but rigid bronchoscopy and/or tracheostomy may be required. Multiple sizes of laryngoscopes, endotracheal tubes, tube exchangers, as well as rigid and flexible bronchoscopes, should be available. Intubation may be accomplished either ante- or retrograde, using Seldinger technique through a limited neck dissection. If the airway cannot be accessed by any of these methods, as in the case of a giant neck mass, aspiration or resection should be undertaken. If an airway cannot be established by any means, or in cases where EXIT is performed to avoid hypoxemia prior to ECMO cannulation, ECMO cannulation may be directly performed. Ventilation is initiated prior to cord division once the airway is secure or the operative procedure completed.

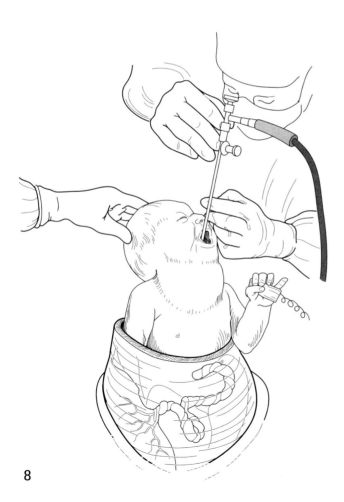

8

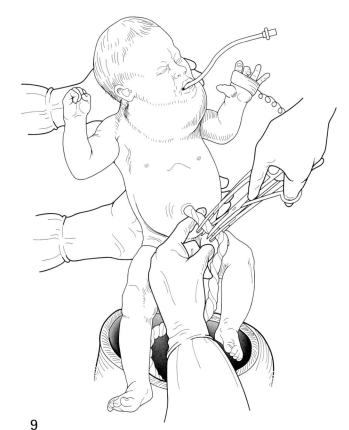

9

DELIVERY

9 Before clamping the cord, umbilical arterial and venous catheters may be placed. Oxytocin should be administered to the mother immediately before delivery, and the child is taken to the resuscitation table once the cord is clamped and divided.

POSTOPERATIVE CARE

Prior to intervention, in addition to the tocolytic regimen described above, uterine activity is monitored by tocodynamometer, and fetal heart rate is followed for any signs of distress. Daily ultrasound assesses for fetal movement, amniotic fluid and membrane status, while echocardiography monitors for indomethacin-related cardiotoxicity, including ductal constriction, oligohydramnios, or tricuspid regurgitation.

During the postoperative period, fluid status must be carefully managed due to the risk of non-cardiogenic pulmonary edema. Empiric furosemide diuresis can be added if signs of pulmonary edema develop. Patients can usually be discharged by postoperative day 4, but should be required to remain on modified bed rest for the first 2 weeks after discharge. Absent uterine irritability, patients can then be allowed moderate activity, but should remain nearby, returning twice weekly for ultrasound and obstetrical assessment. Once the fetus reaches 36 weeks' gestation, lung maturity is assessed by amniocentesis, and Cesarean section is performed.

MATERNAL OUTCOMES

Fortunately, no maternal deaths have been reported, although significant short-term morbidity has been observed. Premature labor is the most common complication, while premature membrane rupture and separation occur frequently. In addition to surgical risks, uterine rupture, chorioamnionitis, placental abruption, amniotic band syndrome, oligohydramnios, and bleeding requiring transfusion have also been observed. In general, reported reproductive outcomes for future pregnancies have been good, with fertility rates similar to background.

FURTHER READING

Adzick NS. Open fetal surgery for life-threatening anomalies. *Seminars in Fetal and Neonatal Medicine* 2010; **15**: 1–8.

Adzick NS, Thom EA, Spong CY *et al.* A randomized trial of prenatal versus postnatal repair of myelomeningocele. *New England Journal of Medicine* 2011; **364**: 993–1004.

Deprest J, Jani J, Lewi L *et al*. Fetoscopic surgery: encouraged by clinical experience and boosted by instrument innovation. *Seminars in Fetal and Neonatal Medicine* 2006; **11**: 398–412.

Leichty K. *Ex utero* intrapartum therapy. *Seminars in Fetal and Neonatal Medicine* 2010; **15**: 34–9.

Senat MV, Deprest J, Boulvain M *et al*. Endoscopic laser surgery versus serial amnioreduction for severe twin-to-twin transfusion syndrome. *New England Journal of Medicine* 2004; **351**: 136–44.

Wilson RD, Lemerand K, Johnson MP *et al*. Reproductive outcomes in subsequent pregnancies after a pregnancy complicated by open maternal-fetal surgery (1996–2007). *American Journal of Obstetrics and Gynecology* 2010; **203**: 209.e1–209.e6.

106

Kidney transplantation

JOHN MAGEE

HISTORY

The first successful kidney transplant was performed between identical twins by Joseph Murray and his colleagues at the Peter Bent Brigham Hospital in 1954. In 1983, the approval of cyclosporine by the Food and Drug Administration ushered in the modern era of transplantation. Over the following decades, improvements have continued in all facets of care including pretransplant management, refinements in surgical technique, improvement in donor selection, perioperative management, and immunosuppression. Currently, there are approximately 800 pediatric kidney transplants performed each year in the United States.

PRINCIPLES AND JUSTIFICATION

Renal transplantation is the treatment of choice for children with end-stage renal disease as it offers the best prospect for health, growth, and development. Absolute contraindications are rare and include ongoing infection and untreated malignancy. Relative contraindications include severe systemic disease that profoundly limits the patient's lifespan or a social situation that makes follow up with post-transplant care and an immunosuppression regimen absolutely impossible.

Concern regarding the appropriate size for a pediatric recipient relates to the ability to fit the donor kidney within the abdomen, the ability to adequately perfuse a kidney from a significantly larger person, and technical constraints related to any caliber mismatch of donor and recipient's vessels that impacts on the construction of the vascular anastomosis. Accordingly, any target size reflects both recipient size as well as the size of potential donors. Typically, this requires the infant to reach a weight of 6–7 kg, but the principle should be to optimize the situation as much as possible and not let an arbitrary weight target compromise the health of the child.

PREOPERATIVE ASSESSMENT AND PREPARATION

All children with chronic kidney disease should be evaluated by a multidisciplinary pediatric transplant team including a transplant surgeon, pediatric nephrologist, social worker, nurse specialist, nutritionist, and psychologist. Efforts to optimize nutrition and dialysis therapy are essential to optimize the child's overall health. When possible, upcoming childhood immunizations should be administered prior to transplantation.

Pediatric candidates are much more likely to have anomalies of the lower urinary tract compared to adults, reflecting the higher incidence of obstructive uropathy or congenital genitourinary abnormalities. An evaluation of the lower urinary system should be completed in such patients, and expertise in these issues or close collaboration with pediatric urology, is critical. In general, the patient's native bladder is the preferred reservoir and will usually be adequate. Select patients may require bladder augmentation or other interventions prior to transplantation.

In smaller children with a history of femoral vein catheterization or a history of intra-abdominal process associated with inflammation (e.g. peritonitis, pancreatitis), it is prudent to image the vena cava and the iliac veins to confirm their patency.

It is also important to evaluate and optimize the overall psychosocial state of the child and caregivers. The stress associated with care of a child with a chronic illness is significant, and adherence to the post-transplant medical regimen is vital for success. Adolescents can be particularly challenging in this regard.

Anesthesia

General anesthesia for renal transplantation follows the principles for major abdominal procedures in children. Attention to intraoperative fluid management and maintenance of core body temperature are particularly critical. In children less than 20 kg, the author establishes central venous access, both for fluid administration and monitoring central venous pressure. In these smaller children, we also place an arterial line for constant blood pressure monitoring. In larger children, two large bore peripheral intravenous lines are sufficient.

Incision

1 The author utilizes a retroperitoneal approach in all children, including small infants, and prefers to place the kidney on the right side as this provides easiest access to the vena cava. A curvilinear incision is made, starting at the midline approximately one finger-breadth superior to the pubic symphysis, extending laterally across the rectus abdominis muscle, and then curving superiorly to about the level of the umbilicus. In small children and infants, the incision must be carried further cephaled to permit adequate exposure as the donor kidney is typically from an adult or a larger adolescent. The significant size mismatch between donor and recipient mandates constant attention to the recipient's hemodynamic profile.

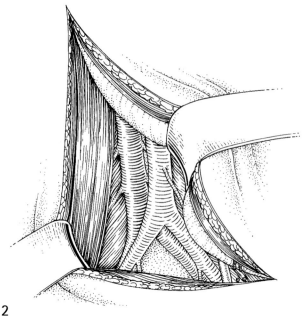

2

OPERATION

Position of patient

Renal transplantation is performed with the patient in the supine position. A prophylactic antibiotic (cefazolin or levofloxacin) with coverage against skin flora is administered. A Foley catheter is placed into the bladder or urinary reservoir and connected to a three-way system to allow for instillation of povidone-iodine (Betadine®) solution to distend the bladder at the time of urinary reconstruction.

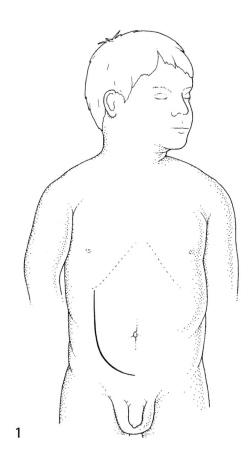

1

Exposure

2 The external oblique, internal oblique, and transversus abdominis muscles are divided, as is the rectus abdominis medially. The preperitoneal space is entered, and the inferior epigastric vessels are typically divided. The peritoneum is swept medially and superiorly to expose the iliac vessels, inferior vena cava, and distal aorta. Care is taken to avoid inadvertent entry into the peritoneal cavity. Any openings in the peritoneum should be noted and closed at the end of the procedure with absorbable sutures to prevent leakage of peritoneal dialysis postoperatively. The spermatic cord should be preserved by careful mobilization and medial retraction. In girls, the round ligament should be divided. At this point, a self-retaining Bookwalter is placed to provide exposure.

Vascular dissection

3 The distal inferior vena cava and aorta are used for vascular reconstruction in children weighing less than approximately 20 kg. Dissection of the distal vena cava is accomplished first. Lumbar veins are divided between fine silk ligatures to free a segment of vena cava approximately 2–3 cm in length. The distal aorta below the inferior mesenteric artery and proximal common iliac arteries are controlled with rubber vessel loops. At least one set of lumbar arteries is generally encountered. These vessels are left intact and controlled with Pott's ties as needed. Care should be exercised during dissection of the aorta to avoid disruption of the abdominal lymphatic trunk. In larger children, the recipient common iliac vessels may be utilized. In choosing the site for the anastomoses, thoughtful consideration needs to be given for the fit of the kidney in the recipient. Particular attention needs to be focused on the length of the renal vessels and their orientation, considering the ultimate position of the kidney after it is perfused, the retractor is removed, and the fascia closed.

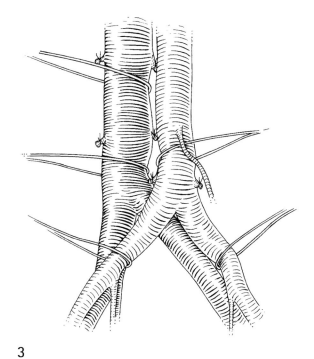

3

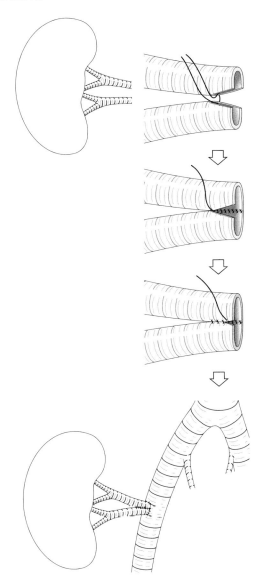

4

Preparation of donor kidney

4 After the recipient dissection is completed, the donor kidney is prepared in a bath of sterile iced saline solution. The renal artery and vein are cleaned of surrounding tissues and side branches are resecured as needed. The renal vein must be kept short, usually not longer than 1–1.5 cm, to prevent kinking. While it is possible to use a Carrel patch of donor aorta if the kidney is from a deceased donor, in practice this usually requires leaving the renal artery too long. Consequently, the renal artery is generally transected to keep it short as well. If multiple renal arteries are present, they are typically syndactylized before reimplantation though they can be implanted separately if necessary. When the vessels are syndactylized, it is important to consider if this will allow the vessels to lie in good position, since syndactylization will fix the vessels relatively firmly in two dimensions. This can limit the options of where the anastomosis can be suitably performed or lead to kinking of one or both of the donor arteries if the final position of the kidney is not anticipated. The kidney may be wrapped in a moistened laparotomy pad with a 'keyhole' fashioned for the vessels. This facilitates keeping the kidney cool as well as handling of the kidney in the wound.

Vascular anastomoses

We do not routinely heparinize most recipients, though we selectively heparinize children less than 20 kg receiving deceased donor grafts. In these select cases, the recipient is given 50 units/kg body weight. Full-dose heparinization is unnecessary, except in cases of known hypercoagulability. Vascular clamps should be carefully chosen to avoid obscuring the field. In infants, tension on double-looped rubber vessel slings is all that is required. Alternatively, low profile gentle vascular spring clips can be used. During construction of the vascular anastomoses, the anesthetic team should volume load the recipient to a central venous pressure of 12–18 cmH$_2$O and administer mannitol, 0.5 g/kg. These maneuvers will counteract the effects of revascularization and its attendant destabilizing effect due to volume shift. A transplanted adult kidney may sequester 20 percent of the circulating blood volume of a 7-kg infant.

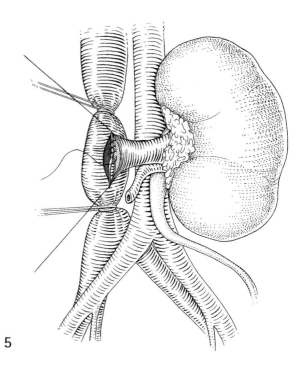

5 A longitudinal incision is made in the anterolateral aspect of the vena cava and 5/0 or 6/0 polypropylene sutures are placed at the apices. The assistant positions the kidney medially in the wound. The anteromedial side of the anastomosis is performed first from within the lumen of the vein, followed by the posterolateral side from the outside. Following completion of the venous anastomosis, the kidney is rotated toward the side of the operating surgeon. In small recipients, the author often places the kidney as it will rest *in situ* from the start, rather than suspend it medially. In this case, the posterolateral side of the anastomosis is performed first from within the lumen.

5

6 The aorta and common iliac arteries are occluded and an aortotomy is made at a site carefully chosen for optimal geometry of the vessels. A 4-mm aortic punch is used to fashion an orifice on the anterolateral aspect of the aorta. This anastomosis is performed with a running 6/0 polypropylene suture, starting at the superior aspect. The 'back wall' of the anastomosis is performed from the inside and the 'front wall' from the outside.

Once the arterial reconstruction is completed, venous outflow is established. We then gently occlude the renal artery with vascular pickups, while restoring distal arterial flow. After several cardiac cycles, inflow to the kidney is established. The kidney should be carefully inspected. Optimally, a uniform pink color and normal turgor are followed promptly by the production of urine. Engorgement of the kidney suggests venous obstruction. This may be due to an imperfect anastomosis, but is more commonly attributable to compression of the vena cava by one of the retractor blades. An excellent pulse should be palpable in the renal hilum and a thrill is quite common. Heparin need not be reversed with protamine sulfate unless troublesome bleeding occurs. Following establishment of hemostasis and assuming satisfactory appearance of the kidney, attention is then turned to the urinary reconstruction.

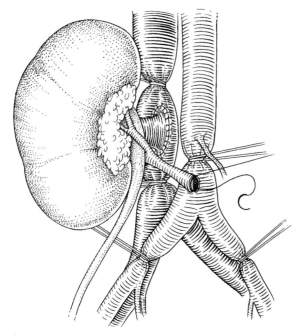

6

External ureteroneocystostomy

When the bladder is to be used for urinary reconstruction, the urinary catheter is clamped and the bladder distended by instilling povidone-iodine solution. The author's preferred technique is an external ureteroneocystostomy. The principles of this technique include direct anastomosis of the ureter to bladder mucosa and construction of a submuscular tunnel of sufficient length to prevent reflux into the transplanted kidney.

A site is chosen anteriorly near the dome of the distended bladder. The choice of site should take into account the course of the transplanted ureter. An appropriate balance must be struck between the need for an adequate ureteric length to reach the anastomotic site when the bladder is empty and the requirement of avoiding excessive redundancy with the attendant risk of ureteric obstruction and distal ureteral ischemia. Given the blood supply to the transplanted ureter is dependent on small branches from the lower pole renal artery, the ureter should be kept as short as possible. In males, the ureter should be brought beneath the spermatic cord to avoid obstruction caused by draping the ureter over the cord.

7 The muscular coat of the bladder is divided, exposing the bladder mucosa for a distance of about 4 cm. An opening is made in the mucosa at the medial aspect of the dissection. The presence of the bladder catheter should be confirmed visually at this time; a thickened peritoneum adjacent to the bladder can fool even the most experienced surgeon.

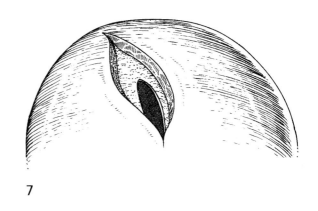

7

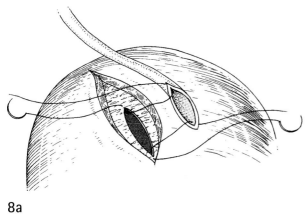

8a

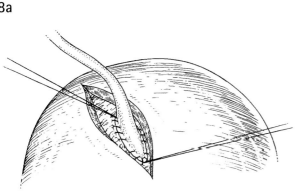

8b

8a,b The ureter is cut to length and spatulated. The anastomosis is performed with running 5/0 monofilament absorbable sutures. Traction sutures are placed at the 'heel' and 'toe' of the anastomosis. Construction of the anastomosis should proceed from 'heel' to 'toe' on the inferior wall and then again 'heel' to 'toe' on the superior wall. This permits precise placement of sutures at the 'heel' where the opportunity for compromising the lumen of the ureter is greatest. Precise attention must be focused on the tension applied to the suture during follow-through and while tying the knot in order to avoid cinching the suture line which will narrow the anastomosis. Careful placement of sutures and avoidance of excessive handling of the ureter are critically important to avoid stenosis or obstruction. A double-J stent may be placed if there is any concern about the quality of the ureter or bladder. It should be placed after the anastomosis is partially completed, with the upper end positioned in the renal pelvis and the lower end passed into the bladder.

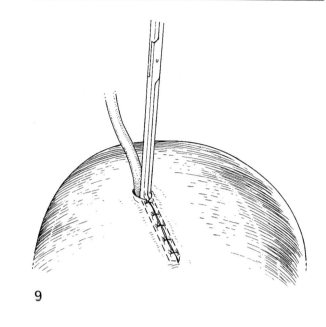

9 After completion of the anastomosis, the ureter is laid in the submuscular space and the muscle wall is approximated over it using interrupted 4/0 monofilament absorbable sutures for a distance extending 2–3 cm beyond the anastomosis. When completed, the tunnel should still admit the end of a right-angled clamp, thus ensuring that the ureter will not be obstructed within the tunnel.

9

Wound closure

The transplanted kidney should lie comfortably within the lower abdomen. No fixation of the kidney allograft is needed. On removal of the self-retaining retractor, the peritoneal contents will hold the kidney against the posterior and lateral side walls. No drains are used. The wound is irrigated and a one-layer fascial closure is completed with running absorbable suture. The skin is closed with a running, absorbable, subcuticular suture.

POSTOPERATIVE CARE

General care and infection prophylaxis

Infants and small children are managed in a pediatric intensive care unit. Although most recipients are extubated in the operating room, a small infant with an adult-sized kidney may require mechanical ventilation for 1–2 days. Urine output is replaced with intravenous fluid milliliter for milliliter for the first 12 hours. Replacement fluids are then gradually tapered. Maintenance of adequate volume status is critical. Any concern regarding graft function should be promptly evaluated via ultrasound with Doppler. The urinary catheter is left in place for 3–4 days. If necessary, satisfactory bladder emptying may be assured with post-micturitional catheterization. Perioperative antibiotic prophylaxis against bacterial infection is given for 24 hours. Prophylaxis is given for 90 days against opportunistic infection including trimethoprim and sulfamethoxazole for *Pneumocystis carinii*, and valganciclovir for *Cytomegalovirus* infection. Nystatin is administered for 30 days for candidiasis. The hospital stay is 5–7 days in most cases.

Immunosuppression

Over the last decade, the introduction of several new agents has permitted several protocol permutations. Immunosuppression protocols tend to be center specific, reflecting local and national experience, and a desire to appropriately balance the risk of rejection with the risks of immunosuppression. Induction immunosuppression is less common in countries where the population is more homogenous and the risk of rejection appears lower. Accordingly, dual agent maintenance therapy is also more common in such settings. Immunosuppressive therapy starts intraoperatively. The author uses induction therapy with polyclonal anti-thymocyte antibody (Thymoglobulin®) for recipients at higher immunologic risk and anti-interleukin-2 receptor monoclonal antibody (basiliximab) for all others. Corticosteroids are also administered intraoperatively. Postoperatively, the calcineurin inhibitor tacrolimus is introduced when renal function is demonstrated. The anti-metabolite, mycophenolate mofetil, completes the standard triple-drug maintenance regimen. Based on recent experience with several multicenter trials, we offer a steroid avoidance protocol where corticosteroids are stopped after 5 days. For patients who are continued on corticosteroids, the dose is rapidly tapered and most patients are maintained on alternate day steroids.

OUTCOME

The overall results of renal transplantation in children have improved steadily. The most important advances have included improvements in pretransplant dialysis and nutritional management, meticulous surgical technique, and management of immunosuppression. Transplant and developmental outcomes have been excellent even among recipients less than one year of age. Graft survival is dependent on donor type and recipient age. For pediatric recipients of living donor kidneys, one- and five-year graft survival ranges from 96 to 99 percent and 76 to 92 percent, respectively. For deceased donor kidneys, one- and five-year graft survival ranges from 92 to 95 percent and 64 to 78 percent, respectively. Adolescent recipients are the population responsible for the lower range of graft outcomes at five years.

FURTHER READING

Gulati A, Sarwal MM. Pediatric renal transplantation: an overview and update. *Current Opinion in Pediatrics* 2010; **22**: 189–96.

LaRosa C, Jorge Baluarte H, Meyers KEC. Outcomes in pediatric solid-organ transplantation. *Pediatric Transplantation* 2011; **15**: 128–41.

Magee JC, Krishnan SM, Benfield MR *et al.* Pediatric transplantation in the United States, 1997–2006. *American Journal of Transplantation* 2008; **8**: 935–45.

Riley P, Marks SD, Desai DY *et al.* Challenges facing renal transplantation in pediatric patients with lower urinary tract dysfunction. *Transplantation* 2010; **89**: 1299–307.

Salvatierra JO, Millan M, Concepcion W. Pediatric renal transplantation with considerations for successful outcomes. *Seminars in Pediatric Surgery* 2006; **15**: 208–17.

Smith JM, Stablein DM, Munoz R *et al.* Contributions of the Transplant Registry: the 2006 annual report of the North American Pediatric Renal Trials and Collaborative Studies (NAPRTCS). *Pediatric Transplantation* 2007; **11**: 366–73.

107

Liver transplantation

RICCARDO A SUPERINA and ALEXANDER DZAKOVIC

HISTORY

Since the first successful human liver transplant performed in 1967 by Thomas Starzl in Denver, Colorado, the field of liver transplantation has undergone significant advances. The most significant changes have been in the refinement of techniques that allow for the reduction in size of an adult liver to accommodate for the smaller size or organ needed in infants and children. This allows for the more timely transplantation of the child waiting for an organ, and has decreased the number of children who die without receiving a liver. Improved immunosuppression with calcineurin inhibitors (CI), such as cyclosporine and more recently, tacrolimus, have improved the long-term survival of transplanted organs. More effective antiviral and antibacterial medications, as well as improved detection techniques for post-transplant lymphoproliferative disease have also contributed to the improved survival. Lastly, more refined techniques of organ procurement, preservation, and implantation, as well as better peri- and postoperative care have all contributed to improve outcomes over the past four decades.

1 The techniques of hepatic size reduction permitting segmental transplantation of the liver, including split, reduced size, and live-donor liver transplantation, require familiarity and understanding of the segmental liver anatomy described by Claude Couinaud. Reduced liver grafts are prepared by cutting down a deceased donor adult liver to produce a left lateral segment (segments II and III), left lobe graft (segments II, III, and IV), or more rarely, the right lobe (segments V–VIII) and were introduced in 1984 by Bismuth. Split-liver transplantation, in which a deceased donor adult liver is divided into two functional grafts, became available in 1988 after its description by Pichlmayer. Pediatric living-donor liver transplantation, in which a healthy adult donates part of his or her liver, followed in 1989 after its first successful execution in Australia. Living-related donation enabled the development of pediatric liver transplant programs in countries without established deceased donor organ systems and has since been extended to both adults and adolescents through the use of right lobe donation.

1

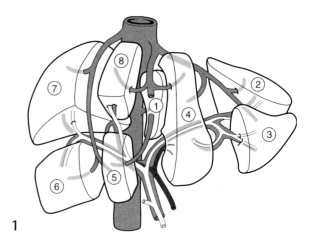

The greatest barrier in survival for children who need a transplant is in organ availability. Since most children awaiting transplantation are infants or small children and the peak age in donors is in the adult ranges of age, attempts at finding age- and size-matched organs for children was associated with a high mortality for those waiting for organs. Size reduction techniques have greatly reduced, although not eliminated the waiting list attrition in lives, particularly in patients under the age of one year.

PRETRANSPLANT CONSIDERATIONS AND MANAGEMENT

Indications

The main indications for pediatric liver transplantation are listed in **Table 107.1**.

The main categories are:

- acute liver failure;
- progressive chronic liver disease;
- chronic liver disease with secondary major morbidity;
- hepatic-based metabolic disorders.

Acute liver failure is not common in children, but the situation may warrant extremely urgent action, and it tests the preparedness of a transplant program to mobilize numerous resources to get a child transplanted. As seen in **Table 107.1**, viral hepatitis is the most common cause of acute liver failure, but the specific virus responsible is

Table 107.1 Indications for pediatric liver transplantation.

Acute liver failure	Viral, e.g. hepatitis A, B, and non-A–E
	Drugs/toxins
	Metabolic
	Autoimmune
Chronic liver disease	
Cholestatic liver disease	Biliary atresia
	Progressive familial intrahepatic cholestasis
	Alagille syndrome
	Sclerosing cholangitis
Metabolic liver disease	α-1-Antitrypsin deficiency
	Wilson's disease
	Cystic fibrosis
	Tyrosinemia
	Crigler–Najjar (type 1) syndrome
	Urea cycle defects
	Hyperoxaluria
	Neonatal hemochromatosis
Autoimmune hepatitis	Liver tumors, e.g. unresectable hepatoblastoma confined to the liver

rarely identified. Drug-related toxicity and some metabolic liver diseases, such as Wilson's disease, can also cause acute decompensation of liver function. Acute liver failure by definition is the onset of encephalopathy within 8 weeks of the appearance of jaundice, and the progression of encephalopathy can be slow or progress to brain death in the patient within 24 hours. Acute liver failure is potentially spontaneously reversible, but most programs proceed with listing of the patient for transplantation with the onset of encephalopathy. Urgent live-donor transplantation has been used in this setting with great success in experienced programs since the wait for a deceased donor organ can be prolonged in a situation where the patient's status may be deteriorating by the hour.

Apart from the onset of encephalopathy, poor prognostic signs include prolongation of the international normalized ratio (INR) above 3, non-acetaminophen-related liver injury, age below ten years, and worsening renal function.

Chronic liver disease with cirrhosis is the most common indication for transplantation in children, and biliary atresia is the most common form of liver disease leading to transplantation, accounting for at least 35–50 percent of cases in large pediatric series and research consortium data. Biliary atresia after a Kasai operation is characterized by progressive jaundice, increasing portal hypertension, ascites, and malnutrition. Even patients with initial clearance of jaundice may require liver transplantation later on in childhood, adolescence, or even adulthood. Chronic liver disease may also lead to progressive encephalopathy, metabolic bone disease, intractable pruritus, pulmonary hypertension and hepatopulmonary syndrome. These are also signs of the need for liver transplantation.

Inborn errors of metabolism resulting from liver enzyme deficiencies or mutations constitute the next most common indication for liver transplantation in children. In many conditions, the disease process damages the liver through the accumulation of toxic metabolites and transplantation is prompted by hepatic decompensation or the development of a malignant tumor. Alpha-1-antitrypsin deficiency or tyrosinemia are examples. Wilson's disease is a genetic disorder of copper metabolism with excessive copper deposition in the liver, basal ganglia, kidney, and other organs. Most cases can be successfully treated medically, but some patients present acutely with liver failure and need an urgent liver transplant. Bile acid transport disorders in progressive familial intrahepatic cholestasis (PFIC) may lead to cirrhosis or secondary hepatocellular carcinoma and may require transplantation in more severe forms of the disease. Byler's disease is the best known example of PFIC. In the future, new specific drug treatments, gene therapy, or hepatocyte transplantation may offer better treatment for some of these hepatic-based metabolic disorders.

Liver tumors, such as hepatoblastoma, that are not safely resectable after neoadjuvant chemotherapy may also be transplanted with good results.

Contraindications to liver transplant include persistent extrahepatic malignant disease, severe extrahepatic disease that cannot be reversed by liver transplantation, such as pulmonary hypertension, uncontrolled systemic sepsis, and severe irreversible neurological injury. Metabolic disorders, such as mitochondriopathies, that affect other organ systems and could lead to death even if the hepatic function is improved, are also contraindications for transplantation.

Timing

Transplantation must be considered in any child with chronic liver disease who is showing signs of decompensated cirrhosis, including growth failure and malnutrition. Portal hypertension alone in a well-compensated cirrhotic may be treated by non-transplant means, but the presence of ascites, non-correctable coagulopathy, hypoalbuminemia, and metabolic bone disease should trigger a transplant evaluation, and quite likely activation on a transplant waiting list. The pediatric and adult end stage liver disease scores (PELD and MELD) were designed to quantify the need for transplantation in an objective manner, and scores above 15 are considered as representing a relatively high risk of dying within a year without a liver transplant. Exceptions to this rule are numerous and lower scores should not exclude a child from being evaluated for liver transplantation.

In children with acute or subacute liver failure, the poor prognostic signs as outlined above should lead to a rapid evaluation of the child for transplantation and once the decision has been made to transplant a child, speed is of the essence since neurological or hemodynamic deterioration may be rapid.

PREOPERATIVE ASSESSMENT AND PREPARATION

Once the decision has been made to evaluate a child for transplantation, the following issues need to be addressed with a multidisciplinary team that includes surgery, hepatology, social work, and other medical specialties as needed (e.g. cardiology):

- Determine the anatomical features of the child that may complicate the transplant. These would include portal vein and arterial anatomy, presence of other anatomical peculiarities, such as situs inversus.

- Exclude comorbidities such as pulmonary hypertension or renal disease.
- Identify and, if possible, correct metabolic, nutritional, and immunization deficiencies. A complete dental examination is also necessary.
- Assess the psychosocial impact of transplantation on the family and educate them about the procedure and the long-term sequelae. This should include educating the family about potential living-donor transplantation and making this option available if it is desired.

A broad range of investigations may be indicated (**Table 107.2**), but the preoperative work up should be customized based on the underlying cause of liver failure. Malnutrition is common because of malabsorption, anorexia, and catabolism. Nutritional status is a major determinant of outcome. Aggressive nutritional support, including nasogastric or even parenteral nutrition, may be needed. Bleeding esophageal varices are treated, preferably by variceal band ligation. Viral screening should include cytomegalovirus (CMV) and Epstein–Barr virus (EBV) serology, both of which are important potential post-transplant pathogens. Patients should be immunized against *Pneumococcus* and hepatitis A and B in addition to routine vaccines. Live vaccines, such as varicella, are best given at least two months before transplant, as they are generally contraindicated in the immunosuppressed patient.

Table 107.2 Investigation of the pediatric liver transplant recipient.

Complete history and physical examination, including assessments of growth, nutrition, development

Hematology – full blood count, clotting, blood group

Biochemistry – urea, electrolytes, creatinine, liver function tests, glucose, lactate, bone profile, magnesium, lipids, vitamin levels, urine biochemistry

Immunology – immunoglobulins, autoantibodies

Microbiology – urine culture, surface swabs

Viral serology – hepatitis A, B, and C, cytomegalovirus, Epstein–Barr virus, herpes simplex virus, Varicella zoster virus, human immunodeficiency virus

Serum α-fetoprotein

Chest x-ray

Abdominal ultrasound scan and Doppler studies of hepatic vessels

Magnetic resonance or computed tomography scan/angiogram (selected cases)

Echocardiogram and ECG

Respiratory function tests ± blood gases

Dental review

2 It is essential to define the vascular anatomy of the liver prior to a transplant. Patients with biliary atresia may have a wide-ranging variety of both congenital and acquired vascular problems. A Doppler ultrasound examination looking for portal vein flow and size is essential. A computed tomography (CT) or magnetic resonance (MR) angiogram may be indicated if other anomalies are suspected. Preoperative demonstration of patent hepatic vasculature is essential to assess the technical feasibility of the operation. Ultrasonography is often sufficient to determining the patency and size of the portal vein and delineate the recipient vascular anatomy. Failure to visualize satisfactory hepatopedal portal blood flow is an indication for CT angiography. In this CT angiogram, one can see a diminutive portal vein (arrow) with the larger coronary going to the left upper quadrant. In this patient, the surgeon should be prepared to reconstruct the portal vein with a vein graft if necessary.

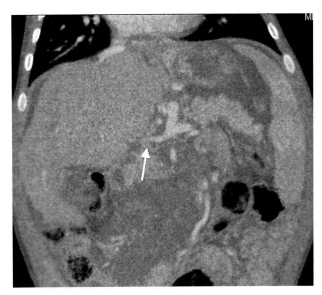

2

Anesthesia

Patients undergoing liver transplantation pose a unique challenge to the anesthesiologist based on the multiple organ systems affected by the failing liver. Management of intracranial pressure in fulminant hepatic failure requires placement of an intracranial monitoring device with the onset of advanced encephalopathy. Maintenance of adequate intra- and perioperative cerebral perfusion and oxygen delivery in order to prevent irreversible effects of cerebral edema requires judicious use of pressors, volume, and anesthetic, and is often challenged by acute blood loss. The cardiopulmonary system is often in a hyperdynamic state characterized by increased cardiac output, peripheral arteriovenous shunting and decreased intravascular resistance and can be complicated by pulmonary hypertension. Severe coagulopathy and thrombocytopenia and the potential for massive blood loss require a large amount of blood products to be readily available. Perioperative broad-spectrum antibiotics, such as ampicillin and cefotaxime, are given. We do not routinely give antifungal prophylaxis unless a predisposition to fungal sepsis exists, such as pretransplant treatment with steroids. Large-bore intravenous access can be established preoperatively through the use of double lumen catheters inserted by radiology.

Given the frequent presence of a distended abdomen, ascites, hepatosplenomegaly, and impaired gastric emptying, rapid sequence induction is used in most patients.

Invasive hemodynamic monitoring and central venous access for rapid infusion are supplemented by a central temperature probe, oximetry, capnography, and a urethral catheter. Invasive right heart catheters are not routinely used but newer, less invasive methods of measuring cardiac output and systemic vascular resistance are gaining popularity.

Blood is analyzed regularly for gases, pH, lactate, hemoglobin and platelet count, prothrombin time, glucose, and electrolytes (including ionized calcium). Thromboelastography is a helpful additional measure of coagulation.

It is essential to insulate the child well and use warming methods in order to prevent the body temperature from falling below 35°C during the anhepatic phase when the cold organ is placed in the body cavity of the child.

During the anhepatic phase, frequent boluses of calcium, bicarbonate, and fresh frozen plasma are necessary to maintain hemodynamic stability. Once the liver has been implanted, calcium requirements drop precipitously due to the metabolism of the calcium bound to bicarbonate in the fresh-frozen plasma by the newly working liver.

3 Venovenous bypass is rarely used in children but may have a place in those who cannot tolerate interruption in venous return from the portal vein and inferior vena cava without becoming hypotensive. Such patients may be those in fulminant failure on vasopressors, or patients with pulmonary hypertension who are extremely preload-dependent in order to maintain cardiac output.

Cannulas are inserted into the portal and femoral veins and diverted blood is pumped through a subclavian catheter into the right atrium. This technique helps to maintain venous return and renal perfusion during caval cross-clamping, reduces portal pressure and blood loss during the recipient hepatectomy, and helps to prevent venous congestion of the gut once the portal vein is divided.

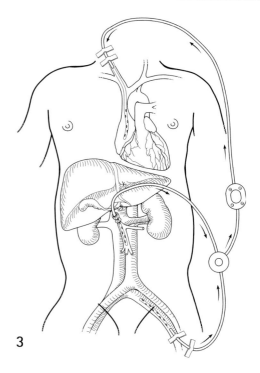

3

DONOR OPERATION

Although livers from donors following cessation of cardiac function have been used in children, this practice is generally avoided due to the high incidence of ischemic cholangioapthy in the recipient. The liver is typically procured from a heart-beating donor in whom brain death has been diagnosed by stringent criteria. Most donors for pediatric liver transplantation are aged between one and 50 years and have died from severe head injury, spontaneous intracranial bleed, or treated bacterial meningitis. More cautiously, deaths from intracranial tumors can also be used.

The donor and recipient should be ABO blood group compatible, but tissue typing is not required. ABO-incompatible donors are justified in urgent situations, particularly for children below the age of one year in whom preformed anti-ABO antibodies are not present.

The donor should have near-normal biochemical liver function, no history of extracranial malignancy, and no evidence of chronic liver disease or past infection with hepatitis B or C, human immunodeficiency virus (HIV), or prions. Donor CMV and EBV serology must be recorded. Most donor livers are removed as part of a multiorgan procurement procedure in which the liver, kidneys, pancreas, heart and/or lungs are removed.

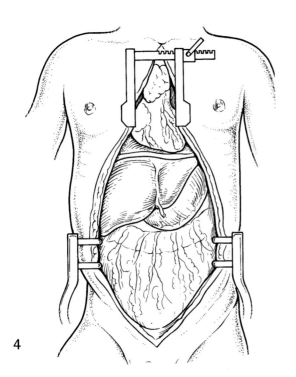

4

4 A midline incision is made from the suprasternal notch to the pubis. The sternum is opened in the midline using a sternal saw and retractor. The authors routinely preserve the falciform ligament and the associated fat pad attached to the graft as an option to pad a potentially redundant arterial reconstruction and prevent kinking. If not needed, this fat pad is tied and resected following reperfusion. The abdominal viscera are carefully inspected to exclude injury or disease. The liver is mobilized by incising its ligamentous attachments. The gastrohepatic ligament is examined for the presence of an accessory/replaced left hepatic artery arising from the left gastric artery, which, if present, must be preserved in continuity with the celiac axis.

5 The porta hepatis is dissected next, checking for an anomalous right hepatic artery arising from the superior mesenteric artery. This usually lies behind the portal vein and must be preserved in continuity with the superior mesenteric artery.

If there is a conventional hepatic arterial supply, the gastroduodenal and right gastric arteries are divided between ligatures followed by ligation of the left gastric and splenic arteries. The common bile duct is divided close to the upper border of the duodenum, the gallbladder is opened and carefully flushed with cold saline. The portal vein is carefully dissected.

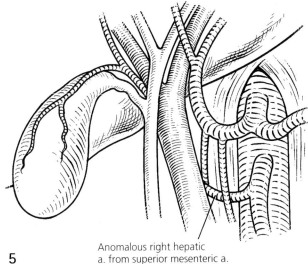

5

Anomalous right hepatic a. from superior mesenteric a.

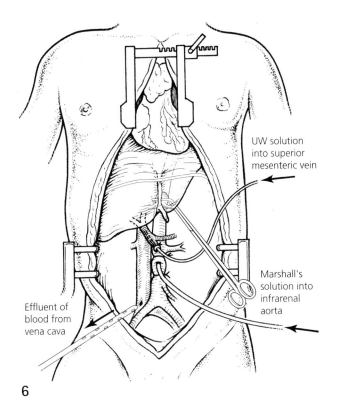

UW solution into superior mesenteric vein

Marshall's solution into infrarenal aorta

Effluent of blood from vena cava

6

6 The distal aorta just above the bifurcation is encircled with two strong tapes and the aorta just above or below the diaphragm is next dissected and encircled with a tape. The superior (or inferior) mesenteric vein at the root of the small bowel mesentery is isolated. At this stage, the cardiac team begins preparing the heart and/or lungs for retrieval, after which the donor is heparinized. A large-bore cannula is then inserted into the distal aorta and used to flush the viscera with 1–4 L of University of Wisconsin (UW) solution. The authors do not routinely use a portal vein flush *in situ*. When all surgical dissection is completed, the diaphragmatic aorta is clamped, the infrarenal vena cava (or intracardiac cava if the heart is not being retrieved) is incised to drain blood from the donor, and cold perfusion begins. Ventilation is stopped. Iced saline slush is poured over the liver and kidneys to provide additional surface cooling.

When the organs are cold and blanched, they are removed. This requires care, as the blanched, non-pulsatile vessels are not so readily identified. The hepatic artery and celiac axis are removed *en bloc* with a small patch of aorta. The portal vein is retrieved with a stump of the splenic and superior mesenteric veins (assuming the pancreas is not being retrieved). The right lobe of the liver and the vena cava are mobilized, retaining the right adrenal gland with the graft. The infrahepatic vena cava is transected just above the renal veins and the suprahepatic vena cava is divided with a cuff of diaphragm.

On the bench, the liver is further perfused with UW solution via the hepatic artery and portal vein. The bile duct is gently irrigated. The liver is packed in sterile plastic bags containing cold UW solution and stored in ice for transportation.

After the kidneys have been removed, the iliac arteries and veins are retrieved for any subsequent vascular reconstruction. Later, during the recipient hepatectomy, the liver is cleaned and prepared on the back bench; redundant tissue is removed and the phrenic and right adrenal veins are ligated. The hepatic artery and portal vein are prepared for implantation. In the rapid perfusion technique, particularly important for unstable donors, the aorta is cannulated quickly, and perfusion of the abdominal viscera is commenced with minimal dissection after administration of heparin. After perfusion, the liver vasculature is quickly divided in the cold with no tying off of branches of the celiac axis. This is done later at the back-table clean up of the liver.

Arterial reconstruction

7 Arterial reconstruction on the back table may be required to simplify implantation of a liver with an anomalous hepatic arterial supply. For example, a right accessory artery arising from the superior mesenteric artery can be anastomosed to the splenic or gastroduodenal stump. An anomalous left artery arising from the left gastric artery requires no particular reconstruction since both the left gastric and common hepatic artery can be revascularized from a Carrel patch on the celiac axis.

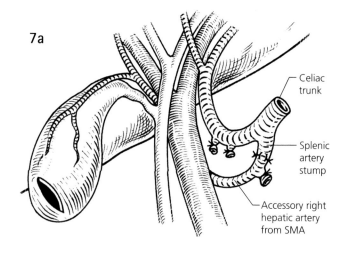

7a

Celiac trunk

Splenic artery stump

Accessory right hepatic artery from SMA

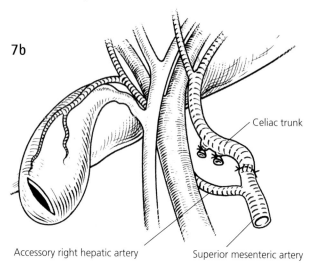

7b

Celiac trunk

Accessory right hepatic artery

Superior mesenteric artery

RECIPIENT OPERATION (ORTHOTOPIC WHOLE GRAFT)

The recipient hepatectomy can be difficult in children with biliary atresia and portal hypertension in whom dense vascular adhesions from previous surgery may make dissection of the portal structures, duodenum, Roux loop, and transverse colon hazardous.

Incision

8 The abdomen is entered through a curved, bilateral subcostal incision and routinely extended vertically in the midline to the xiphoid process for better exposure. The abdominal muscles are divided with cautery to maintain hemostasis. The liver is exposed using an upper abdominal retractor.

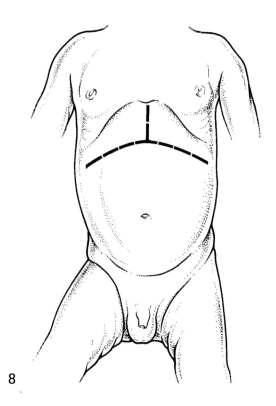

8

Hepatectomy

9 In children who have previously had a portoenterostomy for biliary atresia, the liver is separated from the abdominal wall with cautery, as the normal ligamentous attachments are poorly defined. This dissection becomes easier once freer tissue planes are reached posteriorly. The transverse colon and duodenum are carefully separated from the liver with the aid of precise bipolar cautery. The jejunal Roux loop is identified, divided, and oversewn in two layers close to the liver hilum in order to assure adequate length of the remaining Roux limb. The portal structures can then be dissected. In acute liver failure, the porta hepatis is dissected before mobilizing the liver and the hepatic artery is ligated early to try to minimize hemodynamic instability.

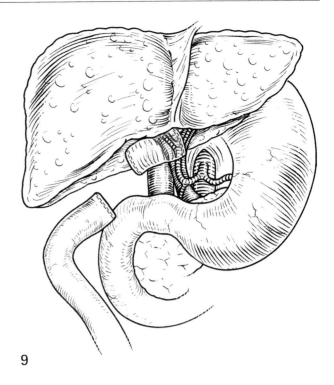

9

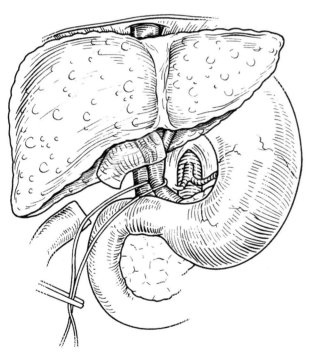

10

10 In patients in whom the bile duct is present, it is divided between ligatures, leaving a good length of common bile duct. The hepatic artery is traced to beyond its segmental branches which are tied individually and divided. This is essential in order to maximize the number of candidate arteries available for possible use at the time of the arterial anastomosis. The portal vein is dissected and isolated; if the portal vein is narrow, either the bifurcation should be preserved or its origin exposed at the confluence of the splenic and superior mesenteric veins. Dividing the gastroduodenal artery helps to expose the proximal aspect of the portal vein, and the confluence of the splenic and mesenteric veins.

11 If not previously divided, the falciform and triangular ligaments are incised. The gastrohepatic ligament is divided between ligatures. The liver is retracted medially and the right lobe is dissected from the diaphragm and retroperitoneum using cautery. The infrahepatic cava is encircled above the renal veins with a tape and, using this plane as a guide, the right adrenal vein is identified and preserved or divided between ligatures if necessary. The plane behind the retrohepatic cava is carefully dissected from both sides until the suprahepatic vena cava can be encircled ready for subsequent clamping.

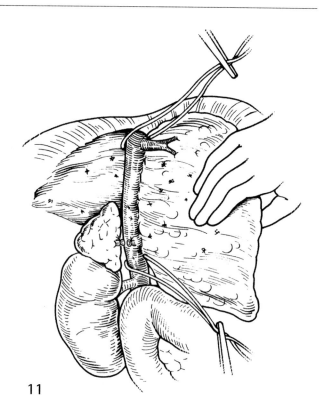

11

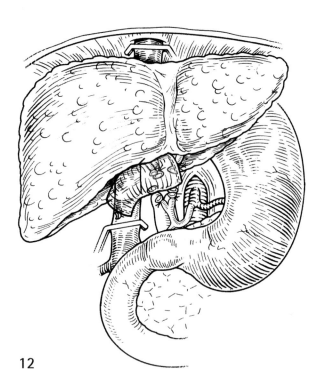

12

12 The portal vein is divided between ligatures or vascular clamps. In some older children, a portal cannula may be inserted for venovenous bypass. Both the suprahepatic and infrahepatic vena cavae are occluded with secure vascular clamps; the former is clamped with a cuff of diaphragm, avoiding the phrenic nerve.

13 Provided the patient is hemodynamically stable, the suprahepatic vena cava is divided – extra length can be obtained by incising the liver at the confluence of the hepatic veins.

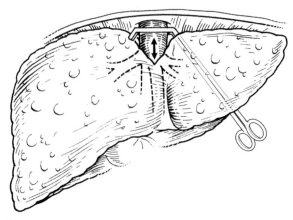

13

14 The infrahepatic vena cava is divided and the liver removed. Meticulous hemostasis of the retroperitoneum should be achieved with a combination of cautery, argon beam coagulation, and suture ligation. Access to this area is more difficult once the donor liver has been implanted.

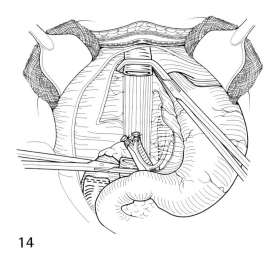

14

15 The inferior vena cava is not always removed with the liver. A piggyback technique has been described which reduces the dissection involved in order to remove the cava. Once the liver is ready for excision, caval clamps are placed above and below the liver, and the liver is dissected sharply off the underlying vena cava. This technique is safer and less prone to bleeding than tying off all the retrohepatic tributaries in these often very hard and cirrhotic livers. Once the liver is mobilized off the inferior vena cava, the right hepatic vein is divided, and then the middle and left together. All venous tributaries on the retrohepatic cava are sutured or ligated. The right hepatic vein may be sutured or left open depending on the size of the liver to be implanted. For segmental II–III grafts or left lobe grafts, it may only be necessary to use the orifices of the left and middle hepatic veins opened together. For right lobe grafts, the right hepatic vein is left open and the left and middle are sutured shut. For whole liver piggybacks, all three hepatic veins are opened and joined together to form a venous cloaca to serve as the site of anastomosis to the donor cava.

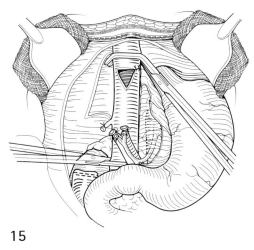

15

Implantation

16 This must be performed expeditiously to minimize the period of warm ischemia of the graft. Implantation begins with the suprahepatic vena caval anastomosis, which is performed with a continuous 3/0 or 4/0 polypropylene suture. A double-ended suture is placed in each corner of the cava and the left side is tied as the liver is placed in the hepatic fossa. The posterior wall of the cava is anastomosed with a continuous everting suture, which ensures endothelial apposition. If the cava is narrow, the anterior wall is closed with interrupted sutures.

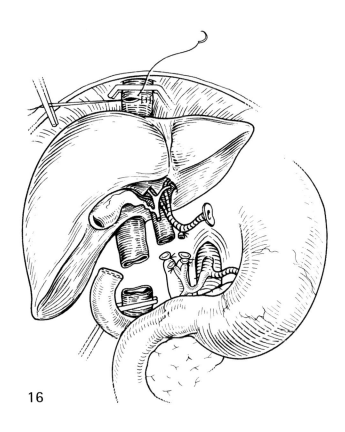

16

17 The infrahepatic vena cava anastomosis is performed next with an everting 4/0 polypropylene suture; the anterior wall is left incomplete. Residual preservative solution rich in potassium is flushed out of the liver with 500 mL of 4.5 percent human albumin solution infused via the portal vein. The effluent flows out of the incompletely anastomosed infrahepatic vena cava, which is then completed.

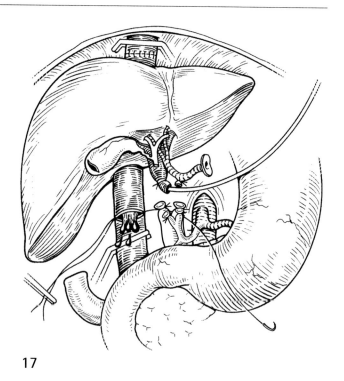

17

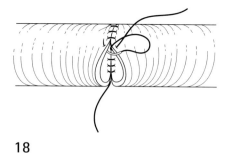

18

18 The portal vein anastomosis is performed next. Care must be taken to avoid redundancy or rotation which might cause kinking. The anastomosis is performed with continuous 6/0 or 7/0 polypropylene or polydioxanone (PDS) sutures. Size discrepancies between the donor and recipient vein must be dealt with by a variety of potential techniques. These include 'cheating' on the larger vein to compensate for the smaller circumference of the smaller vein, spatulation of the smaller vein to increase the effective circumference, fashioning a branch patch from the bifurcation of the smaller recipient vein, or placing an interposition vein graft that is midway in size between the donor and recipient. At the completion of the anastomosis, the knot is tied away from the vein wall allowing the vein wall to expand freely with the influx of blood.

The anesthetist checks the patient for stability and the vascular clamps are removed in sequence. The suprahepatic caval clamp is removed first, followed by the infrahepatic caval clamp. A quick search is made for major bleeding points and the stability of the patient is confirmed before the portal clamp is removed and the liver reperfused. Any major bleeding points are identified and controlled. The gallbladder is removed using cautery and the cystic duct is transfixed and ligated with an absorbable suture.

19 The donor hepatic artery is gently flushed with heparinized saline and a soft bulldog clamp is applied to prevent backflow of blood from the donor liver, which would interfere with the arterial anastomosis. The hepatic artery is anastomosed end-to-end; a branch patch from the recipient hepatic artery bifurcation or gastroduodenal artery can be used if necessary. The anastomosis can be safely performed with a continuous 7/0 or 8/0 polypropylene suture posteriorly and interrupted sutures anteriorly. Magnification (with loupes or a microscope) is essential with small arteries. If the native artery is small or has poor flow, a donor iliac arterial conduit anastomosed to the recipient's infrarenal aorta may be used to arterialize the graft.

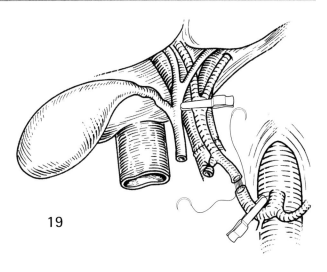

19

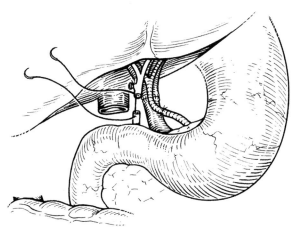

20 A duct-to-duct biliary anastomosis is performed using interrupted 6/0 PDS. The donor duct may require trimming to produce a healthy vascular margin. The posterior row of sutures is placed before the ends of the ducts are approximated and the sutures tied.

A Roux-en-Y hepaticojejunostomy is performed in cases of biliary atresia and sclerosing cholangitis or if the recipient common bile duct is very small. A 40-cm Roux loop of jejunum is prepared and brought up to the porta hepatis in a retrocolic position. A small opening is made in the antimesenteric border close to the tip of the Roux loop and the anastomosis is performed with interrupted 6/0 or 7/0 PDS.

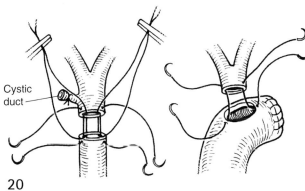

Cystic duct

20

Hemostasis and closure

21 Complete hemostasis is secured. All anastomoses are checked. Bleeding at this stage is often secondary to a coagulopathy, and thromboelastography is useful in guiding the use of blood products. The abdomen is closed en masse with a continuous absorbable suture after placing a soft multi-fenestrated large-bore (20–24 Fr) silicone drain posteriorly in the right upper quadrant. The skin is closed with a subcuticular suture. A prosthetic patch (e.g. Vicryl) or skin closure alone (with delayed muscle closure) may occasionally be necessary to avoid an excessively tight abdominal closure.

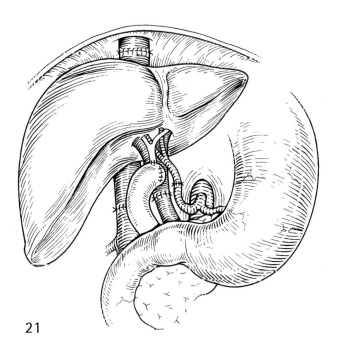

21

TECHNICAL VARIANT GRAFTS

Segmental liver grafts are prepared from whole deceased donor livers and from living donors. In practice, there are three main types of graft: the left lateral segment (segments II and III), the left lobe (segments II–IV), and the right lobe (segments V–VIII). The type of graft is determined by the relative sizes of the donor and recipient and the individual anatomical characteristics of the donor. With cadaveric organs, split-liver grafts are preferable to reduced grafts because this maximizes the donor organ pool. However, when donor anatomy precludes a split-liver transplant, a reduced graft may need to be used. Donor criteria for split or reduced grafts are more stringent than for whole grafts because of the extra insult of the bench procedure: donors under age 50 years, less than 10 percent macrovesicular fat, minimal pressor support, near-normal liver enzymes and bilirubin, and less than 5 days in hospital at the time of the procurement of the organ.

Various size guidelines are helpful in pediatric liver transplantation. As a minimum, the graft weight should be approximately 1 percent of the recipient's body weight in living-related liver transplantation; a greater safety margin is advisable in deceased donor transplantation, especially in small infant recipients. The adult liver usually weighs between 1300 and 1700 g. The left lateral segment comprises approximately 25 percent of the liver weight and the left lobe about 40 percent. The maximum graft size that can be safely accommodated in the child's abdomen depends on the recipient's weight, the presence of ascites and hepatomegaly, and other factors, but, as a rough guide, a donor to recipient weight ratio of up to 1.5:1 is often acceptable for whole livers and right lobe grafts, up to 4:1 for a left lobe graft, up to 13:1 for a left lateral segment graft. However, because of the exceptionally wide variation in the relative size of the segment II–III portion of an adult liver, it must always be necessary to visually inspect the organ prior to deciding on the anatomical unit appropriate for any individual recipient.

Because most donors are adults and most pediatric recipients are infants or small children, the utilization of technical variant transplants has greatly reduced the mortality of children on the transplant waiting list. The mortality in small children still remains unfortunately high.

Reduced grafts

22a Liver reduction is best performed as a bench procedure in the recipient operating suite. The donor liver must be kept totally immersed in cold UW solution at 4°C during the procedure. Care must be taken to avoid excessive traction on the hepatic artery, which could cause intimal injury.

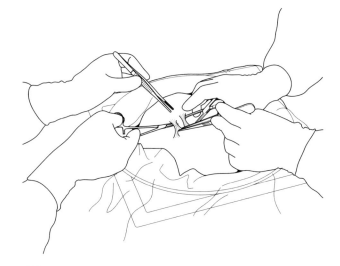

22a

22b–e With right or left lobe grafts, the parenchyma is transected alongside the principal plane slightly to the left or right of the middle hepatic vein, respectively. The interlobar plane is defined by the gall bladder fossa anteriorly and the bed of the inferior vena cava (IVC) posteriorly. Defining the venous drainage is critical. The middle hepatic vein accompanies either the right or left lobe along with either the right or left hepatic vein. The main branches to the lobe that is being discarded are ligated well away from the midline, but outside the parenchyma, so that they are effectively ligated and defined. Bile duct radicles and portal vein branches to the caudate lobe are also divided since the caudate lobe is rarely used in reduced size transplants.

Biliary and vascular branches on the cut surface of the graft are carefully ligated. The vena cava is preserved with the graft but is usually discarded just prior to implantation since most reduced grafts are implanted using the piggyback technique. After division, the cut surface is tested for leaks by gently perfusing UW solution through the portal vein, hepatic artery, and bile duct; these are oversewn. The graft comes with the main portal vein, the celiac axis, the main bile duct, and the IVC, but it can be decided to resect most of these structures and use only the branches to the lobe being used at the time of implantation. In general, preserving the complete vascular structures and using them is unnecessary.

The surface is sprayed with fibrin glue. The lobe is implanted in a similar way to a whole graft.

In preparing a left lateral segment graft, the hilar dissection is very similar to that used for a left lobe graft except that the plane of parenchymal transection is just to the right of the falciform ligament. The right-sided branches of the portal triad are dissected and divided outside the liver; the stump of the right hepatic artery is ligated and the right branch of the portal vein is closed with a continuous polypropylene suture. Portal vein branches to segment IV are divided within the Rex recessus. Caudate branches from the origin of the left portal vein are divided. The left hepatic vein is dissected out and the middle and right hepatic veins are divided and their orifices oversewn. Later, the surgeon may also discard the cava and use only the left hepatic vein orifice with a cuff of cava once it has been ascertained that the recipient vena cava is intact and does not need replacement. The common hepatic artery and main portal trunk are retained with the graft. The main bile duct is preserved in continuity with the left hepatic duct. Care must be taken not to injure the left hepatic duct at the base of segment IV, so the parenchymal division should be away from the hilum as it nears the hilar structures. Afterwards, the surgeon may elect to cut back the duct, and making the biliary anastomosis at the level of the common hepatic duct or even the left hepatic duct. For liver transplantation in small infants, the left lateral segment can be further reduced, creating a monosegmental graft.

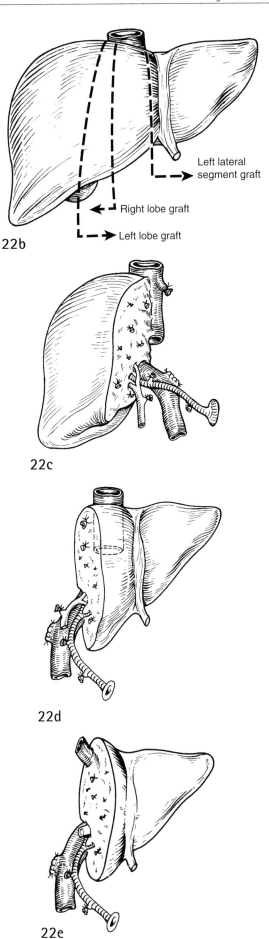

Left lateral segment graft

Right lobe graft

Left lobe graft

22b

22c

22d

22e

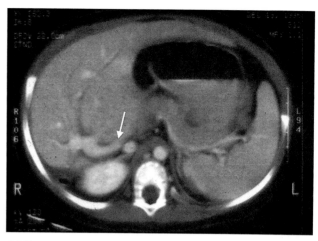

22f

22f In the illustration, it can be seen how the portal vein (arrow) in a size-reduced liver lies transversely across the vena cava and kidney and rotates posteriorly, as the cut surface rotates in a counterclockwise manner. One must compensate for this rotation when planning the hepatic and portal venous anastomoses.

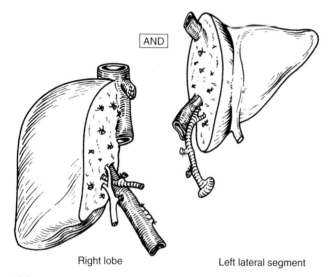

Right lobe   Left lateral segment

23

Split–liver grafts

23 The donor liver is divided into two grafts for transplantation into two recipients. The procedure is more complex than a size reduction since biliary drainage, venous drainage, and portal and arterial supply to both portions of the liver must be preserved intact.

Early assessment of vascular and biliary anatomy is important to ensure that there is no anatomic contraindication to splitting. The gallbladder is removed and the portal vein and hepatic artery carefully dissected to their bifurcations. Arterial anomalies often complicate the split procedure.

Left lobe–right lobe splits are less common than segment II–III/right trisegment grafts, where the right trisegment goes to an adult and the segment II–III graft to a baby or small child.

For the segment II–III/right trisegment grafts split, it is important to try and preserve the arterial supply to segment IV, since the portal blood to segment IV will always be divided. Strict allocation rules have been developed, so that allocation of vessels will be determined primarily by the center to which the primary offer has been made.

If segment IV artery comes off the left hepatic artery, that vessel may be sacrificed rendering segment IV ischemic. The segment II–III/right trisegment graft may still be usable since intraparenchymal collaterals may exist, but the center using the segment II–III/right trisegment graft should realize the risk. The middle hepatic vein goes with the segment II–III/right trisegment graft, as does the bile duct, vena cava, and main portal vein. The celiac axis can go to the primary recipient if a child and then the segment II–III/right trisegment graft will just have the right hepatic artery. When the adult is receiving the primary offer, the child will generally be allocated the left hepatic artery with or without the segment IV vessel. The parenchymal transection is along the same plane as for reduced size livers.

Less commonly, right lobe–left lobe splits are performed. Even though the parenchymal transection is thicker, the hilar dissection is simplified since the arterial supply is always determined by a left–right hepatic artery allocation, with the celiac axis usually going to the graft that has been allocated to the primary recipient. Arterial anomalies complicate any split procedure, and may preclude safe utilization of both pieces. Anomalous left hepatic artery from the left gastric may simplify the arterial division in a segment II–III/right trisegment split, as will an anomalous right hepatic artery coming from the superior mesenteric artery.

Extreme care must be taken in any split procedure in both donor selection and in careful technique during the split procedure since the lives of two recipients will depend on the adequate function of both halves of the split liver.

Most liver splits are performed as a bench procedure after deceased donor organ retrieval (*ex situ* splitting), but many centers advocate for *in situ* split while the organ is still perfused with blood. Where logistic and organizational aspects permit, *in situ* splitting in the donor is an alternative; this facilitates cut-surface hemostasis and minimizes the cold ischemic time, but requires a more experienced retrieval team.

Living related grafts

The greatest experience is with living related donation of the left lateral segment from parent to child but, in recent years, living related donation of the left lobe and adult-to-adult right lobe donation have become increasingly popular. Living related donation has additional ethical and medical issues.

The safety of the donor is paramount. The potential donor should have a compatible blood group and appropriate liver anatomy. In the elective setting, the donor is evaluated for emotional stability and screened for any evidence that he or she may be subject to subtle coercion to donate. Emotionally related donors who do not have any direct family connection to the donor, such as clergy or teachers, may also volunteer to be considered as donors when the parents or direct relatives are not suitable. Last of all, altruistic individuals who step forward as donors for patients they do not know, so-called Good Samaritan donors, must be carefully evaluated both medically and psychologically before being accepted.

Although the live donor liver operation was first conceived of as an elective procedure with adequate time for the prospective donor to come to a full realization of the risks involved, more recent experience has included live donor transplantation for urgent situations, such as fulminant liver failure or acute decompensation of children with chronic liver disease. The familiarity of the public with living donor transplantation has grown to the point where many parents demand to be considered as donors, even in the setting of fulminant failure, if they think that donating will increase their child's chances of surviving.

24 The donor operation is started first. When direct visual confirmation of hepatic suitability is obtained, the recipient operation is started. The authors advocate that the adult operation takes place in an adult-care institution by a team of surgeons separate from the one that will be caring for the child. For a left lateral segmentectomy, an upper midline abdominal incision is used to mobilize the segment II–III graft. The left side of the liver is mobilized by dividing the triangular ligament and the gastroduodenal ligament. The left hepatic vein and left portal triad structures are isolated with slings. The parenchyma is transected at the falciform ligament. Parenchymal transection takes place with Ligasure™ instrumentation.

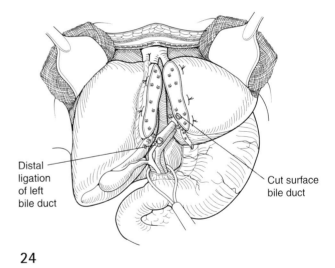

Distal ligation of left bile duct

Cut surface bile duct

24

When the parenchymal division is almost complete, the left portal vein is mobilized (dividing caudate branches) and the hilar plate and left bile duct divided. The segments II and III ducts may be separate at the line of transection.

After completion of the parenchymal section, the left portal vein, hepatic vein, and hepatic artery are divided and the liver graft is removed and perfused with ice-cold UW solution on the bench. A length of the donor inferior mesenteric or ovarian vein may need to be retrieved for use as a vascular conduit.

For left or right lobe grafts, the liver is mobilized laparoscopically, and much of the parenchymal transection is also done laparoscopically with Ligasure. The final division of the vessels is done through a midline incision, and the graft removed.

Laparoscopic mobilization has benefited donors in that the need for a large subcostal incision on both sides of the abdomen has been eliminated and the postoperative recovery is much faster and less painful.

Implantation of the segment II–III or left lobe graft

25 In this figure, the left lobe graft of an older pediatric deceased donor is being implanted into a child with fulminant failure. The orifice of the confluence of the left and middle hepatic veins is seen underneath the suprahepatic vena cava clamp (long arrow). This liver is being piggybacked onto the recipient cava which can be seen as a thin collapsed structure running down from the vena cava clamp (short arrows).

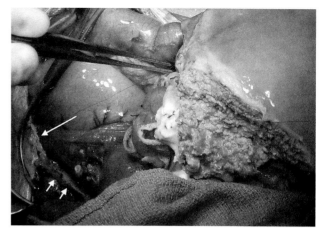

25

A segment II–III graft implantation varies according to whether the graft originates from a live donor or is a reduced graft from a deceased donor. A split liver graft implant is similar to that utilized for a live donor organ. The main difference is in the length of vessels available that would permit reconstructive procedures if necessary. In a live donor or split graft, the length of the portal vein and hepatic artery is quite limited unless the celiac axis is donated with the deceased donor split graft.

Even with a reduced donor graft, the left hepatic vein should be kept short in order to avoid twisting on the venous pedicle. The donor vein is anastomosed to the confluence of the left and middle hepatic veins (see illustration 25) of the recipient and that opening may be further extended onto the ventral surface of the inferior vena cava. The vein must be widely anastomosed and properly oriented to the recipient cava to prevent venous outflow obstruction. The anastomosis is carried out with PDS absorbable monofilament suture. The absorbable suture is thought to prevent fixed anastomotic strictures that may ultimately prevent growth of the anastomosis as the child grows and slowly lead to an outflow obstruction. The anastomosis is started by placing two corner sutures, tying the left superior one, and proceeding by anastomosing the back wall from inside the vein and progressing to the right inferior corner. The front wall is done next from left to right and the liver is flushed through the portal vein with 500 mL of cold lactated Ringer's solution prior to completion of the hepatic vein anastomosis.

The portal vein is done next. Great care must be taken to allow enough vein on the recipient side in order to prevent undue tension in the anastomosis as the suture line falls more posteriorly as the liver is allowed to rotate back into position at the completion of the portal vein suture line.

For living donor and split liver transplants when only a short segment of donor left hepatic artery is available, the hepatic artery anastomosis is done to the recipient vessel at a location that more closely approximates the diameter of the donor artery. When the celiac axis is available, the surgeon may choose to anastomose the entire artery with a Carrel patch directly to the infrarenal aorta of the recipient. Alternately, a donor iliac artery interposition graft may be placed on the recipient aorta and anastomosed to the celiac axis when the length of the celiac axis will not permit direct aortic anastomosis. Interrupted 7/0 or 8/0 sutures are recommended in the smallest arterial reconstructions with 4.5 loupe or operating microscope magnification in living donor and split liver grafts, as the arteries are frequently no more than 2 or 3 mm in diameter.

The Roux loop is anastomosed to the bile duct(s) at the cut surface using interrupted 6/0 PDS sutures with the aid of magnifying loupes. There may often be two ducts in split and live donor grafts, one each from segments II and III. In these cases, there have to be two separate biliary anastomoses. In reduced size grafts, the anastomosis can be anywhere from the common bile duct to the left hepatic duct, but it is advisable to shorten the duct as much as seems convenient in order to reduce the chances of ischemic strictures from developing.

26 A narrow portal vein is frequently found in biliary atresia patients. Alternative methods of reconstruction, with or without a donor venous conduit, may be necessary. If a donor conduit is needed, this can be prepared during the anhepatic phase.

Bleeding from the raw cut surface of the segmental graft is controlled by a combination of fibrin glue and other topical hemostatic agents, superficial sutures, and argon beam coagulation. If bleeding is severe or persistent, venous outflow obstruction must be excluded. Suturing the remnants of donor and recipient falciform ligaments helps to stabilize the graft and reduce the risk of torsion of the left hepatic vein.

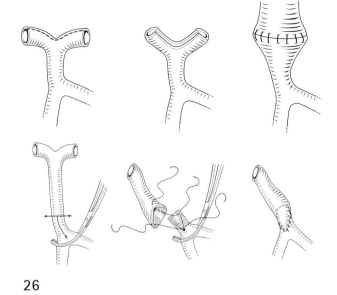

26

Orthotopic auxiliary liver grafts

These have been used in children with acute liver failure where subsequent regeneration of the native liver (and removal of the transplanted graft) is anticipated and also in some children with non-cirrhotic liver-based inborn errors of metabolism, e.g. Crigler–Najjar type 1 and urea cycle defects. The native liver is partially resected and a segmental or whole graft inserted in its place. Auxiliary grafts have a greater risk of technical complications, especially related to portal vein flow. In addition, the stability of the recipient with acute liver failure is a concern. In metabolic conditions, there is the same requirement for long-term immunosuppression as with other transplants. Currently, the application of this technique is very limited.

POSTOPERATIVE CARE

The patient is nursed in intensive care. Early extubation is safe after an uncomplicated transplant provided the patient is clinically stable.

Prostaglandin E infusion as a continuous drip is started immediately after the operation in all split-liver transplants at a dose of 0.01 µg/kg per minute and increased hourly to a maximum of 0.05 as long as the blood pressure is maintained. This decreases ischemic–reperfusion injury and prevents primary non-function of the graft. It is almost never necessary in live donor grafts since the preservation time is quite short.

Arterial blood pressure, temperature, central venous pressure, peripheral perfusion, drain losses, and urine output are closely monitored. The hemoglobin is maintained at 8–10 g/dL. During the first week, frequent abdominal Doppler ultrasound scans help to identify any vascular or biliary complications. CT imaging provides better definition of problems identified with ultrasound screening.

After an initial postoperative chest radiograph, further radiographs are performed only if clinically indicated. A right-sided pleural effusion is common, but typically resolves spontaneously. Paresis of the right hemidiaphragm from a clamp injury to the phrenic nerve may cause prolonged dependence on ventilatory support, but only rarely is a diaphragmatic plication necessary.

The prothrombin time, blood gases, plasma lactate, glucose, and electrolytes are checked regularly and serve as an index of early graft function. Plasma liver function tests, urea and creatinine, calcium, phosphate, and magnesium are recorded daily for the first week. Nasogastric drainage is discontinued as soon as the ileus resolves and enteral feeding is started, usually within 48–72 hours. An acid suppressant is given routinely.

Immunosuppression typically consists of:

- intravenous methylprednisolone given intraoperatively at graft reperfusion and then at 2 mg/kg per day (maximum 40 mg) for 4 days, followed by oral prednisolone tapered progressively to 0.1 mg/kg per day by one month; and
- oral tacrolimus 0.075 mg/kg twice daily or cyclosporine microemulsion 5 mg/kg twice daily (depending on renal function), commencing on day 1 post-transplant and adjusted according to drug levels.

Mycophenolate is started immediately after surgery in order to reduce dependence on calcineurin inhibitors. Rapamycin can be added later.

The advances in surgical techniques and perioperative care yield one-year survival of over 90 percent and the long-term outcomes of pediatric liver transplantation are now mainly affected by successful immunomodulation. While a detailed discussion of all available immunomodulators and their combinations in various regimens is beyond the scope of this chapter, the overall therapeutic strategy remains fairly simple: minimizing adverse effects of immune suppressants, namely bacterial, viral, or fungal infection and malignancy while optimizing graft survival by preventing rejection. There is no universally accepted standard regimen immunomodulation following pediatric liver transplantation and protocols vary widely among institutions. At the authors' center, a single preoperative dose of 10 mg/kg of methylprednisolone is administered. About 12 hours postoperatively, the authors start mycophenolate at 10 mg/kg/dose twice daily and tacrolimus at 0.1 mg/kg/dose twice daily with a goal range of 10–12 ng/mL. Tacrolimus levels, as well as adverse events, are monitored frequently and doses adjusted accordingly. Methylprednisolone is tapered over the following month from 2 to 0.3 mg/kg per day and converted to an oral equivalent after return of bowel function.

Anti-interleukin-2 receptor monoclonal antibodies, such as basiliximab, are sometimes used. Steroid-sparing regimens are becoming increasingly popular, but are not appropriate for patients with a history of autoimmune hepatitis.

Early postoperative complications

BLEEDING

This is more likely with a segmental graft or in the presence of graft dysfunction. Continuing hemorrhage despite correction of coagulopathy warrants early re-exploration, especially if there are signs of a developing abdominal compartment syndrome.

PRIMARY NON-FUNCTION

This occurs in fewer than 5 percent of all transplants and requires emergency retransplantation. In such cases, signs of satisfactory early graft function (hemodynamic stability, early production of bile, normoglycemia, and resolution of lactic acidosis and coagulopathy) are absent. The incidence is higher after split-liver transplantation.

VASCULAR THROMBOSIS

Hepatic artery thrombosis after liver transplantation occurs in 4–8 percent of cases and can be devastating. It is more common in smaller pediatric recipients. Various prophylactic agents, such as low-dose heparin and/or acetylsalicylic acid, are used and the packed cell volume should initially be maintained below 35 percent. Hepatic artery thrombosis may present in several ways: an acute deterioration in liver function progressing to fatal hepatic necrosis, an insidious onset with biliary complications or sepsis, or an absent arterial signal on routine Doppler ultrasound scan. If hepatic artery thrombosis is suspected within days of the transplant, urgent angiography and/or laparotomy are warranted; if revascularization is not possible or unsuccessful, urgent retransplantation is usually required.

Portal vein thrombosis is uncommon, occurring in approximately 2 percent of cases. The narrow portal vein of children with biliary atresia is a risk factor. Early postoperative occlusion may present with acidosis and deranged clotting, gastrointestinal bleeding, ascites, or deteriorating liver function and demands urgent surgical correction. Late portal vein stenosis may cause portal hypertension (splenomegaly, variceal bleeding), but can often be corrected by percutaneous transhepatic balloon angioplasty. In patients in whom percutaneous angioplasty fails to reopen the portal vein, it may be necessary to reconstruct the vein using a meso-Rex bypass vein graft. Less desirable, but often effective, a selective distal splenorenal shunt may be used to treat the complications of portal hypertension in late portal vein thrombosis.

Vena caval occlusion is very rare. Stenosis of the suprahepatic caval anastomosis leading to ascites and lower body edema is uncommon and can usually be treated by percutaneous angioplasty or stenting.

BILIARY COMPLICATIONS

The incidence of biliary leaks and strictures varies between 10 and 30 percent, and is related to the type of graft. Serious biliary complications are less common with whole organ grafts and more common in split liver organs with more than one biliary anastomosis. Hepaticojejunostomies are more prone to leaks because of the relatively smaller size of the bile ducts and the nature of the anastomosis.

Complications can be divided into early leaks or later strictures. Leaks from the cut surface of a reduced size liver may heal spontaneously, but a leak that persists for more than a few days should be repaired operatively and is likely to be either from the anastomosis or a segmental duct that was not seen at the time of the transplant. Strictures generally appear after the first post-transplant month and can usually be dilated percutaneously by the interventional radiologists.

Duct-to-duct anastomoses are more accessible through endoscopic retrograde cholangiopancreatography (ERCP) and both leaks and strictures can be addressed through the enteric route.

Biliary complications are often related to arterial insufficiency. A bile leak that arises secondary to an arterial thrombosis is generally not repairable and requires retransplantation. Ischemic strictures may be isolated to the anastomosis or be widespread in the liver. Bile leaks present in a variety of ways: bile in the drains after surgery, fever abdominal pain, or persistent jaundice. Ultrasound or CT confirms a fluid collection near the cut surface posteriorly, or near the biliary anastomosis in the clinical setting suggestive of a bile leak.

Biliary strictures may be anastomotic or non-anastomotic (when they may reflect ischemia, preservation injury, chronic rejection, etc.). They present with jaundice and/or cholangitis. Strictures may present as Gram-negative sepsis in the absence of any other symptoms.

ACUTE CELLULAR REJECTION

Acute cellular rejection typically manifests as an increase in the plasma levels of transaminases with or without a low-grade fever and irritability. An urgent Doppler ultrasound scan helps to exclude major surgical problems with the graft before performing a percutaneous needle liver biopsy to confirm the diagnosis. Acute rejection is initially treated with three daily doses of 10 mg/kg intravenous methylprednisolone. Most patients respond within 48 hours. A further pulse of steroids may be given and/or other immunosuppressants introduced in resistant cases. Steroid-resistant rejection is treated with an anti-T cell antibody for 5–10 days, and an increase in the baseline immunosuppression.

RENAL COMPLICATIONS

Peritransplant renal dysfunction is common as a result of hepatorenal syndrome, ascites, cardiovascular instability, and nephrotoxic drugs. With good postoperative graft function, most cases recover well, although temporary renal support may be required.

INFECTIONS

Infectious complications are a major cause of mortality and morbidity after liver transplantation because of immunosuppression, indwelling catheters, pre-existing morbidity, malnutrition, and, surgical complications. Early postoperative infections are mostly bacterial or fungal, but viral infections are particularly important later on. Cytomegalovirus infection may cause fever, malaise, diarrhea, gastrointestinal bleeding, abnormal liver function, and pulmonary symptoms. Children are more likely to develop disease if they are primarily infected from a CMV-positive donor than when viral reactivation occurs in a previously immune recipient. Treatment with ganciclovir and reducing the immunosuppression are often effective. Cytomegalovirus prophylaxis is routinely given to naive recipients receiving a CMV-positive graft. Other opportunistic viral infections include herpes simplex, Varicella zoster, adenovirus, and EBV. The last mentioned is a potential cause of post-transplant lymphoproliferative disease. Both CMV and EBV can be monitored by serial estimations of viral load using the polymerase chain reaction.

OUTCOME

Children now enjoy a greater than 90 percent one-year patient survival with graft survival also exceeding 80 percent at one year. Longer-term survival at three and five years is also in excess of 80–90 percent. Children with fulminant failure and encephalopathy or rapid decompensation of chronic liver disease have a worse prognosis primarily because of the comorbidities that accompany rapid decline in liver function. Pre-existing renal failure, pressor dependence, or stage III–IV encephalopathy are markers of worse outcome.

As the survival after liver transplantation now reliably exceeds 90 percent in most pediatric institutions, emphasis has shifted to the quality of life enjoyed by the survivors. Large multi-institutional studies focus on the long-term impact of liver transplantation on school performances, social interactions, and quality of life indices.

United Network for Organ Sharing (UNOS) registry data for the United States indicate that excellent survival of 90 percent at one year is seen in infants as well as older children and adolescents, with diminished survival of 82 percent at one year for children who weigh less than 5 kg at the time of the transplant. Graft availability is often a problem for these small babies and deterioration of other organ functions during the waiting period is a harbinger of a poorer prognosis even for those who are fortunate to receive a graft before dying.

Late complications, including rejection (especially from poor drug compliance), infections, side effects from immunosuppression, and graft dysfunction, continue to pose challenges. It is estimated that about 15 percent of children require retransplantation at some stage.

ACKNOWLEDGMENTS

The author is grateful to Dr Moira O'Meara for her contribution to the section on anesthesia.

FURTHER READING

Broelsch CE, Whitington PF, Emond JC et al. Liver transplantation in children from living related donors. Surgical techniques and results. *Annals of Surgery* 1991; **214**: 428–37.

Deshpande RR, Bowles MJ, Vilca-Melendez H et al. Results of split liver transplantation in children. *Annals of Surgery* 2002; **236**: 248–53.

Emond JC, Heffron TG, Whitington PF, Broelsch CE. Reconstruction of the hepatic vein in reduced size hepatic transplantation. *Surgery, Gynecology and Obstetrics* 1993; **176**: 11–17.

Howard ER, Stringer MD, Colombani PM. *Surgery of the Liver, Bile-Ducts and Pancreas in Children*, 2nd edn. London: Arnold Publishers, 2002.

Shaw BW, Iwatsuki S, Starzl TE. Alternative methods of arterialization of the hepatic graft. *Surgery, Gynecology and Obstetrics* 1984; **159**: 490–3.

108

Small bowel transplantation

KISHORE IYER

History

Intestinal transplantation is a relatively new procedure. As the largest lymphoid organ in the body, transplantation of the intestine presents a significant challenge for immunosuppression. Following animal experiments in the 1960s, notably by Lillehei, and later by Grant, who subsequently performed the first successful liver–intestinal transplant, increasing experience with the procedure has been reported. Deltz reported the first successful long-term small bowel transplant in an adult patient in 1988. In recent years, survival following intestinal transplantation has shown a steadily increasing trend.

PRINCIPLES AND JUSTIFICATION

Parenteral nutrition is life saving in intestinal failure due to short bowel syndrome and a variety of functional causes, such as pseudo-obstruction. The potential of a satisfactory and effective life-saving therapy in the form of parenteral nutrition distinguishes intestinal failure from other forms of end-organ failure. Uncomplicated parenteral nutrition in a stable patient population results in five-year survival of close to 80 percent. A small subset of patients with refractory parenteral nutrition dependence are at risk of significant morbidity and even mortality due to complications that make it potentially dangerous or even impossible to continue this therapy. The most common of these complications is a syndrome of progressive cholestasis that may lead to end-stage liver disease. Despite satisfactory catheter-care techniques, some patients may also suffer inexplicably from central venous catheter-related complications in the form of life-threatening episodes of bacterial or fungal sepsis or loss of venous access due to venous thrombosis. Thus, the fundamental indication for intestinal transplantation is the combined presence of refractory parenteral nutrition dependence and evidence of parenteral nutrition failure with the presence of one of the life-threatening complications of parenteral nutrition.

PREOPERATIVE EVALUATION

A thorough multidisciplinary evaluation is critical prior to a decision to proceed to intestinal transplantation. Key steps in this evaluation are:

- evaluation of residual bowel anatomy;
- evaluation of residual bowel function/motility;
- demonstration of refractory parenteral nutrition dependence and inability to advance enteral feeds;
- evaluation of the presence and extent of liver disease;
- identification of other systemic illnesses/comorbid conditions;
- determination of any significant neurodevelopmental contraindications;
- determination of any psychosocial contraindications.

Following a detailed history and physical examination, it is our practice to carry out abdominal and cervical venous Doppler ultrasound examinations, as well as appropriate gastrointestinal contrast radiographs. Based on the clinical examination and biochemical tests of liver function, a liver biopsy may be required for accurate staging of the extent of liver disease.

Such a detailed evaluation has allowed us to avoid the need for intestinal transplantation and even wean some patients off parenteral nutrition altogether. We also on occasion uncovered previously undiscovered pathology, successful treatment of which has allowed patients to be successfully weaned off parenteral nutrition. On completion of evaluation, the appropriateness of intestinal transplantation for the patient can be determined with a high degree of confidence, and the choice of the type of graft (i.e. isolated small bowel, combined liver–small bowel or multivisceral) can also be made in most cases. It is important to recognize that there is inevitably a long wait for a suitable cadaver donor in most cases (particularly for recipients weighing less than 10 kg) and an accompanying high mortality rate on the waiting list, especially for patients awaiting combined liver–bowel transplantation. Therefore, early referral for patients who appear to be failing parenteral nutrition may be an important step toward improving the outcomes for intestinal transplantation.

The choice of allograft is determined primarily by the presence or absence of advanced liver disease; the presence of cirrhosis with portal hypertension and massive hepatosplenomegaly mandates a combined liver–small bowel transplant. Lesser degrees of liver dysfunction may be reversible with good graft function from an isolated small bowel transplant. The indication for a multivisceral graft is the presence of disease in other organs (e.g. kidney or pancreas) that requires replacement of the organ, or where abdominal exenteration is required for the removal of diseased viscera.

donors who are cytomegalovirus (CMV) positive, except for donors who are below the age of one year and whose CMV positivity may be attributable to passive transfer of maternal antibodies. Donor:recipient size ratios of 0.5–0.6:1 are necessitated by the loss of abdominal domain in the patient with short bowel syndrome who has inevitably had multiple abdominal operations. Patients with functional disorders with few prior operations can accept larger donors. The initial enthusiasm for size-reduction techniques for both isolated bowel and combined liver–bowel grafting have been toned down by the continued challenges of sustaining good outcomes in this patient population, that can be adversely affected by any increase in technical risk.

Routine preoperative antibiotics are administered to the donor. Unlike other groups, we no longer practice any specific intestinal decontamination in the donor, with no apparent increase in complications.

DONOR OPERATIONS

Choice of donor

Hemodynamically stable donors, who are ABO-compatible and ideally about 50–75 percent of recipient weight with evidence of good visceral perfusion (normal liver and renal function) and no acidosis, constitute satisfactory small bowel donors. In recipients who have no evidence of prior exposure to cytomegalovirus, we no longer accept

Organ procurement

ISOLATED SMALL BOWEL GRAFT

The procedure begins with a long midline incision and a median sternotomy. Superficial mesenteric nodes are procured early for tissue typing. An infusion of thymoglobulin, 2 mg/kg, is started at the beginning of the procedure to secure donor lymphocyte depletion after the removal of lymph nodes for tissue typing.

1 We section the falciform ligament and the left triangular ligament, as well as ligamentous attachments to the right lobe of the liver to avoid inadvertent injury to the liver capsule. Mobilization of the right colon along the lateral avascular plane, as well as the root of the mesentery and an extensive Kocherization of the duodenum are carried out. This exposes the aorta to the level of the superior mesenteric artery and the inferior vena cava to the lower aspect of the liver.

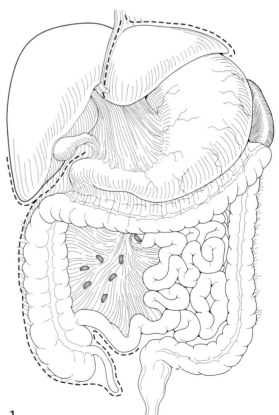

1

2 Attention is turned to hilar dissection. The bile duct is ligated at the superior border of the pancreas, and the duct is divided proximally. Through a small incision in the fundus, the gallbladder is flushed clear of bile with saline. The small venous structures in the hilum, as well as lymphatic and adventitial tissues, are ligated and divided to visualize the anterior surface of the hepatic artery and portal vein. A superficial position of the portal vein may indicate presence of a replaced right hepatic artery arising from the superior mesenteric artery; if identified posterior to the portal vein, the artery should be followed to its origin from the superior mesenteric. The hepatogastric ligament is opened and an exploration for a replaced left hepatic artery from the left gastric artery is made. The gastroduodenal artery at the inferior border of the first part of duodenum is identified and divided. After mobilizing the esophagus to the left, the diaphragmatic crura are sectioned longitudinally and an umbilical tape is passed around the aorta at the level of the hiatus. The anterior surface of the pancreas is exposed by dividing the gastrocolic omentum. The superior mesenteric artery and vein are exposed at the lower border of the pancreas by separating the third part of the duodenum from the mesocolon. The middle colic, right colic, and colonic branches of the ileocolic vessels are divided, unless the colon is also going to be procured for implantation.

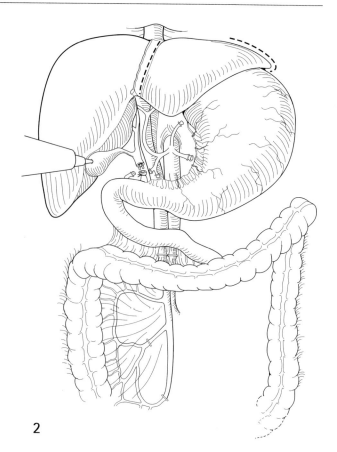

2

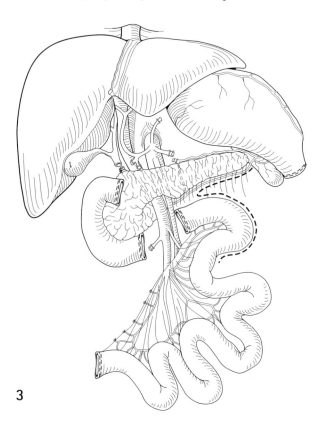

3

3 The small bowel is retracted to the right and the duodenojejunal flexure is fully mobilized. The duodenum just distal to the pylorus is stapled and divided. The stomach is mobilized cephalad and out of the operative field. The small bowel is stapled at the distal ileum. The remaining colonic vessels are divided and the colon is moved out of the field. The retracted colon is omitted and the ostium of the superior mesenteric artery is shown above the pancreas for clarity. The portal vein can be visualized deep to the hepatic artery and bile duct in the hilum of the liver. Note the divided middle colic vessels, gastroduodenal, right gastric, and left gastric artery.

COLD FLUSH

Intravenous heparin (300 IU/kg) is administered by the anesthesiology team. An appropriate-size cannula is placed in the abdominal aorta immediately above the bifurcation.

A second cannula is placed in the inferior mesenteric vein if the size permits. The heart team (for cardiac procurement) sections the inferior vena cava above the diaphragm to vent the blood and clamps the aorta. We simultaneously clamps the supraceliac aorta immediately below the diaphragm. Cold University of Wisconsin (UW) solution is administered via the aortic cannula and, if present, via

the second cannula. The amount of UW solution depends on the size of the donor, and is approximately 50 mL/kg. Cold slush is distributed in the abdominal cavity.

Combined liver–small bowel or multivisceral graft

4 Our technique for combined liver–small bowel or multivisceral grafting avoids any dissection in the porta hepatis. The liver, small bowel, and spleen with stomach and colon if required, are procured *en bloc*. A long segment of thoracic aorta is procured in continuity with the celiac trunk and the superior mesenteric artery. The distal aorta is divided a few millimeters below the superior mesenteric artery, leaving enough aortic length to be oversewn without compromising the flow into the superior mesenteric artery. Aortic (and inferior mesenteric venous) flush with cold UW solution is carried out as before, venting the blood by transecting the inferior vena cava above the diaphragm.

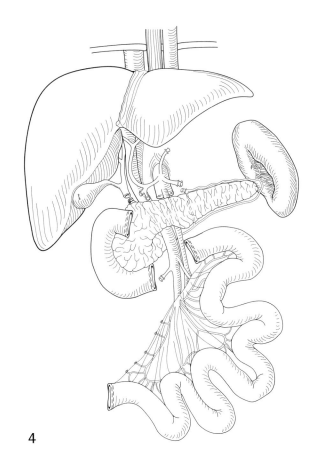

4

Cold dissection and removal of organs (isolated small bowel or combined liver–small bowel)

For small-sized donors or in the presence of technical difficulty, we favor removing the liver and intestine *en bloc* with back table separation of organs in the case of isolated small bowel grafts. Dissection starts with mobilization of the liver. The diaphragm is divided longitudinally anterior to the aorta; dissection continues around the inferior vena cava and then to the right, dividing the right triangular ligament. The dissection is carried through the right adrenal gland, locating the adrenal vein for back-table ligation. The infrahepatic inferior vena cava is divided above the level of the renal veins. The abdominal aorta is divided at the level of the diaphragm and below the origin of the superior mesenteric artery.

The remaining gastrocolic omentum is sectioned with the short gastric vessels. The stomach is retracted further to the left. The lienocolic and lienophrenic ligaments are divided. The spleen is then held as a handle, retracting medially, continuing to dissect medially posterior to the pancreas in a plane anterior to the left kidney and adrenal gland. The inferior mesenteric vein is divided but marked with a ligature to facilitate later identification of the splenic

vein. Transection of the retroaortic tissues completes the maneuver.

As stated earlier, for the combined liver–small bowel allograft, the supraceliac aorta is not isolated, as the whole thoracic aorta will be harvested in continuity with the abdominal segment bearing the celiac trunk and the superior mesenteric artery. There is no dissection in the porta hepatis, except to incise the gallbladder at the fundus and to flush it.

It is routine practice to procure the donor iliac vessels, and in special cases the carotid arteries and jugular veins, in the event that additional vessel length is required in the recipient.

Back-table preparation

If the liver–small bowel–pancreas cluster has been procured for different recipients, the separation of the liver from the pancreas–small bowel graft is carried out on the back table, orientating the viscera in the anatomical position and dividing the portal vein above the superior border of the pancreas. The splenic artery, if not divided earlier, is also divided during this separation. The organs are stored in cold UW solution.

Preparation of the isolated bowel graft

5 The superior mesenteric artery is dissected free from the periadventitial tissue, progressing from its aortic take-off distally. The pancreatic branches are ligated and divided, and dissection is continued until the first jejunal branch. The splenic vein is then dissected to its confluence with the portal vein and superior mesenteric vein; the branches to the head and body of the pancreas are ligated and divided. The pancreas is divided at the isthmus, taking due care to avoid injury to the subjacent portal vein. The pancreas and duodenum can now be safely excised, leaving the small bowel graft on its vascular pedicle based on the portal vein and the superior mesenteric artery. We imbricate the staple lines at either end of the bowel with 5/0 Prolene sutures, and due care is taken to mark the distal end of the bowel with a long tie to ensure accurate positioning in the recipient. It is also our practice to mark the anterior surface of the portal vein with a marking pen and a stay suture to ensure proper orientation at the time of anastomosis.

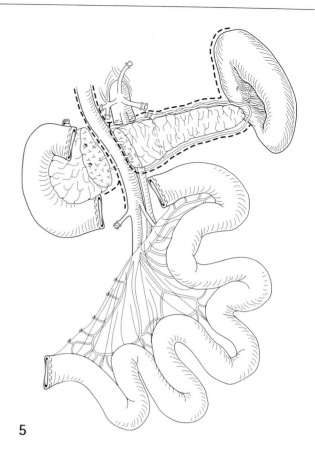

5

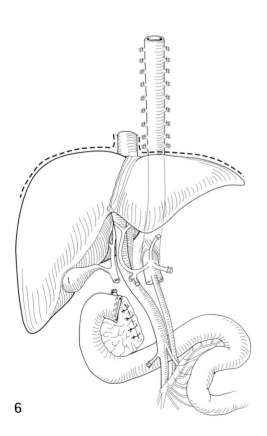

6

Preparation of the liver–small bowel or multivisceral graft

6 The preparation of the liver starts with removal of the diaphragmatic tissue and cleaning around the inferior vena cava. The next step consists of dissection of the thoracic and abdominal aorta with cleaning of the periadventitial tissues and individual ligation of the intercostal arteries. The distal aorta is closed using continuous 6/0 or 7/0 polypropylene sutures, just beyond the take-off of the superior mesenteric artery, taking due care to avoid narrowing the ostium. The celiac trunk is dissected with ligation of the left gastric arteries, except where the stomach is also going to be implanted in the multivisceral recipient; the hepatic artery is dissected to the level of the gastroduodenal artery, which is preserved to vascularize the head of the pancreas and duodenum. The splenic vein is dissected up to the confluence with the superior mesenteric vein. The pancreas is divided to the right of the portal vein. If the pancreatic duct can be identified on the cut surface, it is individually ligated with 5/0 polypropylene suture. In any event, the entire cut surface of the pancreas is oversewn with interrupted 5/0 polypropylene sutures. It must be noted that with forbidding portal hypertension or pancreatic disease, abdominal evisceration including removal of the native pancreas becomes technically simpler or necessary, and in this situation the donor pancreas is left intact with the liver–small bowel graft.

RECIPIENT OPERATION

Isolated small bowel transplant

7 The recipient operation must be timed in concert with the donor operation to keep cold ischemia to the minimum possible.

Abdominal incision can be vertical or horizontal, depending on prior operative scars. A configurable and versatile self-retaining retractor, such as the Thomson abdominal retractor, facilitates exposure. Extensive adhesiolysis is often required. Prior bowel anastomosis between the remnant small bowel and colon is taken down. Obviously non-functional or dilated remnant bowel is excised. The retroperitoneum is exposed, allowing full dissection of the infrarenal abdominal aorta and inferior vena cava up to their pelvic bifurcations. While venous drainage of the graft can be portal or systemic, in the presence of any degree of fibrotic liver disease, systemic venous drainage is preferred. The technical simplicity of the latter has led us to adopt systemic venous drainage of all isolated bowel grafts. Vascular clamps are placed in side-biting fashion when possible, but in the small recipient, these are invariably occlusive. The superior mesenteric artery of the graft is anastomosed initially to the infrarenal aorta of the recipient, followed by anastomosis between the superior mesenteric vein of the graft and the inferior vena cava. Due care must be taken to ensure that the venous anastomosis is cephalad to the arterial anastomosis, and that proper orientation is maintained. On occasion, if graft vessels are unduly short, or if lack of recipient abdominal domain precludes a safe vascular anastomosis, the author has used interposition grafts for both arterial and venous anastomoses as required, as shown in the inset to the figure. Reperfusion starts with release of the venous clamps. Bleeding points in the cut edge of the mesentery are controlled, followed by release of the arterial clamps. Once hemostasis is secured, attention is turned to restoring intestinal continuity. We carry out side–side (functional end–end) anastomosis between the proximal end of the graft and the remnant native proximal jejunum or duodenum. Similarly, distal anastomosis is carried out between the graft ileum and the distal native bowel, whether ileum or colon. We perform anastomoses with a standard two-layered technique due to the theoretically higher risks of poor healing in an immunosuppressed patient. All patients receive a defunctioning distal ileostomy (loop or Bishop–Koop) to allow protocol ileoscopic biopsies for close monitoring of graft histology. It is our practice to leave the skin wound open with dressings to allow healing by secondary intention, in view of the high risk of wound infection.

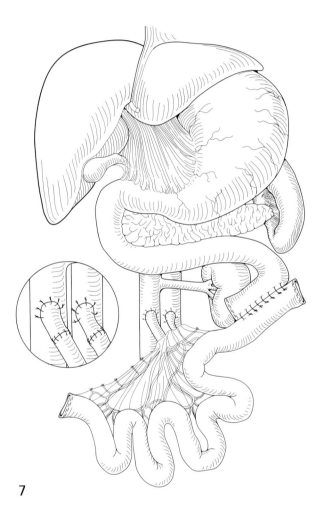

7

Liver–small bowel transplant

8a,b The liver–small bowel transplant recipient tends to be much sicker, and to require even closer intraoperative and perioperative monitoring, than the recipient of an isolated liver transplant. Close anesthesiological monitoring of coagulation, metabolic disturbances (particularly hyperkalemia), and significant blood loss in the face of extensive adhesions and profound portal hypertension require constant vigilance. We employ horizontal or vertical incisions depending on prior operative scars, but on occasion have had to convert to cruciate extensions. Hepatectomy is performed in the usual manner, leaving the native inferior vena cava clamped above and below the liver. The portal vein is ligated, as is the hepatic artery. At this point, the extent of native bowel is also determined, and prior anastomoses are taken down, excising any dysfunctional or dilated bowel. The supraceliac aorta is dissected free and controlled with a sling. The author performs a portocaval shunt between the end of the native portal vein and the infrahepatic inferior vena cava, as shown in the inset; this allows for decompression of all remnant native foregut viscera, such as the stomach, duodenum, and pancreas. Where prior abdominal exenteration removes native foregut in the abdomen, including a near-total gastrectomy prior to a multivisceral transplant, the need for a portocaval shunt is obviated. The inferior vena cava is then reclamped above the shunt.

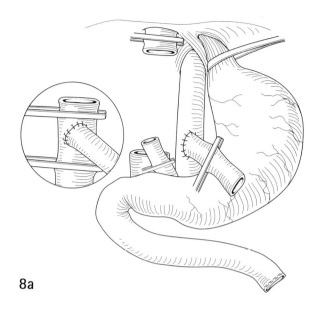

8a

The supraceliac abdominal aorta is then clamped. A segment of donor thoracic aorta is excised and anastomosed in end–side fashion, to be used as an interposition graft, without the composite liver–bowel graft in the way. Aortic flow can be restored immediately after completion of this anastomosis, placing a clamp on the interposition graft. The entire composite graft is then brought into the field.

The anastomoses of the suprahepatic and infrahepatic inferior vena cava are then performed. The donor thoracic aorta (in turn supplying both graft liver and bowel) is then anastomosed to the aortic interposition graft. The use of an interposition graft in this manner allows convenient aortic anastomosis in the depths of the wound, without having the composite allograft in the way, and allowing final arterial anastomosis to the liver–bowel graft at the level of the wound. Reperfusion is carried out by releasing the venous clamps first, followed by the arterial clamps. Bleeding from the mesenteric edge and from the retroperitoneum is controlled, before proceeding with the proximal and distal intestinal anastomoses.

A loop ileostomy or a Bishop–Koop stoma is brought out in all cases, to allow surveillance endoscopic biopsies of the graft. Following fascial closure with a monofilament non-absorbable suture, the skin wound is left open to heal by secondary intention, in view of the high risk of wound infection. (The native stomach, duodenum, and pancreas are omitted from illustration b in the interests of clarity, but the site of the proximal intestinal anastomosis to native proximal bowel remnant is shown.)

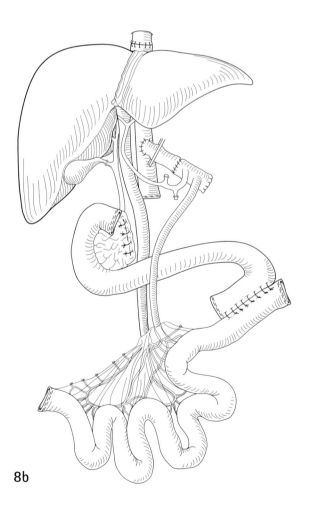

8b

POSTOPERATIVE CARE

Nasogastric decompression is maintained for 5–7 days after transplant, introducing clear liquids, often via a nasojejunal tube, with return of peristaltic activity. Changes in color and appearance of the stoma or its output are a cause for concern and reflect graft vascularity early after transplant. Prophylactic antibiotics are maintained for at least 1 week after transplant. Various prophylactic agents against fungi, viruses such as cytomegalovirus, and opportunist infectious agents such as *Pneumocystis carinii* are routinely prescribed for periods of three months to one year after transplant.

Most centers use an induction regimen with antibody followed by maintenance immunosuppression with tacrolimus and steroids in the long term. Close monitoring of tacrolimus levels is essential for the first few months after transplant to maintain optimal levels.

With satisfactory stomal activity, fat-free enteral formulas are gradually introduced at 1 week after transplant and advanced gradually based on tolerance and stoma outputs. Transition to complete elemental formulas is delayed until 4–6 weeks postoperatively to allow time for lymphatic reconstitution after transplant. Oral aversion is a common obstacle for transitioning to standard diets in the longer term. The ability to remove the central line after demonstrating full enteral tolerance is a major milestone in these patients. Some patients continue to require supplemental intravenous fluids until stoma takedown between six months to one year after transplant.

In the absence of any biochemical markers for rejection, we resort to protocol ileoscopies and biopsies of the allograft to diagnose rejection. Histology remains the gold standard for diagnosis. Rejection may be marked by increased ostomy losses and if diagnosed early, may be reversed by steroid boluses, although on occasion it may require antibody treatment or even graft removal.

COMPLICATIONS AND OUTCOMES

Despite the magnitude of the procedures described above, the postoperative management remains the most challenging aspect of the care of these patients. The high incidence of acute rejection in a lymphoid-rich graft requires very high levels of immunosuppression. This in turn leads to a high incidence of bacterial, viral, and fungal sepsis that requires close monitoring and aggressive early treatment. Bacterial infections, occurring in more than 90 percent of patients, are often due to enteric Gram-negative organisms, which may have to be treated while maintaining significant immunosuppression. In the longer term, complications related to immunosuppression, such as post-transplant lymphoproliferative disease related to Epstein–Barr virus, and chronic rejection continue to pose serious challenges to patient and graft survival. Despite these challenges, the results of intestinal transplantation continue to improve, allowing patient survival at one year of the order of 90 percent and graft survival of 70–75 percent. With improving outcomes, survival even at five years is now greater than 50 percent. When one recognizes that these outcomes are achieved in patients who have 'failed' parenteral nutrition, it is hoped that earlier patient referral before the onset of advanced liver disease and better patient selection may allow continued refinement and even better outcomes.

RECENT DEVELOPMENTS

Our center, along with a few others, has started including the colon as part of the allograft in patients who come to transplant without a colonic remnant. Without an appreciable increase in complication rate, initial impressions suggest a favorable impact on fluid/electrolyte management and preservation of renal function.

Loss of domain in the patient with short bowel with a complex surgical history, remains a major technical challenge. Autologous tissue reconstruction, while desirable, is often not possible and synthetic mesh repairs are accompanied by unacceptable infection rates. Experience with composite abdominal wall transplants remains limited, but there is growing and favorable experience with use of avascular donor abdominal fascia; the key to success with use of fascia appears to be meticulous removal of all fat and muscle and prevention of desiccation of the fascia during the back-table preparation.

Recent success with the use of intravenous fish oil emulsions and other lipid-sparing strategies, and indeed improved understanding of parenteral nutrition-associated liver disease has brought in its wake new challenges for intestinal transplantation. Reversal of biochemical cholestasis in the patient with extreme short bowel who may still have advanced histological liver injury, creates a therapeutic dilemma, in terms of choice of organs for the patient being considered for intestinal transplantation. Current allocation systems do not offer any prioritization for histological liver disease, forcing an often difficult choice between a prolonged wait for a combined liver–bowel graft or an isolated intestinal transplant with unknown but presumably higher risks of liver decompensation.

Among the most exciting developments is the use of the technical principles outlined in this chapter for the management of complex soft tissue tumors at the root of the mesentery. Better understanding of the technical aspects of intestinal allograft procurement, ischemia–reperfusion and transplantation, allows careful planning of *ex-vivo* tumor resections with intestinal autotransplantation, rendering hitherto 'non-resectable' tumors, radically resectable.

FURTHER READING

DeRoover A, Langnas AN. Surgical methods of small bowel transplantation. *Current Opinion in Organ Transplantation* 1999; **4**: 335–42.

Fishbein T. Intestinal transplantation. *New England Journal of Medicine* 2009; **361**: 998–1008.

Grant D, Abu-Elmagd K, Reyes J *et al.* 2003 Report of the Intestine Transplant Registry: a new era has dawned. *Annals of Surgery* 2005; **241**: 607–13.

Langnas AN, Iyer KR. Liver–small bowel transplantation. In: Maddrey C, Schiff ER, Sorrell MF (eds). *Transplantation of the Liver*. Philadelphia, PA: Lippincott, Williams and Wilkins, 2001: 111–19.

Sindhi R, Fox IJ, Heffron T *et al.* Procurement and preparation of human isolated small intestinal grafts for transplantation. *Transplantation* 1995; **60**: 771–3.

Starzl TE, Todo S, Tzakis A *et al.* The many faces of multi-visceral transplantation. *Surgery, Gynecology and Obstetrics* 1991; **172**: 335–44.

Sudan DL. Treatment of intestinal failure: intestinal transplantation. *Nature Clinical Practice. Gastroenterology and Hepatology* 2007; **4**: 503–10.

Sudan DL, Iyer KR, DeRoover A *et al.* A new technique for combined liver–intestinal transplantation. *Transplantation* 2001; **72**: 1846–8.

Todo S, Tzakis AG, Abu-Elmagd K *et al.* Intestinal transplantation in composite visceral grafts or alone. *Annals of Surgery* 1992; **216**: 223–34.

109

Interventional radiology

DEREK J ROEBUCK

BACKGROUND

Interventional radiology (IR) is a rapidly growing field in pediatrics. Most pediatric IR has been adapted from adult practice in an attempt to improve on existing surgical techniques, and radiologists now perform many procedures that were previously exclusively in the domain of pediatric surgery. Continued cooperation between surgeons and radiologists will lead to further improvements.

Most of the following procedures are based on very simple concepts. In one, a structure is first accessed by percutaneous puncture with ultrasound and/or fluoroscopic guidance. A guidewire is inserted, the needle is removed, and a catheter is introduced into the structure over the guidewire (the 'modified Seldinger' technique). This concept is the basis of angiography, abscess drainage, biliary drainage, nephrostomy, cecostomy, and one method of gastrostomy. Another concept is dilation, which is performed by crossing a stenosis with a guidewire followed by a balloon catheter, and inflating the balloon using fluoroscopic guidance. This is the basis of angioplasty (of arteries and veins) and dilation of tracheobronchial, ureteral, and esophageal and other gastrointestinal strictures.

PREOPERATIVE CARE

In general, the perioperative care required for IR is the same as for the corresponding operation in pediatric surgery (see Chapter 1). There are exceptions, however. We do not crossmatch blood for a child of any size for routine central venous access procedures unless there is an uncorrectable coagulopathy. This is because ultrasound-guided central venous access (see Chapter 4) is almost always easy, and bleeding is extremely rare. On the other hand, percutaneous techniques offer less opportunity for intraoperative recognition and treatment of bleeding complications than the corresponding open, endoscopic, or laparoscopic procedure. We therefore check coagulation values and platelet levels before most procedures in the lungs, pleural space, and abdomen, where postoperative bleeding is more likely to be a significant problem.

SEDATION AND ANESTHESIA

Although a wide range of anesthetic practice still exists in pediatric IR, there is a gradual move away from radiologist-managed intravenous sedation towards general anesthesia (GA), which is less unpleasant for the child and may make the procedure safer. GA is of course essential for procedures that are very painful and/or very long.

When GA is not used, topical anesthetic cream is applied before the procedure to the area where local anesthetic will be injected. If the procedure is performed under GA, a longer-acting local anesthetic is used to optimize postoperative pain relief.

For brief but painful procedures, for example renal biopsy or abdominal abscess drainage, older children can breathe an equimolar mixture of oxygen and nitrous oxide (Entonox). This is very effective when used in combination with topical and local anesthetic.

BIOPSY AND DRAINAGE PROCEDURES

1 Image guidance makes percutaneous biopsy and drainage safer and quicker, and blind needle biopsy is now appropriate only for the occasional superficial lesion. Percutaneous biopsies in children are usually performed with semi-automatic core needles. The cutting tip is advanced to expose a slot in which tissue is trapped by an outer sleeve, which advances when the needle is fired. These devices are much easier to use than manual biopsy needles (e.g. Trucut) and biopsy gun systems.

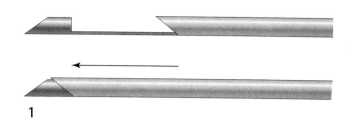

1

Renal biopsy

INDICATIONS

The most common indications for renal biopsy are nephrotic syndrome and impaired function following renal transplantation.

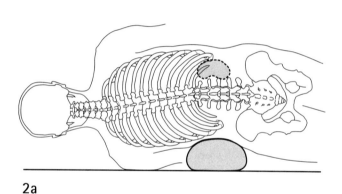

2a

POSITIONING AND ANESTHESIA

2a Renal biopsy is performed under GA in young or uncooperative children, and with sedation or Entonox in older children. Either kidney can be biopsied. The procedure can be performed with the patient prone or seated, but we find it easier to place the patient in a lateral position. This makes it much easier to administer Entonox, and, when GA is used, avoids the need for endotracheal intubation and muscle relaxants. A large pad is placed under the patient's abdomen to increase the convexity of the side to be biopsied. Renal transplant biopsy is performed in the supine position, and does not usually require GA or sedation because it is much less painful than biopsy of a native kidney.

TECHNIQUE

2b The tract is infiltrated with local anesthetic down to the level of the renal capsule. A 16-gauge semi-automatic core biopsy needle is then inserted through a short stab incision. If the child is able to cooperate, he or she is asked to stop breathing as the needle is advanced under real-time ultrasound guidance into the kidney, and the biopsy taken. A shallow or deep trajectory may be appropriate, depending on the size of the kidney and the relationship of its lower pole to the ribs. When the child is under GA, suspension of breathing is not absolutely necessary, and the anesthetist may prefer to allow the patient to breathe spontaneously. A pathology technician is present to examine the core and confirm that sufficient glomeruli are present. If not, another core is taken. Using this method, a definitive histopathology report should be possible for 99 percent of biopsies.

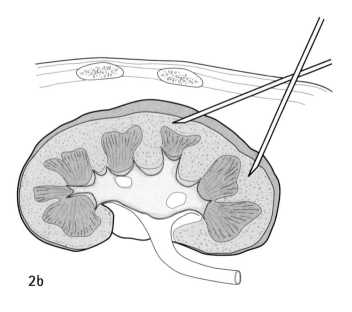

2b

COMPLICATIONS

Significant complications, such as hematuria requiring transfusion, or injury to other organs, should occur in less than 2 percent of biopsies. The most important complication is arteriovenous fistula. These lesions tend to resolve spontaneously, but require embolization (see below) if they are symptomatic.

TECHNIQUE

3a–d A coaxial technique is used for almost all liver biopsies. For generalized liver disease, we use a 17-gauge outer needle, which accepts an 18-gauge biopsy needle. A subcostal approach is almost always possible, and this avoids the risks of pneumothorax and hemothorax associated with the traditional intercostal approach. The outer needle is advanced into the liver under ultrasound guidance, taking care to avoid the gallbladder and major vessels. Its trocar is then removed and replaced with the semi-automated core biopsy needle. After obtaining three or four cores of tissue, the tract is occluded, usually with gelatin foam plugs, in order to prevent intraperitoneal bleeding.

Liver biopsy

INDICATIONS

Percutaneous liver biopsy can be used to evaluate generalized liver disease, large liver masses or small focal lesions. In all these cases, we prefer to use ultrasound guidance.

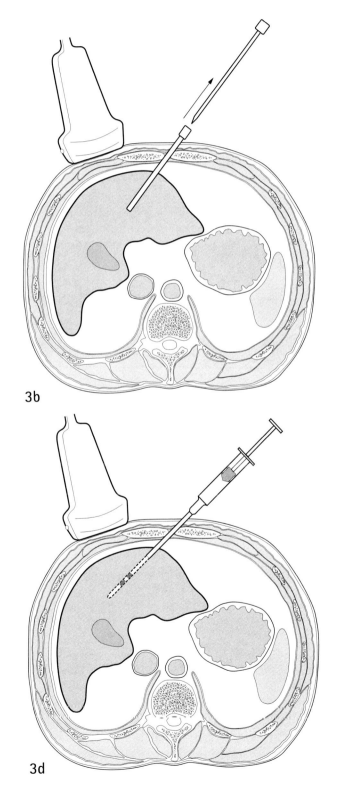

3b

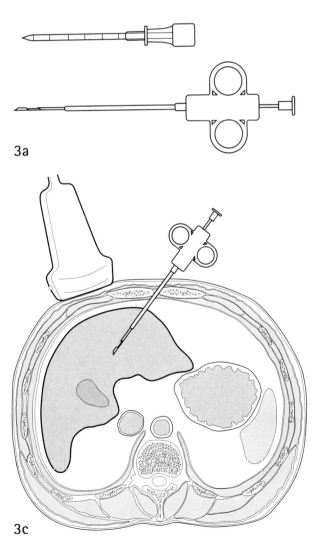

3a

3c

3d

COMPLICATIONS

The most important potential complication of liver biopsy is bleeding, which is occasionally life-threatening. Frequent meticulous postoperative observations are essential, and should be continued for at least 8 hours. Hemorrhage requiring treatment (by blood transfusion, transarterial embolization, or emergency surgery) is rare in children with normal coagulation parameters. It is more common in children with coagulopathy or thrombocytopenia, and those who have undergone bone marrow transplantation. Transjugular biopsy has been recommended in these patients to try to reduce the risk of post-biopsy bleeding, although it has not been proven to be safer than percutaneous biopsy.

Tumor biopsy

INDICATIONS

The histologic diagnosis of most tumors outside the central nervous system is made by ultrasound-guided needle biopsy. Our experience is that needle biopsy is probably safer than, and equally accurate to, open surgical biopsy. The period of convalescence is shorter, and this may allow earlier commencement of chemotherapy. Laparoscopic biopsy is a useful alternative for certain thoracic and abdominal tumors. Open biopsy is performed when it is considered to be safer, or when other techniques have failed.

TECHNIQUE

Ultrasound guidance is best for almost all abdominal and soft tissue biopsies in children. We use computed tomography (CT) mainly for very small retroperitoneal lesions, especially in older children, and lung lesions that do not reach the visceral pleura. Recent advances in pediatric pathology, including immunohistochemical and molecular techniques, have improved the accuracy of needle biopsy. In most patients, ultrasound-guided tumor biopsy can be performed at the same GA as insertion of a central venous access device and, where appropriate, bone marrow aspirates and trephines. The coaxial technique (see above under Liver biopsy) is particularly useful for tumor biopsy, because numerous cores of tissue can be obtained from different parts of the mass, using a single puncture of the tumor capsule. Plugging the tumor biopsy tract may prevent seeding of tumor cells.

COMPLICATIONS

Complications are very rare. Inadequate biopsies can be avoided by careful preoperative imaging, and it is usually worth delaying the biopsy for a day or two to obtain all relevant imaging before the procedure.

Aspiration and drainage of collections

4 Most fluid collections can be drained by IR techniques. In the upper abdomen, most collections are approached through the anterior abdominal wall. Certain lesions, such as urinomas or pancreatic collections, are drained retroperitoneally. Pelvic collections can be approached through the anterior abdominal wall or the rectum using ultrasound guidance, or from the buttock using CT.

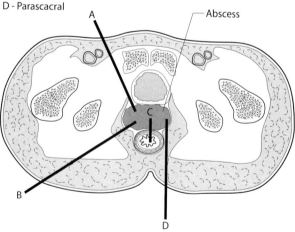

A - Transabdominal
B - Transgluteal
C - Transrectal
D - Parasacral

Abscess

4

TECHNIQUE

5, 6 The usual technique is based on ultrasound-guided puncture of the fluid collection. Guidewire insertion and positioning of the drainage catheter can be monitored with ultrasound or fluoroscopy if necessary. The first step is to select a safe path to the collection by careful ultrasound examination. After injection of local anesthetic, a short stab incision is made in a skin crease, and the collection is punctured using real-time ultrasound guidance. The author uses a trocar needle (usually 18-gauge) for this purpose, because the trocar can be withdrawn slightly into the blunt outer needle, which can then be advanced atraumatically past bowel loops if necessary. When the tip of the needle is in the collection, the trocar is removed and fluid aspirated and saved for culture. A guidewire of appropriate diameter is inserted (see **Table 109.1**). The best guidewire has a stiff shaft, with a floppy segment about 30–60 mm long at its tip. The tip coils in the collection first, and then increased resistance is felt, indicating that the stiff part of the guidewire is in the collection. The needle can then be removed and the tract dilated over the guidewire.

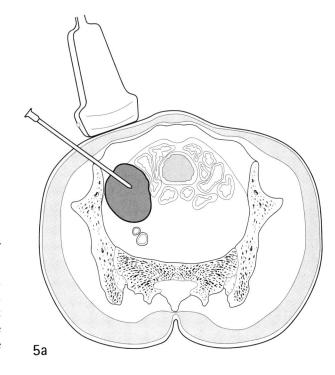

5a

Table 109.1 Guidewires and their diameters.

Needle gauge	Guidewire diameter
21	0.018 inch (0.46 mm)
20	0.025 inch (0.64 mm)
19	0.035 inch (0.89 mm)
18	0.038 inch (0.97 mm)

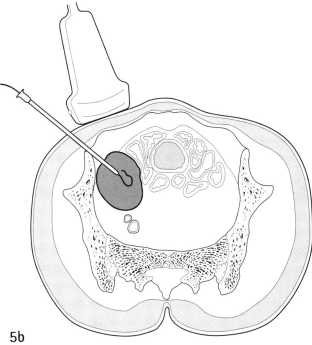

5b

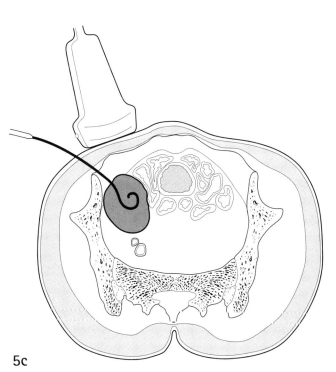

5c

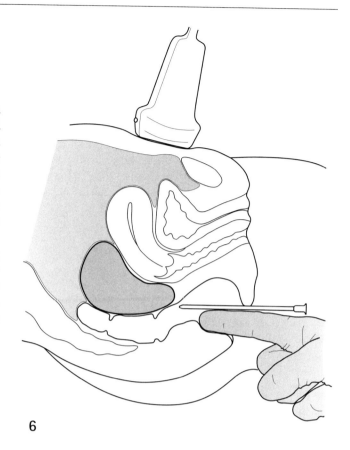

The author often uses a dilator 0.5–1 Fr larger than the intended drainage catheter at this stage. The pigtail catheter (with its internal stiffening cannula) is then advanced over the guidewire and into the collection. The guidewire and stiffener are withdrawn and the pigtail is formed (there are different methods for this, according to the design of the catheter). Fluid is aspirated to confirm adequate position, and a drainage bag is connected. The catheter can be sutured to the skin.

For transrectal drainage, the needle can be laid along the operator's index finger, with the inner trocar partly withdrawn. When the finger is inserted into the patient's rectum, it is easily seen with transabdominal ultrasound, enabling puncture of a pelvic collection with real-time guidance.

6

GASTROINTESTINAL INTERVENTION

Esophageal dilation

Fluoroscopically guided balloon dilation of esophageal strictures is simple and safe, and has almost replaced bougienage. Endoscopy can be regarded as an additional procedure, with certain advantages over a purely fluoroscopic technique, including the ability to inspect and biopsy the esophagus and to evaluate the stomach and proximal small intestine.

INDICATIONS

The common causes of esophageal stenosis in children include congenital and surgical strictures, ingestion of corrosive substances, gastroesophageal reflux, achalasia, and dystrophic epidermolysis bullosa. The natural history, response to treatment, and probability of complications all depend strongly on the underlying cause of the stricture. Repeated dilation is often necessary, especially in children with corrosive injury and epidermolysis bullosa. Resection of esophageal strictures (except for congenital stenosis) is now rarely necessary.

ANESTHESIA

Although it is possible to dilate the esophagus in a sedated child, we prefer to use GA, because it is less distressing for the child and minimizes the risk of a severe vagal reaction. Endotracheal intubation avoids the severe airway compression that may otherwise occur during balloon dilation of strictures in small children.

TECHNIQUE

7 Most strictures can be treated with balloon dilation using an antegrade (transoral) approach. A catheter with a gently curved tip is inserted into the upper esophagus using fluoroscopic guidance, and a contrast study is performed. The stricture is then crossed with a guidewire, which is advanced to the stomach. The catheter is removed, and replaced with an angioplasty catheter with a balloon of appropriate diameter. The angioplasty catheter is advanced over the guidewire until the radio-opaque markers indicate the position of the balloon straddling the stricture. The balloon is then inflated with dilute radiographic contrast. Fluoroscopy is essential at this stage to confirm that the stricture has been successfully dilated, as shown by abolition of the waist on the balloon. The balloon is then deflated, and the catheter and guidewire removed. Occasionally, it is impossible to cross the stricture from above. When this occurs in children who have a gastrostomy, a retrograde (transgastric) approach is almost always successful. In children whose strictures recur relentlessly after dilation, mitomycin application and/or temporary stenting can be tried.

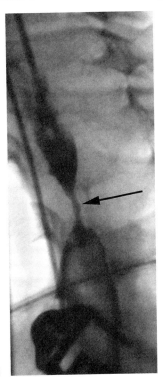

7a

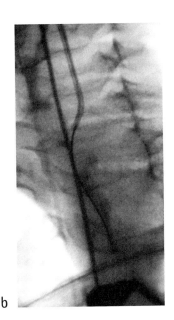

7b

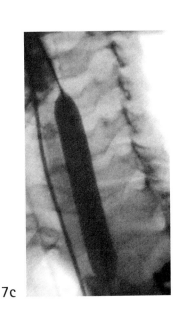

7c

COMPLICATIONS

Complications occur most often during dilation of corrosive strictures, followed by those associated with gastro-esophageal reflux. Three types of esophageal injury occur. Guidewire perforation of the esophagus can be recognized at fluoroscopy and treated conservatively. Submucosal tears of the esophagus are seen as contained extravasation of contrast alongside the inflated balloon. These also seem to do well with conservative treatment. Full-thickness perforation of the esophagus is uncommon. Conservative management, including analgesia, nasojejunal or parenteral feeding, and broad-spectrum antibiotic therapy, is usually successful, but surgical repair is sometimes necessary.

Other gastrointestinal dilation

Balloon dilation may also be used to treat strictures elsewhere in the gastrointestinal tract, including the pylorus, duodenum, colon, and rectum.

Gastrostomy

Radiologic gastrostomy can be performed either by an antegrade technique, in which the gastrostomy tube is pulled down the esophagus into the stomach, or a retrograde technique, in which it is pushed into the stomach through the anterior abdominal wall. The antegrade technique is essentially the same as percutaneous endoscopic gastrostomy, except with fluoroscopic guidance. The retrograde technique may be useful in children with a narrow or diseased esophagus. The perioperative care is the same as for endoscopic gastrostomy.

TECHNIQUE

The antegrade and retrograde techniques are similar. We usually give the child a small amount (2–3 mL/kg) of barium sulfate suspension orally or by nasogastric tube the evening before the procedure, to opacify the colon. Ultrasound is used to mark the position of the left lobe of the liver. A puncture site is selected, where possible lateral to rectus abdominis, about 2 cm from the left costal margin. Occasionally, anatomic considerations (e.g. scoliosis) require the use of a different puncture site. Local anesthetic is infiltrated and a short transverse incision is made in the skin. For antegrade gastrostomy, a snare is passed into the stomach through the mouth. The stomach is then inflated with air. This can be done via the snare catheter or a separate nasogastric tube. In children with esophageal atresia, the stomach can be inflated after percutaneous ultrasound-guided puncture with a fine needle. When the stomach is inflated, an 18-gauge trocar needle is inserted through the incision and used to puncture the stomach. This must be done quickly, before the air escapes from the stomach into the small bowel. The author finds biplane fluoroscopy useful at this point, but it is not essential. Some operators use intravenous glucagon (40 μg/kg, maximum 1 mg) to delay gastric emptying. The snare in the stomach is opened, and a 0.035-inch guidewire is advanced through the needle and grasped with the snare. The wire is then carefully pulled out of the mouth, and the tract dilated to permit the retrograde passage of the snare catheter through the abdominal wall to the mouth. The snare catheter is then used to pull the lubricated gastrostomy tube down the esophagus, and out through the anterior abdominal wall. The procedure is otherwise the same as for endoscopic gastrostomy (Chapter 14).

For retrograde gastrostomy, the stomach is punctured in the same manner as for the antegrade technique, but a needle preloaded with a suture anchor device may be used instead of the trocar needle. These temporary retention devices are used to hold the stomach against the anterior abdominal wall as the tract is dilated. A locking pigtail catheter or balloon device can then be inserted. Although these are more easily dislodged than flanged gastrostomy catheters, they are easier to remove or exchange when the tract is mature. If necessary, a transgastric jejunal feeding catheter may be inserted at the time of creation of the gastrostomy.

COMPLICATIONS

Complications are similar in incidence and nature to those from endoscopic gastrostomy.

Transgastric jejunal intubation

8 This requires the passage of a transpyloric tube through a pre-existing gastrostomy, to a position distal to the duodenojejunal flexure, using fluoroscopic guidance. A stiff dilator (9–15 Fr) is used to engage the pylorus, and a floppy-tipped hydrophilic guidewire is advanced into the duodenum. The dilator is removed, and a long catheter is inserted over the guidewire, and manipulated across the duodenojejunal flexure. The floppy-tipped wire may then be exchanged for a stiff wire, if necessary, and the catheter removed. The transgastric jejunal tube is then lubricated (internally and externally) and inserted over the stiff wire. Injection of contrast through the catheter will confirm its position. Coaxial systems, in which a transpyloric tube can be advanced through a gastrostomy catheter, are also available.

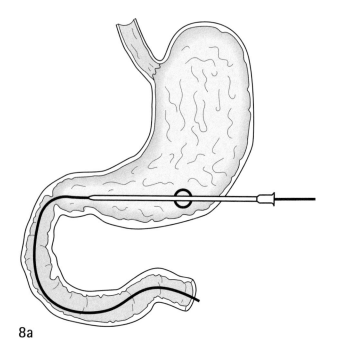

8a

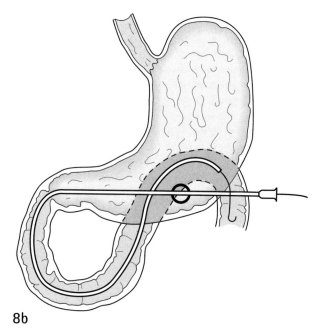

8b

UROLOGIC INTERVENTION

Most urologic interventions are based on nephrostomy. In children, this is usually straightforward when performed with ultrasound guidance, except when the pelvicalyceal system is not dilated. The nephrostomy tract can also be used for other interventions, such as percutaneous stone removal or antegrade ureteral dilation and stenting.

Percutaneous nephrostomy

INDICATIONS

The most common indications for nephrostomy in children are congenital and postoperative obstruction. Intravenous antibiotic prophylaxis is administered to reduce the risk of septicemia.

POSITIONING AND ANESTHESIA

9 Unilateral nephrostomy is best performed with the patient in a semi-prone position, with the affected side tilted up about 20–30°. This facilitates puncture of a posterior lower pole calyx through the relatively avascular zone of Brödel. We prefer to perform bilateral nephrostomy under GA with endotracheal intubation, with the patient prone. This requires angling the needle at about 20–30° to the table top to achieve the same trajectory. In addition, the tip of the needle is angled cranially, to make it easier to see at ultrasound. This technique also facilitates puncture of an interpolar or upper pole calyx, which is sometimes required for ureteral interventions or stone removal.

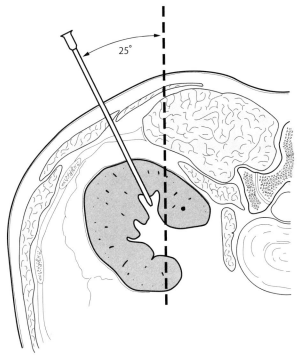

9

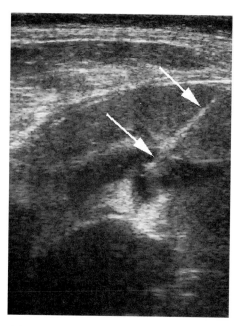

10a

TECHNIQUE

10a–c The exit site and proposed needle tract should be injected with local anesthetic. Using real-time ultrasound guidance, a dilated calyx can almost always be punctured with a single needle pass. Various types of needle are available for this purpose. Trocar or sheathed needles have the advantage that when the trocar is removed, the outer part of the needle (or sheath) has a blunt tip, which is unlikely to damage the collecting system. Needles with echogenic tips are easier to see at ultrasound, but are rarely necessary in children. Once the calyx has been punctured, urine is aspirated for culture, and a smaller volume of dilute contrast (to avoid over-distension of the pelvicalyceal system) is then injected to perform antegrade pyelography.

In general, 6-Fr locking pigtail catheters are appropriate for neonates. In older children, and those with suspected pyonephrosis, larger catheters should be used (typically 8.5 Fr). The use of a stiff wire with a floppy tip is recommended. The largest diameter guidewire that can pass through the stiffener of the pigtail catheter is selected, and the smallest needle that accepts the guidewire is used for the puncture. Once the tip of the guidewire is coiled in the renal pelvis, the tract can be over-dilated by 0.5–1 Fr before inserting the pigtail catheter and stiffener. The author usually sutures the catheter to the skin. Coaxial access sets, which allow puncture with a 21- or 22-gauge needle, are more difficult to use, but may be helpful when the pelvicalyceal system is not dilated. With these systems, a 0.018-inch guidewire is inserted through the thin needle, and is then exchanged for a 0.035-inch wire after insertion of a two-part coaxial dilator.

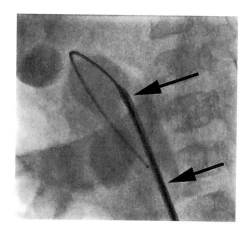

10b

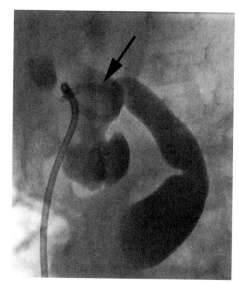

10c

COMPLICATIONS

The most important complication is injury to an intrarenal branch of the renal artery. This may require embolization (see below). Injury to the colon and hemothorax or pneumothorax are unusual.

Ureteral dilation and antegrade stenting

Ureteral dilation is most often required in children who have transplant ureteral strictures. Antegrade access is performed as for nephrostomy, but preferably using a mid-pole (or if possible an upper pole) calyx. The renal pelvis and ureter are opacified with dilute contrast. A peel-away sheath is inserted and the stricture is crossed with a hydrophilic guidewire and a catheter of appropriate shape. With the tip of the guidewire in the bladder, a balloon dilation catheter is positioned across the stricture and inflated with fluoroscopic guidance. A small diameter balloon (3–5 mm, depending on the size of the child) is usually adequate. A cutting balloon may be used if there is a persistent waist.

A double-J stent can be placed in the ureter by pushing it over a guidewire with a pusher catheter. A protective nephrostomy tube is probably not necessary unless there is significant bleeding. Occasionally, transurethral removal of a double-J is difficult, for example when the lower end of the stent migrates up into the ureter. The stent can then be snared and removed percutaneously, after puncture of the pelvicalyceal system.

BILIARY INTERVENTION

Diagnostic percutaneous transhepatic cholangiography (PTC) is obsolescent. One potential indication is sclerosing cholangitis (for example, children with Langerhans' cell histiocytosis), when PTC can be performed at the same time as liver biopsy. When the intrahepatic bile ducts are not dilated, the simplest method is to puncture the gall bladder under ultrasound guidance. PTC, with or without biliary drainage or balloon dilation of biliary strictures, may be required following liver transplantation. Malignant obstructive jaundice is unusual in children; biliary drainage is required in some patients. In these circumstances, ultrasound-guided puncture of a dilated intrahepatic duct allows insertion of an external or internal–external drainage catheter.

VASCULAR INTERVENTION

11a,b Diagnostic arteriography and venography are required much less frequently now than in the past, but interventional angiography is increasing in importance. Arterial embolization is an effective method of controlling iatrogenic or other traumatic hemorrhage. An example is symptomatic arteriovenous or arteriocalyceal fistula following renal biopsy. These lesions may be embolized with metal coils, which are easy to use and very effective. The aim is to preserve as much renal tissue as possible.

Arterial embolization may also be used for the treatment of arteriovenous malformations and tumors. The management of vascular malformations (**Chapter 104**) and arterial interventions, such as angioplasty and stenting, are beyond the scope of this chapter.

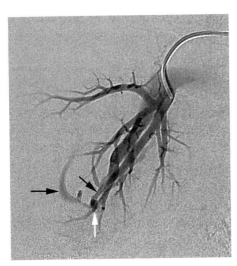

11a

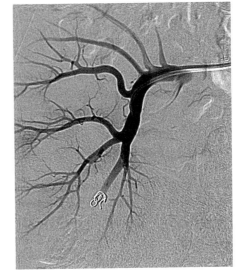

11b

TRACHEOBRONCHIAL INTERVENTION

These techniques are based on bronchography. Balloon dilation of acquired tracheobronchial stenoses is easy and often effective. The procedure is analogous to esophageal dilation. The airway can be accessed through an endotracheal or tracheostomy tube, or a laryngeal mask airway. The measurement facilities on modern angiographic equipment are helpful here, because accurate assessment of the diameter and length of the balloon to be used is very important. Fluoroscopic guidance is useful because it allows accurate positioning of the balloon, as well as confirmation that complete inflation has been achieved. A description of stenting and other pediatric airway intervention is beyond the scope of this chapter.

FURTHER READING

Barnacle AM, Wilkinson AG, Roebuck DJ. Paediatric interventional uroradiology. *Cardiovascular and Interventional Radiology* 2011; **34**: 227–40.

Hogan MJ, Hoffer FA. Biopsy and drainage techniques in children. *Techniques in Vascular and Interventional Radiology* 2010; **13**: 206–13.

Lord DJ. The practice of pediatric interventional radiology. *Techniques in Vascular and Interventional Radiology* 2011; **14**: 2–7.

Marshalleck F. Pediatric arterial interventions. *Techniques in Vascular and Interventional Radiology* 2010; **13**: 238–43.

Roebuck DJ, Hogan MJ, Connolly B, McLaren CA. Interventions in the chest in children. *Techniques in Vascular and Interventional Radiology* 2011; **14**: 8–15.

Roebuck DJ, McLaren CA. Gastrointestinal intervention in children. *Pediatric Radiology* 2011; **41**: 27–41.

110

Exposure for spinal surgery

STEVEN W BRUCH and JAMES D GEIGER

PRINCIPLES AND JUSTIFICATION

Safe exposure of the anterior aspect of the spine allows the orthopedic surgeon to resect, manipulate, and instrument the spine to treat various abnormalities. The role of the pediatric surgeon is to move important structures out of the way to provide adequate and safe exposure for the orthopedic surgeons.

INDICATIONS

The orthopedic indications for procedures requiring anterior spinal exposure are many ranging from deformities (scoliosis and kyphosis), to mass resections, to traumatic injuries. The pediatric surgeons rely on their orthopedic colleagues to ensure that the surgical indications are sound, but should review the imaging studies and have a clear plan with the orthopedic surgeon on the degree of exposure needed.

PREOPERATIVE

The preoperative evaluation should concentrate on co-morbid diseases, neurological examination, and the peripheral vascular examination. These procedures often involve manipulation of the spine, aorta, inferior vena cava, or their major branches, so a baseline vascular and neurological examination is key. It is especially important to obtain preoperative renal function studies since correction of the spinal deformity changes the contour of the aorta and its relationship with the renal artery, which can effect renal blood flow and even cause renal failure postoperatively. In addition, acute changes in the curvature of the spine may compress the spine cord or nerve roots with compromise in nerve function. The chest, abdomen, and flanks should also be evaluated for evidence of previous surgical procedures as they may impact the placement of the incision.

ANESTHESIA

A general anesthesia is required with endotracheal intubation. The degree of monitoring used is determined by the comorbid diseases, and ranges from peripheral intravenous lines, to central venous and arterial lines. Transcranial motor evoked potential and somatosensory evoked potential (SSEP) monitoring of the posterior tibial nerve, with the ulnar nerve as a control, is commonly utilized.

OPERATION

Several approaches are used depending on the target of the orthopedic or neurosurgeon.

C1–C2

A transoral approach is used to gain access to the anterior aspect of C1 and C2. The neck is extended, a Dingmann's clamp is placed in the mouth, and a midline incision is made in the posterior pharyngeal wall. Remaining in the midline will allow separation of the longus capitis and longus colli muscles exposing the anterior longitudinal ligament which is divided in the midline. No neurovascular structures should be encountered by staying midline, thus avoiding injury. The vertebral artery is located about 1 cm lateral to the midline along with the vertebral vein which is a plexus in this area and difficult to control if entered.

C3

1 The anterior aspect of C3 is approached between the carotid sheath which is reflected laterally, and the cervical visceral column which is reflected medially. The approach can be made on either side depending on the pathology. The neck is extended and turned slightly to the contralateral side. An incision is made from the mastoid process passing under the angle of the mandible and continuing anteriorly inferior to the mandible. The platysma is incised in the same direction as the skin incision. The cutaneous sensory branches of the cervical plexus (lesser occipital, greater auricular, and transverse cervical nerves) should be avoided.

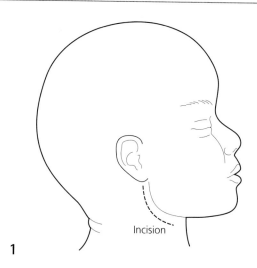

1

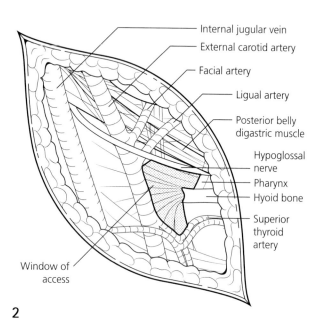

Internal jugular vein
External carotid artery
Facial artery
Ligual artery
Posterior belly digastric muscle
Hypoglossal nerve
Pharynx
Hyoid bone
Superior thyroid artery
Window of access

2

2 The sternocleidomastoid muscle is then retracted laterally and the 'window of access' is opened. This window is bounded by the external carotid artery laterally, the pharynx at the level of the hyoid bone medially, the hypoglossal nerve superiorly, and the superior thyroid artery inferiorly. The pharynx is mobilized medially until the anterior surface of the vertebral column is reached. The use of a nasogastric tube or bougie in the esophagus will help avoid injury during mobilization. The longus colli and longus capitus are separated in the midline, and the prevertebral fascia and anterior longitudinal ligament are divided in the midline to expose the anterior aspect of C3.

C4–T2

3 The anterior surface of the mid- to lower cervical vertebrae can be reached by several methods. The most useful is the anteromedial approach which can be extended up to the level of C1, if necessary. Either side of the neck can be used with this approach, but the left side is preferable for access to vertebral levels C6–T2 to help avoid the recurrent laryngeal nerve which lies more lateral on the right side. The neck is extended with the head turned to the contralateral side opening the space between the neurovascular bundle and the cervical viscera. The skin incision is centered on the anterior aspect of the sternocleidomastoid muscle and placed in the skin lines. The position of the incision depends on the vertebral level of interest. The incision to approach C4–C5 begins at the upper aspect of the thyroid cartilage, for C6 the incision begins at the cricoid cartilage, and for C7–T2 the incision begins a finger's breath above the sternal notch. An incision along the anterior border of the sternocleidomastoid muscle can be used if multiple levels must be approached.

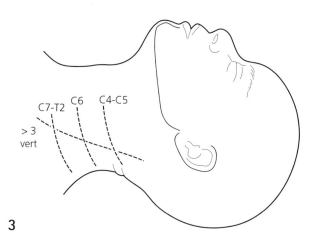

C7–T2   C6   C4–C5

> 3 vert

3

4 The platysma is divided bluntly in the direction of its fibers, and the deep cervical fascia is incised just medial to the sternocleidomastoid muscle. The strap muscles along with the cervical viscera (thyroid gland, larynx, trachea, pharynx, and esophagus) are brought medial, and the neurovascular bundle is retracted laterally to expose the vertebral column. The hypoglossal and recurrent laryngeal nerves must be avoided during this maneuver. Identification of the esophagus is made easier if a nasogastric tube or bougie is inserted, as the decompressed esophagus is a flat structure sometimes difficult to identify and protect from injury. The anterior longitudinal ligament is then opened in the midline at the appropriate level. The prevertebral musculature can be detached laterally, but only for about 1 cm to avoid injury to the vertebral vasculature and the sympathetic trunk.

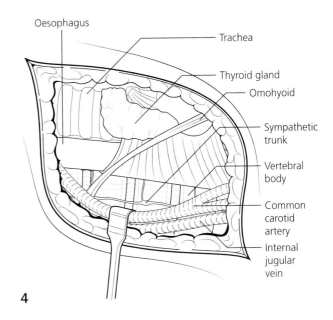

4

T3–T10: OPEN

5 A posterolateral thoracotomy allows access to the anterior vertebral bodies from T3 to T10. The side of the thoracotomy is dictated by the pathology. For kyphoscoliotic disease, in general, the incision is made on the side of the apex of the curve. Since the aorta provides a bit of a challenge on the left, a left-sided approach will be described. The skin incision depends on the level of the target. The incision should be made one rib level higher than the target vertebral level. If in doubt, choose the higher rib since exposure inside the chest is much easier to extend inferiorly than superiorly. A muscle-sparing technique should be used when feasible. The rib that the incision is based on is then resected by incising the periostium and stripping it off the superior aspect of the rib. This is performed using a Freer elevator, as well as a Doyen elevator to circumferentially dissect the periostium. The rib is then divided at the costochondral junction and is divided posteriorly. The rib is preserved for the orthopedic surgeons to use as bone grafts later in the procedure. The chest is then entered through the resected rib bed using an appropriately sized Finochetto for retraction. The mediastinal pleura is incised between the descending aorta and the hemiazygos vein. In certain situations, it may be preferable to stay retropleural. The aorta is rolled medially to expose the vertebral body and intervertebral disks. Segmental vessels give rise to the posterior intercostal vessels and the blood supply to the spinal cord. These vessels should be divided only if necessary, and before they branch and give rise to an anastomotic plexus that feeds the spinal cord. At times, what may predict spinal cord compromise is the testing of each spinal vessel with the use of evoked potentials after the placement of

a vascular clamp (Bulldog) on the selected artery. With continued mobilization, the anterior longitudinal ligament and vertebra are visualized. The thoracic duct should be avoided. It will come into play on the left side in the area of the third and fourth thoracic vertebra where it crosses the midline just ventral to the vertebral column. The duct is present in the right chest inferiorly at the diaphragmatic crura close to the esophagus, coursing superiorly until it crosses the midline. Following the procedure, the chest is closed with a chest tube remaining in place.

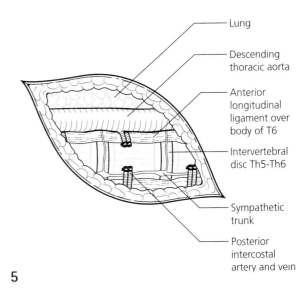

5

T3–T10: THORACOSCOPIC

6 A thoracoscopic approach to the vertebrae in the chest may be appropriate in cases that do not require significant anterior instrumentation. The approach can be from either the right or the left side. The lateral decubitus position is used as in the open technique. Isolation of the ipsilateral lung is imperative for success. The anesthesiologists may use a double-lumen endotracheal tube in larger children, or a bronchial blocker technique in smaller children, and this combined with gentle insufflation provides excellent visualization. The initial Trocar is placed after isolation of the ipsilateral lung in the fifth interspace along the anterior axillary line. The chest is insufflated with CO2 at up to 5 mmHg pressure, and a 5-mm, 30° scope is used. Additional ports and instruments are used to allow dissection for exposure, excision of the disks, and instrumentation, if necessary. The dissection is similar to that in the open description above. The soft tissues are reflected off the anterolateral aspect of the vertebrae after division of segmental vessels if necessary. The segmental vessels are controlled as necessary with electrosurgical instruments, such as the harmonic scalpel or other thermal application devices. Following the procedure, the trocars are removed, the lung re-expanded, and a chest tube is placed through an appropriate Trocar site.

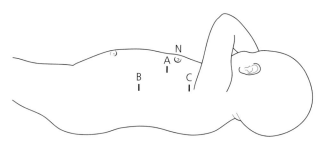

N - Nipple

A - Initial trocar site 5th interspace, anterior axillary line

B - Trocar site - inferior chest in mid axillary line

C - Trocar site - under tip at scapular

6

T11–L1

7 A thoracoabdominal approach through the bed of the tenth rib best exposes the anterior surface of the thoracolumbar junction (T11–L1). The site and type of lesion usually determines the side of the approach, but a left-sided approach would be favored if the lesion does not dictate one side or the other. The reason for the left approach is that the inferior vena cava is more risky to mobilize than the aorta, and the liver is more difficult to retract than is the spleen. The lateral decubitus position with the shoulder rotated back towards the bed allows excellent exposure for both the chest and abdominal portions of the procedure. The skin incision is made along the tenth rib across the costal margin and then inferiorly about 2 cm lateral to the border of the rectus abdominis muscle. The inferior aspect of the incision is determined by the inferior vertebral level required (the body of L2 lies just cranial to the umbilicus). The incision is taken down to the tenth rib incising the latissimus dorsi and external oblique muscles. The tenth rib is removed by incising the periostium and stripping it off the superior aspect of the rib. The rib is then divided at the costochondral junction, elevated, dissected off the neurovascular bundle inferiorly, and divided posteriorly. The rib is saved for bone grafting later. The bed of the tenth rib is opened to gain access to the pleural cavity. The retroperitoneal space is entered by cutting the cartilage of the tenth rib and the underlying diaphragm and transversus abdominis

musculature. This allows visualization of the peritoneum and the fatty tissue associated with it. The diaphragm is opened in a radial fashion leaving a 2-cm edge to allow adequate reconstruction. Sutures are placed on each side of the diaphragm incision at intervals to allow accurate realignment of the muscle.

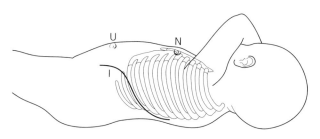

U - Umbilicus

N - Nipple

I - Incision (over 10th rib extending on to abdomen along lateral border of rectus muscle)

7

8 While dividing the diaphragm, the peritoneum is reflected anteriorly and inferiorly off the diaphragm and the lateral and posterior abdominal walls. To gain access to the vertebral column, the mediastinal pleura is opened just lateral to the thoracic aorta, and the left diaphragmatic crus is divided. The aorta then must be mobilized to the right to gain access to the anterior longitudinal ligament and the anterior surface of the vertebral column. If division of segmental vessels is required, they should be divided next to the aortic wall to preserve spinal blood flow. The thoracic duct passes behind the aorta at this level and should be avoided.

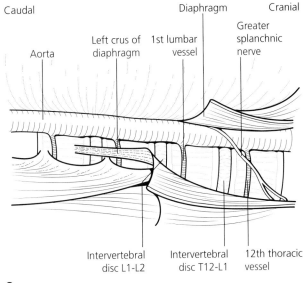

8

L2–L4

9 The lateral extraperitoneal approach allows excellent exposure to the mid-lumbar vertebral column. Again, a left-sided approach is preferable, but the pathology will determine the side of the exposure. A semi-lateral position with the table flexed using the kidney rest between the iliac crest and costal margin allows excellent exposure with the surgeon standing in front of the patient. The skin incision starts at the mid-point between the costal margin and the iliac crest at the mid-axillary line, extends toward the umbilicus, and ends at different points along the edge of the rectus muscle depending on the target level. For L2, the incision ends just superior to the umbilicus. For L3, the incision ends at the level of the umbilicus. And for L4, the incision ends just inferior to the umbilicus. There are three muscle layers to divide before getting to the level of the peritoneum. The external oblique, internal oblique, and transversus abdominis muscle layers should all be bluntly separated in the direction of their fibers to gain access to the peritoneum. A large blunt hemostat is useful for splitting the muscle layers without entering the peritoneum. An alternative approach creates a longitudinal incision from the costal margin to the anterior superior iliac spine. After the fascia of the external oblique is divided, the internal oblique and transversalis muscles are bluntly opened to gain access to the retroperitoneal space. The anterior dissection of the peritoneum should begin as far posterior as possible where there is more extraperitoneal fat making this dissection easier and less likely to enter the peritoneal cavity. If the peritoneum is entered, it should be immediately closed to minimize the extent of the hole.

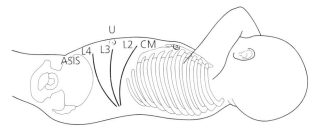

U - Umblicus

ASIS - Anterior superior iliac spine

CM - Costal margin

L2,3,4 - Lines of incision for lumar vertebrae

9

10 A hole in the peritoneum allows the extruded bowel to significantly compromise the exposure. The tissues above the psoas muscle, including the ureter, are mobilized medially to gain access to the vertebral column. The aorta on the left and the inferior vena cava on the right are then mobilized medially to expose the lumbar vertebrae. There are lumbar arteries and veins that tether the aorta and inferior vena cava to the vertebral column and require division to gain exposure to the anterior aspect of the vertebral column. At the L5 area, the segmental veins enter the common or internal iliac vein on the left, called the iliolumbar vein. If this is not controlled prior to mobilization of the vessels, it can easily tear and be difficult to control. The dissection is completed by sweeping off the remainder of the prevertebral connective tissue which may lead to bleeding from the prevertebral venous plexus. The L5 region, due to take off of the iliac vessels may be challenging, and an anterior approach (see below) may be the most optimal approach.

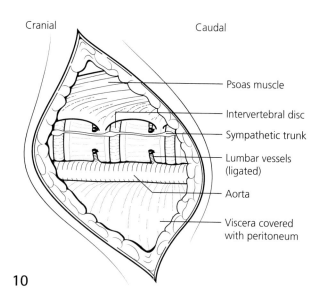

10

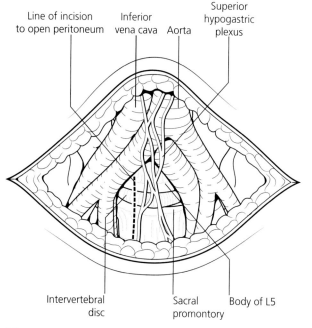

11

L5–S1

11 A transperitoneal approach provides the best exposure for the lumbosacral junction. In the supine position, a Pfannenstiel incision opening the midline from the symphysis to the umbilicus provides the required exposure. A Foley catheter decompresses the bladder. With the help of Trendelenburg positioning, the small intestine is mobilized superiorly, and the sigmoid colon to the left allowing visualization of the sacral promontory, and the aortic and inferior vena cava bifurcations. A self-retaining retractor facilitates exposure. The middle sacral vessels require division. The iliac arteries and veins may or may not require mobilization depending on their location. The iliolumbar vein must be divided if significant mobilization of the left iliac vein is required to prevent troublesome bleeding if it is avulsed. The superior hypogastric plexus of nerves, an autonomic nerve plexus that controls the ejaculatory mechanism, lies distal to the inferior mesenteric artery over the aorta and extends over the left common iliac vein and L5, and L5–S1. At the level of S1, it divides into the right and left hypogastric nerves. It lies close to the midline, but often somewhat to the left of midline. To preserve this nerve plexus, the posterior peritoneum overlying the L5–S1 area should be opened to the right of midline medial to the ureter, and the medial tissue should be bluntly (without the use of electrocautery) dissected to the left to lift the superior hypogastric nerve plexus off the vertebra and preserve it while gaining access to the anterior aspect of the lumbosacral junction.

POSTOPERATIVE CARE

The postoperative care differs depending on the location of the exposure and is shared with the orthopedic surgeon. The exposures of C1–T2 involve transoral or neck incisions. These patients are often left intubated overnight and observed for bleeding and airway issues. Their diets can then be advanced following extubation. The exposures of T3–L1 involve a thoracotomy, thoracoabdominal, or thoracoscopic approach, all of which require chest tube drainage. The chest tube should be left to suction for 48 hours and then removed if there is no air leak or significant fluid output (less than 1 mL/kg per 8-hour shift). Early removal of chest tubes is especially important when anterior hardware has been placed to reduce the risk of infection. The diet can be advanced on the first postoperative day. The patients who require a thoracoabdominal approach may experience an early postoperative ileus, especially if the duodenum is mobilized, and should have their diets advanced accordingly. The exposures of L2–S1 require retroperitoneal mobilization or a transperitoneal approach and may experience a postoperative ileus. The diet is advanced as the ileus resolves. The thoracoabdominal cases and children with severe comorbid illness often require an initial postoperative stay in the intensive care unit.

COMPLICATIONS

Intraoperative

Intraoperative complications vary depending on the level of the exposure. The majority of intraoperative complications relate to vessel injury. Paraplegia is a concern especially when the exposure requires the division of multiple segmental arteries to the spine. The mid-thoracic spine (T4–T9) is at greatest risk for ischemia leading to paralysis. If these segmental vessels require division, it should take place as close to the aorta as possible, and be limited to one side of the spine to retain the collateral circulation. Test occlusion with somatosensory evoked potential monitoring should guide division. Injuries to nerves can occur in different areas. The recurrent laryngeal nerve can be injured directly or secondary to a stretch injury from retraction when exposing the cervical and upper thoracic spine. The hypogastric plexus of nerves must be avoided when exposing the lower lumbar and sacral spinal levels. Injury to this plexus can result in retrograde ejaculation. An injury to the thoracic duct can result in a chylothorax.

Postoperative

The majority of postoperative complications are related to the respiratory system. A review of 505 children who had an anterior spinal exposure reported a 9.8 percent overall complication rate with half of the complications being respiratory in nature, including effusions, pneumothoraces, atelectasis, and respiratory failure. Gastrointestinal complications included superior mesenteric artery syndrome, which resolved in every case with conservative management (parenteral nutrition or use of a nasojejunal feeding tube), and gastrointestinal bleeding. The other complications reported in this review were vessel injuries at the time of the exposure and urinary tract infections.

FURTHER READING

Crawford BK, Morgan JA. Thoracic exposures for spinal deformity surgery. In: Errico TJ (ed.). *Surgical Management of Spinal Deformities*, 1st edn. Philadelphia: Saunders , 2009: 503–10.

Fasel JHD. *Anterior Approaches to the Vertebral Column*. Toronto: Hogrefe & Huber, 1991: 11–49.

Gardocki RJ. Spinal anatomy and surgical approaches. In: Canale ST, Beaty JH (eds). *Campbell's Operative Orthopedics*, 11th edn. St Louis: Mosby, 2007: 1735–51.

Janik JS, Burrington JD, Janik JE *et al.* Anterior exposure of spinal deformities and tumors: a 20 year experience. *Journal of Pediatric Surgery* 1997; **32**: 852–9.

111

Conjoined twins

LEWIS SPITZ, EDWARD KIELY and AGOSTINO PIERRO

HISTORICAL HIGHLIGHTS

The earliest example of conjoined twins is a 17-cm marble statuette portraying parapagus twins, 'the double goddess', dating from the sixth millennium BC. The statue of the sisters of Catathoyuk is housed in the Anatolian Civilisation Museum in Ankara, Turkey. Another early example is a stone carving of pygopagus twins dated to BC80 in the St Marco Museum, Florence, Italy. The earliest attempt at separation of conjoined twins occurred in Kappadokia, Armenia, in AD970. When one of the male ischiopagus twins died, aged 30 years, an attempt was made to save the surviving twin by separating him from his dead brother, but he died 3 days later.

The first well-documented case is that of the Biddenden maids born in Kent, England, in AD1100 who were joined at the hips and the shoulders. They lived together for 34 years. When Mary fell ill and died, Eliza was advised to be separated but absolutely refused saying, 'as we came together we will also go together'. She died 6 hours later.

The first successful separation of conjoined twins took place in 1689. The surgeon, Johannes Fatio, separated omphalopagus twins in Basel, Switzerland, by 'tracing the umbilical vessels to the navel where he tied them separately. He then transfixed and tied the bridge between the two infants with a silken cord and cut the isthmus.' The ligature fell off on the ninth postoperative day and both children survived.

The most celebrated pair of conjoined twins was Chang and Eng, born on a river boat in Siam in 1911. They were joined at the xiphisternum by a short bridge that stretched so they were eventually able to stand side by side. They were taken to the United States where they were exhibited by the showman, Phineas Barnum. They married sisters, lived in North Carolina, and had 21 children between them. They lived together for 63 years.

INCIDENCE AND ETIOLOGY

The frequency of conjoined twins has been estimated at 1 in 250 000 live births. Sixty percent of conjoined twins die during gestation or at birth. Females predominate with a ratio of 3:1.

The most widely held theory of their occurrence is that secondary fusion occurs between two originally separate monovular embryonic disks at around 13–15 days' gestation ('fusion' theory of Spencer). An alternative theory is that of failure of complete separation of the embryonic disc ('fission' theory).

CLASSIFICATION

Conjoined twins are classified on the basis of the site of union, with the suffix 'pagus' meaning fixed or fastened (**Table 111.1**). The twins can have four (tetrapus), three (tripus), or two (bipus) legs.

Table 111.1 Classification of conjoined twins.

Classification	Percent occurrence
Thoracopagus	40
Omphalopagus	33
Pygopagus	19
Ischiopagus	6
Craniopagus	2

Thoracopagus

The twins lie face to face (**Figure 111.1**) and share the sternum, diaphragm, upper abdomen wall and liver and have an exomphalos.

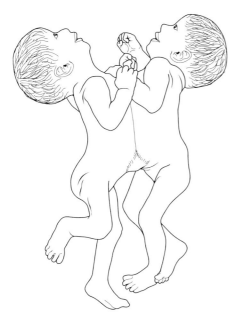

Figure 111.1 Thoracopagus.

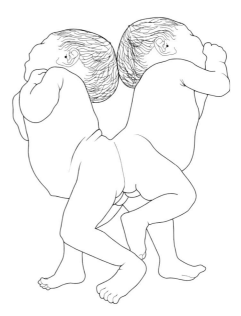

Figure 111.2 Pygopagus.

In the majority of the cases, they share the pericardium (90 percent) and heart (85 percent). They may have a common small intestine (50 percent) which joins at the duodenum and separates at ileum; the biliary tree can be joined in 25 percent of patients. There may be associated cardiac anomalies, such as ventricular septal defect, atrial septal defect, and tetralogy of Fallot.

Omphalopagus

The heart is never fused. The liver is joined in 80 percent of cases and there is an exomphalos. The stomach and proximal small bowel are usually separate, and each twin has a rectum. In up to one-third of omphalopagus twins, the intestine usually join at Meckel's diverticulum, the terminal ileum and colon are shared, and may also have a dual blood supply. There is usually no union of the genitourinary tract.

Pygopagus

The twins are joined dorsally (**Figure 111.2**), sharing the sacrococcygeal and perineal regions. They face away from each other, and share the sacrum, coccyx and part of the pelvic bones. The spinal cords are usually separate. Twenty-five percent share the lower gastrointestinal (GI) tract and have a single anus and one or two rectums. In 15 percent of cases, there is a single bladder. There is an increased incidence of vertebral anomalies, including hemivertebrae, hemisacral agenesis, and thoracic anomalies.

Although the pelvic conjunction is fundamentally different than in ischiopagus twinning, the types are similar insofar as numerous other associated orthopedic anomalies have been reported in association with pelvic conjunction,

such as hip subluxation or dislocation, congenital vertical talus, talipes equinovarus, Sprengel shoulder, and scoliosis.

There can also be a variable degree of spinal and cord fusion. Although there may be only one anus and rectum, the remainder of the intestines are usually separate. The upper bodies are not fused and there are four arms and four legs.

Parapagus

This is a relatively new term denoting extensive side-to-side fusion (**Figure 111.3**). The twins share the umbilicus, lower abdomen, pelvis (single symphysis pubis), and the genitourinary (GU) tract. They can have anorectal anomaly and colovesical fistula and may be at risk of anencephaly.

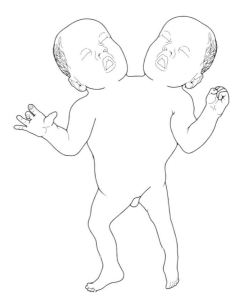

Figure 111.3 Parapagus.

Craniopagus

The conjoined twins share the skull, meninges and the venous sinuses (**Figure 111.4**). The brains are usually separate, although some cortical fusion can occur in 33 percent of cases.

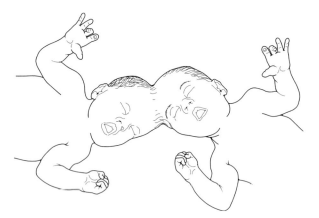

Figure 111.4 Craniopagus.

Cephalopagus

The twins often have a fused thorax in addition to a fused head. The single fused head may have two faces (janiceps) facing away from each other; one face may be rudimentary. These twins are terminated or die *in utero*. They are nonviable.

Rachipagus

The twins have generally vertebral anomalies and neural tube defects.

Ischiopagus

The twins may lie face to face or end to end (**Figure 111.5**). They have two sacra or two symphysis pubis. They may share the lower gastrointestinal tract (70 percent) and/ or the genitourinary tract (50 percent) and may have crossing ureters. The twins can be tetrapus, tripus, or bipus, although the most common arrangement is the presence of four legs. Pelvic conjunction leads to complex urogenital and orthopedic anatomy. The kidneys usually function normally, but are often malrotated or ectopic in location. When two bladders are present, they lie side by side in a collateral position or they may lie in a sagittal midline location with one bladder draining into the other. The ureters frequently cross over and insert into a contralateral bladder, such that they will need to be rerouted during separation. Partial urethral duplication is possible, but a single urethral orifice is typical. The distal gastrointestinal tract is often shared, with anorectal agenesis and rectovesical fistula. Contrast studies are necessary to delineate distal bowel anatomy. Urogenital sinus or cloaca may be present. In boys, there is an increased incidence of undescended testes.

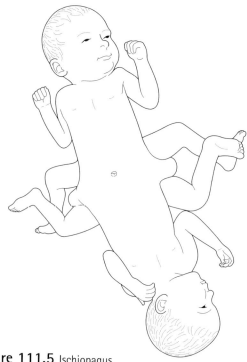

Figure 111.5 Ischiopagus.

PRENATAL DIAGNOSIS

The diagnosis of conjoined twins should be considered in any twin pregnancy that has a single placenta and no visible separating amniotic membrane. Polyhydramnios occurs in as many as 50 percent of conjoined twin pregnancies compared with 10 percent of normal twins and 2 percent of singleton pregnancies.

Prenatal ultrasonography is capable of diagnosing conjoined twin pregnancies as early as 12 weeks' gestation. The sonographic findings include inseparable fetal bodies and skin contours, an unchanged relative position of the fetuses, both fetal heads persistently at the same level, and a single umbilical cord containing more than three vessels. Detailed scanning at around 20 weeks' gestation will accurately define the extent of the conjoined area and provide an assessment of which viscera are shared. Fetal echocardiography is mandatory, as twins with a complex shared heart have an extremely poor prognosis and termination of the pregnancy is invariably recommended. Computed tomography (CT) and magnetic resonance imaging (MRI) may be performed at 32–34 weeks' gestation, but once the decision has been made to proceed with the pregnancy, these investigations can be carried out with greater accuracy after delivery. An additional advantage of prenatal diagnosis is that the time, place, and mode of delivery can be planned. The delivery should take place at or close to the surgical unit where separation will be performed. Delivery must always be by Cesarean section at 36–38 weeks' gestation.

MANAGEMENT

The management of conjoined twins can be divided into four separate time frames.

Prenatal

Once the diagnosis of conjoined twins is suspected on prenatal scan at 12 weeks' gestation, it is important to define the anatomy of the union. Termination of the pregnancy is recommended where there is complex cardiac fusion or extensive cerebral fusion. Detailed echocardiography and accurate ultrasonography is essential. The extent of deformity expected following possible subsequent separation must be carefully and accurately explained so that an informed decision can be made either to terminate or to proceed with the pregnancy.

Non-operative treatment

No attempt at surgical separation should be considered in the presence of complex cardiac or cerebral fusion or where the expected deformity following separation is unacceptable to the parents.

Emergency separation

This procedure is undertaken when one twin is dead or dying and threatening the survival of the remaining twin, or where a life-threatening correctable congenital abnormality (e.g. intestinal atresia, malrotation with or without volvulus, ruptured omphalocele, or anorectal agenesis) is present in one or both twins. Under these circumstances, the only chance of saving one or both infants lies in immediate separation. Emergency separation carries a significantly higher mortality rate compared with elective procedures.

Elective separation

This will normally take place between two and four months of age. It allows the twins to stabilize and thrive, and provides time to carry out detailed investigations to define the nature and the extent of union. It also allows the application of methods to be carried out to achieve primary closure of the wound, such as tissue expansion. Detailed planning of the operative procedure with all members of the operating team should take place before the separation. The survival rate for elective separation is in excess of 80 percent.

INVESTIGATIONS

The choice of imaging study will depend on the site of union. For thoraco-omphagopagus twins, essential investigations include echocardiogram, CT (**Figure 111.6**),

and MRI scans with particular attention directed to the anatomy of the hearts, livers, and genitourinary systems. Where the livers are fused, it is important to document the presence of separate gallbladders and hepatic veins. Gastrointestinal contrast studies are useful in showing separate gastrointestinal systems. MRI angiography has superseded percutaneous angiography to define vascular anatomy. Bony anatomy is best demonstrated on plain x-ray and MRI scan.

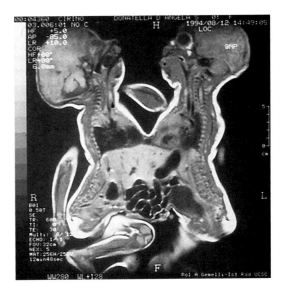

Figure 111.6 Computed tomography scan of omphalo-thoracopagus twins.

ANESTHETIC MANAGEMENT

Two sets of anesthesiologists, one for each infant, are essential, as each has to be separately monitored throughout the procedure. Essential monitoring consists of arterial and central venous catheters, electrocardiogram, pulse oximetry, capnography, and urinary output. All lines need to be color coded for individual infants to avoid confusion when their position is changed. Regular blood gas analyses are undertaken throughout the procedure. All drugs and intravenous fluids are calculated on a total weight basis, with half being delivered to each twin. Because of the cross-circulation, drugs given intravenously may have an unpredictable effect. Thus, particular care is essential when administering drugs such as opioids, which should be given incrementally.

OPERATIVE PROCEDURE

Technical details of the operative procedure will be dictated by the anatomy of the junction and by the organs and structures shared.

In thoracopagus, the liver is invariably shared. In 90 percent of cases, there is a common pericardium which can be separated to provide an individual pericardial sac for each twin. Major myocardial connections are present in 75 percent of cases and only a few attempts have been made at separation. The upper gastrointestinal tract is common in 50 percent of cases with a shared biliary system in 25 percent.

In omphalopagus, the liver is shared in 80 percent of cases and in 33 percent the intestines join at the level of the Meckel's diverticulum and the common terminal ileum and colon have a dual blood supply. The lower intestinal tract is common in both pygopagus and ischiopagus and the genitourinary tract is shared in 15 percent of the former and 50 percent of the latter. It is not uncommon for the ureters in these situations to cross over from one twin and enter the contralateral bladder (**Figure 111.7**).

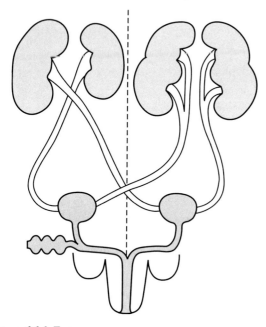

Figure 111.7 Urological anatomy in one set of conjoined twins.

The high mortality rate associated with craniopagus is almost entirely due to cerebral fusion, which is also responsible for the neurodevelopmental sequelae in survivors.

Blood loss may be a major intraoperative problem, especially where there is pelvic bony fusion. Blood loss occurring during division of the liver should be minimized by using ultrasonic dissection, meticulously ligating major connecting vessels, and coagulating minor vessels, and by applying fibrin glue (Tisseel®) to the raw surface, postoperative ooze of blood and leakage of bile may be prevented. Despite every attempt to define as accurately

as possible all anatomical connections prior to surgery, 'unexpected events' are frequently encountered during the operation. Examples in our experience include abnormal vascular communications, and previously unidentified intestinal and genitourinary anomalies.

The surgical team should be aware of these variations in anatomy and be prepared to vary the operative procedure accordingly.

When, despite all possible maneuvers, primary closure of the defect proves impossible, it will be necessary to insert prosthetic material (polypropylene mesh, Silastic sheet, Gore-Tex®) as a temporary measure. The insertion of a prosthetic patch in closure of the abdomen is preferable to 'closure under tension' which may embarrass respiration or inhibit venous return.

POSTOPERATIVE MANAGEMENT

Postoperatively, the surviving infant/s are extremely fragile.

All intraoperative monitoring must be continued postoperatively in the intensive care unit and because of the prolonged duration of surgery, the infants are electively paralyzed and mechanically ventilated for a variable period of time.

Meticulous attention should be directed at monitoring fluid and electrolyte balance, and in particular avoiding over-hydration which may precipitate cardiovascular instability. Sepsis is a major cause of mortality and morbidity and strict infectious precautions must be exercised, particularly where large skin defects are present. Late unexpected deaths following separation are unfortunately not uncommon.

OUTCOME FOR CONJOINED TWINS TREATED AT GREAT ORMOND STREET HOSPITAL

Since 1985, at Great Ormond Street Hospital in London, we have had experience with 31 pairs of conjoined twins:

- **Nonoperative treatment** was carried out in seven sets, all of whom died within a short period of time.
- **Emergency separation** was attempted in eight sets with four survivors (25 percent).
- **Planned separation** was performed in 14 sets with 25 long-term survivors (89 percent). Of the three deaths, two occurred many months after successful separation.

Comparison with other series in the literature is shown in **Table 111.2**.

Table 111.2 Outcome of management of conjoined twins in the major series.

Authors	Year	No.	No operation	Emergency separation (survivors (%))	Planned separation (survived (%))
O'Neill (United States)	1988	18	5	5 sets (1 (10%) survived)	8 sets (13 survived (81%))
Cywes/Rode (South Africa)	2006	33	16	None	17 sets (22 survived (65%))
Al Rabeeah (Saudi Arabia)	2006	29	19 (1 abandoned operation)	None	10 sets (19 survived (95%))
Saguil (Philippines)	2009	22	6	6 sets (1 (8%) survived)	9 sets (15 survived (83%))
Spitz/Kiely/Pierro (UK)	2010	31	9	8 sets (4 (25%) survived)	14 sets (25 survived (89%))

FURTHER READING

Kingston CA, McHugh K, Kumaradevan J et al. Imaging in the preoperative assessment of conjoined twins. *RadioGraphics 2001*; **21**: 1187–208.

Spitz L, Kiely EM. Experience in the management of conjoined twins. *British Journal of Surgery 2002*; **89**: 1188–92.

Spitz L, Kiely EM. Conjoined twins. *Journal of the American Medical Association 2002*; **289**: 1307–10.

Wilcox DT, Quinn SM, Spitz L et al. Urological problems in conjoined twins. *British Journal of Urology 1998*; **81**: 905–10.

Index

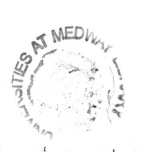